metoclopramide HCl	morphine sulfate	nalbuphine HCl	pentazocine lactate	pentobarbital Na	perphenazine	phenobarbital Na	prochlorperazine edisylate	promazine HCl	promethazine HCl	ranitidine HCl	scopolamine HBr	secobarbital Na	sodium bicarbonate	thiethylperazine maleate	thiopental Na	
P	P	Y	P	P	Y		P	P	P	Y	P					atropine sulfate
	Y		Y	N		N					Y	N			N	benzquinamide HCl
	Y		Y	N	Y		Y		Y		Y			Y		butorphanol tartrate
P	P		P	N	Y		Y	P	P	Y	P				N	chlorpromazine HCl
	Y	Y	Y	N	Y		Y	Y	Y		Y	N				cimetidine HCl
																codeine phosphate
P	P		P	N	Y		N	N	N	Y	P				N	dimenhydrinate
Y	P		P	N	Y		P	P	P	Y	P				N	diphenhydramine HCl
P	P	Y	P	N	Y		P	P	P		P					droperidol
P	P		P	N	Y		P	P	P	Y	P					fentanyl citrate
	Y		N	N		Y	Y	Y	Y	Y	Y	N	N		N	glycopyrrolate
P(5)	N*		N		P(5)		N									heparin Na
		Y	Y			N*		Y	Y	Y				Y		hydromorphone HCl
P	Y	Y	Y	N			P	P	P	N	Y					hydroxyzine HCl
P	N		P	N	P		P	P	Y	Y	P				N	meperidine HCl
■	P		P		P		P	P	P	Y	P		N		N	metoclopramide HCl
P	■		P	N*	Y		P*	P	P*	Y	P				N	morphine sulfate
		■	N		Y		Y	Y	Y		Y			Y		nalbuphine HCl
P	P		■	N	Y		P	Y	Y	Y	Y	P				pentazocine lactate
	N*	N	N	■	N		N	N	N		Y		Y		Y	pentobarbital Na
P	Y		Y	N	■		P			Y						perphenazine
						■					N					phenobarbital Na
P	P*	Y	P	N	Y		■	P	P	Y	P				N	prochlorperazine edisylate
P	P		Y	N			P	■	P	P						promazine HCl
P	P*	Y	Y	N			P	P	■	Y	P				N	promethazine HCl
Y	Y	Y	Y		Y	N	Y	P	Y	■	Y			Y		ranitidine HCl
P	P	Y	P	Y			P		P	Y	■				Y	scopolamine HBr
												■				secobarbital Na
N			Y										■		N	sodium bicarbonate
		Y									Y			■		thiethylperazine maleate
	N			Y			N		N		Y		N		■	thiopental Na

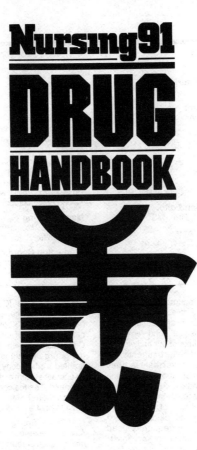

Nursing91 DRUG HANDBOOK

NURSING91 BOOKS™
SPRINGHOUSE CORPORATION
SPRINGHOUSE, PENNSYLVANIA

NURSING91 DRUG HANDBOOK™

Staff

Executive Director, Editorial
Stanley Loeb

Editorial Director
Helen Klusek Hamilton

Clinical Director
Barbara F. McVan, RN

Art Director
John Hubbard

Clinical Editor
Joanne Patzek DaCunha, RN, BS

Drug Information Editor
George J. Blake, RPh, MS

Editorial Assistants
Maree DeRosa, Beverly Lane

Copy Editors
Jane V. Cray, Traci A. Ginnona

Designers
Stephanie Peters (associate art director),
Matie Patterson

Art Production
Robert Perry (manager), Anna Brindisi,
Donald Knauss, Catherine Mace, Bob
Wieder

Typography
David C. Kosten (director), Diane Paluba
(manager), Elizabeth Bergman, Joyce
Rossi Biletz, Phyllis Marron, Robin Rantz,
Valerie Rosenberger

Manufacturing
Deborah C. Meiris (manager), T.A. Landis, Jennifer Suter

Production Coordination
Aline S. Miller (manager), Colleen M.
Hayman

The clinical procedures described and recommended in this publication are based on research and consultation with nursing, medical, and legal authorities. To the best of our knowledge, these procedures reflect currently accepted practice; nevertheless, they can't be considered absolute and universal recommendations. For individual application, all recommendations must be considered in light of the patient's clinical condition and, before administration of new or infrequently used drugs, in light of latest package-insert information. The authors and the publisher disclaim responsibility for any adverse effects resulting directly or indirectly from the suggested procedures, from any undetected errors, or from the reader's misunderstanding of the text.

NGDH-020291
ISSN 0273-320X
ISBN 0-87434-322-4

CONTENTS

Anesthetic Agents

Nutritional Agents

Miscellaneous Drug Categories

Appendices and Index

CONSULTANTS, REVIEWERS, AND ADVISORS

At the time of publication, the clinical consultants, pharmacy reviewers, and advisors held the following positions:

Clinical Consultants

Catharine Keenan Bean, RN, BSN, OCN, Interim Co-Assistant Director of Nursing Education, Dana Farber Cancer Institute, Boston

Michael J. Booth, RN, MA, CRNA, Co-Director, Graduate Program of Nurse Anesthesia; Assistant Professor, Department of Anesthesiology, Medical College of Pennsylvania and Medical College of Pennsylvania Hospital, Philadelphia

Charmaine J. Cummings, RN, MSN, Director, Nursing Education, National Institutes of Health, Clinical Center, Bethesda, Md.

Walter Carl Faubion, RN, MS, Manager, Parenteral and Enteral Nutrition Team, University of Michigan Medical Center, Ann Arbor

Roseann Hendrickson, RN, Staff Nurse, Emergency Department, Underwood Memorial Hospital, Woodbury, N.J.

Marcia Jo Hill, RN, MSN, Manager, Dermatologic Therapeutics, The Methodist Hospital, Houston; Clinical Assistant Professor, Department of Dermatology, Baylor College of Medicine, Tex.

Karen Landis, RN, MS, CCRN, Pulmonary Clinical Nurse Specialist, Lehigh Valley Hospital Center, Allentown, Pa.

Meredith Ann McCord, RN, MS, Assistant Professor, Oregon Health Sciences University School of Nursing, Portland

Chris Platt Moldovanyi, RN, MSN, CDE, Staff Nurse, Operating Room, Endocrinology Clinical Specialist, Cleveland (Ohio) Clinic Foundation

Sandra Ludwig Nettina, RNC, MSN, CRNP, Adult Nurse Practitioner, Department of Emergency Medicine, Temple University Hospital, Philadelphia

Margaret A. Smellie-Belfield, RN, BSN, CCRN, Clinical Services Director, SICU/PACU, Veterans Administration Medical Center, San Diego

Marilyn Sawyer Sommers, RN, MA, CCRN, Nurse Consultant, Instructor, College of Nursing and Health, University of Cincinnati

Nancy Baptie Walrath, RN, BSN, CGC, Director, Gastroenterology Department, Daniel Freeman Memorial and Marina Hospitals, Inglewood, Calif.

Special thanks to the following, who contributed to past editions: Wendy L. Baker, RN, MS, CCRN; Beverly A. Baldwin, RN, MA; Heather Boyd-Monk, SRN, RN, BSN; Paula Brammer-Vetter, RN, BSN, CCRN; Karen E. Burgess, RN, MSN; Nancy Burns, RN, PhD; Carla J. Burton, RN, BS; Maribel J. Clements, RN, MA; Elizabeth R. DiMeo, RN, MSN; Judy Donlen, RNC, MSN; Gail D'Onofrio, RN, MS; DeAnn M. Englert, RN, MSN; Margarethe Hawken, RN, MA, CNRN; Kathleen M. Hawkins, RN; Denise A. Hess, RN, BS; Tobie Hittle, RN, CCRN, BSN; Carolyn Holt, RN, BSEd; Maureen L. Metters, BSN; Margaret E. Miller, RN, MSN; John Nagelhout, CRNA, PhD; Helene K. Nawrocki, RN, MSN; Brenda Marion Nevidson, RN, MSN; Elizabeth A. Phillips, RN, BA, BSN; Judith M. Rohde, RN, MS, CNP, CNRN; Dale Elizabeth Schreffler, RN, BSN; Roberta Seifer, RN, CNP, BS; Despina Seremelis, RN, BSN; Barbara Solomon, RN, MS; Robin Tourigian, RN, MSN; Carmen Brochu Wohrle, RN, MS

Pharmacy Reviewers

Bruce M. Frey, BS, RPh, PharmD, Clinical Pharmacist in Pediatrics, Thomas Jefferson University Hospital, Philadelphia

Joel Glucroft, PhD, Director, J. Glucroft & Associates, Canoga Park, Calif.

David W. Hawkins, PharmD, Associate Professor and Assistant Dean of Pharmacy, College of Pharmacy, University of Georgia, Athens

Alan W. Hopefl, PharmD, Associate Professor of Pharmacy Practice, St. Louis College of Pharmacy; Assistant Professor of Pharmacy in Internal Medicine, St. Louis University School of Medicine

Nina E. Jakobowski, PharmD, Clinical Pharmacist in Medicine/ Oncology, Thomas Jefferson University Hospital, Philadelphia

1

How to use Nursing91 Drug Handbook

Nursing91 Drug Handbook is meant to fill a very special need. It represents a joint effort by pharmacists and nurses to provide the nursing profession with drug information that focuses on what nurses need to know. With this in mind, it emphasizes clinical aspects and does not attempt to replace detailed pharmacology texts. Also, the information is arranged in a format designed to make it readily accessible.

Introductory information
Following this chapter, Chapter 2 explains, in a general way, how drugs work. It also tells about side effects and adverse reactions and gives general guidelines about drug use in pregnancy and the presence of drugs in breast milk. Chapters 3 and 4 discuss the unique problems of administering drugs to children and elderly patients and offer guidelines to minimize problems in these areas. Chapter 5 discusses drug therapy as it relates to the nursing process.

In the remaining chapters, all drugs are classified according to their approved therapeutic uses. Drugs that have multiple therapeutic uses are classified according to their most common use; they are also listed (with a cross-reference to the major drug entry) in drug groups that share their secondary applications. For example, nadolol, a beta-adrenergic blocker, is described in the chapter that covers antianginals because its major therapeutic application is the management of angina pectoris; because it is less commonly used to treat hypertension, it is listed among the generic drugs grouped as antihypertensives with a cross-reference to Chapter 21, Antianginals.

Such classification by therapeutic use offers several advantages. It helps the reader identify an unknown drug by its clinical application alone. At the same time, it automatically identifies all other drugs that share the same use and provides easy comparison of their dosages and effects. Thereby, it quickly identifies potential pharmacotherapeutic alternatives for patients who cannot tolerate or fail to respond to a particular drug.

Drug information
Each chapter, representing a major therapeutic use, begins with an alphabetically arranged list of the generic names of drugs described in that chapter. This is followed by a list of selected combination products in which these drugs are found. Specific information on each drug is arranged under the following headings: *How Supplied, Mechanism of Action; Indications & Dosage; Adverse Reactions; Interactions;* and *Nursing Considerations.*

In each drug entry, the drug's generic name is immediately followed by an alphabetic list of its brand names. A trade name followed by an open diamond indicates a drug that is available in preparations that do not require a prescription (◇). Brands available *only* in Canada are designated with a dagger (†); those available *only* in Australia, with a double dagger (‡). A brand name with no symbol after it is available in the United States, Canada, and possibly Australia. If a drug is a controlled substance, that too is clearly indicated (example: Controlled Substance Schedule II). Products listed, although generally available, may not be approved by the Food and Drug Administration. The mention of a brand name in no way implies endorsement of that product or guarantees its legality.

Each systemically absorbed drug has been assigned a pregnancy risk category based upon available clinical and preclinical information. The Pregnancy Risk Category parallels the five Pregnancy Categories (A, B, C, D, and X) assigned by the Food and Drug Administration to reflect a drug's potential to cause birth defects. Although it is generally accepted that no drugs should be used during pregnancy, this rating system permits rapid assessment of the risk-benefit ratio should drug administration to a pregnant woman become necessary. Drugs in category A are generally considered safe to use in pregnancy; drugs in category X are generally contraindicated.

• A: Adequate studies in pregnant women have failed to show a risk to the fetus in the first trimester of pregnancy—and there is no evidence of risk in later trimesters.

• B: Animal studies have not shown a risk to the fetus, but there are no adequate clinical studies in pregnant women; or, animal studies have shown an adverse effect on the fetus, but adequate studies in pregnant women have not shown a risk to the fetus during the first trimester of pregnancy and there is no evidence of risk in later trimesters.

• C: Animal studies *have* shown an adverse effect on the fetus, but there are no adequate studies in humans. The benefits from use in pregnant women may be acceptable despite potential risks; or, there are no animal reproduction studies or adequate human studies. Pregnancy risk is unknown.

• D: There is evidence of risk to the human fetus, but the potential benefits of use in pregnant women may be acceptable despite risks.

• X: Studies in animals or humans show fetal abnormalities, or adverse reaction reports indicate evidence of fetal risk. The risks involved clearly outweigh potential benefits.

• NR: Not rated.

In this volume, the Pregnancy Risk Category has been omitted if the drug is not rated and if such rating is not applicable.

The section titled *How Supplied* lists the preparations available for each drug (for example, tablets, capsules, solutions for injection), specifying available dosage forms and strengths. Preparations that do not require a prescription are marked with an open diamond (◊).

The section titled *Mechanism of Action* succinctly describes *how* each specific drug provides its therapeutic effect. For example, although all antihypertensives lower blood pressure, they don't all do this by the same pharmacologic process.

The section titled *Indications & Dosage* lists general dosage information for adults (including recommended geriatric dosages, when available) and children, as applicable. Children's dosages are usually indicated in terms of mg/kg daily. Dosage instructions reflect current clinical trends in therapeutics and can't be considered as absolute and universal recommendations. For individual application, dosage instructions must be considered in light of the patient's clinical condition.

The section titled *Adverse Reactions* lists each drug's commonly observed adverse reactions (and selected rare ones if life-threatening). The most common and life-threatening adverse reactions are italicized for easy reference. An exception to this rule is an adverse reaction that, although normally considered hazardous, has been reported to be mild and reversible with the drug in question. For example, thrombocytopenia is considered a life-threatening adverse reaction to plicamycin but a mild and reversible reaction to methyldopa. Hence, thrombocytopenia listed as an adverse reaction to plicamycin is italicized, whereas the same reaction under methyldopa is not. Adverse reactions are grouped according to the body system in which they appear.

The next section, *Interactions,* lists each drug's confirmed, *clinically significant* interactions with other drugs (additive effects, potentiated effects, and antagonistic effects) with specific suggestions for avoiding dangerous drug interactions (for example, by reducing doses). Drug interactions are listed under the drug that is adversely affected. For example, magnesium trisilicate, an ingredient in antacids, interacts with tetracycline to cause decreased absorption of tetracycline. Therefore, this interaction is listed under tetracycline. To check on the possible effects of using two or more drugs simultaneously, refer to the interaction entry for *each* of the drugs in question.

The final section, *Nursing Considerations,* lists other useful information, starting with contraindications and precautions, followed by monitoring techniques and suggestions for prevention and treatment of adverse reactions. Also included are suggestions for patient comfort, for patient teaching, and for preparing, administering, and storing each drug.

Alcohol and tartrazine content
Many liquid drug preparations for oral use contain alcohol. Although

the slight sedative effect that alcohol produces is not harmful in most patients—and can sometimes be beneficial—alcohol ingestion can be undesirable and even dangerous in some circumstances. So, alcohol-containing oral drugs should be given very cautiously, if at all, to patients who are:
• concomitantly taking potent CNS depressants, such as barbiturates.
• taking drugs that may produce a disulfiram-type reaction (such as chlorpropamide, metronidazole, and moxalactam).
• taking disulfiram (Antabuse) as part of a treatment program for their alcoholism. Such patients, upon ingestion of alcohol, will exhibit severe symptoms that may include blurred vision, confusion, dyspnea, flushing, sweating, and tachycardia.

To help prevent inadvertent exposure to alcohol, this volume signals alcohol content with a single asterisk (*) after each brand of a liquid preparation that may contain it. In many of the preparations so marked, the alcohol content is small. Nevertheless, these drugs should be avoided in patients who are susceptible to adverse effects upon exposure to alcohol.

Tartrazine dye, also known as FD&C Yellow No. 5, is a common coloring agent in some foods and drugs. Usually harmless, it can provoke a severe allergic reaction in susceptible persons. For this reason, most drug manufacturers have begun to eliminate tartrazine from their products, but many drugs still contain it.

The incidence of tartrazine sensitivity is estimated at approximately 1 in 10,000 in the general population but somewhat higher in persons with asthma and/or sensitivity to aspirin. Why this is so is unknown. The most common symptoms of tartrazine sensitivity are urticaria, rhinorrhea, asthma, and angioedema. Acutely sensitive persons may develop allergic vascular purpura, tachycardia, dyspnea, and chest pain. These allergic symptoms generally subside spontaneously upon discontinuation of the tartrazine-containing drug but occasionally require treatment with antihistamines or epinephrine.

Avoiding exposure to tartrazine is not simply a matter of avoiding yellow-colored drugs because this substance may be present in many other color blends, such as turquoise, green, and maroon. To prevent exposure to tartrazine, this volume signals possible tartrazine content with a double asterisk (**) after each brand that may contain it. If you suspect tartrazine sensitivity in a patient receiving such a drug, inform the doctor and contact the manufacturer to determine which dosage forms contain tartrazine.

A guide to abbreviations

AIDS	acquired immunodeficiency syndrome
ALT	alanine aminotransferase
AST	aspartate aminotransferase
AV	atrioventricular
b.i.d.	twice daily
BUN	blood urea nitrogen
CBC	complete blood count
CHF	congestive heart failure
CMV	cytomegalovirus
CNS	central nervous system
COPD	chronic obstructive pulmonary disease
CPK	creatine phosphokinase
CV	cardiovascular
CVA	cerebrovascular accident
DNA	deoxyribonucleic acid
ECG	electrocardiogram
EENT	eyes, ears, nose, throat
FDA	Food and Drug Administration
g	gram
G	gauge
GI	gastrointestinal
GFR	glomerular filtration rate
GU	genitourinary
G6PD	glucose-6-phosphate dehydrogenase
h.s.	at bedtime
I.M.	intramuscular
IND	investigational new drug
IPPB	intermittent positive pressure breathing
ID	intradermal
IU	international unit
I.V.	intravenous
kg	kilogram
M	molar
m^2	square meter
MAO	monoamine oxidase
mcg	microgram
mEq	milliequivalent
mg	milligram
ml	milliliter
Na	sodium
NaCl	sodium chloride
NSAID	nonsteroidal anti-inflammatory drug

OTC	over the counter
PABA	para-aminobenzoic acid
P.O.	by mouth
P.R.	by rectum
p.r.n.	as needed
q	every
q.d.	every day
q.i.d.	four times daily
q.o.d.	every other day
RBC	red blood cell
RDA	recommended daily allowance
REM	rapid eye movement
RNA	ribonucleic acid
RSV	respiratory syncytial virus
SA	sinoatrial
S.C.	subcutaneous
SIADH	syndrome of inappropriate antidiuretic hormone
S.L.	sublingual
t.i.d.	three times daily
UCE	urea cycle enzymopathy
USP	United States Pharmacopeia
WBC	white blood cell

2

Drug actions, reactions, and interactions explained

Administration of any drug provokes a series of physiochemical events within the body. The first event, when a drug combines with cell drug receptors, is known as the drug action. What follows as a result of this action of the drug is known as the drug effect. Depending on the number of different cellular drug receptors affected by a given drug, a drug effect can be local, systemic, or both. For example, the antipeptic ulcer drug cimetidine (Tagamet) acts solely by blocking histamine receptor cells in the parietal cells of the stomach. This is known as a local drug effect because the drug action is sharply limited to one area and does not spread to other parts of the body. On the other hand, diphenhydramine (Benadryl) produces a systemic effect in that it blocks histamine receptors in widespread areas of the body. In other words, local drug effects are specific to a limited number of organ systems, whereas systemic drug effects are generalized and affect different and diverse organ systems.

Three factors modify drug action
1. Absorption
Before a drug can act within the body, it must be absorbed into the bloodstream—usually after oral administration, the most frequently used route. Before a drug contained in a tablet or capsule can be absorbed, the dosage form must disintegrate, that is, break into smaller particles. Then, these smaller particles can dissolve in

gastric juices. Only after so dissolving can a drug be absorbed into the bloodstream. Once absorbed and circulated in the bloodstream, it is said to be bioavailable, or ready to produce a drug effect. Whether such absorption is complete or partial depends on several factors: the drug's physiochemical effects, its dosage form, its route of administration, its interactions with other substances in the GI tract, and various patient characteristics. These same factors also determine the speed of absorption. Thus, oral solutions and elixirs, which bypass the need for disintegration and dissolution, are usually absorbed more rapidly. Some tablets have special (enteric) coatings that prevent disintegration in the acidic environment of the stomach; other may have coatings of varying thickness that delay release of the drug.

Drugs administered intramuscularly must first be absorbed through the muscle into the bloodstream. Rectal suppositories must dissolve to be absorbed through the rectal mucosa. Drugs administered intravenously, which are placed directly into the bloodstream, are completely and immediately bioavailable.
2. Distribution
After absorption, a drug moves from the bloodstream into various fluids and tissues within the body; this is distribution. Individual patient variations can greatly alter the amount of drug that is distributed throughout the

body. For example, in an edematous patient, a given dose must be distributed to a larger volume than in a nonedematous patient; the amount of drug must sometimes be increased to account for this. Remember, the dosage should be decreased when the edema is corrected. Conversely, in an extremely dehydrated patient, the drug will be distributed to a much smaller volume, so the dose must then be decreased. The total area to which a drug is distributed is known as volume of distribution. Patients who are particularly obese may present another problem when considering drug distribution. Some drugs—such as digoxin, gentamicin, and tobramycin—are not well distributed to fatty tissue. Therefore, dosing based on actual body weight may lead to overdose and serious toxicity. In some cases, dosing must be based on lean body weight, which may be estimated from actuarial tables that give average weight range for height.

3. Metabolism and excretion (drug elimination)

Most drugs are metabolized in the liver and excreted by the kidneys. Hepatic diseases may affect one or more of the metabolic functions of the liver. Therefore, in patients with hepatic disease, the metabolism of a drug may be increased, decreased, or unchanged. Clearly, all patients with hepatic disease must be monitored closely for drug effect and toxicity. Some drugs (digoxin, gentamicin) are eliminated almost unchanged by the kidneys. For safe use of such drugs, renal function must be adequate or the drug will accumulate, producing toxic effects. Some drugs can alter the effect and excretion of other drugs. For example, they can stimulate hepatic metabolizing enzymes to speed up the rate of metabolism and change the drug effect. Or they can block or promote renal excretion of other drugs, causing them to accumulate and enhance their effects or causing them to be too rapidly excreted and so diminish their effects. Some slight elimination takes place by way of perspiration, saliva, breast milk, and so on. Certain volatile anesthetics, however—halothane, for instance—are eliminated primarily by exhalation.

The rate at which a drug is metabolized varies with the individual. In some patients, drugs are metabolized so quickly that their blood and tissue levels prove therapeutically inadequate. In others, the rate of metabolism is so slow that ordinary doses can produce toxic results.

Other modifying factors

An important factor that influences a drug's action and effect is its *binding to plasma proteins,* especially albumin, and other tissue components. Because only a free, unbound drug can act in the body, such binding greatly influences effectiveness and duration of effect.

The *patient's age* is another important factor. Elderly patients usually have decreased hepatic function, less muscle mass, and diminished renal function. Consequently, they need lower doses and sometimes longer dosage intervals to avoid toxicity. With similar consequences, neonates have underdeveloped metabolic enzyme systems and inadequate renal function. They need highly individualized dosage and careful monitoring.

Underlying disease can also markedly affect drug action and effect. For example, acidosis may cause insulin resistance. Genetic diseases, such as glucose-6-phosphate dehydrogenase (G6PD) deficiency and hepatic porphyria, may turn drugs into toxins with serious consequences. Patients with G6PD deficiency may develop hemolytic anemia when given sulfonamides or a number of other drugs. A genetically susceptible patient can develop an acute porphyria attack if given a barbiturate. Also, patients who have highly active hepatic enzyme systems (for example, rapid acetylators), when treated with isoniazid, can develop hepatitis from the rapid intrahepatic buildup of a toxic metabolite.

Things to consider about administration

1. *Dosage forms do matter.* Some tablets and capsules are too large to be readily swallowed by very ill patients. You may then request an oral solution or elixir of the same drug, but bear in mind that because a liquid is more easily and completely absorbed, it produces higher blood levels than a tablet. When a potentially toxic drug (such as digoxin) is given, the increased amount absorbed could cause toxicity. Sometimes a change in dosage form requires a change in dosage.

2. *Routes of administration are not therapeutically interchangeable.* For example, phenytoin (Dilantin) is readily absorbed orally but is slowly and erratically absorbed intramuscularly. On the other hand, carbenicillin must be given parenterally because oral administration yields inadequate blood levels to treat systemic infections. However, it can be given orally to treat urinary tract infections because it concentrates in the urine.

3. *Improper storage can alter a drug's potency.* Most drugs should be stored in tight containers protected from direct sunlight and extremes in temperature and humidity which can cause them to deteriorate. Some may require special storage conditions (such as refrigeration).

4. *The timing of drug administration can be important.* Sometimes giving an oral drug during or shortly after mealtime decreases the amount of drug absorbed. This is not clinically significant with most drugs and may in fact be desirable with irritating drugs such as aspirin or phenylbuta-

zone. But penicillins and tetracyclines should not be scheduled for administration at mealtimes because certain foods can inactivate them. If in doubt about the effect of food on a certain drug, check with the pharmacist.

5. *Consider the patient's age, height, and weight.* The doctor will need this information when calculating the dose for many drugs. It should be accurately recorded on the patient's chart. This chart should also include current laboratory data, especially kidney and liver function studies, so the doctor can adapt dosage as needed.

6. *Watch for metabolic changes.* Monitor for any physiologic change that might alter drug effect (examples: depressed respiratory function and the development of acidosis or alkalosis).

7. *Know the patient's history.* Whenever possible, obtain a comprehensive family history from the patient or his family. Ask about past reactions to drugs, possible genetic traits that might alter drug response, and the current use of other drugs. Multiple drug therapy can cause drug interactions that can dramatically change the effects of many drugs.

Drug interactions

When one drug administered in combination with or shortly after another drug alters the effect of one or both drugs, this is known as a drug interaction. Usually, the effect of one drug is increased or decreased. For instance, one drug may inhibit or stimulate the metabolism or excretion of the other; or it may release another from plasma protein-binding sites, freeing it for further action.

Combination therapy is based upon drug interaction. One drug, for example, may be given to potentiate another. Probenecid, which blocks the excretion of penicillin, is sometimes given with penicillin to maintain adequate blood levels of penicillin for a longer period. Often two drugs with similar action are given together precisely because of the additive effect that results. Aspirin and codeine, for instance, both analgesics, are often given in combination because together they provide greater relief from pain than either alone.

Drug interactions are sometimes used to prevent or antagonize certain adverse reactions. Hydrochlorothiazide and spironolactone, both diuretics, are often administered in combination, because the former is potassium-depleting, while the latter is potassium-sparing.

But not all drug interactions are beneficial. Multiple drugs can interact to produce effects that are often undesirable and sometimes hazardous. Harmful drug interactions decrease efficacy or increase toxicity. A hypertensive patient well controlled with guanethidine may see his blood pressure rise to its former high level if he takes the antidepressant amitriptyline (Elavil) at the same time. Such a drug effect is known as antagonism. Drug combinations that produce these effects should be avoided if possible. Another kind of inhibiting effect occurs when a tetracycline drug is administered with calcium- or magnesium-containing drugs or foods (such as antacids or milk). These combine with tetracycline in the GI tract and cause inadequate absorption of tetracycline.

Adverse reactions

Any drug effect other than what is therapeutically intended can be called an adverse reaction. It may be expected and benign, or unexpected and potentially harmful. Mild, but *predictable,* adverse reactions are sometimes called side effects. Drowsiness caused by antihistamines is an example of this. During hay fever season, a patient may have to contend with this drowsiness to get relief from hay fever symptoms. In such a case, the dosage

may be adjusted up or down to balance therapeutic effects with side effects.

An adverse reaction may be tolerated for a necessary therapeutic effect, or it may be hazardous and unacceptable and require discontinuation of the drug. Some adverse reactions subside with continued use. As an example, the drowsiness associated with methyldopa (Aldomet) and the orthostatic hypotension associated with prazosin (Minipress) usually subside after several days, as the patient develops a tolerance to these effects. But many adverse reactions are dosage-related and lessen or disappear only if dosage is reduced. Although most adverse reactions are not therapeutically desirable, an occasional one can be put to clinical use. An outstanding example of this is the drowsiness associated with diphenhydramine (Benadryl), which makes it clinically useful as a mild hypnotic.

Hypersensitivity, a term sometimes used interchangeably with drug allergy, is the result of an antigen-antibody immune reaction that occurs in the body when a drug is given to a susceptible patient. One of the most dangerous of all drug hypersensitivities is penicillin allergy. In its severest form, penicillin anaphylaxis can rapidly become fatal.

Rarely, idiosyncratic reactions occur. These are highly unpredictable, individual, and unusual. Probably the best known idiosyncratic drug reaction is the aplastic anemia caused by the antibiotic chloramphenicol (Chloromycetin). This reaction appears in only 1 out of 40,000 patients, but when it does, it is often fatal. A more common idiosyncratic reaction is extreme sensitivity to very low doses of a drug, or insensitivity to higher-than-normal doses.

To deal with adverse reactions correctly, you need to be alert to even minor changes in the patient's clinical status. Such minor changes may be an early warning of pending toxicity. Listen to the patient's complaints about his reactions to a drug, and consider each complaint objectively. You may be able to reduce adverse reactions in several ways. Obviously, dosage reduction often helps. But often so does a simple rescheduling of the same dose. For example, pseudoephedrine (Sudafed) may produce stimulation that will be no problem if it's given early in the day; similarly, the drowsiness that occurs with antihistamines or tranquilizers can be totally harmless if the dose is given at bedtime. Most important, your patient needs to be told what adverse reactions to expect so he won't become worried or even stop taking the drug on his own. Of course, the patient should report any unusual or unexpected adverse reactions to the doctor.

Recognizing drug allergies or serious idiosyncratic reactions can sometimes be lifesaving. Ask each patient about drugs he is taking or has taken in the past and what, if any, unusual effects he experienced from taking them. If a patient claims to be allergic to a drug, ask him to tell you exactly what happens when he takes it. He may be calling a harmless side effect such as upset stomach an allergic reaction, or he may have a true tendency to anaphylaxis. In either case, you and the doctor need to know this. Of course, you must record and report any clinical changes throughout the patient's hospital stay. If you suspect a severe adverse reaction, withhold the drug until you can check with the pharmacist and the doctor.

Toxic reactions
Chronic drug toxicities are generally due to the cumulative effect and resulting buildup of the drug in the body. These effects may be extensions of the desired therapeutic effect. For example, guanethidine-induced nor-

epinephrine depletion produces a desired antihypertensive effect, but in larger doses, this action often produces orthostatic hypotension.

Drug toxicities usually occur when drug blood levels rise due to impaired metabolism or excretion. For example, blood levels of theophylline rise when hepatic dysfunction impairs metabolism of the drug. Similarly, digoxin toxicity can follow impaired renal function because digoxin is eliminated from the body almost exclusively by the kidneys (via glomerular filtration). Of course, toxic blood levels also follow excessive dosage. Aspirin tinnitus (ringing in ears) is usually a sign that the safe dose has been exceeded.

Most drug toxicities are predictable and dosage-related; fortunately, most are also readily reversible upon dosage adjustment. So it's essential to monitor patients carefully for physiologic changes that might alter drug effect. Watch especially for impaired hepatic and renal function. Warn the patient about signs of pending toxicity, and tell him what to do if a toxic reaction occurs. Also, be sure to emphasize the importance of taking a drug exactly as prescribed. Warn the patient about serious problems that could arise if he changes the dosage or the schedule for taking it.

Drugs and pregnancy
Ever since the thalidomide tragedy of the late 1950s—when thousands of malformed infants were born after their mothers used this mild sedative-hypnotic during pregnancy—use of drugs during pregnancy has been a source of serious medical concern and controversy. To identify drugs that may cause such teratogenic effects, preclinical drug studies always include tests on pregnant laboratory animals. These tests point out gross teratogenicity but do not clearly establish safety. Because different species

react to drugs in different ways, animal studies do not rule out possible teratogenic effects in humans. For example, the preliminary studies on thalidomide gave no warning of teratogenic effects, and it was subsequently released for general use in Europe.

What about the placental barrier? Once thought to protect the fetus from drug effects, the placenta isn't actually much of a barrier at all. Except for drugs with exceptionally large molecular structure, almost every drug administered to a pregnant woman crosses the placenta and enters the fetal circulation. An example of such large molecular size is heparin, the injectable anticoagulant. Theoretically, then, heparin could be used in a pregnant woman without fear of harming the fetus—but even heparin carries a warning for cautious use in pregnancy. Conversely, just because a drug crosses the placenta doesn't necessarily mean it's harmful to the fetus.

Actually, only one factor—stage of fetal development—seems clearly related to exaggerated risk during pregnancy. During two stages of pregnancy—the first and the third trimesters—the fetus is especially vulnerable to damage from maternal use of drugs. During these times, *all* drugs should be given with extreme caution.

The most sensitive period for drug-induced fetal malformation is the first trimester, when fetal organs are differentiating (organogenesis). During this time, *all* drugs should be withheld unless doing so would jeopardize the mother's health. Theoretically, during this sensitive time, even aspirin could harm the fetus. So, strongly advise your patient to avoid *all* self-prescribed drugs during early pregnancy.

The other time of special fetal sensitivity to drugs is the last trimester. The reason? At birth, when separated from his mother, the newborn must rely on his own metabolism to eliminate any remaining drug. Because his detoxifying systems are not fully developed, any residual drug may take a long time to be metabolized—and thus may induce prolonged toxic reactions. Consequently, drugs should be used only when absolutely necessary during the last 3 months of pregnancy.

Of course, in many circumstances, pregnant women must continue to take certain drugs. For example, a woman with a seizure disorder who is well controlled with an anticonvulsant should continue to take it even during pregnancy. Or a pregnant woman with a bacterial infection must receive antibiotics. In such cases, the potential risk to the fetus is overbalanced by the mother's need. The relative risk to the fetus is expressed by the drug's pregnancy risk category (see Chapter 1).

Following these general guidelines can prevent indiscriminate and potentially harmful use of drugs in pregnancy:

• Before a drug is prescribed for a woman of childbearing age, she should be asked the date of her last menstrual period and whether there is a possibility she is pregnant. If a drug is a known teratogen (for example, isotretinoin), some manufacturers may recommend special precautions to ensure that the drug not be given to a female of childbearing age until pregnancy is ruled out.

• Especially during the first and the third trimesters, a pregnant patient should avoid *all* drugs except those *essential* to maintain the pregnancy or maternal health.

• Topical drugs are not exempt from the warning against indiscriminate use during pregnancy. Many topically applied drugs can be absorbed in large enough amounts to be harmful to the fetus.

• When a pregnant patient needs *any* drug, the doctor should prescribe the *safest* possible drug in the *lowest* possible dose to minimize any harmful effect to the fetus.

• Every pregnant patient should check with her doctor before taking *any* drug.

Drugs and lactation

Most drugs a nursing mother takes appear in breast milk. Drug levels in breast milk tend to be high when blood levels are high—generally, shortly after taking each dose. Therefore, the mother should be advised to breast-feed *before* taking medication, not *after*.

Nevertheless, with very few exceptions, a mother who wishes to breast-feed may continue to do so with her doctor's permission. However, breast-feeding should be temporarily interrupted and replaced with bottle-feeding when the mother must take:

• tetracyclines
• chloramphenicol
• sulfonamides (during first 2 weeks postpartum)
• oral anticoagulants
• iodine-containing drugs
• antineoplastics.

To protect her infant, a nursing mother should avoid taking drugs indiscriminately. If she needs to take a drug to maintain her own health, she should first check with her doctor to be sure of taking the safest drug at the safest dose.

What to teach patients about proper use of drugs

Store drugs in their original containers, at room temperature, in places that are not accessible to children or exposed to sunlight. Avoid storage in the bathroom medicine cabinet or the glove compartment or trunk of an automobile, where extremes of temperature and humidity will cause them to deteriorate. Never share prescription drugs with others.

Learn the trade name and generic name of any drug you are taking. Be

sure to tell doctors, dentists, or other health care professionals you see regularly that you are taking it. Before taking any drug, be sure you have informed your doctor, nurse, or pharmacist about any unusual reactions you've had to drugs in the past and about your allergies to foods and other substances, any special medical problems, and any drugs you've taken over the last few weeks, including any nonprescription drugs.

Always take any drug exactly as prescribed, at the recommended dosage schedule and duration of treatment.

To avoid hazardous mistakes, always read the label before taking any drug. When using a drug prescribed for occasional or prolonged use, check the container for an expiration date (if available).

To avoid potentially harmful changes in effectiveness, do not change brands of a drug required for long-term use without medical approval. Certain generic preparations are not precisely equivalent in effect to brand-name preparations of the same drug.

Never mix different drugs in a single container, and don't remove any drug from its original container or remove the label. Relying on your memory to identify a drug and specific directions for its use is extremely hazardous.

Discard any drugs that are outdated or no longer needed.

Before you have any surgery (including dental surgery), tell the doctor about all of the drugs that you have been taking.

Be sure to tell the doctor, nurse, or pharmacist about any side effects or unpleasant effects you've experienced while taking a drug. Such effects may require medical attention.

If you suspect that you or someone else has taken an overdose, call your doctor, poison control center, or pharmacist immediately. Keep syrup of ipecac in your home to induce vomiting, but induce vomiting only if one of these professionals has advised you to do so.

Drug therapy in children

A child's absorption, distribution, metabolism, and excretion processes undergo profound changes that affect drug dosage. To ensure optimal drug effect and minimal toxicity, consider these factors when administering drugs to a child.

Absorption

Drug absorption in children depends on the form of the drug; its physical properties; other drugs or substances, such as food, taken simultaneously; physiologic changes; and concurrent disease.

• The pH of neonatal gastric fluid is neutral or slightly acidic and becomes more acidic as the infant matures. This affects drug absorption. For example, nafcillin and penicillin G, erratically absorbed or malabsorbed in an adult due to degradation by gastric acid, are better absorbed in an infant due to low gastric acidity.

• Various infant formulas or milk products may increase gastric pH and impede absorption of acidic drugs. So, if possible, give a child oral medications when his stomach is empty.

• Gastric emptying time and transit time through the small intestine—which is longer in children than in adults—can affect absorption. Also, intestinal hypermotility (as in diarrhea) can diminish the drug's absorption.

• A child's comparatively thin epidermis allows increased absorption of topical drugs.

Distribution

As with absorption, changes in body weight and physiology during childhood can significantly influence a drug's distribution and effects. In a premature infant, body fluid makes up about 85% of total body weight; in a full-term infant, 55% to 70%; and in an adult, 50% to 55%. Extracellular fluid (mostly blood) constitutes 40% of a neonate's body weight, compared with 20% in an adult. Intracellular fluid remains fairly constant throughout life and has little effect on drug dosage.

Since most drugs travel through extracellular fluid to reach their receptors, however, extracellular fluid volume influences a water-soluble drug's concentration and effect. Children have a larger proportion of fluid to solid body weight, so their distribution area is proportionately greater.

Because the proportion of fat to lean body mass increases with age, the distribution of fat-soluble drugs is more limited in children than in adults. As a result, a drug's lipid- or water-solubility affects the dosage for a child.

Binding to plasma proteins

As the result of a decrease in albumin concentration or intermolecular attraction between drug and plasma protein, many drugs are less bound to plasma proteins in infants than in adults.

Furthermore, preparations that bind plasma proteins may displace endogenous compounds, such as bilirubin or free fatty acids. Conversely, an endogenous compound may displace a weakly bound drug. For example, displacement of bound bilirubin can cause a rise in unbound bilirubin, which can lead to increased risk of kernicterus at normal bilirubin levels.

Since only an unbound, or free, drug has a pharmacologic effect, any alteration in ratio of a protein-bound to an unbound active drug can greatly influence its effect.

Several diseases and disorders, such as nephrotic syndrome and malnutrition, can also decrease plasma protein and increase the concentration of an unbound drug, intensifying the drug's effect or producing toxicity.

Metabolism

A newborn's ability to metabolize a drug depends on the integrity of his hepatic enzyme system, his intrauterine exposure to the drug, and the nature of the drug itself.

Certain metabolic mechanisms are underdeveloped in neonates. Glucuronidation is a metabolic process that renders most drugs more water soluble, thereby facilitating renal excretion. This process is insufficiently developed to permit full pediatric doses until the infant is 1 month old. Because of this, the use of chloramphenicol in a newborn may cause gray baby syndrome, illustrating the newborn's inability to metabolize the drug. Use of chloramphenicol in neonates, therefore, requires decreased dosage (25 mg/kg/day) and monitoring of blood levels.

Conversely, intrauterine exposure to drugs may induce precocious development of hepatic enzyme mechanisms, increasing the infant's capacity to metabolize potentially harmful substances.

Older children can metabolize some drugs (theophylline, for example) more rapidly than adults. This ability may be due to their increased hepatic metabolic activity. Larger doses than those recommended for adults may be required.

Also, preparations given concurrently to a child may alter hepatic metabolism and induce production of hepatic enzymes. Phenobarbital, for example, can induce hepatic enzyme production and accelerate metabolism of drugs given concurrently.

Excretion

Renal excretion of a drug is the net effect of glomerular filtration, active tubular secretion, and passive tubular reabsorption. Because so many drugs are excreted in the urine, the degree of renal development or presence of renal disease can profoundly affect a child's dosage requirements.

If a child is unable to excrete a drug renally, drug accumulation and possible toxicity may result unless dosage is reduced.

Physiologically, an infant's kidneys differ from an adult's in that they have:
• high resistance to blood flow and receive a smaller proportion of cardiac output
• incomplete glomerular and tubular development and short, incomplete loops of Henle (A child's glomerular filtration reaches adult values by age 2½ to 5 months; his tubular secretion may reach adult values by age 7 to 12 months.)
• low glomerular filtration rate (Penicillins are eliminated by this route.)
• decreased ability to concentrate urine or reabsorb various filtered compounds
• reduced ability by the proximal tubules to secrete organic acids.

Both children and adults have diurnal variations in urine pH that correlate with sleep-wake patterns.

Calculating and monitoring pediatric dosages

When calculating pediatric dosages,

don't use formulas that modify adult dosages: a child is not a scaled-down version of an adult. Pediatric dosages should be calculated on the basis of either body weight (mg/kg) or body surface area (mg/m²).

• Reevaluate dosages at regular intervals to ensure necessary adjustments as the child develops.

• Although useful for adults and older children, don't use dosages based on body surface area in premature or full-term infants. Use the body weight method instead.

• Don't exceed the maximum adult dosage when calculating amounts per kilogram of body weight (except with certain drugs, such as theophylline, if indicated).

• Obtain an accurate maternal drug history—prescription and nonprescription drugs, vitamins, and herbs or other health foods taken during pregnancy.

• Drugs passed through breast milk can also have adverse effects on the nursing infant. Before a drug is prescribed for a breast-feeding mother, the potential effects on the infant should be investigated. For example, sulfonamides given to a breast-feeding mother for a urinary tract infection appear in breast milk and may cause kernicterus at lower-than-normal levels of unconjugated bilirubin. Also, high concentrations of isoniazid appear in breast milk. Since this drug is metabolized by the liver, an infant's immature hepatic enzyme mechanisms cannot metabolize the drug, and the infant may suffer central nervous system (CNS) toxicity.

Oral medications

• *When giving oral medication to an infant,* administer it in liquid form if possible. For accuracy, measure and give the preparation by syringe; never use a vial or cup.

• Lift the patient's head to prevent aspiration of the medication, and press down on his chin to prevent choking.

• You may also place the drug in a nipple and allow the infant to suck the contents.

• *If the patient is a toddler,* explain how you're going to give him the medication. If possible, have the parents enlist the child's cooperation.

• Don't mix medication with food or call it "candy" even if it has a pleasant taste.

• Let the child drink liquid medication from a calibrated medication cup rather than from a spoon: it's easier and more accurate. If the preparation is available only in tablet form, crush it and mix it with a compatible syrup. (Check with the pharmacist to make sure the tablet can be crushed without losing its effectiveness.)

• *If the patient's an older child* who can swallow a tablet or capsule by himself, have him place the medication on the back of his tongue and swallow it with water or fruit juice. Remember, milk or milk products may interfere with drug absorption.

Intravenous infusions

When administering I.V. infusions to children, note the following special considerations.

Protecting the insertion site
In infants, use a peripheral vein or a scalp vein in the temporal region for I.V. infusions. The scalp vein is safest in that the needle is not likely to be dislodged; however, the head must be shaved around the site. Temporary disfigurement may also result from the needle and infiltrated fluids. For these reasons, the scalp veins are not used as frequently today as they were in the past.

The extremities are the most accessible insertion sites; however, since patients tend to move about, take these precautions:

• Protect the insertion site to prevent catheter or needle dislodgment.
• Use a padded arm board to minimize dislodgment. Remove the arm board during range-of-motion exercises.
• Place the clamp out of the child's reach; if extension tubing is used to allow the child greater mobility, securely tape the connection.
• Restrain the child only when necessary.
• To allay anxiety, give a simple explanation to the child who must be restrained while asleep.

Maintaining flow rate and fluid balance
While administering a continuous I.V. infusion to a child, monitor flow rate and check the patient's condition and insertion site at least hourly—more frequently when giving drug intermittently.
   Adjust the flow rate only while the patient is composed; crying and emotional upset can constrict blood vessels. Flow rate may vary if a pump isn't used. Flow should be adequate because some drugs (calcium, for example) can be very irritating at low flow rates.

Making dilutions
Some drugs are hyperosmolar; in infants, these drugs must be diluted to prevent radical changes in fluid that might induce CNS hemorrhage. Sodium bicarbonate, for example, must be diluted to half-strength to lower osmolality and lessen the risk of CNS bleeding.
   In general, however, use the minimum amount of compatible fluid over the shortest recommended period of time. Remember also to check the total daily fluid intake and the amount allotted to medication.

Intramuscular injections
Intramuscular injections are preferred when the drug cannot be given by other parenteral routes and rapid absorption is necessary.
• In children under 2 years, the vastus lateralis muscle is the preferred injection site; in older children, either the ventrogluteal area or the gluteus medius muscle can be used.
• To determine correct needle size, consider the patient's age, muscle mass, and nutritional status and the drug's viscosity; record and rotate injection sites.
• Explain to the patient that the injection will hurt, but that the medication will help him. Restrain him during the injection, if needed, and comfort him afterward.

Dermatomucosal medications
• Use eardrops warmed to room temperature; cold drops can cause considerable pain and possibly vertigo.
• To administer drops, turn the patient on his side, with the affected ear up. If he is younger than 3 years, pull the pinna down and back; if he is older than 3 years, pull the pinna up and back.
• Avoid using inhalants in very young children: obtaining their cooperation is difficult.
• Before attempting to administer medication through a metered-dose nebulizer to an older child, explain the inhaler to him. Then have him hold the nebulizer upside down and close his lips around the mouthpiece. Have him exhale; pinch his nostrils shut; and when he starts to inhale, release one dose of medication into his mouth. Tell the patient to continue inhaling until his lungs feel full.
• Most inhaled agents are not useful if taken orally; therefore, if you doubt the patient's ability to use the inhalant correctly, don't use it.
• Use topical corticosteroids with caution, because chronic steroid use in children has been associated with delayed growth. When topical corti-

costeroids are used on the diaper area of infants, avoid covering this area with plastic or rubber pants, which will act as an occlusive dressing and enhance systemic absorption.

Parenteral nutrition

Intravenous nutrition is given to patients who can't or won't take adequate food orally and patients with hypermetabolic conditions who need I.V. supplementation. The latter group includes premature infants and children who have burns or other major trauma, intractable diarrhea, malabsorption syndromes, gastrointestinal abnormalities, emotional disorders (such as anorexia nervosa), and congenital abnormalities.

Before fat emulsions are administered to infants and children, however, potential benefits must be weighed against possible risks.

Fats—supplied as 10% or 20% emulsions—are administered both peripherally and centrally. Their use is limited by the child's ability to metabolize them. An infant or child with a diseased liver cannot efficiently metabolize fats, for example.

Some fats, however, must be supplied both to prevent essential fatty acid deficiency and to permit normal growth and development. A minimum of calories (2% to 4%) must be supplied as linoleic acid—an essential fatty acid found in lipids. In infants, fats are essential for normal neurologic development.

Nevertheless, fat solutions may decrease oxygen perfusion and may adversely affect children with pulmonary disease. This risk can be minimized by supplying only the minimum fat needed for essential fatty acid requirements and not the usual intake of 40% to 50% of the child's total calories.

Fatty acids can also displace bilirubin bound to serum albumin, causing a rise in free, unconjugated bilirubin and an increased risk of kernicterus. However, fat solutions may interfere with some bilirubin assays and cause falsely elevated levels. To avoid this complication, a blood sample should be drawn 4 hours after infusion of the lipid emulsion; or if the emulsion is introduced over 24 hours, the blood sample should be centrifuged before the assay is performed.

4

Drug therapy in elderly patients

If you're providing drug therapy for elderly patients, you'll want to understand physiologic and pharmacokinetic changes that may alter drug dosage, common adverse reactions, and compliance problems in elderly patients.

Physiologic changes affecting drug action

As a person ages, gradual physiologic changes occur. Some of these age-related changes may alter the therapeutic and toxic effects of medications.

Body composition
Proportions of fat, lean tissue, and water in the body change with age. Total body mass and lean body mass tend to decrease; the proportion of body fat tends to increase.

Varying from person to person, these changes in body composition affect the relationship between a drug's concentration and distribution in the body.

For example, a water-soluble drug, such as gentamicin, is not distributed to fat. Since there's relatively less lean tissue in an elderly person, more drug remains in the blood.

Gastrointestinal function
In elderly patients, decreases in gastric acid secretion and GI motility slow the emptying of stomach contents and the movement of intestinal contents through the entire tract. Furthermore, inconclusive research shows that elderly patients may have more difficulty absorbing medica-

tions. This is a particularly significant problem with drugs having a narrow therapeutic range, such as digoxin, in which any change in absorption can be crucial.

Hepatic function
The liver's ability to metabolize certain drugs decreases with age. This is due to diminished blood flow to the liver, which results from the age-related decrease in cardiac output and from the diminished activity of certain liver enzymes. When an elderly patient takes certain sleep medications, such as secobarbital, his liver's reduced ability to metabolize the drug may produce a hangover effect the next morning.

Decreased hepatic function may cause:
• more intense drug effects due to higher blood levels
• longer-lasting drug effects due to prolonged blood concentrations
• greater incidence of drug toxicity.

Renal function
Although an elderly person's renal function is usually sufficient to eliminate excess body fluid and waste, his ability to eliminate some medications may be reduced by 50% or more.

Many medications commonly used by elderly patients, such as digoxin, are excreted primarily through the kidneys. If the kidneys' ability to excrete the drug is decreased, high blood concentrations may result. Digoxin toxicity, therefore, is relatively common in elderly patients who are not receiving a reduced digoxin dosage to account for their decreased renal function.

Drug dosages can be modified to compensate for age-related decreases in renal function. Aided by laboratory tests, such as blood urea nitrogen and serum creatinine, clinical pharmacists may recommend a change and doctors may adjust medication dosages so the patient receives the expected therapeutic benefits without the risk of toxicity. Observe your patient for signs of toxicity. A patient taking digoxin, for example, may experience anorexia, nausea, vomiting, or confusion.

Adverse drug reactions

As compared with younger people, elderly patients experience twice as many adverse drug reactions relating to greater drug consumption, poor compliance, and physiologic changes.

Signs and symptoms of adverse drug reactions—confusion, weakness, and lethargy—are often mistakenly attributed to senility or disease. If the adverse reaction isn't identified, the patient may continue to receive the drug. Furthermore, he may receive unnecessary additional medication to treat complications caused by the original medication. This can sometimes result in the pattern of inappropriate and excessive medication use referred to as "polypharmacy."

Although any medication can cause adverse reactions, most of the serious reactions in the elderly are caused by relatively few medications. Be particularly alert for toxicities resulting from diuretics, antihypertensives, digoxin, corticosteroids, sleeping aids, and nonprescription drugs.

Diuretic toxicity
Because total body water content decreases with age, normal dosages of potassium-wasting diuretics, such as hydrochlorothiazide and furosemide,
may result in fluid loss and even dehydration in an elderly patient.

These diuretics may deplete serum potassium, causing weakness in the patient; and they may raise blood uric acid and glucose levels, complicating preexisting gout and diabetes mellitus.

Antihypertensive toxicity
Many elderly people experience lightheadedness or fainting when using antihypertensive medications. This is partially due to the fact that hypertension in elderly patients is partly a response to such changes as atherosclerosis and decreased elasticity of the blood vessels. Antihypertensive drugs lower blood pressure too rapidly, resulting in insufficient blood flow to the brain. This may cause dizziness, fainting, or even stroke.

Consequently, dosages of antihypertensive drugs must be carefully individualized for each patient. In elderly patients, overaggressive treatment of high blood pressure may clearly do more harm than good, so treatment goals should be reasonable. While it may be appropriate to bring blood pressure down to 120/85 mm Hg for a young hypertensive patient, a more reasonable goal for some elderly hypertensive patients might be 150/95 mm Hg.

Digoxin toxicity
As the body's renal function and rate of excretion decline, digoxin concentrations in the blood may build to toxic levels, causing nausea, vomiting, diarrhea, and—most serious—cardiac arrhythmias. Try to prevent severe toxicity by observing your patient for early signs, such as appetite loss, confusion, or depression.

Corticosteroid toxicity
Elderly patients on corticosteroids may experience short-term effects, including fluid retention and psycholog-

ical manifestations ranging from mild euphoria to acute psychotic reactions. Long-term toxic effects, such as osteoporosis, can be especially severe in elderly patients who have been taking prednisone or related steroidal compounds for months or even years. To prevent serious toxicity, carefully monitor patients on long-term regimens. Observe them for subtle changes in appearance, mood, and mobility, as well as for signs of impaired healing and fluid and electrolyte disturbances.

Sleeping aid toxicity
Sedatives or sleeping aids, such as flurazepam, may cause excessive sedation or residual drowsiness.

Nonprescription drug toxicity
When aspirin and aspirin-containing analgesics are used in moderation, toxicity is minimal, but prolonged ingestion may cause GI irritation and gradual blood loss resulting in severe anemia. Although anemia from chronic aspirin consumption can affect all age-groups, elderly patients may be less able to compensate because of their already reduced iron stores.

Laxatives may cause diarrhea in elderly patients who are extremely sensitive to drugs such as bisacodyl. Chronic oral use of mineral oil as a lubricating laxative may result in lipid pneumonia due to aspiration of small residual oil droplets in the patient's mouth.

Patient noncompliance
Poor compliance is a problem with patients of all ages. However, in elderly patients, specific factors linked to aging—such as diminished visual acuity, hearing loss, forgetfulness, the common need for multiple drug therapy, and various socioeconomic factors—combine to make compliance a special problem. Approximately one-third of elderly patients fail to comply with their prescribed drug therapy. They may fail to take prescribed doses or to follow the correct schedule; they may take medications prescribed for previous disorders, discontinue medications prematurely, or use p.r.n. medications indiscriminately.

Review your patient's medication regimen with him. Be sure he understands the medication amount and the time and frequency of doses. Also, explain how he should take each medication, that is, with food or water or by itself.

Give your patient whatever help you can to avoid drug therapy problems, and refer him to the doctor or pharmacist if he needs further information.

Drug therapy and the nursing process

The nursing process guides nursing decisions about drug administration to ensure the patient's safety and meet medical and legal standards. This process, in five steps, provides thorough assessment, appropriate nursing diagnosis, purposeful planning, appropriate interventions, and constant evaluation.

First step: Assessment
During assessment, the nurse focuses on direct data collection by:
• obtaining a drug history from the patient, parent, spouse, or significant other
• reviewing the patient's previous medical history
• performing a physical examination of the patient
• obtaining relevant laboratory or diagnostic test results.

Drug history
Data collection begins at admission to the hospital or in an outpatient setting with specific questions about the patient's background, including allergies, medical history, habits, socioeconomic status, life-style and beliefs, and sensory deficits. These aspects of the patient's background can have significant influence on drug therapy.

Allergies
The patient's allergy profile includes the patient's reactions to both drugs and food. Information about allergic reactions to drugs must specify the drug, when the allergic reaction oc-

curred, the situation and setting at the time of the reaction, a description of the reaction, and any contributing factors. Examples of contributing factors might include the concurrent use of stimulants, tobacco, alcohol, or illicit drugs, or a significant change in nutritional patterns. Asking the patient to describe his allergic reaction is especially important to help determine whether the patient actually reacts adversely to a drug or simply dislikes taking it.

Allergies to foods can also affect a drug therapy. For example, allergies to shellfish can contraindicate use of drugs that contain iodine or are by-products of shellfish. Allergies to eggs are significant in patients who are to receive vaccines, which are commonly derived from chick embryos.

Prescription drugs
The patient's drug history should explore the following:
• the reason for using the drug
• the patient's knowledge of the appropriate dosage and schedule of administration
• the patient's knowedge about determining effectiveness of the drug (if appropriate), adverse effects the drug might cause, what to do about adverse effects, and when to contact the doctor
• route of administration
• the pattern of administration at home
• use of OTC drugs
• cognitive status.

Note any special monitoring the patient must perform, such as blood glucose monitoring before insulin administration or checking radial pulse rate before taking digoxin. Make sure the patient is performing such procedures correctly and that the results are within acceptable limits.

Discuss the effects of drug therapy with the patient and determine if new symptoms or unpredicted adverse effects have developed. Noting the patient's pattern of administration may provide insight into why a particular drug regimen succeeds or fails.

Over-the-counter drugs
A comprehensive drug history should also list any OTC drugs the patient is taking. Many OTC drugs can inhibit or potentiate the effects of a prescribed drug. For example, aspirin potentiates the anticoagulant effects of warfarin.

OTC drugs include a wide range of products from common aspirin and nutritional supplements to various sprays and cleansing agents. The patient may not think of all of these products as drugs, so the nurse may have to suggest a general list of products to get an accurate response.

Dosage and frequency of use are just as important as the type of the OTC product the patient is using. One tablet of aspirin taken once a day may have no effect on concomitant drug therapy; however, a higher dosage (such as that used for arthritis) could influence it profoundly.

Medical history
In gathering the medical history, note any chronic diseases or disorders the patient may have and record the following information for each:
• date of diagnosis
• initial prescribed treatment
• current treatment
• the doctor in charge.

Careful attention to this part of the medical history can uncover one of the most important problems with drug therapy—conflicting and incompatible drug regimens. The patient who does not have a family physician to oversee and coordinate all care may seek the care of several specialists who may prescribe drug treatment without knowing what other drugs the patient is taking. A carefully detailed medical history can uncover such problems. The nurse who identifies such conflicting or overlapping drug therapy must call them to the appropriate doctor's attention and then teach the patient about the importance of informing all care-givers about all drugs he is taking.

Habits
Carefully consider dietary habits and the nontherapeutic use of drugs.

Certain foods can directly affect the effectiveness of many drugs. For example, a person who is taking the anticoagulant warfarin (Coumadin) should not increase his intake of green leafy vegetables because they contain significant levels of vitamin K that can antagonize the drug's anticoagulant effect.

Nontherapeutic use of drugs can profoundly affect a patient's health and impair the effectiveness of a drug therapy. Consider the possible use of alcohol, tobacco, caffeine, and illicit drugs, such as marijuana, cocaine, and heroin. For example, if the patient uses alcohol, note the frequency of use, the amount, and the type of alcohol consumed. Carefully document the intake of stimulants, such as caffeine, because they significantly affect a patient's cardiovascular status and nervous system. Record the type of stimulant (coffee, tea, soda, or chocolate), the frequency of intake, and the amount consumed.

For the patient who smokes, document the following information:

• the length of time the patient has smoked

• what the patient smokes (cigarettes, cigar, or pipe)

• how many cigarettes or cigars the patient smokes per day

• the brand of cigarettes or cigars the patient smokes

• the brand of tobacco and how much he chews per day, if he chews it.

Defining the patient's use of illicit drugs may be difficult. However, the nurse who suspects such use should encourage the patient to discuss it honestly, emphasizing that these drugs have profound effects that may cause serious drug interactions. If the patient admits using illicit drugs, document the drug, the amount and frequency of use, and the route of administration.

Socioeconomic status
Note the patient's age, educational level, occupation, and insurance coverage. These factors may be significant to compliance and to an effective care plan. The patient's age, for example, can determine whom to include in the care plan (parents or other family members) and the level of information that is appropriate for teaching the patient.

Knowing the patient's educational background and occupation helps the nurse select interventions at an appropriate level, plan a drug regimen that fits the patient's daily routine, and encourage compliance. Knowing the patient's insurance status may help you anticipate the patient's need for financial assistance and counseling. Remember that noncompliance frequently results from inability to afford costly medications.

Life-style and beliefs
Support systems, marital status, childbearing status, attitudes toward health and health care, use of the health care system, and daily patterns

of activities all affect the plan of care and patient compliance. For example, an 18-year-old single parent, who is a high-school dropout on medical assistance and has no family support, will probably require more extensive teaching and support to gain a commitment and compliance to drug therapy than a 40-year-old affluent professional, with a lot of family support who can understand why she needs the drug and can readily pay for it.

Sensory deficits
Any sensory deficit can significantly shape an appropriate care plan. For example, impaired vision, paralysis of one or more extremities, loss of a limb, or loss of sensation in an extremity can impair the patient's ability to administer a subcutaneous injection, break a scored tablet, or open a medication container. Color blindness may cause difficulty in distinguishing between two medications. Hearing impairment can prevent effective patient instruction. Any sensory deficit requires careful consideration in any plan of prescribed drug therapy.

Clinical status
Two other factors can profoundly influence drug therapy: the patient's cognitive status and systemic effects of the prescribed drugs. A patient's intact cognitive abilities ensure that he can understand and implement the actions necessary for compliance. During the interview, note if the patient is alert and oriented, if he is able to interact appropriately with people, and if his conversation is appropriate to the subject being discussed. Consider whether the patient can think clearly, and express his thoughts coherently. Finally, check both short-term and long-term memory because the patient needs both to follow a specified drug regimen. If such evaluation identifies a cognitive deficit, de-

termine the probable cause, which can range from a transient drug-related effect to permanent neurologic impairment, and then determine whether or not the patient can carry out the prescribed drug regimen. If not, the nurse must find another way to ensure that the patient receives the prescribed therapy.

After completing the drug history, perform a physical examination to assess those body systems that may be affected by a particular drug the patient is taking or that may be prescribed. Every drug has a desired effect on a body system but it may have an undesired effect on another. For example, chemotherapeutic agents destroy cancerous cells but they also affect normal cells and often cause the patient to experience hair loss, diarrhea, or nausea. Therefore, examine the patient for expected drug effects; also closely monitor the patient for potentially harmful adverse effects.

Second step: Formulating a nursing diagnosis
Using information gathered during assessment, define any potential or actual drug-related problems by formulating each in a relevant nursing diagnosis. The most common problem statements related to drug therapy are "Knowledge deficit," "Noncompliance," and "Alteration in Health Maintenance."

Third step: Planning
Nursing diagnoses provide the framework for planning interventions and outcome criteria (patient goals).

Outcome criteria
Outcome criteria state the desired patient behaviors or responses that should result from nursing care. Outcome criteria should be measurable and objective, concise, realistic for the patient, and attainable by nursing management; they should express pa-

tient behavior in terms of expectations and specify a time frame. A typical outcome statement is "The patient verbalizes major adverse effects related to his chemotherapy drugs prior to discharge."

Fourth step: Intervention
After developing the outcome criteria, the nurse determines the interventions needed to help the patient reach the desired behavior or goals. Drug-related interventions may focus on patient teaching for a drug's action, adverse effects, scheduling, steps to avoid or treat a drug reaction, or drug administration techniques.

Appropriate interventions related to drug therapy will also include administration procedures, administration techniques, legal and ethical concerns, patient teaching, and any special concerns related to special groups of patients (geriatric, pediatric, and pregnant or breast-feeding patients). Such interventions may be independent nursing actions, such as turning a bedridden patient every 2 hours, or may be nursing actions that require a doctor's order.

Fifth step: Evaluation
The final component of the nursing process, evaluation, is a formal and systematic process for determining the effectiveness of nursing care. This process enables the nurse to determine whether outcome criteria were met, and thereby make informed decisions about subsequent interventions. For example, if the patient experienced relief of headache within 1 hour after the nurse administered a p.r.n. analgesic, the outcome criterion was met. If the headache was the same or worse, the outcome criterion was not met and requires reassessment, which may require replanning or may yield new data that invalidates the nursing diagnosis or suggests new nursing interventions that are more specific or

more acceptable to the patient. Such reassessment could lead to a higher dosage, a different analgesic, or a re-evaluation of the cause.

Evaluation enables the nurse to design and implement a revised care plan, to continuously reevaluate outcome criteria, and to replan until each nursing diagnosis is resolved.

Amebicides and trichomonacides

carbarsone
chloroquine hydrochloride
  (See Chapter 9, ANTIMALARIALS.)
chloroquine phosphate
  (See Chapter 9, ANTIMALARIALS.)
emetine hydrochloride
iodoquinol
metronidazole
metronidazole hydrochloride
paromomycin sulfate

COMBINATION PRODUCTS
None.

---

carbarsone
Carbarsone Pulvules

Pregnancy Risk Category: D

HOW SUPPLIED
Capsules: 250 mg

MECHANISM OF ACTION
An organic arsenic derivative with
amebicidal activity in the intestinal
lumen, probably by causing enzyme
inhibition following combination with
sulfhydryl groups.

INDICATIONS & DOSAGE
Intestinal amebiasis—
Adults: 250 mg P.O. b.i.d. or t.i.d.
for 10 days. Rectal (as retention
enema): 2 g dissolved in 200 ml warm
2% sodium bicarbonate solution, every other night for five doses. Solution should be retained overnight.
Discontinue oral therapy when enema
is given.
Children: average total dosage is 75
mg/kg P.O. daily in three divided

doses over 10-day period. Recommended total dosage varies according
to age—2 to 4 years, 2 g total; 5 to 8
years, 3 g total; 9 to 12 years, 4 g total; and over 12 years, 5 g total.

ADVERSE REACTIONS
Blood: *agranulocytosis.*
CNS: neuritis, seizures, *hemorrhagic
encephalitis.*
EENT: sore throat, retinal edema, visual disturbances.
GI: epigastric pain and burning, irritation, *nausea, vomiting,* diarrhea,
anorexia, constipation, increased motility, abdominal cramps.
GU: polyuria, albuminuria, kidney
damage.
Hepatic: hepatomegaly, jaundice,
hepatitis.
Skin: eruptions, *exfoliative dermatitis,* pruritus.
Other: edema of wrists, ankles, and
knees; weight loss; splenomegaly.

INTERACTIONS
None significant.

NURSING CONSIDERATIONS
• Contraindicated as initial treatment
in hepatic or renal disease; in patients
with contracted visual or color fields;
and in patients with known hypersensitivity or intolerance to any arsenical
treatment.
• Don't exceed recommended dose;
toxicity may result. If second treatment is needed, allow at least 10 days
between courses.
• Monitor for signs of acute arsenic
toxicity: sore throat; edema of wrists,

ankles, and knees; nausea and vomiting. Acute toxicity may be treated with dimercaprol.
• Divide carbarsone capsule to obtain required dose. Give in ½ glass orange juice or milk, in small amount of 1% sodium bicarbonate solution, or in jelly or other food.
• Discontinue upon first sign of intolerance or toxicity. Fatal exfoliative dermatitis has been reported.
• Tell patient to report any unusual symptoms, even post-treatment.
• Liver function tests should precede therapy. Careful inspection of skin, vision testing, and palpation of liver and spleen should be repeated regularly.
• Monitor intake/output. Record number, frequency, and character of stools.
• If ordered, give a cleansing enema of 2% sodium bicarbonate before giving carbarsone enema.
• All members of household may need to have stools examined.
• Deliver stool specimen to lab promptly; movements of parasites are seen only when stool is warm. Amebic cysts in stool indicate need for additional therapy. Stool specimen should be studied 1 week after stopping therapy and monthly for 1 year.
• To help prevent reinfestation, teach-patient about the need for good personal hygiene, especially handwashing technique. Patient should refrain from preparing food until stools are negative.

emetine hydrochloride
Pregnancy Risk Category: X

HOW SUPPLIED
Injection: 65 mg/ml

MECHANISM OF ACTION
Kills *Entamoeba histolytica* by a mechanism related to the inhibition of protein synthesis.

INDICATIONS & DOSAGE
Acute fulminating amebic dysentery—
Adults: 1 mg/kg daily up to 60 mg daily (one or two doses) deep S.C. or I.M. 3 to 5 days (only until symptoms are under control). Give another antiamebic drug simultaneously.
Children: 1 mg/kg daily in two doses I.M. for up to 5 days.
Amebic hepatitis and abscess—
Adults: 60 mg daily (one or two doses) deep S.C. or I.M. for 10 days.

ADVERSE REACTIONS
CNS: dizziness, headache, mild sensory disturbances, central or peripheral nerve function changes, neuromuscular symptoms (weakness, aching, stiffness, tenderness, pain, tremors).
CV: *acute toxicity*—can occur at any dose (hypotension, tachycardia, precordial pain, dyspnea, *ECG abnormalities,* gallop rhythm, cardiac dilatation, severe acute degenerative myocarditis, pericarditis, congestive failure).
GI: *nausea, vomiting, diarrhea,* abdominal cramps, loss of sense of taste.
Metabolic: decreased serum potassium levels.
Skin: eczematous, urticarial purpuric lesions.
Local: skeletal muscle stiffness, aching, tenderness, *muscle weakness at injection site, cellulitis.*
Other: edema.

INTERACTIONS
None significant.

NURSING CONSIDERATIONS
• Contraindicated in cardiac or renal disease, except with amebic abscess or hepatitis not controlled by chloroquine or metronidazole; in patients who have received a course of emetine less than 6 to 8 weeks previously; in children, except for those with severe dysentery unresponsive to other

---

Italicized adverse reactions are common or life-threatening.
*Liquid form contains alcohol.   **May contain tartrazine.

amebicides; and in patients with poly-neuropathy or muscle disease. Use with caution and in reduced dosage in elderly or debilitated patients, patients with hypotension, or those about to undergo surgery.
• Record pulse rate and blood pressure 2 to 3 times daily. Discontinue use if drug produces tachycardia, precipitous fall in blood pressure, neuromuscular symptoms, marked gastrointestinal effects, or considerable weakness. Weakness and muscle symptoms usually precede more serious symptoms and serve as a guide for avoiding toxicity.
• Because of potential for cardiovascular toxicity, don't exceed recommended dose or extend therapy beyond 10 days. Impose bed rest during treatment and for several days thereafter.
• Drug may alter ECG tracings for 6 weeks. ECG should be taken before therapy, after fifth dose, upon completion, and 1 week after therapy. Patterns can resemble those of myocardial infarction. First and most consistent change is T wave inversion.
• Deep S.C. administration is preferred; I.M. is acceptable, but I.V. route can be cardiotoxic and is contraindicated. Rotate sites and apply warm soaks.
• Record intake/output; odor and consistency of stools; and presence of mucus, blood, or other foreign matter. Send warm specimens to lab for analysis. Repeat fecal examinations at 3-month intervals to assure elimination of amebae. Patients with acute amebic dysentery often become asymptomatic carriers. Check family members and suspected contacts.
• Suspect emetine-induced reaction if stools increase in number following initial relief of diarrhea.
• To help prevent reinfestation, teach patient about the need for good personal hygiene, especially handwashing technique. Patient should refrain from preparing food until stools are negative.
• Drug is very irritating. Avoid contact with eyes and mucous membranes.

iodoquinol
(diiodohydroxyquin)
Diodoquin†, Moebiquin, Yodoxin
Pregnancy Risk Category: C

HOW SUPPLIED
Tablets: 210 mg, 650 mg

MECHANISM OF ACTION
An iodine derivative with amebicidal activity in the intestinal lumen. Its precise mechanism of action is unknown.

INDICATIONS & DOSAGE
Intestinal amebiasis—
Adults: 630 to 650 mg P.O. t.i.d. for 20 days. Total daily dosage should not exceed 2 g.
Children: usual dosage 30 to 40 mg/kg of body weight daily in two to three divided doses for 20 days.
Additional courses of iodoquinol therapy should not be repeated before a resting interval of 2 to 3 weeks.

ADVERSE REACTIONS
Blood: *agranulocytosis.*
CNS: neurotoxicity (dose-related), dysesthesia, weakness, vertigo, malaise, headache, agitation, retrograde amnesia, ataxia, *peripheral neuropathy.*
EENT: *optic neuritis,* optic atrophy, loss of vision.
GI: anorexia, nausea, vomiting, abdominal cramps, diarrhea, increased motility, constipation, epigastric burning and pain, gastritis, anal irritation and itching.
Skin: pruritus, hives, papular and pustular eruptions, urticaria, discoloration of hair and nails.

Other: thyroid enlargement, fever, chills, generalized furunculosis, hair loss.

INTERACTIONS
None significant.

NURSING CONSIDERATIONS
• Contraindicated in patients with known hypersensitivity to 8-hydroxyquinoline derivatives or iodine-containing preparations. Iodoquinol causes hepatic damage in such patients. Also contraindicated in hepatic or renal disease or preexisting optic neuropathy.
• Patient should have periodic ophthalmologic examinations during treatment.
• Give after meals. Crush tablets and mix with applesauce or chocolate syrup.
• Record intake/output and color and amount of stool. Send warm specimens to lab for analysis.
• Watch for diarrhea during the first 2 or 3 days of treatment. Notify doctor if it continues past 3 days.
• Advise patient not to discontinue the medication prematurely. Tell him to notify doctor if skin rash occurs.
• May interfere with thyroid function tests for up to 6 months after discontinuation of drug.
• To help prevent reinfestation, teach patient about the need for good personal hygiene, especially handwashing technique. Patient should refrain from preparing food until stools are negative.

metronidazole
Apo-Metronidazole†, Flagyl, Metizol, Metric 21, Metrogyl‡, Metrozine‡, Metryl, Neo-Metric†, Novonidazol†, PMS Metronidazole†, Protostat

metronidazole hydrochloride
Flagyl I.V., Flagyl I.V. RTU, Metro I.V., Novonidazol†

Pregnancy Risk Category: B

HOW SUPPLIED
Tablets: 200 mg‡, 250 mg, 400 mg‡, 500 mg
Oral suspension (benzoyl metronidazole): 200 mg/5 ml‡
Injection: 500 mg/100 ml ready to use
Powder for injection: 500-mg single-dose vials

MECHANISM OF ACTION
A direct-acting trichomonacide and amebicide that works at both intestinal and extraintestinal sites.

INDICATIONS & DOSAGE
Amebic hepatic abscess—
Adults: 500 to 750 mg P.O. t.i.d. for 5 to 10 days.
Children: 35 to 50 mg/kg daily (in three doses) for 10 days.
Intestinal amebiasis—
Adults: 750 mg P.O. t.i.d. for 5 to 10 days.
Children: 35 to 50 mg/kg daily (in three doses) for 10 days. Follow this therapy with oral iodoquinol.
Trichomoniasis—
Adults (both male and female): 250 mg P.O. t.i.d. for 7 days or 2 g P.O. in single dose; 4 to 6 weeks should elapse between courses of therapy.
Refractory trichomoniasis—
Women: 250 mg P.O. b.i.d. for 10 days.
Treatment of bacterial infections caused by anaerobic microorganisms—

Italicized adverse reactions are common or life-threatening.
*Liquid form contains alcohol.   **May contain tartrazine.

Adults: Loading dose is 15 mg/kg I.V. infused over 1 hour (approximately 1 g for a 70-kg adult). Maintenance dose is 7.5 mg/kg I.V. or P.O. q 6 hours (approximately 500 mg for a 70-kg adult). The first maintenance dose should be administered 6 hours following the loading dose. Maximum dosage not to exceed 4 g daily.

Giardiasis—
Adults: 250 mg P.O. t.i.d. for 5 days.
Children: 5 mg/kg P.O. t.i.d. for 5 days.

Prevention of postoperative infection in contaminated or potentially contaminated colorectal surgery—
Adults: 15 mg/kg infused over 30 to 60 minutes and completed approximately 1 hour before surgery. Then, 7.5 mg/kg infused over 30 to 60 minutes at 6 and 12 hours after the initial dose.

ADVERSE REACTIONS
Blood: transient leukopenia, neutropenia.
CNS: vertigo, headache, ataxia, incoordination, confusion, irritability, depression, restlessness, weakness, fatigue, drowsiness, insomnia, sensory neuropathy, paresthesias of extremities, psychic stimulation, neuromyopathy.
CV: ECG change (flattened T wave), edema (with I.V. RTU preparation).
GI: abdominal cramping, stomatitis, *nausea, vomiting, anorexia,* diarrhea, constipation, proctitis, dry mouth.
GU: darkened urine, polyuria, dysuria, pyuria, incontinence, cystitis, decreased libido, dyspareunia, dryness of vagina and vulva, sense of pelvic pressure.
Skin: pruritus, flushing.
Local: *thrombophlebitis after I.V. infusion.*
Other: overgrowth of nonsusceptible organisms, especially *Candida* (glossitis, furry tongue), metallic taste, fever, gynecomastia.

INTERACTIONS
Alcohol: disulfiram-like reaction (nausea, vomiting, headache, cramps, flushing). Don't use together.
Disulfiram: acute psychoses and confusional states. Don't use together.

NURSING CONSIDERATIONS
Warning: This drug has been shown to be carcinogenic in mice and possibly rats. Unnecessary use should be avoided.
• If indicated during pregnancy for trichomoniasis, the 7-day regimen is preferred over the 2-g single-dose regimen.
• Use cautiously in patients with a history of blood dyscrasia or CNS disorder, and in patients with retinal or visual field changes. Use with caution in hepatic disease or alcoholism and in conjunction with known hepatotoxic drugs.
• Tell patient to avoid alcohol or alcohol-containing medications during therapy and for at least 48 hours after therapy is completed.
• Give oral form with meals to minimize GI distress.
• Tell patient metallic taste and dark or red-brown urine may occur.
• Record number and character of stools when used in the treatment of amebiasis. Metronidazole should be used only after *Trichomonas vaginalis* has been confirmed by wet smear or culture or *Entamoeba histolytica* has been identified. Asymptomatic sexual partners of patients being treated for *T. vaginalis* infection should be treated simultaneously to avoid reinfection. Instruct patient in proper hygiene.
• The I.V. form should be administered by slow infusion only. Don't give I.V. push.
• Follow package instructions carefully when mixing the I.V. solution.
• Don't refrigerate Flagyl I.V. RTU
• Flagyl I.V. RTU may cause sodium retention. Observe carefully for

edema, especially in patients also receiving corticosteroids.

---

paromomycin sulfate
Humatin

Pregnancy Risk Category: C

HOW SUPPLIED
Capsules: 250 mg

MECHANISM OF ACTION
Acts as an intestinal amebicide. Its specific mechanism of action is unknown.

INDICATIONS & DOSAGE
Intestinal amebiasis, acute and chronic—
Adults and children: 25 to 35 mg/kg daily P.O. in three doses for 5 to 10 days after meals.
Tapeworms (fish, beef, pork, dog)—
Adults: 1 g P.O. q 15 minutes for 4 doses.
Children: 11 mg/kg P.O. q 15 minutes for 4 doses.

ADVERSE REACTIONS
Blood: eosinophilia.
CNS: headache, vertigo.
EENT: ototoxicity.
GI: anorexia, *nausea, vomiting, epigastric pain and burning, abdominal cramps,* diarrhea, constipation, increased motility, steatorrhea, pruritus ani, malabsorption syndrome.
GU: hematuria, nephrotoxicity.
Skin: rash, exanthema, pruritus.
Other: overgrowth of nonsusceptible organisms.

INTERACTIONS
None significant.

NURSING CONSIDERATIONS
• Contraindicated in patients with impaired renal function or intestinal obstruction. Use with caution in patients with ulcerative lesions of the bowel to avoid inadvertent absorption and resulting renal toxicity. Poorly absorbed orally, but will accumulate with renal impairment or ulcerative lesions.
• Ask about history of sensitivity to drug before giving first dose.
• Administer after meals.
• To help prevent reinfestation, teach patient about the need for good personal hygiene, especially handwashing technique. Patient should refrain from preparing food until stools are negative.
• Criterion of cure is absence of amebae in stools examined weekly for 6 weeks after treatment and thereafter at monthly intervals for 2 years. Examine feces of family members or suspected contacts.
• Avoid high doses or prolonged therapy.
• Watch for signs of superinfection (continued fever and other signs of new infections, especially monilial infections).

Anthelmintics

mebendazole
niclosamide
oxamniquine
piperazine adipate
piperazine citrate
praziquantel
pyrantel embonate
pyrantel pamoate
quinacrine hydrochloride
thiabendazole

COMBINATION PRODUCTS
None.

mebendazole
Vermox

Pregnancy Risk Category: C

HOW SUPPLIED
Tablets (chewable): 100 mg
Oral suspension: 100 mg/5 ml‡

MECHANISM OF ACTION
Selectively and irreversibly inhibits
uptake of glucose and other nutrients
in susceptible helminths.

INDICATIONS & DOSAGE
Pinworm—
Adults and children over 2 years:
100 mg P.O. as a single dose. If infection persists 3 weeks later, repeat
treatment.
Roundworm, whipworm, hookworm—
Adults and children over 2 years:
100 mg P.O. b.i.d. for 3 days. If infection persists 3 weeks later, repeat
treatment.

ADVERSE REACTIONS
GI: occasional, transient abdominal
pain and diarrhea in massive infection
and expulsion of worms.

INTERACTIONS
None significant.

NURSING CONSIDERATIONS
• Tablets may be chewed, swallowed
whole, or crushed and mixed with
food.
• No dietary restrictions, laxatives, or
enemas are necessary.
• Treat all family members.
• Teach patient about the need for
good personal hygiene, especially
good handwashing technique. To
avoid reinfection, teach him to wash
perianal area daily. Change undergarments and bedclothes daily. Wash
hands and clean fingernails before
meals and after bowel movements.
Advise patient to refrain from preparing food during infestation.

niclosamide
Niclocide, Yomesan‡

Pregnancy Risk Category: B

HOW SUPPLIED
Tablets (chewable): 500 mg

MECHANISM OF ACTION
Inhibits the metabolic process of oxi-
dative phosphorylation in tapeworms.

INDICATIONS & DOSAGE
Tapeworms (fish, beef, and pork)—

Adults: 4 tablets (2 g) chewed thoroughly as a single dose.
Children (more than 34 kg): 3 tablets (1.5 g) chewed thoroughly as a single dose.
Children (11 to 34 kg): 2 tablets (1 g) chewed thoroughly as a single dose.
Dwarf tapeworm—
Adults: 4 tablets chewed thoroughly as a single daily dose for 7 days.
Children over age 2 (more than 34 kg): 3 tablets chewed thoroughly on the first day, then 2 tablets for the next 6 days.
Children over age 2 (11 to 34 kg): 2 tablets chewed thoroughly on the first day, then 1 tablet daily for the next 6 days.

ADVERSE REACTIONS
CNS: drowsiness, dizziness, headache.
EENT: oral irritation, bad taste in mouth.
GI: *nausea, vomiting, anorexia,* diarrhea.
Skin: rash, pruritus ani.

INTERACTIONS
None reported.

NURSING CONSIDERATIONS
• Instruct patient to chew tablets thoroughly and wash down with water; for smaller children, the tablets can be crushed and mixed with water or applesauce.
• Tablets should be taken as a single dose after breakfast.
• A mild laxative should be administered to cleanse the bowel prior to initiation of niclosamide therapy in patients who are constipated.
• When treating dwarf tapeworms, urge patient to drink fruit juices. This helps to eliminate the accumulated intestinal mucus under which they lodge.
• Teach patient about the need for good personal hygiene, especially good handwashing technique. Advise

patient to refrain from preparing food during infestation.
• Patient is not considered cured until the stool has been negative for tapeworms for at least 3 months.

oxamniquine
Vansil

Pregnancy Risk Category: C

HOW SUPPLIED
Capsules: 250 mg

MECHANISM OF ACTION
Reduces the egg load of *Schistosoma mansoni,* but its exact mechanism of action is unknown.

INDICATIONS & DOSAGE
Treatment of schistosomiasis caused by Schistosoma mansoni, Western Hemisphere strains—
Adults and children (more than 30 kg): 12 to 15 mg/kg given as a single oral dose.
Children (less than 30 kg): 10 mg/kg P.O., followed by 10 mg/kg P.O. 2 to 8 hours later.

ADVERSE REACTIONS
CNS: seizures, *dizziness, drowsiness, headache.*
GI: nausea, vomiting, abdominal pain, anorexia.
Skin: urticaria.

INTERACTIONS
None significant.

NURSING CONSIDERATIONS
• Use cautiously in patients with a history of seizure disorders. Epileptiform seizures have rarely been observed within the first few hours after ingestion. Patients with a history of seizures should be kept under medical supervision.
• Instruct patient to avoid driving and other hazardous activities if he's dizzy or drowsy.

Italicized adverse reactions are common or life-threatening.
*Liquid form contains alcohol.   **May contain tartrazine.

• GI tolerance is improved if the drug is given after meals.

• Although *S. mansoni* infection is rare in the United States and Canada, travelers or immigrants from such areas as Puerto Rico, Latin America, and Africa may have contracted the infection from contaminated water.

---

piperazine adipate
Entacyl†

piperazine citrate
Antepar, Bryrel, Pin-Tega Tabs, Pipril, Ta-Verm, Veriga†, Vermirex†, Vermizine

Pregnancy Risk Category: B

HOW SUPPLIED
adipate
Oral suspension: 600 mg/5 ml
Granules: 2 g/packet
citrate
Tablets: 250 mg
Syrup: 500 mg/5 ml

MECHANISM OF ACTION
Blocks neuromuscular action, paralyzing the worm and causing its expulsion by normal peristalsis.

INDICATIONS & DOSAGE
Pinworm—
Adults and children: 65 mg/kg P.O. daily 7 to 8 days. Maximum daily dosage is 2.5 g.
Roundworm—
Adults: 3.5 g P.O. in single doses for 2 consecutive days.
Children: 75 mg/kg P.O. daily in single doses for 2 consecutive days. Maximum daily dosage is 3.5 g.

ADVERSE REACTIONS
CNS: ataxia, tremors, choreiform movements, muscular weakness, myoclonus, hyporeflexia, paresthesias, seizures, sense of detachment, EEG abnormalities, memory defect, *headache, vertigo*.

EENT: nystagmus, blurred vision, paralytic strabismus, cataracts with visual impairment, lacrimation, difficulty in focusing, rhinorrhea.
GI: *nausea, vomiting,* diarrhea, abdominal cramps.
Skin: urticaria, photodermatitis, *erythema multiforme,* purpura, eczematous skin reactions.
Other: arthralgia, fever, bronchospasm, hemolytic anemia.

INTERACTIONS
Pyrantel pamoate: possible pharmacologic antagonism. Don't administer together.

NURSING CONSIDERATIONS
• Contraindicated in hepatic and/or renal impairment, or seizure disorders. Use with caution in severe malnutrition or anemia.
• Discontinue if CNS or significant GI reactions occur.
• Because of potential neurotoxicity, avoid prolonged or repeated treatment, especially in children.
• No dietary restrictions, laxatives, or enemas are necessary.
• May be taken with food; but, for best absorption, tell patient to take on empty stomach.
• Mix powder for oral suspension in 57 ml water, milk, or fruit juice.
• Treat all family members.
• Teach patient about the need for good personal hygiene, especially good handwashing technique. To avoid reinfection, teach him to wash perianal area, to change undergarments and bedclothes daily, and to wash hands and clean fingernails before meals and after bowel movements. Advise patient to refrain from preparing food during infestation.
• Mix powder for oral suspension in 57 ml water, milk, or fruit juice.

---

praziquantel
Biltricide

Pregnancy Risk Category: B

HOW SUPPLIED
Tablets: 600 mg

MECHANISM OF ACTION
Causes a contraction of schistosomes by a specific effect on the permeability of the cell membrane.

INDICATIONS & DOSAGE
Treatment of schistosomiasis caused by Schistosoma mekongi, S. japonicum, S. mansoni, *and* S. haematobium—

Adults and children 4 years and older: 20 mg/kg P.O. t.i.d. as a 1-day treatment. The interval between doses should be between 4 and 6 hours.

ADVERSE REACTIONS
CNS: *drowsiness, malaise,* headache, dizziness.
GI: abdominal discomfort, nausea.
Hepatic: minimal increase in liver enzymes.
Skin: urticaria.
Other: fever.

INTERACTIONS
None significant.

NURSING CONSIDERATIONS
• Contraindicated with ocular cysticercosis.
• May produce drowsiness. Tell patient to avoid hazardous activities that require alertness on the day of treatment and the day after treatment.
• Adverse effects may be more frequent or serious in patients with a heavy worm burden.
• In the event of overdose, give a fast-acting laxative.
• Advise patient to take the tablet during meals and to wash down the unchewed tablet with a liquid.
• Tablets taste very bitter. Keeping them in the mouth may cause gagging or vomiting.
• Praziquantel is effective for several different species of *Schistosoma*.
• May also be effective against liver flukes.

pyrantel embonate
Anthel‡, Combantrin‡, Early Bird‡

pyrantel pamoate
Antiminth, Combantrin†

Pregnancy Risk Category: C

HOW SUPPLIED
embonate
Tablets: 125 mg‡, 250 mg‡
Oral suspension: 50 mg/ml‡
Granules: 100 mg/g‡
Squares (chocolate-flavored): 100 mg‡
pamoate
Tablets: 125 mg†
Oral suspension: 50 mg/ml

MECHANISM OF ACTION
Blocks neuromuscular action, paralyzing the worm and causing its expulsion by normal peristalsis.

INDICATIONS & DOSAGE
Roundworm and pinworm—
Adults and children over 2 years: single dosage of 11 mg/kg P.O. Maximum dosage 1 g. For pinworm, dosage should be repeated in 2 weeks.

ADVERSE REACTIONS
CNS: headache, dizziness, drowsiness, insomnia.
GI: anorexia, nausea, vomiting, gastralgia, cramps, diarrhea, tenesmus.
Hepatic: transient elevation of AST (SGOT).
Skin: rashes.
Other: fever, weakness.

INTERACTIONS
Piperazine salts: Possible pharmaco-

Italicized adverse reactions are common or life-threatening.
*Liquid form contains alcohol.   **May contain tartrazine.

logic antagonism. Don't administer together.

NURSING CONSIDERATIONS
• Use cautiously in severe malnutrition or anemia, or in hepatic dysfunction. Treat for anemia, dehydration, or malnutrition before giving drug.
• No dietary restrictions, laxatives, or enemas are necessary.
• May be taken with food, milk, or fruit juices. Shake suspension well before pouring.
• Treat all family members.
• Teach patient about the need for good personal hygiene, especially good handwashing technique. To avoid reinfection, teach him to wash perianal area daily, to change undergarments and bedclothes daily, and to wash hands and clean fingernails before meals and after bowel movements. Advise patient to refrain from preparing food during infestation.
• Protect drug from light. Store below 30° C. (86° F.).

---

quinacrine hydrochloride (mepacrine hydrochloride)
Atabrine

Pregnancy Risk Category: C

HOW SUPPLIED
Tablets: 100 mg

MECHANISM OF ACTION
Inhibits DNA metabolism in susceptible parasites.

INDICATIONS & DOSAGE
Treatment of giardiasis—
Adults: 300 mg P.O. in 3 divided doses for 5 to 7 days.
Children: 7 mg/kg/day P.O. given in 3 divided doses after meals for 5 days. Maximum 300 mg/day. If necessary, the dosage may be repeated in 2 weeks.
Tapeworms (beef, pork, and fish)—
Adults and children over 14 years: 4 doses of 200 mg P.O. given 10 minutes apart (800 mg total).
Children 11 to 14 years: 600 mg P.O. total dosage, administered in 3 or 4 divided doses, 10 minutes apart.
Children 5 to 10 years: 400 mg P.O. total dosage, administered in 3 or 4 divided doses, 10 minutes apart.

ADVERSE REACTIONS
CNS: *headache, dizziness, nervousness, vertigo, mood shifts, nightmares, seizures.*
GI: *diarrhea, anorexia, nausea, abdominal cramps,* vomiting.
GU: yellow urine.
Skin: pleomorphic skin eruptions, yellow discoloration.

INTERACTIONS
None significant.

NURSING CONSIDERATIONS
• Contraindicated if patient is taking primaquine since primaquine toxicity could be increased.
• Use with extreme caution in porphyria or psoriasis; may exacerbate these conditions.
• Use with caution in hepatic disease, alcoholism, severe renal or cardiac disease, psychosis, and G6PD deficiency, and in those over 60 years or under 1 year.
• Give after meals with large glass of water, tea, or fruit juice to reduce GI irritation. Bitter taste may be disguised by jam or honey.
• Nausea and vomiting after large doses may be lessened by taking sodium bicarbonate with each dose.
• Administer a saline cathartic 1 to 2 hours after drug is given, to expel the worm.
• Collect all of stool after treatment. Don't put toilet paper in bedpan. Look for the scolex (attachment organ), which will be stained yellow from drug.
• Warn patient about temporary yel-

low color of skin and urine—it is not jaundice.
• Patient should be on a bland, non-fat, semisolid diet for 24 hours, and should fast after the evening meal before treatment.

---

thiabendazole
Mintezol

Pregnancy Risk Category: C

HOW SUPPLIED
Tablets (chewable): 500 mg
Oral suspension: 500 mg/5 ml

MECHANISM OF ACTION
Unknown.

INDICATIONS & DOSAGE
Systemic infection with pinworm, roundworm, threadworm, whipworm, cutaneous larva migrans, and trichinosis—
Adults or children: 25 mg/kg P.O. in two doses daily for 2 successive days. Maximum dosage is 3 g daily.
Cutaneous infestations with larva migrans (creeping eruption)—
Adults and children: 25 mg/kg P.O. b.i.d. for 2 to 5 days. Maximum 3 g daily. If lesions persist after 2 days, repeat course.
*Pinworm—*two doses daily for 1 day; repeat in 7 days.
*Roundworm, threadworm, whipworm—*two doses daily for 2 successive days.
*Trichinosis—*two doses daily for 2 to 4 successive days.

ADVERSE REACTIONS
CNS: impaired mental alertness, impaired physical coordination, *drowsiness, giddiness,* headache, dizziness.
GI: *anorexia, nausea, vomiting,* diarrhea, epigastric distress.
Skin: rash, pruritus, *erythema multiforme.*
Other: lymphadenopathy, fever, flushing, chills.

INTERACTIONS
None significant.

NURSING CONSIDERATIONS
• Use with caution in hepatic or renal dysfunction, severe malnutrition, and anemia, and in patients who are vomiting. Supportive therapy indicated for anemic, dehydrated, or malnourished patients. In children under 15 kg, weigh benefits of therapy against risks.
• Warn that medication may cause drowsiness and dizziness.
• Give after meals. Shake suspension before measuring; chew tablets before swallowing.
• No dietary restrictions, laxatives, or enemas are necessary.
• Treat all family members.
• Teach patient about the need for good personal hygiene, especially good handwashing technique. To avoid reinfection, teach him to wash perianal area daily, to change undergarments and bedclothes daily, and to wash hands and clean fingernails before meals and after bowel movements. Advise patient to refrain from preparing food during infestation.

Italicized adverse reactions are common or life-threatening.
*Liquid form contains alcohol.   **May contain tartrazine.

8

Antifungals

amphotericin B
fluconazole
flucytosine
griseofulvin microsize
griseofulvin ultramicrosize
ketoconazole
miconazole
nystatin

COMBINATION PRODUCTS
None.

---

amphotericin B
Fungilin Oral‡, Fungizone
Pregnancy Risk Category: B

HOW SUPPLIED
Tablets: 100 mg‡
Oral suspension: 100 mg/ml‡
Lozenges: 10 mg‡
Injection: 50-mg lyophilized cake

MECHANISM OF ACTION
Probably acts by binding to sterols in the fungal cell membrane, altering cell permeability and allowing leakage of intracellular components.

INDICATIONS & DOSAGE
Systemic fungal infections (histoplasmosis, coccidioidomycosis, blastomycosis, cryptococcosis, disseminated moniliasis, aspergillosis, phycomycosis), meningitis—
Adults: initially, 1 mg in 250 ml of dextrose 5% in water infused over 2 to 4 hours; or 0.25 mg/kg daily by slow infusion over 6 hours. Increase daily dosage gradually as patient tolerance develops to maximum 1 mg/kg daily.

Therapy must not exceed 1.5 mg/kg. If drug is discontinued for 1 week or more, administration must resume with initial dose and again increase gradually.
Intrathecal: 25 mcg/0.1 ml diluted with 10 to 20 ml of cerebrospinal fluid and administered by barbotage 2 or 3 times weekly. Initial dose should not exceed 100 mcg.
Treatment of Candida albicans *infections involving the GI tract—*
Adults: 100 mg P.O. q.i.d. for 2 weeks.
Oral and perioral candidal infections—
Adults: 1 lozenge q.i.d. for 7 to 14 days. The lozenge should be sucked and allowed to dissolve slowly in the mouth.

ADVERSE REACTIONS
Blood: normochromic, normocytic anemia.
CNS: headache, peripheral neuropathy; with intrathecal administration—peripheral nerve pain, paresthesias.
CV: hypotension, *cardiac arrhythmias, asystole.*
GI: *anorexia, weight loss, nausea,* vomiting, dyspepsia, diarrhea, epigastric cramps.
GU: abnormal renal function with *hypokalemia, azotemia, hyposthenuria,* renal tubular acidosis, nephrocalcinosis; with large doses—permanent renal impairment, anuria, oliguria.
Local: burning, stinging, irritation, tissue damage with extravasation, *thrombophlebitis,* pain at site of injection.

Other: arthralgia, myalgia, muscle weakness secondary to hypokalemia, *fever, chills,* malaise, generalized pain.

INTERACTIONS

Other nephrotoxic antibiotics: may cause additive kidney toxicity. Administer very cautiously.

NURSING CONSIDERATIONS

• Use cautiously in patients with impaired renal function.
• Use parenterally only in hospitalized patients, under close supervision, when diagnosis of potentially fatal fungal infection has been confirmed.
• Oral form is not available in the United States.
• Monitor vital signs; fever and hypotension may appear 1 to 2 hours after start of I.V. infusion and should subside within 4 hours of discontinuation.
• Monitor intake/output; report change in urine appearance or volume. Monitor BUN and serum creatine (or creatinine clearance) at least weekly during therapy. Renal damage usually reversible if drug is stopped at first sign of dysfunction.
• Obtain liver and renal function studies weekly. If BUN exceeds 40 mg/100 ml, or if serum creatinine exceeds 3 mg/100 ml, doctor may reduce or stop drug until renal function improves. Monitor CBC weekly. Stop drug if alkaline phosphatase or bilirubin levels become elevated.
• Monitor potassium levels closely. Report any signs of hypokalemia. Check calcium and magnesium levels twice weekly. Perform liver and renal function studies and monitor CBCs weekly.
• In the dry state, store at 2° to 8° C. (35.6° to 46.4° F.). Protect from light. Reconstitute with 10 ml sterile water only. Mixing with solutions containing sodium chloride, other electrolytes, or bacteriostatic agents, such as benzyl alcohol, causes precipitation. Do not use if solution contains precipitate or foreign matter.
• Severity of some adverse reactions can be reduced by premedication with aspirin, antihistamines, antiemetics, or small doses of corticosteroids; addition of phosphate buffer and heparin to the solution; and alternate-day dose schedule. For severe reactions, drug may have to be discontinued for varying intervals.
• Appears to be compatible with limited amounts of heparin sodium, hydrocortisone sodium succinate, and methylprednisolone sodium succinate.
• Reconstituted solution is stable for 1 week under refrigeration or 24 hours at room temperature. It has 24-hour stability in room light.
• An initial test dose may be prescribed: 1 mg is added to 50 to 250 ml of dextrose 5% in water and infused over 20 to 30 minutes and the patient's pulse, respiratory rate, temperature, and blood pressure are monitored for at least 4 hours. Some clinicians give this test dose more slowly (over a 4 hour period).
• For I.V. infusion, an in-line filter with mean pore diameter larger than 1 micron can be used. Infuse very slowly; rapid infusion may result in cardiovascular collapse. Warn patient of possible discomfort at infusion site and other potential side effects. Advise patient that several months of therapy may be needed to assure adequate response.
• Administer in distal veins. If veins become thrombosed, doctor can change to every-other-day regimen.
• Antibiotics should be given separately; don't mix or piggyback with amphotericin B.

Italicized adverse reactions are common or life-threatening.
*Liquid form contains alcohol.   **May contain tartrazine.

fluconazole
Diflucan

Pregnancy Risk Category: C

HOW SUPPLIED
Tablets: 50 mg, 100 mg, 200 mg
Injection: 200 mg/100 ml, 400 mg/
200 ml

MECHANISM OF ACTION
Inhibits fungal cytochrome P-450, an
enzyme responsible for fungal sterol
synthesis. This results in weakening
of fungal cell walls.

INDICATIONS & DOSAGE
Oropharyngeal candidiasis—
Adults: 200 mg P.O. or I.V. on the
first day, followed by 100 mg once
daily. Therapy should continue for 2
weeks.
Esophageal candidiasis—
Adults: 200 mg P.O. or I.V. on the
first day, followed by 100 mg once
daily. Higher doses (up to 400 mg
daily) have been used, depending
upon the patient's condition and tolerance of treatment. Patients should receive the drug for at least 3 weeks and
for 2 weeks after symptoms resolve.
Systemic candidiasis—
Adults: 400 mg P.O. or I.V. on the
first day, followed by 200 mg once
daily. Treatment should continue for
at least 4 weeks or for 2 weeks after
symptoms resolve.
Cryptococcal meningitis—
Adults: 400 mg P.O. or I.V. on the
first day, followed by 200 mg once
daily. Higher doses (up to 400 mg
daily) may be used. Treatment should
continue for 10 to 12 weeks after cultures of the cerebrospinal fluid are
negative.
*Suppression of relapse of cryptococcal
meningitis in patients with AIDS—*
Adults: 200 mg P.O. or I.V. daily.

ADVERSE REACTIONS
CNS: headache.
GI: *nausea,* vomiting, abdominal
pain, diarrhea.
Skin: rash, Stevens-Johnson syn-
drome (rare).
Other: hepatotoxicity (rare), elevated
liver enzymes.

INTERACTIONS
*Cyclosporine, phenytoin, oral antidi-
abetic agents (tolbutamide, glyburide,
glipizide):* may cause increased
plasma concentrations of these drugs.
*Isoniazid, phenytoin, rifampin, val-
proic acid, oral sulfonylureas:* increased incidence of abnormally elevated hepatic transaminases.
Rifampin: enhanced metabolism of
fluconazole.
Warfarin: increased prothrombin
time.

NURSING CONSIDERATIONS
• Contraindicated in patients hypersensitive to the drug. Use cautiously
in patients hypersensitive to other antifungal azole compounds because
there is no information regarding
cross-sensitivity.
• The incidence of adverse reactions
appears to be greater in human immunodeficiency virus (HIV)–infected
patients.
• Because the drug is excreted unchanged by the kidneys, dosage
should be adjusted in patients with
renal failure. If creatinine clearance is
21 to 50 ml/minute, dosage should be
reduced 50%. If creatinine clearance
is 11 to 20 ml/minute, reduce dosage
by 75%. Patients receiving regular hemodialysis treatment should receive
the usual dose after each dialysis session.
• Oral bioavailability of fluconazole
is greater than 90% and is unaffected
by gastric pH. Dosage is the same for
oral or I.V. use.
• I.V. fluconazole may be administered by continuous infusion at a rate
not to exceed 200 mg/hour. Do not
connect in series with other infusions

---

†Available in Canada only.　　　‡Available in Australia only.　　　◇Available OTC.

to prevent air embolism. Do not add any other drugs to the solution.
• I.V. bags of fluconazole are shipped with a protective overwrap that should not be removed until just before use. This helps ensure product sterility. The plastic container may show some opacity from moisture absorbed during sterilization. This is normal, will not affect the drug, and will diminish over time.
• Safety and effectiveness in children have not been established, but a few children 3 to 13 years have received 3 to 6 mg/kg/day.

flucytosine (5-FC)
Ancobon

Pregnancy Risk Category: C

HOW SUPPLIED
Capsules: 250 mg, 500 mg

MECHANISM OF ACTION
Appears to penetrate fungal cells, where it is converted to fluorouracil, a known metabolic antagonist. Causes defective protein synthesis.

INDICATIONS & DOSAGE
For severe fungal infections caused by susceptible strains of Candida *(including septicemia, endocarditis, urinary tract and pulmonary infections) and* Cryptococcus *(meningitis, pulmonary infection, and possible urinary tract infections)*—
Adults and children weighing more than 50 kg: 50 to 150 mg/kg daily q 6 hours P.O.
Adults and children weighing less than 50 kg: 1.5 to 4.5 g/m²/day in four divided doses P.O.
  Severe infections, such as meningitis, may require doses up to 250 mg/kg.

ADVERSE REACTIONS
Blood: anemia, *leukopenia,* bone marrow suppression, *thrombocytopenia.*
CNS: dizziness, drowsiness, confusion, headache, vertigo.
GI: *nausea, vomiting, diarrhea,* abdominal bloating.
Hepatic: elevated AST (SGOT), ALT (SGPT).
Metabolic: elevated serum alkaline phosphatase, BUN, serum creatinine.
Skin: occasional rash.

INTERACTIONS
None significant.

NURSING CONSIDERATIONS
• Use with extreme caution in patients with impaired hepatic or renal function or bone marrow depression.
• Hematologic tests and renal and liver function studies should precede therapy and should be repeated at frequent intervals thereafter. Before treatment, susceptibility tests should establish that organism is flucytosine-sensitive. Tests should be repeated weekly to monitor drug resistance.
• GI adverse reactions are reduced if capsules are given over a 15-minute period.
• Monitor intake/output; report any marked change.
• If possible, blood level assays of drug should be performed regularly to maintain flucytosine at therapeutic level (25 to 120 mcg/ml). Higher blood levels may be toxic.
• Drug is usually combined with amphotericin because they are synergistic.
• Inform patient that adequate therapeutic response may take weeks or months.

griseofulvin microsize
Fulcin‡, Fulvicin-U/F, Grifulvin V, Grisactin, Grisovin‡, Grisovin 500‡, Grisovin-FP

griseofulvin ultramicrosize
Fulvicin P/G, Grisactin Ultra, Griseostatin‡, Gris-PEG

Pregnancy Risk Category: C

HOW SUPPLIED
microsize
Tablets: 125 mg, 250 mg, 500 mg
Capsules: 125 mg, 250 mg
Oral suspension: 125 mg/5ml
ultramicrosize
Tablets: 125 mg, 165 mg, 250 mg, 330 mg

MECHANISM OF ACTION
Arrests fungal cell activity by disrupting its mitotic spindle structure.

INDICATIONS & DOSAGE
Ringworm infections of skin, hair, nails (tinea corporis, tinea pedis, tinea capitis) when caused by Trichophyton, Microsporum, *or* Epidermophyton—
Adults: 500 mg (microsize) P.O. daily in single or divided doses. Severe infections may require up to 1 g daily. Alternatively, may give 330 to 375 mg ultramicrosize in single or divided doses.
Tinea pedis and tinea unguium—
Adults: 0.75 to 1 g (microsize) P.O. daily. Alternatively, may give 660 to 750 mg ultramicrosize P.O. daily.
Children: 11 mg/kg/day (microsize) P.O. Alternatively, may give 7.3 mg/kg/day of the ultramicrosize.

ADVERSE REACTIONS
Blood: leukopenia, *granulocytopenia* (requires discontinuation of drug).
CNS: headaches (in early stages of treatment), transient decrease in hearing, fatigue with large doses, occasional mental confusion, impaired performance of routine activities, psychotic symptoms, dizziness, insomnia.
GI: nausea, vomiting, excessive thirst, flatulence, diarrhea.
Metabolic: porphyria.
Skin: rash, urticaria, photosensitivity (may aggravate lupus erythematosus).
Other: estrogen-like effects in children, oral thrush.

INTERACTIONS
Alcohol: may cause tachycardia, diaphoresis, and flushing. Avoid alcohol.
Barbiturates: decreased griseofulvin blood levels due to decreased absorption or increased metabolism. Avoid using together or administer griseofulvin t.i.d.
Coumarin anticoagulants: decreased effectiveness. Monitor prothrombin times when used concurrently.
Oral contraceptives: decreased effectiveness. Suggest alternate methods of contraception.

NURSING CONSIDERATIONS
• Contraindicated in porphyria or hepatocellular failure. Since griseofulvin is a penicillin derivative, cross-sensitivity is possible. Use cautiously in penicillin-sensitive patients. Use only when topical treatment fails to arrest mycotic disease.
• CBC should be repeated regularly.
• Advise patient that prolonged treatment may be needed to control infection and prevent relapse, even if symptoms abate in first few days of therapy. Tell patient to keep skin clean and dry and to maintain good hygiene. Caution him to avoid intense sunlight.
• Most effectively absorbed and causes least GI distress when given after high-fat meal.
• Effective treatment of tinea pedis may require concomitant use of topical agent.
• Diagnosis of infecting organism should be verified in lab. Continue drug until clinical and laboratory ex-

---

aminations confirm complete eradication.
- Because griseofulvin ultramicrosize is dispersed in polyethylene glycol (PEG), it is absorbed more rapidly and completely than microsize preparations and is effective at one half to two thirds the usual griseofulvin dose.
- Advise patient to avoid alcoholic beverages.

ketoconazole
Nizoral

Pregnancy Risk Category: C

HOW SUPPLIED
Tablets: 200 mg
Oral suspension: 100 mg/5 ml

MECHANISM OF ACTION
Inhibits purine transport and DNA, RNA, and protein synthesis; increases cell wall permeability, making the fungus more susceptible to osmotic pressure.

INDICATIONS & DOSAGE
Treatment of systemic candidiasis, chronic mucocandidiasis, oral thrush, candiduria, coccidioidomycosis, histoplasmosis, chromomycosis, and paracoccidioidomycosis; severe cutaneous dermatophyte infections resistant to therapy with topical or oral griseofulvin—
Adults and children over 40 kg: initially, 200 mg P.O. daily single dose. Dosage may be increased to 400 mg once daily in patients who don't respond to lower dosage.
Children less than 20 kg: 50 mg (¼ tablet) daily single dose.
Children 20 to 40 kg: 100 mg (½ tablet) daily single dose.

ADVERSE REACTIONS
CNS: headache, nervousness, dizziness.
GI: *nausea, vomiting,* abdominal pain, diarrhea, constipation.

Hepatic: elevated liver enzymes, *fatal hepatotoxicity.*
Skin: itching.
Other: gynecomastia with breast tenderness in males.

INTERACTIONS
Antacids, anticholinergics, H₂ blockers: decreased absorption of ketoconazole. Wait at least 2 hours after ketoconazole dose before administering these drugs.
Rifampin, isoniazid: increases ketoconazole metabolism. Monitor for decreased antifungal effect.

NURSING CONSIDERATIONS
- Ketoconazole is not effective in patients with achlorhydria because drug requires acidity for dissolution and absorption. Instruct such patients to dissolve each tablet in 4 ml aqueous solution of 0.2 N hydrochloric acid; and, to avoid contact with teeth, to sip the mixture through a straw (glass or plastic). Tell patient to follow with a glass of water.
- Make sure patient understands that treatment should be continued until all clinical and laboratory tests indicate that active fungal infection has subsided. If drug is discontinued too soon, infection will recur. Minimum treatment for candidiasis is 7 to 14 days. Minimum treatment for other systemic fungal infections is 6 months. Minimum treatment for resistant dermatophyte infections is at least 4 weeks.
- Reassure patient that, although nausea is common early in therapy, it will subside. To minimize nausea, you may, with doctor's permission, divide the daily dosage into 2 doses. Taking with meals also helps to decrease nausea.
- Monitor for elevated liver enzymes and nausea that does not subside, as well as unusual fatigue, jaundice, dark urine, or pale stools. May be signs of hepatotoxicity.

Italicized adverse reactions are common or life-threatening.
*Liquid form contains alcohol.   **May contain tartrazine.

- Much larger doses (up to 800 mg/day) can be used to effectively treat fungal meningitis and intracerebral fungal lesions.
- Ketoconazole is the most effective oral antifungal drug available.
- Because of the potential of serious liver toxicity, ketoconazole should not be prescribed or used for such less serious conditions as fungus infections of the skin or nails.

miconazole
Monistat I.V.

Pregnancy Risk Category: B

HOW SUPPLIED
Injection: 10 mg/ml

MECHANISM OF ACTION
Inhibits purine transport and DNA, RNA, and protein synthesis; increases cell wall permeability, making the fungus more susceptible to osmotic pressure.

INDICATIONS & DOSAGE
Treatment of systemic fungal infections (coccidioidomycosis, candidiasis, cryptococcosis, paracoccidioidomycosis), chronic mucocutaneous candidiasis—
Adults: 200 to 3,600 mg/day. Dosages may vary with diagnosis and with infective agent. May divide daily dosage over 3 infusions, 200 to 1,200 mg per infusion. Dilute in at least 200 ml of 0.9% sodium chloride. Repeated courses may be needed because of relapse or reinfection.
Children 1 year and older: 20 to 40 mg/kg/day. Do not exceed 15 mg/kg per infusion.
Fungal meningitis—
Adults: 20 mg intrathecally as an adjunct to intravenous administration, q 3 to 7 days.

ADVERSE REACTIONS
Blood: transient decreases in hematocrit, thrombocytopenia.
CNS: dizziness, drowsiness.
GI: *nausea, vomiting,* diarrhea.
Metabolic: *transient decrease in serum sodium.*
Skin: *pruritic rash.*
Local: *phlebitis at injection site.*

INTERACTIONS
None significant.

NURSING CONSIDERATIONS
- Rapid injection of undiluted miconazole may produce arrhythmias. Dilute infusion in at least 200 ml of 0.9% sodium chloride and infuse over 30 to 60 minutes.
- Acute cardiorespiratory arrest has occurred with the first dose. The first dose should be given under continuous medical supervision with emergency resuscitative equipment immediately available.
- Premedication with antiemetic may lessen nausea and vomiting.
- Avoid administration at mealtime in order to lessen GI adverse reactions.
- Lesser incidence and severity of adverse reactions with this drug may offer a significant advantage over other antifungals.
- Pruritic rash may persist for weeks after drug is discontinued. Pruritus may be controlled with oral or I.V. diphenhydramine.
- In treatment of fungal meningitis and urinary bladder infections, must be supplemented with intrathecal administration and bladder irrigation, respectively.
- Inform patient that adequate therapeutic response may take weeks or months.
- Monitor levels of hemoglobin, hematocrit, electrolytes, and lipids regularly. Transient elevations in serum cholesterol and triglycerides may be due to castor oil vehicle.

nystatin

Mycostatin*, Nadostine†, Nilstat,
Nystex*

Pregnancy Risk Category: B

HOW SUPPLIED

Tablets: 500,000 units
Oral suspension: 100,000 units/ml
Vaginal suppositories: 100,000 units

MECHANISM OF ACTION

Probably acts by binding to sterols in
the fungal cell membrane, altering
cell permeability and allowing leakage of intracellular components.

INDICATIONS & DOSAGE

Gastrointestinal infections—
Adults: 500,000 to 1 million units as
oral tablets, t.i.d.
*Treatment of oral, vaginal, and intes-
tinal infections caused by* Candida albicans (Monilia) *and other* Candida
species—
Adults: 400,000 to 600,000 units oral
suspension q.i.d. for oral candidiasis.
**Children and infants over 3
months:** 250,000 to 500,000 units
oral suspension q.i.d.
Newborn and premature infants:
100,000 units oral suspension q.i.d.
Vaginal infections—
Adults: 100,000 units, as vaginal tablets, inserted high into vagina, daily
or b.i.d. for 14 days.

ADVERSE REACTIONS

GI: *transient nausea, vomiting, diarrhea* (usually with large oral dosage).

INTERACTIONS

None significant.

NURSING CONSIDERATIONS

• Nystatin is virtually nontoxic and
nonsensitizing when used orally, vaginally, or topically, but advise patient
to report redness, swelling, or irritation.
• Vaginal tablets can be used by preg-

nant women up to 6 weeks before
term to treat maternal infection that
may cause thrush in newborns.
• Continue therapy during menstruation.
• Instruct patient to wash applicator
thoroughly after each use.
• Explain that use of antibiotics, oral
contraceptives, and corticosteroids;
diabetes; reinfection by sexual partner; and tight-fitting panty hose are
predisposing factors of vaginal infection.
• For treatment of oral candidiasis
(thrush): Be sure the mouth is clean of
food debris before administering
drug, then tell patient to hold suspension in mouth for several minutes before swallowing. When treating infants, swab medication on oral mucosa. Instruct patient in good oral hygiene techniques. Tell patient overuse
of mouthwash or poorly fitting dentures, especially in older patients,
may alter flora and promote infection.
• Advise patient to continue medication for 1 to 2 weeks after symptomatic improvement to ensure against
reinfection. Consult doctor for exact
length of therapy.
• For treatment of oral candidiasis,
immunosuppressed patients sometimes take vaginal tablets (100,000
units) by mouth since this provides
prolonged contact with oral mucosa.
• Instruct patient in careful hygiene
for affected areas.
• Not effective against systemic infections.

Italicized adverse reactions are common or life-threatening.
*Liquid form contains alcohol.   **May contain tartrazine.

Antimalarials

chloroquine hydrochloride
chloroquine phosphate
chloroquine sulphate
hydroxychloroquine sulfate
mefloquine hydrochloride
primaquine phosphate
pyrimethamine
pyrimethamane with sulfadoxine
quinine bisulfate
quinine sulfate

COMBINATION PRODUCTS
ARALEN PHOSPHATE WITH PRIMA-
QUINE PHOSPHATE: chloroquine phosphate 500 mg (300 mg base) and primaquine phosphate 79 mg (45 mg
base).
M-KYA, Q-VEL: quinine sulfate 64.8
mg and vitamin E 400 U (as d,l alpha-
tocopheryl acetate).

chloroquine hydrochloride
Aralen HCl, Chlorquin‡

chloroquine phosphate
Aralen Phosphate, Chlorquin‡

chloroquine sulphate
Nivaquine‡

Pregnancy Risk Category: C

HOW SUPPLIED
hydrochloride
Injection: 50 mg/ml (40-mg/ml base)
phosphate
Tablets: 250 mg (150-mg base), 500
mg (300-mg base)
sulphate
Tablets: 200 mg (150-mg base)
Syrup: 68 mg (50-mg base)/5ml

MECHANISM OF ACTION
As an antimalarial, may bind to and
alter the properties of DNA in susceptible parasites. As an amebicide,
mechanism of action is unknown.

INDICATIONS & DOSAGE
*Suppressive prophylaxis and treatment
of acute attacks of malaria due to*
Plasmodium vivax, P. malariae, P.
ovale, *and susceptible strains of* P.
falciparum—
Adults: initially, 600 mg (base) P.O.,
then 300 mg P.O. at 6, 24, and 48
hours. Or 160 to 200 mg (base) I.M.
initially; repeat in 6 hours if needed.
Switch to oral therapy as soon as possible.
Children: initially, 10 mg (base)/kg
P.O., then 5 mg (base)/kg dose P.O. at
6, 24, and 48 hours (do not exceed
adult dose). Or 5 mg (base)/kg I.M.
initially; repeat in 6 hours if needed.
Switch to oral therapy as soon as possible.
Malaria suppressive treatment—
Adults and children: 5 mg (base)/kg
P.O. (not to exceed 300 mg) weekly
on same day of the week (begin 2
weeks before entering endemic area
and continue for 8 weeks after leaving). If treatment begins after exposure, double the initial dose (600 mg
for adults, 10 mg/kg for children) in 2
divided doses P.O. 6 hours apart.
Extraintestinal amebiasis—
Adults: 160 to 200 mg chloroquine
(hydrochloride) base I.M. daily for no
more than 12 days. As soon as possible, substitute 1 g (600 mg base)
chloroquine phosphate P.O. daily for

2 days; then 500 mg (300 mg base) daily for at least 2 to 3 weeks. Treatment is usually combined with an effective intestinal amebicide.
Children: 10 mg/kg of chloroquine (hydrochloride) base for 2 to 3 weeks. Maximum 300 mg daily.
Rheumatoid arthritis and lupus erythematosus—
250 mg chloroquine phosphate daily with evening meal.

ADVERSE REACTIONS
Blood: *agranulocytosis, aplastic anemia,* hemolytic anemia, thrombocytopenia.
CNS: mild and transient headache, neuromyopathy, psychic stimulation, fatigue, irritability, nightmares, seizures, dizziness.
CV: hypotension, ECG changes.
EENT: *visual disturbances* (blurred vision; difficulty in focusing; reversible corneal changes; generally irreversible, sometimes progressive or delayed, retinal changes, such as narrowing of arterioles; macular lesions; pallor of optic disk; optic atrophy; patchy retinal pigmentation, often leading to blindness); ototoxicity (nerve deafness, vertigo, tinnitus).
GI: anorexia, abdominal cramps, diarrhea, nausea, vomiting, stomatitis.
Skin: pruritus, lichen planus-like eruptions, skin and mucosal pigmentary changes, pleomorphic skin eruptions.

INTERACTIONS
Magnesium and aluminum salts, kaolin: Decreased GI absorption. Separate administration times.

NURSING CONSIDERATIONS
• Contraindicated in retinal or visual field changes or porphyria. Use with extreme caution in presence of severe GI, neurologic, or blood disorders. Drug concentrates in liver; use cautiously in patients with hepatic dis-

ease or alcoholism. Use with caution in patients with G6PD deficiency or psoriasis; drug may exacerbate these conditions.
• Complete blood cell counts and liver function studies should be made periodically during prolonged therapy; if severe blood disorder appears that is not attributable to disease under treatment, drug may need to be discontinued.
• Overdosage can quickly lead to toxic symptoms: headache, drowsiness, visual disturbances, cardiovascular collapse, and seizures, followed by respiratory and cardiac arrest. Children are extremely susceptible to toxicity; avoid long-term treatment.
• Baseline and periodic ophthalmologic examinations needed. Tell patient to report blurred vision, increased sensitivity to light, or muscle weakness. Check periodically for ocular muscle weakness after long-term use. Audiometric examinations recommended before, during, and after therapy, especially if long term.
• Drug should be taken immediately before or after meals on same day each week.
• To avoid exacerbated drug-induced dermatoses, warn patient to avoid excessive exposure to sun.

hydroxychloroquine sulfate
Plaquenil
Pregnancy Risk Category: C

HOW SUPPLIED
Tablets: 200 mg (150-mg base)

MECHANISM OF ACTION
May bind to and alter the properties of DNA.

INDICATIONS & DOSAGE
Suppressive prophylaxis of attacks of malaria due to Plasmodium vivax, P. malariae, P. ovale, *and susceptible strains of* P. falciparum—

Italicized adverse reactions are common or life-threatening.
*Liquid form contains alcohol.   **May contain tartrazine.

Adults and children: for suppression: 5 mg (base)/kg body weight P.O. (not to exceed 310 mg) weekly on same day of the week (begin 2 weeks prior to entering and continue for 8 weeks after leaving endemic area). If not started prior to exposure, double initial dose (620 mg for adults, 10 mg/kg for children) in 2 divided doses P.O. 6 hours apart.

Treatment of acute malarial attacks—
Adults and children over 15 years: initially, 800 mg (sulfate) P.O., then 400 mg after 6 to 8 hours, then 400 mg daily for 2 days (total 2 g sulfate salt).

Children 11 to 15 years: 600 mg (sulfate) P.O. stat, then 200 mg 8 hours later, then 200 mg 24 hours later (total 1 g sulfate salt).

Children 6 to 10 years: 400 mg (sulfate) P.O. stat, then 2 doses of 200 mg at 8-hour intervals (total 800 mg sulfate salt).

Children 2 to 5 years: 400 mg (sulfate) P.O. stat, then 200 mg 8 hours later (total 600 mg sulfate salt).

Children under 1 year: 100 mg (sulfate) P.O. stat; then 3 doses of 100 mg 6 to 9 hours apart (total 400 mg sulfate salt).

Lupus erythematosus (chronic discoid and systemic)—
Adults: 400 mg P.O. daily or b.i.d., continued for several weeks or months, depending on response. Prolonged maintenance dosage—200 to 400 mg P.O. daily.

Rheumatoid arthritis—
Adults: initially, 400 to 600 mg P.O. daily. When good response occurs (usually in 4 to 12 weeks), cut dosage in half.

ADVERSE REACTIONS

Blood: *agranulocytosis, leukopenia,* thrombocytopenia, hemolysis in patients with G6PD deficiency, *aplastic anemia.*
CNS: irritability, nightmares, ataxia, seizures, psychic stimulation, toxic psychosis, vertigo, tinnitus, nystagmus, lassitude, fatigue, dizziness, hypoactive deep tendon reflexes, skeletal muscle weakness.
EENT: visual disturbances (blurred vision; difficulty in focusing; reversible corneal changes; generally irreversible, sometimes progressive or delayed, retinal changes, e.g., narrowing of arterioles; macular lesions; pallor of optic disk; optic atrophy; visual field defects; patchy retinal pigmentation, often leading to blindness), ototoxicity (irreversible nerve deafness, tinnitus, labyrinthitis).
GI: anorexia, abdominal cramps, diarrhea, nausea, vomiting.
Skin: pruritus, lichen planus-like eruptions, skin and mucosal pigmentary changes, pleomorphic skin eruptions.
Other: weight loss, alopecia, bleaching of hair.

INTERACTIONS

Magnesium and aluminum salts, kaolin: Decreased GI absorption. Separate administration times.

NURSING CONSIDERATIONS

• Contraindicated in patients with retinal or visual field changes, or porphyria. Use with extreme caution in presence of severe GI, neurologic, or blood disorders. Drug concentrates in the liver; use cautiously in patients with hepatic disease or alcoholism. Use with caution in patients with G6PD deficiency or psoriasis; drug may exacerbate these conditions.
• Complete blood cell counts and liver function studies should be made periodically during prolonged therapy; if severe blood disorder appears that is not attributable to disease under treatment, consider discontinuing.
• Overdosage can quickly lead to toxic symptoms: headache, drowsiness, visual disturbances, cardiovascular collapse, and seizures, followed by respiratory and cardiac arrest.

Children are extremely susceptible to toxicity; avoid long-term treatment.
• Baseline and periodic ophthalmologic examinations needed. Tell patient to report blurred vision, increased sensitivity to light, or muscle weakness. Check periodically for ocular muscle weakness after long-term use. Audiometric examinations recommended before, during, and after therapy, especially if long term.
• Drug should be taken immediately before or after meals on same day of each week.

mefloquine hydrochloride
Lariam
Pregnancy Risk Category: C

HOW SUPPLIED
Tablets: 250 mg

MECHANISM OF ACTION
Exact mechanism unknown. Mefloquine is a structural analog of quinine. Antimalarial activity may be related to its ability to form complexes with hemin.

INDICATIONS & DOSAGE
Treatment of acute malaria infections caused by mefloquine-sensitive strains of Plasmodium falciparum *or* Plasmodium vivax—
Adults: 1,250 mg P.O. as a single dose. Patients with *P. vivax* infections should receive subsequent therapy with primaquine or other 8-aminoquinolones to avoid relapse after treatment of the initial infection.
Malaria prophylaxis—
Adults: 250 mg P.O. once weekly for 4 weeks, then 250 mg every other week. Initiate prophylaxis 1 week before entering endemic area, and continue prophylaxis for 4 weeks after return from such areas. When returning to an area without malaria after a prolonged stay in an endemic area, prophylaxis ends after three doses.

ADVERSE REACTIONS
CNS: dizziness, syncope, headache, transient emotional disturbances (rare).
CV: extrasystoles.
EENT: tinnitus.
GI: loss of appetite, vomiting, *nausea,* loose stools, diarrhea, GI discomfort.
Skin: rash.
Other: fatigue, fever, chills.

INTERACTIONS
Quinine, chloroquine: increased risk of seizures.
Quinine, quinidine, beta-adrenergic blocking agents: ECG abnormalities and cardiac arrest may occur.
Valproic acid: decreased valproic acid blood levels and loss of seizure control at start of mefloquine therapy. Monitor anticonvulsant blood levels.

NURSING CONSIDERATIONS
• Contraindicated in patients hypersensitive to mefloquine or related compounds.
• Use cautiously in patients with cardiac disease.
• Advise the patient to take the drug on the same day of the week when using it for prophylaxis.
• Tell the patient not to take the drug on an empty stomach and always to take it with a full glass (at least 8 oz [240 ml]) of water.
• Because the health risks from concomitant administration of quinine and mefloquine are great, mefloquine therapy should not begin sooner than 12 hours after the last dose of quinine or quinidine.
• Advise patients to use caution when performing hazardous activities that require alertness and good coordination because there have been reports of dizziness, a disturbed sense of balance, and neuropsychiatric reactions.
• In cases of suspected overdose, induce vomiting and seek medical advice immediately because there is po-

tential for cardiotoxicity. Animal studies reveal that mefloquine has cardiac actions similar to quinidine and quinine.
• Patients taking mefloquine prophylaxis should discontinue the drug if they notice signs or symptoms of unexplained anxiety, depression, confusion, or restlessness. These symptoms may indicate impending toxicity.
• Periodic ophthalmic examinations are recommended in patients undergoing long-term therapy because ocular lesions have been noted in laboratory animals.
• Periodic liver function tests are recommended.
• Patients with infections caused by *P. vivax* are at high risk of relapse because the drug does not eliminate the hepatic phase (exoerythrocytic parasites). Follow-up therapy is advisable.

primaquine phosphate
Pregnancy Risk Category: C

HOW SUPPLIED
Tablets: 7.5 mg (base)‡, 15 mg (base)

MECHANISM OF ACTION
A gametocidal drug that destroys exoerythrocytic forms and prevents delayed primary attack. Its precise mechanism of action is unknown.

INDICATIONS & DOSAGE
Radical cure of relapsing vivax malaria, eliminating symptoms and infection completely; prevention of relapse—
Adults: 15 mg (base) P.O. daily for 14 days. (26.3 mg tablet = 15 mg of base).

ADVERSE REACTIONS
Blood: leukopenia, hemolytic anemia in G6PD deficiency, methemoglobinemia in NADH methemoglobin reductase deficiency, leukocytosis, mild anemia, *granulocytopenia, agranulocytosis.*
CNS: headache.
EENT: disturbances of visual accommodation.
GI: nausea, vomiting, epigastric distress, abdominal cramps.
Skin: urticaria.

INTERACTIONS
Magnesium and aluminum salts: Decreased GI absorption. Separate administration times.

NURSING CONSIDERATIONS
• Contraindicated in lupus erythematosus and rheumatoid arthritis; in patients taking bone marrow suppressants and potentially hemolytic drugs.
• Use with a fast-acting antimalarial, such as chloroquine. Use full dose to reduce possibility of drug-resistant strains.
• Light-skinned patients taking more than 30 mg (base) daily, dark-skinned patients taking more than 15 mg (base) daily, and patients with severe anemia or suspected sensitivity should have frequent blood studies and urine examinations. Sudden fall in hemoglobin concentration, erythrocyte or leukocyte count, or marked darkening of the urine suggests impending hemolytic reactions.
• Observe closely for tolerance in patients with previous idiosyncrasy (manifested by hemolytic anemia, methemoglobinemia, or leukopenia); family or personal history of favism; erythrocytic G6PD deficiency or NADH methemoglobin reductase deficiency.
• Administer drug with meals or with antacids.

---

pyrimethamine
Daraprim

pyrimethamine with sulfadoxine
Fansidar

Pregnancy Risk Category: C

HOW SUPPLIED
pyrimethamine
Tablets: 25 mg
pyrimethamine with sulfadoxine
Tablets: pyrimethamine 25 mg, sulfadoxine 500 mg

MECHANISM OF ACTION
Inhibits the enzyme dihydrofolate reductase, thereby impeding reduction of dihydrofolic acid to tetrahydrofolic acid.

INDICATIONS & DOSAGE
Malaria prophylaxis and transmission control (pyrimethamine)—
Adults and children over 10 years: 25 mg P.O. weekly.
Children 4 to 10 years: 12.5 mg P.O. weekly.
Children under 4 years: 6.25 mg P.O. weekly.
Continue in all age groups at least 10 weeks after leaving endemic areas.
Acute attacks of malaria (Fansidar)—
Adults: 2 to 3 tablets as a single dose, either alone or in sequence with quinine or primaquine.
Children 9 to 14 years: 2 tablets.
Children 4 to 8 years: 1 tablet.
Children under 4 years: ½ tablet.
Malaria prophylaxis (Fansidar)—
Adults: 1 tablet weekly, or 2 tablets q 2 weeks.
Children 9 to 14 years: ¾ tablet weekly, or 1½ tablets q 2 weeks.
Children 4 to 8 years: ½ tablet weekly, or 1 tablet q 2 weeks.
Children under 4 years: ¼ tablet weekly, or ½ tablet q 2 weeks.
Acute attacks of malaria (pyrimethamine)—

Not recommended alone in nonimmune persons; use with faster-acting antimalarials, such as chloroquine, for 2 days to initiate transmission control and suppressive cure.
Adults and children over 15 years: 25 mg P.O. daily for 2 days.
Children under 15 years: 12.5 mg P.O. daily for 2 days.
Toxoplasmosis (pyrimethamine)—
Adults: initially, 100 mg P.O., then 25 mg P.O. daily for 4 to 5 weeks; during same time give 1 g sulfadiazine P.O. q 6 hours.
Children: initially, 1 mg/kg P.O., then 0.25 mg/kg daily for 4 to 5 weeks, along with 100 mg sulfadiazine/kg P.O. daily, divided q 6 hours.

ADVERSE REACTIONS
Blood: *agranulocytosis, aplastic anemia,* megaloblastic anemia, bone marrow suppression, leukopenia, thrombocytopenia, pancytopenia.
CNS: stimulation and seizures (acute toxicity).
GI: anorexia, vomiting, diarrhea, atrophic glossitis.
Skin: rashes, *erythema multiforme (Stevens-Johnson syndrome), toxic epidermal necrolysis.*

INTERACTIONS
Folic acid and para-aminobenzoic acid: decreased antitoxoplasmic effects. May require dosage adjustment.
Sulfonamides, co-trimoxazole: increased adverse effects. Use together cautiously.

NURSING CONSIDERATIONS
• Sulfadoxine, an ingredient in Fansidar, is a sulfonamide; therefore, this combination is contraindicated in porphyria. Use cautiously in impaired hepatic or renal function, severe allergy or bronchial asthma, or G6PD deficiency.
• Contraindicated in chloroquine-resistant malaria. Use cautiously in

seizure disorders; smaller doses may be needed. Also use cautiously following treatment with chloroquine.
• Warn patient taking Fansidar to stop drug and notify doctor at first sign of skin rash.
• Dosages required to treat toxoplasmosis approach toxic levels. Twice-weekly blood counts, including platelets, are required. If signs of folic or folinic acid deficiency develop, dosage should be reduced or discontinued while patient receives parenteral folinic acid (leucovorin) until blood counts become normal.
• Give with meals to minimize GI distress.
• The first dose of Fansidar, when taken prophylactically, should be taken 1 to 2 days before traveling to an endemic area.
• Because of the possibility of severe skin reactions, Fansidar should be used only in regions where chloroquine-resistant malaria is prevalent and only when the traveler plans to stay in the region longer than 3 weeks.

---

quinine bisulfate (quinine bisulphate)
Bi-Chinine‡, Biquinate‡, Myoquin‡, Quinbisul‡

quinine sulfate (quinine sulphate)
Chinine‡, Legatrin, Novoquinine†, Quinamm, Quinate‡, Quindan, Quine-200◇, Quine-300, Quinoctal‡, Quiphile, Strema, Sulquin‡

Pregnancy Risk Category: X

HOW SUPPLIED
bisulphate
Tablets: 100 mg, 300 mg
sulfate
Tablets: 260 mg, 325 mg◇
Capsules: 130 mg◇, 195 mg◇, 200 mg◇, 260 mg, 300 mg◇, 325 mg◇

MECHANISM OF ACTION
Mechanism of antiprotozoal action is unknown, but the drug is often referred to as a generalized protoplasmic poison. As a muscle relaxant, quinine appears to have a direct effect on muscle fibers that decreases their response to repetitive stimulation.

INDICATIONS & DOSAGE
Malaria due to Plasmodium falciparum *(chloroquine-resistant)—*
Adults: 650 mg P.O. q 8 hours for 10 days, with 25 mg pyrimethamine q 12 hours for 3 days, and with 500 mg sulfadiazine q.i.d. for 5 days.
Nocturnal leg cramps—
Adults: 260 to 300 mg P.O. at bedtime or after the evening meal.

ADVERSE REACTIONS
Blood: hemolytic anemia, thrombocytopenia, *agranulocytosis,* hypoprothrombinemia.
CNS: severe headache, apprehension, excitement, confusion, delirium, syncope, hypothermia, seizures (with toxic doses).
CV: hypotension, *cardiovascular collapse* with overdosage or rapid I.V. administration.
EENT: altered color perception, photophobia, blurred vision, night blindness, amblyopia, scotoma, diplopia, mydriasis, optic atrophy, tinnitus, impaired hearing.
GI: epigastric distress, diarrhea, nausea, vomiting.
GU: renal tubular damage, anuria.
Skin: rashes, pruritus.
Local: thrombosis at infusion site.
Other: asthma, flushing.

INTERACTIONS
Sodium bicarbonate: elevates quinine levels by decreasing quinine excretion. Use together cautiously.

NURSING CONSIDERATIONS
• Contraindicated in G6PD defi-

---

ciency. Use with caution in cardiovascular conditions.

• Discontinue if any signs of idiosyncrasy or toxicity occur.

• Quinine is no longer used for acute attacks of malaria due to *Plasmodium vivax* or for suppression of malaria due to organism resistance.

• Administer after meals to minimize GI distress. Do not crush tablets, as the drug is irritating to gastric mucosa.

• When parenteral therapy is necessary or when oral therapy is not feasible, quinine dihydrochloride may be obtained from the Centers for Disease Control. Administer by slow infusion (over at least 1 hour).

10

Antituberculars and antileprotics

capreomycin sulfate
clofazimine
cycloserine
dapsone
ethambutol hydrochloride
ethionamide
isoniazid
pyrazinamide
rifampin
streptomycin sulfate
  (See Chapter 11, AMINOGLYCOSIDES.)

COMBINATION PRODUCTS
P-I-N FORTE: isoniazid 100 mg and pyridoxine hydrochloride 5 mg.
RIFAMATE: isoniazid 150 mg and rifampin 300 mg.
RIMACTANE/INH DUAL PACK: thirty 300-mg isoniazid tablets and sixty 300-mg rifampin capsules.

---

capreomycin sulfate
Capastat

Pregnancy Risk Category: C

HOW SUPPLIED
Injection: 1 g/vial

MECHANISM OF ACTION
Unknown (bactericidal).

INDICATIONS & DOSAGE
Adjunctive treatment in pulmonary tuberculosis—
Adults: 15 mg/kg/day up to 1 g I.M. daily injected deeply into large muscle mass for 60 to 120 days; then 1 g 2 to 3 times weekly for a period of 18 to 24 months. Maximum dosage should not exceed 20 mg/kg daily. Must be given in conjunction with another antitubercular drug.

ADVERSE REACTIONS
Blood: eosinophilia, leukocytosis, leukopenia.
CNS: headache.
EENT: *ototoxicity* (tinnitus, vertigo, hearing loss).
GU: *nephrotoxicity* (elevated BUN and nonprotein nitrogen, casts, red blood cells, leukocytes; tubular necrosis; proteinuria; decreased creatinine clearance).
Metabolic: hypokalemia, alkalosis, hepatotoxicity.
Local: pain, induration, excessive bleeding and sterile abscesses at injection site.
Other: neuromuscular blockade

INTERACTIONS
None significant.

NURSING CONSIDERATIONS
• Contraindicated in patients receiving other ototoxic or nephrotoxic drugs. Use cautiously in patients with impaired renal function, history of allergies, or hearing impairment.
• Considered a "second-line" drug in the treatment of tuberculosis.
• Drug is never given I.V. Intravenous use may cause neuromuscular blockade.
• Administer deep into large muscle mass to minimize local reactions. If approved by the doctor, reconstitute I.M. dose with 0.5% lidocaine hydrochloride without epinephrine. Apply ice to injection site p.r.n. for pain.

• Evaluate patient's hearing before and every 1 to 2 weeks during therapy. Notify doctor if patient complains of tinnitus, vertigo, or hearing impairment.
• Monitor renal function (output, specific gravity, urinalysis, BUN, and serum creatinine) before and during therapy; notify doctor of decreasing renal function. Dose must be reduced in renal impairment.
• Straw- or dark-colored solution does not indicate a loss in potency. Do not administer solutions that contain a precipitate.

---

clofazimine
Lamprene

Pregnancy Risk Category: C

HOW SUPPLIED
Capsules: 50 mg, 100 mg

MECHANISM OF ACTION
Inhibits mycobacterial growth by binding preferentially to mycobacterial DNA. Also has anti-inflammatory effects that suppress skin reactions of erythema nodosum leprosum.

INDICATIONS & DOSAGE
Treatment of dapsone-resistant leprosy—
Adults: 100 mg P.O. daily in combination with other antileprotics for 3 years. Then, clofazimine *alone,* 100 mg daily.
Erythema nodosum leprosum—
Adults: 100 to 200 mg P.O. daily for up to 3 months. Taper dosage to 100 mg daily as soon as possible. Dosages above 200 mg daily are not recommended.

ADVERSE REACTIONS
EENT: conjunctival and corneal pigmentation.
GI: *epigastric pain, diarrhea, nausea, vomiting, GI intolerance, bowel obstruction, GI bleeding.*

Skin: *Pink to brownish black pigmentation, ichthyosis and dryness,* rash, itching.
Other: *Splenic infarction,* discolored body fluids and excrement.

INTERACTIONS
None significant.

NURSING CONSIDERATIONS
• Use cautiously in GI dysfunction, such as abdominal pain and diarrhea.
• Advise patient to take the drug with meals.
• Doses that exceed 100 mg daily should be given for as short a period as possible and only under close medical supervision.
• If patient complains of colicky or burning abdominal pain or of any other GI symptom, report this to the doctor, who may reduce the dose or increase the interval between doses.
• Warn patient that clofazimine may discolor skin, body fluids, and excrement. The color ranges from red to brownish black. Reassure patient that the unsightly skin discoloration is reversible but may not disappear until several months or years after drug treatment ends.
• Recommend application of skin oil or cream to help reverse skin dryness or ichthyosis.

---

cycloserine
Seromycin

Pregnancy Risk Category: C

HOW SUPPLIED
Capsules: 250 mg

MECHANISM OF ACTION
Inhibits cell wall biosynthesis by inhibiting the utilization of amino acids (bacteriostatic).

INDICATIONS & DOSAGE
Adjunctive treatment in pulmonary or extrapulmonary tuberculosis—

Italicized adverse reactions are common or life-threatening.
*Liquid form contains alcohol.   **May contain tartrazine.

Adults: initially, 250 mg P.O. q 12 hours for 2 weeks; then, if blood levels are below 25 to 30 mcg/ml and there are no clinical signs of toxicity, dosage is increased to 250 mg P.O. q 8 hours for 2 weeks. If optimum blood levels are still not achieved, and there are no signs of clinical toxicity, then dosage is increased to 250 mg P.O. q 6 hours. Maximum dosage is 1 g/day. If CNS toxicity occurs, drug is discontinued for 1 week, then resumed at 250 mg daily for 2 weeks. If no serious toxic effects occur, dosage is increased by 250-mg increments q 10 days until blood level of 25 to 30 mcg/ml is obtained.

ADVERSE REACTIONS
CNS: drowsiness, headache, tremor, dysarthria, vertigo, confusion, loss of memory, *possible suicidal tendencies and other psychotic symptoms, nervousness, hallucinations, depression,* hyperirritability, paresthesias, paresis, hyperreflexia.
Other: hypersensitivity (allergic dermatitis).

INTERACTIONS
Ethanol or ethionamide: increased risk of CNS toxicity (seizures).
Isoniazid: monitor for CNS toxicity (dizziness or drowsiness).

NURSING CONSIDERATIONS
● Contraindicated in seizure disorders, depression or severe anxiety, severe renal insufficiency, or chronic alcoholism. Use cautiously in impaired renal function; reduced dosage required.
● Considered a "second-line" drug in the treatment of tuberculosis.
● Obtain specimen for culture and sensitivity tests before therapy begins and periodically thereafter to detect possible resistance.
● Serious neurologic effects can be precipitated by ingestion of alcohol; warn patient to avoid alcohol.

● Toxic reactions may occur with blood levels above 30 mcg/ml.
● Pyridoxine, anticonvulsants, tranquilizers, or sedatives may help to relieve adverse reactions.
● Observe for psychiatric symptoms.
● Monitor hematologic tests and renal and liver function studies.
● Instruct patient to take drug exactly as prescribed; warn against discontinuing use without doctor's approval.

---

dapsone
Avlosulfon†, Dapsone 100‡
Pregnancy Risk Category: A

HOW SUPPLIED
Tablets: 25 mg, 100 mg

MECHANISM OF ACTION
Inhibits folic acid biosynthesis in susceptible organisms (bactericidal).

INDICATIONS & DOSAGE
All forms of leprosy (Hansen's disease)—
Adults: 100 mg P.O. daily for indefinite period, plus rifampin 600 mg daily for 6 months.
Children: 1.4 mg/kg P.O. daily.
Prophylaxis for leprosy patient's close contacts—
Adults: 50 mg P.O. daily.
Children age 6 to 12: 25 mg P.O. daily.
Children age 2 to 5: 25 mg P.O. three times weekly.
Infants age 6 to 23 months: 12 mg P.O. three times weekly.
Children under age 6 months: 6 mg P.O. three times weekly.
Dermatitis herpetiformis—
Adults: 50 mg. P.O. daily; may increase to 400 mg. daily.
Malaria suppression or prophylaxis due to chloroquine-resistant Plasmodium falciparum *when other agents aren't available—*
Adults: 100 mg. P.O. weekly; usually

given with pyrimethimine 12.5 mg.
P.O. weekly.
Children: 2 mg/kg P.O. weekly, with
pyrimethamine 0.25 mg/kg weekly.
   Continue prophylaxis during exposure and for 6 months after exposure.
Treatment of Pneumocystis carinii
pneumonia in patients with AIDS—
Adults: 100 mg P.O. daily in conjunction with trimethoprim 20 mg/kg P.O.
daily (usually divided q.i.d.).
Actinomycotic mycetoma—
Adults: 100 mg P.O. b.i.d. Treatment
is usually continued for months after
clinical symptoms abate.

ADVERSE REACTIONS

Blood: *aplastic anemia, agranulocytosis, hemolytic anemia;* methemoglobinemia; possible leukopenia.
CNS: psychosis, headache, dizziness,
lethargy, severe malaise, paresthesias.
EENT: tinnitus, allergic rhinitis.
GI: anorexia, abdominal pain, nausea, vomiting.
Hepatic: hepatitis, cholestatic jaundice.
Skin: allergic dermatitis (generalized
or fixed maculopapular rash).

INTERACTIONS

Probenecid: elevates levels of dapsone. Use together with extreme caution.

NURSING CONSIDERATIONS

• Use cautiously in chronic renal, hepatic, or cardiovascular disease or refractory types of anemia.
• Use cautiously in G6PD deficiency.
• Therapy should be interrupted if
generalized, diffuse dermatitis occurs.
• Dapsone dosage should be reduced
or temporarily discontinued if hemoglobin falls below 9 g/dl; if leukocyte
count falls below 5,000/mm³; if
erythrocyte count falls below 2.5 mil-
lion/mm³ or remains low.

• Antihistamines may help to combat
dapsone-induced allergic dermatitis.
• Erythema nodosum type of lepra reaction may occur during therapy as a
result of *Mycobacterium leprae* bacilli
(malaise, fever, painful inflammatory
induration in the skin and mucosa, iritis, and neuritis). In severe cases,
therapy should be stopped and glucocorticoids given cautiously.
• Obtain CBC before treatment and
monitor frequently throughout therapy (weekly for the first month,
monthly for 6 months, and semiannu-
ally thereafter).
• Also used to treat relapsing poly-
chondritis and as prophylaxis against
malaria. Has been used investigationally to treat rheumatoid arthritis, allergic vasculitis, relapsing polychon-
dritis, and postular and inflammatory
dermatoses.
• Instruct breast-feeding mothers to
report cyanosis in infants, as this indicates high sulfone level.

ethambutol hydrochloride
Etibi†, Myambutol

Pregnancy Risk Category: B

HOW SUPPLIED
Tablets: 100 mg, 400 mg

MECHANISM OF ACTION
Interferes with the synthesis of RNA,
thus inhibiting protein metabolism
(bacteriostatic).

INDICATIONS & DOSAGE
*Adjunctive treatment in pulmonary tu-
berculosis*—
Adults and children over 13 years:
initial treatment for patients who have
not received previous antitubercular
therapy is 15 mg/kg P.O. daily single
dose.
Re-treatment: 25 mg/kg P.O. daily
single dose for 60 days with at least
one other antitubercular drug; then

Italicized adverse reactions are common or life-threatening.
*Liquid form contains alcohol.   **May contain tartrazine.

decrease to 15 mg/kg P.O. daily single dose.

ADVERSE REACTIONS
CNS: headache, dizziness, mental confusion, possible hallucinations, peripheral neuritis (numbness and tingling of extremities).
EENT: optic neuritis (vision loss and loss of color discrimination, especially red and green).
GI: anorexia, nausea, vomiting, abdominal pain.
Metabolic: *elevated uric acid.*
Other: anaphylactoid reactions, fever, malaise, bloody sputum.

INTERACTIONS
None significant.

NURSING CONSIDERATIONS
• Contraindicated in optic neuritis and in children under 13 years. Use cautiously in impaired renal function, cataracts, recurrent eye inflammations, gout, and diabetic retinopathy.
• Dose must be reduced in renal impairment.
• Perform visual acuity and color discrimination tests before and during therapy.
• Always monitor serum uric acid; observe patient for symptoms of gout.
• Reassure patient that visual disturbances will disappear several weeks to months after drug is stopped.

---

ethionamide
Trecator-SC
Pregnancy Risk Category: D

HOW SUPPLIED
Tablets: 250 mg

MECHANISM OF ACTION
Unknown (bacteriostatic).

INDICATIONS & DOSAGE
Adjunctive treatment in pulmonary or extrapulmonary tuberculosis (when primary therapy with streptomycin or isoniazid cannot be used or has failed)—
Adults: 500 mg to 1 g P.O. daily in divided doses. Concomitant administration of other effective antitubercular drugs and pyridoxine recommended.
Children: 12 to 15 mg/kg P.O. daily in 3 to 4 doses. Maximum dosage is 750 mg.

ADVERSE REACTIONS
Blood: thrombocytopenia.
CNS: *peripheral neuritis,* psychic disturbances (especially mental depression).
CV: postural hypotension.
GI: *anorexia,* metallic taste in mouth, nausea, vomiting, sialorrhea, *epigastric distress,* diarrhea, stomatitis, weight loss.
Hepatic: jaundice, hepatitis, elevated AST (SGOT) and ALT (SGPT).
Skin: rash, *exfoliative dermatitis.*

INTERACTIONS
None significant.

NURSING CONSIDERATIONS
• Contraindicated in severe hepatic damage. Use cautiously in diabetes mellitus.
• Culture and sensitivity tests should be performed before starting therapy. Stop drug if skin rash occurs; may progress to exfoliative dermatitis.
• Monitor hepatic function every 2 to 4 weeks.
• Give with meals or antacids to minimize GI effects. Patient may require antiemetic.
• Pyridoxine may be ordered to prevent neuropathy.
• Instruct patient to take this drug exactly as prescribed; warn against discontinuing drug without doctor's consent.
• Warn patient to avoid excess alcohol ingestion because it may make him more vulnerable to liver damage.

isoniazid (INH)

DOW-Isoniazid, Isotamine†,
Laniazid, Nydrazid**, PMS-
Isoniazid†

Pregnancy Risk Category: C

HOW SUPPLIED

Tablets: 50 mg, 100 mg, 300 mg
Oral solution: 50 mg/5 ml
Injection: 100 mg/ml

MECHANISM OF ACTION

Inhibits cell wall biosynthesis by interfering with lipid and DNA synthesis (bactericidal).

INDICATIONS & DOSAGE

Primary treatment against actively growing tubercle bacilli—
Adults: 5 mg/kg P.O. or I.M. daily single dose, up to 300 mg/day, continued for 6 months to 2 years.
Infants and children: 10 to 20 mg/kg P.O. or I.M. daily single dose, up to 300 to 500 mg/day, continued for 18 months to 2 years. Concomitant administration of at least one other effective antitubercular drug is recommended.
Preventive therapy against tubercle bacilli of those closely exposed or those with positive skin test whose chest X-rays and bacteriologic studies are consistent with nonprogressive tuberculous disease—
Adults: 300 mg P.O. daily single dose, continued for 1 year.
Infants and children: 10 mg/kg P.O. daily single dose, up to 300 mg/day, continued for 1 year.

ADVERSE REACTIONS

Blood: *agranulocytosis,* hemolytic anemia, *aplastic anemia,* eosinophilia, leukopenia, neutropenia, thrombocytopenia, methemoglobinemia, pyridoxine-responsive hypochromic anemia.
CNS: *peripheral neuropathy* (especially in the malnourished, alcoholics, diabetics, and slow acetylators), usually preceded by paresthesias of hands and feet, psychosis.
GI: nausea, vomiting, epigastric distress, constipation, dryness of the mouth.
Hepatic: *hepatitis, occasionally severe and sometimes fatal, especially in elderly patients.*
Metabolic: hyperglycemia, metabolic acidosis.
Local: irritation at injection site.
Other: rheumatic syndrome and systemic lupus erythematosus–like syndrome; hypersensitivity (fever, rash, lymphadenopathy, vasculitis).

INTERACTIONS

Aluminum-containing antacids and laxatives: may decrease the rate and amount of isoniazid absorbed. Give isoniazid at least 1 hour before antacid or laxative.
Carbamazepine: increased risk of isoniazid hepatotoxicity. Use together very cautiously.
Corticosteroids: may decrease therapeutic effectiveness. Monitor need for larger isoniazid dose.
Disulfiram: neurologic symptoms, including changes in behavior and coordination, may develop with concomitant isoniazid use. Avoid concomitant use.

NURSING CONSIDERATIONS

• Contraindicated in acute hepatic disease or isoniazid-associated hepatic damage. Use cautiously in chronic non-isoniazid-associated hepatic disease, seizure disorders (especially those taking phenytoin), severe renal impairment, chronic alcoholism; and in elderly patients.
• Isoniazid pharmacokinetics may vary among patients, since its metabolism occurs in the liver by genetically controlled acetylation. Fast acetylators metabolize the drug up to five times as fast as slow acetylators. About 50% of blacks and whites are

---

Italicized adverse reactions are common or life-threatening.
*Liquid form contains alcohol.   **May contain tartrazine.

slow acetylators; over 80% of Chinese, Japanese, and Eskimos are fast acetylators.
• Monitor hepatic function. Tell patient to notify doctor immediately if symptoms of hepatic impairment occur (loss of appetite, fatigue, malaise, jaundice, dark urine).
• Alcohol may be associated with increased incidence of isoniazid-related hepatitis. Advise against use.
• Pyridoxine should be given to prevent peripheral neuropathy, especially in malnourished patients.
• Instruct patient to take this drug exactly as prescribed; warn against discontinuing drug without doctor's consent.
• Encourage patient to fully comply with treatment, which may take months or years.
• Advise patient to take with food if GI irritation occurs.
• Reportedly effective when used investigationally to treat arthritis and action tremor in multiple sclerosis.

---

pyrazinamide
PMS Pyrazinamide†, Tebrazid†, Zinamide‡

Pregnancy Risk Category: C

HOW SUPPLIED
Tablets: 500 mg

MECHANISM OF ACTION
Unknown (bactericidal).

INDICATIONS & DOSAGE
Adjunctive treatment of tuberculosis (when primary and secondary antitubercular drugs cannot be used or have failed)—
Adults: 20 to 35 mg/kg P.O. daily, divided in 3 to 4 doses. Maximum dosage is 3 g daily.

ADVERSE REACTIONS
Blood: sideroblastic anemia, possible bleeding tendency due to thrombocytopenia.
GI: anorexia, nausea, vomiting.
GU: dysuria.
Hepatic: hepatitis.
Metabolic: interference with control in diabetes mellitus, *hyperuricemia.*
Other: malaise, fever, arthralgia.

INTERACTIONS
None significant.

NURSING CONSIDERATIONS
• Contraindicated in severe hepatic disease. Use cautiously in diabetes mellitus or gout.
• Nearly 100% excreted in urine; reduced dose needed in patients with renal impairment.
• Perform liver function studies and examination for jaundice, liver tenderness, or enlargement before and frequently during therapy.
• Watch closely for signs of gout and of hepatic impairment (loss of appetite, fatigue, malaise, jaundice, dark urine, and liver tenderness). Notify doctor at once.
• Question doses that exceed 35 mg/ kg, as they may cause liver damage.
• Monitor hematopoietic studies and serum uric acid.
• When used with surgical management of tuberculosis, start pyrazinamide 1 to 2 weeks before surgery and continue for 4 to 6 weeks postoperatively.

---

rifampin (rifampicin)
Rifadin, Rimactane, Rimycin‡, Rofact†

Pregnancy Risk Category: C

HOW SUPPLIED
Capsules: 150 mg, 300 mg
Kit: 60 capsules, 300 mg

MECHANISM OF ACTION
Inhibits DNA-dependent RNA poly-

---

merase, thus impairing RNA synthesis (bactericidal).

INDICATIONS & DOSAGE

Primary treatment in pulmonary tuberculosis—
Adults: 600 mg P.O. daily single dose 1 hour before or 2 hours after meals.
Children over 5 years: 10 to 20 mg/kg P.O. daily single dose 1 hour before or 2 hours after meals. Maximum dosage is 600 mg daily. Concomitant administration of other effective antitubercular drugs is recommended.
Meningococcal carriers—
Adults: 600 mg P.O. b.i.d. for 2 days.
Children 1 to 12 years: 10 mg/kg P.O. b.i.d. or 2 days, not to exceed 600 mg/dose.
Infants 3 months to 1 year: 5 mg/kg P.O. b.i.d. for 2 days.
Prophylaxis of Hemophilus influenza type b—
Adults and children: 20 mg/kg P.O. once daily for 4 days. Do not exceed 600 mg/day.

ADVERSE REACTIONS

Blood: thrombocytopenia, transient leukopenia, hemolytic anemia.
CNS: headache, fatigue, *drowsiness,* ataxia, dizziness, mental confusion, generalized numbness.
GI: epigastric distress, anorexia, nausea, vomiting, abdominal pain, diarrhea, flatulence, sore mouth and tongue.
Metabolic: hyperuricemia.
Hepatic: *serious hepatotoxicity as well as transient abnormalities in liver function tests.*
Skin: pruritus, urticaria, rash.
Other: flu-like syndrome, discoloration of body fluids.

INTERACTIONS

Alcohol: may increase risk of hepatotoxicity.
Para-aminosalicylate sodium, ketoconazole: may interfere with absorption of rifampin. Give these drugs 8 to 12 hours apart.
Probenecid: may increase rifampin levels. Use cautiously.

NURSING CONSIDERATIONS

• Contraindicated in clinically active hepatitis.
• Use cautiously in hepatic disease or in those receiving other hepatotoxic drugs.
• Monitor hepatic function, hematopoietic studies, and serum uric acid.
• Watch closely for signs of hepatic impairment (loss of appetite, fatigue, malaise, jaundice, dark urine, liver tenderness). Notify doctor if these occur.
• Warn patient about drowsiness and the possibility of red-orange discoloration of urine, feces, saliva, sweat, sputum, and tears. Soft contact lenses may be permanently stained.
• Rifampin is not considered a teratogen. However, it may cause hemorrhaging in the newborns of rifampin-treated mothers.
• Advise patient to avoid alcoholic beverages while taking this drug. May increase risk of hepatotoxicity.
• Give 1 hour before or 2 hours after meals for optimal absorption; however, if GI irritation occurs, patient may take rifampin with meals.
• Increases enzyme activity of liver; may require increased doses of warfarin, corticosteroids, oral contraceptives, and oral hypoglycemics. See each drug entry for specific drug interactions.
• Concomitant treatment with at least one other antitubercular drug is recommended.

Italicized adverse reactions are common or life-threatening.
*Liquid form contains alcohol.   **May contain tartrazine.

11

Aminoglycosides

amikacin sulfate
gentamicin sulfate
kanamycin sulfate
neomycin sulfate
netilmicin sulfate
streptomycin sulfate
tobramycin sulfate

COMBINATION PRODUCTS
NEOSPORIN G.U. IRRIGANT: 40 mg
neomycin sulfate and 200,000 units
polymixin B sulfate/ml.

amikacin sulfate
Amikin

Pregnancy Risk Category: C

HOW SUPPLIED
Injection: 50 mg/ml, 250 mg/ml

MECHANISM OF ACTION
Inhibits protein synthesis by binding
directly to the 30S ribosomal subunit.
Generally bactericidal.

INDICATIONS & DOSAGE
Serious infections caused by sensitive
Pseudomonas aeruginosa, Escherichia coli, Proteus, Klebsiella, Serratia, Enterobacter, Acinetobacter,
Providencia, Citrobacter, Staphylococcus—
**Adults and children with normal
renal function:** 15 mg/kg/day divided q 8 to 12 hours I.M. or I.V. infusion (in 100 to 200 ml dextrose 5%
in water run in over 30 to 60 minutes). May be given by direct I.V.
push if necessary.
Neonates with normal renal func-

tion: initially, 10 mg/kg I.M. or I.V.
infusion (in dextrose 5% in water run
in over 1 to 2 hours), then 7.5 mg/kg
q 12 hours I.M. or I.V. infusion.
Meningitis—
Adults: systemic therapy as above;
may also use up to 20 mg intrathecally or intraventricularly daily.
Children: systemic therapy as above;
may also use 1 to 2 mg intrathecally
daily.
*Uncomplicated urinary tract infec-
tions—*
Adults: 250 mg I.M. or I.V. b.i.d.
**Adults with impaired renal func-
tion:** initially, 7.5 mg/kg. Subsequent
doses and frequency determined by
blood amikacin levels and renal function studies.

ADVERSE REACTIONS
CNS: headache, lethargy, *neuromuscular blockade.*
EENT: *ototoxicity (tinnitus, vertigo,
hearing loss).*
GU: *nephrotoxicity (cells or casts in
urine, oliguria, proteinuria, decreased creatinine clearance, increased BUN and serum creatinine
levels).*
Other: hypersensitivity reactions, hepatic necrosis.

INTERACTIONS
Cephalothin: increased nephrotoxicity. Use together cautiously.
Dimenhydrinate: may mask symptoms of ototoxicity. Use with caution.
*General anesthetics, neuromuscular
blocking agents:* may potentiate neuromuscular blockade.

I.V. loop diuretics (e.g. furosemide): increase ototoxicity. Use cautiously.
Other aminoglycosides, amphotericin B, cisplatin, methoxyflurane: increases nephrotoxicity. Use together cautiously.
Parenteral penicillins (e.g. carbenicillin, ticarcillin): amikacin inactivation in vitro. Don't mix together in I.V.

NURSING CONSIDERATIONS

• Use cautiously in impaired renal function, in neonates and infants, and in elderly patients.
• Obtain specimen for culture and sensitivity tests before first dose. Therapy may begin pending test results.
• Weigh patient and obtain baseline renal function studies before therapy begins.
• Monitor renal function (output, specific gravity, urinalysis, BUN and creatinine levels, and creatinine clearance). Notify doctor of signs of decreasing renal function.
• Patient should be well hydrated while taking drug to minimize chemical irritation of the renal tubules.
• Evaluate patient's hearing before and during therapy. Notify doctor if patient complains of tinnitus, vertigo, or hearing loss.
• Watch for superinfection (continued fever and other signs of new infections, especially of upper respiratory tract).
• Usual duration of therapy is 7 to 10 days. If no response after 3 to 5 days, therapy may be stopped and new specimens obtained for culture and sensitivity.
• Peak blood levels that are above 35 mcg/ml and trough levels that are above 10 mcg/ml may be associated with higher incidence of toxicity.
• After I.V. infusion, flush line with normal saline solution or dextrose 5% in water.
• Draw blood for peak amikacin level 1 hour after I.M. injection and 30

minutes to 1 hour after infusion ends; for trough levels, draw blood just before next dose. Don't collect blood in a heparinized tube because heparin is incompatible with aminoglycosides.
• Potency of drug is not affected if solution turns light yellow.

---

gentamicin sulfate
Cidomycin†‡, Garamycin, Gentafair, Jenamicin

Pregnancy Risk Category: C

HOW SUPPLIED
Injection: 40 mg/ml (adult), 10 mg/ml (pediatric), 2 mg/ml (intrathecal)

MECHANISM OF ACTION
Inhibits protein synthesis by binding directly to the 30S ribosomal subunit. Generally bactericidal.

INDICATIONS & DOSAGE
Serious infections caused by sensitive Pseudomonas aeruginosa, Escherichia coli, Proteus, Klebsiella, Serratia, Enterobacter, Citrobacter, Staphylococcus—
Adults with normal renal function: 3 mg/kg daily in divided doses q 8 hours I.M. or I.V. infusion (in 50 to 200 ml of normal saline solution or dextrose 5% in water infused over 30 minutes to 2 hours). May be given by direct I.V. push if necessary. For life-threatening infections, patient may receive up to 5 mg/kg daily in 3 to 4 divided doses.
Children with normal renal function: 2 to 2.5 mg/kg I.M. or I.V. infusion q 8 hours.
Infants and neonates over 1 week with normal renal function: 2.5 mg/kg q 8 hours I.M. or I.V. infusion.
Neonates under 1 week: 2.5 mg/kg I.V. q 12 hours. For I.V. infusion, dilute in normal saline solution or dextrose 5% in water and infuse over 30 minutes to 2 hours.
Meningitis—

Italicized adverse reactions are common or life-threatening.
*Liquid form contains alcohol.   **May contain tartrazine.

Adults: systemic therapy as above; may also use 4 to 8 mg intrathecally daily.

Children: systemic therapy as above; may also use 1 to 2 mg intrathecally daily.

Endocarditis prophylaxis for GI or GU procedure or surgery—

Adults: 1.5 mg/kg I.M. or I.V. 30 to 60 minutes before procedure or surgery and q 8 hours after, for 2 doses. Given with aqueous penicillin G or ampicillin.

Children: 2.5 mg/kg I.M. or I.V. 30 to 60 minutes before procedure or surgery and q 8 hours after, for 2 doses. Given with aqueous penicillin G or ampicillin.

Patients with impaired renal function: initial dose is same as for those with normal renal function. Subsequent doses and frequency determined by renal function studies and serum concentrations of gentamicin.

Posthemodialysis to maintain therapeutic blood levels—

Adults: 1 to 1.7 mg/kg I.M. or I.V. infusion after each dialysis.

Children: 2 mg/kg I.M. or I.V. infusion after each dialysis.

ADVERSE REACTIONS

CNS: headache, lethargy, *neuromuscular blockade*.

EENT: *ototoxicity (tinnitus, vertigo, hearing loss)*.

GU: *nephrotoxicity (cells or casts in the urine; oliguria; proteinuria; decreased creatinine clearance; increased BUN, nonprotein nitrogen, and serum creatinine levels)*.

Other: hypersensitivity reactions, hepatic necrosis.

INTERACTIONS

Cephalothin: increases nephrotoxicity. Use together cautiously.

Dimenhydrinate: may mask symptoms of ototoxicity. Use with caution.

General anesthetics, neuromuscular

blocking agents: may potentiate neuromuscular blockade.

I.V. loop diuretics (e.g. furosemide): increase ototoxicity. Use cautiously.

Other aminoglycosides, methoxyflurane: increase ototoxicity and nephrotoxicity. Use together cautiously.

Parenteral penicillins (e.g. carbenicillin and ticarcillin): gentamicin inactivation in vitro. Don't mix together in I.V.

NURSING CONSIDERATIONS

• Use cautiously in impaired renal function, and in neonates, infants, and elderly patients.

• Obtain specimen for culture and sensitivity tests before first dose. Therapy may begin pending test results.

• Weigh patient and obtain baseline renal function studies before therapy begins.

• Monitor renal function (output, specific gravity, urinalysis, BUN and creatinine levels, and creatinine clearance). Notify doctor of signs of decreasing renal function.

• Patient should be well hydrated while taking drug to minimize chemical irritation of the renal tubules.

• After completing I.V. infusion, flush the line with normal saline solution or dextrose 5% in water.

• Evaluate patient's hearing before and during therapy. Notify doctor if patient complains of tinnitus, vertigo, or hearing loss.

• Watch for superinfection (continued fever and other signs of new infections, especially of upper respiratory tract).

• Usual duration of therapy is 7 to 10 days. If no response in 3 to 5 days, therapy may be stopped and new specimens obtained for culture and sensitivity.

• Peak blood levels above 12 mcg/ml and trough levels (those drawn just before next dose) above 2 mcg/ml

---

may be associated with higher incidence of toxicity.

• Draw blood for peak gentamicin level 1 hour after I.M. injection and 30 minutes to 1 hour after infusion ends; for trough levels, draw blood just before next dose.Don't collect blood in a heparinized tube because heparin is incompatible with aminoglycosides.

• Hemodialysis (8 hours) removes up to 50% of drug from blood.

• Intrathecal form (without preservatives) should be used when intrathecal administration is indicated.

kanamycin sulfate
Kanasig‡, Kantrex, Klebcil

Pregnancy Risk Category: D

HOW SUPPLIED
Capsules: 500 mg
Injection: 37.5 mg/ml (pediatric), 250 mg/ml, 333 mg/ml

MECHANISM OF ACTION
Inhibits protein synthesis by binding directly to the 30S ribosomal subunit. Generally bactericidal.

INDICATIONS & DOSAGE
Serious infections caused by sensitive Escherichia coli, Proteus, Enterobacter aerogenes, Klebsiella pneumoniae, Serratia marcescens, Acinetobacter—
Adults and children with normal renal function: 15 mg/kg daily divided q 8 to 12 hours deep I.M. into upper outer quadrant of buttocks or I.V. infusion (diluted 500 mg/200 ml of normal saline solution or dextrose 5% in water infused at 60 to 80 drops/minute). Maximum daily dosage is 1.5 g.
Neonates: 15 mg/kg daily I.M. or I.V. divided q 12 hours.
Adjunctive treatment in hepatic coma—
Adults: 8 to 12 g daily P.O. in divided doses.

Preoperative bowel sterilization—
Adults: 1 g P.O. q 1 hour for 4 doses, then q 4 hours for 4 doses; or 1 g P.O. q 1 hour for 4 doses, then q 6 hours for 36 to 72 hours.
Intraperitoneal irrigation—
500 mg in 20 ml sterile distilled water instilled via catheter into wound after patient is fully recovered from anesthesia and neuromuscular blocking agent effects.
Wound irrigation—
Up to 2.5 mg/ml in normal saline solution irrigant.

ADVERSE REACTIONS
CNS: headache, lethargy, *neuromuscular blockade.*
EENT: o*totoxicity (tinnitus, vertigo, hearing loss).*
GU: *nephrotoxicity (cells or casts in the urine, oliguria, proteinuria, decreased creatinine clearance, increased BUN and serum creatinine levels).*
Other: hypersensitivity reactions.

INTERACTIONS
Cephalothin: increases nephrotoxicity. Use together cautiously.
Dimenhydrinate: may mask symptoms of ototoxicity. Use with caution.
General anesthetics, neuromuscular blocking agents: may potentiate neuromuscular blockade.
I.V. loop diuretics (e.g., furosemide): increase ototoxicity. Use cautiously.
Other aminoglycosides, amphotericin B, cisplatin, methoxyflurane: increases nephrotoxicity. Don't use together.
Parenteral penicillins (e.g., carbenicillin, ticarcillin): kanamycin inactivation in vitro. Don't mix together in I.V.

NURSING CONSIDERATIONS
• Oral use contraindicated in intestinal obstruction and treatment of systemic infection. Use cautiously in pa-

---

Italicized adverse reactions are common or life-threatening.
*Liquid form contains alcohol.   **May contain tartrazine.

tients with impaired renal function and in the elderly.

• Obtain specimen for culture and sensitivity tests before first dose. Therapy may begin pending test results.

• Weigh patient and obtain baseline renal function studies before therapy begins.

• Monitor renal function (output, specific gravity, urinalysis, BUN and creatinine levels, and creatinine clearance). Notify doctor of signs of decreasing renal function.

• Patient should be well hydrated while taking drug to minimize chemical irritation of the renal tubules.

• Evaluate patient's hearing before and during therapy. Notify doctor if patient complains of tinnitus, vertigo, or hearing loss.

• Watch for superinfection (continued fever and other signs of new infection, especially of upper respiratory tract).

• If no response in 3 to 5 days, therapy may be stopped and new specimens obtained for culture and sensitivity.

• Peak blood levels over 30 mcg/ml and trough levels over 10 mcg/ml may be associated with increased incidence of toxicity.

---

neomycin sulfate
Mycifradin, Neosulf‡

Pregnancy Risk Category: C

HOW SUPPLIED
Tablets: 500 mg
Oral solution: 125 mg/ml

MECHANISM OF ACTION
Inhibits protein synthesis by binding directly to the 30S ribosomal subunit. Generally bactericidal.

INDICATIONS & DOSAGE
Infectious diarrhea caused by enteropathogenic Escherichia coli—

Adults: 50 mg/kg daily P.O. in four divided doses for 2 to 3 days.
Children: 50 to 100 mg/kg daily P.O. divided q 4 to 6 hours for 2 to 3 days.
Suppression of intestinal bacteria preoperatively—
Adults: 1 g P.O. q 1 hour for four doses, then 1 g q 4 hours for the balance of the 24 hours. A saline cathartic should precede therapy.
Children: 40 to 100 mg/kg daily P.O. divided q 4 to 6 hours. First dose should be preceded by saline cathartic.
Adjunctive treatment in hepatic coma—
Adults: 1 to 3 g P.O. q.i.d. for 5 to 6 days; or 200 ml of 1% or 100 ml of 2% solution as enema retained for 20 to 60 minutes q 6 hours.

ADVERSE REACTIONS
CNS: headache, lethargy.
EENT: *ototoxicity (tinnitus, vertigo, hearing loss).*
GI: nausea, vomiting.
GU: *nephrotoxicity (cells or casts in the urine, oliguria, proteinuria, decreased creatinine clearance, increased BUN and serum creatinine levels).*
Skin: rash, urticaria.
Other: hypersensitivity reactions.

INTERACTIONS
Cephalothin: Increases nephrotoxicity. Use together cautiously.
Dimenhydrinate: may mask symptoms of ototoxicity. Use with caution.
I.V. loop diuretics (e.g. furosemide): increase ototoxicity. Use cautiously.
Oral anticoagulants: oral neomycin inhibits vitamin K–producing bacteria and may potentiate anticoagulant effect.
Other aminoglycosides, amphotericin B, cisplatin, methoxyflurane: increases nephrotoxicity. Use together cautiously.

NURSING CONSIDERATIONS
• Contraindicated in intestinal obstruction. Use cautiously in impaired renal function, ulcerative bowel lesions, and in elderly patients.
• The ototoxic and nephrotoxic properties of neomycin limit its usefulness. Limited absorption prevents substantial systemic effects.
• Nonabsorbable at recommended dosage. However, more than 4 g/day may be systemically absorbed and lead to nephrotoxicity.
• Weigh patient and obtain baseline renal function studies before therapy begins.
• Obtain specimen for culture and sensitivity tests before first dose. Therapy may begin pending test results.
• Watch for superinfection (fever or other signs of new infection).
• Monitor renal function (output, specific gravity, urinalysis, BUN and creatinine levels, and creatinine clearance). Notify doctor of signs of decreasing renal function.
• Patient should be well hydrated while taking drug to minimize chemical irritation of the renal tubules.
• Watch for respiratory depression in patients with renal disease, hypocalcemia, or neuromuscular diseases, such as myasthenia gravis.
• Evaluate hearing of patient with hepatic or renal disease before and during prolonged therapy. Notify doctor if patient complains of tinnitus, vertigo, or hearing loss. Onset of deafness may occur several weeks after drug is stopped.
• An adjunctive treatment of hepatic coma, neomycin is used to decrease ammonia-producing flora in the GI tract. During such treatment, decrease patient's dietary protein and assess neurologic status frequently.
• For preoperative disinfection, provide a low-residue diet and a cathartic immediately before oral administration of neomycin.

• Available in combination with polymyxin B as a urinary bladder irrigant.

---

netilmicin sulfate
Netromycin

Pregnancy Risk Category: C

HOW SUPPLIED
Injection: 10 mg/ml, 25 mg/ml, 100 mg/ml

MECHANISM OF ACTION
Inhibits protein synthesis by binding directly to the 30S ribosomal subunit. Generally bactericidal.

INDICATIONS & DOSAGE
Serious infections caused by sensitive Pseudomonas aeruginosa, Escherichia coli, Proteus, Klebsiella, Serratia, Enterobacter, Citrobacter, Staphylococcus—
Adults and children over 12 years: 3 to 6.5 mg/kg/day by I.M. injection or I.V. infusion. May be given q 12 hours to treat serious urinary tract infections and q 8 to 12 hours to treat serious systemic infections.
Infants and children 6 weeks to 12 years: 5.5 to 8 mg/kg/day by I.M. injection or I.V. infusion given either as 1.8 to 2.7 mg/kg q 8 hours or as 2.7 to 4 mg/kg q 12 hours.
Neonates under 6 weeks: 4 to 6.5 mg/kg/day by I.M. injection or I.V. infusion given as 2 to 3.25 mg/kg q 12 hours.
Patients with impaired renal function: Initial dose is the same as for patients with normal renal function. Subsequent doses and frequency are determined by renal function studies and serum concentration of netilmicin.

ADVERSE REACTIONS
CNS: headache, lethargy, *neuromuscular blockade*.
EENT: *ototoxicity (tinnitus, vertigo, hearing loss)*.

GU: *nephrotoxicity (cells or casts in the urine; oliguria; proteinuria; decreased creatinine clearance; increased BUN, nonprotein nitrogen, and serum creatinine levels).*
Other: hypersensitivity reactions.

INTERACTIONS
Cephalothin: increases nephrotoxicity. Use together cautiously.
Dimenhydrinate: may mask symptoms of ototoxicity. Use with caution.
General anesthetics, neuromuscular blocking agents: may potentiate neuromuscular blockade.
I.V. loop diuretics (e.g. furosemide): increase ototoxicity. Use cautiously.
Other aminoglycosides, amphotericin B, cisplatin, methoxyflurane: increases nephrotoxicity. Use together cautiously.
Parenteral penicillins (e.g., carbenicillin, ticarcillin): netilmicin inactivation. Don't mix together in I.V.

NURSING CONSIDERATIONS
• Use cautiously in impaired renal function and in neonates, infants, and elderly patients.
• Obtain specimen for culture and sensitivity tests before first dose. Therapy may begin pending test results.
• Weigh patient and obtain baseline renal function studies before therapy begins.
• Monitor renal function (output, specific gravity, urinalysis, BUN and creatinine levels, and creatinine clearance). Notify doctor of signs of decreasing renal function.
• Patient should be well hydrated while taking drug to minimize chemical irritation of the renal tubules.
• After completing I.V. infusion, flush the line with normal saline solution or dextrose 5% in water.
• Evaluate patient's hearing before and during therapy. Notify doctor if patient complains of tinnitus, vertigo, or hearing loss.

• Watch for superinfection (continued fever and other signs of new infections, especially of upper respiratory tract).
• Usual duration of therapy is 7 to 10 days. If no response in 3 to 5 days, therapy may be stopped and new specimens obtained for culture and sensitivity.
• Peak blood levels above 16 mcg/ml and trough levels (those drawn just before next dose) above 4 mcg/ml may be associated with higher incidence of toxicity.
• Draw blood for peak netilmicin level 1 hour after I.M. injection and 30 minutes to 1 hour after infusion ends; for trough levels, draw blood just before next dose. Don't draw blood in a heparinized tube because heparin is incompatible with aminoglycosides.
• Netromycin is the newest aminoglycoside. Some studies show that this drug is less ototoxic than other drugs in its class.

---

streptomycin sulfate
Pregnancy Risk Category: D

HOW SUPPLIED
Injection: 400 mg/ml, 500 mg/ml, 1-g vial, 5-g vial

MECHANISM OF ACTION
Inhibits protein synthesis by binding directly to the 30S ribosomal subunit. Generally bactericidal.

INDICATIONS & DOSAGE
Streptococcal endocarditis—
Adults: 10 mg/kg I.M. (maximum 0.5 g) q 12 hours for 2 weeks with penicillin.
Primary and adjunctive treatment in tuberculosis—
Adults: with normal renal function, 1 g I.M. daily for 2 to 3 months, then 1 g 2 or 3 times a week. Inject deeply into upper outer quadrant of buttocks.

Children: with normal renal function, 20 mg/kg daily in divided doses injected deeply into large muscle mass. Give concurrently with other antitubercular agents, but *not* with capreomycin, and continue until sputum specimen becomes negative.
Patients with impaired renal function: initial dose is same as for those with normal renal function. Subsequent doses and frequency determined by renal function study results.
Enterococcal endocarditis—
Adults: 1 g I.M. q 12 hours for 2 weeks, then 500 mg I.M. q 12 hours for 4 weeks with penicillin.
Tularemia—
Adults: 1 to 2 g I.M. daily in divided doses injected deep into upper outer quadrant of buttocks. Continue until patient is afebrile for 5 to 7 days.

ADVERSE REACTIONS
CNS: *neuromuscular blockade.*
EENT: *ototoxicity (tinnitus, vertigo, hearing loss).*
GU: some nephrotoxicity (not nearly as frequent as with other aminoglycosides).
Local: pain, irritation, and sterile abscesses at injection site.
Skin: *exfoliative dermatitis.*
Other: *hypersensitivity* (rash, fever, urticaria, and angioneurotic edema), headache, transient agranulocytosis.

INTERACTIONS
Cephalothin: increases nephrotoxicity. Use together cautiously.
Dimenhydrinate: may mask symptoms of streptomycin-induced ototoxicity. Use together cautiously.
General anesthetics, neuromuscular blocking agents: may potentiate neuromuscular blockade.
I.V. loop diuretics (e.g. furosemide): increase ototoxicity. Use cautiously.

NURSING CONSIDERATIONS
• Contraindicated in labyrinthine disease. Use cautiously in impaired renal function and in the elderly.
• Obtain specimen for culture and sensitivity tests before first dose except when treating tuberculosis. Therapy may begin pending test results.
• Patient should be well hydrated while taking drug to minimize chemical irritation of the renal tubules.
• Evaluate patient's hearing before, during, and 6 months after therapy. Notify doctor if patient complains of hearing loss, roaring noises, or fullness in ears.
• Watch for superinfection (continued fever and other signs of new infections).
• Protect hands when preparing. Drug is irritating.
• Endocarditis prophylaxis is recommended for all patients with rheumatic or congenital heart disease or with prosthetic heart valve. Patients should receive prophylactic antibiotics during GI or GU procedures or surgery.
• In primary treatment of tuberculosis, streptomycin is discontinued when sputum becomes negative.
• Draw blood for peak streptomycin level 1 to 2 hours after I.M. injection; for trough levels, draw blood just before next dose. Don't use a heparinized tube because heparin is incompatible with aminoglycosides.

---

tobramycin sulfate
Nebcin
Pregnancy Risk Category: D

HOW SUPPLIED
Injection: 40 mg/ml, 10 mg/ml (pediatric)

MECHANISM OF ACTION
Inhibits protein synthesis by binding directly to the 30S ribosomal subunit. Generally bactericidal.

Italicized adverse reactions are common or life-threatening.
*Liquid form contains alcohol.   **May contain tartrazine.

INDICATIONS & DOSAGE

Serious infections caused by sensitive strains of Escherichia coli, Proteus, Klebsiella, Enterobacter, Serratia, Staphylococcus aureus, Pseudomonas, Citrobacter, Providencia—
Adults and children with normal renal function: 3 mg/kg I.M. or I.V. daily divided q 8 hours. Up to 5 mg/kg I.M. or I.V. daily divided q 6 to 8 hours for life-threatening infections.
Neonates under 1 week: up to 4 mg/kg I.M. or I.V. daily divided q 12 hours. For I.V. use, dilute in 50 to 100 ml normal saline solution or dextrose 5% in water for adults and in less volume for children. Infuse over 20 to 60 minutes.
Patients with impaired renal function: initial dose is same as for those with normal renal function. Subsequent doses and frequency determined by renal function study results and serum concentrations of tobramycin.

ADVERSE REACTIONS

CNS: headache, lethargy, *neuromuscular blockade.*
EENT: *ototoxicity (tinnitus, vertigo, hearing loss).*
GU: *nephrotoxicity (cells or casts in the urine, oliguria, proteinuria, decreased creatinine clearance, increased BUN and serum creatinine levels).*
Other: hypersensitivity reactions.

INTERACTIONS

Cephalothin: increase nephrotoxicity. Use together cautiously.
Dimenhydrinate: may mask symptoms of ototoxicity. Use with caution.
General anesthetics, neuromuscular blocking agents: may potentiate neuromuscular blockade.
I.V. loop diuretics (e.g., furosemide): increase ototoxicity. Use cautiously.
Other aminoglycosides, amphotericin B, cisplatin, methoxyflurane: in-
creases nephrotoxicity. Use together cautiously.
Parenteral penicillins (e.g., carbenicillin and ticarcillin): tobramycin inactivation in vitro. Don't mix together in I.V.

NURSING CONSIDERATIONS

• Use cautiously in impaired renal function and in the elderly.
• Obtain specimen for culture and sensitivity tests before first dose. Therapy may begin pending test results.
• Weigh patient and obtain baseline renal function studies before starting therapy.
• Usual duration of therapy is 7 to 10 days.
• Monitor renal function (output, specific gravity, urinalysis, BUN and creatinine levels, and creatinine clearance). Notify doctor of signs of decreasing renal function.
• Patient should be well hydrated while taking drug to minimize chemical irritation of the renal tubules.
• Evaluate patient's hearing before and during therapy. Notify doctor if patient complains of tinnitus, vertigo, or hearing loss.
• Watch for superinfection (continued fever and other signs of new infections).
• Peak blood levels over 12 mcg/ml and trough levels above 2 mcg/ml may be associated with increased incidence of toxicity.
• Draw blood for peak tobramycin level 1 hour after I.M. injection and 30 minutes to 1 hour after infusion ends; draw blood for trough level just before next dose. Don't collect blood in a heparinized tube because heparin is incompatible with aminoglycosides.
• After I.V. infusion, flush line with normal saline solution or dextrose 5% in water.

---

†Available in Canada only. ‡Available in Australia only. ◊ Available OTC.

12

Penicillins

amdinocillin
amoxicillin/clavulanate
  potassium
amoxicillin trihydrate amoxycillin
  trihydrate)
ampicillin
ampicillin sodium
ampicillin trihydrate
ampicillin sodium/sulbactam
  sodium
azlocillin sodium
bacampicillin hydrochloride
carbenicillin disodium
carbenicillin indanyl sodium
cloxacillin sodium
cyclacillin
dicloxacillin sodium
methicillin sodium
mezlocillin sodium
nafcillin sodium
oxacillin sodium
penicillin G benzathine
penicillin G potassium
penicillin G procaine
penicillin G sodium
penicillin V
penicillin V potassium
piperacillin sodium
ticarcillin disodium
ticarcillin disodium/clavulanate
  potassium

COMBINATION PRODUCTS

AUGMENTIN, CLAVULIN†: amoxicillin
250 mg and clavulanate potassium
125 mg per tablet; amoxicillin 500 mg
and clavulanate potassium 125 mg per
tablet; amoxicillin 125 mg and potassium clavulanate 31.5 mg per 5 ml
oral suspension; amoxicillin 250 mg
and potassium clavulanate 31.5 mg
per 5 ml oral suspension; amoxicillin
125 mg and potassium clavulanate
31.5 mg per chewable tablet; amoxicillin 250 mg and potassium clavulanate 31.5 mg per chewable tablet.
POLYCILLIN-PRB: ampicillin trihydrate 3.5 g and probenecid 1g per bottle.
PRINCIPEN WITH PROBENECID: ampicillin trihydrate 3.5g and probenecid
1g per 9-capsule regimen.
TIMENTIN INJECTION: ticarcillin disodium 3 g and clavulanate potassium
100 mg per vial.
UNASYN INJECTION: ampicillin sodium 1 g and sulbactam sodium 500
mg per vial; ampicillin sodium 2 g
and sulbactam sodium 1 g per vial.

---

amdinocillin
Coactin

Pregnancy Risk Category: B

HOW SUPPLIED
Injection: 500-mg, 1,000-mg vials

MECHANISM OF ACTION
Although classified as a penicillin,
amdinocillin differs structurally and
in mechanism of action. It binds to a
minor penicillin-binding protein (PPB
2) and prevents the bacterial cell from
elongating. Generally considered bacteriostatic.

INDICATIONS & DOSAGE
*Treatment of complicated and uncom-
plicated urinary tract infections due to
susceptible strains of* Escherichia coli,
Klebsiella, *and* Enterobacter—

Italicized adverse reactions are common or life-threatening.
*Liquid form contains alcohol.   **May contain tartrazine.

Adults: 10 mg/kg I.M. or I.V. q 4 to 6 hours.

ADVERSE REACTIONS
Blood: *eosinophilia; thrombocytosis.*
CNS: dizziness.
GI: diarrhea, nausea, vomiting.
Local: thrombophlebitis.
Other: *hypersensitivity (erythematous maculopapular rash, urticaria, anaphylaxis),* overgrowth of nonsusceptible organisms.

INTERACTIONS
Probenecid: increases blood levels of amdinocillin and other penicillins. Probenecid may be used for this purpose.

NURSING CONSIDERATIONS
• Use cautiously in patients with other drug allergies, especially to cephalosporins (possible cross-allergenicity).
• Obtain specimen for culture and sensitivity tests before first dose. Therapy may begin pending test results.
• Watch for superinfection (fever or other signs of new infection).
• Before giving amdinocillin, ask patient about any allergic reactions to penicillin. However, a negative history doesn't rule out future penicillin allergy.
• Amdinocillin may act synergistically with other penicillins and cephalosporins and is frequently prescribed in combination with these drugs. May be a less toxic alternative to aminoglycosides.
• Dosage should be decreased in patients with moderate-to-severe renal failure.

amoxicillin/clavulanate potassium (amoxycillin/ clavulanate potassium)
Augmentin, Clavulin†

Pregnancy Risk Category: B

HOW SUPPLIED
Tablets (chewable): 125 mg amoxicillin trihydrate, 31.25 mg clavulanic acid; 250 mg amoxicillin trihydrate, 62.5 mg clavulanic acid
Tablets (film-coated): 250 mg amoxicillin trihydrate, 125 mg clavulanic acid; 500 mg amoxicillin trihydrate, 125 mg clavulanic acid
Oral suspension: 125 mg amoxicillin trihydrate and 31.25 mg clavulanic acid/5 ml (after reconstitution); 250 mg amoxicillin trihydrate and 62.5 mg clavulanic acid/5 ml (after reconstitution)

MECHANISM OF ACTION
An aminopenicillin that acts by preventing bacterial cell wall synthesis during active replication. Clavulanic acid increases amoxicillin effectiveness by inactivating beta lactamases, which destroy amoxicillin.

INDICATIONS & DOSAGE
Lower respiratory infections, otitis media, sinusitis, skin and skin structure infections, and urinary tract infections caused by susceptible strains of gram-positive and gram-negative organisms—
Adults: 250 mg (based on the amoxicillin component) P.O. q 8 hours. For more severe infections, 500 mg q 8 hours.
Children: 20 to 40 mg/kg (based on the amoxicillin component) P.O. daily given in divided doses q 8 hours.

ADVERSE REACTIONS
Blood: anemia, thrombocytopenia, thrombocytopenic purpura, eosinophilia, leukopenia.
GI: *nausea,* vomiting, *diarrhea.*

Other: *hypersensitivity (erythematous maculopapular rash, urticaria, anaphylaxis),* overgrowth of nonsusceptible organisms.

INTERACTIONS
Allopurinol: increased incidence of skin rash.
Probenecid: increases blood levels of amoxicillin and other penicillins. Probenecid may be used for this purpose.

NURSING CONSIDERATIONS
• Use cautiously in patients with other drug allergies, especially to cephalosporins (possible cross-allergenicity), and in mononucleosis (high incidence of maculopapular rash).
• Before giving, ask patient about any allergic reactions to penicillin. However, a negative history doesn't rule out future penicillin allergy.
• Obtain specimen for culture and sensitivity tests before first dose. Therapy may begin pending test results.
• Tell patient to take drug exactly as prescribed, even after he feels better. Patient should take entire quantity prescribed.
• Give with food to prevent GI distress.
• Incidence of diarrhea is greater than with amoxicillin alone.
• With large doses and prolonged therapy, bacterial and fungal superinfection may occur, especially in elderly, debilitated, or immunosuppressed patients. Close observation is essential.
• Both the "250" and "500" tablets contain the same amount of clavulanic acid (125 mg). Therefore, two "250" tablets are not equivalent to one "500" tablet.
• Particularly useful in clinical settings with high prevalence of amoxicillin-resistant organisms.
• Give amoxacillin/potassium clavulanate least 1 hour before bacteriostatic antibiotics.

amoxicillin trihydrate (amoxycillin trihydrate)
Alphamox‡, Amoxil‡, Apo-Amoxi†, Axicillin†, Cilamox‡, Ibiamox‡, Moxacin‡, Novamoxin†, Polymox†, Trimox, Utimox, Wymox
Pregnancy Risk Category: B

HOW SUPPLIED
Tablets (chewable): 125 mg, 250 mg
Capsules: 250 mg, 500 mg
Oral suspension: 50 mg/5 ml (pediatric drops), 125 mg/5 ml, 250 mg/5 ml (after reconstitution)

MECHANISM OF ACTION
An aminopenicillin that is bactericidal against microorganisms by inhibiting cell wall synthesis during active multiplication. Bacteria resist amoxicillin by producing penicillinases—enzymes that hydrolyze amoxicillin.

INDICATIONS & DOSAGE
Systemic infections, acute and chronic urinary tract infections caused by susceptible strains of gram-positive and gram-negative organisms—
Adults: 750 mg to 1.5 g P.O. daily in divided doses given q 8 hours.
Children: 20 to 40 mg/kg P.O. daily in divided doses given q 8 hours.
Uncomplicated gonorrhea—
Adults: 3 g P.O. with 1 g probenecid given as a single dose.
Uncomplicated urinary tract infections caused by susceptible organisms—
Adults: 3 g P.O. given as a single dose.

ADVERSE REACTIONS
Blood: anemia, thrombocytopenia, thrombocytopenic purpura, eosinophilia, leukopenia.
GI: *nausea,* vomiting, *diarrhea.*
Other: *hypersensitivity (erythematous maculopapular rash, urticaria, ana-*

Italicized adverse reactions are common or life-threatening.
*Liquid form contains alcohol.   **May contain tartrazine.

phylaxis), overgrowth of nonsusceptible organisms.

INTERACTIONS
Allopurinol: increased incidence of skin rash.
Probenecid: increases blood levels of amoxicillin and other penicillins. Probenecid may be used for this purpose.

NURSING CONSIDERATIONS
• Use cautiously in patients with other drug allergies, especially to cephalosporins (possible cross-allergenicity), and in mononucleosis—high incidence of maculopapular rash in those receiving amoxicillin.
• Obtain specimen for culture and sensitivity tests before first dose. Therapy may begin pending test results.
• Before giving amoxicillin, ask patient if he's had any allergic reactions to penicillin. However, a negative history of penicillin allergy is no guarantee against a future allergic reaction.
• Tell patient to take medication exactly as prescribed, even after he feels better. Entire quantity prescribed should be taken.
• Give with food to prevent GI distress.
• With large doses and prolonged therapy, bacterial and fungal superinfections may occur, especially in elderly, debilitated, or immunosuppressed patients. Close observation is essential.
• Warn patient never to use leftover amoxicillin for a new illness or to share it with family and friends.
• Trimox oral suspension may be stored at room temperature for up to 2 weeks. Be sure to check individual product labels for storage information.
• Tell patient to call the doctor if rash, fever, or chills develop. A rash is the most common allergic reaction. The rash is most common if the patient is also taking allopurinol.

• Amoxicillin and ampicillin have similar clinical applications.
• Urine glucose determinations may be false-positive with copper sulfate tests (Clinitest); glucose enzymatic tests (Clinistix, Tes-Tape) are not affected.
• Give amoxicillin at least 1 hour before bacteriostatic antibiotics.

ampicillin
Amcill, Ampicin†, Ampilean†, Apo-Ampi†, Novo Ampicillin†, Omnipen, Penbritin†, Principen

ampicillin sodium
Ampicyn Injection‡, Omnipen-N, Polycillin-N, Totacillin-N

ampicillin trihydrate
Amcill, Ampicyn Oral‡, D-Amp, Omnipen, Penamp-250, Penamp-500, Penbritin‡, Polycillin, Principen-250, Principen-500, Totacillin

Pregnancy Risk Category: B

HOW SUPPLIED
Capsules: 250 mg, 500 mg
Oral suspension: 100 mg/ml (pediatric drops), 125 mg/5 ml, 250 mg/5 ml, 500 mg/5 ml (after reconstitution)
Injection: 125 mg, 250 mg, 500 mg, 1 g, 2 g
Infusion: 500 mg, 1 g, 2 g
Pharmacy bulk package: 10-g vial

MECHANISM OF ACTION
An aminopenicillin that is bactericidal against microorganisms by inhibiting cell wall synthesis during active multiplication. Bacteria resist ampicillin by producing penicillinases—enzymes that hydrolyze ampicillin.

INDICATIONS & DOSAGE
Systemic infections, acute and chronic urinary tract infections caused by sus-

ceptible strains of gram-positive and gram-negative organisms—
Adults: 1 to 4 g P.O. daily, divided into doses given q 6 hours; 2 to 12 g I.M. or I.V. daily, divided into doses given q 4 to 6 hours.
Children: 50 to 100 mg/kg P.O. daily, divided into doses given q 6 hours; or 100 to 200 mg/kg I.M. or I.V. daily, divided into doses given q 6 hours.
Meningitis—
Adults: 8 to 14 g I.V. daily for 3 days, then I.M. divided q 3 to 4 hours.
Children: up to 300 mg/kg I.V. daily for 3 days, then I.M. divided q 4 hours.
Uncomplicated gonorrhea—
Adults: 3.5 g P.O. with 1 g probenecid given as a single dose.

ADVERSE REACTIONS
Blood: anemia, thrombocytopenia, thrombocytopenic purpura, eosinophilia, leukopenia.
GI: *nausea*, vomiting, *diarrhea*, glossitis, stomatitis.
Local: pain at injection site, vein irritation, thrombophlebitis.
Other: *hypersensitivity (erythematous maculopapular rash, urticaria, anaphylaxis), overgrowth of nonsusceptible organisms.*

INTERACTIONS
Allopurinol: increased incidence of skin rash.
Probenecid: increases blood levels of ampicillin and other penicillins. Probenecid may be used for this purpose.

NURSING CONSIDERATIONS
• Use cautiously in patients with other drug allergies, especially to cephalosporins (possible cross-allergenicity), and in mononucleosis—high incidence of maculopapular rash in those receiving ampicillin.
• Obtain specimen for culture and sensitivity tests before first dose.

Therapy may begin pending test results.
• Before giving ampicillin, ask patient if he's had any allergic reactions to penicillin. However, a negative history of penicillin allergy is no guarantee against a future allergic reaction.
• Tell patient to take medication exactly as prescribed, even after he feels better. Entire quantity prescribed should be taken.
• Tell the patient to call the doctor if rash, fever, or chills develop. A rash is the most common allergic reaction. Rash is most common if the patient is also taking allopurinol.
• When given orally, drug may cause GI disturbances. Food may interfere with absorption, so give 1 to 2 hours before meals or 2 to 3 hours after.
• Don't give I.M. or I.V. unless infection is severe or patient can't take oral dose.
• Dosage should be altered in patients with impaired renal functions.
• When giving I.V., mix with dextrose 5% in water or a saline solution. Don't mix with other drugs or solutions: they might be incompatible.
• Give I.V. intermittently to prevent vein irritation. Change site every 48 hours.
• With large doses or prolonged therapy, bacterial or fungal superinfections may occur, especially in elderly, debilitated, or immunosuppressed patients. Close observation is essential.
• Warn patient never to use leftover ampicillin for a new illness or to share it with family and friends.
• Initial dilution in vial is stable for 1 hour. Follow manufacturer's direction for stability data when ampicillin is further diluted for I.V. infusion.
• In pediatric meningitis, may be given concurrently with parenteral chloramphenicol for 24 hours pending cultures.
• Urine glucose determinations may be false-positive with copper sulfate tests (Clinitest); glucose enzymatic

---

Italicized adverse reactions are common or life-threatening.
*Liquid form contains alcohol.   **May contain tartrazine.

tests (Clinistix, Tes-Tape) are not affected.

• Give ampicillin at least 1 hour before bacteriostatic antibiotics.

---

ampicillin sodium/ sulbactam sodium
Unasyn

Pregnancy Risk Category: C

HOW SUPPLIED
Injection: vials and piggyback vials containing 1.5 g (1 g ampicillin sodium with 500 mg sulbactam sodium) and 3 g (2 g ampicillin sodium with 1 g sulbactam sodium)

MECHANISM OF ACTION
Ampicillin (an aminopenicillin) inhibits cell wall synthesis during active multiplication. Sulbactam inactivates bacterial beta-lactamase, the enzyme that inactivates ampicillin and provides bacterial resistance to it.

INDICATIONS & DOSAGE
Intraabdominal, gynecologic, and integumentary infections caused by susceptible strains of bacteria—
Adults: dosage expressed as total drug (each 1.5-g vial contains 1 g ampicillin sodium and 0.5 g sulbactam sodium): 1.5 to 3 g I.M. or I.V. q 6 hours. Maximum daily dose is 4 g sulbactam (12 g of the combined drugs).

ADVERSE REACTIONS
CNS: fatigue, malaise, headache, chills.
CV: edema, erythema.
GI: diarrhea, nausea, vomiting, flatulence, abdominal distention.
GU: dysuria, urine retention.
Local: pain at injection site, thrombophlebitis.
Other: rash, itching, candidiasis, *anaphylaxis.*

INTERACTIONS
Allopurinol: increased incidence of skin rash.
Probenecid: increased levels of ampicillin. Probenecid may be used for this purpose.

NURSING CONSIDERATIONS
• Use cautiously in patients with other drug allergies, especially to cephalosporins (possible cross-allergenicity), and in mononucleosis— high incidence of maculopapular rash in those receiving ampicillin.
• Obtain specimen for culture and sensitivity tests before first dose. Therapy may begin pending test results.
• Before giving ampicillin, ask patient if he's had any allergic reactions to penicillin. However, a negative history of penicillin allergy is no guarantee against a future allergic reaction.
• When preparing I.V. injection, reconstitute powder with any of the following diluents: normal saline solution, dextrose 5% in water, lactated Ringer's injection, ⅙ M sodium lactate, dextrose 5% and 0.45% saline injection, and 10% invert suger. Stability varies with diluent, temperature, and concentration of solution.
• After reconstitution, allow vials to stand for a few minutes to allow foam to dissipate. This will permit visual inspection of contents for particles.
• Give I.V. dose by slow injection (over 10 to 15 minutes), or dilute in 50 to 100 ml of a compatible diluent and infuse over 15 to 30 minutes.
• When administering I.M., give by deep injection. Drug may be reconstituted with sterile water for injection, or 0.5% or 2% lidocaine hydrochloride injection. Add 3.2 ml to a 1.5-g vial (or 6.4 ml to a 3-g vial) to yield a concentration of 375 mg/ml.
• Tell the patient to call the doctor if rash, fever, or chills develop. A rash is the most common allergic reaction.

- Dosage should be altered in patients with impaired renal functions.
- When giving I.V., mix with dextrose 5% in water or saline solution. Don't mix with other drugs or solutions: they might be incompatible.
- Give I.V. intermittently to prevent vein irritation. Change site every 48 hours.
- With large doses and prolonged therapy, bacterial and fungal superinfections may occur, especially in elderly, debilitated, or immunosuppressed patients. Close observation is essential.
- Urine glucose determinations may be false-positive with copper sulfate tests (Clinitest); glucose enzymatic tests (Clinistix, Tes-Tape) are not affected.
- Give ampicillin/sulbactam at least 1 hour before bacteriostatic antibiotics.

azlocillin sodium
Azlin, Securopen‡

Pregnancy Risk Category: B

HOW SUPPLIED
Injection: 2 g, 3 g, 4 g per vial

MECHANISM OF ACTION
An extended-spectrum penicillin that is bactericidal against microorganisms by inhibiting cell wall synthesis during active multiplication. Bacteria resist azlocillin by producing penicillinases—enzymes that hydrolyze azlocillin.

INDICATIONS & DOSAGE
Serious infections caused by susceptible strains of gram-negative organisms, including Pseudomonas aeruginosa—

Adults: 200 to 350 mg/kg daily I.V. given in four to six divided doses. Usual dose is 3 g q 4 hours (18 g daily). Maximum daily dosage is 24 g. May be administered by I.V. intermittent infusion or by direct slow I.V. injection.

Children with acute exacerbation of cystic fibrosis: 75 mg/kg q 4 hours (450 mg/kg daily). Maximum daily dosage is 24 g.

Azlocillin should not be used in neonates.

ADVERSE REACTIONS
Blood: *bleeding with high doses,* neutropenia, eosinophilia, leukopenia, *thrombocytopenia.*
CNS: neuromuscular irritability, headache, dizziness.
GI: nausea, diarrhea.
Metabolic: *hypokalemia.*
Local: pain at injection site, vein irritation, phlebitis.
Other: *hypersensitivity (edema, fever, chills, rash, pruritus, urticaria, anaphylaxis), overgrowth of nonsusceptible organisms.*

INTERACTIONS
Aminoglycoside antibiotics (e.g., gentamicin, tobramycin): chemically incompatible. Don't mix together in I.V. solution.
Probenecid: increased levels of azlocillin. Probenecid may be used for this purpose.

NURSING CONSIDERATIONS
- Use cautiously in patients hypersensitive to drugs, especially to cephalosporins (possible cross-allergenicity), and in bleeding tendencies, uremia, or hypokalemia.
- Obtain specimen for culture and sensitivity tests before first dose. Therapy may begin pending test results.
- Before giving azlocillin, ask patient if he's had allergic reactions to penicillin. A negative history of penicillin allergy, however, is no guarantee against future allergic reactions.
- Dosage should be altered in patients with impaired renal functions.
- Check CBC and platelets fre-

Italicized adverse reactions are common or life-threatening.
*Liquid form contains alcohol.   **May contain tartrazine.

quently. Drug may cause thrombocytopenia.
- Monitor serum potassium level.
- Patient with high serum level of azlocillin may have seizures. Institute seizure precautions.
- When giving I.V., mix with dextrose 5% in water or other suitable I.V. fluids.
- Give I.V. intermittently to prevent vein irritation. Change site every 48 hours.
- Rapid administration may cause chest discomfort. Don't infuse over a period of less than 5 minutes.
- Almost always used with another antibiotic, such as gentamicin.
- With large doses and prolonged therapy, bacterial and fungal superinfections may occur, especially in elderly, debilitated, or immunosuppressed patients. Monitor patient closely.
- Azlocillin is less likely to cause hypokalemia than similar antibiotics, such as carbenicillin and ticarcillin.
- Drug may be better suited to patients on salt-free diets than carbenicillin and ticarcillin (contains 2.17 mEq Na^+/g of azlocillin).
- Give azlocillin at least 1 hour before bacteriostatic antibiotics.

---

bacampicillin hydrochloride
Penglobe†, Spectrobid

Pregnancy Risk Category: B

HOW SUPPLIED
Tablets: 400 mg
Oral suspension: 125 mg/5 ml (after reconstitution)

MECHANISM OF ACTION
An aminopenicillin that is converted to ampicillin in vivo, each mg of bacampicillin yields 623 to 727 mcg ampicillin. It is bactericidal against microorganisms by inhibiting cell wall synthesis during active multiplication. Bacteria resist bacampicillin by producing penicillinases—enzymes that hydrolyze its active form (ampicillin).

INDICATIONS & DOSAGE
Upper and lower respiratory tract infections due to streptococci, pneumococci, staphylococci, and Hemophilus influenzae; urinary tract infections due to Escherichia coli, Proteus mirabilis, and Streptococcus faecalis; skin infections due to streptococci and susceptible staphylococci—
Adults and children weighing more than 25 kg: 400 to 800 mg P.O. q 12 hours.
Gonorrhea—
Usual dosage is 1.6 g plus 1 g probenecid given as a single dose.
   Not recommended for children under 25 kg.

ADVERSE REACTIONS
Blood: anemia, thrombocytopenia, thrombocytopenic purpura, eosinophilia, leukopenia.
GI: *nausea,* vomiting, *diarrhea,* glossitis, stomatitis.
Other: *hypersensitivity (erythematous maculopapular rash, urticaria, anaphylaxis),* overgrowth of nonsusceptible organisms.

INTERACTIONS
Allopurinol: increased incidence of skin rash.
Probenecid: increases blood levels of bacampicillin or other penicillins. Probenecid may be used for this purpose.

NURSING CONSIDERATIONS
- Use cautiously in patients with other drug allergies, especially to cephalosporins (possible cross-allergenicity), and in mononucleosis. This drug, like ampicillin, is linked to a high incidence of maculopapular rash.
- Obtain specimen for culture and sensitivity tests before first dose.

Therapy may begin pending test results.

• Before giving bacampicillin, ask patient if he's had any previous allergic reactions to penicillin. However, a negative history of penicillin allergy is no guarantee against a future allergic reaction.

• Bacampicillin is especially formulated to produce high blood levels of antibiotic when administered twice daily.

• Diarrhea may occur less frequently with bacampicillin than with ampicillin.

• Tell patient to take medication even after he feels better. Entire quantity prescribed should be taken.

• Tell patient to call the doctor if rash, fever, or chills develop. A rash is the most common allergic reaction.

• With large doses and prolonged therapy, bacterial or fungal superinfections may occur, especially in elderly, debilitated, or immunosuppressed patients. Monitor closely.

• Warn patient never to use leftover bacampicillin for a new illness or to share it with family and friends.

• Unlike ampicillin, bacampicillin tablets may be taken with meals without fear of diminished drug absorption. Give with food to prevent GI distress. However, bacampicillin suspension should be taken on an empty stomach.

• Administer bacampicillin at least 1 hour before bacteriostatic antibiotics.

---

carbenicillin disodium
Carbapen‡, Geopen, Pyopen

Pregnancy Risk Category: B

HOW SUPPLIED
Injection: 1 g, 2 g, 5 g per vial
I.V. infusion piggyback: 2 g, 5 g, 10 g
Pharmacy bulk package: 10 g, 20 g, 30 g per vial

MECHANISM OF ACTION
Bactericidal against microorganisms by inhibiting cell wall synthesis during active multiplication. Bacteria resist carbenicillin by producing penicillinases—enzymes that hydrolyze its active form.

INDICATIONS & DOSAGE
Systemic infections caused by susceptible strains of gram-positive and especially gram-negative organisms (including Proteus, Pseudomonas aeruginosa)—
Adults: 30 to 40 g daily I.V. infusion, divided into doses given q 4 to 6 hours.
Children: 300 to 500 mg/kg daily I.V. infusion, divided into doses given q 4 to 6 hours.
Urinary tract infections—
Adults: 200 mg/kg daily I.M. or I.V. infusion, divided into doses given q 4 to 6 hours.
Children: 50 to 200 mg/kg daily I.M. or I.V. infusion, divided into doses given q 4 to 6 hours.

ADVERSE REACTIONS
Blood: *bleeding with high doses,* neutropenia, eosinophilia, leukopenia, *thrombocytopenia.*
CNS: neuromuscular irritability, seizures.
GI: nausea, vomiting.
Metabolic: *hypokalemia.*
Local: pain at injection site, vein irritation, phlebitis.
Other: *hypersensitivity (edema, fever, chills, rash, pruritus, urticaria, anaphylaxis),* overgrowth of nonsusceptible organisms.

INTERACTIONS
Aminoglycoside antibiotics (e.g., gentamicin, tobramycin): chemically incompatible. Don't mix together in I.V.
Probenecid: increases blood levels of carbenicillin and other penicillins. Probenecid may be used for this purpose.

Italicized adverse reactions are common or life-threatening.
*Liquid form contains alcohol.   **May contain tartrazine.

NURSING CONSIDERATIONS
• Use cautiously in patients with other drug allergies, especially to cephalosporins (possible cross-allergenicity), and in bleeding tendencies, uremia, and hypokalemia. Use cautiously in patients on sodium-restricted diets; contains 4.7 mEq sodium/g.
• Obtain specimen for culture and sensitivity tests before first dose. Therapy may begin pending test results.
• Before giving carbenicillin, ask patient if he's had any allergic reactions to penicillin. However, a negative history of penicillin allergy is no guarantee against a future allergic reaction.
• Dosage should be altered in patients with impaired renal function. Patients with impaired renal function are susceptible to nephrotoxicity. Monitor intake/output.
• Check CBC and platelets frequently. Drug may cause thrombocytopenia.
• Monitor serum potassium level. Patients may develop hypokalemia due to large amount of sodium in the preparation.
• If patient has high blood level of this drug, he may have seizures. Institute seizure precautions.
• When giving I.V., mix with dextrose 5% in water or other suitable I.V. fluids.
• Give I.V. intermittently to prevent vein irritation. Change site every 48 hours.
• Almost always used with another antibiotic, such as gentamicin.
• With large doses and prolonged therapy, bacterial and fungal superinfections may occur, especially in elderly, debilitated, or immunosuppressed patients. Close observation is essential.
• Give carbenicillin at least 1 hour before bacteriostatic antibiotics.

carbenicillin indanyl sodium
Geocillin, Geopen Oral†
Pregnancy Risk Category: B

HOW SUPPLIED
Tablets: 382 mg

MECHANISM OF ACTION
Bactericidal against microorganisms by inhibiting cell wall synthesis during active multiplication. Bacteria resist carbenicillin by producing penicillinases—enzymes that hydrolyze its active form.

INDICATIONS & DOSAGE
Urinary tract infection and prostatitis caused by susceptible strains of gram-negative organisms—
Adults: 382 to 764 mg P.O. q.i.d.
    Not recommended for children.

ADVERSE REACTIONS
Blood: leukopenia, neutropenia, eosinophilia, anemia, thrombocytopenia.
GI: *nausea,* vomiting, *diarrhea, flatulence, abdominal cramps, unpleasant taste.*
Other: *hypersensitivity (rash, chills, fever, urticaria, pruritus, anaphylaxis),* overgrowth of nonsusceptible organisms.

INTERACTIONS
None significant.

NURSING CONSIDERATIONS
• Use cautiously in patients with other drug allergies, especially to cephalosporins (possible cross-allergenicity).
• Obtain specimen for culture and sensitivity tests before first dose. Therapy may begin pending test results.
• Before giving carbenicillin, ask patient if he's had any allergic reactions to penicillin. However, a negative his-

tory of penicillin allergy is no guarantee against a future allergic reaction.
• Tell patient to take medication exactly as prescribed, even after he feels better. Entire quantity prescribed should be taken.
• Tell patient to call the doctor if he develops rash, fever, or chills. A rash is the most common allergic reaction.
• When given orally, drug may cause GI disturbances. Food may interfere with absorption, so give 1 to 2 hours before meals or 2 to 3 hours after.
• With large doses or prolonged therapy, bacterial or fungal superinfections may occur, especially in elderly, debilitated, or immunosuppressed patients. Close observation is essential.
• Warn patient never to use leftover carbenicillin for a new illness or to share it with family and friends.
• Use only in patients whose creatinine clearance is 10 ml/minute or more.
• Excellent treatment for *Pseudomonas* urinary tract infections in ambulatory patients.
• May be useful in treatment of cystitis, but not pyelonephritis.
• Not effective for any systemic infection because blood levels are nil.

---

cloxacillin sodium
Alclox‡, Apo-Cloxi†, Austrastaph‡, Bactopen†, Cloxapen, Novocloxin†, Orbenin†, Orbenin Injection‡, Tegopen

Pregnancy Risk Category: B

HOW SUPPLIED
Capsules: 250 mg, 500 mg
Oral solution: 125 mg/5 ml (after reconstitution)
Injection: 500 mg/vial‡

MECHANISM OF ACTION
Bactericidal against microorganisms by inhibiting cell wall synthesis during active multiplication. Bacteria resist penicillins by producing penicilli-

nases—enzymes that convert penicillins to inactive penicilloic acis. Cloxacillin resists these enzymes.

INDICATIONS & DOSAGE
Systemic infections caused by penicillinase-producing staphylococci—
Adults: 2 to 4 g P.O. daily, divided into doses given q 6 hours.
Children: 50 to 100 mg/kg P.O. daily, divided into doses given q 6 hours.

ADVERSE REACTIONS
Blood: eosinophilia.
GI: *nausea,* vomiting, *epigastric distress, diarrhea.*
Other: *hypersensitivity (rash, urticaria, chills, fever, sneezing, wheezing, anaphylaxis),* intrahepatic cholestasis, overgrowth of nonsusceptible organisms.

INTERACTIONS
Probenecid: increases blood levels of cloxacillin and other penicillins. Probenecid may be used for this purpose.

NURSING CONSIDERATIONS
• Use with caution in patients with other drug allergies, especially to cephalosporins (possible cross-allergenicity).
• Obtain specimen for culture and sensitivity tests before first dose. Therapy may begin pending test results.
• Before giving cloxacillin, ask patient if he's had any allergic reactions to penicillin. However, a negative history of penicillin allergy is no guarantee against a future allergic reaction.
• Tell patient to take medication exactly as prescribed, even if he feels better. Entire quantity prescribed should be taken.
• Tell patient to call the doctor if rash, fever, or chills develop. A rash is the most common allergic reaction.
• When given orally, drug may cause GI disturbances. Food may interfere

---

Italicized adverse reactions are common or life-threatening.
*Liquid form contains alcohol.   **May contain tartrazine.

with absorption, so give 1 to 2 hours before meals or 2 to 3 hours after.
- Patient should take each dose with a full glass of water, not fruit juice or carbonated beverage, because acid will inactivate the drug.
- With large doses and prolonged therapy, bacterial and fungal superinfections may occur, especially in the elderly, debilitated, or immunosuppressed patients. Close observation is essential.
- Warn patient never to use leftover cloxacillin for a new illness or to share it with family and friends.
- Give cloxacillin at least 1 hour before bacteriostatic antibiotics.

cyclacillin
Cyclapen-W

Pregnancy Risk Category: B

HOW SUPPLIED
Tablets: 250 mg, 500 mg
Oral suspension: 125 mg/5 ml, 250 mg/5 ml (after reconstitution)

MECHANISM OF ACTION
Bactericidal against microorganisms by inhibiting cell wall synthesis during active multiplication. Bacteria resist cyclacillin by producing penicillinases—enzymes that hydrolyze cyclacillin to an inactive form.

INDICATIONS & DOSAGE
Systemic and urinary tract infections caused by susceptible strains of gram-positive and gram-negative organisms—
Adults: 250 to 500 mg P.O. q.i.d. in equally spaced doses.
Children: 50 to 100 mg/kg P.O. daily t.i.d. in equally divided doses.

ADVERSE REACTIONS
Blood: anemia, thrombocytopenia, thrombocytopenic purpura, leukopenia, neutropenia, eosinophilia.
GI: *nausea,* vomiting, diarrhea.

Other: *hypersensitivity (edema, fever, chills, rash, pruritus, urticaria, anaphylaxis),* overgrowth of nonsusceptible organisms.

INTERACTIONS
Probenecid: increases blood levels of cyclacillin. Probenecid may be used for this purpose.

NURSING CONSIDERATIONS
- Contraindicated in patients allergic to other penicillins.
- Obtain specimen for culture and sensitivity tests before first dose. Therapy may begin pending test results.
- Before giving cyclacillin, ask patient if he's had any allergic reactions to penicillin. However, a negative history of penicillin allergy is no guarantee against a future allergic reaction.
- Tell patient he must take all medication exactly as prescribed, for as long as ordered, even after he feels better.
- Patients with renal insufficiency should receive less drug in accordance with their creatinine clearance level.
- With large doses and prolonged therapy, bacterial and fungal superinfections may occur, especially in elderly, debilitated, or immunosuppressed patients. Close observation is essential.
- Warn patient never to use leftover cyclacillin for a new illness or to share it with family and friends.
- Tell patient to call the doctor if he develops rash, fever, or chills. A rash is the most common allergic reaction.
- Studies show that cyclacillin is as effective as amoxicillin in treating acute otitis media and causes less diarrhea.
- Give cyclacillin at least 1 hour before bacteriostatic antibiotics.

dicloxacillin sodium
Dycill, Dynapen, Pathocil

Pregnancy Risk Category: B

HOW SUPPLIED
Capsules: 125 mg, 250 mg, 500 mg
Oral suspension: 62.5 mg/5 ml (after reconstitution)

MECHANISM OF ACTION
Bactericidal against microorganisms by inhibiting cell wall synthesis during active multiplication. Bacteria resist penicillins by producing penicillinases—enzymes that convert penicillins to inactive penicilloic acid. Dicloxacillin resists these enzymes.

INDICATIONS & DOSAGE
Systemic infections caused by penicillinase-producing staphylococci—
Adults: 1 to 2 g daily P.O., divided into doses given q 6 hours.
Children: 25 to 50 mg/kg P.O. daily, divided into doses given q 6 hours.

ADVERSE REACTIONS
Blood: eosinophilia.
CNS: neuromuscular irritability, seizures.
GI: *nausea*, vomiting, *epigastric distress*, flatulence, *diarrhea*.
Other: *hypersensitivity (pruritus, urticaria, rash, anaphylaxis)*, overgrowth of nonsusceptible organisms.

INTERACTIONS
Probenecid: increases blood levels of dicloxacillin and other penicillins. Probenecid may be used for this purpose.

NURSING CONSIDERATIONS
• Use cautiously in patients allergic to cephalosporins (possible cross-allergenicity).
• Obtain specimen for culture and sensitivity tests before first dose. Therapy may begin pending test results.
• Before giving dicloxacillin, ask patient if he's had any allergic reactions to penicillin. However, a negative history of penicillin allergy is no guarantee against a future allergic reaction.
• Tell patient to take medication exactly as prescribed, even if he feels better. Entire quantity prescribed should be taken.
• Tell patient to call the doctor if rash, fever, or chills develop. A rash is the most common allergic reaction.
• Drug may cause GI disturbances. Food may interfere with absorption, so give 1 to 2 hours before meals or 2 to 3 hours after.
• With large doses and prolonged therapy, bacterial and fungal superinfections may occur, especially in elderly, debilitated, or immunosuppressed patients. Close observation is essential.
• Periodic assessments of renal, hepatic, and hematopoietic function should be made when therapy is prolonged.
• Warn patient never to use leftover dicloxacillin for a new illness or to share it with family and friends.
• Give dicloxacillin at least 1 hour before bacteriostatic antibiotics.

methicillin sodium
Metin‡, Staphcillin

Pregnancy Risk Category: B

HOW SUPPLIED
Injection: 1 g, 4 g, 6 g
I.V. infusion piggyback: 1 g, 4 g
Pharmacy bulk package: 10 g

MECHANISM OF ACTION
Bactericidal against microorganisms by inhibiting cell wall synthesis during active multiplication. Bacteria resist penicillins by producing penicillinases—enzymes that convert penicillins to inactive penicilloic acids. Methicillin resists these enzymes.

INDICATIONS & DOSAGE

Systemic infections caused by penicillinase-producing staphylococci—
Adults: 4 to 12 g I.M. or I.V. daily, divided into doses given q 4 to 6 hours.
Children: 100 to 200 mg/kg I.M. or I.V. daily, divided into doses given q 4 to 6 hours.

ADVERSE REACTIONS

Blood: *agranulocytosis, eosinophilia,* hemolytic anemia, transient neutropenia.
CNS: neuropathy, seizures with high doses.
GI: glossitis, stomatitis.
GU: interstitial nephritis.
Local: *vein irritation, thrombophlebitis.*
Other: *hypersensitivity (chills, fever, edema, rash, urticaria, anaphylaxis),* overgrowth of nonsusceptible organisms.

INTERACTIONS

Probenecid: increases blood levels of methicillin and other penicillins. Probenecid may be used for this purpose.

NURSING CONSIDERATIONS

• Use cautiously in patients with other drug allergies, especially to cephalosporins (possible cross-allergenicity), and in infants.
• Obtain specimen for culture and sensitivity tests before first dose. Therapy may begin pending test results.
• Methicillin-resistant strains of Staphylococci should be treated with vancomycin.
• Before giving methicillin, ask patient if he's had any allergic reactions to penicillin. However, a negative history of penicillin allergy is no guarantee against a future allergic reaction.
• If ordered 4 times a day, be sure to give every 6 hours—even during the night.
• Closely monitor renal function. Urinalysis should be done frequently to detect interstitial nephritis.
• If patient has high blood level of this drug, he may have seizures. Institute seizure precautions.
• When giving I.V., mix with a normal saline solution. Don't mix with others because methicillin may be inactivated. Initial dilution must be made with sterile water for injection.
• Give I.V. intermittently to prevent vein irritation. Change site every 48 hours.
• With large doses and prolonged therapy, bacterial and fungal superinfections may occur, especially in elderly, debilitated, or immunosuppressed patients. Close observation is essential.
• Periodic assessment of hepatic, renal, and hematopoietic function is required during prolonged therapy.
• Give methicillin at least 1 hour before bacteriostatic antibiotics.

---

mezlocillin sodium
Mezlin

Pregnancy Risk Category: B

HOW SUPPLIED
Injection: 1 g, 2 g, 3 g, 4 g

MECHANISM OF ACTION
Bactericidal against microorganisms by inhibiting cell wall synthesis during active multiplication. Bacteria resist mezlocillin by producing penicillinases—enzymes that hydrolyze mezlocillin.

INDICATIONS & DOSAGE
Systemic infections caused by susceptible strains of gram-positive and especially gram-negative organisms (including Proteus, Pseudomonas aeruginosa)—
Adults: 200 to 300 mg/kg daily I.V. or I.M. given in 4 to 6 divided doses. Usual dose is 3 g q 4 hours or 4 g q 6

hours. For very serious infections, up to 24 g daily may be administered.
Children to age 12: 50 mg/kg q 4 hours by I.V. infusion or direct I.V. injection.

ADVERSE REACTIONS
Blood: *bleeding with high doses,* neutropenia, eosinophilia, leukopenia, *thrombocytopenia.*
CNS: neuromuscular irritability.
GI: nausea, diarrhea.
Metabolic: *hypokalemia.*
Local: pain at injection site, vein irritation, phlebitis.
Other: *hypersensitivity (edema, fever, chills, rash, pruritus, urticaria, anaphylaxis), overgrowth of nonsusceptible organisms.*

INTERACTIONS
Aminoglycoside antibiotics (e.g., gentamicin, tobramycin): chemically incompatible. Don't mix together in I.V. solution. Give 1 hour apart, especially in patients with renal insufficiency.
Probenecid: increases blood levels of mezlocillin. Probenecid may be used for this purpose.

NURSING CONSIDERATIONS
● Use cautiously in patients hypersensitive to drugs, especially to cephalosporins (possible cross-hypersensitivity), and in bleeding tendencies, uremia, and hypokalemia.
● Obtain specimen for culture and sensitivity tests before first dose. Therapy may begin pending test results.
● Before giving mezlocillin, ask patient if he's had any allergic reactions to penicillin. A negative history of penicillin allergy, however, is no guarantee against future allergic reaction.
● Dosage should be altered in patients with impaired renal function.
● Check CBC and platelets frequently. Drug may cause thrombocytopenia.

● Monitor serum potassium level.
● Patient with high serum level of this drug may have seizures. Institute seizure precautions.
● When giving I.V., mix with dextrose 5% in water or other suitable I.V. fluids.
● Give I.V. intermittently to prevent vein irritation. Change site every 48 hours.
● Almost always used with another antibiotic, such as gentamicin.
● With large doses and prolonged therapy, bacterial and fungal superinfections may occur, especially in elderly, debilitated, or immunosuppressed patients. Monitor patient closely.
● Compared with similar antibiotics, such as carbenicillin and ticarcillin, mezlocillin is less likely to cause hypokalemia.
● Drug may be better suited to patients on salt-free diets than carbenicillin and ticarcillin (contains 1.85 mEq Na/g of mezlocillin).
● Give mezlocillin at least 1 hour before bacteriostatic antibiotics.

nafcillin sodium
Nafcil, Nallpen, Unipen
Pregnancy Risk Category: B

HOW SUPPLIED
Tablets: 500 mg
Capsules: 250 mg
Oral solution: 250 mg/5 ml (after reconstitution)
Injection: 500 mg, 1 g, 2 g
I.V. infusion piggyback: 1 g, 1.5 g, 2 g, 4 g
Pharmacy bulk package: 10 g

MECHANISM OF ACTION
Bactericidal against microorganisms by inhibiting cell wall synthesis during active multiplication. Bacteria resist nafcillin by producing penicillinases—enzymes that hydrolyze nafcillin.

Italicized adverse reactions are common or life-threatening.
*Liquid form contains alcohol.   **May contain tartrazine.

INDICATIONS & DOSAGE
Systemic infections caused by penicillinase-producing staphylococci—
Adults: 2 to 4 g P.O. daily, divided into doses given q 6 hours; 2 to 12 g I.M. or I.V. daily, divided into doses given q 4 to 6 hours.
Children: 50 to 100 mg/kg P.O. daily, divided into doses given q 4 to 6 hours; or 100 to 200 mg/kg I.M. or I.V. daily, divided into doses given q 4 to 6 hours.

ADVERSE REACTIONS
Blood: transient leukopenia, neutropenia, granulocytopenia, thrombocytopenia with high doses.
GI: *nausea,* vomiting, diarrhea.
Local: *vein irritation, thrombophlebitis.*
Other: *hypersensitivity (chills, fever, rash, pruritus, urticaria, anaphylaxis).*

INTERACTIONS
None significant.

NURSING CONSIDERATIONS
• Use cautiously in patients with other drug allergies, especially to cephalosporins (possible cross-allergenicity), and in GI distress.
• Obtain specimen for culture and sensitivity tests before first dose. Therapy may begin pending test results.
• Before giving nafcillin, ask patient if he's had any allergic reactions to penicillin. However, a negative history of penicillin allergy is no guarantee against a future allergic reaction.
• Tell patient to take medication exactly as prescribed, even if he feels better. Entire quantity prescribed should be taken.
• Tell patient to call the doctor if rash, fever, or chills develop. A rash is the most common allergic reaction.
• When given orally, drug may cause GI disturbances. Food may interfere

with absorption, so give 1 to 2 hours before meals or 2 to 3 hours after.
• When giving I.V., mix with dextrose 5% in water or a saline solution.
• Give I.V. intermittently to prevent vein irritation. Change site every 48 hours.
• With large doses and prolonged therapy, bacterial and fungal superinfections may occur, especially in elderly, debilitated, or immunosuppressed patients. Close observation is essential.
• Give nafcillin at least 1 hour before bacteriostatic antibiotics.

oxacillin sodium
Bactocill, Prostaphlin

Pregnancy Risk Category: B

HOW SUPPLIED
Capsules: 250 mg, 500 mg
Oral solution: 250 mg/5 ml (after reconstitution)
Injection: 250 mg, 500 mg, 1 g, 2 g, 4 g, 10 g
I.V. infusion: 1 g, 2 g, 4 g
Pharmacy bulk package: 4 g, 10 g

MECHANISM OF ACTION
Bactericidal against microorganisms by inhibiting cell wall synthesis during active multiplication. Bacteria resist penicillins by producing penicillinases—enzymes that convert penicillins to inactive penicilloic acids. Oxacillin resists these enzymes.

INDICATIONS & DOSAGE
Systemic infections caused by penicillinase-producing staphylococci—
Adults: 2 to 4 g P.O. daily, divided into doses given q 6 hours; 2 to 12 g I.M. or I.V. daily, divided into doses given q 4 to 6 hours.
Children: 50 to 100 mg/kg P.O. daily, divided into doses given q 6 hours; 100 to 200 mg/kg I.M. or I.V. daily, divided into doses given q 4 to 6 hours.

ADVERSE REACTIONS
Blood: granulocytopenia, thrombocytopenia, eosinophilia, hemolytic anemia, transient neutropenia.
CNS: neuropathy, neuromuscular irritability, seizures.
GI: oral lesions.
GU: interstitial nephritis, transient hematuria, proteinuria.
Hepatic: hepatitis, elevated enzymes.
Local: *thrombophlebitis.*
Other: *hypersensitivity (fever, chills, rash, urticaria, anaphylaxis),* overgrowth of nonsusceptible organisms.

INTERACTIONS
Probenecid: increases blood levels of oxacillin and other penicillins. Probenecid may be used for this purpose.

NURSING CONSIDERATIONS
• Use cautiously in patients with other drug allergies, especially to cephalosporins (possible cross-allergenicity), in premature newborns, and in infants.
• Obtain specimen for culture and sensitivity tests before first dose. Therapy may begin pending test results.
• Before giving oxacillin, ask patient if he's had any allergic reactions to penicillin. However, a negative history of penicillin allergy is no guarantee against a future allergic reaction.
• Tell the patient to take medication exactly as prescribed, even if he feels better. The entire quantity prescribed should be taken.
• Tell patient to call the doctor if rash, fever, or chills develop. A rash is the most common allergic reaction.
• When given orally, drug may cause GI disturbances. Food may interfere with absorption, so give 1 to 2 hours before meals or 2 to 3 hours after.
• Don't give I.M. or I.V. unless infection is severe or patient can't take oral dose.
• Periodic liver function studies are

indicated; watch for elevated AST (SGOT) and ALT (SGPT).
• When giving I.V., mix with dextrose 5% in water or a saline solution.
• Give I.V. intermittently to prevent vein irritation. Change site every 48 hours.
• With large doses and prolonged therapy, bacterial and fungal superinfections may occur, especially in elderly, debilitated, or immunosuppressed patients. Close observation is essential.
• Give oxacillin at least 1 hour before bacteriostatic antibiotics.

penicillin G benzathine (benzylpenicillin benzathine)
Bicillin L-A, Megacillin
Pregnancy Risk Category: B

HOW SUPPLIED
Tablets: 200,000 units
Injection: 300,000 units/ml, 600,000 units/ml

MECHANISM OF ACTION
Bactericidal against microorganisms by inhibiting cell wall synthesis during active multiplication. Bacteria resist penicillin by producing penicillinases—enzymes that convert penicillin to inactive penicilloic acid.

INDICATIONS & DOSAGE
Congenital syphilis—
Children under age 2: 50,000 units/kg I.M. as a single dose.
Group A streptococcal upper respiratory infections—
Adults: 1.2 million units I.M. in a single injection.
Children over 27 kg: 900,000 units I.M. in a single injection.
Children under 27 kg: 300,000 to 600,000 units I.M. in a single injection.
Prophylaxis of poststreptococcal rheumatic fever—

Italicized adverse reactions are common or life-threatening.
*Liquid form contains alcohol.   **May contain tartrazine.

Adults and children: 1.2 million units I.M. once a month or 600,000 units twice a month.
Syphilis of less than 1 year's duration—
Adults: 2.4 million units I.M. in a single dose.
Syphilis of more than 1 year's duration—
Adults: 2.4 million units I.M. weekly for 3 successive weeks.

ADVERSE REACTIONS
Blood: eosinophilia, hemolytic anemia, thrombocytopenia, leukopenia.
CNS: neuropathy, seizures with high doses.
Local: pain and sterile abscess at injection site.
Other: *hypersensitivity (maculopapular and exfoliative dermatitis, chills, fever, edema, anaphylaxis).*

INTERACTIONS
Probenecid: increases blood levels of penicillin. Probenecid may be used for this purpose.

NURSING CONSIDERATIONS
• Use cautiously in patients with other drug allergies, especially to cephalosporins (possible cross-allergenicity).
• Obtain specimen for culture and sensitivity tests before first dose. Therapy may begin pending test results.
• Before giving penicillin, ask patient if he's had any allergic reactions to this drug. However, a negative history of penicillin allergy is no guarantee against a future allergic reaction.
• Tell patient to call the doctor if rash, fever, or chills develop. Fever and eosinophilia are the most common allergic reactions.
• With large doses and prolonged therapy, bacterial and fungal superinfections may occur, especially in elderly, debilitated, or immunosuppressed patients.

• Shake medication well before injection.
• Never give I.V.—inadvertent I.V. administration has caused cardiac arrest and death.
• Very slow absorption time makes allergic reactions difficult to treat.
• Inject deeply into upper outer quadrant of buttocks in adults; in midlateral thigh in infants and small children.
• Give penicillin G benzathine at least 1 hour before bacteriostatic antibiotics.

---

penicillin G potassium (benzylpenicillin potassium)
Megacillin†, NovoPen-G†, P-50†, Pentids**, Pfizerpen
Pregnancy Risk Category: B

HOW SUPPLIED
Tablets: 200,000 units, 250,000 units, 400,000 units, 500,000 units, 800,000 units
Oral suspension: 200,000 units/5 ml, 250,000 units/5 ml, 400,000 units/5 ml (after reconstitution)
Injection: 200,000 units, 500,000 units, 1 million units, 5 million units, 10 million units, 20 million units

MECHANISM OF ACTION
Bactericidal against microorganisms by inhibiting cell wall synthesis during active multiplication. Bacteria resist penicillin by producing penicillinases—enzymes that convert penicillin to inactive penicilloic acid.

INDICATIONS & DOSAGE
Moderate to severe systemic infections—
Adults: 1.6 to 3.2 million units P.O. daily in divided doses given q 6 hours (1 mg = 1,600 units); 1.2 to 24 million units I.M. or I.V. daily in divided doses given q 4 hours.
Children: 25,000 to 100,000 units/kg

P.O. daily in divided doses given q 6 hours; or 25,000 to 300,000 units/kg I.M. or I.V. daily in divided doses given q 4 hours.

ADVERSE REACTIONS

Blood: hemolytic anemia, leukopenia, thrombocytopenia.
CNS: neuropathy, seizures with high doses.
Metabolic: possible severe potassium poisoning with high doses (hyperreflexia, seizures, coma).
Local: *thrombophlebitis, pain at injection site.*
Other: *hypersensitivity (rash, urticaria, maculopapular eruptions, exfoliative dermatitis, chills, fever, edema, anaphylaxis),* overgrowth of nonsusceptible organisms.

INTERACTIONS

Probenecid: increases blood levels of penicillin. Probenecid may be used for this purpose.

NURSING CONSIDERATIONS

• Use cautiously in patients with other drug allergies, especially to cephalosporins (possible cross-allergenicity).
• Obtain specimen for culture and sensitivity tests before first dose. Therapy may begin pending test results.
• Before giving penicillin, ask patient if he's had any allergic reactions to this drug. However, a negative history of penicillin allergy is no guarantee against a future allergic reaction.
• Tell patient to take medication exactly as prescribed, even if he feels better, and to take entire amount prescribed.
• Tell patient to call the doctor if rash, fever, or chills develop. A rash is the most common allergic reaction.
• When given orally, drug may cause GI disturbances. Food may interfere with absorption, so give 1 to 2 hours before meals or 2 to 3 hours after.

• Extremely painful when given I.M. Inject deep into large muscle.
• Patients with poor renal function are predisposed to high blood levels. Monitor renal function closely.
• If patient has high blood level of this drug, he may have seizures. Institute seizure precautions.
• When giving I.V., mix with dextrose 5% in water or a saline solution.
• Give I.V. intermittently to prevent vein irritation. Change site every 48 hours.
• With large doses and prolonged therapy, bacterial and fungal superinfections may occur, especially in elderly, debilitated, or immunosuppressed patients. Close observation is essential.
• Warn patient never to use leftover penicillin for a new illness or to share penicillin with family and friends.
• Give penicillin G potassium at least 1 hour before bacteriostatic antibiotics.

penicillin G procaine (benzylpenicillin procaine)

Ayercillin†, Crysticillin A.S., Duracillin A.S., Pfizerpen-AS, Wycillin

Pregnancy Risk Category: B

HOW SUPPLIED

Injection: 300,000 units/ml, 500,000 units/ml, 600,000 units/ml

MECHANISM OF ACTION

Bactericidal against microorganisms by inhibiting cell wall synthesis during active multiplication. Bacteria resist penicillin by producing penicillinases—enzymes that convert penicillin to inactive penicilloic acid.

INDICATIONS & DOSAGE

Moderate to severe systemic infections—
Adults: 600,000 to 1.2 million units I.M. daily given as a single dose.

Italicized adverse reactions are common or life-threatening.
*Liquid form contains alcohol.   **May contain tartrazine.

Children: 300,000 units I.M. daily given as a single dose.

Uncomplicated gonorrhea—
Adults and children over 12 years: give 1 g probenecid; then 30 minutes later give 4.8 million units of penicillin G procaine I.M., divided into two injection sites.

Pneumococcal pneumonia—
Adults and children over 12 years: 300,000 to 600,000 units I.M. daily q 6 to 12 hours.

ADVERSE REACTIONS
Blood: thrombocytopenia, hemolytic anemia, leukopenia.
CNS: arthralgia, seizures.
Other: *hypersensitivity (rash, urticaria, chills, fever, edema, prostration, anaphylaxis)*, overgrowth of nonsusceptible organisms.

INTERACTIONS
Probenecid: increases blood levels of penicillin. Probenecid may be used for this purpose.

NURSING CONSIDERATIONS
• Contraindicated in patients with hypersensitivity to procaine. Use cautiously in patients with other drug allergies, especially to cephalosporins (possible cross-allergenicity).
• Obtain specimen for culture and sensitivity tests before first dose. Therapy may begin pending test results.
• Before giving penicillin, ask patient if he's had any allergic reactions to this drug. However, a negative history of penicillin allergy is no guarantee against a future allergic reaction.
• Tell patient to call doctor if rash, fever, or chills develop. A rash is the most common allergic reaction.
• Give deep I.M. in upper outer quadrant of buttocks in adults; in midlateral thigh in small children. Do not give subcutaneously. Don't massage injection site.
• Never give I.V.—inadvertent I.V.

administration has caused death, due to CNS toxicity from procaine.
• Due to slow absorption rate, allergic reactions are hard to treat.
• With large doses and prolonged therapy, bacterial and fungal superinfections may occur, especially in elderly, debilitated, or immunosuppressed patients. Close observation is essential.
• Periodic evaluations of renal and hematopoietic function are recommended.
• Give penicillin G procaine at least 1 hour before bacteriostatic antibiotics.

penicillin G sodium (benzylpenicillin sodium)
Crystapen†
Pregnancy Risk Category: B

HOW SUPPLIED
Injection: 5 million units

MECHANISM OF ACTION
Bactericidal against microorganisms by inhibiting cell wall synthesis during active multiplication. Bacteria resist penicillin by producing penicillinases—enzymes that convert penicillin to inactive penicilloic acid.

INDICATIONS & DOSAGE
Moderate to severe systemic infections—
Adults: 1.2 to 24 million units daily I.M. or I.V., divided into doses given q 4 hours.
Children: 25,000 to 300,000 units/kg daily I.M. or I.V., divided into doses given q 4 hours.
Endocarditis prophylaxis for dental surgery—
Adults: 2 million units I.V. or I.M. 30 to 60 minutes before procedure, then 1 million units 6 hours later.

ADVERSE REACTIONS
Blood: hemolytic anemia, leukopenia, thrombocytopenia.

CNS: arthralgia, neuropathy, seizures.
CV: *congestive heart failure with high doses.*
Local: *vein irritation, pain at injection site, thrombophlebitis.*
Other: *hypersensitivity (chills, fever, edema, maculopapular rash, exfoliative dermatitis, urticaria, anaphylaxis)*, overgrowth of nonsusceptible organisms.

INTERACTIONS
Probenecid: increases blood levels of penicillin. Probenecid may be used for this purpose.

NURSING CONSIDERATIONS
• Contraindicated in patients on sodium restriction. Use cautiously in patients with other drug allergies, especially to cephalosporins (possible cross-allergenicity).
• Obtain specimen for culture and sensitivity tests before first dose. Therapy may begin pending test results.
• Before giving penicillin, ask patient if he's had any allergic reactions to this drug. However, a negative history of penicillin allergy is no guarantee against a future allergic reaction.
• If patient has high blood level of this drug, he may have seizures. Institute seizure precautions.
• Give I.V. intermittently to prevent vein irritation. Change site every 48 hours.
• With large doses and prolonged therapy, bacterial or fungal superinfections may occur, especially in elderly, debilitated, or immunosuppressed patients. Close observation is essential.
• Give penicillin G sodium at least 1 hour before bacteriostatic antibiotics.

penicillin V (phenoxymethyl penicillin)

penicillin V potassium (phenoxymethylpenicillin potassium)
Abbocillin VK‡, Apo-Pen-VK†, Beepen-VK, Betapen-VK, Cilicane VK‡, Ledercillin VK, Nadopen-V†, NovoPen-VK†, PVK‡, Penapar VK, Pen Vee K, PVF K†, Robicillin VK, V-Cillin K, VC-K, Veetids**

Pregnancy Risk Category: B

HOW SUPPLIED
penicillin V
Tablets: 250 mg, 500 mg
Oral suspension: 125 mg/5 ml, 250 mg/5 ml (after reconstitution)
penicillin V potassium
Tablets: 125 mg, 250 mg, 500 mg
Tablets (film-coated): 250 mg, 500 mg
Capsules: 250 mg‡
Oral suspension: 125 mg/5 ml, 250 mg/5 ml (after reconstitution)

MECHANISM OF ACTION
Bactericidal against microorganisms by inhibiting cell wall synthesis during active multiplication. Bacteria resist penicillin by producing penicillinases—enzymes that convert penicillin to inactive penicilloic acid.

INDICATIONS & DOSAGE
Mild to moderate systemic infections—
Adults: 250 to 500 mg (400,000 to 800,000 units) P.O. q 6 hours.
Children: 15 to 50 mg/kg (25,000 to 90,000 units/kg) P.O. daily, divided into doses given q 6 to 8 hours.
Endocarditis prophylaxis for dental surgery—
Adults: 2 g P.O. 30 to 60 minutes before procedure, then 1 g 6 hours after.
Children under 30 kg: half of the adult dose.

ADVERSE REACTIONS
Blood: eosinophilia, hemolytic anemia, leukopenia, thrombocytopenia.
CNS: neuropathy.
GI: *epigastric distress*, vomiting, diarrhea, *nausea*.
Other: *hypersensitivity (rash, urticaria, chills, fever, edema, anaphylaxis)*, overgrowth of nonsusceptible organisms.

INTERACTIONS
Neomycin: decreases absorption of penicillin. Give penicillin by injection.
Probenecid: increases blood levels of penicillin. Probenecid may be used for this purpose.

NURSING CONSIDERATIONS
• Use cautiously in patients with other drug allergies, especially to cephalosporins (possible cross-allergenicity), and in GI disturbances.
• Obtain specimen for culture and sensitivity tests before first dose. Therapy may begin pending test results.
• Before giving penicillin, ask patient if he's had any allergic reactions to this drug. However, a negative history of penicillin allergy is no guarantee against a future allergic reaction.
• Tell patient to take medication exactly as prescribed, even if he feels better. Entire quantity prescribed should be taken.
• Tell patient to call the doctor if rash, fever, or chills develop. A rash is the most common allergic reaction.
• May cause GI disturbances. Food may interfere with absorption, so give 1 to 2 hours before meals or 2 to 3 hours after.
• Patient should take each dose with a full glass of water, not fruit juice or a carbonated beverage, because acid will inactivate the drug.
• Patients being treated for streptococcal infections should take the drug

until the full 10-day course is completed.
• With large doses and prolonged therapy, bacterial and fungal superinfections may occur, especially in elderly, debilitated, or immunosuppressed patients. Close observation is essential.
• Periodic renal and hematopoietic function studies are recommended in patients receiving prolonged therapy.
• Warn patient never to use leftover penicillin for a new illness or to share penicillin with family and friends.
• Give penicillin V at least 1 hour before bacteriostatic antibiotics.

---

piperacillin sodium
Pipracil, Pipril‡
Pregnancy Risk Category: B

HOW SUPPLIED
Injection: 2 g, 3 g, 4 g
Pharmacy bulk package: 40 g

MECHANISM OF ACTION
Bactericidal against microorganisms by inhibiting cell wall synthesis during active multiplication. Bacteria resist penicillin by producing penicillinases—enzymes that convert penicillin to inactive penicilloic acid.

INDICATIONS & DOSAGE
Systemic infections caused by susceptible strains of gram-positive and especially gram-negative organisms (including Proteus, Pseudomonas aeruginosa)—
Adults and children over 12 years: 100 to 300 mg/kg daily divided q 4 to 6 hours I.V. or I.M. Doses for children under 12 years not established.
Prophylaxis of surgical infections—
Adults: 2 g I.V., given 30 to 60 minutes before surgery. Depending on type of surgery, dose may be repeated during surgery, and once or twice more after surgery.

ADVERSE REACTIONS
Blood: *bleeding with high doses,* neutropenia, eosinophilia, leukopenia, *thrombocytopenia.*
CNS: neuromuscular irritability, seizures, headache, dizziness.
GI: nausea, diarrhea.
Local: pain at injection site, vein irritation, phlebitis.
Metabolic: *hypokalemia.*
Other: *hypersensitivity (edema, fever, chills, rash, pruritus, urticaria, anaphylaxis),* overgrowth of nonsusceptible organisms.

INTERACTIONS
Aminoglycoside antibiotics (e.g., gentamicin, tobramycin): chemically incompatible.
Probenecid: increases blood levels of piperacillin. Probenecid may be used for this purpose.

NURSING CONSIDERATIONS
• Use cautiously in patients hypersensitive to drugs, especially to cephalosporins (possible cross-hypersensitivity), and in bleeding tendencies, uremia, and hypokalemia.
• Cystic fibrosis patients tend to be most susceptible to fever or rash.
• Obtain specimen for culture and sensitivity tests before first dose. Therapy may begin pending test results.
• Before giving piperacillin, ask patient if he's had any allergic reactions to penicillin. A negative history of penicillin allergy, however, is no guarantee against future allergic reaction.
• Dosage should be altered in patients with impaired renal function.
• Check CBC and platelets frequently. Drug may cause thrombocytopenia.
• Monitor serum potassium level.
• Patient with high serum level of this drug may have seizures. Institute seizure precautions.
• Give I.V. intermittently to prevent

vein irritation. Change site every 48 hours.
• Almost always used with another antibiotic, such as gentamicin.
• With large doses and prolonged therapy, bacterial and fungal superinfections may occur, especially in elderly, debilitated, or immunosuppressed patients. Monitor patient closely.
• Drug may be better suited to patients on salt-free diets than carbenicillin and ticarcillin (contains 1.98 mEq Na/g of piperacillin).
• Piperacillin has shown greater activity against *Pseudomonas aeruginosa* than carbenicillin, ticarcillin, or mezlocillin.
• Give piperacillin at least 1 hour before bacteriostatic antibiotics.

ticarcillin disodium
Ticar, Ticillin‡

Pregnancy Risk Category: B

HOW SUPPLIED
Injection: 1 g, 3 g, 6 g
I.V. infusion: 3 g
Pharmacy bulk package: 20 g, 30 g

MECHANISM OF ACTION
Bactericidal against microorganisms by inhibiting cell wall synthesis during active multiplication. Bacteria resist penicillin by producing penicillinases—enzymes that convert penicillin to inactive penicilloic acid.

INDICATIONS & DOSAGE
Severe systemic infections caused by susceptible strains of gram-positive and especially gram-negative organisms (including Pseudomonas, Proteus)—
Adults: 18 g I.V. or I.M. daily, divided into doses given q 4 to 6 hours.
Children: 200 to 300 mg/kg I.V. or I.M. daily, divided into doses given q 4 to 6 hours.

Italicized adverse reactions are common or life-threatening.
*Liquid form contains alcohol.   **May contain tartrazine.

ADVERSE REACTIONS
Blood: leukopenia, neutropenia, eosinophilia, *thrombocytopenia,* hemolytic anemia.
CNS: seizures, neuromuscular excitability.
GI: nausea, diarrhea.
Metabolic: *hypokalemia.*
Local: pain at injection site, vein irritation, phlebitis.
Other: *hypersensitivity (rash, pruritus, urticaria, chills, fever, edema, anaphylaxis),* overgrowth of nonsusceptible organisms.

INTERACTIONS
Aminoglycoside antibiotics (e.g., gentamicin, tobramycin): chemically incompatible. Don't mix together in I.V.
Probenecid: increases blood levels of ticarcillin and other penicillins. Probenecid may be used for this purpose.

NURSING CONSIDERATIONS
• Use cautiously in other drug allergies, especially to cephalosporins (possible cross-allergenicity), and in impaired renal function, hemorrhagic conditions, hypokalemia, or sodium restrictions (contains 5.2 mEq Na/g).
• Obtain specimen for culture and sensitivity tests before first dose. Therapy may begin pending test results.
• Before giving ticarcillin, ask patient if he's had any allergic reactions to penicillin. However, a negative history of penicillin allergy is no guarantee against a future allergic reaction.
• Dosage should be decreased in patients with impaired renal functions.
• Check CBC and platelets frequently. Drug may cause thrombocytopenia.
• If patient has high blood level of this drug, he may develop seizures. Institute seizure precautions.
• When giving I.V., mix with dextrose 5% in water or other suitable I.V. fluids.
• Give I.V. intermittently to prevent vein irritation. Change site every 48 hours.
• Administer deep I.M. into large muscle.
• Almost always used with another antibiotic, such as gentamicin.
• With large doses and prolonged therapy, bacterial and fungal superinfections may occur, especially in elderly, debilitated, or immunosuppressed patients. Close observation is essential.
• Monitor serum potassium.
• Give ticarcillin at least 1 hour before bacteriostatic antibiotics.

ticarcillin disodium/ clavulanate potassium
Timentin
Pregnancy Risk Category: B

HOW SUPPLIED
Injection: 3 g ticarcillin and 100 mg clavulanic acid

MECHANISM OF ACTION
Clavulanic acid increases ticarcillin's effectiveness by inactivating beta lactamases, which destroy ticarcillin.

INDICATIONS & DOSAGE
Treatment of infections of the lower respiratory tract, urinary tract, bones and joints, skin and skin structure, and septicemia when caused by beta-lactamase–producing strains of bacteria or by ticarcillin-susceptible organisms—
Adults: 3.1-g vial (contains ticarcillin 3 g and clavulanate potassium 0.1 g) administered by I.V. infusion q 4 to 6 hours.

ADVERSE REACTIONS
Blood: leukopenia, neutropenia, eosinophilia, *thrombocytopenia,* hemolytic anemia.
CNS: seizures, neuromuscular excitability.
GI: nausea, diarrhea.

Metabolic: *hypokalemia.*
Local: pain at injection site, vein irritation, phlebitis.
Other: *hypersensitivity (rash, pruritus, urticaria, chills, fever, edema, anaphylaxis),* overgrowth of nonsusceptible organisms.

INTERACTIONS
Probenecid: increases blood levels of ticarcillin. Probenecid may be used for this purpose.
Aminoglycoside antibiotics (e.g., gentamicin, tobramycin): chemically incompatible. Don't mix together in I.V.

NURSING CONSIDERATIONS
• Use cautiously in patients with other drug allergies, especially to cephalosporins (possible cross-allergenicity), and in impaired renal function, hemorrhagic conditions, hypokalemia, or sodium restrictions.
• Obtain specimen for culture and sensitivity tests before first dose. Therapy may begin pending test results.
• Before giving Timentin, ask patient if he's had any allergic reactions to penicillin. However, a negative history of penicillin allergy is no guarantee against a future allergic reaction.
• Dosage should be decreased in patients with impaired renal functions.
• With large doses and prolonged therapy, bacterial and fungal superinfections may occur, especially in elderly, debilitated, or immunosuppressed patients. Close observation is essential.
• Check CBC and platelets frequently. Drug may cause thrombocytopenia.
• Monitor serum potassium.
• Administer by I.V. infusion over 30 minutes. Don't give by I.V. push or I.M.
• Particularly useful in clinical settings with a high prevalence of ticarcillin-resistant organisms.
• Give ticarcillin disodium/clavulanate potassium at least 1 hour before bacteriostatic antibiotics.

Italicized adverse reactions are common or life-threatening.
*Liquid form contains alcohol.   **May contain tartrazine.

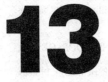

Cephalosporins

cefaclor
cefadroxil monohydrate
cefamandole nafate
cefazolin sodium
cefixime
cefmetazole sodium
cefonicid sodium
cefoperazone sodium
ceforanide
cefotaxime sodium
cefotetan disodium
cefoxitin sodium
ceftazidime
ceftizoxime sodium
ceftriaxone sodium
cefuroxime axetil
cefuroxime sodium
cephalexin monohydrate
cephalothin sodium
cephapirin sodium
cephradine
moxalactam disodium

COMBINATION PRODUCTS
None.

cefaclor
Ceclor

Pregnancy Risk Category: B

HOW SUPPLIED
Capsules: 250 mg, 500 mg
Oral suspension: 125 mg/5 ml, 250 mg/5 ml

MECHANISM OF ACTION
Inhibits cell wall synthesis, promoting osmotic instability. Usually bactericidal.

INDICATIONS & DOSAGE
Treatment of infections of respiratory or urinary tracts, skin, and soft tissue; and otitis media due to Hemophilus influenzae, Streptococcus pneumoniae, S. pyogenes, Escherichia coli, Proteus mirabilis, Klebsiella *species, and staphylococci*—
Adults: 250 to 500 mg P.O. q 8 hours. Total daily dose should not exceed 4 g.
Children: 20 mg/kg daily P.O. in divided doses q 8 hours. In more serious infections, 40 mg/kg daily are recommended, not to exceed 1 g per day.

ADVERSE REACTIONS
Blood: transient leukopenia, lymphocytosis, anemia, eosinophilia.
CNS: dizziness, headache, somnolence.
GI: *nausea,* vomiting, *diarrhea,* anorexia, *pseudomembranous colitis.*
GU: red and white cells in urine, vaginal moniliasis, vaginitis.
Skin: *maculopapular rash,* dermatitis.
Other: hypersensitivity, fever, cholestatic jaundice.

INTERACTIONS
Probenecid: may inhibit excretion and increase blood levels of cefaclor.

NURSING CONSIDERATIONS
• Contraindicated in hypersensitivity to other cephalosporins. Use cautiously in impaired renal function and in those with history of sensitivity to penicillin. Ask patient if he's had any

---

†Available in Canada only.   ‡Available in Australia only.   ◊Available OTC.

reaction to previous cephalosporin or penicillin therapy before administering first dose.

• Obtain specimen for culture and sensitivity tests before first dose. Therapy may begin pending test results.

• Major clinical use appears to be in treating otitis media caused by *H. influenzae* when resistant to ampicillin or amoxicillin. Drug is a second-generation cephalosporin.

• Tell patient to take medication exactly as prescribed, even after he feels better, and to take entire amount prescribed.

• Call doctor if skin rash develops.

• With large doses or prolonged therapy, monitor for superinfection, especially in high-risk patients.

• Store reconstituted suspension in refrigerator. Stable for 14 days if refrigerated. Shake well before using.

• Drug may be taken with meals.

• Cefaclor is a relatively expensive antibiotic and should be used only when the organism is resistant to other agents.

• If ordered, total daily dose of cefaclor may be administered twice daily rather than 3 times daily with similar therapeutic results.

• Urine glucose determinations may be false-positive with copper sulfate tests (Clinitest); glucose enzymatic tests (Clinistix, Tes-Tape) are not affected.

---

cefadroxil monohydrate
Duricef, Ultracef

Pregnancy Risk Category: B

HOW SUPPLIED
Tablets: 1 g
Capsules: 500 mg
Oral suspension: 125 mg/5 ml, 250 mg/5 ml, 500 mg/5 ml

MECHANISM OF ACTION
Inhibits cell wall synthesis, promoting osmotic instability. Usually bactericidal.

INDICATIONS & DOSAGE
Treatment of urinary tract infections caused by Escherichia coli, Proteus mirabilis, *and* Klebsiella *species; infections of skin and soft tissue; and streptococcal pharyngitis—*
Adults: 500 mg to 2 g P.O. per day, depending on the infection being treated. Usually given in once-daily or b.i.d. dosage.
Children: 30 mg/kg P.O. daily in 2 divided doses.

ADVERSE REACTIONS
Blood: transient neutropenia, eosinophilia, leukopenia, anemia.
CNS: dizziness, headache, malaise, paresthesias.
GI: *pseudomembranous colitis, nausea,* anorexia, vomiting, *diarrhea,* glossitis, *dyspepsia,* abdominal cramps, anal pruritus, tenesmus, oral candidiasis (thrush).
GU: genital pruritus, moniliasis.
Skin: *maculopapular and erythematous rashes.*
Other: dyspnea.

INTERACTIONS
Probenecid: may inhibit excretion and increase blood levels of cefadroxil.

NURSING CONSIDERATIONS
• Contraindicated in patients with hypersensitivity to other cephalosporins. Use cautiously in impaired renal function and in those with history of sensitivity to penicillin. Ask patient if he's had any reaction to previous cephalosporin or penicillin therapy before administering first dose.

• Obtain specimen for culture and sensitivity tests before first dose. Therapy may begin pending test results.

• If creatinine clearance is below 50 ml/minute, dosage interval should be

---

Italicized adverse reactions are common or life-threatening.
*Liquid form contains alcohol.　　**May contain tartrazine.

lengthened so drug doesn't accumulate.
• Tell patient to take medication exactly as prescribed, even after he feels better, and to take entire amount prescribed.
• Call doctor if skin rash develops.
• Since absorption not delayed by presence of food, tell the patient to take with food or milk to lessen GI discomfort.
• Longer half-life permits once- or twice-daily dosing.
• Urine glucose determinations may be false-positive with copper sulfate tests (Clinitest); glucose enzymatic tests (Clinistix, Tes-Tape) are not affected.
• With large doses or prolonged therapy, monitor for superinfection, especially in high-risk patients.

cefamandole nafate
Mandol

Pregnancy Risk Category: B

HOW SUPPLIED
Injection: 500 mg, 1 g, 2 g, 10 g
Pharmacy bulk package: 10 g

MECHANISM OF ACTION
Inhibits cell wall synthesis, promoting osmotic instability. Usually bactericidal.

INDICATIONS & DOSAGE
Treatment of serious infections of respiratory and genitourinary tracts, skin and soft-tissue infections, bone and joint infections, septicemia, and peritonitis due to Escherichia coli *and other coliform bacteria,* S. aureus *(penicillinase- and nonpenicillinase-producing),* S. epidermidis, *group A beta-hemolytic streptococci,* Klebsiella, Hemophilus influenzae, Proteus mirabilis, *and* Enterobacter—
Adults: 500 mg to 1 g q 4 to 8 hours. In life-threatening infections, up to 2 g q 4 hours may be needed.

Infants and children: 50 to 100 mg/kg daily in equally divided doses q 4 to 8 hours. May be increased to total daily dose of 150 mg/kg (not to exceed maximum adult dose) for severe infections.
Total daily dosage is same for I.M. or I.V. administration and depends on susceptibility of organism and severity of infection. In patients with impaired renal function, doses or frequency of administration must be modified according to degree of renal impairment, severity of infection, and susceptibility of organism. Should be injected deep I.M. into a large muscle mass, such as gluteus or lateral aspect of thigh.

ADVERSE REACTIONS
Blood: transient neutropenia, eosinophilia, hemolytic anemia, *hypoprothrombinemia,* bleeding.
CNS: headache, malaise, paresthesias, dizziness.
GI: *pseudomembranous colitis,* nausea, anorexia, vomiting, *diarrhea,* glossitis, dyspepsia, abdominal cramps, tenesmus, anal pruritus, oral candidiasis (thrush).
GU: genital pruritus and moniliasis.
Skin: *maculopapular and erythematous rashes, urticaria.*
Local: *at injection site—pain, induration, sterile abscesses,* temperature elevation, tissue sloughing; *phlebitis and thrombophlebitis with I.V. injection.*
Other: *hypersensitivity,* dyspnea.

INTERACTIONS
Ethyl alcohol: may cause a disulfiram-like reaction. Warn patients not to drink alcohol for several days after discontinuing cefamandole.
Oral anticoagulants, aspirin: increased risk of bleeding.
Probenecid: may inhibit excretion and increase blood levels of cefamandole.

NURSING CONSIDERATIONS
• Contraindicated in patients with hypersensitivity to other cephalosporins. Use cautiously in impaired renal function and in those with history of sensitivity to penicillin. Ask patient if he's had any reaction to previous cephalosporin or penicillin therapy before administering first dose.
• Obtain specimen for culture and sensitivity tests before first dose. Therapy may begin pending test results.
• Not as effective as cefoxitin in treating anaerobic infections.
• For most cephalosporin-sensitive organisms, cefamandole offers little advantage over previously available agents.
• For I.V. use, reconstitute 1 g with 10 ml of sterile water for injection, dextrose 5% or 0.9% sodium chloride for injection.
• Don't mix with I.V. infusions containing magnesium or calcium ions; chemically incompatible.
• I.M. cefamandole is not as painful as cefoxitin. Does not require addition of lidocaine.
• After reconstitution, drug remains stable for 24 hours at room temperature or 96 hours under refrigeration.
• The chemical structure of this drug includes the methylthiotetrazole (MTT) side chain that has been associated with bleeding disorders. If bleeding occurs, it can be promptly reversed with administration of vitamin K.
• With large doses or prolonged therapy, monitor for superinfection, especially in high-risk patients.
• Urine glucose determinations may be false-positive with copper sulfate tests (Clinitest); glucose enzymatic tests (Clinistix, Tes-Tape) are not affected.

cefazolin sodium
Ancef, Kefzol

Pregnancy Risk Category: B

HOW SUPPLIED
Injection (parenteral): 250 mg, 500 mg, 1 g, 5 g, 10 g
Infusion: 500 mg/100 ml vial, 500-mg or 1-g Redi Vials, Faspaks, or ADD-Vantage vials

MECHANISM OF ACTION
Inhibits cell wall synthesis, promoting osmotic instability. Usually bactericidal.

INDICATIONS & DOSAGE
Treatment of serious infections of respiratory and genitourinary tracts, skin and soft-tissue infections, bone and joint infections, septicemia, and endocarditis due to Escherichia coli, *Enterobacteriaceae, gonococci,* Hemophilus influenzae, Klebsiella, Proteus mirabilis, Staphylococcus aureus, Streptococcus pneumoniae, *and group A beta-hemolytic streptococci; and perioperative prophylaxis—*
Adults: 250 mg I.M. or I.V. q 8 hours to 1 g q 6 hours. Maximun 12g/day in life-threatening situations.
Children over 1 month: 8 to 16 mg/kg I.M. or I.V. q 8 hours, or 6 to 12 mg/kg q 6 hours.

Total daily dosage is same for I.M. or I.V. administration and depends on susceptibility of organism and severity of infection. In patients with impaired renal function, doses or frequency of administration must be modified according to degree of renal impairment, severity of infection, and susceptibility of organism. Should be injected deep I.M. into a large muscle mass, such as gluteus or lateral aspect of thigh.

ADVERSE REACTIONS
Blood: transient neutropenia, leukopenia, eosinophilia, anemia.

CNS: dizziness, headache, malaise, paresthesias.

GI: *pseudomembranous colitis,* nausea, anorexia, vomiting, *diarrhea,* glossitis, dyspepsia, abdominal cramps, anal pruritus, tenesmus, oral candidiasis (thrush).

GU: genital pruritus and moniliasis, vaginitis.

Skin: *maculopapular and erythematous rashes, urticaria.*

Local: *at injection site—pain, induration, sterile abscesses, tissue sloughing; phlebitis and thrombophlebitis with I.V. injection.*

Other: *hypersensitivity,* dyspnea.

INTERACTIONS
Probenecid: may inhibit excretion and increase blood levels of cefazolin.

NURSING CONSIDERATIONS
• Use cautiously in impaired renal function and in those with history of sensitivity to penicillin. Ask patient if he's ever had any reaction to cephalosporin or penicillin therapy before administering first dose.

• Avoid doses greater than 4 g daily in patients with severe renal impairment.

• Obtain specimen for culture and sensitivity tests before first dose. Therapy may begin pending test results.

• Because of long duration of effect, most infections can be treated with a dose q 8 hours.

• For I.M. administration, reconstitute with sterile water, bacteriostatic water, or 0.9% sodium chloride solution as follows: 2 ml to 250-mg vial; 2 ml to 500-mg vial; 2.5 ml to 1-g vial. Shake well until dissolved. Resultant concentration: 125 mg/ml, 225 mg/ml, 330 mg/ml, respectively.

• Not as painful as other cephalosporins when given I.M.

• Alternate injection sites if I.V. therapy lasts longer than 3 days. Use of small I.V. needles in the larger available veins may be preferable.

• Reconstituted cefazolin sodium is stable for 24 hours at room temperature or 96 hours under refrigeration.

• About 40% to 75% of patients receiving cephalosporins show a false-positive direct Coombs' test; only a few of these indicate hemolytic anemia.

• With large doses or prolonged therapy, monitor for superinfection, especially in high-risk patients.

• Considered the first-generation cephalosporin of choice by most authorities.

• Urine glucose determinations may be false-positive with copper sulfate tests (Clinitest); glucose enzymatic tests (Clinistix, Tes-Tape) are not affected.

---

cefixime
Suprax

Pregnancy Risk Category: B

HOW SUPPLIED
Tablets: 200 mg, 400 mg
Oral suspension: 100 mg/5 ml (after reconstitution)

MECHANISM OF ACTION
Inhibits cell wall synthesis, promoting osmotic instability. Usually bactericidal.

INDICATIONS & DOSAGE
Treatment of uncomplicated urinary tract infections caused by Escherichia coli *and* Proteus mirabilis; *otitis media caused by* Hemophilus influenzae *(beta-lactam positive and negative strains,* Moraxella (Branhamella) catarrhalis, *and* Streptococcus pyogenes; *pharyngitis and tonsillitis caused by* S. pyogenes; *acute bronchitis and acute exacerbations of chronic bronchitis caused by* S. pneumoniae *and* H. influenzae *(beta-lactamase positive and negative strains)—*

Adults: 400 mg/day orally as a single 400-mg tablet or 200 mg q 12 hours.
Children: 8 mg/kg/day suspension orally as a single daily dose or 4 mg/kg orally q 12 hours.

Treat children over age 12 and those who weigh more than 50 kg with the recommended adult dose.

ADVERSE REACTIONS
Blood: thrombocytopenia, leukopenia, eosinophilia.
CNS: headaches, dizziness.
GI: *diarrhea,* loose stools, abdominal pain, nausea, vomiting, dyspepsia, flatulence, pseudomembranous colitis.
GU: genital pruritus, vaginitis, genital candidiasis.
Skin: pruritus, rash, urticaria.
Other: drug fever, hypersensitivity reactions.

INTERACTIONS
None significant.

NURSING CONSIDERATIONS
• Contraindicated in patients with hypersensitivity to other cephalosporins. Use cautiously and with reduced dosage in patients with renal dysfunction. Use cautiously in patients with a history of sensitivity to penicillin. Ask patients if they have had any reactions to previous cephalosporin or penicillin therapy before administering the first dose.
• Obtain specimen for culture and sensitivity tests before first dose. Therapy may begin pending test results.
• If creatinine clearance is less than 60 ml/minute, dosage should be reduced to avoid drug accumulation.
• Call doctor is skin rash develops.
• Preparation of oral suspension: add required amount of water to powder in two portions. Shake well after each addition. After mixing, suspension is stable for 14 days. It does not require

refrigeration, but keep tightly closed. Shake well before using.
• With large doses or prolonged therapy, monitor for superinfection, especially in high-risk patients.
• About 40% to 75% of patients receiving cephalosporins show a false-positive direct Coombs' test, but only a few of these tests indicate hemolytic anemia.
• Urine glucose determinations may be false-positive with copper sulfate tests (Clinitest); glucose enzymatic tests (Clinistix, Tes-Tape) are not affected.

cefmetazole sodium
Zefazone
Pregnancy Risk Category: B

HOW SUPPLIED
Injection: 1 g, 2 g

MECHANISM OF ACTION
Inhibits cell wall synthesis, promoting osmotic instability. Usually bactericidal.

INDICATIONS & DOSAGE
Lower respiratory tract infections caused by Streptococcus pneumoniae, Staphylococcus aureus *(penicillinase- and nonpenicillinase-producing strains),* Escherichia coli, *and* Hemophilus influenzae *(nonpenicillinase-producing strains); intraabdominal infections caused by* E. coli *or* Bacteroides fragilis; *skin and skinstructure infections caused by* S. aureus *(penicillinase- and nonpenicillinase-producing strains),* Staphylococcus epidermidis, Streptococcus pyogenes, Streptococcus agalactiae, E. coli, Proteus mirabilis, Klebsiella pneumoniae, *and* B. fragilis—
Adults: 2 g I.V. q 6 to 12 hours for 5 to 14 days.
Urinary tract infections caused by E. coli—
Adults: 2 g I.V. q 12 hours.

Prophylaxis in patients undergoing vaginal hysterectomy—
Adults: 2 g I.V. 30 to 90 minutes before surgery as a single dose; or 1 g I.V. 30 to 90 minutes before surgery, repeated in 8 and 16 hours.

Prophylaxis in patients undergoing abdominal hysterectomy—
Adults: 1 g I.V. 30 to 90 minutes before surgery, repeated in 8 and 16 hours.

Prophylaxis in patients undergoing cesarean section—
Adults: 2 g I.V. as a single dose after clamping cord; or 1 g I.V. after clamping cord, repeated in 8 and 16 hours.

Prophylaxis in patients undergoing colorectal surgery—
Adults: 2 g I.V. as a single dose 30 to 90 minutes before surgery. Some clinicians follow with additional 2-g doses in 8 and 16 hours.

Prophylaxis in patients undergoing cholecystectomy (high risk)—
Adults: 1 g I.V. 30 to 90 minutes before surgery, repeated in 8 and 16 hours.

ADVERSE REACTIONS
CNS: headache.
CV: shock, hypotension.
EENT: epistaxis.
GI: nausea, vomiting, *diarrhea,* epigastric pain, pseudomembranous colitis.
GU: vaginitis.
Respiratory: pleural effusion, dyspnea, respiratory distress.
Skin: rash, pruritus, generalized erythema.
Local: pain at injection site, phlebitis.
Other: fever, bacterial or fungal superinfection, hypersensitivity, altered color perception.

INTERACTIONS
Alcohol: disulfiram-like reaction. Alcohol should be avoided within 24 hours of administration.

Aminoglycosides: increased risk of nephrotoxicity.

NURSING CONSIDERATIONS
• Contraindicated in patients with a history of hypersensitivity to cephalosporins. Ask patient if he's had any reaction to previous cephalosporin or penicillin therapy before administering first dose.
• Obtain specimen for culture and sensitivity before first dose. Therapy may begin pending test results.
• Prolonged use may result in overgrowth of nonsusceptible organisms. Monitor patient for bacterial and fungal superinfections.
• The chemical structure of this drug includes the methylthiotetrazole (MTT) side chain that has been associated with bleeding disorders. However, such bleeding has not been reported with this drug. Monitor prothrombin time and administer vitamin K as ordered.
• Cephalosporins may cause false-positive results for urine glucose with copper sulfate tests (Clinitest). Glucose enzymatic tests (Clinistix, Tes-Tape) are not affected.
• Reconstitute with bacteriostatic water for injection, sterile water for injection, or 0.9% sodium chloride for injection. Following reconstitution, the drug may be further diluted to concentrations ranging from 1 to 20 mg/ml by adding it to 0.9% sodium chloride injection, 5% dextrose in water, or lactated Ringer's injection. Reconstituted or dilute solutions are stable for 24 hours at room temperature (77° F. [25° C.]) or 1 week if refrigerated (46° F. [8° C.]).

---

cefonicid sodium
Monocid

Pregnancy Risk Category: B

HOW SUPPLIED
Injection: 500 mg, 1 g

Infusion: 1 g/100 ml
Pharmacy bulk package: 10 g

MECHANISM OF ACTION
Inhibits cell wall synthesis, promoting osmotic instability. Usually bactericidal.

INDICATIONS & DOSAGE
Treatment of serious infections of the lower respiratory and urinary tract; skin and skin structure infections; septicemia; and bone and joint infections. Susceptible microorganisms include Streptococcus pneumoniae, Klebsiella pneumoniae, Escherichia coli, Hemophilus influenzae, Proteus mirabilis, Staphyloccus aureus and epidermidis, *and* Streptococcus pyogenes—
Adults: usual dosage is 1 g I.V. or I.M. q 24 hours. In life-threatening infections, 2 g q 24 hours.

Total daily dosage is same for I.M. or I.V. administration and depends on susceptibility of organism and severity of infection. In patients with impaired renal function, doses or frequency of administration must be modified according to degree of renal impairment, severity of infection, and susceptibility of organism. Should be injected deep I.M. into a large muscle mass, such as gluteus or lateral aspect of thigh.

ADVERSE REACTIONS
Blood: transient neutropenia, leukopenia, eosinophilia, anemia.
CNS: dizziness, headache, malaise, paresthesias.
GI: *pseudomembranous colitis,* nausea, anorexia, vomiting, diarrhea, glossitis, dyspepsia, abdominal cramps, anal pruritus, tenesmus, oral candidiasis (thrush).
GU: genital pruritus and moniliasis, vaginitis.
Skin: *maculopapular and erythematous rashes, urticaria.*
Local: *at injection site—pain, indura-*
tion, sterile abscesses, tissue sloughing; phlebitis and thrombophlebitis with I.V. injection.
Other: hypersensitivity, dyspnea.

INTERACTIONS
Probenecid: may inhibit excretion and increase blood levels of cefonicid.

NURSING CONSIDERATIONS
• Contraindicated in patients with hypersensitivity to other cephalosporins. Use cautiously in impaired renal function and in those with history of sensitivity to penicillin. Ask patient if he's had any reaction to previous cephalosporin or penicillin therapy before administering first dose.
• Obtain specimen for culture and sensitivity tests before first dose. Therapy may begin pending test results.
• When administering 2-g I.M. doses once daily, one-half the dose should be administered in different large muscle masses.
• With large doses or prolonged therapy, monitor for superinfection, especially in high-risk patients.
• Has been promoted as a cost-effective agent for surgical prophylaxis.

cefoperazone sodium
Cefobid

Pregnancy Risk Category: B

HOW SUPPLIED
Infusion: 1 g, 2 g piggyback
Parenteral: 1 g, 2 g

MECHANISM OF ACTION
Inhibits cell wall synthesis, promoting osmotic instability. Usually bactericidal.

INDICATIONS & DOSAGE
Treatment of serious infections of the respiratory tract; intraabdominal, gynecologic, and skin infections; bacteremia, septicemia. Susceptible micro-

organisms include Streptococcus pneumoniae and pyogenes; Staphylococcus aureus *(penicillinase and non-penicillinase-producing)* and epidermidis; *enterococcus;* Escherichia coli; Klebsiella; Hemophilus influenzae; Enterobacter; Citrobacter; Proteus; *some* Pseudomonas, *including* Pseudomonas aeruginosa; *and* Bacteroides fragilis—

Adults: Usual dosage is 1 to 2 g q 12 hours I.M. or I.V. In severe infections, or infections caused by less sensitive organisms, the total daily dosage or frequency may be increased up to 16 g/day in certain situations.

No dosage adjustment is usually necessary in patients with renal impairment. However, doses of 4 g/day should be given very cautiously in patients with hepatic disease. Should be injected deep I.M. into a large muscle mass, such as gluteus or lateral aspect of the thigh.

ADVERSE REACTIONS

Blood: transient neutropenia, eosinophilia, hemolytic anemia, *hypoprothrombinemia, bleeding.*
CNS: headache, malaise, paresthesias, dizziness.
GI: *pseudomembranous colitis,* nausea, anorexia, vomiting, *diarrhea,* glossitis, dyspepsia, abdominal cramps, tenesmus, anal pruritus, oral candidiasis (thrush).
Hepatic: mildly elevated liver enzymes.
GU: genital pruritus and moniliasis.
Skin: *maculopapular and erythematous rashes, urticaria.*
Local: *at injection site—pain, induration, sterile abscesses, temperature elevation, tissue sloughing; phlebitis and thrombophlebitis with I.V. injection.*
Other: hypersensitivity, dyspnea.

INTERACTIONS

Ethyl alcohol: may cause a disulfiram-like reaction. Warn patients not to drink alcohol for several days after discontinuing cefoperazone.
Oral anticoagulants, aspirin: increased risk of bleeding.
Probenecid: may inhibit excretion and increase blood levels of cefoperazone.

NURSING CONSIDERATIONS

• Contraindicated in patients with hypersensitivity to other cephalosporins. Use cautiously in impaired renal function and in those with history of sensitivity to penicillin. Ask patient if he's had any reaction to previous cephalosporin or penicillin therapy before administering first dose.
• Obtain specimen for culture and sensitivity tests before first dose. Therapy may begin pending test results.
• Cefoperazone is one of the third-generation cephalosporins. It has greater activity than first-generation cephalosporins against gram-negative organisms, but less activity against gram-positive organisms.
• Because of high degree of biliary excretion, may cause more diarrhea than other cephalosporins.
• The chemical structure of this drug includes the methylthiotetrazole (MTT) side chain that has been associated with bleeding disorders. If bleeding occurs, it can be promptly reversed with administration of vitamin K. Monitor prothrombin time regularly.
• With large doses or prolonged therapy, monitor for superinfection, especially in high-risk patients.
• Urine glucose determinations may be false-positive with copper sulfate tests (Clinitest); glucose enzymatic tests (Clinistix, Tes-Tape) are not affected.

ceforanide
Precef

Pregnancy Risk Category: B

HOW SUPPLIED
Injection: 500 mg, 1 g
Infusion: 500 mg, 1 g piggyback

MECHANISM OF ACTION
Inhibits cell wall synthesis, promoting osmotic instability. Usually bactericidal.

INDICATIONS & DOSAGE
Treatment of serious infections of the lower respiratory and urinary tract, skin and skin structure infections, endocarditis, septicemia, and bone and joint infections. Susceptible microorganisms include Streptococcus pneumoniae and pyogenes, Klebsiella pneumoniae, Escherichia coli, Hemophilus influenzae, Proteus mirabilis, and Staphylococcus aureus *and* epidermidis—
Adults: 0.5 to 1 g I.V. or I.M. q 12 hours.
Children: 20 to 40 mg/kg/day in equally divided doses q 12 hours.
Prophylaxis of surgical infections—
Adults: 0.5 to 1 g I.M. or I.V. 1 hour prior to surgery.

Total daily dosage is same for I.M. or I.V. administration and depends on susceptibility of organism and severity of infection. In patients with impaired renal function, doses or frequency of administration must be modified according to degree of renal impairment, severity of infection, and susceptibility of organism. Should be injected deep I.M. into a large muscle mass, such as gluteus or lateral aspect of thigh.

ADVERSE REACTIONS
Blood: transient neutropenia, leukopenia, eosinophilia, thrombocytopenia.
CNS: confusion, headache, lethargy.

GI: *pseudomembranous colitis,* nausea, anorexia, vomiting, diarrhea, glossitis, dyspepsia, abdominal cramps, oral candidiasis (thrush).
GU: genital pruritus and moniliasis, vaginitis.
Hepatic: transient elevation in liver enzymes.
Skin: *maculopapular and erythematous rashes, urticaria.*
Local: *at injection site—pain, induration, sterile abscesses, tissue sloughing; phlebitis and thrombophlebitis with I.V. injection.*
Other: hypersensitivity, dyspnea.

INTERACTIONS
Probenecid: may inhibit excretion and increase blood levels of ceforanide.

NURSING CONSIDERATIONS
• Contraindicated in patients with hypersensitivity to other cephalosporins. Use cautiously in impaired renal function and in those with history of sensitivity to penicillin. Ask patient if he's had a previous reaction to cephalosporin or penicillin therapy before administering first dose.
• Obtain specimen for culture and sensitivity tests before first dose. Therapy may begin pending test results.
• Upon reconstitution, ceforanide injection may appear cloudy. Let stand briefly to allow solution to deaerate and clarify.
• With large doses or prolonged therpay, monitor for superinfection, especially in high-risk patients.
• Ceforanide is a second-generation cephalosporin which may be administered twice daily.

cefotaxime sodium
Claforan

Pregnancy Risk Category: B

HOW SUPPLIED
Injection: 500 mg, 1 g, 2 g

Italicized adverse reactions are common or life-threatening.
*Liquid form contains alcohol.   **May contain tartrazine.

Infusion: 1 g, 2 g
Pharmacy bulk package: 10-g vial

MECHANISM OF ACTION
Inhibits cell wall synthesis, promoting osmotic instability. Usually bactericidal.

INDICATIONS & DOSAGE
Treatment of serious infections of the lower respiratory and urinary tracts, CNS infections, gynecologic infections, bacteremia, septicemia, and skin infections. Among susceptible microorganisms are streptococci, including Streptococcus pneumoniae *and* pyogenes; Staphylococcus aureus *(penicillinase- and nonpenicillinase-producing)* and epidermidis; Escherichia coli; Klebsiella; Hemophilus influenzae; Enterobacter; Proteus; *and* Peptostreptococcus—
Adults: usual dose is 1 g I.V. or I.M. q 6 to 8 hours. Up to 12 g daily can be administered in life-threatening infections.

Total daily dosage is same for I.M. or I.V. administration and depends on susceptibility of organism and severity of infection. In patients with impaired renal function, doses or frequency of administration must be modified according to degree of renal impairment, severity of infection, and susceptibility of organism. Should be injected deep I.M. into a large muscle mass, such as gluteus or lateral aspect of thigh.
Children 1 month to 12 years: 50 to 180 mg/kg/day I.M. or I.V. in 4 to 6 divided doses.
Neonates to 1 week: 50 mg/kg I.V. q 12 hours.
Neonates 1 to 4 weeks: 50 mg/kg I.V. q 8 hours.

ADVERSE REACTIONS
Blood: transient neutropenia, eosinophilia, hemolytic anemia.
CNS: headache, malaise, paresthesias, dizziness.
GI: *pseudomembranous colitis,* nausea, anorexia, vomiting, *diarrhea,* glossitis, dyspepsia, abdominal cramps, tenesmus, anal pruritus, oral candidiasis (thrush).
GU: genital pruritus and moniliasis.
Skin: *maculopapular and erythematous rashes, urticaria.*
Local: *at injection site—pain, induration, sterile abscesses, temperature elevation, tissue sloughing; phlebitis and thrombophlebitis with I.V. injection.*
Other: hypersensitivity, dyspnea, elevated temperature.

INTERACTIONS
Probenecid: may inhibit excretion and increase blood levels of cefotaxime. Use together cautiously.

NURSING CONSIDERATIONS
• Contraindicated in patients with hypersensitivity to other cephalosporins. Use cautiously in impaired renal function and in those with history of sensitivity to penicillin. Ask patient if he's had any reaction to previous cephalosporin or penicillin therapy before administering first dose.
• Obtain specimen for culture and sensitivity tests before first dose. Therapy may begin pending test results.
• With large doses or prolonged therapy, monitor for superinfection, especially in high-risk patients.
• Cefotaxime was the first of the so-called third-generation cephalosporins. It has increased antibacterial activity against gram-negative microorganisms.
• Some doctors may prescribe cefotaxime in clinical situations in which they formerly prescribed aminoglycosides. However, this drug is usually not effective against infections caused by *Pseudomonas* organisms.
• Urine glucose determinations may be false-positive with copper sulfate tests (Clinitest); glucose enzymatic

---

tests (Clinistix, Tes-Tape) are not affected.

cefotetan disodium
Cefotan

Pregnancy Risk Category: B

HOW SUPPLIED
Injection: 1 g, 2 g
Infusion: 1 g, 2 g piggyback

MECHANISM OF ACTION
Inhibits cell wall synthesis, promoting osmotic instability. Usually bactericidal.

INDICATIONS & DOSAGE
Treatment of serious infections of the urinary and lower respiratory tracts, and gynecologic, skin and skin structure, intraabdominal, and bone and joint infections. Among susceptible microorganisms are streptococci, Staphylococcus aureus *(penicillinase- and nonpenicillinase-producing)* and epidermidis, Escherichia coli, Klebsiella, Enterobacter, Proteus, Hemophilus influenzae, Neisseria gonorrhoeae, *and* Bacteroides, including B. fragilis.
Adults: 1 to 2 g I.V. or I.M. q 12 hours for 5 to 10 days. Up to 6 g daily in life-threatening infections.

Total daily dosage is same for I.M. or I.V. administration and depends on susceptibility of organism and severity of infection. In patients with impaired renal function, doses or frequency of administration must be modified according to degree of renal impairment, severity of infection, and susceptibility of organism. Should be injected deep I.M. into a large muscle mass, such as gluteus or lateral aspect of thigh.

ADVERSE REACTIONS
Blood: transient neutropenia, eosinophilia, hemolytic anemia, hypoprothrombinemia, bleeding.

CNS: headache, malaise, paresthesias, dizziness.
GI: *pseudomembranous colitis,* nausea, anorexia, vomiting, *diarrhea,* glossitis, dyspepsia, abdominal cramps, tenesmus, anal pruritus.
GU: genital pruritus and moniliasis.
Skin: *maculopapular and erythematous rashes, urticaria.*
Local: *at injection site—pain, induration, sterile abscesses, tissue sloughing; phlebitis and thrombophlebitis with I.V. injection.*
Other: *hypersensitivity,* dyspnea, elevated temperature.

INTERACTIONS
Ethyl alcohol: may cause a disulfiram-like reaction. Warn patients not to drink alcohol for several days after discontinuing cefotetan.
Oral anticoagulants, aspirin: increased risk of bleeding.
Probenecid: may inhibit excretion and increase blood levels of cefotetan.

NURSING CONSIDERATIONS
• Contraindicated in patients with hypersensitivity to other cephalosporins. Use cautiously in impaired renal status and in those with history of sensitivity to penicillin. Ask patient if he's had any reaction to previous cephalosporin or penicillin therapy before administering first dose.
• Obtain specimen for culture and sensitivity tests before first dose. Therapy may begin pending test results.
• For I.V. use, reconstitute with sterile water for injection. Then, may be mixed with 50 to 100 ml of dextrose 5% in water or 0.9% sodium chloride solution.
• I.M. injection may be reconstituted with sterile water or bacteriostatic water for injection, normal saline, 0.5% or 1% lidocaine hydrochloride. Shake to dissolve and let stand until clear.
• Reconstituted solution remains sta-

Italicized adverse reactions are common or life-threatening.
*Liquid form contains alcohol.   **May contain tartrazine.

ble for 24 hours at room temperature or 96 hours when refrigerated.
• The chemical structure of this drug includes the methylthiotetrazole (MTT) side chain that has been associated with bleeding disorders. However, such bleeding has not been reported with this drug.
• With large doses or prolonged therapy, monitor for superinfection, especially in high-risk patients.
• Cefotetan is similar to cefoxitin in that it's particularly useful in intraabdominal and gynecologic infection (highly active against *B. fragilis*).

cefoxitin sodium
Mefoxin

Pregnancy Risk Category: B

HOW SUPPLIED
Injection: 1 g, 2 g
Infusion: 1 g, 2 g in 50-ml or 100-ml container
Pharmacy bulk package: 10 g

MECHANISM OF ACTION
Inhibits cell wall synthesis, promoting osmotic instability. Usually bactericidal.

INDICATIONS & DOSAGE
Treatment of serious infection of respiratory and genitourinary tracts, skin and soft-tissue infections, bone and joint infections, bloodstream and intra-abdominal infections caused by Escherichia coli *and other coliform bacteria,* Staphylcoccus aureus *(penicillinase- and nonpenicillinase-producing) and* epidermidis, *streptococci,* Klebsiella, Hemophilus influenzae, *and* Bacteroides, *including* B. fragilis—
Adults: 1 to 2 g q 6 to 8 hours for uncomplicated forms of infection. Up to 12 g daily in life-threatening infections.
Children: 80 to 160 mg/kg daily given in 4 to 6 equally divided doses.

Total daily dosage is same for I.M. or I.V. administration and depends on susceptibility of organism and severity of infection. In patients with impaired renal function, doses or frequency of administration must be modified according to degree of renal impairment, severity of infection, and susceptibility of organism. Should be injected deep I.M. into a large muscle mass, such as gluteus or lateral aspect of thigh.

ADVERSE REACTIONS
Blood: transient neutropenia, eosinophilia, hemolytic anemia.
CNS: headache, malaise, paresthesias, dizziness.
GI: *pseudomembranous colitis,* nausea, anorexia, vomiting, *diarrhea,* glossitis, dyspepsia, abdominal cramps, tenesmus, anal pruritus, oral candidiasis (thrush).
GU: genital pruritus and moniliasis.
Skin: *maculopapular and erythematous rashes, urticaria.*
Local: *at injection site—pain, induration, sterile abscesses, tissue sloughing; phlebitis and thrombophlebitis with I.V. injection.*
Other: *hypersensitivity,* dyspnea, elevated temperature.

INTERACTIONS
Probenecid: may inhibit excretion and increase blood levels of cefoxitin.

NURSING CONSIDERATIONS
• Contraindicated in patients with hypersensitivity to other cephalosporins. Use cautiously in impaired renal status and in those with history of sensitivity to penicillin. Ask patient if he's had any reaction to previous cephalosporin or penicillin therapy before administering first dose.
• Obtain specimen for culture and sensitivity tests before first dose. Therapy may begin pending test results.
• A very useful cephalosporin when

anaerobic or mixed aerobic-anaerobic infection is suspected, especially *B. fragilis*.
• Associated with development of thrombophlebitis. Assess I.V. site frequently.
• For I.V. use, reconstitute 1 g with at least 10 ml of sterile water for injection, and 2 g with 10 to 20 ml. Solutions of dextrose 5% and 0.9% sodium chloride for injection can also be used.
• I.M. injection can be reconstituted with 0.5% or 1% lidocaine HCl (without epinephrine) to minimize pain.
• After reconstitution, remains stable for 24 hours at room temperature or 1 week under refrigeration.
• With large doses or prolonged therapy, monitor for superinfection, especially in high-risk patients.
• Urine glucose determinations may be false-positive with copper sulfate tests (Clinitest); glucose enzymatic tests (Clinistix, Tes-Tape) are not affected.

ceftazidime
Fortaz, Magnacef†, Tazicef, Tazidime

Pregnancy Risk Category: B

HOW SUPPLIED
Injection: 500 mg, 1 g, 2 g
Infusion: 1 g, 2 g in 100-ml vials and bags
Pharmacy bulk package: 6 g

MECHANISM OF ACTION
Inhibits cell wall synthesis, promoting osmotic instability. Usually bactericidal.

INDICATIONS & DOSAGE
Treatment of serious infections of the lower respiratory and urinary tracts, gynecologic infections, bacteremia, septicemia, intraabdominal infections, CNS infections, and skin infec-tions. Among susceptible microorganisms are streptococci, including Streptococcus pneumoniae *and* pyogenes; Staphylococcus aureus *(penicillinase- and nonpenicillinase-producing);* Escherichia coli; Klebsiella; Proteus; Enterobacter; Hemophilus influenzae; Pseudomonas; *and some strains of* Bacteroides—
Adults: 1 g I.V. or I.M. q 8 to 12 hours; up to 6 g daily in life-threatening infections.
Children 1 month to 12 years: 30 to 50 mg/kg I.V. q 8 hours.
Neonates 0 to 4 weeks: 30 mg/kg I.V. q 12 hours.
   Total daily dosage is same for I.M. or I.V. administration and depends on susceptibility of organism and severity of infection. In patients with impaired renal function, doses or frequency of administration must be modified according to degree of renal impairment, severity of infection, and susceptibility of organism. Should be injected deep I.M. into a large muscle mass, such as gluteus or lateral aspect of thigh.

ADVERSE REACTIONS
Blood: *eosinophilia; thrombocytosis,* leukopenia.
CNS: headache, dizziness.
GI: *pseudomembranous enterocolitis,* nausea, vomiting, diarrhea, dysgeusia, abdominal cramps.
GU: genital pruritus and moniliasis.
Hepatic: transient elevation in liver enzymes.
Skin: *maculopapular and erythematous rashes, urticaria.*
Local: *at injection site—pain, induration, sterile abscesses, tissue sloughing; phlebitis and thrombophlebitis with I.V. injection.*
Other: *hypersensitivity,* dyspnea, elevated temperature.

INTERACTIONS
Sodium bicarbonate–containing solu-

Italicized adverse reactions are common or life-threatening.
*Liquid form contains alcohol.   **May contain tartrazine.

tions: make ceftazidime unstable.
Don't mix together.

NURSING CONSIDERATIONS
• Contraindicated in patients with hypersensitivity to other cephalosporins. Use cautiously in patients with history of sensitivity to penicillin. Ask patient if he's had any previous reaction to cephalosporin or penicillin therapy before administering first dose.
• Obtain specimen for culture and sensitivity tests before first dose. Therapy may begin pending test results.
• The vials of ceftazidime are supplied under reduced pressure. When the antibiotic is dissolved, carbon dioxide is released and a positive pressure develops. Each brand of ceftazidime includes specific instructions for reconstitution. Read and follow these instructions carefully.
• This third-generation cephalosporin has excellent activity against infections caused by *Pseudomonas aeruginosa.* May be prescribed for these infections, especially when aminoglycosides are potentially too dangerous.
• With large doses or prolonged therapy, monitor for superinfection, especially in high-risk patients.

ceftizoxime sodium
Cefizox

Pregnancy Risk Category: B

HOW SUPPLIED
Injection: 1 g, 2 g
Infusion: 1 g, 2 g in 100-mg vials, or 50 ml in D₅W

MECHANISM OF ACTION
Inhibits cell wall synthesis, promoting osmotic instability. Usually bactericidal.

INDICATIONS & DOSAGE
Treatment of serious infections of the lower respiratory and urinary tracts, *gynecologic infections, bacteremia, septicemia, meningitis, intraabdominal infections, bone and joint infections, and skin infections. Among susceptible microorganisms are streptococci, including* Streptococcus pneumoniae *and* pyogenes; Staphylococcus aureus *(penicillinase- and nonpenicillinase-producing)* and epidermidis; Escherichia coli; Klebsiella; Hemophilus influenzae; Enterobacter; Proteus; *some* Pseudomonas; and Peptostreptococcus—
Adults: usual dosage is 1 to 2 g I.V. or I.M. q 8 to 12 hours. In life-threatening infections, up to 2 g q 4 hours.

Total daily dosage is same for I.M. or I.V. administration and depends on susceptibility of organism and severity of infection. In patients with impaired renal function, doses or frequency of administration must be modified according to degree of renal impairment, severity of infection, and susceptibility of organism. Should be injected deep I.M. into a large muscle mass, such as gluteus or lateral aspect of thigh.

ADVERSE REACTIONS
Blood: transient neutropenia, eosinophilia, hemolytic anemia.
CNS: headache, malaise, paresthesias, dizziness.
GI: *pseudomembranous colitis,* nausea, anorexia, vomiting, *diarrhea,* glossitis, dyspepsia, abdominal cramps, tenesmus, anal pruritus.
GU: genital pruritus and moniliasis.
Skin: *maculopapular and erythematous rashes, urticaria.*
Local: *at injection site—pain, induration, sterile abscesses, tissue sloughing; phlebitis and thrombophlebitis with I.V. injection.*
Other: hypersensitivity, dyspnea, elevated temperature.

INTERACTIONS
Probenecid: may inhibit excretion and increase blood levels of ceftizoxime.

NURSING CONSIDERATIONS

• Contraindicated in patients with hypersensitivity to other cephalosporins. Use cautiously in impaired renal function and in those with history of sensitivity to penicillin. Ask patient if he's had any reaction to previous cephalosporin or penicillin therapy before administering first dose.

• Obtain specimen for culture and sensitivity tests before first dose. Therapy may begin pending test results.

• With large doses or prolonged therapy, monitor for superinfection, especially in high-risk patients.

• Ceftizoxime is a third-generation cephalosporin, which is comparable in activity to cefotaxime, moxalactam, ceftriaxone and cefoperazone. No significant degree of bleeding or disulfiram-type reaction has been reported with its use.

---

ceftriaxone sodium
Rocephin

Pregnancy Risk Category: B

HOW SUPPLIED
Injection: 250 mg, 500 mg, 1 g, 2 g
Infusion: 1 g, 2 g
Pharmacy bulk package: 10 g

MECHANISM OF ACTION
Inhibits cell wall synthesis, promoting osmotic instability. Usually bactericidal.

INDICATIONS & DOSAGE
Treatment of serious infections of the CNS (meningitis), lower respiratory and urinary tracts, gynecological infections, bacteremia, septicemia, intraabdominal infections, and skin infections and Lyme disease. Susceptible microorganisms are streptococci, including Streptococcus pneumoniae *and* pyogenes; Staphylococcus aureus *(penicillinase- and nonpenicillinase-producing)* and epidermidis; Escherichia coli; Klebsiella; Hemophilus influenzae; Neisseria meningitidis; Enterobacter; Proteus; Pseudomonas; Peptostreptococcus *and* Serratia marcescens—

Adults: 1 to 2 g I.M. or I.V. once daily or in equally divided doses twice daily. Total daily dose should not exceed 4 g.
Children: 50 to 75 mg/kg, given in divided doses q 12 hours.
Treatment of meningitis—
Adults and children: 100 mg/kg given in divided doses q 12 hours. May give loading dose of 75 mg/kg.

Total daily dose is same for I.M. or I.V. administration and depends on susceptibility of organism and severity of infection. Should be injected deep I.M. into a large muscle mass, such as gluteus or lateral aspect of thigh.

ADVERSE REACTIONS
Blood: *eosinophilia; thrombocytosis,* leukopenia.
CNS: headache, dizziness.
GI: *pseudomembranous enterocolitis,* nausea, vomiting, diarrhea, dysgeusia, abdominal cramps.
GU: genital pruritus and moniliasis.
Hepatic: transient elevation in liver enzymes.
Skin: *maculopapular and erythematous rashes, urticaria.*
Local: *at injection site—pain, induration, sterile abscesses, tissue sloughing; phlebitis and thrombophlebitis with I.V. injection.*
Other: hypersensitivity, dyspnea, elevated temperature.

INTERACTIONS
None significant.

NURSING CONSIDERATIONS
• Contraindicated in patients with hypersensitivity to other cephalosporins. Use cautiously in history of sensitivity to penicillin. Ask patient if he's had any previous reaction to cephalospo-

---

Italicized adverse reactions are common or life-threatening.
*Liquid form contains alcohol.   **May contain tartrazine.

rin or penicillin therapy before administering first dose.
• Obtain specimen for culture and sensitivity tests before first dose. Therapy may begin pending test results.
• A third-generation cephalosporin with the longest half-life of any available cephalosporin. Allows once-daily dose regimen.
• Dosage adjustment generally not needed in patients with renal insufficiency.
• Commonly used in home antibiotic programs for outpatient treatment of serious infections, such as osteomyelitis.
• With large doses or prolonged therapy, monitor for superinfection, especially in high-risk patients.

cefuroxime axetil
Ceftin

cefuroxime sodium
Kefurox, Zinacef

Pregnancy Risk Category: B

HOW SUPPLIED
axetil
Tablets: 125 mg, 250 mg, 500 mg
sodium
Injection: 750 mg, 1.5 g
Infusion: 750 mg, 1.5 g premixed, frozen solution

MECHANISM OF ACTION
Inhibits cell wall synthesis, promoting osmotic instability. Usually bactericidal.

INDICATIONS & DOSAGE
Treatment of serious infections of the lower respiratory and urinary tract; skin and skin structure infections; septicemia, meningitis, and gonorrhea. Among susceptible organisms are Streptococcus pneumoniae and pyogenes, Hemophilus influenzae, Klebsiella, Staphylococcus aureus,

Escherichia coli, Enterobacter, *and* Neisseria gonorrhoeae—
Adults: Usual dosage of cefuroxime sodium is 750 mg to 1.5 g I.M. or I.V. q 8 hours, usually for 5 to 10 days. For life-threatening infections and infections caused by less susceptible organisms, 1.5 g I.M. or I.V. q 6 hours; for bacterial meningitis, up to 3 g I.V. q 6 hours.
Alternatively, administer cefuroxime axetil 250 mg P.O. q 12 hours. For severe infections or less susceptible organisms, dosage may be increased to 500 mg P.O. q 12 hours.
Children and infants over 3 months: 50 to 100 mg/kg/day cefuroxime sodium I.M. or I.V. Higher doses are administered when treating meningitis. Alternatively, give cefuroxime axetil 125 mg P.O. q 12 hours.
Uncomplicated urinary tract infections—
Adults: 125 to 250 mg P.O. q 12 hours.
Otitis media—
Children under 2 years: 125 mg P.O. q 12 hours.
Children 2 years and over: 250 mg P.O. q 12 hours.

ADVERSE REACTIONS
Blood: transient neutropenia, eosinophilia, hemolytic anemia, decrease in hemoglobin and hematocrit.
CNS: headache, malaise, paresthesias, dizziness.
GI: *pseudomembranous colitis,* nausea, anorexia, vomiting, *diarrhea,* glossitis, dyspepsia, abdominal cramps, tenesmus, anal pruritus.
GU: genital pruritus and moniliasis.
Skin: *maculopapular and erythematous rashes, urticaria.*
Local: *at injection site—pain, induration, sterile abscesses, temperature elevation, tissue sloughing; phlebitis and thrombophlebitis with I.V. injection.*
Other: hypersensitivity, dyspnea.

INTERACTIONS
Probenecid: may inhibit excretion and increase blood levels of cefuroxime.

NURSING CONSIDERATIONS
• Contraindicated in hypersensitivity to other cephalosporins. Use cautiously in patients with impaired renal function and in those with history of sensitivity to penicillin. Ask patient if he's had any reaction to previous cephalosporin or penicillin therapy before administering first dose.
• Total daily dosage is same for I.M. or I.V. administration and depends on susceptibility of organism and severity of infection. In patients with impaired renal function, doses or frequency of administration must be modified according to degree of renal impairment, severity of infection, and susceptibility of organism. Should be injected deep I.M. into a large muscle mass, such as gluteus or lateral aspect of thigh.
• Absorption of cefuroxime axetil is enhanced by food.
• Cefuroxime axetil is available only in tablet form, which may be crushed for patients who cannot swallow tablets. However, it has a bitter taste that is difficult to mask, even with food. Alternative therapy may be necessary.
• Obtain specimen for culture and sensitivity tests before first dose. Therapy may begin pending test results.
• With large doses or prolonged therapy, monitor for superinfection, especially in high-risk patients.
• Cefuroxime is a second-generation cephalosporin similar to cefamandole. However, cefuroxime has not been associated with prothrombin deficiency and bleeding as are some of the other cephalosporins. Advantage over some other cephalosporins is that cefuroxime is useful in treating meningitis.

cephalexin monohydrate
Ceporex†‡, Keflet, Keflex, Keftab, Novolexin†

Pregnancy Risk Category: B

HOW SUPPLIED
Tablets: 250 mg, 500 mg, 1 g
Capsules: 500 mg, 1,250 mg
Oral suspension: 100 mg/5 ml, 125 mg/5 ml, 250 mg/5 ml

MECHANISM OF ACTION
Inhibits cell wall synthesis, promoting osmotic instability. Usually bactericidal.

INDICATIONS & DOSAGE
Treatment of infections of respiratory or genitourinary tract, skin and soft-tissue infections, bone and joint infections, and otitis media due to Escherichia coli *and other coliform bacteria,* group A beta-hemolytic streptococci, Hemophilus influenzae, Klebsiella, Proteus mirabilis, Streptococcus pneumoniae, *and staphylococci—*
Adults: 250 mg to 1 g P.O. q 6 hours.
Children: 6 to 12 mg/kg P.O. q 6 hours. Maximum 25 mg/kg q 6 hours.

ADVERSE REACTIONS
Blood: transient neutropenia, eosinophilia, anemia.
CNS: dizziness, headache, malaise, paresthesias.
GI: *pseudomembranous colitis, nausea, anorexia,* vomiting, *diarrhea,* glossitis, dyspepsia, abdominal cramps, anal pruritus, tenesmus, oral candidiasis (thrush).
GU: genital pruritus and moniliasis, vaginitis.
Skin: *maculopapular and erythematous rashes, urticaria.*
Other: *hypersensitivity,* dyspnea.

INTERACTIONS
Probenecid: may increase blood levels of cephalosporins.

Italicized adverse reactions are common or life-threatening.
*Liquid form contains alcohol.   **May contain tartrazine.

NURSING CONSIDERATIONS

• Use cautiously in impaired renal function and in those with history of sensitivity to penicillin. Ask patient if he's had any reaction to previous cephalosporin or penicillin therapy before administering first dose.
• Obtain specimen for culture and sensitivity tests before first dose. Therapy may begin pending test results.
• Tell patient to take medication exactly as prescribed, even after he feels better. Group A beta-hemolytic streptococcal infections should be treated for a minimum of 10 days.
• Tell patient to take with food or milk to lessen GI discomfort.
• Call doctor if skin rash develops.
• Preparation of oral suspension: add required amount of water to powder in two portions. Shake well after each addition. After mixing, store in refrigerator. Stable for 14 days without significant loss of potency. Keep tightly closed and shake well before using.
• With large doses or prolonged therapy, monitor for superinfection, especially in high-risk patients.
• About 40% to 75% of patients receiving cephalosporins show a false-positive direct Coombs' test, but only a few of these indicate hemolytic anemia.
• Urine glucose determinations may be false-positive with copper sulfate tests (Clinitest); glucose enzymatic tests (Clinistix, Tes-Tape) are not affected.

cephalothin sodium
Ceporacin†‡ ,Keflin

Pregnancy Risk Category: B

HOW SUPPLIED
Injection: 1 g, 2 g, 4 g
Infusion: 1 g/50 ml, 2 g/50 ml, 1 g/dl, 2 g/dl
Pharmacy bulk package: 10 g, 20 g

MECHANISM OF ACTION
Inhibits cell wall synthesis, promoting osmotic instability. Usually bactericidal.

INDICATIONS & DOSAGE
Treatment of serious infections of respiratory, genitourinary, or gastrointestinal tract; skin and soft-tissue infections (including peritonitis); bone and joint infections; septicemia; and endocarditis due to Escherichia coli *and other coliform bacteria, Enterobacteriaceae, enterococci, gonococci, group A beta-hemolytic streptococci,* Hemophilus influenzae, Klebsiella, Proteus mirabilis, Salmonella, Staphylococcus aureus, Shigella, Streptococcus pneumoniae and viridans, and *staphylococci*—
Adults: 500 mg to 1 g I.M. or I.V. (or intraperitoneally) q 4 to 6 hours; in life-threatening infections, up to 2 g q 4 hours.
Children: 14 to 27 mg/kg I.V. q 4 hours, or 20 to 40 mg/kg q 6 hours; dose should be proportionately less in accordance with age, weight, and severity of infection.

Dosage schedule is determined by degree of renal impairment, severity of infection, and susceptibility of causative organism. Should be injected deep I.M. into a large muscle mass, such as gluteus or lateral aspect of thigh. I.V. route is preferable in severe or life-threatening infections.

ADVERSE REACTIONS
Blood: transient neutropenia, eosinophilia, hemolytic anemia.
CNS: headache, malaise, paresthesias, dizziness.
GI: *pseudomembranous colitis*, nausea, anorexia, vomiting, *diarrhea*, glossitis, dyspepsia, abdominal cramps, tenesmus, anal pruritus, oral candidiasis (thrush).
GU: *nephrotoxicity*, genital pruritus and moniliasis.

Skin: *maculopapular and erythematous rashes, urticaria.*
Local: *at injection site—pain, induration, sterile abscesses, tissue sloughing; phlebitis and thrombophlebitis with I.V. injection.*
Other: *hypersensitivity,* dyspnea, fever.

INTERACTIONS
Aminoglycosides: increased nephrotoxicity. Monitor kidney function tests carefully.
Probenecid: may increase blood levels of cephalosporins. Use together cautiously.

NURSING CONSIDERATIONS
• Use cautiously in impaired renal function and in those with history of sensitivity to penicillin. Ask patient if he's had any reaction to previous cephalosporin or penicillin therapy before administering first dose.
• Obtain specimen for culture and sensitivity tests before first dose. Therapy may begin pending test results.
• Drug causes severe pain when administered I.M.; avoid this route if possible.
• When giving this drug I.V., check frequently for vein irritation and phlebitis. Alternate injection sites if I.V. therapy lasts longer than 3 days. Use of small I.V. needle in the larger available veins may be preferable. Addition of a small concentration of heparin (100 units) or hydrocortisone (10 to 25 mg) may reduce incidence of phlebitis.
• For I.M. administration, reconstitute each gram of cephalothin sodium with 4 ml of sterile water for injection, providing 500 mg in each 2.2 ml. If vial contents do not dissolve completely, add an additional 0.2 to 0.4 ml diluent, and warm contents slightly.
• For I.V. administration, dilute contents of 4-g vial with at least 20 ml of sterile water for injection, dextrose 5% injection, or 0.9% sodium chloride injection and add to one of following I.V. solutions: acetated Ringer's injection, dextrose 5% injection, dextrose 5% in lactated Ringer's injection, Ionosol B in dextrose 5% in water, lactated Ringer's injection, Normosol-N in dextrose 5% in water, Plasma-Lyte injection, Plasma-Lyte-N injection in dextrose 5%, Ringer's injection, or 0.9% sodium chloride injection. Choose solution and fluid volume according to patient's fluid and electrolyte status.
• With large doses or prolonged therpay, monitor for superinfection, especially in high-risk patients.
• About 40% to 75% of patients receiving cephalosporins show a false-positive direct Coombs' test; only a few of these indicate hemolytic anemia.
• Urine glucose determinations may be false-positive with copper sulfate tests (Clinitest); glucose enzymatic tests (Clinistix, Tes-Tape) are not affected.

cephapirin sodium
Cefadyl
Pregnancy Risk Category: B

HOW SUPPLIED
Injection: 500-mg, 1-g, 2-g vials; 1-g, 2-g, 4-g piggyback vials; 20-g pharmacy bulk package

MECHANISM OF ACTION
Inhibits cell wall synthesis, promoting osmotic instability. Usually bactericidal.

INDICATIONS & DOSAGE
Serious infections of respiratory, genitourinary, or gastrointestinal tract; skin and soft-tissue infections; bone and joint infections (including osteomyelitis); septicemia; endocarditis due to Streptococcus pneumoniae, Esche-

---

richia coli, *group A beta-hemolytic streptococci,* Hemophilus influenzae, Klebsiella, Proteus mirabilis, Staphylococcus aureus, *and* Streptococcus viridans—

Adults: 500 mg to 1 g I.V. or I.M. q 4 to 6 hours up to 12 g daily.

Children over 3 months: 10 to 20 mg/kg I.V. or I.M. q 6 hours; dose depends on age, weight, and severity of infection.

Should be injected deep I.M. into a large muscle mass, such as gluteus or lateral aspect of thigh. Depending on causative organism and severity of infection, patients with reduced renal function may be treated adequately with a lower dose (7.5 to 15 mg/kg q 12 hours). Patients with severely reduced renal function and who are to be dialyzed should receive same dose just before dialysis and q 12 hours thereafter.

ADVERSE REACTIONS

Blood: transient neutropenia, eosinophilia, anemia.
CNS: dizziness, headache, malaise, paresthesias.
GI: *pseudomembranous colitis,* nausea, anorexia, vomiting, *diarrhea,* glossitis, dyspepsia, abdominal cramps, tenesmus, anal pruritus, oral candidiasis (thrush).
GU: genital pruritus and moniliasis, vaginitis.
Skin: *maculopapular and erythematous rashes, urticaria.*
Local: *at injection site—pain, induration, sterile abscesses, tissue sloughing; phlebitis and thrombophlebitis with I.V. injection.*
Other: *hypersensitivity,* dyspnea.

INTERACTIONS

Probenecid: may increase blood levels of cephalosporins.

NURSING CONSIDERATIONS

• Use cautiously in impaired renal function and in those with a history of sensitivity to penicillin. Ask patient if he's had any reaction to previous cephalosporin or penicillin therapy before administering first dose.
• Obtain specimen for culture and sensitivity tests before first dose. Therapy may begin pending test results.
• For I.M. administration, reconstitute 1-g vial with 2 ml sterile water for injection or bacteriostatic water for injection so that 1.2 ml contains 500 mg of cephapirin. I.M. injection is painful; prepare patient for this.
• When giving this drug I.V., check frequently for vein irritation and phlebitis. Alternate injection sites if I.V. therapy lasts longer than 3 days. Use of small I.V. needles in the larger available veins may be preferable.
• Prepare I.V. infusion using dextrose injection, sodium chloride injection, or bacteriostatic water for injection as diluent: 20 ml yields 1 g per 10 ml; 50 ml yields 1 g per 25 ml; 100 ml yields 1 g per 50 ml.
• I.V. infusion with Y-tubing: during infusion of cephapirin solution, it is desirable to stop other solution. Check volume of cephapirin solution carefully so that calculated dose is infused. When Y-tubing is used, dilute 4-g vial with 40 ml of diluent.
• Reconstituted cephapirin is stable and compatible for 10 days under refrigeration and for 24 hours at room temperature.
• With large doses or prolonged therapy, monitor for superinfection, especially in high-risk patients.
• About 40% to 75% of patients receiving cephalosporins show a false-positive direct Coombs' test, but only a few indicate hemolytic anemia.
• Urine glucose determinations may be false-positive with copper sulfate tests (Clinitest); glucose enzymatic tests (Clinistix, Tes-Tape) are not affected.

---

cephradine
Anspor, Velosef**

Pregnancy Risk Category: B

HOW SUPPLIED
Capsules: 250 mg, 500 mg
Oral suspension: 125 mg/5 ml, 250 mg/5 ml
Injection: 250 mg, 500 mg, 1 g, 2 g, 4 g
Infusion: 2 g

MECHANISM OF ACTION
Inhibits cell wall synthesis, promoting osmotic instability. Usually bactericidal.

INDICATIONS & DOSAGE
Serious infection of respiratory, genitourinary, or gastrointestinal tract; skin and soft-tissue infections; bone and joint infections; septicemia; endocarditis; and otitis media due to Escherichia coli *and other coliform bacteria,* group A beta-hemolytic streptococci, Hemophilus influenzae, Klebsiella, Proteus mirabilis, Staphylococcus aureus, Streptococcus pneumoniae and viridans, and *staphylococci—*
Adults: 500 mg to 1 g I.M. or I.V. 2 to 4 times daily; do not exceed 8 g daily. Or 250 to 500 mg P.O. q 6 hours. Severe or chronic infections may require larger and/or more frequent doses (up to 1 g P.O. q 6 hours).
Children over 1 year: 6 to 12 mg/kg P.O. q 6 hours. 12 to 25 mg/kg I.M. or I.V. q 6 hours.
Otitis media—19 to 25 mg/kg P.O. q 6 hours. Do not exceed 4 g daily.

All patients, regardless of age and weight: larger doses (up to 1 g q.i.d.) may be given for severe or chronic infections. Parenteral therapy may be followed by oral. Injections should be given deep I.M. into a large muscle mass, such as gluteus or lateral aspect of thigh.

ADVERSE REACTIONS
Blood: transient neutropenia, eosinophilia.
CNS: dizziness, headache, malaise, paresthesias.
GI: *pseudomembranous colitis, nausea, anorexia,* vomiting, heartburn, glossitis, dyspepsia, abdominal cramping, *diarrhea,* tenesmus, anal pruritus, oral candidiasis (thrush).
GU: genital pruritus and moniliasis, vaginitis.
Skin: *maculopapular and erythematous rashes, urticaria.*
Local: *at injection site—pain, induration, sterile abscesses, tissue sloughing; phlebitis and thrombophlebitis with I.V. injection.*
Other: *hypersensitivity,* dyspnea.

INTERACTIONS
Probenecid: may increase blood levels of cephalosporins.

NURSING CONSIDERATIONS
• Contraindicated in patients with hypersensitivity to other cephalosporins.
• Use cautiously in impaired renal function and in those with a history of sensitivity to penicillin. Ask patient if he's had any reaction to previous cephalosporin or penicillin therapy before administering first dose.
• Obtain specimen for culture and sensitivity tests before first dose. Therapy may begin pending test results.
• When giving this drug I.V., check frequently for vein irritation and phlebitis. Alternate injection sites if I.V. therapy lasts longer than 3 days. Use of small I.V. needle in the larger available veins may be preferable.
• Tell patient to take medication exactly as prescribed, even after he feels better. Group A beta-hemolytic streptococcal infections should be treated for a minimum of 10 days.
• Tell patient to take the oral dosage form with food or milk to lessen GI discomfort.

Italicized adverse reactions are common or life-threatening.
*Liquid form contains alcohol.   **May contain tartrazine.

- I.M. injection is painful.
- For I.M. administration, reconstitute with sterile water for injection or with bacteriostatic water for injection as follows: 1.2 ml to 250-mg vial; 2 ml to 500-mg vial; 4 ml to 1-g vial. I.M. solutions must be used within 2 hours if kept at room temperature and within 24 hours if refrigerated. Solutions may vary in color from light straw to yellow without affecting potency.
- When preparing cephradine for intravenous administration, when available, use preparation specifically supplied for infusion. Follow specific product directions carefully when reconstituting.
- With large doses or prolonged therapy, monitor for superinfection, especially in high-risk patients.
- About 40% to 75% of patients receiving cephalosporins show a false-positive direct Coombs' test, but only a few indicate hemolytic anemia.
- Urine glucose determinations may be false-positive with copper sulfate tests (Clinitest); glucose enzymatic tests (Clinistix, Tes-Tape) are not affected.
- Cephradine is the only cephalosporin available in both oral and injectable forms.

---

moxalactam disodium (latamoxef disodium)

Moxalactam‡, Moxam

Pregnancy Risk Category: C

HOW SUPPLIED
Parenteral: 1 g, 2 g

MECHANISM OF ACTION
Inhibits cell wall synthesis, promoting osmotic instability. Usually bactericidal.

INDICATIONS & DOSAGE
Treatment of serious infections of lower respiratory and urinary tract, *CNS infections, intraabdominal infections, gynecologic infections, bacteremia, septicemia, and skin infections. Susceptible microorganisms include* Streptococcus pneumoniae *and* pyogenes; Staphylococcus aureus *(penicillinase- and nonpenicillinase-producing)* and epidermidis; Escherichia coli; Klebsiella; Hemophilus influenzae; Enterobacter; Proteus; *some* Pseudomonas; *and* Peptostreptococcus—

Adults: Usual daily dose is 2 to 6 g I.M. or I.V. administered in divided doses q 8 hours for 5 to 10 days, or up to 14 days. Up to 12 g daily may be needed in life-threatening infections or in infections due to less susceptible organisms.

Children: 50 mg/kg I.M. or I.V. q 6 to 8 hours.

Neonates: 50 mg/kg I.M. or I.V. q 8 to 12 hours.

Total daily dosage is same for I.M. or I.V. administration and depends on susceptibility of organism and severity of infection. In patients with impaired renal function, doses or frequency of administration must be modified according to degree of impairment, severity of infection, and susceptibility of organism. Should be injected deep I.M. into the gluteus or lateral aspect of thigh.

ADVERSE REACTIONS
Blood: transient neutropenia, eosinophilia, hemolytic anemia, *hypoprothrombinemia, bleeding.*

CNS: headache, malaise, paresthesias, dizziness.

GI: *pseudomembranous colitis,* nausea, anorexia, vomiting, *diarrhea,* glossitis, dyspepsia, abdominal cramps, tenesmus, pruritus ani, oral candidiasis (thrush).

GU: genital moniliasis.

Skin: *maculopapular and erythematous rashes,* urticaria.

Local: *pain at injection site, induration, sterile abscesses, tissue slough-*

---

*ing; phlebitis and thrombophlebitis
with I.V. injection.*
Other: *hypersensitivity,* dyspnea, elevated temperature.

INTERACTIONS
Ethyl alcohol: may cause a disulfiram-like reaction. Warn patients not to drink alcohol for several days after discontinuing moxalactam.
Oral anticoagulants, aspirin: increased risk of bleeding.

NURSING CONSIDERATIONS
• Contraindicated in patients with hypersensitivity to other cephalosporins. Use cautiously in impaired renal function and in those with history of sensitivity to penicillin. Before giving first dose, ask patient if he's had any reaction to penicillin.
• Obtain specimen for culture and sensitivity tests before first dose. Therapy may begin pending test results.
• For direct intermittent I.V. administration, add 10 ml of sterile water for injection, dextrose 5% injection, or 0.9% NaCl injection/g of moxalactam.
• With large doses or prolonged therapy, monitor for superinfection, especially in high-risk patients.
• Bleeding associated with hypoprothrombinemia can be prevented with vitamin K. Doctor may order 10 mg vitamin K per week to be given prophylactically.
• The chemical structure of this drug includes the methylthiotetrazole (MTT) side chain that has been associated with bleeding disorders. If bleeding occurs, it can be promptly reversed with the administration of vitamin K. Monitor prothrombin times regularly.
• Moxalactam does not interefere with urine glucose determinations.
• Moxalactam is a third-generation cephalosporin.

Italicized adverse reactions are common or life-threatening.
*Liquid form contains alcohol.   **May contain tartrazine.

14

Tetracyclines

demeclocycline hydrochloride
doxycycline
doxycycline hyclate
doxycycline hydrochloride
minocycline hydrochloride
oxytetracycline hydrochloride
tetracycline hydrochloride

COMBINATION PRODUCTS
None.

---

demeclocycline hydrocholoride
Declomycin, Ledermycin‡

Pregnancy Risk Category: D

HOW SUPPLIED
Tablets: 150 mg, 300 mg
Capsules: 150 mg

MECHANISM OF ACTION
Exerts bacteriostatic effect by binding to the 30S ribosomal subunit of microorganisms, thus inhibiting protein synthesis.

INDICATIONS & DOSAGE
Infections caused by susceptible gram-negative and gram-positive organisms, trachoma, rickettsiae—
Adults: 150 mg P.O. q 6 hours or 300 mg P.O. q 12 hours.
Children over 8 years: 6 to 12 mg/kg P.O. daily, divided q 6 to 12 hours.
Gonorrhea—
Adults: 600 mg P.O. initially, then 300 mg P.O. q 12 hours for 4 days (total 3 g).
Uncomplicated urethral, endocervi-cal, or rectal infection caused by Chlamydia trachomatis—
Adults: 300 mg P.O. q.i.d. for at least 7 days.
Syndrome of inappropriate antidiuretic hormone (a hyposmolar state)—
Adults: 600 to 1,200 mg P.O. daily in divided doses.

ADVERSE REACTIONS
Blood: neutropenia, eosinophilia.
CV: pericarditis.
EENT: dysphagia, glossitis.
GI: anorexia, *nausea, vomiting, diarrhea*, enterocolitis, anogenital inflammation.
Metabolic: *increased BUN*, diabetes insipidus syndrome (polyuria, polydipsia, weakness).
Skin: *maculopapular and erythematous rashes, photosensitivity, increased pigmentation, urticaria.*
Other: hypersensitivity.

INTERACTIONS
Antacids (including sodium bicarbonate) and laxatives containing aluminum, magnesium, or calcium; food, milk, or other dairy products: decrease antibiotic absorption. Give antibiotic 1 hour before or 2 hours after any of the above.
Ferrous sulfate and other iron products, zinc: decrease antibiotic absorption. Give demeclocycline 3 hours after or 2 hours before iron administration.
Methoxyflurane: may cause nephrotoxicity with tetracyclines. Monitor carefully.
Oral contraceptives: decreased con-

traceptive effectiveness and increased risk of breakthrough bleeding.

NURSING CONSIDERATIONS
• Use with extreme caution in impaired renal or hepatic function. Use of these drugs during last half of pregnancy and in children under 8 years may cause permanent discoloration of teeth, enamel defects, and retardation of bone growth.
• Obtain specimen for culture and sensitivity tests before first dose. Therapy may begin pending test results.
• Check expiration date. Outdated or deteriorated demeclocycline has been associated with reversible nephrotoxicity (Fanconi's syndrome).
• Do not expose these drugs to light or heat; store in tight container.
• With large doses or prolonged therapy, monitor for superinfection, especially in high-risk patients.
• Check patient's tongue for signs of monilia infection. Stress good oral hygiene.
• Warn patient to avoid direct sunlight and ultraviolet light. A sunscreen may help prevent photosensitivity reactions. Photosensitivity persists for some time after discontinuation of drug.
• Effectiveness is reduced when taken with milk or other dairy products, food, antacids, or iron products. Explain this to patient. Tell patient to take each dose with a full glass of water on an empty stomach, at least 1 hour before meals or 2 hours afterward. Give at least 1 hour before bedtime to prevent esophagitis.
• Instruct patient to take medication for as long as prescribed, exactly as prescribed, even after he feels better, and to take entire amount prescribed.
• May cause false-negative reading of Clinistix or Tes-Tape.

doxycycline
Doxylin‡

doxycycline hyclate
Doxy-100, Doxy-200, Doxy-Caps, Doxychel, Doxy-Lemmon, Doxy-Tabs, Vibramycin, Vibra-Tabs

doxycycline hydrochloride
Cyclidox‡, Doryx‡, Vibramycin‡, Vibramycin IV‡, Vibra-Tabs 50‡

Pregnancy Risk Category: D

HOW SUPPLIED
doxycycline
Tablets: 50 mg‡, 100 mg‡
doxycycline hyclate
Tablets: 50 mg, 100 mg
Capsules: 50 mg, 100 mg
Injection: 100 mg, 200 mg
doxycycline hydrochloride
Tablets: 50 mg‡, 100 mg‡
Capsules: 50 mg‡, 100 mg‡, 250 mg‡
Injection: 100 mg‡

MECHANISM OF ACTION
Exerts bacteriostatic effect by binding to the 30S ribosomal subunit of microorganisms, thus inhibiting protein synthesis.

INDICATIONS & DOSAGE
Infections caused by sensitive gram-negative and gram-positive organisms, trachoma, rickettsiae, Myco-plasma, Chlamydia, and Lyme disease—
Adults: 100 mg P.O. q 12 hours on first day, then 100 mg P.O. daily; or 200 mg I.V. on first day in one or two infusions, then 100 to 200 mg I.V. daily.
Children over 8 years (under 45 kg): 4.4 mg/kg P.O. or I.V. daily, divided q 12 hours first day, then 2.2 to 4.4 mg/kg daily. For children over 45 kg, dosage is same as adults.
  Give I.V. infusion slowly (minimum 1 hour). Infusion must be completed within 12 hours (within 6 hours

---

Italicized adverse reactions are common or life-threatening.
*Liquid form contains alcohol.   **May contain tartrazine.

in lactated Ringer's solution or dextrose 5% in lactated Ringer's solution).

Gonorrhea in patients allergic to penicillin—
Adults: 200 mg P.O. initially, followed by 100 mg P.O. at bedtime, and 100 mg P.O. b.i.d. for 3 days; or 300 mg P.O. initially and repeat dose in 1 hour.

Primary or secondary syphilis in patients allergic to penicillin—
Adults: 300 mg P.O. daily in divided doses for 10 days.

Uncomplicated urethral, endocervical or rectal infections caused by Chlamydia trachomatis *or* Ureaplasma urealyticum—
Adults: 100 mg P.O. b.i.d. for at least 7 days.

To prevent "traveler's diarrhea" commonly caused by enterotoxigenic Escherichia coli—
Adults: 100 mg P.O. daily.

ADVERSE REACTIONS
Blood: neutropenia, eosinophilia.
CNS: intracranial hypertension.
CV: pericarditis.
EENT: sore throat, glossitis, dysphagia.
GI: anorexia, *epigastric distress, nausea*, vomiting, *diarrhea*, enterocolitis, anogenital inflammation.
Skin: *maculopapular and erythematous rashes, photosensitivity, increased pigmentation, urticaria*.
Local: thrombophlebitis.
Other: hypersensitivity.

INTERACTIONS
Antacids (including sodium bicarbonate) and laxatives containing aluminum, magnesium, or calcium: decrease antibiotic absorption. Give antibiotic 1 hour before or 2 hours after any of the above.
Ferrous sulfate and other iron products, zinc: decrease antibiotic absorption. Give doxycycline 3 hours after or 2 hours before iron administration.

Oral contraceptives: decreased contraceptive effectiveness and increased risk of breakthrough bleeding.
Phenobarbital, carbamazepine, alcohol: decrease antibiotic effect. Avoid if possible.

NURSING CONSIDERATIONS
• Use of these drugs during last half of pregnancy and in children under 8 years may cause permanent discoloration of teeth, enamel defects, and retardation of bone growth.
• Patient may develop thrombophlebitis with I.V. administration.
• Obtain specimen for culture and sensitivity tests before first dose. Therapy may begin pending test results.
• Don't expose drug to light or heat. Protect from sunlight during infusion.
• With large doses or prolonged therapy, monitor for superinfection, especially in high-risk patients.
• Check patient's tongue for signs of monilia infection. Stress good oral hygiene.
• May be taken with milk or food if GI adverse effects develop.
• Do not give with antacids.
• Tell patient to take medication exactly as prescribed, even after he feels better, and to take entire amount prescribed.
• Reconstitute powder for injection with sterile water for injection. Use 10 ml in 100-mg vial and 20 ml in 200-mg vial. Dilute solution to 100 to 1,000 ml for I.V. infusion. Do not infuse solutions more concentrated than 1 mg/ml.
• Reconstituted solution is stable for 72 hours refrigerated.
• Doxycycline may be used in patients with renal impairment; does not accumulate or cause a significant rise in BUN.
• Parenteral form may cause false-positive reading of Clinitest. All forms may cause false-negative reading of Clinistix or Tes-Tape.

- Should not be taken within 1 hour of bedtime because of increased incidence of dysphagia.
- Check expiration date. Outdated or deteriorated tetracyclines have been associated with reversible nephrotoxicity (Fanconi's syndrome).

minocycline hydrochloride
Minocin*, Minomycin‡, Minomycin IV‡

Pregnancy Risk Category: D

HOW SUPPLIED
Tablets: 50 mg, 100 mg
Capsules: 50 mg, 100 mg
Oral suspension: 50 mg/5 ml
Injection: 100 mg‡

MECHANISM OF ACTION
Exerts bacteriostatic effect by binding to the 30S ribosomal subunit of microorganisms, thus inhibiting protein synthesis.

INDICATIONS & DOSAGE
Infections caused by sensitive gram-negative and gram-positive organisms, trachoma, amebiasis—
Adults: 200 mg I.V., then 100 mg I.V. q 12 hours. Do not exceed 400 mg/day. Or, give 200 mg P.O. initially, then 100 mg P.O. q 12 hours. Some clinicians use 100 or 200 mg P.O. initially, followed by 50 mg q.i.d.
Children over 8 years: initially, 4 mg/kg P.O. or I.V., followed by 2 mg/kg q 12 hours.
Give I.V. in 500- to 1,000-ml solution without calcium, and administer over 6 hours.
Gonorrhea in patients sensitive to penicillin—
Adults: initially, 200 mg P.O., then 100 mg q 12 hours for 4 days.
Syphilis in patients sensitive to penicillin—
Adults: initially, 200 mg P.O., then 100 mg q 12 hours for 10 to 15 days.
Meningococcal carrier state—

100 mg P.O. q 12 hours for 5 days.
Uncomplicated urethral, endocervical, or rectal infection caused by Chlamydia trachomatis *or* Ureaplasma urealyticam—
Adults: 100 mg P.O. b.i.d. for at least 7 days.
Uncomplicated gonoccocal urethritis in men—
Adults: 100 mg P.O. b.i.d. for 5 days.

ADVERSE REACTIONS
Blood: neutropenia, eosinophilia.
CNS: *light-headedness, dizziness from vestibular toxicity.*
CV: pericarditis.
EENT: dysphagia, glossitis.
GI: *anorexia,* epigastric distress, *nausea,* vomiting, *diarrhea,* enterocolitis, inflammatory lesions in anogenital region.
Metabolic: increased BUN.
Skin: *maculopapular and erythematous rashes, photosensitivity, increased pigmentation, urticaria.*
Local: *thrombophlebitis.*
Other: hypersensitivity.

INTERACTIONS
Antacids (including sodium bicarbonate) and laxatives containing aluminum, magnesium, or calcium: decrease antibiotic absorption. Give antibiotic 1 hour before or 2 hours after any of the above.
Ferrous sulfate and other iron products, zinc: decrease antibiotic absorption. Tetracyclines should be given 3 hours after or 2 hours before iron administration.
Methoxyflurane: may cause severe nephrotoxicity with tetracyclines. Monitor carefully.
Oral contraceptives: decreased contraceptive effectiveness and increased risk of breakthrough bleeding.

NURSING CONSIDERATIONS
- Use with extreme caution in impaired renal or hepatic function. Use during last half of pregnancy and in

---

Italicized adverse reactions are common or life-threatening.
*Liquid form contains alcohol.   **May contain tartrazine.

children under 8 years may cause permanent discoloration of teeth, enamel defects, and retardation of bone growth.
• Patient may develop thrombophlebitis with I.V. administration of this drug. Avoid extravasation.
• Obtain specimen for culture and sensitivity tests before first dose. Therapy may begin pending test results.
• Do not expose these drugs to light or heat. Keep cap tightly closed.
• With large doses or prolonged therapy, monitor for superinfection, especially in high-risk patients.
• Check patient's tongue for signs of monilia infection. Stress good oral hygiene.
• May be taken with food. Tell patient to take medication exactly as prescribed, even after he feels better, and to take entire amount prescribed.
• May cause tooth discoloration in young adults. Observe for brown pigmentation and inform doctor if it occurs.
• Reconstitute 100 mg powder with 5 ml sterile water for injection, with further dilution of 500 to 1,000 ml for I.V. infusion. Stable for 24 hours at room temperature.
• Parenteral form may cause false-positive reading of Clinitest. All forms may cause false-negative reading of Clinistix or Tes-Tape.
• Check expiration date. Outdated or deteriorated tetracyclines have been associated with reversible nephrotoxicity (Fanconi's syndrome).

---

oxytetracycline hydrochloride
E.P. Mycin, Terramycin

Pregnancy Risk Category: D

HOW SUPPLIED
Tablets: 250 mg
Capsules: 250 mg
Injection: (I.V.) 250 mg, 500 mg; (I.M.) 50 mg/ml, 125 mg/ml (with lidocaine 2%)

MECHANISM OF ACTION
Exerts bacteriostatic effect by binding to the 30S ribosomal subunit of microorganisms, thus inhibiting protein synthesis.

INDICATIONS & DOSAGE
Infections caused by sensitive gram-negative and gram-positive organisms, trachoma, rickettsiae—
Adults: 250 mg P.O. q 6 hours; 100 mg I.M. q 8 to 12 hours; 250 mg I.M. as a single dose.
Children over 8 years: 25 to 50 mg/kg P.O. daily, divided q 6 hours; 15 to 25 mg/kg I.M. daily, divided q 8 to 12 hours
Brucellosis—
Adults: 500 mg P.O. q.i.d. for 3 weeks with streptomycin 1 g I.M. q 12 hours first week, once daily second week.
Syphilis in patients sensitive to penicillin—
Adults: 30 to 40 g total dosage P.O., divided equally over 10 to 15 days.
Gonorrhea in patients sensitive to penicillin—
Adults: initially, 1.5 g P.O. followed by 0.5 g q.i.d. for a total of 9 g.

ADVERSE REACTIONS
Blood: neutropenia, eosinophilia.
CNS: intracranial hypertension.
CV: pericarditis.
EENT: dysphagia, glossitis.
GI: *anorexia, nausea,* vomiting, *diarrhea,* enterocolitis, anogenital inflammation.
Metabolic: *increased BUN.*
Skin: *maculopapular and erythematous rashes, urticaria, photosensitivity, increased pigmentation.*
Local: *irritation after I.M. injection, thrombophlebitis.*
Other: hypersensitivity.

INTERACTIONS

Antacids (including sodium bicarbonate) and laxatives containing aluminum, magnesium, or calcium; food, milk, or other dairy products: decrease antibiotic absorption. Give antibiotic 1 hour before or 2 hours after.
Ferrous sulfate and other iron products, zinc: decrease antibiotic absorption. Give tetracyclines 3 hours after or 2 hours before iron administration.
Methoxyflurane: may cause severe nephrotoxicity with tetracyclines.
Oral contraceptives: decreased contraceptive effectiveness and increased risk of breakthrough bleeding.

NURSING CONSIDERATIONS

• Use with extreme caution in impaired renal or hepatic function. Use during last half of pregnancy and in children under 8 years may cause permanent discoloration of teeth, enamel defects, and retardation of bone growth.
• Obtain specimen for culture and sensitivity tests before first dose. Therapy may begin pending test results.
• Check expiration date. Outdated or deteriorated oxytetracyclines have been associated with reversible nephrotoxicity (Fanconi's syndrome).
• Do not expose these drugs to light or heat.
• Inject I.M. dose deeply. Warn that it may be painful. Rotate sites. I.M. preparations contain a local anesthetic; ask patient about hypersensitivity to local anesthetics.
• With large doses or prolonged therapy, monitor for superinfections, especially in high-risk patients.
• Check patient's tongue for signs of monilia infection. Stress good oral hygiene.
• Warn patient to avoid direct sunlight and ultraviolet light. A sunscreen may help prevent photosensitivity reactions. Photosensitivity persists for considerable time after discontinuation of drug.
• Effectiveness is reduced when taken with milk or other dairy products, food, antacids, or iron products. Explain this to patient. Tell patient to take each dose with a full glass of water on an empty stomach, at least 1 hour before meals or 2 hours afterward. Give at least 1 hour before bedtime to prevent esophagitis.
• Tell patient to take medication exactly as prescribed, even after he feels better, and to take entire amount prescribed.
• For I.V. use, reconstitute 250 mg and 500 mg powder for injection with 10 ml sterile water.
• Dilute to at least 100 ml in dextrose 5% in water, normal saline solution, or Ringer's solution. Do not mix with any other drug.
• Store reconstituted solutions in refrigerator. Stable for 48 hours.
• Parenteral form may cause false-positive reading of Clinitest. All forms may cause false-negative reading of Clinistix or Tes-Tape.

---

tetracycline hydrochloride

Achromycin, Achromycin V, Apo-Tetra†, Austramycin V‡, Bristacycline, Cyclopar, Hostacycline P‡, Kesso-Tetra, Nor-Tet, Novotetra†, Panmycin**, Panmycin P‡, Robitet, Sarocycline, Sumycin, Tetracap, Tetracyn, Tetralan, Tetralean†

Pregnancy Risk Category: D

HOW SUPPLIED

Tablets: 250 mg, 500 mg
Capsules: 250 mg, 500 mg
Oral suspension: 125 mg/5 ml
Injection: 100 mg, 250 mg, 500 mg

MECHANISM OF ACTION

Exerts bacteriostatic effect by binding to the 30S ribosomal subunit of mi-

---

Italicized adverse reactions are common or life-threatening.
*Liquid form contains alcohol.   **May contain tartrazine.

croorganisms, thus inhibiting protein synthesis.

INDICATIONS & DOSAGE

Infections caused by sensitive gram-negative and gram-positive organisms, trachoma, rickettsiae, Mycoplasma, *and* Chlamydia—
Adults: 250 to 500 mg P.O. q 6 hours; 250 mg I.M. daily or 150 mg I.M. q 12 hours; or 250 to 500 mg I.V. q 8 to 12 hours (I.M. and I.V. hydrochloride salt only).
Children over 8 years: 25 to 50 mg/kg P.O. daily, divided q 6 hours; 15 to 25 mg/kg daily (maximum 250 mg) I.M. single dose or divided q 8 to 12 hours; or 10 to 20 mg/kg I.V. daily, divided q 12 hours.
Uncomplicated urethral, endocervical, or rectal infection caused by Chlamydia trachomatis—
Adults: 500 mg P.O. q.i.d. for at least 7 days.
Brucellosis—
Adults: 500 mg P.O. q 6 hours for 3 weeks with streptomycin 1 g I.M. q 12 hours week 1 and daily week 2.
Gonorrhea in patients sensitive to penicillin—
Adults: initially, 1.5 g P.O., then 500 mg q 6 hours for 7 days.
Syphilis in patients sensitive to penicillin—
Adults: 30 to 40 g P.O. total in equally divided doses over 10 to 15 days.
Acne—
Adults and adolescents: initially, 250 mg P.O. q 6 hours, then 125 to 500 mg P.O. daily or every other day.
Shigellosis—
Adults: 2.5 g P.O. in 1 dose.

ADVERSE REACTIONS

Blood: neutropenia, eosinophilia.
CNS: dizziness, headache, intracranial hypertension.
CV: pericarditis.
EENT: sore throat, glossitis, dysphagia.
GI: anorexia, *epigastric distress, nausea,* vomiting, *diarrhea,* stomatitis, enterocolitis, inflammatory lesions in anogenital region.
Hepatic: hepatotoxicity with large doses given I.V.
Metabolic: *increased BUN.*
Skin: *maculopapular and erythematous rashes, urticaria, photosensitivity, increased pigmentation.*
Local: *irritation after I.M. injection, thrombophlebitis.*

INTERACTIONS

Antacids (including sodium bicarbonate) and laxatives containing aluminum, magnesium, or calcium; food, milk, or other dairy products: decrease antibiotic absorption. Give antibiotic 1 hour before or 2 hours after any of the above.
Ferrous sulfate and other iron products, zinc: decrease antibiotic absorption. Give tetracyclines 3 hours after or 2 hours before iron administration.
Lithium carbonate: may alter serum lithium levels.
Methoxyflurane: may cause severe nephrotoxicity with tetracyclines.
Oral contraceptives: decreased contraceptive effectiveness and increased risk of breakthrough bleeding.

NURSING CONSIDERATIONS

• Use with extreme caution in impaired renal or hepatic function. Use during last half of pregnancy and in children under 8 years may cause permanent discoloration of teeth, enamel defects, and retardation of bone growth.
• Obtain specimen for culture and sensitivity tests before first dose. Therapy may begin pending test results.
• Effectiveness reduced when taken with milk or other dairy products, food, antacids, or iron products. Explain this to patient. Tell patient to take each dose with a full glass of water on an empty stomach, at least 1

hour before meals or 2 hours afterward. Give at least 1 hour before bedtime to prevent esophagitis.

• Patient may develop thrombophlebitis with I.V. administration. Avoid extravasation.

• Check expiration date. Outdated or deteriorated tetracyclines have been associated with reversible nephrotoxicity (Fanconi's syndrome).

• Discard I.M. solutions after 24 hours because they deteriorate. Exception: discard Achromycin solution in 12 hours.

• Do not expose to light or heat.

• Inject I.M. dose deeply. Warn patient that it may be painful. Rotate sites. I.M. preparations often contain a local anesthetic; ask patient about hypersensitivity to local anesthetics.

• With large doses or prolonged therapy, monitor for superinfection, especially in high-risk patients.

• Check patient's tongue for signs of monilia infection. Stress good oral hygiene.

• Warn patient to avoid direct sunlight and ultraviolet light. A sunscreen may help prevent photosensitivity reactions. Photosensitivity persists after discontinuation of drug.

• Tell patient to take drug exactly as prescribed, even after he feels better, and to take entire amount prescribed.

• For I.V. use, reconstitute 100 mg and 250 mg powder for injection with 5 ml sterile water; with 10 ml for 500 mg. Further dilute in 100 to 1,000 ml volume of dextrose 5% in 0.9% saline solution. Refrigerate diluted solution for I.V. use and use within 24 hours. Exception: use Achromycin solution immediately.

• Do not mix tetracycline solution with any other I.V. additive.

• For I.M. use, reconstitute 100 mg powder for injection with 2 ml sterile water for injection. Concentration will be 50 mg/ml. Amount of diluent for 250-mg injection varies according to brand. Check with pharmacy or follow manufacturer's instructions.

• Parenteral form may cause false-positive reading of Clinitest. All forms may cause false-negative reading of Clinistix or Tes-Tape.

• Tetracycline may be used as a pleural sclerosing agent in malignant pleural effusions. Instilled through chest tube.

Italicized adverse reactions are common or life-threatening.
*Liquid form contains alcohol.   **May contain tartrazine.

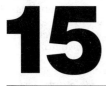

15

Sulfonamides

co-trimoxazole
sulfadiazine
sulfamethoxazole
sulfasalazine
sulfisoxazole

COMBINATION PRODUCTS
AZO GANTANOL, AZO SULFAMETHOX-
AZOLE†, URO GANTANOL†: sulfamethoxazole 500 mg and phenazopyridine hydrochloride 100 mg.
AZO GANTRISIN: sulfisoxazole 500
mg and phenazopyridine hydrochloride 50 mg.
NEOTRIZINE: sulfadiazine 167 mg,
sulfamerazine 167 mg, and sulfa-
methazine 167 mg.
PEDIAZOLE: sulfisoxazole 600 mg and
erythromycin ethylsuccinate 200 mg
per 5 ml.
TERFONYL: sulfadiazine 167 mg, sulfamerazine 167 mg, and sulfametha-
zine 167 mg.
THIOSULFIL-A: sulfamethizole 250
mg and phenazopyridine hydrochloride 50 mg.
TRIPLE SULFA: sulfadiazine 167 mg,
sulfamerazine 167 mg, and sulfa-
methazine 167 mg.
UROBIOTIC-250: sulfamethizole 250
mg, oxytetracycline (as the hydrochloride) 250 mg, and phenazopyridine hydrochloride 50 mg.

co-trimoxazole
(sulfamethoxazole-
trimethoprim)
Apo-Sulfatrim†, Apo-Sulfatrim DS†,
Bactrim*, Bactrim DS, Bactrim I.V.
Infusion, Cotrim, Cotrim D.S.,
Novotrimel†, Novotrimel DS†,
Protrin†, Protrin DF†, Resprim‡,
Roubac†, Roubac DS†, Septra*,
Septra DS, Septra I.V. Infusion,
Septrin‡, SMZ-TMP,
Sulfamethoprim, Sulfamethoprim
DS, Sulmeprim, Trib‡, Uroplus DS,
Uroplus SS

*Pregnancy Risk Category: C (D if
near term)*

HOW SUPPLIED
Tablets: trimethoprim 80 mg and sulfamethoxazole 400 mg; trimethoprim
160 mg and sulfamethoxazole 800 mg
Oral suspension: trimethoprim 40 mg
and sulfamethoxazole 200 mg/5 ml
Injection: trimethoprim 16 mg and
sulfamethoxazole 80 mg/ml (5ml/am-
pule)

MECHANISM OF ACTION
The sulfamethoxazole component inhibits the formation of dihydrofolic
acid from para-aminobenzoic acid
(PABA). The trimethoprim component inhibits dihydrofolate reductase.
Both decrease bacterial folic acid synthesis.

INDICATIONS & DOSAGE
*Urinary tract infections and shigel-
losis—*
Adults: 160 mg trimethoprim/800 mg

sulfa (double strength tablet) P.O. q 12 hours for 10 to 14 days in urinary tract infections and for 5 days in shigellosis. For simple cystitis or acute urethral syndrome, may give one to three double strength tablets as a single dose. If indicated, give by I.V. infusion 8 to 10 mg/kg/day (based upon trimethoprim component) in two to four divided doses q 6, 8, or 12 hours for up to 14 days.

Children: 8 mg/kg trimethoprim/40 mg/kg sulfa P.O. per 24 hours, in two divided doses q 12 hours (10 days for urinary tract infections; for 5 days in shigellosis).

Otitis media—

Children: 8 mg/kg trimethoprim/40 mg/kg sulfa P.O. per 24 hours, in two divided doses q 12 hours for 10 days. Pneumocystis carinii *pneumonitis—*

Adults and children: 20 mg/kg trimethoprim/100 mg/kg sulfa P.O. per 24 hours, in equally divided doses q 6 hours for 14 days. If indicated, give by I.V. infusion 15 to 20 mg/kg/day (based upon trimethoprim component) in three or four divided doses q 6 to 8 hours for up to 14 days.

Chronic bronchitis—

Adults: 160 mg trimethoprim/800 mg sulfa P.O. q 12 hours for 10 to 14 days. Not recommended for infants under 2 months old.

ADVERSE REACTIONS

Blood: *agranulocytosis, aplastic anemia,* megaloblastic anemia, thrombocytopenia, leukopenia, hemolytic anemia.

CNS: headache, mental depression, seizures, hallucinations.

GI: *nausea, vomiting, diarrhea,* abdominal pain, anorexia, stomatitis.

GU: toxic nephrosis with oliguria and anuria, crystalluria, hematuria.

Hepatic: jaundice.

Skin: *erythema multiforme (Stevens-Johnson syndrome), generalized skin eruption, epidermal necrolysis, exfoli-ative dermatitis,* photosensitivity, urticaria, pruritus.

Other: *hypersensitivity, serum sickness, drug fever, anaphylaxis.*

INTERACTIONS

Ammonium chloride, ascorbic acid: doses sufficient to acidify urine may cause precipitation of sulfonamide and crystalluria. Don't use together.

Oral anticoagulants: increased anticoagulant effect.

Oral contraceptives: decreased contraceptive effectiveness and increased risk of breakthrough bleeding.

Oral hypoglycemic agents: increased hypoglycemic effect.

NURSING CONSIDERATIONS

• Contraindicated in porphyria. Use cautiously and in reduced dosages in impaired hepatic or renal function and in those with severe allergy or bronchial asthma, G6PD deficiency, and blood dyscrasias.

• Adverse reactions, especially hypersensitivity reactions, rash, and fever, occur much more frequently in AIDS patients.

• I.V. infusion must be diluted in dextrose 5% in water prior to administration. Don't mix with other drugs or solutions.

• I.V. infusion must be infused slowly over 60 to 90 minutes. Don't give by rapid infusion or bolus injection. Must be used within 2 hours of mixing. Do not refrigerate.

• This combination is often used in extremely ill immunosuppressed patients when prescribed for treatment of *Pneumocystis carinii* pneumonia.

• Note that the "DS" or "DF" product name means "double strength."

• Promptly report skin rash, sore throat, fever, or mouth sores—early signs of blood dyscrasias.

• Watch for superinfection (fever or other signs of new infection).

• Obtain specimen for culture and sensitivity tests before first dose.

Italicized adverse reactions are common or life-threatening.
*Liquid form contains alcohol.   **May contain tartrazine.

Therapy may begin pending test results.

• Tell patient to take medication exactly as prescribed, even if he feels better, and to take entire amount prescribed.

• Used effectively for treatment of chronic bacterial prostatitis.

• Used prophylactically for recurrent urinary tract infections in women and for "traveler's diarrhea."

---

sulfadiazine
Microsulfon

Pregnancy Risk Category: B (D if near term)

HOW SUPPLIED
Tablets: 500 mg

MECHANISM OF ACTION
Inhibits formation of dihydrofolic acid from para-aminobenzoic acid (PABA), decreasing bacterial folic acid synthesis.

INDICATIONS & DOSAGE
Urinary tract infection—
Adults: initially, 2 to 4 g P.O., then 500 mg to 1 g P.O. q 6 hours.
Children: initially, 75 mg/kg or 2 g/m² P.O., then 150 mg/kg or 4 g/m² P.O. in 4 to 6 divided doses daily. Maximum daily dosage is 6 g.
Rheumatic fever prophylaxis, as an alternative to penicillin—
Children over 30 kg: 1 g P.O. daily.
Children under 30 kg: 500 mg P.O. daily.
Adjunctive treatment in toxoplasmosis—
Adults: 4 g P.O. in divided doses q 6 hours for 3 to 4 weeks, discontinued for 1 week; given with pyrimethamine 25 mg P.O. daily for 3 to 4 weeks.
Children: 100 mg/kg P.O. in divided doses q 6 hours for 3 to 4 weeks; given with pyrimethamine 2 mg/kg daily for 3 days, then 1 mg/kg daily for 3 to 4 weeks.

ADVERSE REACTIONS
Blood: *agranulocytosis, aplastic anemia,* megaloblastic anemia, thrombocytopenia, leukopenia, hemolytic anemia.
CNS: headache, mental depression, convulsions, hallucinations.
GI: *nausea, vomiting, diarrhea,* abdominal pain, anorexia, stomatitis.
GU: toxic nephrosis with oliguria and anuria, crystalluria, hematuria.
Hepatic: jaundice.
Skin: *erythema multiforme (Stevens-Johnson syndrome), generalized skin eruption, epidermal necrolysis, exfoliative dermatitis,* photosensitivity, urticaria, pruritus.
Local: irritation, extravasation.
Other: *hypersensitivity, serum sickness, drug fever, anaphylaxis.*

INTERACTIONS
Ammonium chloride, ascorbic acid: doses sufficient to acidify urine may cause precipitation of sulfonamide and crystalluria. Don't use together.
Oral anticoagulants: increased anticoagulant effect.
Oral contraceptives: decreased contraceptive effectiveness and increased risk of breakthrough bleeding.
Oral hypoglycemic agents: increased hypoglycemic effect.
PABA-containing drugs: inhibit antibacterial action. Don't use together.

NURSING CONSIDERATIONS
• Contraindicated in porphyria or in infants under 2 months (except in congenital toxoplasmosis). Use cautiously in reduced doses in impaired hepatic or renal function, bronchial asthma, history of multiple allergies, G6PD deficiency, and blood dyscrasias.
• Tell patient to drink a full glass of water with each dose and to drink plenty of water throughout the day to prevent crystalluria. Monitor input/output. Intake should be sufficient to produce output of 1,500 ml daily (be-

---

† Available in Canada only.   ‡ Available in Australia only.   ◇ Available OTC.

tween 3,000 and 4,000 ml daily for adults). To aid in prevention of crystalluria, sodium bicarbonate may be administered to alkalinize urine. Monitor urine pH daily.
• Watch for superinfection (fever or other signs of new infection).
• Obtain specimen for culture and sensitivity tests before first dose. Therapy may begin pending test results.
• Tell patient to take medication exactly as prescribed, even if he feels better, and to take entire amount prescribed.
• Warn patient to avoid direct sunlight and ultraviolet light to prevent photosensitivity reaction.
• Give drug on schedule to maintain constant blood level.
• Monitor for signs of blood dyscrasias (purpura, ecchymosis, sore throat, fever, and pallor). Report them immediately.
• Monitor urine cultures, CBCs, and urinalyses before and during therapy.
• Folic or folinic acid may be used during rest periods in toxoplasmosis therapy to reverse hematopoietic depression and/or anemia associated with pyrimethamine and sulfadiazine.
• Protect drug from light.

sulfamethoxazole (sulphamethoxazole)

Apo-Sulfamethoxazole†, Gantanol, Gantanol DS

Pregnancy Risk Category: B (D if near term)

HOW SUPPLIED
Tablets: 500 mg, 1,000 mg
Oral suspension: 500 mg/5 ml

MECHANISM OF ACTION
Inhibits formation of dihydrofolic acid from para-aminobenzoic acid (PABA), decreasing bacterial folic acid synthesis.

INDICATIONS & DOSAGE
Urinary tract and systemic infections—
Adults: initially, 2 g P.O., then 1 g P.O. b.i.d. up to t.i.d. for severe infections.
Children and infants over 2 months: initially, 50 to 60 mg/kg P.O., then 25 to 30 mg/kg b.i.d. Maximum dosage should not exceed 75 mg/kg daily.
Lymphogranuloma venereum (genital, inguinal, or anorectal infection)—
Adults: 1 g P.O. daily for at least 2 weeks.

ADVERSE REACTIONS
Blood: *agranulocytosis, aplastic anemia,* megaloblastic anemia, thrombocytopenia, leukopenia, hemolytic anemia.
CNS: headache, mental depression, seizures, hallucinations.
GI: *nausea, vomiting, diarrhea,* abdominal pain, anorexia, stomatitis.
GU: toxic nephrosis with oliguria and anuria, crystalluria, hematuria.
Hepatic: jaundice.
Skin: *erythema multiforme (Stevens-Johnson syndrome), generalized skin eruption, epidermal necrolysis, exfoliative dermatitis,* photosensitivity, urticaria, pruritus.
Other: *hypersensitivity, serum sickness, drug fever, anaphylaxis.*

INTERACTIONS
Ammonium chloride, ascorbic acid: doses sufficient to acidify urine may cause precipitation of sulfonamide and crystalluria. Don't use together.
Oral anticoagulants: increased anticoagulant effect.
Oral contraceptives: decreased contraceptive effectiveness and increased risk of breakthrough bleeding.
Oral hypoglycemic agents: increased hypoglycemic effect.
PABA-containing drugs: inhibit antibacterial action. Don't use together.

Italicized adverse reactions are common or life-threatening.
*Liquid form contains alcohol.   **May contain tartrazine.

NURSING CONSIDERATIONS

• Contraindicated in porphyria or in infants under 2 months (except in congenital toxoplasmosis). Use cautiously and in reduced dosages in impaired hepatic or renal function and in those with severe allergy or bronchial asthma, G6PD deficiency, and blood dyscrasias.

• Tell patient to drink a full glass of water with each dose and to drink plenty of water during the day to prevent crystalluria. Monitor fluid intake/output. Intake should be sufficient to produce output of 1,500 ml daily (between 3,000 and 4,000 ml daily for adults). To aid in prevention of crystalluria, sodium bicarbonate may be administered to alkalinize urine. Monitor urine pH daily.

• Watch for superinfection (fever or other signs of new infection).

• Obtain specimen for culture and sensitivity tests before first dose. Therapy may begin pending test results.

• Tell patient to take medication exactly as prescribed, even if he feels better, and to take entire amount prescribed.

• Warn patient to avoid direct sunlight and ultraviolet light to prevent photosensitivity reaction.

• Monitor urine cultures, CBCs, and urinalyses before and during therapy.

• Sulfamethoxazole is also used in adjunctive therapy for treatment of toxoplasmosis.

• Instruct patient to report early signs of blood dyscrasias (sore throat, fever, and pallor) to doctor immediately.

sulfasalazine (salazosulfapyridine, sulphasalazine)

Azulfidine, Azulfidine EN-Tabs, PMS Sulfasalazine E.C.†, Salazopyrin†‡, Salazopyrin EN-Tabs†‡, S.A.S., S.A.S.-Enteric

Pregnancy Risk Category: B (D if near term)

HOW SUPPLIED
Tablets: 500 mg with or without enteric coating
Oral suspension: 250 mg/5 ml

MECHANISM OF ACTION
Inhibits formation of dihydrofolic acid from para-aminobenzoic acid (PABA), decreasing bacterial folic acid synthesis.

INDICATIONS & DOSAGE
Mild to moderate ulcerative colitis, adjunctive therapy in severe ulcerative colitis—
Adults: initially, 3 to 4 g P.O. daily in evenly divided doses; usual maintenance dosage is 1.5 to 2 g P.O. daily in divided doses q 6 hours. May need to start with 1 to 2 g initially, with a gradual increase in dosage to minimize adverse effects.
Children over 2 years: initially, 40 to 60 mg/kg P.O. daily, divided into 3 to 6 doses; then 30 mg/kg daily in 4 doses. May need to start at lower dose if GI intolerance occurs.

ADVERSE REACTIONS
Blood: *agranulocytosis, aplastic anemia,* megaloblastic anemia, thrombocytopenia, leukopenia, hemolytic anemia.
CNS: headache, mental depression, seizures, hallucinations.
GI: *nausea, vomiting, diarrhea,* abdominal pain, anorexia, stomatitis.
GU: toxic nephrosis with oliguria and anuria, crystalluria, hematuria.
Hepatic: jaundice, hepatotoxicity.

Skin: *erythema multiforme (Stevens-Johnson syndrome), generalized skin eruption, epidermal necrolysis, exfoliative dermatitis,* photosensitivity, urticaria, pruritus.
Other: *hypersensitivity, serum sickness, drug fever, anaphylaxis,* oligospermia, infertility.

INTERACTIONS
Folic acid: absorption may be decreased.
Oral anticoagulants: increased anticoagulant effect.
Oral contraceptives: decreased contraceptive effectiveness and increased risk of breakthrough bleeding.
Oral hypoglycemic agents: increased hypoglycemic effect.

NURSING CONSIDERATIONS
• Contraindicated in porphyria. Use cautiously and in reduced dosages in impaired hepatic or renal function and in those with severe allergy, bronchial asthma, and G6PD deficiency. Also contraindicated in intestinal and urinary obstruction, and in patients allergic to salicylates.
• Watch for superinfection (fever or other signs of new infection).
• Obtain specimen for culture and sensitivity tests before first dose. Therapy may begin pending test results.
• Tell patient to take medication exactly as prescribed, even if he feels better, and to take entire amount prescribed.
• Warn patient to avoid direct sunlight and ultraviolet light to prevent photosensitivity reaction.
• Colors alkaline urine orange-yellow.
• Adverse reactions are usually those affecting GI tract. Minimize symptoms by spacing doses evenly and administering after food intake.

sulfisoxazole (sulfafurazole, sulphafurazole)
Azo-Sulfisoxazole†‡, Gantrisin, Lipo Gantrisin, Novosoxazole†

Pregnancy Risk Category: B (D if near term)

HOW SUPPLIED
Tablets: 500 mg
Liquid: 500 mg/5 ml
Long-acting emulsion: 0.5 g/5 ml

MECHANISM OF ACTION
Inhibits formation of dihydrofolic acid from para-aminobenzoic acid (PABA), decreasing bacterial folic acid synthesis.

INDICATIONS & DOSAGE
Urinary tract and systemic infections—
Adults: initially, 2 to 4 g P.O., then 1 to 2 g P.O. q.i.d.; extended-release suspension 4 to 5 g P.O. q 12 hours.
Children over 2 months: initially, 75 mg/kg P.O. daily or 2 g/m² P.O. daily in divided doses q 6 hours, then 150 mg/kg or 4 g/m² P.O. daily in divided doses q 6 hours; extended-release suspension 60 to 70 mg/kg P.O. q 12 hours.

ADVERSE REACTIONS
Blood: *agranulocytosis, aplastic anemia,* megaloblastic anemia, thrombocytopenia, leukopenia, hemolytic anemia.
CNS: headache, mental depression, seizures, hallucinations.
GI: *nausea, vomiting, diarrhea,* abdominal pain, anorexia, stomatitis.
GU: toxic nephrosis with oliguria and anuria, crystalluria, hematuria.
Hepatic: jaundice.
Skin: *erythema multiforme (Stevens-Johnson syndrome), generalized skin eruption, epidermal necrolysis, exfoliative dermatitis,* photosensitivity, urticaria, pruritus.

Italicized adverse reactions are common or life-threatening.
*Liquid form contains alcohol.   **May contain tartrazine.

Other: *hypersensitivity, serum sickness, drug fever, anaphylaxis.*

INTERACTIONS

Ammonium chloride, ascorbic acid: doses sufficient to acidify urine may cause crystalluria and precipitation of sulfonamide. Don't use together.
Oral anticoagulants: increased anticoagulant effect.
Oral contraceptives: decreased contraceptive effectiveness and increased risk of breakthrough bleeding.
Oral hypoglycemic agents: increased hypoglycemic effect.
PABA-containing drugs: inhibit antibacterial action. Don't use together.

NURSING CONSIDERATIONS

• Contraindicated in porphyria and in infants under 2 months (except in congenital toxoplasmosis). Use cautiously in impaired hepatic or renal function, severe allergy or bronchial asthma, and G6PD deficiency.
• Tell patient to drink a full glass of water with each dose and to drink plenty of water throughout the day to prevent crystalluria. Monitor intake/output. Intake should be sufficient to produce output of 1,500 ml daily (between 3,000 and 4,000 ml daily for adults). To aid in prevention of crystalluria, sodium bicarbonate may be administered to alkalinize urine. Monitor urine pH daily.
• Watch for superinfection (fever or other signs of new infection).
• Obtain specimen for culture and sensitivity tests before first dose. Therapy may begin pending test results.
• Tell patient to take medication exactly as prescribed, even if he feels better, and to take entire amount prescribed.
• Warn patient to avoid direct sunlight and ultraviolet light to prevent photosensitivity reaction.
• Monitor urine cultures, CBCs, pro-thrombin time, and urinalyses before and during therapy.
• Gantrisin suspension and Lipo Gantrisin suspension cannot be interchanged, since the latter is an extended-release preparation.
• Sulfisoxazole-pyrimethamine combination is used to treat toxoplasmosis.
• Tell patient to report early signs of blood dyscrasias (sore throat, fever, and pallor) immediately to doctor.
• When given preoperatively, the patient should receive a low-residue diet and a minimal number of enemas and cathartics.
• Although often given, initial loading dose is not necessary.

16

Urinary tract antiseptics

cinoxacin
methenamine hippurate
methenamine mandelate
methylene blue
nalidixic acid
nitrofurantoin microcrystals
nitrofurantoin macrocrystals
norfloxacin

COMBINATION PRODUCTS

CYSTEX: methenamine 165 mg, salicylamide 65 mg, sodium salicylate 97 mg, and benzoic acid 32 mg.
HEXALOL: methenamine 40.8 mg, phenyl salicylate 18.1 mg, atropine sulfate 0.03 mg, hyoscyamine 0.03 mg, benzoic acid 4.5 mg, and methylene blue 5.4 mg.
URO-PHOSPHATE: methenamine 300 mg and sodium acid phosphate 500 mg. Sugar coated.
UROQUID-ACID: methenamine mandelate 350 mg and sodium acid phosphate 200 mg.
UROQUID-ACID NO. 2: methenamine mandelate 500 mg and sodium acid phosphate 500 mg.

---

cinoxacin
Cinobac

Pregnancy Risk Category: B

HOW SUPPLIED
Capsules: 250 mg, 500 mg

MECHANISM OF ACTION
Inhibits microbial DNA synthesis.

INDICATIONS & DOSAGE
Treatment of initial and recurrent urinary tract infections caused by susceptible strains of Escherichia coli, Klebsiella, Enterobacter, Proteus mirabilis, Proteus vulgaris, *and* Proteus morgani, Serratia, *and* Citrobacter—*
Adults and children over 12 years: 1 g P.O. daily, in two to four divided doses for 7 to 14 days.
   Not recommended for children under 12 years.

ADVERSE REACTIONS
CNS: *dizziness, headache,* drowsiness, insomnia, seizures.
EENT: photosensitivity, tinnitus.
GI: *nausea, vomiting, abdominal pain,* diarrhea.
Skin: rash, urticaria, pruritus, photosensitivity.

INTERACTIONS
Probenecid: may decrease urine levels of cinoxacin by inhibiting renal tubular secretion. Monitor for increased toxicity and reduced antibacterial effectiveness.

Italicized adverse reactions are common or life-threatening.
*Liquid form contains alcohol.   **May contain tartrazine.

NURSING CONSIDERATIONS
- Contraindicated in patients with hypersensitivity to nalidixic acid. Use cautiously in patients with impaired renal and hepatic function.
- Not effective against *Pseudomonas*, enterococci, or staphylococci.
- Obtain clean-catch urine specimen for culture and sensitivity before starting therapy and repeat p.r.n. Therapy may begin pending test results.
- Remind patient to continue taking this drug, even when he feels better, and to take entire amount prescribed.
- High urine levels permit twice-daily dosing.
- Report CNS adverse reactions to doctor immediately. They indicate serious toxicity and usually mean that administration of drug should be stopped.
- Cinoxacin should be taken with meals to help decrease GI adverse reactions.
- Warn patient about photosensitizing effects of the drug, and advise him to avoid very bright sunlight and use sunblock.

---

methenamine hippurate
Hiprex**, Hip-Rex†, Urex

methenamine mandelate
Mandameth, Mandelamine, Sterine†

Pregnancy Risk Category: C

HOW SUPPLIED
hippurate
Tablets: 1 g
mandelate
Tablets: 500 mg, 1 g
Tablets (enteric-coated): 250 mg, 500 mg, 1 g
Tablets (film-coated): 500 mg, 1 g
Oral suspension: 250 mg/5 ml
Granules: 500 mg, 1 g

MECHANISM OF ACTION
In acid urine, methenamines are hydrolyzed to ammonia and to formaldehyde, which is responsible for antibacterial action against gram-positive and gram-negative organisms. Mandelic and hippuric acids, with which methenamines are combined, are also antibacterial by unknown mechanisms.

INDICATIONS & DOSAGE
Long-term prophylaxis or suppression of chronic urinary tract infections—
Adults and children over 12 years: 1 g (hippurate) P.O. q 12 hours.
Children 6 to 12 years: 500 mg to 1 g (hippurate) P.O. q 12 hours.
Urinary tract infections, infected residual urine in patients with neurogenic bladder—
Adults: 1 g (mandelate) P.O. q.i.d. after meals.
Children 6 to 12 years: 500 mg (mandelate) P.O. q.i.d. after meals.
Children under 6 years: 50 mg/kg (mandelate) P.O. divided in four doses after meals.

ADVERSE REACTIONS
GI: nausea, vomiting, diarrhea.
GU: with high doses, urinary tract irritation, dysuria, frequency, albuminuria, hematuria.
Hepatic: elevated liver enzymes.
Skin: rashes.

INTERACTIONS
Acetazolamide: antagonizes methenamine effect. Use together cautiously.
Urine alkalinizing agents: inhibit methenamine action. Don't use together.

NURSING CONSIDERATIONS
- Contraindicated in renal insufficiency, severe hepatic disease, or severe dehydration.
- Ineffective against *Candida* infection.
- Oral suspension contains vegetable oil. Administer cautiously to elderly

---

or debilitated patients, because aspiration could cause lipid pneumonia.
• Monitor intake/output. Intake should be at least 1,500 to 2,000 ml daily.
• Obtain a clean-catch urine specimen for culture and sensitivity tests before starting therapy, and repeat p.r.n. Therapy may begin pending test results.
• Limit intake of alkaline foods, such as vegetables, milk, and peanuts. May drink cranberry, plum, and prune juices. These juices or ascorbic acid may be used to acidify urine.
• Warn patient not to take antacids, including Alka-Seltzer and sodium bicarbonate.
• For best results, maintain urine pH at 5.5 or below. Use Nitrazine paper to check pH. Large doses of ascorbic acid (12 g/day) may be necessary to effectively acidify urine.
• *Proteus* and *Pseudomonas* tend to raise urine pH; urine acidifiers are usually necessary when treating these infections.
• Obtain liver function studies periodically during long-term therapy.
• Administer after meals to minimize GI upset.
• If rash appears, withhold dose and contact doctor.

---

methylene blue
Urolene Blue

Pregnancy Risk Category: C (D if injected intra-amniotically)

HOW SUPPLIED
Tablets: 55 mg, 65 mg
Injection: 10 mg/ml

MECHANISM OF ACTION
Methylene blue is a mildly antiseptic dye. High concentrations convert the ferrous iron of reduced hemoglobin to ferric iron to form methemoglobin. This mechanism is the basis for its use as an antidote in cyanide poisoning. Low concentrations of methylene blue can hasten conversion of methemoglobin to hemoglobin.

INDICATIONS & DOSAGE
Cystitis, urethritis—
Adults: 55 to 130 mg P.O. b.i.d. or t.i.d. after meals with glass of water.
Methemoglobinemia and cyanide poisoning—
Adults and children: 1 to 2 mg/kg of 1% sterile solution slow I.V.

ADVERSE REACTIONS
Blood: anemia (long-term use).
GI: nausea, vomiting, diarrhea, blue-green stool.
GU: dysuria, bladder irritation, blue-green urine.
Other: fever (large doses).

INTERACTIONS
None significant.

NURSING CONSIDERATIONS
• Contraindicated in renal insufficiency.
• Monitor intake/output carefully. Intake should be at least 2,000 ml daily.
• Monitor hemoglobin; possibility of anemia from accelerated destruction of erythrocytes.
• Turns urine and stool blue-green.
• Seldom used as urinary tract antiseptic.
• I.V. form has been used to treat nitrite intoxication.
• Use caution when handling injectable form, since the liquid can stain the skin. Avoid extravasation. S.C. injection can cause necrotic abcess formation.

---

nalidixic acid
NegGram

Pregnancy Risk Category: B

HOW SUPPLIED
Tablets: 250 mg, 500 mg, 1 g
Oral suspension: 250 mg/5 ml

MECHANISM OF ACTION
Inhibits microbial DNA synthesis.

INDICATIONS & DOSAGE
Acute and chronic urinary tract infections caused by susceptible gram-negative organisms (Proteus, Klebsiella, Enterobacter, *and* Escherichia coli)—
Adults: 1 g P.O. q.i.d. for 7 to 14 days; 2 g daily for long-term use.
Children over 3 months: 55 mg/kg P.O. daily divided q.i.d. for 7 to 14 days; 33 mg/kg daily for long-term use.

ADVERSE REACTIONS
Blood: eosinophilia.
CNS: drowsiness, weakness, headache, dizziness, vertigo, seizures in epileptics, confusion, hallucinations.
EENT: sensitivity to light, change in color perception, diplopia, blurred vision.
GI: *abdominal pain, nausea, vomiting,* diarrhea.
Skin: pruritus, photosensitivity, urticaria, rash.
Other: angioedema, fever, chills, increased intracranial pressure and bulging fontanelles in infants and children.

INTERACTIONS
Oral anticoagulants: Increased anticoagulant effect.

NURSING CONSIDERATIONS
• Contraindicated in seizure disorders. Use with caution in impaired hepatic or renal function, or severe cerebral arteriosclerosis. Should be used very cautiously in prepubertal children; erosion of cartilage of immature animals has been reported.
• Not effective against *Pseudomonas* or infections outside of the urinary tract.
• Tell the patient to report visual disturbances; these usually disappear with reduced dose.

• Obtain specimen for culture and sensitivity tests before starting therapy and repeat p.r.n. Therapy may begin pending test results.
• Obtain CBC, renal and liver function studies during long-term therapy.
• Resistant bacteria may emerge within the first 48 hours of therapy.
• May cause a false-positive Clinitest reaction. Use Clinistix or Tes-Tape to monitor urine glucose. Also gives false elevations in urine vanillylmandelic acid (VMA) and 17-ketosteroids. Repeat tests after therapy is completed.
• Avoid undue exposure to sunlight due to photosensitivity. Patient may continue to be photosensitive for as long as 3 months after drug is discontinued.

nitrofurantoin microcrystals
Apo-Nitrofurantoin†, Furadantin, Furalan, Furan, Furanite, Macrodantin, Nephronex†, Nitrofan, Novofuran†

nitrofurantoin macrocrystals
Macrodantin

Pregnancy Risk Category: B

HOW SUPPLIED
microcrystals
Tablets: 50 mg, 100 mg
Capsules: 50 mg, 100 mg
Oral suspension: 25 mg/5 ml
macrocrystals
Capsules: 25 mg, 50 mg, 100 mg
Oral suspension: 25 mg/5 ml

MECHANISM OF ACTION
Bacteriostatic in low concentration and possibly bactericidal in high concentration. Interferes with bacterial enzyme systems.

INDICATIONS & DOSAGE
Pyelonephritis, pyelitis, and cystitis

---

†Available in Canada only.   ‡Available in Australia only.   ◇Available OTC.

due to susceptible Escherichia coli, Staphylococcus aureus, *enterococci; certain strains of* Klebsiella, Proteus, *and* Enterobacter—
Adults and children over 12 years: 50 to 100 mg P.O. q.i.d. with milk or meals.
Children 1 month to 12 years: 5 to 7 mg/kg P.O. daily, divided q.i.d.
Long-term suppression therapy—
Adults: 50 to 100 mg P.O. daily at bedtime.
Children: 1 to 2 mg/kg P.O. daily at bedtime.

ADVERSE REACTIONS
Blood: hemolysis in patients with G6PD deficiency (reversed after stopping drug), *agranulocytosis,* thrombocytopenia.
CNS: peripheral neuropathy, headache, dizziness, drowsiness, *ascending polyneuropathy with high doses or renal impairment.*
GI: *anorexia, nausea, vomiting,* abdominal pain, *diarrhea.*
Hepatic: hepatitis.
Skin: maculopapular, erythematous, or eczematous eruption; pruritus; urticaria; *exfoliative dermatitis; Stevens-Johnson syndrome.*
Other: asthmatic attacks in patients with history of asthma; *anaphylaxis;* hypersensitivity; transient alopecia; drug fever; overgrowth of nonsusceptible organisms in the urinary tract; *pulmonary sensitivity reactions (cough, chest pains, fever, chills, dyspnea).*

INTERACTIONS
Magnesium-containing antacids: decreased nitrofurantoin absorption. Separate administration times by 1 hour.
Nalidixic acid, norfloxacin: possible decreased effectiveness. Avoid using together.
Probenecid, sulfinpyrazone: increased blood levels and decreased urine levels. May result in increased toxicity and lack of therapeutic effect. Don't use together.

NURSING CONSIDERATIONS
• Contraindicated in moderate to severe renal impairment, anuria, oliguria, or creatinine clearance under 40 ml/minute; use cautiously in G6PD deficiency.
• Hypersensitivity may develop when used for long-term therapy.
• Obtain specimen for culture and sensitivity tests before starting therapy and repeat p.r.n. Therapy may begin pending test results.
• Monitor CBC regularly.
• Give with food or milk to minimize GI distress.
• Some patients may experience fewer GI adverse effects with nitrofurantoin macrocrystals.
• Monitor intake/output carefully. May turn urine brown or darker.
• Store in amber container. Keep away from metals other than stainless steel or aluminum to avoid precipitate formation. Warn patients not to use pillboxes made of these materials.
• Continue treatment for 3 days after sterile urine specimens have been obtained.
• Monitor pulmonary status.
• Has no effect in blood or tissue outside the urinary tract.
• Monitor for superinfection. Use of nitrofurantoin may result in growth of nonsusceptible organisms, especially *Pseudomonas.*
• May cause false-positive results with urine sugar test using copper sulfate reduction method (Clinitest) but not with glucose oxidase tests (Tes-Tape, Diastix, Clinistix).

norfloxacin
Noroxin
Pregnancy Risk Category: C

HOW SUPPLIED
Tablets: 400 mg

Italicized adverse reactions are common or life-threatening.
*Liquid form contains alcohol. **May contain tartrazine.

MECHANISM OF ACTION
Inhibits bacterial DNA synthesis, mainly by inhibiting DNA gyrase. Bactericidal.

INDICATIONS & DOSAGE
Treatment of complicated or uncomplicated urinary tract infections caused by susceptible strains of Escherichia coli, Klebsiella, Enterobacter, Proteus, Pseudomonas aeruginosa, Citrobacter, Staphylococcus aureus *(and* epidermidis*), and group D streptococci—*
Adults: For uncomplicated infections, 400 mg P.O. b.i.d. for 7 to 10 days. For complicated infections, 400 mg b.i.d. for 10 to 21 days.

ADVERSE REACTIONS
CNS: fatigue, somnolence, headache, dizziness.
GI: nausea, constipation, flatulence, heartburn, dry mouth.
Hepatic: transient elevations of AST (SGOT) and ALT (SGPT).
Skin: rash.

INTERACTIONS
Antacids: may hinder absorption.
Nitrofurantoin: decreases norfloxacin's effectiveness. Don't use together.
Probenecid: may increase serum levels of norfloxacin by decreasing its excretion.

NURSING CONSIDERATIONS
• Contraindicated in patients with hypersensitivity to nalidixic acid and cinoxacin.
• Warn patients not to exceed the recommended dosages. Advise them to drink several glasses of water throughout the day to maintain hydration and adequate urine output.
• Advise patients to take the drug 1 hour before or 2 hours after meals since the presence of food may hinder absorption.
• Because norfloxacin may cause dizziness, patients should avoid hazardous activities that require alertness and good coordination until the CNS effects of the drug are known.

17

Antivirals

acyclovir sodium
amantadine hydrochloride
ganciclovir
ribavirin
vidarabine monohydrate
zidovudine

COMBINATION PRODUCTS
None.

---

acyclovir sodium
Zovirax

Pregnancy Risk Category: C

HOW SUPPLIED
Capsules: 200 mg
Injection: 500 mg/vial

MECHANISM OF ACTION
Becomes incorporated into viral DNA and inhibits viral multiplication.

INDICATIONS & DOSAGE
Treatment of initial and recurrent episodes of mucocutaneous herpes simplex virus (HSV-1 and HSV-2) infections in immunocompromised patients; severe initial episodes of herpes genitalis in patients who are not immunocompromised—
Adults and children over 11 years: 5 mg/kg, given at a constant rate over a period of 1 hour by I.V. infusion q 8 hours for 7 days (5 days for herpes genitalis).
Children under 12 years: 250 mg/ m², given at a constant rate over a period of 1 hour by I.V. infusion q 8 hours for 7 days (5 days for herpes genitalis).

Treatment of initial genital herpes—
Adults: 200 mg P.O. q 4 hours while awake (a total of 5 capsules daily). Treatment should continue for 10 days.
Intermittent therapy for recurrent genital herpes—
Adults: 200 mg P.O. q 4 hours while awake (a total of 5 capsules daily). Treatment should continue for 5 days. Initiate therapy at the first sign of recurrence.
Chronic suppressive therapy for recurrent genital herpes—
Adults: 200 mg P.O. t.i.d. for up to 6 months.

ADVERSE REACTIONS
CNS: (associated with I.V. dosage): *headache, encephalopathic changes (lethargy, obtundation, tremors, confusion, hallucinations, agitation, seizures, coma).*
CV: hypotension.
GI: (associated with P.O. dosage): *nausea, vomiting,* diarrhea.
GU: *transient elevations of serum creatinine,* hematuria.
Skin: rash, itching.
Local: *inflammation, vesicular eruptions and phlebitis at injection site.*

INTERACTIONS
Probenecid: increased acyclovir blood levels. Monitor for possible toxicity.

NURSING CONSIDERATIONS
For I.V. form:
• Don't administer topically, intramuscularly, orally, subcutaneously, or ophthalmically.

Italicized adverse reactions are common or life-threatening.
*Liquid form contains alcohol.   **May contain tartrazine.

- Don't give by bolus injection.
- Infusion must be administered over at least 1 hour to prevent renal tubular damage. Bolus injection, dehydration (decreased urine output), preexisting renal disease, and the concomitant use of other nephrotoxic drugs increase the risk of renal toxicity.
- Notify doctor if serum creatinine level does not return to normal within a few days. He may increase hydration, adjust dose, or discontinue acyclovir.
- Encephalopathic changes are more likely in patients with neurologic disorders or in those who have had neurologic reactions to cytotoxic drugs.
- Patient must be adequately hydrated during acyclovir infusion.

For P.O. form:
- Teach patient that drug is effective in managing the disease but does not eliminate or cure it.
- Instruct patient that acyclovir will not prevent spread of infection to others.
- Urge patient to recognize the early symptoms of infection (such as tingling, itching, or pain) so he can take acyclovir before the infection fully develops.

amantadine hydrochloride
Antadine‡, Symadine, Symmetrel
Pregnancy Risk Category: C

HOW SUPPLIED
Capsules: 100 mg
Syrup: 50 mg/5 ml

MECHANISM OF ACTION
Interferes with influenza A virus penetration into susceptible cells. Its action in the treatment of parkinsonism is unknown.

INDICATIONS & DOSAGE
Prophylaxis or symptomatic treatment of influenza type A virus, respiratory tract illnesses—

Adults to 64 years and children 10 years and over: 200 mg P.O. daily in a single dose or divided b.i.d.
Children 1 to 9 years: 4.4 to 8.8 mg/kg P.O. daily, divided b.i.d. or t.i.d. Don't exceed 150 mg daily.
Adults over 64 years: 100 mg P.O. once daily.

Treatment should continue for 24 to 48 hours after symptoms disappear. Prophylaxis should start as soon as possible after initial exposure and continue for at least 10 days after exposure. May continue prophylactic treatment up to 90 days for repeated or suspected exposures if influenza vaccine unavailable. If used with influenza vaccine, continue dose for 2 to 3 weeks until protection from vaccine develops.
To treat drug-induced extrapyramidal reactions—
Adults: 100 mg P.O. b.i.d., up to 300 mg daily in divided doses. Patient may benefit from as much as 400 mg daily, but dosages over 200 mg must be closely supervised.
To treat idiopathic parkinsonism, parkinsonian syndrome—
Adults: 100 mg P.O. b.i.d.; in patients who are seriously ill or receiving other antiparkinsonism drugs, 100 mg daily for at least 1 week, then 100 mg b.i.d., p.r.n.

ADVERSE REACTIONS
CNS: depression, fatigue, confusion, dizziness, psychosis, hallucinations, anxiety, *irritability,* ataxia, *insomnia,* weakness, headache, light-headedness, difficulty concentrating.
CV: peripheral edema, orthostatic hypotension, CHF.
GI: anorexia, nausea, constipation, vomiting, dry mouth.
GU: urine retention.
Skin: *livedo reticularis* (with prolonged use).

INTERACTIONS
None significant.

NURSING CONSIDERATIONS
- Use cautiously in epilepsy, congestive heart failure, peripheral edema, hepatic disease, mental illness, eczematoid rash, renal impairment, orthostatic hypotension, and cardiovascular disease, and in elderly patients.
- For best absorption, drug should be taken after meals.
- Instruct patient to report adverse reactions to the doctor, especially dizziness, depression, anxiety, nausea, and urine retention.
- Elderly patients are more susceptible to neurological adverse effects. Taking the drug in two daily doses rather than single dose may reduce their incidence.
- If orthostatic hypotension occurs, instruct patient not to stand or change positions too quickly.
- If insomnia occurs, dose should be taken several hours before bedtime.
- When prescribed for parkinsonism, warn patient against discontinuing drug abruptly since this might precipitate a parkinsonian crisis.

---

ganciclovir
Cytovene

Pregnancy Risk Category: C

HOW SUPPLIED
Injection: 500 mg/vial

MECHANISM OF ACTION
Inhibits viral DNA synthesis of the cytomegalovirus (CMV).

INDICATIONS & DOSAGE
CMV retinitis treatment of immunocompromised individuals, including patients with acquired immunodeficiency syndrome (AIDS)—
Adults: induction treatment: initially, 5 mg/kg I.V. q 12 hours for 14 to 21 days (normal renal function); maintenance treatment: 5 mg/kg I.V. once daily, for 7 days each week, or 6 mg/kg once daily, for 5 days each week.

ADVERSE REACTIONS
Blood: *granulocytopenia, thrombocytopenia.*
CNS: altered dreams, confusion, ataxia, dizziness, headache.
CV: arrhythmias, hypotension, hypertension.
GI: nausea, vomiting, diarrhea, anorexia.
GU: hematuria.
Local: injection site inflammation, pain, phlebitis.
Other: retinal detachment in CMV retinitis patients.

INTERACTIONS
Cytotoxic agents: additive toxic effects, especially hematologic effects and stomatitis.
Imipenem/cilastatin: reports of seizure activity with concomitant use.
Probenecid: increased ganciclovir blood levels.
Zidovudine: increased incidence of granulocytopenia with concurrent use.

NURSING CONSIDERATIONS
- Dosage of ganciclovir should be reduced in patients with renal dysfunction.
- Ganciclovir should not be administered to patients with an absolute neutrophil count below 500/mm³ or a platelet count below 25,000/mm³.
- Do not administer ganciclovir subcutaneously or intramuscularly.
- Infusion must take place over at least **1 hour.** Do not administer as an I.V. bolus. Infusions faster than 60 minutes will result in increased toxicity.
- Ganciclovir infusion therapy should be accompanied by adequate hydration.
- Due to the frequency of granulocytopenia and thrombocytopenia, neutrophil and platelet counts should be obtained every 2 days during twice-daily ganciclovir dosing and at least weekly thereafter.

• Use caution when preparing ganciclovir solution, which is alkaline.

---

ribavirin
Virazole

Pregnancy Risk Category: X

HOW SUPPLIED
Powder to be reconstituted for inhalation: 6 g in 100-ml glass vial

MECHANISM OF ACTION
Inhibits viral activity by an unknown mechanism. Thought to inhibit RNA and DNA synthesis by depleting intracellular nucleotide pools.

INDICATIONS & DOSAGE
Treatment of hospitalized infants and young children infected by respiratory syncytial virus (RSV)—
Infants and young children: solution in concentration of 20 mg/ml delivered via the Viratek Small Particle Aerosol Generator (SPAG-2). Treatment is carried out for 12 to 18 hours/day for at least 3, and no more than 7, days.

ADVERSE REACTIONS
Blood: anemia, reticulocytosis.
EENT: conjunctivitis.
Respiratory: worsening of respiratory state.
Other: rash or erythema of eyelids.

INTERACTIONS
None significant.

NURSING CONSIDERATIONS
• Contraindicated in females who are or may become pregnant during treatment with drug.
• Ribavirin aerosol is indicated only for severe lower respiratory tract infection due to respiratory syncytial virus (RSV). Although treatment may be started while awaiting diagnostic test results, existence of RSV infection must be eventually documented.

• Most infants and children with RSV infection don't require treatment because the disease is often mild and self-limiting. Infants with underlying conditions, such as prematurity or cardiopulmonary disease get RSV in its severest form, and benefit most from treatment with ribavirin aerosol.
• This treatment must be accompanied by, and does not replace, supportive respiratory and fluid management.
• Ribavirin aerosol *must* be administered by the Viratek Small Particle Aerosol Generator (SPAG-2). Don't use any other aerosol generating device.
• Ribavarin may precipitate in ventilator apparatus which may result in equipment malfunction with serious consequences. The use of ribavirin in ventilator dependent patients is not recommended.
• The water used to reconstitute this drug must not contain any antimicrobial agent. Use sterile USP water for injection, *not* bacteriostatic water.
• Discard solutions placed in the SPAG-2 unit at least every 24 hours before adding newly reconstituted solution.
• Store reconstituted solutions at room temperature for 24 hours.

---

vidarabine monohydrate (adenine arabinoside, ara-A)
Vira-A

Pregnancy Risk Category: C

HOW SUPPLIED
Concentrate for I.V. infusion: 200 mg/ml in 5-ml vial (equivalent to 187.4 mg vidarabine)

MECHANISM OF ACTION
Becomes incorporated into viral DNA and inhibits viral multiplication.

---

†Available in Canada only.   ‡Available in Australia only.   ◊Available OTC.

INDICATIONS & DOSAGE

Herpes simplex virus encephalitis—
Adults and children (including neonates): 15 mg/kg I.V. daily for 10 days. Slowly infuse the total daily dose by I.V. infusion at a constant rate over 12-to 24-hour period. Avoid rapid or bolus injection.

ADVERSE REACTIONS

Blood: anemia, neutropenia, thrombocytopenia.
CNS: tremor, dizziness, hallucinations, confusion, psychosis, ataxia.
GI: *anorexia, nausea,* vomiting, diarrhea.
Hepatic: elevated AST (SGOT), bilirubin.
Skin: pruritus, rash.
Local: pain at injection site.
Other: weight loss.

INTERACTIONS

Allopurinol: concurrent therapy reduces metabolism of vidarabine and increases risk of CNS adverse effects.

NURSING CONSIDERATIONS

• Will reduce mortality caused by herpes simplex virus encephalitis from 70% to 28%. No evidence that vidarabine is effective in encephalitis due to other viruses.
• Don't give I.M. or subcutaneously because of low solubility and poor absorption.
• Monitor hematologic tests, such as hemoglobin, hematocrit, WBC, and platelets during therapy. Also monitor renal and liver function studies.
• Patient with impaired renal function may need dosage adjustment.
• Once in solution, vidarabine is stable at room temperature for at least 2 weeks.
• Use with an I.V. filter of 0.45 μm or smaller.
• Must be diluted to a concentration of less than 0.5 mg/ml.
• Any I.V. solution is suitable as a diluent.

zidovudine (azidothymidine, AZT)

Retrovir

Pregnancy Risk Category: C

HOW SUPPLIED

Capsules: 100 mg
Syrup: 50 mg/5 ml
Injection: 20 mg/ml

MECHANISM OF ACTION

Prevents replication of the human immunodeficiency virus (HIV) by inhibiting the enzyme reverse transcriptase.

INDICATIONS & DOSAGE

Patients with AIDS or advanced AIDS-related complex (ARC) who have a history of Pneumocystis carinii *pneumonia or a CD_4 lymphocyte count below 200 cells/mm[2]—*
Adults: initially, 200 mg P.O. q 4 hours around the clock for 1 month, then 100 mg P.O. q 4 hours around the clock.
Children: dosage is individualized and will vary according to treatment IND protocol. Early studies have employed doses between 0.9 and 1.4 mg/kg/hour by continuous I.V. infusion; others have used 100 mg/m[2] I.V. or P.O. q 6 hours.
Postexposure prophylaxis—
Adults: dosage will vary according to study protocol, but most studies use 200 mg P.O. q 4 hours around the clock for 6 to 8 weeks. Some investigators attempt to initiate therapy within 1 hour of exposure.

ADVERSE REACTIONS

Blood: *Severe bone marrow depression (resulting in anemia), granulocytopenia, thrombocytopenia.*
CNS: *headache,* agitation, restlessness, insomnia, confusion, anxiety.
GI: nausea, anorexia.
Skin: rash, itching.
Other: myalgia.

Italicized adverse reactions are common or life-threatening.
*Liquid form contains alcohol. **May contain tartrazine.

INTERACTIONS

Acyclovir: possible lethargy and fatigue. Use together cautiously.

Co-trimoxazole, acetaminophen: may impair hepatic metabolism of zidovudine, increasing the drug's toxicity.

Other cytotoxic drugs: additive adverse effects on the bone marrow.

Pentamidine, dapsone, flucytosine, amphotericin B: increased risk of nephrotoxicity.

Probenecid: may decrease the renal clearance of zidovidine.

NURSING CONSIDERATIONS

• Zidovudine frequently causes a low red blood cell count by suppressing the bone marrow. Advise patients that they may need blood transfusions during treatment with zidovudine.

• Frequent monitoring of blood studies (every 2 weeks) is recommended to detect anemia or granulocytopenia. Patients may require dosage reduction or temporary discontinuation of the drug.

• Remind patients that they *must* comply with the every-4-hour dosage schedule. Suggest ways to avoid missing doses, such as the use of alarm clocks.

• Warn patients not to take any other drugs for AIDS (especially from the "street") unless their doctors have approved them. Some purported AIDS "cures" may interfere with zidovudine's effectiveness.

• The drug has been shown to temporarily decrease morbidity and mortality in certain patients with AIDS or AIDS-related complex.

• The optimum duration of treatment, as well as the dosage for optimum effectiveness and minimum toxicity, is not yet known.

• Health-care workers who consider zidovudine prophylaxis following occupational exposure (after needlestick injury, for example) should understand that animal and human studies are insufficient to judge the drug's safety or efficacy. These persons should consider the potential toxicity of the drug, as well as the risk of acquiring HIV following occupational exposure. Some clinicians do not advocate such use of zidovudine.

18

Miscellaneous anti-infectives

aztreonam
bacitracin
chloramphenicol
chloramphenicol palmitate
chloramphenicol sodium
   succinate
ciprofloxacin
clindamycin hydrochloride
clindamycin palmitate
   hydrochloride
clindamycin phosphate
erythromycin base
erythromycin estolate
erythromycin ethylsuccinate
erythromycin gluceptate
erythromycin lactobionate
erythromycin stearate
imipenem/cilastatin sodium
lincomycin hydrochloride
pentamidine isethionate
polymyxin B sulfate
spectinomycin dihydrochloride
trimethoprim
vancomycin hydrochloride

COMBINATION PRODUCTS
None.

---

aztreonam
Azactam

Pregnancy Risk Category: B

HOW SUPPLIED
Injection: 500-mg, 1-g, 2-g vials

MECHANISM OF ACTION
Inhibits bacterial cell wall synthesis,
ultimately causing cell wall destruction. Bactericidal.

INDICATIONS & DOSAGE
*Treatment of urinary tract infections,
lower respiratory tract infections, septicemia, skin and skin structure infections, intraabdominal infections, and
gynecologic infections caused by various gram-negative organisms—*
Adults: 500 mg to 2 g I.V. or I.M. q 8
to 12 hours. For severe systemic or
life-threatening infections, 2 g q 6 to
8 hours may be given. Maximum dosage is 8 g daily.

ADVERSE REACTIONS
Blood: neutropenia, anemia.
CNS: seizures, headache, insomnia.
CV: hypotension.
GI: diarrhea, nausea, vomiting.
Hepatic: transient elevations of AST
(SGOT) and ALT (SGPT).
Local: thrombophlebitis at I.V. site,
discomfort and swelling at I.M. injec-
tion site.

INTERACTIONS
Furosemide, probenecid: increased
serum aztreonam levels.
Other: hypersensitivity, *anaphylaxis,*
altered taste, halitosis.

NURSING CONSIDERATIONS
• Use cautiously in elderly patients
and in impaired renal function.
• Aztreonam is a narrow-spectrum
antibiotic, effective solely against
gram-negative organisms. Because it
is ineffective against gram-positive
and anaerobic organisms, aztreonam
must be used with other antibiotics
for immediate treatment of life-
threatening illnesses.

Italicized adverse reactions are common or life-threatening.
*Liquid form contains alcohol.   **May contain tartrazine.

• Patients who are allergic to penicillins or cephalosporins may not be allergic to aztreonam since there is no cross-allergenicity.

• To administer a bolus of aztreonam, inject it slowly (over 3 to 5 minutes) directly into a vein or I.V. tubing.

• I.M. injections should be given deep into a large muscle mass, such as the upper outer quadrant of the gluteus maximus or the lateral part of the thigh.

• Obtain specimen for culture and sensitivity tests before first dose. Therapy may begin pending test results.

• Watch for superinfection (fever or other signs of new infection).

• Aztreonam is the first commercially available member of a new antibiotic family, the monobactams. Its effectiveness against gram-negative organisms is comparable to that of the aminoglycoside antibiotics, without the ototoxicity or nephrotoxicity usually associated with the aminoglycosides.

---

bacitracin
Pregnancy Risk Category: C

HOW SUPPLIED
Injection: 10,000-unit, 50,000-unit vials

MECHANISM OF ACTION
Hinders bacterial cell wall synthesis, damaging the bacterial plasma membrane and making the cell more vulnerable to osmotic pressure.

INDICATIONS & DOSAGE
Pneumonia or empyema caused by susceptible staphylococci—
Infants over 2.5 kg: 1,000 units/kg I.M. daily, divided q 8 to 12 hours.
Infants under 2.5 kg: 900 units/kg I.M. daily, divided q 8 to 12 hours.

Although the FDA approves the use of bacitracin in infants only, adults with susceptible staphylococcal infections may receive 10,000 to 25,000 units I.M. q 6 hours (maximum 25,000 units/dose, 100,000 units daily).

ADVERSE REACTIONS
Blood: blood dyscrasias, eosinophilia.
EENT: ototoxicity.
GI: nausea, vomiting, anorexia, diarrhea, rectal itching or burning.
GU: *nephrotoxicity (albuminuria,* cylindruria, oliguria, anuria, increased BUN, tubular and glomerular necrosis).
Skin: urticaria, rash.
Local: *pain at injection site.*
Other: superinfection, fever, *anaphylaxis,* neuromuscular blockade.

INTERACTIONS
None significant.

NURSING CONSIDERATIONS
• Contraindicated in impaired renal function. Use cautiously in myasthenia gravis and neuromuscular disease.

• Obtain specimen for culture and sensitivity tests before first dose. Therapy may begin pending test results.

• For I.M. administration only. Give deep I.M.; injection may be painful; dilute in solution containing sodium chloride and 2% procaine hydrochloride (if hospital policy permits). Do not dilute in procaine hydrochloride if patient is sensitive to procaine or PABA derivatives.

• Maintain adequate fluid intake, and monitor urine output closely. If intake or output decreases, notify the doctor.

• Obtain baseline renal function studies before starting therapy. Monitor daily during therapy. Notify doctor of any change.

• Concentration of bacitracin should be between 5,000 and 10,000 units/

---

ml. Store in refrigerator. Drug is inactivated if stored at room temperature.
• Report adverse effects to the doctor immediately.
• May be used with neomycin as a bowel preparation, or in solution as a wound irrigating agent.
• Urine pH should be kept above 6.0 to reduce the risk of nephrotoxicity.
• Prolonged therapy may result in overgrowth of nonsusceptible organisms, especially *Candida albicans*.
• Don't administer by I.V. route; drug is irritating to vein and predisposes patient to severe thrombophlebitis.

---

chloramphenicol
Chloromycetin, Novochlorocap†

chloramphenicol palmitate
Chloromycetin Palmitate

chloramphenicol sodium succinate
Chloromycetin, Pentamycetin†, Sodium Succinate

Pregnancy Risk Category: C

HOW SUPPLIED
Capsules: 250 mg, 500 mg
Oral suspension: 150 mg/5 ml
Injection: 1-g, 10-g vials

MECHANISM OF ACTION
Inhibits bacterial protein synthesis by binding to the 50S subunit of the ribosome.

INDICATIONS & DOSAGE
Hemophilus influenzae *meningitis, acute* Salmonella typhi *infection, and meningitis, bacteremia, or other severe infections caused by sensitive* Salmonella *species,* Rickettsia, *lymphogranuloma, psittacosis, or various sensitive gram-negative organisms—*
Adults and children: 50 to 100 mg/ kg P.O. or I.V. daily, divided q 6 hours. Maximum dosage is 100 mg/ kg daily.

Premature infants and neonates 2 weeks or younger: 25 mg/kg P.O. or I.V. daily, divided q 6 hours. I.V. route must be used to treat meningitis.

ADVERSE REACTIONS
Blood: *aplastic anemia,* hypoplastic anemia, *granulocytopenia,* thrombocytopenia.
CNS: headache, mild depression, confusion, delirium, peripheral neuropathy with prolonged therapy.
EENT: optic neuritis (in patients with cystic fibrosis), glossitis, decreased visual acuity.
GI: nausea, vomiting, stomatitis, diarrhea, enterocolitis.
Other: infections by nonsusceptible organisms, hypersensitivity reaction (fever, rash, urticaria, *anaphylaxis*), jaundice, *gray baby syndrome in premature and newborn infants (abdominal distention, gray cyanosis, vasomotor collapse, respiratory distress, death within a few hours of onset of symptoms).*

INTERACTIONS
Acetaminophen: elevates chloramphenicol levels. Monitor for chloramphenicol toxicity.
Chlorpropamide, dicumarol, phenobarbital, phenytoin, tolbutamide: blood levels of these agents may be increased by chloramphenicol.

NURSING CONSIDERATIONS
• Use cautiously in impaired hepatic or renal function, and with other drugs causing bone marrow depression or blood disorders. *Don't use for infections caused by organisms susceptible to other agents or for trivial infections; use only when clearly indicated for severe infection.*
• Obtain specimen for culture and sensitivity tests before first dose. Therapy may begin pending test results.
• Monitor CBC, platelets, serum iron, and reticulocytes before and ev-

---

Italicized adverse reactions are common or life-threatening.
*Liquid form contains alcohol.   **May contain tartrazine.

ery 2 days during therapy. Stop drug immediately if anemia, reticulocytopenia, leukopenia, or thrombocytopenia develops.
• Instruct patient to report adverse reactions to the doctor, especially nausea, vomiting, diarrhea, fever, confusion, sore throat, or mouth sores.
• Tell patient to take medication for as long as prescribed, exactly as directed, even after he feels better.
• Give I.V. slowly over 1 minute. Check injection site daily for phlebitis and irritation.
• Reconstitute 1-g vial of powder for injection with 10 ml sterile water for injection. Concentration will be 100 mg/ml. Stable for 30 days at room temperature, but refrigeration recommended. Do not use cloudy solutions.
• Monitor for evidence of superinfection by nonsusceptible organisms.
• Therapeutic plasma concentrations are 5 to 25 mcg/ml.

---

ciprofloxacin
Cipro, Ciproxin‡

Pregnancy Risk Category: C

HOW SUPPLIED
Tablets: 250 mg, 500 mg, 750 mg

MECHANISM OF ACTION
A broad-spectrum quinolone antibiotic. Exact mechanism is unknown, but bactericidal effects may result from drug's ability to inhibit bacterial DNA gyrase and to prevent DNA replication in susceptible bacteria.

INDICATIONS & DOSAGE
Mild to moderate urinary tract infections—
Adults: 250 mg P.O. q 12 hours.
Severe or complicated urinary tract infections; mild to moderate bone and joint infections; mild to moderate respiratory tract infections; mild to
moderate skin and skin structure infections; infectious diarrhea—
Adults: 500 mg P.O. q 12 hours.
Severe or complicated bone or joint infections; severe respiratory tract infections; severe skin and skin structure infection—
Adults: 750 mg P.O. q 12 hours.

ADVERSE REACTIONS
CNS: headache, restlessness, tremor, light-headedness, confusion, hallucinations, *seizures.*
GI: nausea, diarrhea, vomiting, abdominal pain or discomfort, oral candidiasis.
GU: crystalluria.
Other: rash.

INTERACTIONS
Antacids containing magnesium hydroxide or aluminum hydroxide: decreased ciprofloxacin absorption. Separate administration by at least 2 hours.
Probenecid: may elevate serum level of ciprofloxacin.
Theophylline: increased plasma theophylline concentrations and prolonged theophylline half-life.

NURSING CONSIDERATIONS
• Contraindicated in patients sensitive to quinolone antibiotics, in pregnant or breast-feeding women, and in children. Quinolone antibiotics have been shown to produce arthropathy in young laboratory animals.
• Obtain specimen for culture and sensitivity tests before first dose. Therapy may begin pending test results.
• The preferred time for dosing is 2 hours after a meal. Food does not affect absorption but may delay peak serum levels.
• May cause CNS stimulation. Use with caution in CNS disorders, such as severe cerebral arteriosclerosis or epilepsy, and in other patients who are at an increased risk of seizures.

- May cause dizziness or light-headedness. Warn patient to avoid hazardous tasks that require alertness, such as driving, until CNS effects of the drug are known.
- Advise patient to drink plenty of fluids to reduce the risk of crystalluria.
- Dosage adjustments may be necessary in patients with renal dysfunction.
- Prolonged use may result in overgrowth of organisms that are resistant to ciprofloxacin.

---

clindamycin hydrochloride
Cleocin HCl, Dalacin C†‡

clindamycin palmitate hydrochloride
Cleocin Pediatric, Dalacin C Palmitate†‡

clindamycin phosphate
Cleocin, Cleocin Phosphate, Dalacin C†‡, Dalacin C Phosphate

Pregnancy Risk Category: C

HOW SUPPLIED
Capsules: 75 mg, 150 mg
Oral solution: 75 mg/5 ml
Injection: 150 mg/ml

MECHANISM OF ACTION
Inhibits bacterial protein synthesis by binding to the 50S subunit of the ribosome.

INDICATIONS & DOSAGE
Infections caused by sensitive staphylococci, streptococci, pneumococci, Bacteroides, Fusobacterium, *Clostridium perfringens, and other sensitive aerobic and anaerobic organisms—*
Adults: 150 to 450 mg P.O. q 6 hours; or 300 mg I.M. or I.V. q 6, 8, or 12 hours. Up to 2,700 mg I.M. or I.V. daily, divided q 6, 8, or 12 hours.
   May be used for severe infections.

Children over 1 month: 8 to 25 mg/ kg P.O. daily, divided q 6 to 8 hours; or 15 to 40 mg/kg I.M. or I.V. daily, divided q 6 hours.

ADVERSE REACTIONS
Blood: transient leukopenia, eosinophilia, thrombocytopenia.
GI: *nausea,* vomiting, abdominal pain, *diarrhea, pseudomembranous enterocolitis,* esophagitis, flatulence, anorexia, *bloody or tarry stools, dysphagia.*
Hepatic: elevated AST (SGOT), alkaline phosphatase, bilirubin.
Skin: maculopapular rash, urticaria.
Local: *pain,* induration, *sterile abscess with I.M. injection;* thrombophlebitis, erythema, and pain after I.V. administration.
Other: unpleasant or bitter taste, *anaphylaxis.*

INTERACTIONS
Erythromycin: antagonist that may block access of clindamycin to its site of action; don't use together.
Kaolin: decreased absorption of oral clindamycin.
Neuromuscular blocking agents: clindamycin may potentiate neuromuscular blockade.

NURSING CONSIDERATIONS
- Contraindicated in patients with known hypersensitivity to the antibiotic congener lincomycin; also in patients with history of GI disease, especially colitis. Use cautiously in newborns and patients with renal or hepatic disease, asthma, or significant allergies.
- Monitor renal, hepatic, and hematopoietic functions during prolonged therapy.
- Obtain specimen for culture and sensitivity tests before first dose. Therapy may begin pending test results.
- Don't use in meningitis. Drug does not penetrate blood/brain barrier.

Italicized adverse reactions are common or life-threatening.
*Liquid form contains alcohol.   **May contain tartrazine.

• Don't refrigerate reconstituted oral solution, as it will thicken. Drug is stable for 2 weeks at room temperature.

• Instruct patient to report adverse reactions to the doctor, especially diarrhea. Warn patient not to treat such diarrhea himself.

• Advise patients taking the capsule form to take with a full glass of water to prevent dysphagia.

• Don't give diphenoxylate compound (Lomotil) to treat drug-induced diarrhea. May prolong and worsen diarrhea.

• Give deep I.M. Rotate sites. Warn that I.M. injection may be painful. Doses greater than 600 mg per injection are not recommended.

• When giving I.V., check site daily for phlebitis and irritation. For I.V. infusion, dilute each 300 mg in 50 ml solution, and give no faster than 30 mg/minute.

• Watch for superinfection (fever or other signs of new infection).

• I.M. injection may cause creatinine phospokinase level to rise due to muscle irritation.

erythromycin base
Apo-Erythro base†, EMU-V‡, E-Mycin, Eryc, Eryc Sprinkle, Ery-Tab, Erythromid†, Ilotycin, Novorythro†, PCE Dispersatabs, Robimycin

erythromycin estolate
Ilosone, Novorythro†

erythromycin ethylsuccinate
Apo-Erythro-ES†, E.E.S., E-Mycin E, EryPed, Erythrocin, Pediamycin, Wyamycin E

erythromycin gluceptate
Ilotycin

erythromycin lactobionate
Erythrocin

erythromycin stearate
Apo-Erythro-S†, Erypar, Erythrocin, Novorythro†, Wyamycin S

Pregnancy Risk Category: B

HOW SUPPLIED
base
Tablets (enteric-coated): 250 mg, 330 mg, 500 mg
Pellets (enteric-coated): 250 mg
Oral suspension: 125 mg/5 ml, 200 mg/5 ml, 400 mg/5 ml
estolate
Tablets: 250 mg, 500 mg
Tablets (chewable): 125 mg, 250 mg
Capsules: 125 mg, 250 mg
Oral suspension: 125 mg/5 ml, 250 mg/5 ml
Drops: 100 mg/ml
ethylsuccinate
Tablets (chewable): 200 mg, 400 mg
gluceptate
Injection: 250-mg, 500-mg, 1-g vials
lactobionate
Injection: 500-mg, 1-g vials
stearate
Tablets (film-coated): 250 mg, 500 mg

MECHANISM OF ACTION
Inhibits bacterial protein synthesis by binding to the 50S subunit of the ribosome.

INDICATIONS & DOSAGE
Acute pelvic inflammatory disease caused by Neisseria gonorrhoeae—
Women: 500 mg I.V. (erythromycin glucceptate, lactobionate) q 6 hours for 3 days, then 250 mg (erythromycin base, estolate, stearate) or 400 mg (erythromycin ethylsuccinate) P.O. q 6 hours for 7 days.
Endocarditis prophylaxis for dental procedures in patients allergic to penicillin—
Adults: 1 g (erythromycin base, estolate, stearate) P.O. 1 hour before procedure, then 500 mg P.O. 6 hours later.
Intestinal amebiasis—
Adults: 250 mg (erythromycin base, estolate, stearate) P.O. q 6 hours for 10 to 14 days.
Children: 30 to 50 mg/kg (erythromycin base, estolate, stearate) P.O. daily, divided q 6 hours for 10 to 14 days.
Mild-to-moderately severe respiratory tract, skin, and soft tissue infections caused by sensitive group A beta-hemolytic streptococci, Diplococcus pneumoniae, Mycoplasma pneumoniae, Corynebacterium diphtheriae, Bordetella pertussis, Listeria monocytogenes—
Adults: 250 to 500 mg (erythromycin base, estolate, stearate) P.O. q 6 hours; or 400 to 800 mg (erythromycin ethylsuccinate) P.O. q 6 hours; or 15 to 20 mg/kg I.V. daily, as continuous infusion or divided q 6 hours.
Children: 30 mg/kg to 50 mg/kg (oral erythromycin salts) P.O. daily, divided q 6 hours; or 15 to 20 mg/kg I.V. daily, divided q 4 to 6 hours.
Syphilis—
Adults: 500 mg (erythromycin base, estolate, stearate) P.O. q.i.d. for 15 days.

Legionnaire's Disease—
Adults: 500 mg to 1 g I.V. or P.O. q 6 hours for 21 days.
Uncomplicated urethral, endocervical, or rectal infections where tetracyclines are contraindicated—
Adults: 500 mg P.O. q.i.d. for at least 7 days.
Urogenital Chlamydia trachomatis *infections during pregnancy—*
Adults: 500 mg P.O. q.i.d. for at least 7 days or 250 mg P.O. q.i.d. for at least 14 days.
Conjunctivitis caused by Chlamydia trachomatis *in newborns—*
Newborns: 50 mg/kg P.O. daily in four divided doses for at least 2 weeks.
Pneumonia of infancy due to Chlamydia trachomatis—
Infants: 50 mg/kg/day in four divided doses for at least 3 weeks.

ADVERSE REACTIONS
EENT: hearing loss with high I.V. doses.
GI: *abdominal pain and cramping, nausea, vomiting, diarrhea.*
Hepatic: cholestatic jaundice (with erythromycin estolate).
Skin: urticaria, rashes.
Local: *venous irritation, thrombophlebitis following I.V. injection.*
Other: overgrowth of nonsusceptible bacteria or fungi; *anaphylaxis;* fever.

INTERACTIONS
Clindamycin, lincomycin: may be antagonistic. Don't use together.
Oral anticoagulants: increased anticoagulant effects.
Theophylline: decreased erythromycin blood level and increased theophylline toxicity. Use together cautiously.

NURSING CONSIDERATIONS
• Erythromycin estolate contraindicated in hepatic disease. Use other erythromycin salts cautiously in impaired hepatic function.
• Obtain specimen for culture and

Italicized adverse reactions are common or life-threatening.
*Liquid form contains alcohol.   **May contain tartrazine.

sensitivity tests before first dose. Therapy may begin pending test results.

• For best absorption, instruct patient to take oral form of drug with a full glass of water 1 hour before or 2 hours after meals. If tablets are coated, they may be taken with meals. Tell patient not to drink fruit juice with medication. Chewable erythromycin tablets should not be swallowed whole.

• Coated forms of erythromycin are associated with lower incidence of GI problems. May be more tolerable in patients who cannot easily tolerate erythromycin.

• When administering suspension, be sure to note the concentration.

• May cause overgrowth of nonsusceptible bacteria or fungi. Monitor for signs and symptoms of superinfection.

• Tell patient to take medication for as long as prescribed, exactly as directed, even after he feels better, and to take entire amount prescribed. Treat streptococcal infections for 10 days.

• Report adverse reactions, especially nausea, abdominal pain, and fever.

• Erythromycin estolate may cause serious hepatotoxicity in adults (reversible cholestatic jaundice). Monitor hepatic function (increased levels of bilirubin, AST [SGOT], ALT [SGPT], and alkaline phosphatase may occur). Other erythromycin salts cause hepatotoxicity to a lesser degree. Patients who develop hepatotoxicity from estolate may react similarly to treatment with any erythromycin preparation.

• I.V. dose should be administered over 60 minutes. Reconstitute according to manufacturer's directions and dilute each 250 mg in at least 100 ml 0.9% normal saline solution.

• Erythromycin lactobionate should not be administered with other drugs.

imipenem/cilastatin sodium
Primaxin

Pregnancy Risk Category: C

HOW SUPPLIED
Injection: 250-ml, 500-ml vials

MECHANISM OF ACTION
Imipenem is bactericidal and inhibits bacterial cell wall synthesis. Cilastatin inhibits the enzymatic breakdown of imipenem in the kidney, making it effective in the urinary tract.

INDICATIONS & DOSAGE
Treatment of serious infections of the lower respiratory and urinary tracts, intraabdominal and gynecologic infections, bacterial septicemia, bone and joint infections, skin and soft tissue infections, and endocarditis. Most known microorganisms susceptible: Staphylococcus, Streptococcus, Escherichia coli, Klebsiella, Proteus, Enterobacter, Pseudomonas aeruginosa, *and* Bacteroides, *including* B. fragilis—

Adults: 250 mg to 1 g by I.V. infusion q 6 to 8 hours. Maximum daily dosage is 50 mg/kg/day or 4 g/day, whichever is less.

ADVERSE REACTIONS
CNS: *seizures,* dizziness.
CV: hypotension.
GI: nausea, vomiting, diarrhea, *pseudomembranous colitis.*
Skin: rash, urticaria, pruritus.
Local: *thrombophlebitis, pain at injection site.*
Other: *hypersensitivity.*

INTERACTIONS
None significant.

NURSING CONSIDERATIONS
• Use cautiously in patients allergic to penicillins or cephalosporins because this drug is chemically similar. Ask patient if he's had a hypersensi-

tivity reaction to either of these drugs before administering first dose of imipenem.
• Use cautiously in patients who have a history of seizure disorders, especially if they also have compromised renal function. If patient develops seizures that persist despite anticonvulsant therapy, notify doctor. The drug should then be discontinued.
• Don't administer by direct I.V. bolus injection. Each 250- or 500-mg dose should be given by I.V. infusion over 20 to 30 minutes. Each 1-g dose should be infused over 40 to 60 minutes. If nausea occurs, the infusion may be slowed.
• When reconstituting powder, shake until the solution is clear. Solutions may range from colorless to yellow and variations of color within this range don't affect the drug's potency. After reconstitution, solution is stable for 10 hours at room temperature and for 48 hours when refrigerated.
• Imipenem/cilastatin has the broadest antibacterial spectrum of any available antibiotic. The drug is most valuable for empiric treatment of infections and for mixed infections that would otherwise require a combination of antibiotics, often including an aminoglycoside.
• Patients with impaired renal function may need lower dosage or longer intervals between doses.
• Obtain specimen for culture and sensitivity tests before first dose. Therapy may begin pending test results.
• Monitor patient for bacterial or fungal superinfections and resistant infections during and after therapy.

lincomycin hydrochloride
Lincocin

Pregnancy Risk Category: B

HOW SUPPLIED
Capsules: 500 mg
Pediatric capsules: 250 mg
Syrup: 250 mg/5 ml
Injection: 300 mg/ml in 2-ml and 10-ml vials and 2-ml U-Ject

MECHANISM OF ACTION
Inhibits bacterial protein synthesis by binding to the 50S subunit of the ribosome.

INDICATIONS & DOSAGE
Respiratory tract, skin and soft tissue, and urinary tract infections; osteomyelitis, septicemia caused by sensitive group A beta-hemolytic streptococci, pneumococci, and staphylococci—
Adults: 500 mg P.O. q 6 to 8 hours (not to exceed 8 g daily); or 600 mg I.M. daily or q 12 hours; or 600 mg to 1 g I.V. q 8 to 12 hours (not to exceed 8 g daily).
Children over 1 month: 30 to 60 mg/kg P.O. daily, divided q 6 to 8 hours; or 10 mg/kg I.M. daily or divided q 12 hours; or 10 to 20 mg/kg I.V. daily, divided q 6 to 8 hours. For I.V. infusion, dilute to 100 ml; infuse over 1 hour to avoid hypotension.

ADVERSE REACTIONS
Blood: *neutropenia, leukopenia,* thrombocytopenia, purpura.
CNS: dizziness, headache.
CV: hypotension with rapid I.V. infusion.
EENT: glossitis, tinnitus.
GI: nausea, vomiting, *pseudomembranous colitis, persistent diarrhea,* abdominal cramps, stomatitis, pruritus ani.
GU: vaginitis.
Hepatic: cholestatic jaundice.
Skin: rashes, urticaria.
Local: pain at injection site.
Other: hypersensitivity, angioedema.

INTERACTIONS
Antidiarrheal medication (kaolin, pectin, attapulgite): reduce oral absorption of lincomycin by as much as 90%. Antidiarrheals should be

---

Italicized adverse reactions are common or life-threatening.
*Liquid form contains alcohol.   **May contain tartrazine.

avoided or given at least 2 hours before lincomycin.
Neuromuscular blocking agents: lincomycin may potentiate neuromuscular blockade.

NURSING CONSIDERATIONS
• Contraindicated in patients with hypersensitivity to clindamycin. Use cautiously in GI disorders (especially colitis), asthma or significant allergies, hepatic or renal disease, and endocrine or metabolic disorders.
• Obtain specimen for culture and sensitivity tests before first dose. Therapy may begin pending test results.
• For best absorption, instruct patient to take drug with a full glass of water 1 hour before or 2 hours after meals.
• Tell patient to take medication exactly as directed, even after he feels better, and to take entire amount prescribed.
• Tell patient to report adverse reactions to doctor, especially diarrhea. Warn him not to treat diarrhea himself because it may reflect the onset of antibiotic associated pseudomembraneous colitis.
• Monitor for signs of bacterial and fungal superinfection, especially when therapy exceeds 10 days.
• Give deep I.M. Rotate sites. Warn that I.M. injection may be painful.
• When giving I.V., check site daily for phlebitis and irritation. Rotate infusion sites regularly.
• Rapid I.V. infusion may cause hypotension and syncope. Monitor blood pressure in patients receiving the drug parenterally.
• Monitor hepatic function (increased levels of alkaline phosphatase, AST (SGOT), ALT (SGPT), bilirubin may occur).
• Monitor CBC and platelets. Stop drug immediately if neutropenia, leukopenia, or other blood disorders develop.

pentamidine isethionate
NebuPent, Pentam 300
Pregnancy Risk Category: C

HOW SUPPLIED
Injection: 300-mg vials

MECHANISM OF ACTION
Interferes with biosynthesis of DNA, RNA, phospholipids, and proteins in susceptible organisms.

INDICATIONS & DOSAGE
Treatment of pneumonia due to Pneumocystis carinii—
Adults and children: 4 mg/kg I.V. or I.M. once a day for 14 days.
Prevention of Pneumocystis carinii *pneumonia in high-risk individuals—*
Adults: 300 mg by inhalation (using a Respirgard II nebulizer) once every 4 weeks.

ADVERSE REACTIONS
Blood: *leukopenia,* thrombocytopenia, anemia.
CNS: confusion, hallucinations.
CV: *hypotension,* tachycardia.
Endocrine: *hypoglycemia,* hyperglycemia, hypocalcemia.
GI: nausea, anorexia, metallic taste.
GU: *elevated serum creatinine,* renal toxicity.
Hepatic: elevated liver enzymes.
Local: *sterile abscess, pain or induration at injection site.*
Skin: rash, facial flushing, pruritus.
Other: fever.

INTERACTIONS
Aminoglycosides, amphotericin B, cisplatin, vancomycin, zidovudine: increased risk of nephrotoxicity.

NURSING CONSIDERATIONS
• Once the diagnosis of *Pneumocystis carinii* pneumonia has been firmly established, there are no absolute contraindications to pentamidine therapy.
• Use cautiously in hypertension, hy-

potension, hypoglycemia, hypocalcemia, leukopenia, thrombocytopenia, anemia, and hepatic or renal dysfunction.

• Patient should be lying down when receiving the drug because sudden, severe hypotension may develop. Monitor blood pressure during administration and several times thereafter until blood pressure is stable.

• When administering I.V., infuse over 60 minutes to minimize risk of hypotension.

• Monitor blood glucose, serum creatinine, and BUN daily. After parenteral administration, blood glucose may decrease initially; hypoglycemia may be severe in 5% to 10% of patients. This may be followed by hyperglycemia and insulin-dependant diabetes mellitus (which may be permanent).

• Pain and induration occur universally with I.M. injection. Administer by deep I.M. injection.

• In patients with AIDS, pentamidine may produce less severe adverse reactions than the alternative treatment co-trimoxazole.Therefore, in some AIDS patients, pentamidine is considered the treatment of choice.

polymyxin B sulfate
Aerosporin

Pregnancy Risk Category: B

HOW SUPPLIED
Powder for injection: 500,000-unit vials

MECHANISM OF ACTION
Hinders bacterial cell wall synthesis, damaging the bacterial plasma membrane and making the cell more vulnerable to osmotic pressure.

INDICATIONS & DOSAGE
Acute urinary tract infections or septicemia caused by sensitive Pseudomonas aeruginosa, *or when other antibiotics are ineffective or contraindicated; bacteremia caused by sensitive* Enterobacter aerogenes *and* Klebsiella pneumoniae, *or acute urinary tract infections caused by* Escherichia coli—
Adults and children: 15,000 to 25,000 units/kg daily I.V. infusion, divided q 12 hours; or 25,000 to 30,000 units/kg daily, divided q 4 to 8 hours. I.M. not advised due to severe pain at injection site.
Meningitis caused by sensitive P. aeruginosa *or* Hemophilus influenzae *when other antibiotics ineffective or contraindicated*—
Adults and children over 2 years: 50,000 units intrathecally once daily for 3 to 4 days, then 50,000 units every other day for at least 2 weeks after cerebrospinal fluid tests are negative and cerebrospinal fluid sugar is normal.
Children under 2 years: 20,000 units intrathecally once daily for 3 to 4 days, then 25,000 units every other day for at least 2 weeks after cerebrospinal fluid tests are negative and cerebrospinal fluid sugar is normal.

ADVERSE REACTIONS
CNS: irritability, drowsiness, facial flushing, weakness, ataxia, respiratory paralysis, headache and meningeal irritation with intrathecal administration, peripheral and perioral paresthesias, seizures, *coma.*
EENT: blurred vision.
GU: *nephrotoxicity* (albuminuria, cylindruria, hematuria, proteinuria, decreased urine output, increased BUN).
Skin: urticaria.
Local: *pain at I.M. injection site.*
Other: hypersensitivity reactions with fever, *anaphylaxis.*

INTERACTIONS
• *Aminoglycosides, amphotericin B, cisplatin, vancomycin, zidovudine:* increased risk of nephrotoxicity.

Italicized adverse reactions are common or life-threatening.
*Liquid form contains alcohol.   **May contain tartrazine.

- *Neuromuscular blocking agents:* polymyxin B may potentiate neuromuscular blockade.

NURSING CONSIDERATIONS
- Use cautiously in impaired renal function or myasthenia gravis.
- Give only to hospitalized patients under constant medical supervision.
- For meningitis, must give intrathecally to achieve adequate cerebrospinal fluid levels.
- Give deep I.M. Warn that injection may be painful. If patient isn't allergic to procaine, use 1% procaine (if hospital policy permits) as diluent to decrease pain. Rotate sites.
- Don't give solution containing local anesthetics I.V. or intrathecally.
- When giving I.V., check site daily for phlebitis and irritation. Dilute each 500,000 units in 300 to 500 ml dextrose 5% in water; infuse over 60 to 90 minutes. Rotate I.V. sites regularly.
- Parenteral solutions should be refrigerated and used within 72 hours.
- Monitor renal function (BUN, serum creatinine, creatinine clearance, urine output) before and during therapy. Intake should be sufficient to maintain output at 1,500 ml/day (between 3,000 and 4,000 ml/day for adults).
- Obtain specimen for culture and sensitivity tests before first dose. Therapy may begin pending test results.
- Notify doctor immediately if patient develops fever, CNS adverse effects, rash, or symptoms of nephrotoxicity.
- If patient is scheduled for surgery, notify anesthesiologist of preoperative treatment with this drug since it may prolong neuromuscular blockade.

spectinomycin dihydrochloride
Trobicin

Pregnancy Risk Category: B

HOW SUPPLIED
Injection: 2-g vial with 3.2-ml diluent; 4-g vial with 6.2-ml diluent
Powder for injection: 2 g, 4 g

MECHANISM OF ACTION
Inhibits protein synthesis by binding to the 30S subunit of the ribosome.

INDICATIONS & DOSAGE
Gonorrhea—
Adults: 2 to 4 g I.M. single dose injected deeply into the upper outer quadrant of the buttock.

ADVERSE REACTIONS
CNS: insomnia, dizziness.
GI: nausea.
GU: decreased urine output.
Skin: urticaria.
Local: pain at injection site.
Other: fever, chills (may mask or delay symptoms of incubating syphilis).

INTERACTIONS
None significant.

NURSING CONSIDERATIONS
- Not effective in the treatment of syphilis.
- Serologic test for syphilis should be done before treatment dose and 3 months after.
- Use 20G needle to administer drug. The 4-g dose (10 ml) should be divided into two 5-ml injections—one in each buttock.
- Shake vial vigorously after reconstitution and before withdrawing dose. Store at room temperature after reconstitution and use within 24 hours.
- Should be reserved for penicillin-resistant strains of gonorrhea.

---

trimethoprim
Alprin‡, Proloprim, Trimpex,
Triprim‡

Pregnancy Risk Category: C

HOW SUPPLIED
Tablets: 100 mg, 200 mg

MECHANISM OF ACTION
Interferes with the action of dihydrofolate reductase, inhibiting bacterial
synthesis of folic acid.

INDICATIONS & DOSAGE
*Treatment of uncomplicated urinary
tract infections caused by susceptible
strains of* Escherichia coli, Proteus
mirabilis, Klebsiella, *and* Enterobacter—
Adults: 100 mg P.O. every 12 hours
for 10 days.
   Not recommended for children under 12 years.

ADVERSE REACTIONS
Blood: thrombocytopenia, leukopenia, megaloblastic anemia, methemoglobinemia.
GI: *epigastric distress, nausea, vomiting,* glossitis.
Skin: *rash, pruritus, exfoliative dermatitis.*
Other: fever.

INTERACTIONS
Phenytoin: trimethoprim may decrease phenytoin metabolism and increase serum levels of phenytoin.

NURSING CONSIDERATIONS
• Contraindicated in documented
megaloblastic anemia due to folate
deficiency.
• Clinical signs such as sore throat,
fever, pallor, or purpura may be early
indications of serious blood disorders.
Complete blood counts should be
done routinely. Prolonged use of trimethoprim at high doses may cause
bone marrow suppression.

• Dosage should be decreased in patients with severely impaired renal
function. Give cautiously to patients
with impaired hepatic function.
• Obtain specimen for culture and
sensitivity tests before first dose.
Therapy may begin pending test results.
• Instruct patient to continue taking
the drug, even if he feels better, and
to take entire amount prescribed.

vancomycin hydrochloride
Vancocin

Pregnancy Risk Category: C

HOW SUPPLIED
Powder for oral solution: 1-g, 10-g
bottles
Powder for injection: 500-mg, 1-g
vials

MECHANISM OF ACTION
Hinders bacterial cell wall synthesis,
damaging the bacterial plasma membrane and making the cell more vulnerable to osmotic pressure.

INDICATIONS & DOSAGE
*Severe staphylococcal infections when
other antibiotics ineffective or contraindicated—*
Adults: 500 mg I.V. q 6 hours, or 1 g q
12 hours.
Children: 44 mg/kg I.V. daily, divided q 6 hours.
Neonates: 10 mg/kg I.V. daily, divided q 6 to 12 hours.
*Antibiotic-associated pseudomem-
branous and staphylococcal enterocolitis—*
Adults: 125 to 500 mg P.O. q 6 hours
for 7 to 10 days.
Children: 44 mg/kg P.O. daily, divided q 6 hours.
*Endocarditis prophylaxis for dental
procedures—*
Adults: 1 g I.V. slowly over 1 hour,
starting 1 hour before procedure. No
repeat dose is necessary.

Italicized adverse reactions are common or life-threatening.
*Liquid form contains alcohol.   **May contain tartrazine.

ADVERSE REACTIONS
Blood: transient eosinophilia, leukopenia.
EENT: tinnitus, ototoxicity (deafness).
GI: nausea.
Skin: "red-neck" syndrome with rapid I.V. infusion (maculopapular rash on face, neck, trunk, and extremities).
Local: pain or thrombophlebitis with I.V. administration, necrosis.
Other: chills, fever, *anaphylaxis,* overgrowth of nonsusceptible organisms.

INTERACTIONS
Aminoglycosides, amphotericin B, cisplatin, pentamidine: increased risk of nephrotoxicity.

NURSING CONSIDERATIONS
• Use cautiously in patients receiving other neurotoxic, nephrotoxic, or ototoxic drugs. Use cautiously in impaired hepatic or renal function; also in those with preexisting hearing loss; in patients over 60 years; and in patients with allergies to other antibiotics. Patients with renal dysfunction require adjustment of dosage or dosing interval.
• Obtain specimen for culture and sensitivity tests before first dose. Therapy may begin pending test results.
• Tell patient to take medication exactly as directed, even after he feels better, and to take entire amount prescribed. Treat staphylococcal endocarditis for at least 4 weeks.
• Patients should receive auditory function tests before and during prolonged therapy.
• Tell patient to report adverse reactions at once, especially fullness or ringing in ears. Stop drug immediately if these occur.
• Do not give drug I.M.
• For I.V. infusion, dilute in 200 ml sodium chloride injection or 5% glucose solution and infuse over 60 minutes. Check site daily for phlebitis and irritation. Report pain at infusion site. Avoid extravasation. Severe irritation and necrosis can result.
• Monitor patient carefully for "red-neck" syndrome. Stop infusion and notify doctor promptly if you see this reaction.
• Refrigerate I.V. solution after reconstitution and use within 96 hours.
• Monitor renal function (BUN, serum creatinine, urinalysis, creatinine clearance, and urine output) before and during therapy. Also monitor for signs of superinfection.
• Oral preparation stable for 2 weeks if refrigerated.

Cardiac glycosides and amrinone

amrinone lactate
deslanoside
digitoxin
digoxin

COMBINATION PRODUCTS
None.

amrinone lactate
Inocor

Pregnancy Risk Category: C

HOW SUPPLIED
Injection: 5 mg/ml

MECHANISM OF ACTION
Produces inotropic action by increasing cellular levels of cyclic adenosine monophosphate. Produces vasodilation through a direct relaxant effect on vascular smooth muscle.

INDICATIONS & DOSAGE
Short-term management of CHF—
Adults: initially, 0.75 mg/kg I.V. bolus over 2 to 3 minutes. Then begin maintenance infusion of 5 to 10 mcg/kg/minute. Additional bolus of 0.75 mg/kg may be given 30 minutes after start of therapy. Total daily dosage should not exceed 10 mg/kg.

ADVERSE REACTIONS
Blood: *thrombocytopenia* (dose-dependent).
CV: *arrhythmias,* hypotension.
GI: nausea, vomiting, cramps, dyspepsia, diarrhea.

Hepatic: elevated enzymes, rarely hepatotoxicity.
Local: burning at site of injection.
Other: hypersensitivity reactions (pericarditis, ascites, myositis vasculitis, pleuritis).

INTERACTIONS
Digitalis glycosides: Enhanced inotropic effect. Beneficial drug interaction.
Disopyramide: excessive hypotension. Don't administer concurrently.

NURSING CONSIDERATIONS
• Don't use in severe aortic or pulmonic valvular disease. Use cautiously in idiopathic hypertrophic subaortic stenosis. Not recommended during acute phase of myocardial infarction.
• Dosage should be based on clinical response, including assessment of pulmonary artery pressures and cardiac output. Cardiovascular effects begin within 2 to 5 minutes after starting infusion, and may last for 30 minutes to 2 hours after infusion is discontinued.
• Amrinone may be added to digitalis glycoside therapy in atrial fibrillation and flutter since it enhances AV conduction and increases ventricular response rate.
• Amrinone should be administered with a continuous infusion pump.
• Monitor blood pressure and heart rate throughout the infusion. Slow or stop infusion and notify doctor if patient's blood pressure falls.
• Monitor platelet count. Platelet

count below 150,000/mm^3 usually requires a decreased dosage.
• Administer amrinone as supplied, or dilute in 0.45% or 0.9% saline solution to a concentration of 1 to 3 mg/ml. Use diluted solution within 24 hours. Don't mix other drugs into this solution.
• Furosemide will form a precipitate with amrinone solutions. Don't mix together.
• Don't dilute with solutions containing dextrose because a slow chemical reaction occurs over 24 hours. However, amrinone can be injected into running dextrose infusions through a Y connector or directly into the tubing.
• Amrinone is primarily prescribed for patients who have not responded to therapy with digitalis, diuretics, and vasodilators.

deslanoside (desacetyl-lanatoside C)
Cedilanid†, Cedilanid-D
Pregnancy Risk Category: C

HOW SUPPLIED
Injection: 0.2 mg/ml

MECHANISM OF ACTION
Promotes movement of calcium from extracellular to intracellular cytoplasm and inhibits sodium-potassium activated adenosine triphosphatase. These actions strengthen myocardial contraction.

INDICATIONS & DOSAGE
CHF, paroxysmal atrial tachycardia, atrial fibrillation and flutter—
Adults: loading dose is 1.2 to 1.6 mg I.M. or slow I.V. in two divided doses over 24 hours; for maintenance, use another glycoside. Not recommended for children.

ADVERSE REACTIONS
The following are signs of toxicity that may occur with all cardiac glycosides:
CNS: *fatigue, generalized muscle weakness, agitation,* hallucinations, headache, malaise, dizziness, vertigo, stupor, paresthesias.
CV: *increased severity of CHF, arrhythmias (most commonly conduction disturbances with or without AV block, premature ventricular contractions, and supraventricular arrhythmias),* hypotension.
Toxic effects on heart may be life-threatening and require immediate attention.
EENT: *yellow-green halos around visual images, blurred vision,* light flashes, photophobia, diplopia.
GI: *anorexia, nausea,* vomiting, diarrhea.

INTERACTIONS
Amphotericin B, carbenicillin, ticarcillin, corticosteroids, and diuretics (including loop diuretics, chlorthalidone, metolazone, and thiazides): hypokalemia, predisposing patient to digitalis toxicity. Monitor serum potassium.
Parenteral calcium, thiazides: hypercalcemia and hypomagnesemia, predisposing patient to digitalis toxicity. Monitor serum calcium and serum magnesium.

NURSING CONSIDERATIONS
• Contraindicated in presence of any digitalis-induced toxicity; ventricular fibrillation; ventricular tachycardia unless caused by CHF. Administering calcium salts to digitalized patient is contraindicated. Calcium affects cardiac contractility and excitability in much the same way as glycosides and may lead to serious arrhythmias in digitalized patient. Use with extreme caution in elderly patients, and in those with acute myocardial infarction, incomplete AV block, chronic constrictive pericarditis, idiopathic

hypertrophic subaortic stenosis, renal insufficiency, severe pulmonary disease, or hypothyroidism.

• Use only for rapid digitilization, not maintenance therapy. Deslanoside has a low therapeutic index, and its dosage should be based upon patient response.

• Maintenance therapy with an oral digitalis glycoside is usually initiated within 12 to 24 hours.

• Hypothyroid patients are sensitive to effects of glycosides; hyperthyroid patients may need larger doses.

• Obtain baseline data (heart rate and rhythm, blood pressure, and electrolytes) before giving first dose. Monitor ECG continuously.

• Question patient about recent use of cardiac glycosides (within the previous 2 to 3 weeks) before administering a loading dose. Always divide loading dose over first 24 hours unless clinical situation indicates otherwise.

• Dosage is adjusted to patient's clinical condition and is monitored by serum levels of cardiac glycoside, calcium, potassium, magnesium, and by ECG.

• Take apical-radial pulse for a full minute. Record and report to doctor any significant changes (sudden increase or decrease in rate, pulse deficit, irregular beats, and particularly regularization of a previously irregular rhythm). Check blood pressure and obtain 12-lead ECG with these changes.

• Excessive slowing of the pulse rate (60 beats/minute or less) may be a sign of digitalis toxicity. Withhold drug and notify doctor.

• I.M. injection is painful; give I.V. if possible. I.V. administration also provides for a more rapid effect.

• Monitor serum potassium carefully. Take corrective action *before* hypokalemia occurs.

digitoxin
Crystodigin

Pregnancy Risk Category: C

HOW SUPPLIED
Tablets: 0.05 mg, 0.1 mg, 0.15 mg, 0.2 mg

MECHANISM OF ACTION
Promotes movement of calcium from extracellular to intracellular cytoplasm and inhibits sodium-potassium activated adenosine triphosphatase. These actions strengthen myocardial contraction.

INDICATIONS & DOSAGE
CHF, paroxysmal atrial tachycardia, atrial fibrillation and flutter—
Adults: loading dose is 1.2 to 1.6 mg P.O. in divided doses over 24 hours; average maintenance dosage is 0.15 mg daily (range: 0.05 to 0.3 mg daily).
Children 2 to 12 years: loading dose is 0.03 mg/kg or 0.75 mg/m² P.O. in divided doses over 24 hours; maintenance dosage is one-tenth of loading dose or 0.003 mg/kg or 0.075 mg/m² daily. Monitor closely for toxicity.
Children 1 to 2 years: loading dose is 0.04 mg/kg P.O. over 24 hours in divided doses; maintenance dosage is 0.004 mg/kg daily. Monitor closely for toxicity.
Children 2 weeks to 1 year: loading dose is 0.045 mg/kg P.O. in divided doses over 24 hours; maintenance dosage is 0.0045 mg/kg daily. Monitor closely for toxicity.
Premature infants, neonates, severely ill older infants: loading dose is 0.022 mg/kg P.O. in divided doses over 24 hours; maintenance dosage is 0.0022 mg/kg daily. Monitor closely for toxicity.

ADVERSE REACTIONS
The following are signs of toxicity that may occur with all cardiac glycosides:

Italicized adverse reactions are common or life-threatening.
*Liquid form contains alcohol.   **May contain tartrazine.

CNS: *fatigue, generalized muscle weakness, agitation, hallucinations,* headache, malaise, dizziness, vertigo, stupor, paresthesias.
CV: *increased severity of CHF, arrhythmias (most commonly conduction disturbances with or without AV block, premature ventricular contractions, and supraventricular arrhythmias),* hypotension.
Toxic effects on heart may be life-threatening and require immediate attention.
EENT: *yellow-green halos around visual images, blurred vision,* light flashes, photophobia, diplopia.
GI: *anorexia, nausea,* vomiting, diarrhea.

INTERACTIONS

Amphotericin B, carbenicillin, ticarcillin, corticosteroids, and diuretics (including loop diuretics, chlorthalidone, metolazone, and thiazides): hypokalemia, predisposing patient to digitalis toxicity. Monitor serum potassium.
Antacids, kaolin-pectin: decreased absorption of oral digitoxin. Schedule doses as far as possible from oral digitoxin administration.
Cholestyramine, colestipol, metoclopramide: decreased absorption of oral digitoxin. Monitor for decreased effect and low blood levels. Dosage may have to be increased.
Cimetidine: decreased digitoxin metabolism. Monitor for digitoxin toxicity.
Parenteral calcium, thiazides: hypercalcemia and hypomagnesemia, predisposing patient to digitalis toxicity. Monitor serum calcium and serum magnesium.
Phenylbutazone, phenobarbital, phenytoin, rifampin: faster metabolism and shorter duration of digitoxin. Observe for underdigitalization.
Quinidine, verapamil: Possible increased serum digitoxin levels. Monitor patient closely.

NURSING CONSIDERATIONS

• Contraindicated in presence of any digitalis-induced toxicity; ventricular fibrillation; ventricular tachycardia unless caused by CHF. Administering calcium salts to digitalized patient is contraindicated. Calcium affects cardiac contractility and excitability in much the same way as glycosides and may lead to serious arrhythmias in digitalized patient. Use with extreme caution in acute myocardial infarction, incomplete AV block, chronic constrictive pericarditis, idiopathic hypertrophic subaortic stenosis, severe pulmonary disease, and hypothyroidism; and in elderly patients.
• Hypothyroid patients are very sensitive to glycosides; hyperthyroid patients may need larger doses.
• Obtain baseline data (heart rate and rhythm, blood pressure, and electrolytes) and question patient about recent use of cardiac glycosides (within the previous 2 to 3 weeks) before administering a loading dose. Always divide loading dose over first 24 hours unless clinical situation indicates otherwise.
• Dosage is adjusted to patient's clinical condition and is monitored by serum levels of cardiac glycoside, calcium, potassium, magnesium, and by ECG.
• Take apical-radial pulse for a full minute. Record and report to doctor any significant changes (sudden increase or decrease in rate, pulse deficit, irregular beats, and particularly regularization of a previously irregular rhythm). Check blood pressure and obtain 12-lead ECG with these changes.
• Excessive slowing of the pulse rate (60 beats/minute or less) may be a sign of digitalis toxicity. Withhold drug and notify doctor.
• Monitor serum potassium carefully. Take corrective action *before* hypokalemia occurs.

- Encourage the patient to eat potassium-rich foods.
- I.M. injection is painful and poorly absorbed; give I.V. if parenteral route is necessary.
- Digitoxin is a long-acting drug; watch for cumulative effects and signs of toxicity, especially in children and elderly patients. Ask patient about nausea, vomiting, anorexia, visual disturbances, and other symptoms of toxicity.
- Protect solution from light.
- Instruct patient and responsible family member about drug action, dosage regimen, how to take pulse, reportable signs, and follow-up plans.
- Don't substitute one brand for another.
- Therapeutic blood levels of digitoxin range from 25 to 35 ng/ml.
- Digitoxin toxicity may be treated by administering agents that bind the drug in the intestine (for example, colestipol and cholestyramine). Dysrhythmias may be treated with phenytoin I.V. Potentially life-threatening toxicity may be treated by specific antigen-binding fragments (such as digoxin immune FAB).

digoxin
Lanoxicaps, Lanoxin*, Novodigoxin†

Pregnancy Risk Category: C

HOW SUPPLIED
Tablets: 0.125 mg, 0.25 mg, 0.5 mg
Capsules: 0.05 mg, 0.1 mg, 0.2 mg
Elixir: 0.05 mg/ml
Injection: 0.05 mg/ml†, 0.1 mg/ml (pediatric), 0.25 mg/ml

MECHANISM OF ACTION
Promotes movement of calcium from extracellular to intracellular cytoplasm and inhibits sodium-potassium activated adenosine triphosphatase. These actions strengthen myocardial contraction.

INDICATIONS & DOSAGE
CHF, paroxysmal atrial tachycardia, atrial fibrillation and flutter—
Adults: loading dose is 0.5 to 1 mg I.V. or P.O. in divided doses over 24 hours; maintenance dosage is 0.125 to 0.5 mg I.V. or P.O. daily (average 0.25 mg). Larger doses are often needed for treatment of arrhythmias, depending on patient response. Smaller loading and maintenance doses should be given in patients with impaired renal function.
Adults over 65 years: 0.125 mg P.O. daily as maintenance dose. Frail or underweight elderly patients may require only 0.0625 mg daily or 0.125 mg every other day.
Children over 2 years: loading dose is 0.02 to 0.04 mg/kg P.O. divided q 8 hours over 24 hours; I.V. loading dose is 0.015 to 0.035 mg/kg; maintenance dosage is 0.012 mg/kg P.O. daily divided q 12 hours.
Children 1 month to 2 years: loading dose is 0.035 to 0.06 mg/kg P.O. in three divided doses over 24 hours; I.V. loading dose is 0.03 to 0.05 mg/kg; maintenance dosage is 0.01 to 0.02 mg/kg P.O. daily divided q 12 hours.
Neonates under 1 month: loading dose is 0.035 mg/kg P.O. divided q 8 hours over 24 hours; I.V. loading dose is 0.02 to 0.03 mg/kg; maintenance dosage is 0.01 mg/kg P.O. daily divided q 12 hours.
Premature infants: loading dose is 0.025 mg/kg I.V. in three divided doses over 24 hours; maintenance dosage is 0.01 mg/kg I.V. daily divided q 12 hours.

ADVERSE REACTIONS
The following are signs of toxicity that may occur with all cardiac glycosides:
CNS: *fatigue, generalized muscle weakness, agitation, hallucinations,* headache, malaise, dizziness, vertigo, stupor, paresthesias.
CV: *increased severity of CHF, ar-*

Italicized adverse reactions are common or life-threatening.
*Liquid form contains alcohol.   **May contain tartrazine.

rhythmias (*most commonly conduction disturbances with or without AV block, premature ventricular contractions, and supraventricular arrhythmias*), hypotension.

Toxic effects on heart may be life-threatening and require immediate attention.

EENT: *yellow-green halos around visual images, blurred vision,* light flashes, photophobia, diplopia.

GI: *anorexia, nausea,* vomiting, diarrhea.

INTERACTIONS

Amiloride: inhibits and increases digoxin excretion. Monitor for altered digoxin effect.

Amphotericin B, carbenicillin, ticarcillin, corticosteroids, and diuretics (including loop diuretics, chlorthalidone, metolazone, and thiazides): hypokalemia, predisposing patient to digitalis toxicity. Monitor serum potassium.

Antacids, kaolin-pectin: decreased absorption of oral digoxin. Schedule doses as far as possible from oral digoxin administration.

Anticholinergics: may increase digoxin absorption of oral tablets. Monitor blood levels and observe for toxicity.

Cholestyramine, colestipol, metoclopramide: decreased absorption of oral digoxin. Monitor for decreased effect and low blood levels. Dosage may have to be increased.

Parenteral calcium, thiazides: hypercalcemia and hypomagnesemia, predisposing patient to digitalis toxicity. Monitor serum calcium and serum magnesium.

Quinidine, diltiazem, amiodarone, nifedipine, verapamil: increased digoxin blood levels. Monitor for toxicity.

NURSING CONSIDERATIONS

• Contraindicated in presence of any digitalis-induced toxicity; ventricular fibrillation; ventricular tachycardia unless caused by CHF. Administering calcium salts to digitalized patient is contraindicated. Calcium affects cardiac contractility and excitability in much the same way as glycosides and may lead to serious arrhythmias in digitalized patient. Use with extreme caution in elderly patients, and in those with acute myocardial infarction, incomplete AV block, chronic constrictive pericarditis, idiopathic hypertrophic subaortic stenosis, renal insufficiency, severe pulmonary disease, or hypothyroidism. Dosage must be reduced in renal impairment.

• Infuse I.V. dose slowly over at least 5 minutes.

• Hypothyroid patients are very sensitive to glycosides; hyperthyroid patients may need larger doses.

• Obtain baseline data (heart rate and rhythm, blood pressure, and electrolytes) before giving first dose.

• Question patient about recent use of cardiac glycosides (within the previous 2 to 3 weeks) before administering a loading dose. Always divide loading dose over first 24 hours unless clinical situation indicates otherwise.

• Dose is adjusted to patient's clinical condition and is monitored by serum levels of cardiac glycoside, calcium, potassium, magnesium, and by ECG. Obtain blood for digoxin levels 8 hours after last P.O. dose.

• Take apical-radial pulse for a full minute. Record and report to doctor any significant changes (sudden increase or decrease in rate, pulse deficit, irregular beats, and particularly regularization of a previously irregular rhythm). Check blood pressure and obtain 12-lead ECG with these changes.

• Excessive slowing of the pulse rate (60 beats/minute or less) may be a sign of digitalis toxicity. Withhold drug and notify doctor.

• Ask patient about nausea, vomiting, anorexia, visual disturbances, and other symptoms of toxicity.

• Monitor serum potassium carefully. Take corrective action *before* hypokalemia occurs. Encourage patient to eat potassium-rich foods.
• Withhold drug for 1 to 2 days before elective electrocardioversion. Adjust dose after cardioversion.
• Instruct patient and responsible family member about drug action, dosage regimen, how to take pulse, reportable signs, and follow-up plans.
• Don't substitute one brand for another.
• When changing from oral tablets or elixir to parenteral therapy, dosage should be reduced by 20% to 25%. When changing from liquid-filled capsules to parenteral therapy, dosage is about equivalent because absorption is best using liquid-filled capsules. Therefore, when changing from oral tablets or elixir to liquid-filled capsules, reduce dose by 20% to 25%.
• Therapeutic blood levels of digoxin range from 0.5 to 2.0 ng/ml.

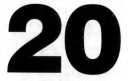

Antiarrhythmics

adenosine
amiodarone hydrochloride
atropine sulfate
bretylium tosylate
disopyramide
disopyramide phosphate
encainide hydrochloride
esmolol hydrochloride
flecainide acetate
indecainide hydrochloride
lidocaine hydrochloride
mexiletine hydrochloride
phenytoin
(See Chapter 29, ANTICONVULSANTS.)
phenytoin sodium
(See Chapter 29, ANTICONVULSANTS.)
procainamide hydrochloride
propafenone hydrochloride
propranolol hydrochloride
(See Chapter 21, ANTIANGINALS.)
quinidine bisulfate
quinidine gluconate
quinidine polygalacturonate
quinidine sulfate
tocainide hydrochloride

COMBINATION PRODUCTS
None.

---

adenosine
Adenocard

Pregnancy Risk Category: C

HOW SUPPLIED
Injection: 3 mg/ml in 2-ml vials

MECHANISM OF ACTION
Adenosine is a naturally occurring nucleoside. In the heart, it acts on the AV node to slow conduction and in-
hibit reentry pathways. Adenosine is also useful for the treatment of paroxysmal supraventricular tachycardia (PSVT) associated with accessory bypass tracts (Wolff-Parkinson-White syndrome).

INDICATIONS & DOSAGE
Conversion of PSVT to sinus rhythm—
Adults: 6 mg I.V. by rapid bolus injection (over 1 to 2 seconds). If PSVT is not eliminated in 1 to 2 minutes, give 12 mg by rapid I.V. push. Repeat 12-mg dose if necessary. Single doses over 12 mg are not recommended.

ADVERSE REACTIONS
CNS: apprehension, back pain, blurred vision, burning sensation, dizziness, heaviness in arms, lightheadedness, neck pain, numbness, tingling in arms.
CV: chest pain, *facial flushing,* headache, hypotension, palpitations, sweating.
GI: metallic taste, nausea.
Respiratory: *chest pressure, dyspnea, shortness of breath,* hyperventilation.
Other: *tightness in throat, groin pressure.*

INTERACTIONS
Carbamazepine: higher degrees of heart block may occur.
Dipyridamole: may potentiate the drug's effects. Smaller doses may be necessary.
Methylxanthines: antagonism of the drug's effects. Patients receiving the-ophylline or caffeine may require

---

higher doses or may not respond to adenosine therapy.

NURSING CONSIDERATIONS
• Contraindicated in patients with atrial flutter, atrial fibrillation, and ventricular tachycardia because the drug is ineffective in the treatment of these arrhythmias. It is also contraindicated in patients allergic to the drug. Because it decreases conduction through the AV node, adenosine may produce a transient first-, second-, or third-degree heart block. For this reason, it is contraindicated in patients with second- or third-degree heart block or sick sinus syndrome, unless the patient has an artificial pacemaker. Because the drug has a very short half-life, these effects are usually transient; however, patients who develop significant block after a dose of adenosine should not receive additional doses.
• In clinical trials, more than half of the patients exhibited new arrhythmias when adenosine was used to convert to normal sinus rhythm. They are usually transient, but may include sinus bradycardia or tachycardia, atrial premature contractions, various degrees of AV block, premature ventricular contractions, and skipped beats.
• Inhaled adenosine will cause bronchoconstriction in asthmatic patients. Asthma attacks have not been reported, but the potential for bronchoconstriction exists.
• There is experimental evidence that high concentrations of adenosine may induce chromosomal damage. The clinical significance of this property is not known.
• Rapid I.V. injection is necessary for drug action. Administer directly into a vein if possible; if an I.V. line is used, employ the most proximal port and follow with a rapid saline flush to ensure that the drug reaches the systemic circulation quickly.

• Check solution for crystals, which may occur if solution is cold. If crystals are visible, gently warm solution to room temperature. Do not use solutions that aren't clear.
• Because it contains no preservatives, unused drug should be discarded.

---

amiodarone hydrochloride
Cordarone, Cordarone X‡
Pregnancy Risk Category: C

HOW SUPPLIED
Tablets: 100 mg†‡, 200 mg

MECHANISM OF ACTION
A Group III antiarrhythmic that prolongs the refractory period and action potential duration and decreases repolarization.

INDICATIONS & DOSAGE
Ventricular and supraventricular arrhythmias, including recurrent supraventricular tachycardia (Wolff-Parkinson-White syndrome), atrial fibrillation and flutter, and ventricular tachycardia refractory to other antiarrhythmics—
Adults: loading dose is 5 to 10 mg/kg by I.V. infusion via central line, followed by I.V. infusion of 10 mg/kg/day for 3 to 5 days. (*Note:* I.V. use of amiodarone is investigational.) Or, give loading dose of 800 to 1,600 mg P.O. daily for 1 to 3 weeks until initial therapeutic response occurs. Maintenance dosage is 200 to 600 mg P.O. daily.

ADVERSE REACTIONS
CNS: peripheral neuropathy, extrapyramidal symptoms, headache, *malaise, fatigue.*
CV: bradycardia, hypotension, *arrhythmias, CHF.*
EENT: *corneal microdeposits,* visual disturbances.

Italicized adverse reactions are common or life-threatening.
*Liquid form contains alcohol.   **May contain tartrazine.

Endocrine: hypothyroidism, hyperthyroidism, gynecomastia.
GI: *nausea, vomiting,* constipation.
Hepatic: *altered liver enzymes,* hepatic dysfunction.
Respiratory: *severe pulmonary toxicity (pneumonitis/alveolitis).*
Skin: *photosensitivity,* blue-gray skin pigmentation.
Other: muscle weakness.

INTERACTIONS

Antiarrhythmic agents: use with amiodarone may induce torsade de pointes; amiodarone may reduce the hepatic or renal clearance of flecainide, procainamide, and quinidine.
Antihypertensives: increased hypotensive effect. Use together cautiously.
Beta blockers, calcium channel blockers: increased cardiac depressant effects; may potentiate slowing of sinus node and AV conduction. Use together cautiously.
Digitalis glycosides: increased serum digoxin levels.
Phenytoin: phenytoin metabolism may be decreased.
Warfarin: increased anticoagulant effect. Monitor patient closely.

NURSING CONSIDERATIONS

• Use cautiously in preexisting bradycardia or sinus node disease; conduction disturbances; severely depressed ventricular function; and marked cardiomegaly. Use cautiously (if at all) in patients receiving Class I antiarrhythmics.
• Amiodarone is often effective for treatment of arrhythmias resistant to other drug therapy. However, large incidence of adverse reactions limits its use.
• Most patients treated show corneal microdeposits upon slit-lamp ophthalmologic examination. Onset of this effect from 1 to 4 months after beginning amiodarone therapy. However, only 2% to 3% have actual visual disturbances. To minimize this compli-

cation, recommend instillation of methylcellulose ophthalmic solution during amiodarone therapy.
• Monitor carefully for pulmonary toxicity, which can be fatal. Incidence increases in patients receiving more than 400 mg/day.
• Monitor for symptoms of pneumonitis—exertional dyspnea, nonproductive cough, and pleuritic chest pain. Monitor pulmonary function tests and chest X-ray.
• Monitor blood pressure and heart rate and rhythm frequently. Continuous ECG monitoring should be performed during initiation and alteration of dosage. Notify doctor of any significant change.
• Monitor hepatic and thyroid function tests. Monitor serum electrolytes, particularly potassium and magnesium levels.
• Divide oral loading dose into three equal doses and give with meals to decrease GI intolerance. Maintenance dosage may be given once daily, but may be divided into two doses taken with meals if GI intolerance occurs.
• Advise patient to use a sunscreen to prevent photosensitivity. Monitor for burning or tingling skin followed by erythema and possible skin blistering.
• Amiodarone's adverse reactions are more prevalent at high doses but are generally reversible when drug therapy is stopped. Resolution of adverse reactions may take up to 4 months.

---

atropine sulfate
Pregnancy Risk Category: C

HOW SUPPLIED
Tablets: 0.4 mg, 0.6 mg, 0.6 mg
Injection: 0.05 mg/ml, 0.1 mg/ml, 0.3 mg/ml, 0.4 mg/ml, 0.5 mg/ml, 0.6 mg/ml, 0.8 mg/ml, 1 mg/ml, 1.2 mg/ml

MECHANISM OF ACTION
An anticholinergic, it inhibits acetyl-

choline at the parasympathetic neuroeffector junction, blocking vagal effects on the sinoatrial node; this enhances conduction through the AV node and speeds heart rate.

INDICATIONS & DOSAGE
Symptomatic bradycardia, bradyarrhythmia (junctional or escape rhythm)—
Adults: usually 0.5 to 1 mg I.V. push; repeat q 5 minutes, to maximum of 2 mg. Lower doses (less than 0.5 mg) can cause bradycardia.
Children: 0.01 mg/kg I.V. dose up to maximum of 0.4 mg; or 0.3 mg/m^2 dose; may repeat q 4 to 6 hours.
Antidote for anticholinesterase insecticide poisoning—
Adults and children: 2 mg I.M. or I.V. repeated hourly until muscarinic symptoms disappear. Severe cases may require up to 6 mg I.M. or I.V. q 1 hour.
Preoperatively for diminishing secretions and blocking cardiac vagal reflexes—
Adults: 0.4 to 0.6 mg I.M. 45 to 60 minutes before anesthesia.
Children: 0.01 mg/kg I.M. up to a maximum dose of 0.4 mg 45 to 60 minutes before anesthesia.
Adjunctive treatment of peptic ulcer disease; treatment of functional GI disorders such as irritable bowel syndrome—
Adults: 0.4 to 0.6 mg P.O. q 4 to 6 hours.
Children: 0.01 mg/kg or 0.3 mg/m^2 (not to exceed 0.4 mg) q 4 to 6 hours.

ADVERSE REACTIONS
Blood: leukocytosis.
CNS: *headache, restlessness,* ataxia, disorientation, hallucinations, delirium, coma, *insomnia, dizziness;* excitement, agitation, and confusion (especially in elderly patients).
CV: 1 to 2 mg—*tachycardia, palpitations;* greater than 2 mg—*extreme tachycardia, angina.*

EENT: 1 mg—*slight mydriasis,* photophobia; 2 mg—*blurred vision, mydriasis.*
GI: *dry mouth (common even at low doses),* thirst, *constipation,* nausea, vomiting.
GU: urine retention.
Skin: hot, flushed skin.

INTERACTIONS
Methotrimeprazine: may produce extrapyramidal symptoms. Monitor patient carefully.

NURSING CONSIDERATIONS
• Contraindicated in narrow-angle glaucoma, obstructive uropathy, obstructive disease of GI tract, myasthenia gravis, paralytic ileus, intestinal atony, unstable cardiovascular status in acute hemorrhage, and toxic megacolon. Use cautiously in patients with Down's syndrome.
• Adverse reactions vary considerably with dose. Most common is dry mouth.
• Many of the adverse reactions (such as dry mouth and constipation) are an extension of the drug's pharmacologic activity and may be expected.
• Watch for tachycardia in cardiac patients.
• Antidote for atropine overdose is physostigmine salicylate.
• Other anticholinergic drugs may increase vagal blockage.
• When given I.V., may cause paradoxical initial bradycardia. Usually disappears within 2 minutes.
• Monitor intake/output. Drug causes urine retention and urinary hesitancy; have patient void before receiving the drug.
• Monitor closely for urine retention in elderly men with benign prostatic hypertrophy.

Italicized adverse reactions are common or life-threatening.
*Liquid form contains alcohol.   **May contain tartrazine.

bretylium tosylate
Bretylate†‡, Bretylol

Pregnancy Risk Category: C

HOW SUPPLIED
Injection: 50 mg/ml

MECHANISM OF ACTION
A Group III antiarrhythmic that initially exerts transient adrenergic stimulation through release of norepinephrine. Subsequent depletion of norepinephrine causes adrenergic blocking actions to predominate. Repolarization is prolonged; duration of action potential and effective refractory period are increased.

INDICATIONS & DOSAGE
Ventricular fibrillation—
Adults: 5 mg/kg by I.V. push over 1 minute. If necessary, increase dose to 10 mg/kg and repeat q 15 to 30 minutes until 30 mg/kg have been given.
Children: safety and efficacy have not been established, but some clinicians use 2 to 5 mg/kg I.M. as a single dose, or 5 mg/kg I.V. followed by 10 mg/kg I.V. if fibrillation persists.
Other ventricular arrhythmias—
Adults: initially, 500 mg diluted to 50 ml with dextrose 5% in water or normal saline solution and infused I.V. over more than 8 minutes at 5 to 10 mg/kg. Dose may be repeated in 1 to 2 hours. Thereafter, repeat q 6 to 8 hours.
I.V. maintenance—
Adults: infused in diluted solution of 500 ml dextrose 5% in water or normal saline solution at 1 to 2 mg/minute.
I.M. injection—
Adults: 5 to 10 mg/kg undiluted. Repeat in 1 to 2 hours if needed. Thereafter, repeat q 6 to 8 hours.

ADVERSE REACTIONS
CNS: *vertigo, dizziness, light-headedness, syncope* (usually secondary to hypotension).
CV: *severe hypotension (especially orthostatic), bradycardia,* anginal pain, transient arrhythmias.
GI: severe nausea, vomiting (with rapid infusion).

INTERACTIONS
All antihypertensives: may potentiate hypotension. Monitor blood pressure.
Other antiarrhythmics: additive or antagonistic antiarrhythmic effects. Monitor for additive toxicity.

NURSING CONSIDERATIONS
• There are no contraindications to the use of bretylium in the treatment of ventricular fibrillation or life-threatening arrhythmias; however, patients who are hypersensitive to corn or corn products should not receive the commercially available preparation mixed in dextrose 5% in water.
• Use cautiously in patients with fixed cardiac output, aortic stenosis, and pulmonary hypertension to avoid severe and sudden drop in blood pressure.
• Avoid initiating bretylium therapy concomitantly with digitalis glycoside therapy. Do not use in digitalized patients unless the arrhythmia is life-threatening, not caused by digitalis, and is unresponsive to other drugs.
• Monitor blood pressure and heart rate and rhythm continuously. Notify doctor immediately of any significant change. If supine systolic blood pressure falls below 75 mm Hg, notify doctor; he may order norepinephrine, dopamine, or volume expanders to raise blood pressure.
• The initial release of norepinephrine caused by bretylium may induce transient hypertension and arrhythmias. Monitor patient closely.
• Keep patient in the supine position until tolerance to hypotension develops. Tell patient to avoid sudden postural changes.

- Follow dosage directions carefully to avoid nausea and vomiting.
- Rotate I.M. injection sites to prevent tissue damage, and don't exceed 3-ml volume in any one site.
- To be used with other cardiopulmonary resuscitative measures, such as CPR, countershock, epinephrine, sodium bicarbonate, and lidocaine.
- Avoid subtherapeutic doses (less than 5 mg/kg), because such doses may cause hypotension.
- Ventricular tachycardia and other ventricular arrhythmias respond less rapidly to treatment than ventricular fibrillation.
- Dosage should be decreased in renal impairment.
- Monitor carefully if pressor amines (sympathomimetics) are given to correct hypotension, because bretylium potentiates pressor amines.
- Ineffective treatment for atrial arrhythmias.
- Has been used investigationally to treat hypertension.
- Observe for increased anginal pain in susceptible patients.
- Observe patient for adverse reactions and notify doctor if any occur.

---

disopyramide
Rythmodan†

disopyramide phosphate
Napamide, Norpace, Norpace CR, Rythmodan LA†

Pregnancy Risk Category: C

HOW SUPPLIED
disopyramide
Capsules: 100 mg†, 150 mg†
disopyramide phosphate
Tablets (sustained-release): 250 mg†
Capsules: 100 mg, 150 mg
Capsules (controlled-release): 100 mg, 150 mg
Injection: 10 mg/ml†

MECHANISM OF ACTION
A Class Ia antiarrhythmic that depresses phase O. It prolongs the action potential. All Class I drugs have membrane stabilizing effects.

INDICATIONS & DOSAGE
Premature ventricular contractions (unifocal, multifocal, or coupled); ventricular tachycardia not severe enough to require electrocardioversion; to convert atrial fibrillation or flutter to normal sinus rhythm—
Adults: usual maintenance dosage 150 to 200 mg P.O. q 6 hours; for patients who weigh less than 50 kg or those with renal, hepatic, or cardiac impairment—100 mg P.O. q 6 hours. May give sustained-release capsule q 12 hours.

Recommended dosages in advanced renal insufficiency: creatinine clearance 15 to 40 ml/minute—100 mg q 10 hours; creatinine clearance 5 to 15 ml/minute—100 mg q 20 hours; creatinine clearance 1 to 5 ml/minute—100 mg q 30 hours.

Children 12 to 18 years: 6 to 15 mg/kg P.O. daily.
Children 4 to 12 years: 10 to 15 mg/kg P.O. daily.
Children 1 to 4 years: 10 to 20 mg/kg P.O. daily.
Children less than 1 year: 10 to 30 mg/kg P.O. daily.

All children's dosages should be divided into equal amounts and given q 6 hours.

ADVERSE REACTIONS
CNS: dizziness, agitation, depression, fatigue, muscle weakness, syncope.
CV: *hypotension, CHF, heart block, edema, weight gain, arrhythmias.*
EENT: *blurred vision, dry eyes, dry nose.*
GI: nausea, vomiting, anorexia, bloating, abdominal pain, *constipation, dry mouth.*

Italicized adverse reactions are common or life-threatening.
*Liquid form contains alcohol.   **May contain tartrazine.

GU: urine retention and urinary hesitancy.
Hepatic: cholestatic jaundice.
Metabolic: hypoglycemia.
Skin: rash in 1% to 3% of patients.

INTERACTIONS
Antiarrhythmics: possible additive or antagonized antiarrhythmic effects.
Phenytoin: increases disopyramide's metabolism. Monitor for decreased antiarrhythmic effect.

NURSING CONSIDERATIONS
• Contraindicated in cardiogenic shock or second- or third-degree heart block with no pacemaker. Use very cautiously, and avoid, if possible, in CHF. Use cautiously in underlying conduction abnormalities, urinary tract diseases (especially prostatic hypertrophy), hepatic or renal impairment, myasthenia gravis, or narrow-angle glaucoma. Adjust dosage in renal insufficiency.
• Don't give sustained-release capsule for rapid control of ventricular arrhythmias; when therapeutic blood levels must be rapidly attained; in cardiomyopathy or possible cardiac decompensation; or in severe renal impairment.
• When transferring patient from immediate-release to sustained-release capsules, advise him to begin a sustained-release capsule 6 hours after the last immediate-release capsule was taken.
• Discontinue if heart block develops, if QRS complex widens by more than 25%, or if Q-T interval lengthens by more than 25% above baseline.
• Correct any underlying electrolyte abnormalities before use.
• Watch for recurrence of arrhythmias and check for adverse reactions; notify doctor if any occur.
• Check apical pulse before administering drug. Notify doctor if pulse rate is slower than 60 beats/minute or faster than 120 beats/minute.

• Teach patient the importance of taking drug on time, exactly as prescribed. To do this, he may have to use an alarm clock for night doses.
• Relieve discomfort of dry mouth by chewing gum or hard candy.
• Manage constipation with proper diet or bulk laxatives.
• Use of disopyramide with other antiarrhythmics may cause further myocardial depression.
• Most doctors prefer to prescribe disopyramide for patients not in heart failure who can't tolerate quinidine or procainamide.
• Pharmacist may prepare disopyramide suspension from 100-mg capsules using cherry syrup. Protect suspension from light. It should be dispensed in amber glass bottles. May be best for young children.

encainide hydrochloride
Enkaid
Pregnancy Risk Category: C

HOW SUPPLIED
Capsules: 25 mg, 35 mg, 50 mg

MECHANISM OF ACTION
A Class Ic antiarrhythmic that depresses phase O and fast sodium channel activity. Unlike Class Ia and Ib agents, it does not prolong or shorten the action potential. All Class I drugs have membrane-stabilizing effects.

INDICATIONS & DOSAGE
Treatment of life-threatening ventricular arrhythmias, such as sustained ventricular tachycardia—
Adults: initially, 25 mg P.O. t.i.d. at approximately 8-hour intervals. After 3 to 5 days, dosage may be increased to 35 mg t.i.d. if necessary. After an additional 3 to 5 days, dosage may be increased to 50 mg t.i.d. Maximum daily dosage is 75 mg q.i.d.

ADVERSE REACTIONS
CNS: *dizziness, blurred vision, insomnia, headache,* tremor.
CV: *new or worsened arrhythmias, palpitations,* edema, *chest pains, cardiac arrest.*
EENT: tinnitus.
GI: dry mouth, constipation, nausea, vomiting.
Other: dyspnea, weakness.

INTERACTIONS
Cimetidine: may increase encainide blood levels. Use together cautiously.

NURSING CONSIDERATIONS
• Contraindicated in preexisting second- or third-degree AV block or right bundle branch block when associated with a left hemiblock, unless a pacemaker is present; in cardiogenic shock and severe hypokalemia.
• Use cautiously in cardiomyopathy or sick sinus syndrome.
• Findings from the Cardiac Arrhythmia Suppression Trial (CAST) include a greater-than-twofold increase in the number of deaths and in nonfatal cardiac arrest in patients treated with encainide. Therefore, it should be used only in immediately life-threatening arrhythmias.
• Patients with a history of sustained ventricular tachycardia or fibrillation taking more than 200 mg daily may be at a higher risk of developing new or worsened arrhythmias, especially during the first week of therapy.
• Patients who receive encainide dosage of 200 mg/day or more should be hospitalized.
• Encainide may induce several ECG changes, including prolonged PR and QRS intervals; however, ECG changes are not good predictors of effectiveness, overdose, or toxicity.
• Allowing at least 3 days to adjust to the dosage before increasing it significantly reduces the risk of proarrhythmia. Warn patient of the risk of increasing his own encainide dosage.

• Some patients who are well controlled on 50 mg t.i.d. or less may be treated as effectively with a 12-hour dosage schedule to ease compliance. Discuss this possibility with the doctor.

---

esmolol hydrochloride
Brevibloc

Pregnancy Risk Category: C

HOW SUPPLIED
Injection: 10 mg/ml in 10-ml vials; 250 mg/ml in 10-ml ampules

MECHANISM OF ACTION
A Class II antiarrhythmic, esmolol is an ultrashort-acting beta-adrenergic blocking agent. Decreases heart rate, myocardial contractility, and blood pressure.

INDICATIONS & DOSAGE
Supraventricular tachycardia—
Adults: loading dose is 500 mcg/kg/minute by I.V. infusion over 1 minute, followed by a 4-minute maintenance infusion of 50 mcg/kg/minute. If adequate response does not occur within 5 minutes, repeat the loading dose followed by a maintenance infusion of 100 mcg/kg/minute for 4 minutes. Maximum maintenance infusion is 200 mcg/kg/minute.

ADVERSE REACTIONS
CNS: dizziness, somnolence, headache, agitation, fatigue.
CV: *hypotension* (sometimes with diaphoresis).
GI: *nausea,* vomiting.
Local: inflammation and induration at infusion site.
Other: bronchospasm.

INTERACTIONS
Digoxin: esmolol may increase serum digoxin levels by 10% to 20%.
Morphine: may increase esmolol

Italicized adverse reactions are common or life-threatening.
*Liquid form contains alcohol.   **May contain tartrazine.

blood levels. Titrate esmolol carefully.

Reserpine (and other catecholamine-depleting drugs): may cause additive bradycardia and hypotension. Titrate esmolol carefully.

Succinylcholine: esmolol may prolong neuromuscular blockade.

NURSING CONSIDERATIONS
• Contraindicated in sinus bradycardia, heart block greater than first degree, cardiogenic shock, or overt heart failure.
• Use cautiously in impaired renal function, diabetes, or bronchospasm.
• Monitor continuous ECG and blood pressure during infusion. Up to 50% of all patients treated with esmolol develop hypotension. Monitor closely, especially if patient's pretreatment blood pressure was low.
• Hypotension can usually be reversed within 30 minutes by decreasing the dose or, if necessary, by stopping the infusion.
• Esmolol is recommended only for short-term use, no longer than 48 hours.
• If a local reaction develops at the infusion site, change to another site. Avoid butterfly needles.
• Don't give esmolol by I.V. push; use a controlled infusion device. Drug must be diluted before infusion.
• Esmolol solutions are incompatible with diazepam, furosemide, sodium bicarbonate, and thiopental sodium.
• When patient's heart rate becomes stable, esmolol will be replaced by alternative (longer-acting) antiarrhythmics, such as propranolol, digoxin, or verapamil. As the replacement drug is started, the esmolol infusion should be gradually reduced over 1 hour.
• Esmolol has an ultrashort duration of action and can be accurately titrated. Therefore, it has advantages over other beta blockers in treating cardiac arrhythmias.

flecainide acetate
Tambocor
Pregnancy Risk Category: C

HOW SUPPLIED
Tablets: 100 mg
Injection: 10 mg/ml‡

MECHANISM OF ACTION
A Class Ic antiarrhythmic that depresses phase O. Unlike Class Ia and Ib agents, however, it does not prolong or shorten the action potential. All Class I drugs have membrane stabilizing effects.

INDICATIONS & DOSAGE
Treatment of life-threatening ventricular arrhythmias, such as sustained ventricular tachycardia—
Adults: 100 mg P.O. q 12 hours. May be increased in increments of 50 mg b.i.d. q 4 days until efficacy is achieved. Maximum dosage is 400 mg daily for most patients.
   Initial dosage for patients with CHF is 50 mg q 12 hours.
   Where available, flecainide may be given by I.V. injection—
Adults: 2 mg/kg I.V. push over not less than 10 minutes; or the dose may be diluted with dextrose 5% in water and administered as an infusion. Do not use any other solutions for infusion.

ADVERSE REACTIONS
CNS: *dizziness, headache,* fatigue, tremor.
CV: *new or worsened arrhythmias,* chest pain, *CHF, cardiac arrest.*
EENT: *blurred vision and other visual disturbances.*
GI: nausea, constipation, abdominal pain.
Other: *dyspnea,* edema, skin rash.

INTERACTIONS
Amiodarone, cimetidine, digoxin,

propranolol: altered pharmacokinetics. Monitor for toxicity.

Digitalis glycosides: flecainide may increase plasma digoxin levels by 15% to 25%.

Propranolol, beta-adrenergic blocking agents: both flecainide and propranolol plasma levels increase by 20% to 30%.

Urine acidifying and alkalinizing agents: extremes of urine pH may substantially alter excretion of flecainide.

NURSING CONSIDERATIONS

• Contraindicated in preexisting second- or third-degree AV block or right bundle branch block when associated with a left hemiblock, unless a pacemaker is present; contraindicated in cardiogenic shock.

• Findings from the Cardiac Arrhythmia Suppression Trial (CAST) include a greater-than-twofold increase in the number of deaths and nonfatal cardiac arrest in patients treated with flecainide. Therefore, it should be used only in immediately life-threatening arrhythmias, such as sustained ventricular tachycardia.

• Flecainide can alter endocardial pacing thresholds. Determine pacing threshold 1 week before and after initiating therapy in patients with pacemakers.

• Use cautiously in preexisting CHF, cardiomyopathy, severe renal or hepatic disease, prolonged Q-T interval, sick sinus syndrome, or blood dyscrasias.

• Hypokalemia or hyperkalemia may alter the effect of flecainide and should be corrected before this drug is given.

• Incidence of adverse effects increases when trough blood levels exceed 1 mcg/ml. Periodically monitor blood levels, especially in patients with renal failure or CHF.

• Most patients can be adequately maintained on an every-12-hour dosage schedule, but some need to receive flecainide every 8 hours.

• Full therapeutic effect of flecainide may take 3 to 5 days. The doctor may order I.V. lidocaine while awaiting full effect.

• Loading doses may aggravate arrhythmias and are therefore not recommended.

• Twice-daily dosing for flecainide aids patient compliance.

• Therapeutic serum levels of flecainide range from 0.2 to 1 mcg/ml.

indecainide hydrochloride
Decabid

Pregnancy Risk Category: B

HOW SUPPLIED
Tablets: 50 mg, 75 mg, 100 mg

MECHANISM OF ACTION
A Group Ic antiarrhythmic that blocks the inward sodium current in myocardial and Purkinge fibers. It stabilizes the cardiac cell membrane and slows the conduction of an impulse.

INDICATIONS & DOSAGE
Treatment of life-threatening ventricular arrhythmias, such as sustained ventricular tachycardia—
Adults: initially, 50 mg P.O. q 12 hours. If necessary, increase the dosage to 75 mg q 12 hours, but only after at least 4 days of treatment at initial dosage. After an additional 4 days, the dosage may then be increased to 100 mg q 12 hours if necessary. Some patients may require higher dosages (up to 400 mg/day).

Patients with renal failure (creatinine clearance <30 ml/minute, or serum creatinine of 3 mg/dl or more) should begin therapy at 50 mg once a day. After at least 7 days of monitoring, dosage may be increased to 75 mg daily if necessary, but monitoring of trough blood levels should show

---

Italicized adverse reactions are common or life-threatening.
*Liquid form contains alcohol.   **May contain tartrazine.

that the plasma level is no higher than 900 mcg/liter. Further gradual increases may be made, to 50 mg b.i.d. or 100 mg daily, but only with close monitoring of renal function, clinical response, and trough blood levels.

ADVERSE REACTIONS
CNS: *dizziness*, nervousness, anxiety, headache, insomnia, *asthenia*.
CV: *new or worsened arrhythmias, prolongation of the PR or QRS interval, chest pain,* angina, bundle branch block, CHF, first-degree AV block, hypertension, hypotension, palpitations.
EENT: blurred vision.
GI: abdominal pain, constipation, diarrhea, dyspepsia, dry mouth, nausea.
Respiratory: *dyspnea*, cough.
Other: back pain, fever, circumoral paresthesia.

INTERACTIONS
Antiarrhythmic agents: additive pharmacologic effects.
Cimetidine: increased plasma levels of indecainide. Use together cautiously; monitor plasma levels closely.

NURSING CONSIDERATIONS
• Contraindicated in patients hypersensitive to the drug; in patients with cardiogenic shock; and in those with preexisting second- or third-degree AV block or bifascicular block (right bundle branch block associated with a left hemiblock) unless a pacemaker is present.
• Other class Ic antiarrhythmic agents have been associated with a higher incidence of mortality or nonfatal cardiac arrest.
• Like other antiarrhythmic agents, indecainide can cause new or worsened arrhythmias ("proarrhythmic events"). Most occur during the first 2 weeks of therapy or when dosage is increased; they occur more frequently when total dosage exceeds 200 mg

daily or when predose (trough) blood levels exceed 900 mcg/liter.
• Close monitoring of serum levels may be necessary in elderly patients and those with renal failure or severe CHF.
• Hypokalemia or hyperkalemia may alter the effects of the drug. Monitor serum electrolytes and administer potassium as ordered.
• Administration with food will not affect the absorption of indecainide.
• Because higher doses increase the risk of serious toxicity (including proarrhythmic events), dosage alterations should be made gradually (allowing at least 4 days between adjustments) to prevent adverse reactions.
• Patients with CHF have altered indecainide pharmacokinetics. Temporary hospitalization with close monitoring is required when initiating therapy in these patients and when adjusting dosage beyond 200 mg/day.
• Little information is available regarding transfer of patients from therapy with other drugs to indecainide. Withdraw the first antiarrhythmic for 16 to 40 hours (2 to 5 half-lives) before initiating indecainide; if such withdrawal can be potentially life-threatening, the patient must be hospitalized.

---

lidocaine hydrochloride (lignocaine hydrochloride)
Lido Pen Auto-Injector, Xylocaine, Xylocard†‡

Pregnancy Risk Category: B

HOW SUPPLIED
Injection (for direct I.V. use): 1% (10 mg/ml) in 5-ml (50-mg), 10-ml (100-mg) syringes; 2% (20 mg/ml) in 5-ml (100-mg) vials, syringes, and ampules
Injection (for I.M. use): 10% (100 mg/ml) in 3-ml automatic injection device or 5-ml ampules
Injection (for I.V. admixtures): 4% (40 mg/ml) in 25-ml (1-g) vials and

syringes and 50-ml (2-g) vials and syringes; 10% (100 mg/ml) in 10-ml
(1-g) vials; 20% (200 mg/ml) in 5-ml
(1-g) vials and syringes and 10-ml
(2-g) vials and syringes
Infusion (premixed): 0.2% (2 mg/ml)
in 500-ml vials; 0.4% (4 mg/ml) in
250-ml, 500-ml, 1,000-ml vials;
0.8% (8 mg/ml) in 250-ml, 500-ml
vials

MECHANISM OF ACTION
A Class Ib antiarrhythmic that depresses phase O. It shortens the action
potential. All Class I drugs have
membrane stabilizing effects.

INDICATIONS & DOSAGE
*Ventricular arrhythmias from myocar-
dial infarction, cardiac manipulation,
or cardiac glycosides; ventricular
tachycardia—*
Adults: 50 to 100 mg (1 to 1.5 mg/
kg) I.V. bolus at 25 to 50 mg/minute.
Give half this amount to elderly patients or patients under 50 kg, and to
those with CHF or hepatic disease.
Repeat bolus q 3 to 5 minutes until arrhythmias subside or adverse reactions develop. Don't exceed 300-mg
total bolus during a 1-hour period. Simultaneously, begin constant infusion
of 1 to 4 mg/minute. If single bolus
has been given, repeat smaller bolus
15 to 20 minutes after start of infusion to maintain therapeutic serum
level. After 24 hours of continuous
infusion, decrease rate by half.
I.M. administration: 200 to 300 mg in
deltoid muscle only.
Children: 1mg/kg by I.V. bolus, followed by infusion of 30 mcg/kg/min-
ute.

ADVERSE REACTIONS
CNS: *confusion, tremors,* lethargy,
somnolence, *stupor, restlessness,*
slurred speech, euphoria, depression,
light-headedness, paresthesias, muscle twitching, *seizures.*

CV: *hypotension,* bradycardia, further arrhythmias.
EENT: *tinnitus, blurred or double vision.*
Other: *anaphylaxis,* soreness at injection site, sensations of cold, diaphoresis.

INTERACTIONS
Cimetidine, beta blockers: decreased
metabolism of lidocaine. Monitor for
toxicity.
Phenytoin: additive cardiac depressant effects. Monitor carefully.

NURSING CONSIDERATIONS
• Contraindicated in patients who are
allergic to related local anesthetics of
the amide type, such as Nupercaine.
• Use cautiously in complete or
second-degree heart block. Use of lidocaine with epinephrine (for local
anesthesia) to treat arrhythmias is
contraindicated. Use with caution in
elderly patients, those with CHF,
renal or hepatic disease, or those who
weigh less than 50 kg. Such patients
will need a reduced dose.
• In many severely ill patients, seizures may be the first clinically apparent sign of toxicity. However, severe reactions usually are preceded by
somnolence, confusion, and parethe-
sias.
• If toxic signs (such as dizziness) occur, stop drug at once and notify doctor. Continued infusion could lead to
seizures and coma. Give oxygen via
nasal cannula, if not contraindicated.
Keep oxygen and CPR equipment
readily available.
• Patients receiving infusions must be
attended *at all times,* and be on a cardiac monitor. Use a continuous infusion pump for administering infusion
precisely. Do not exceed an infusion
rate of 4 mg/minute. A faster rate
greatly increases risk of toxicity.
• Monitor patient's response, especially blood pressure and serum electrolytes, BUN, and creatinine. Notify

doctor promptly if abnormalities develop.

• Discontinue infusion and notify doctor if arrhythmias worsen or ECG changes, such as widening QRS complex or substantially prolonged PR interval, are evident.

• A bolus dose not followed by infusion will have a short-lived effect.

• A patient who has received lidocaine I.M. will show a sevenfold increase in serum creatinine phosphokinase (CPK) level. Such CPK originates in the skeletal muscle, not the heart. Test isoenzymes if using I.M. route.

• Used investigationally to treat refractory status epilepticus.

• Therapeutic serum levels are 2 to 5 mcg/ml.

mexiletine hydrochloride
Mexitil

Pregnancy Risk Category: C

HOW SUPPLIED
Capsules: 50 mg‡, 100 mg†, 150 mg, 200 mg, 250 mg
Injection: 250 mg/10 ml‡

MECHANISM OF ACTION
A Class Ib antiarrhythmic that depresses phase O. It shortens the action potential. All Group I drugs have membrane stabilizing effects.

INDICATIONS & DOSAGE
Treatment of refractory ventricular arrhythmias, including ventricular tachycardia and premature ventricular contractions—
Adults: 200 to 400 mg P.O. followed by 200 mg q 8 hours. May increase dose to 400 mg q 8 hours if satisfactory control is not obtained. Some patients may respond well to an every-12-hour schedule. May give up to 450 mg q 12 hours.

Where available, mexiletine may be given I.V.—

Adults: following a loading dose of 200 to 250 mg I.V. at a rate of 25 mg/minute, prepare an infusion solution of 250 mg mexiletine/500 ml dextrose 5% in water. Administer the first 120 ml (60 mg) over 1 hour. If clinical response is inadequate, give another bolus of 200 mg over 10 to 20 minutes. Maintenance dose is 0.5 mg/minute (1 ml/minute of prepared solution).

ADVERSE REACTIONS
CNS: *tremor, dizziness,* blurred vision, ataxia, diplopia, confusion, nystagmus, nervousness, headache.
CV: hypotension, bradycardia, widened QRS complex, arrhythmias.
GI: nausea, vomiting.
Skin: rash.

INTERACTIONS
Cimetidine: increased mexiletine blood levels. Monitor carefully.
Phenytoin, rifampin, phenobarbital: decreased mexiletine blood levels. Monitor carefully.

NURSING CONSIDERATIONS
• Contraindicated in cardiogenic shock or preexisting second- or third-degree AV block (if pacemaker is not present).

• Early sign of mexiletine toxicity is tremor, usually a fine tremor of the hands. This progresses to dizziness and later to ataxia and nystagmus as the drug's blood level increases. Question your patient about these symptoms.

• When changing from lidocaine to mexiletine, stop the infusion when the first mexiletine dose is given. Keep the infusion line open, however, until the arrhythmia appears to be satisfactorily controlled.

• May administer oral dose with meals to lessen GI distress.

• Therapeutic levels range from 0.75 to 2 mcg/ml.

• Monitor blood pressure and heart

rate and rhythm frequently. Notify doctor of any significant change.
• Patients who respond well to mexiletine can often be maintained on a q 12 hour schedule. Notify doctor if you feel the patient is a good candidate for q 12 hour therapy. Twice-daily dosage eases compliance.
• Mexiletine injection is compatible with 0.99% sodium chloride, 5% dextrose in water, 5% sodium bicarbonate, 1/6 M sodium lactate, and 10% fructose (laevulose).

procainamide hydrochloride
Procan SR, Promine, Pronestyl**, Pronestyl-SR, Rhythmin

Pregnancy Risk Category: C

HOW SUPPLIED
Tablets: 250 mg, 375 mg, 500 mg
Tablets (sustained-release): 250 mg, 500 mg, 750 mg, 1,000 mg
Capsules: 250 mg, 375 mg, 500 mg
Injection: 100 mg/ml, 500 mg/ml

MECHANISM OF ACTION
A Class Ia antiarrhythmic that depresses phase O. It prolongs the action potential. All Class I drugs have membrane stabilizing effects.

INDICATIONS & DOSAGE
Premature ventricular contractions, ventricular tachycardia, atrial arrhythmias unresponsive to quinidine, paroxysmal atrial tachycardia—
Adults: 100 mg q 5 minutes slow I.V. push, no faster than 25 to 50 mg/minute until arrhythmias disappear, adverse reactions develop, or 1 g has been given. (Usual effective dose is 500 to 600 mg.) When arrhythmias disappear, give continuous infusion of 2 to 6 mg/minute. If arrhythmias recur, repeat bolus as above and increase infusion rate; 0.5 to 1 g I.M. q 4 to 8 hours until oral therapy begins.

Loading dose for atrial fibrillation or paroxysmal atrial tachycardia—
Adults: 1 to 1.25 g P.O. If arrhythmias persist after 1 hour, give additional 750 mg. If no change occurs, give 500 mg to 1 g q 2 hours until arrhythmias disappear or adverse reactions occur.
Loading dose for ventricular tachycardia—
Adults: 1 g P.O. Maintenance dosage is 50 mg/kg daily q 3 hours; average is 250 to 500 mg q 3 hours.
Note: Sustained-release tablet may be used for maintenance dosing when treating ventricular tachycardia, atrial fibrillation, and paroxysmal atrial tachycardia. Dose is 500 mg to 1 g q 6 hours.

ADVERSE REACTIONS
Blood: thrombocytopenia, *neutropenia* (especially with sustained-release forms), *agranulocytosis,* hemolytic anemia, *increased antinuclear antibodies titer.*
CNS: hallucinations, confusion, seizures, depression.
CV: *severe hypotension, bradycardia,* AV block, ventricular fibrillation (after parenteral use).
GI: *nausea, vomiting, anorexia, diarrhea, bitter taste.*
Skin: *maculopapular rash.*
Other: *fever, lupus erythematosus syndrome (especially after prolonged administration),* myalgia.

INTERACTIONS
Amiodarone: increased procainamide levels and possible drug toxicity.
Anticholinergics: additive anticholinergic effects.
Anticholinesterase agents: anticholinesterase dosage may need to be increased.
Cimetidine: may increase procainamide blood levels. Monitor for toxicity.
Neuromuscular blocking agents: in-

Italicized adverse reactions are common or life-threatening.
*Liquid form contains alcohol. **May contain tartrazine.

creased skeletal muscle relaxant effects. Monitor patient closely.

NURSING CONSIDERATIONS
• Contraindicated in patients with hypersensitivity to procaine and related drugs; with complete, second-, or third-degree heart block unassisted by electrical pacemaker; or with myasthenia gravis. Use with caution in CHF or other conduction disturbances, such as bundle branch block or cardiac glycoside intoxication, or with hepatic or renal insufficiency.
• Patients receiving infusions must be *attended at all times.* Use a continuous infusion pump to administer the infusion precisely.
• Monitor serum electrolytes, especially potassium level. Hypokalemia predisposes patients to arrhythmias.
• Monitor blood pressure and ECG continuously during I.V. administration. Watch for prolonged Q-T and QRS intervals, heart block, or increased arrhythmias. If these occur, withhold drug, obtain rhythm strip, and notify doctor immediately.
• Keep patient supine for I.V. administration if hypotension occurs.
• If procainamide is administered too rapidly, I.V. hypotension can occur. Watch closely for adverse reactions and notify doctor if they occur. Instruct patient to report fever, rash, muscle pain, diarrhea, bleeding, bruises, or pleuritic chest pain.
• Procainamide solution for injection may become discolored. If so, check with pharmacy and prepare to discard.
• Monitor CBC frequently during first 3 months of therapy, particularly in patients taking sustained-release dosage forms.
• Decrease dose in hepatic and renal dysfunction, and give over 6 hours. Half-life of procainamide is increased as much as threefold in these states.
• N-acetylprocainamide (NAPA), an active metabolite, may accumulate

when renal function is decreased. This may add to toxicity.
• Patient with CHF has a lower volume of distribution and can be treated with lower doses.
• Positive antinuclear antibody titer is common in about 60% of patients who don't have symptoms of lupus erythematosus syndrome. This response seems related to prolonged use, not dosage.
• After prolonged atrial fibrillation, restoration of normal rhythm may result in thromboembolism, due to dislodgment of thrombi from atrial wall. Anticoagulation usually advised before restoration of normal sinus rhythm.
• Stress importance of taking drug exactly as prescribed. Patient may have to set an alarm clock for night doses.
• Reassure patients who are taking the extended-release form of procainamide that a wax matrix 'ghost' from the tablet may be passed in the stool. The drug is completely absorbed before this occurs.
• Elderly patients may be more likely to develop hypotension. Monitor blood pressure carefully.

propafenone hydrochloride
Rythmol

Pregnancy Risk Category: C

HOW SUPPLIED
Tablets: 150 mg, 300 mg

MECHANISM OF ACTION
A Class Ic antiarrhythmic agent that stabilizes cardiac cell membranes, probably by decreasing sodium influx. It also has weak beta-adrenergic blocking properties.

INDICATIONS & DOSAGE
Suppression of life-threatening ventricular arrhythmias, such as episodic ventricular tachycardia—

Adults: initially, 150 mg P.O. q 8 hours. Dosage may be increased to 225 mg q 8 hours after 3 or 4 days; if necessary, increase dosage to 300 mg q 8 hours. Maximum daily dosage is 900 mg.

ADVERSE REACTIONS
CNS: anorexia, anxiety, ataxia, dizziness, drowsiness, fatigue, headache, insomnia, syncope, tremor, weakness.
CV: angina, atrial fibrillation, bradycardia, bundle branch block, *CHF,* chest pain, edema, first-degree AV block, hypotension, increased QRS duration, intraventricular conduction delay, palpitations, *proarrhythmic events (ventricular tachycardia, premature ventricular contractions).*
EENT: blurred vision.
GI: abdominal pain or cramps, constipation, diarrhea, dyspepsia, flatulence, nausea, vomiting, dry mouth, unusual taste.
Respiratory: dyspnea.
Skin: rash.
Other: diaphoresis, joint pain.

INTERACTIONS
Antiarrhythmics: increased potential for CHF.
Cimetidine: decreased metabolism of propafenone.
Digitalis glycosides, oral anticoagulants: propafenone may increase serum levels of these agents, resulting in toxicity.
Local anesthetics: increased risk of CNS toxicity.
Propranolol, metoprolol: propafenone slows the metabolism of these agents. Dosage adjustments may be necessary.
Quinidine: slows the metabolism of propafenone. Avoid concomitant use.

NURSING CONSIDERATIONS
• Contraindicated in severe or uncontrolled CHF; cardiogenic shock; SA, AV, or intraventricular disorders of impulse conduction; sinus node dys-

function in the absence of a pacemaker; severe bradycardia (50 beats/minute or less); marked hypotension; bronchospastic disorders; severe obstructive pulmonary disease; severe electrolyte imbalance; severe hepatic failure; and known hypersensitivity to the drug.
• Use cautiously in patients with CHF because propafenone can exert a negative inotropic effect on the heart. Use cautiously with other cardiac depressant drugs and in hepatic or renal failure.
• Because plasma levels do not increase linearly with dose, dosage should be increased stepwise at 3- to 4-day intervals.
• Some patients metabolize propafenone rapidly, and early studies indicate that the drug may have a plasma half-life of 5 to 6 hours in fast metabolizers and 17 hours or more in slow metabolizers.
• Continuous cardiac monitoring is recommended during initiation of therapy and during dosage adjustments. If PR interval or QRS duration increase by more than 25%, a reduction in dosage may be necessary.
• Administer drug with food to minimize adverse GI reactions.
• During concomitant use with digoxin, frequently monitor ECG and serum digoxin levels because propafenone increases serum digoxin levels by 35% to 85%.

quinidine bisulfate
(66.4% quinidine base)
Biquin Durules†, Kinidin Durules‡

quinidine gluconate
(62% quinidine base)
Duraquin, Quinaglute Dura-Tabs,
Quinalan, Quinate†

quinidine polygalacturonate
(60.5% quinidine base)
Cardioquin

quinidine sulfate
(83% quinidine base)
Apo-Quinidine†, CinQuin,
Novoquindin†, Quine, Quinidex
Extentabs, Quinora

Pregnancy Risk Category: C

HOW SUPPLIED
bisulfate
Tablets: 250 mg†‡
gluconate
Tablets (sustained-release): 324 mg,
325 mg†, 330 mg
Injection: 80 mg/ml
polygalacturonate
Tablets: 275 mg
sulfate
Tablets: 100 mg, 200 mg, 300 mg
Tablets (sustained-release): 300 mg
Capsules: 200 mg, 300 mg
Injection: 200 mg/ml

MECHANISM OF ACTION
A Class Ia antiarrhythmic that depresses phase O. It prolongs the action
potential. All Class I drugs have
membrane stabilizing effects.

INDICATIONS & DOSAGE
Atrial flutter or fibrillation—
Adults: 200 mg quinidine sulfate or
equivalent base P.O. q 2 to 3 hours for
5 to 8 doses with subsequent daily increases until sinus rhythm is restored
or toxic effects develop. Administer
quinidine only after digitalization to
avoid increasing AV conduction.
Maximum dosage is 3 to 4 g daily.
*Paroxysmal supraventricular tachy-
cardia—*
Adults: 400 to 600 mg I.M. gluconate q 2 to 3 hours until toxic adverse
reactions develop or arrhythmia subsides.
*Premature atrial and ventricular con-
tractions; paroxysmal atrioventricular
junctional rhythm; paroxysmal atrial
tachycardia; paroxysmal ventricular
tachycardia; maintenance after cardioversion of atrial fibrillation or flutter—*
Adults: test dose is 50 to 200 mg
P.O., then monitor vital signs before
beginning therapy. Quinidine sulfate
or equivalent base 200 to 400 mg P.O.
q 4 to 6 hours; or initially, quinidine
gluconate 600 mg I.M., then up to
400 mg q 2 hours, p.r.n.; or quinidine
gluconate 800 mg (10 ml of the commercially available solution) added to
40 ml dextrose 5% in water, infused
I.V. at 16 mg (1 ml)/minute.
Children: test dose is 2 mg/kg; 3 to 6
mg/kg q 2 to 3 hours for 5 doses P.O.
daily.

ADVERSE REACTIONS
Blood: *hemolytic anemia, thrombocytopenia, agranulocytosis.*
CNS: *vertigo, headache, light-
headedness,* confusion, restlessness,
cold sweat, pallor, fainting, dementia.
CV: *premature ventricular contractions; severe hypotension; SA and AV
block; ventricular fibrillation, tachycardia; aggravated CHF; ECG
changes (particularly widening of
QRS complex, notched P waves, widened Q-T interval, ST segment depression).*
EENT: *tinnitus,* excessive salivation,
blurred vision.
GI: *diarrhea, nausea, vomiting,* anorexia, abdominal pains.
Hepatic: hepatotoxicity including
granulomatous hepatitis.

Skin: rash, petechial hemorrhage of buccal mucosa, pruritus.
Other: angioedema, acute asthmatic attack, respiratory arrest, *fever, cinchonism.*

INTERACTIONS

Acetazolamide, antacids, sodium bicarbonate: may increase quinidine blood levels due to alkaline urine. Monitor for increased effect.
Barbiturates, phenytoin, rifampin: may antagonize quinidine activity. Monitor for decreased quinidine effect.
Cimetidine: increased serum quinidine levels. Monitor for increased effect.
Digoxin: increased serum digoxin levels after initiating quinidine therapy. Monitor closely.
Nifedipine: may decrease quinidine blood levels. Monitor carefully.
Verapamil: may result in hypotension. Monitor blood pressure.
Warfarin: increased anticoagulant effect. Monitor closely.

NURSING CONSIDERATIONS

• Contraindicated in cardiac glycoside toxicity when AV conduction is grossly impaired and in complete AV block with AV nodal or idioventricular pacemaker. Use with caution in myasthenia gravis. Anticholinesterase drug doses may have to be increased.
• May increase toxicity of digitalis derivatives. Use with caution in patients previously digitalized. Monitor digoxin levels.
• Monitor liver function tests during the first 4 to 8 weeks of therapy.
• The I.V. route should only be used to treat acute arrhythmias. For maintenance, give only by oral or I.M. route.
• Dosage varies—some patients may require drug q 4 hours; others, q 6 hours. Titrate dose by both clinical response and blood levels.
• When changing route of administra-

tion, alter dosage to compensate for variations in quinidine base content.
• Dosage should be decreased in CHF and hepatic disease.
• Check apical pulse rate and blood pressure before starting therapy. If you detect extremes in pulse rate, withhold drug and notify doctor at once.
• Lidocaine may be effective in treating quinidine-induced arrhythmias, because it increases AV conduction.
• GI adverse reactions, especially diarrhea, are signs of toxicity. Notify doctor. Check quinidine blood levels, which are toxic when greater than 8 mcg/ml. GI symptoms may be decreased by giving with meals. Monitor patient response carefully.
• Instruct patient to notify doctor if skin rash, fever, unusual bleeding, bruising, ringing in ears, or visual disturbance occurs.
• After long-standing atrial fibrillation, restoration of normal sinus rhythm may result in thromboembolism due to dislodgment of thrombi from atrial wall. Anticoagulation often advised before restoration of normal atrial rhythm.
• Never use discolored (brownish) quinidine solution.
• Store away from heat and direct light.
• The Centers for Disease Control (CDC) is investigating the use of quinidine gluconate for the treatment of severe *Plasmodium falciparum* malaria when quinine dihydrochloride is unavailable. Contact the CDC malaria branch for further information.

---

tocainide hydrochloride
Tonocard

Pregnancy Risk Category: C

HOW SUPPLIED
Tablets: 400 mg, 600 mg

Italicized adverse reactions are common or life-threatening.
*Liquid form contains alcohol.   **May contain tartrazine.

MECHANISM OF ACTION
A Class Ib antiarrhythmic that depresses phase O. It shortens the action potential. All Class I drugs have membrane stabilizing effects.

INDICATIONS & DOSAGE
Suppression of symptomatic ventricular arrhythmias, including frequent premature ventricular contractions and ventricular tachycardia—
Adults: initially, 400 mg P.O. q 8 hours. Usual dosage is between 1,200 and 1,800 mg daily in three divided doses.

ADVERSE REACTIONS
Blood: aplastic anemia.
CNS: *light-headedness, tremors,* restlessness, paresthesias, confusion, dizziness.
CV: hypotension, arrhythmias, *CHF.*
EENT: blurred vision.
GI: *nausea, vomiting, epigastric pain,* constipation, diarrhea, anorexia.
Hepatic: hepatitis.
Respiratory: *respiratory arrest,* pulmonary fibrosis, pneumonitis, *pulmonary edema.*
Skin: rash.

INTERACTIONS
Beta blockers: decreased myocardial contractility; increased CNS toxicity.

NURSING CONSIDERATIONS
• Contraindicated in patients who are hypersensitive to lidocaine or other amide-type local anesthetics and inpatients with second- or third-degree AV block in the absence of a ventricular pacemaker.
• Use cautiously in CHF or diminished cardiac reserve.
• Use cautiously in hepatic or renal impairment. These patients may often be treated effectively with a lower dose.
• Therapeutic blood levels range from 4 to 10 mcg/ml.

• Adverse reactions are generally mild, transient, and reversible by reducing dosage. GI reactions can be minimized by taking the drug with food.
• Dizziness and falling are more likely to occur in elderly patients.
• Monitor patient for tremor. This may indicate the approaching of maximum dose.
• Considered by cardiologists as an "oral lidocaine." May ease transition from I.V. lidocaine to oral antiarrhythmic therapy. Monitor patient carefully during this transition period.

21

Antianginals

diltiazem hydrochloride
erythrityl tetranitrate
isosorbide dinitrate
nadolol
nicardipine
nifedipine
nitroglycerin
pentaerythritol tetranitrate
propranolol hydrochloride
verapamil hydrochloride

COMBINATION PRODUCTS
ANGIJEN NO. 1: pentaerythritol tetranitrate 20 mg and phenobarbital sodium 15 mg.
ARCOTRATE NO. 3: pentaerythritol tetranitrate 20 mg and phenobarbital sodium 8 mg.
BITRATE: pentaerythritol tetranitrate 15 mg and phenobarbital sodium 20 mg.
DIMYCOR: pentaerythritol tetranitrate 10 mg and phenobarbital sodium 15 mg.
NITROTYM-PLUS: nitroglycerin 2.5 mg and butabarbital sodium 48 mg.
PERBUZEM: pentaerythritol tetranitrate 10 mg and butabarbital sodium 15 mg.

---

diltiazem hydrochloride
Cardizem, Cardizem SR

Pregnancy Risk Category: C

HOW SUPPLIED
Tablets: 30 mg, 60 mg, 90 mg, 120 mg
Capsules (sustained-release): 60 mg, 90 mg, 120 mg

MECHANISM OF ACTION
Inhibits calcium ion influx across cardiac and smooth muscle cells, decreasing myocardial contractility and oxygen demand, and dilates coronary arteries and peripheral arterioles.

INDICATIONS & DOSAGE
Management of vasospastic (also called Prinzmetal's or variant) angina and classic chronic stable angina pectoris—
Adults: 30 mg P.O. t.i.d. or q.i.d. before meals and at bedtime. Dosage may be gradually increased to a maximum of 360 mg/day, in divided doses.
Hypertension—
Adults: 60 mg P.O. b.i.d. (sustained-release capsule). Titrate dosage to effect. Maximum recommended dosage is 360 mg/day.

ADVERSE REACTIONS
CNS: *headache, fatigue, drowsiness,* dizziness, nervousness, depression, insomnia, confusion.
CV: *edema, arrhythmias,* flushing, bradycardia, hypotension, conduction abnormalities, CHF.
GI: *nausea,* vomiting, diarrhea.
GU: nocturia, polyuria.
Hepatic: transient elevation of liver enzymes.
Skin: *rash,* pruritus.
Other: photosensitivity.

INTERACTIONS
Cimetidine: may inhibit diltiazem metabolism. Monitor for toxicity.
Digoxin: diltiazem may increase

Italicized adverse reactions are common or life-threatening.
*Liquid form contains alcohol.   **May contain tartrazine.

serum levels of digoxin. Monitor for toxicity.

Propranolol (and other beta blockers): may prolong cardiac conduction time. Use together cautiously.

NURSING CONSIDERATIONS
• Contraindicated in sick sinus syndrome, unless a functioning ventricular pacemaker is present; hypotension when systolic blood pressure is less than 90 mm Hg; and second- or third-degree AV block.
• Use cautiously in elderly patients because duration of action may be prolonged.
• Use cautiously in impaired ventricular function or conduction abnormalities.
• Use cautiously in impaired hepatic or renal function.
• Monitor blood pressure during initiation of therapy and dosage adjustments. Assist patients with ambulation during initiation of diltiazem therapy because dizziness may occur.
• If systolic pressure is less than 90 mm Hg, or heart rate is less than 60 beats/minute, withhold dose and notify doctor.
• If nitrate therapy is prescribed during titration of diltiazem dosage, urge patient to continue compliance. Sublingual nitroglycerin, especially, may be taken concomitantly as needed when anginal symptoms are acute.
• Of the available calcium antagonists, diltiazem may offer the lowest risk of adverse reactions.
• Used investigationally to treat supraventricular tachycardia.
• May be useful as migraine prophylaxis in some patients. However, diltiazem itself may cause headaches.

erythrityl tetranitrate
Cardilate

Pregnancy Risk Category: C

HOW SUPPLIED
Tablets (chewable): 10 mg
Tablets (oral, sublingual, buccal): 5 mg, 10 mg

MECHANISM OF ACTION
Reduces cardiac oxygen demand by decreasing left ventricular end-diastolic pressure (preload) and, to a lesser extent, systemic vascular resistance (afterload). Also increases blood flow through the collateral coronary vessels.

INDICATIONS & DOSAGE
Prophylaxis and long-term management of frequent or recurrent anginal pain, reduced exercise tolerance associated with angina pectoris—
Adults: 5 mg orally, sublingually, or buccally t.i.d., increasing in 2 to 3 days if needed.

ADVERSE REACTIONS
CNS: *headache, sometimes with throbbing; dizziness;* weakness.
CV: *orthostatic hypotension, tachycardia, flushing, palpitations,* fainting.
GI: nausea, vomiting.
Skin: cutaneous vasodilation.
Local: sublingual burning.
Other: hypersensitivity reactions.

INTERACTIONS
None significant.

NURSING CONSIDERATIONS
• Contraindicated in hypersensitivity to nitrites, head trauma, cerebral hemorrhage, or severe anemia. Use with caution in hypotension.
• Monitor blood pressure and intensity and duration of response to drug.
• May cause headaches, especially at first. Treat headache with aspirin or

acetaminophen. Dosage may need to be reduced temporarily, but tolerance usually develops.

• Tell patient to take medication regularly, even long-term, if ordered, and to keep it easily accessible at all times. Physiologically necessary but not habit-forming.

• Additional dose may be taken before anticipated stress or at bedtime if angina is nocturnal.

• Advise patient to avoid alcoholic beverages; may produce increased hypotension.

• May cause orthostatic hypotension. To minimize it, patient should change to upright position slowly. He should go up and down stairs carefully, and lie down at the first sign of dizziness.

• Teach patient to take sublingual tablet at first sign of attack. He should wet the tablet with saliva, place it under the tongue until completely absorbed, and sit down and rest. Dose may be repeated every 10 to 15 minutes for a maximum of three doses. If no relief, patient should call doctor or go to hospital emergency room. If patient complains of tingling sensation with drug placed sublingually, he may try holding tablet in buccal pouch.

• Teach patient to take oral tablet on empty stomach, either half an hour before or 1 to 2 hours after meals, and to swallow oral tablets whole.

• Drug should not be discontinued abruptly—coronary vasospasm may occur.

• Store drug in cool place, in a tightly closed container, away from light. To ensure freshness, replace supply every 3 months. Remove cotton from container, since it absorbs drug.

isosorbide dinitrate
Apo-ISDN†, Cedocard-SR†, Coronex†, Dilatrate-SR, Iso-Bid, Isonate, Isorbid Isordil, Isotrate, Nitro-Spray‡, Novosorbide†, Sorbitrate, Sorbitrate SA

Pregnancy Risk Category: C

HOW SUPPLIED
Tablets: 5 mg, 10 mg, 20 mg, 30 mg, 40 mg
Tablets (chewable): 5 mg, 10 mg
Tablets (sublingual): 2.5 mg, 5 mg, 10 mg
Tablets (sustained-release): 40 mg
Capsules: 40 mg
Capsules (sustained-release): 40 mg
Topical spray: 10% w/w‡, 12.5 mg/metered spray‡

MECHANISM OF ACTION
Reduces cardiac oxygen demand by decreasing left ventricular end-diastolic pressure (preload) and, to a lesser extent, systemic vascular resistance (afterload). Also increases blood flow through the collateral coronary vessels.

INDICATIONS & DOSAGE
Treatment of acute anginal attacks (sublingual and chewable tablets only); prophylaxis in situations likely to cause anginal attacks; treatment of chronic ischemic heart disease (by preload reduction)—
Adults: *Sublingual form—*2.5 to 10 mg under the tongue for prompt relief of anginal pain, repeated q 5 to 10 minutes (maximum of three doses per 30-minute period). For prophylaxis, 2.5 to 10 mg under the tongue q 2 to 3 hours.
*Chewable form—*5 to 10 mg, p.r.n., for acute attack or q 2 to 3 hours for prophylaxis but only after initial test dose of 5 mg to determine risk of severe hypotension.
*Oral form—*5 to 30 mg P.O. q.i.d. for prophylaxis only (use smallest effec-

tive dose); sustained-release forms 40 mg P.O. q 6 to 12 hours.
Topical form (where available)—initially, 2 sprays to the chest in the morning from a distance of about 20 cm. Rub solution in. Dosage is gradually increased as needed to 2 to 5 sprays, daily or b.i.d. (in the morning and h.s.).
Adjunct with other vasodilators, such as hydralazine and prazosin, in treatment of severe chronic CHF—
Adults: *Oral or chewable form*—20 to 40 mg q 4 hours.

ADVERSE REACTIONS
CNS: *headache, sometimes with throbbing; dizziness;* weakness.
CV: *orthostatic hypotension, tachycardia, palpitations, ankle edema,* fainting.
GI: nausea, vomiting.
Skin: cutaneous vasodilation, *flushing.*
Local: sublingual burning.
Other: hypersensitivity reactions.

INTERACTIONS
Antihypertensives: possibly increased hypotensive effects. Monitor closely during initial therapy.

NURSING CONSIDERATIONS
• Contraindicated in hypersensitivity to nitrites, head trauma, cerebral hemorrhage, or severe anemia. Use with caution in hypotension.
• Monitor blood pressure and intensity and duration of response to drug.
• May cause headaches, especially at first. Treat headache with aspirin or acetaminophen. Dosage may need to be reduced temporarily, but tolerance usually develops.
• Tell patient to take medication regularly, even long-term, if ordered, and to keep it easily accessible at all times. Physiologically necessary but not habit-forming.
• Additional dose may be taken be-

fore anticipated stress or at bedtime if angina is nocturnal.
• Advise patient to avoid alcoholic beverages; they may produce increased hypotension.
• May cause orthostatic hypotension. To minimize it, patient should change to upright position slowly. He should go up and down stairs carefully, and lie down at the first sign of dizziness.
• Teach patient to take sublingual tablet at first sign of attack. He should wet the tablet with saliva, place it under the tongue until completely absorbed, and sit down and rest. Dose may be repeated every 10 to 15 minutes for a maximum of three doses. If no relief, patient should call doctor or go to hospital emergency room. If patient complains of tingling sensation with drug placed sublingually, he may try holding tablet in buccal pouch.
• Warn patient not to confuse sublingual with oral form.
• Teach patient to take oral tablet on empty stomach, either half an hour before or 1 to 2 hours after meals; to swallow oral tablets whole; and to chew chewable tablets thoroughly before swallowing.
• Drug should not be discontinued abruptly—coronary vasospasm may occur.
• Store in cool place, in tightly closed container, away from light.
• Has been used investigationally in treatment of congestive heart failure and diffuse esophageal spasms.

nadolol
Corgard
Pregnancy Risk Category: C

HOW SUPPLIED
Tablets: 20 mg, 40 mg, 80 mg, 120 mg, 160 mg

MECHANISM OF ACTION
A beta-adrenergic blocker that reduces cardiac oxygen demand by

blocking catecholamine-induced increases in heart rate, blood pressure, and force of myocardial contraction. Depresses renin secretion.

INDICATIONS & DOSAGE
Management of angina pectoris—
Adults: 40 mg P.O. once daily, initially. Dosage may be increased in 40- to 80-mg increments until optimum response occurs. Usual maintenance dosage range is 40 to 240 mg once daily.
Treatment of hypertension—
Adults: 40 mg P.O. once daily, initially. Dosage may be increased in 40- to 80-mg increments until optimum response occurs. Usual maintenance dosage range is 40 to 320 mg once daily. Doses of 640 mg may be necessary in rare cases.

ADVERSE REACTIONS
CNS: fatigue, lethargy.
CV: *bradycardia, hypotension, CHF,* peripheral vascular disease.
GI: nausea, vomiting, diarrhea.
Metabolic: hypoglycemia without tachycardia.
Skin: rash.
Other: *increased airway resistance,* fever.

INTERACTIONS
Antihypertensive agents: enhanced antihypertensive effect.
Cardiac glycosides: excessive bradycardia and increased depressant effect on myocardium. Use together cautiously.
Epinephrine: severe vasoconstriction and reflex bradycardia. Monitor blood pressure and observe patient carefully.
Indomethacin: decreased antihypertensive effect. Monitor blood pressure and adjust dosage.
Insulin, hypoglycemic drugs (oral): can alter dosage requirements in previously stabilized diabetics. Observe patient carefully.

NURSING CONSIDERATIONS
• Contraindicated in bronchial asthma, sinus bradycardia and greater than first-degree conduction block, and cardiogenic shock.
• Elderly patients may experience enhanced adverse reactions. Dose may need to be adjusted.
• Use cautiously in patients with heart failure, chronic bronchitis, renal or hepatic insufficiency, or emphysema.
• Always check patient's apical pulse before giving this drug. If slower than 60 beats/minute, withhold drug and call doctor.
• Monitor blood pressure frequently. If patient develops severe hypotension, administer a vasopressor as ordered.
• Don't discontinue abruptly; can exacerbate angina and myocardial infarction. Gradually reduce dosage over 1 to 2 weeks.
• Teach patient about his disease and therapy. Explain the importance of taking this drug as prescribed, even when he's feeling well. Tell outpatient not to discontinue drug suddenly, but to call doctor if unpleasant adverse reactions occur.
• Has been used in a limited number of patients with atrial flutter or fibrillation. Also has been used for a few patients in the treatment of migraine headaches.
• This drug masks common signs of shock, hyperthyroidism, and hypoglycemia.
• May be given without regard to meals.

---

nicardipine
Cardene
Pregnancy Risk Category: C

HOW SUPPLIED
Capsules: 20 mg, 30 mg

MECHANISM OF ACTION
Inhibits calcium ion influx across cardiac and smooth muscle cells, thus decreasing myocardial contractility and oxygen demand, and dilates coronary arteries and arterioles.

INDICATIONS & DOSAGE
Chronic stable angina (used alone or in combination with beta blockers)—
Adults: initially, 20 mg P.O. t.i.d. Titrate dosage according to patient response. Usual dosage range is 20 to 40 mg P.O. t.i.d.
Hypertension—
Adults: initially, 20 to 40 mg P.O. t.i.d. Increase dosage according to patient response.

ADVERSE REACTIONS
CNS: dizziness or light-headedness, headache, paresthesias, drowsiness, asthenia.
CV: peripheral edema, palpitations, angina, tachycardia.
GI: nausea, abdominal discomfort, dry mouth.
Skin: rash, flushing.

INTERACTIONS
Antihypertensive agents: enhanced antihypertensive effect.
Beta-adrenergic blocking agents: may increase cardiac depressant effects. Monitor patient closely.
Cimetidine: may decrease metabolism of calcium channel blocking agents. Monitor for increased pharmacologic effect.
Cyclosporine: nicardipine may increase plasma levels of cyclosporine. Monitor for toxicity.
Theophylline: pharmacologic effects of theophylline may be enhanced. Monitor for toxicity.

NURSING CONSIDERATIONS
• Contraindicated in patients with hypersensitivity to nicardipine, and in advanced aortic stenosis. Use cautiously in cardiac conduction disturbances, hypotension, and CHF.
• Some patients may experience increased frequency, severity, or duration of chest pain at beginning of therapy or during dosage adjustments. The mechanism for this adverse reaction is not known. Advise patient to report chest pain immediately.
• Patients with renal impairment should be titrated slowly to optimal response. Begin therapy with 20 mg P.O. t.i.d.
• Patients with hepatic impairment should receive lower initial doses (20 mg P.O. b.i.d.) and be carefully titrated to optimal response.
• Allow at least 3 days between dosage adjustments to achieve steady plasma levels.
• Measure blood pressure frequently during initial therapy. Maximum blood pressure response occurs about 1 hour after dosing. Check for potential orthostatic hypotension 1 to 2 hours after first dose. Because large swings in blood pressure may occur depending upon blood level of drug, assess adequacy of antihypertensive effect 8 hours after dosing.

---

nifedipine
Adalat, Adalat P.A.†, Apo-Nifed, Novo-Nifedin, Procardia, Procardia XL

Pregnancy Risk Category: C

HOW SUPPLIED
Tablets (sustained-release): 30 mg, 60 mg, 90 mg
Capsules: 10 mg, 20 mg

MECHANISM OF ACTION
Inhibits calcium ion influx across cardiac and smooth muscle cells, decreasing myocardial contractility and oxygen demand, and dilates coronary arteries and arterioles.

INDICATIONS & DOSAGE

Management of vasospastic (also called Prinzmetal's or variant) angina and classic chronic stable angina pectoris; Raynaud's disease—
Adults: starting dose is 10 mg P.O. t.i.d. Usual effective dose range is 10 to 20 mg t.i.d. Some patients may require up to 30 mg q.i.d. Maximum daily dosage is 180 mg.
Hypertension—
Adults: 30 or 60 mg P.O. (sustained release form only) once daily. Titrate over a 7- to 14-day period.

ADVERSE REACTIONS

CNS: *dizziness, light-headedness, flushing, headache,* weakness, syncope.
CV: peripheral edema, hypotension, palpitations.
EENT: nasal congestion.
GI: *nausea, heartburn,* diarrhea.
Metabolic: hypokalemia.
Other: muscle cramps, dyspnea.

INTERACTIONS

Cimetidine, ranitidine: decreased nifedipine metabolism.
Propranolol (and other beta blockers): may cause hypotension and heart failure. Use together cautiously.

NURSING CONSIDERATIONS

• Use cautiously in CHF or hypotension.
• Monitor blood pressure regularly, especially in patients who are also taking beta blockers or antihypertensives.
• Use cautiously in elderly patients because duration of action may be prolonged.
• Monitor serum potassium level regularly.
• Patient may briefly develop anginal exacerbation when beginning drug therapy or when dosage is increased. Reassure him that this symptom is temporary.
• Although rebound effect hasn't been observed when drug is stopped, dosage should still be reduced slowly under doctor's supervision.
• If patient is kept on nitrate therapy while drug dosage is being titrated, urge him to continue his compliance. Sublingual nitroglycerin, especially, may be taken as needed when anginal symptoms are acute.
• Instruct patient to swallow the capsule whole without breaking, crushing, or chewing it. The sustained-release tablets should never be chewed, crushed, or broken.
• There's no sublingual form of nifedipine available. However, the liquid in the oral capsule can be withdrawn by puncturing the capsule with a needle. Instill the drug into the buccal pouch.
• Sublingual nifedipine may be useful in decreasing blood pressure during hypertensive emergencies. Continuous blood pressure and ECG monitoring is recommended.
• Protect capsules from direct light and moisture and store at room temperature.

nitroglycerin (glyceryl trinitrate)

Deponit, Klavikordal, Niong, Nitradisc‡, Nitro-Bid, Nitro-Bid I.V., Nitrocap, Nitrocap T.D., Nitrocine, Nitrodisc, Nitro-Dur, Nitro-Dur II, Nitrogard, Nitrogard SR, Nitrol, Nitrolate Ointment‡, Nitrolin, Nitrolingual, Nitrol TSAR, Nitronet, Nitrong, Nitrong S.R., Nitrospan, Nitrostat, Nitrostat I.V., NTS, Transderm-Nitro, Tridil

Pregnancy Risk Category: C

HOW SUPPLIED

Tablets (buccal): 1 mg, 2 mg, 3 mg
Tablets (sublingual): 0.15 mg (1/400 gr), 0.3 mg (1/200 gr), 0.4 mg (1/150 gr), 0.6 mg (1/100 gr)
Tablets (sustained-release): 2.6 mg, 6.5 mg, 9 mg

Italicized adverse reactions are common or life-threatening.
*Liquid form contains alcohol.   **May contain tartrazine.

Capsules (sustained-release): 6.5 mg, 9 mg
I.V.: 0.5 mg/ml, 0.8 mg/ml, 5 mg/ml
Aerosol (translingual): 0.4 mg/metered spray
Topical: 2% ointment
Transdermal: 2.5 mg, 5 mg, 7.5 mg, 10 mg, 15 mg/24 hour systems

MECHANISM OF ACTION

Reduces cardiac oxygen demand by decreasing left ventricular end-diastolic pressure (preload) and, to a lesser extent, systemic vascular resistance (afterload). Also increases blood flow through the collateral coronary vessels.

INDICATIONS & DOSAGE

Prophylaxis against chronic anginal attacks—
Adults: 2.5 mg sustained-release (capsule) q 8 to 12 hours; or 2% ointment: Start with ½″ ointment, increasing by ½″ increments until headache occurs, then decreasing to previous dose. Range of dosage with ointment is 2″ to 5″. Usual dose is 1″ to 2″. Alternatively, transdermal disc or pad (Nitrodisc, Nitro-Dur, or Transderm-Nitro) may be applied to hairless site once daily.
Relief of acute angina pectoris, prophylaxis to prevent or minimize anginal attacks when taken immediately before stressful events—
Adults: 1 sublingual tablet (gr ¼₀₀, ¹⁄₂₀₀, ¹⁄₁₅₀, ¹⁄₁₀₀) dissolved under the tongue or in the buccal pouch immediately upon indication of anginal attack. May repeat q 5 minutes for 15 minutes. Or, using Nitrolingual spray, spray one or two doses into mouth, preferably onto or under the tongue. May repeat q 3 to 5 minutes to a maximum of 3 doses within a 15-minute period. Or, transmucosally, 1 to 3 mg q 3 to 5 hours during waking hours.
To control hypertension associated with surgery; to treat CHF associated with myocardial infarction; to relieve angina pectoris in acute situations; to produce controlled hypotension during surgery (by I.V. infusion)—
Adults: initial infusion rate is 5 mcg/minute. May be increased by 5 mcg/minute q 3 to 5 minutes until a response is noted. If a 20 mcg/minute rate doesn't produce a response, dosage may be increased by as much as 20 mcg/minute q 3 to 5 minutes.

ADVERSE REACTIONS

CNS: *headache, sometimes with throbbing; dizziness;* weakness.
CV: *orthostatic hypotension, tachycardia, flushing, palpitations,* fainting.
GI: nausea, vomiting.
Skin: cutaneous vasodilation.
Local: sublingual burning.
Other: hypersensitivity reactions.

INTERACTIONS

Antihypertensives: possibly enhanced hypotensive effect. Monitor closely.

NURSING CONSIDERATIONS

• Contraindicated in hypersensitivity to nitrites, head trauma, cerebral hemorrhage, hypertrophic cardiomyopathy, or severe anemia. Use with caution in hypotension.
• Monitor blood pressure and intensity and duration of response to drug.
• May cause headaches, especially at first. Treat headache with aspirin or acetaminophen. Dosage may need to be reduced temporarily, but tolerance usually develops.
• Tell patient to take medication regularly, even long-term, if ordered, and to keep it easily accessible at all times. Physiologically necessary but not habit-forming.
• Additional dose may be taken before anticipated stress or at bedtime if angina is nocturnal.
• Advise patient to avoid alcoholic beverages; may produce increased hypotension.
• May cause orthostatic hypotension.

---

†Available in Canada only.   ‡Available in Australia only.   ◊ Available OTC.

To minimize it, patient should change to upright position slowly. He should go up and down stairs carefully, and lie down at the first sign of dizziness.

• Teach patient to take sublingual tablet at first sign of attack. He should wet the tablet with saliva, place it under the tongue until completely absorbed, and sit down and rest. Dose may be repeated every 10 to 15 minutes for a maximum of three doses. If no relief, patient should call doctor or go to hospital emergency room. If patient complains of tingling sensation with drug placed sublingually, he may try holding tablet in buccal pouch.

• Although a burning sensation used to be an indication of tablet potency, today many brands don't produce this sensation.

• Store drug in cool, dark place in a tightly closed container. To ensure freshness, replace supply of sublingual tablets every 3 months. Remove cotton from container, since it absorbs drug.

• Tell patient to store nitroglycerin sublingual tablets in original container or other container specifically approved for this use.

• Advise patient not to carry bottle close to body. Patient should carry it in jacket pocket or purse.

• Teach patient to take oral tablet on empty stomach, either half an hour before or 1 to 2 hours after meals; to swallow oral tablets whole; and to chew chewable tablets thoroughly before swallowing.

• To apply ointment, spread uniform, thin layer on any nonhairy area. Do not rub in. Cover with plastic film to aid absorption and to protect clothing. If using Tape-Surrounded Appli-Ruler (TSAR) system, keep the TSAR on skin to protect patient's clothing and to ensure that ointment remains in place.

• Be sure to remove all excess ointment from previous site before applying the next dose.

• Avoid getting ointment on fingers.

• Transdermal dosage forms can be applied to any hairless part of the skin except distal parts of the arms or legs, because absorption will not be maximal at these sites.

• Be sure to remove transdermal patch before defibrillation. Because of its aluminum backing, the electric current may cause the patch to explode.

• When terminating transdermal treatment of angina, gradually reduce the dosage and frequency of application over 4 to 6 weeks.

• Instruct patient to use caution when wearing transdermal patch near microwave oven. Leaking radiation may heat patch's metallic backing and cause burns.

• The various brands of transdermal nitroglycerin products can be interchanged to achieve the prescribed dose. Now, standardized labels specify the amount of nitroglycerin released over 24 hours.

• If nitroglycerin lingual aerosol (Nitrolingual) has been prescribed for patient, instruct him how to use this device correctly. Remind him he should *not* inhale the spray, but should release the spray onto or under the tongue. Also tell him not to swallow immediately after administering the spray—wait about 10 seconds or so before swallowing.

• The transmucosal dosage form may be used to provide relief from an acute anginal attack as well as for prophylaxis.

• Tell patient to place the transmucosal tablet between lip and gum above the incisors, or between cheek and gum. Tell him not to swallow or chew tablet; this will make it ineffective.

• When administering as an I.V. infusion, be sure to use the special nonabsorbing tubing supplied by the manufacturer, because up to 80% of the drug can be absorbed by regular plas-

---

Italicized adverse reactions are common or life-threatening.
*Liquid form contains alcohol.   **May contain tartrazine.

tic tubing. Also, be sure to prepare in a glass bottle or container, and use a controlled infusion pump.
• Closely monitor vital signs during infusion.

pentaerythritol tetranitrate
Dilar, Duotrate, Naptrate, Pentritol, Pentylan, Peritrate, Peritrate Forte†, Peritrate SA, PETN

Pregnancy Risk Category: C

HOW SUPPLIED
Tablets: 10 mg, 20 mg, 40 mg, 80 mg
Tablets (sustained-release): 80 mg
Capsules (sustained-release): 30 mg, 45 mg, 80 mg

MECHANISM OF ACTION
Reduces cardiac oxygen demand by decreasing left ventricular end-diastolic pressure (preload) and, to a lesser extent, systemic vascular resistance (afterload). Also increases blood flow through the collateral coronary vessels.

INDICATIONS & DOSAGE
Prophylaxis against angina pectoris—
Adults: 10 to 20 mg P.O. q.i.d.; may be titrated upward to 40 mg P.O. q.i.d. half an hour before or 1 hour after meals and h.s.; 80 mg sustained-release preparations P.O. b.i.d.

ADVERSE REACTIONS
CNS: *headache, sometimes with throbbing; dizziness;* weakness.
CV: *orthostatic hypotension, tachycardia, flushing, palpitations,* fainting.
GI: nausea, vomiting.
Skin: cutaneous vasodilation.
Other: hypersensitivity reactions.

INTERACTIONS
None significant.

NURSING CONSIDERATIONS
• Contraindicated in head trauma, cerebral hemorrhage, or severe anemia. Use with caution in hypotension and glaucoma.
• Monitor blood pressure and intensity and duration of response to drug.
• May cause headaches, especially at first. Treat with aspirin or acetaminophen. Dosage may need to be reduced temporarily, but tolerance usually develops.
• Medication should be taken regularly, even long-term, if ordered. Physiologically necessary but not habit-forming.
• Additional doses may be taken before anticipated stress or at bedtime for nocturnal angina.
• Not to be used for relief of acute anginal attacks.
• May cause orthostatic hypotension. To minimize it, patient should change to upright position slowly. He should go up and down stairs carefully, and lie down at the first sign of dizziness.
• Advise patient to avoid alcoholic beverages; may exacerbate hypotension.
• Drug should not be discontinued abruptly—coronary vasospasm may occur.
• Store in cool place, in a tightly covered container away from light.

propranolol hydrochloride
Apo-Propranolol†, Deralin‡, Detensol†, Inderal, Inderal LA, Ipran, Novopranol†, PMS-Propranolol†

Pregnancy Risk Category: C

HOW SUPPLIED
Tablets: 10 mg, 20 mg, 40 mg, 60 mg, 80 mg, 90 mg
Capsules (sustained-release): 60 mg, 80 mg, 120 mg, 160 mg
Oral solution: 4 mg/ml, 8 mg/ml, 80 mg/ml (concentrate)
Injection: 1 mg/ml

MECHANISM OF ACTION

A beta-adrenergic blocker that reduces cardiac oxygen demand by blocking catecholamine-induced increases in heart rate, blood pressure, and force of myocardial contraction. Depresses renin secretion. Also prevents vasodilation of the cerebral arteries.

INDICATIONS & DOSAGE

Management of angina pectoris—
Adults: 10 to 20 mg P.O. t.i.d. or q.i.d. Or, 1 80-mg sustained-release capsule daily. Dosage may be increased at 7- to 10-day intervals. The average optimum dosage is 160 mg daily.
To reduce mortality following myocardial infarction—
Adults: 180 to 240 mg P.O. daily in divided doses. Usually administered t.i.d. to q.i.d.
Supraventricular, ventricular, and atrial arrhythmias; tachyarrhythmias caused by excessive catecholamine action during anesthesia, hyperthyroidism, and pheochromocytoma—
Adults: 1 to 3 mg I.V. diluted in 50 ml dextrose 5% in water or normal saline solution infused slowly, not to exceed 1 mg/minute. After 3 mg have been infused, another dose may be given in 2 minutes; subsequent doses no sooner than q 4 hours. Usual maintenance dosage is 10 to 80 mg P.O. t.i.d. or q.i.d.
Hypertension—
Adults: initial treatment of hypertension: 80 mg P.O. daily in two to four divided doses or the sustained-release form once daily. Increase at 3- to 7-day intervals to maximum daily dosage of 640 mg. Usual maintenance dosage for hypertension is 160 to 480 mg daily.
Prevention of frequent, severe, uncontrollable, or disabling migraine or vascular headache—
Adults: initially, 80 mg P.O. daily in divided doses or 1 sustained-release capsule daily. Usual maintenance dosage is 160 to 240 mg daily, divided t.i.d. or q.i.d.

ADVERSE REACTIONS

CNS: *fatigue, lethargy,* vivid dreams, hallucinations.
CV: *bradycardia, hypotension, CHF,* peripheral vascular disease.
GI: nausea, vomiting, diarrhea.
Metabolic: hypoglycemia without tachycardia.
Skin: rash.
Other: *increased airway resistance,* fever, arthralgia.

INTERACTIONS

Aminophylline: antagonized beta-blocking effects of propranolol. Use together cautiously.
Cardiac glycosides, verapamil: excessive bradycardia and increased depressant effect on myocardium. Use together cautiously.
Cimetidine: inhibits propranolol's metabolism. Monitor for greater beta-blocking effect.
Epinephrine: severe vasoconstriction. Monitor blood pressure and observe patient carefully.
Insulin, hypoglycemic drugs (oral): can alter requirements for these drugs in previously stabilized diabetics. Monitor for hypoglycemia.
Isoproterenol, glucagon: antagonized propranolol effect. May be used therapeutically and in emergencies.

NURSING CONSIDERATIONS

• Contraindicated in diabetes mellitus, asthma, or allergic rhinitis; during ethyl ether anesthesia; with sinus bradycardia and in heart block greater than first degree; in cardiogenic shock; and with right ventricular failure secondary to pulmonary hypertension. Use with caution in patients with CHF or respiratory disease, and in patients taking other antihypertensive drugs.
• Elderly patients may experience en-

Italicized adverse reactions are common or life-threatening.
*Liquid form contains alcohol.   **May contain tartrazine.

hanced adverse reactions. Dosage may need to be adjusted.
- Always check patient's apical pulse before giving this drug. If you detect extremes in pulse rates, withhold drug and call the doctor immediately.
- Monitor blood pressure, ECG, and heart rate and rhythm frequently, especially during I.V. administration. If patient develops severe hypotension, notify doctor. He may prescribe a vasopressor.
- After prolonged atrial fibrillation, restoration of normal sinus rhythm may result in thromboembolism due to dislodgment of thrombi from atrial wall. Anticoagulation often advised before restoration of normal atrial rhythm.
- Teach patient about his disease and therapy. Explain the importance of taking this drug as prescribed, even when he's feeling well. Tell outpatient not to discontinue his drug suddenly; abrupt discontinuation can exacerbate angina and myocardial infarction. Tell patient to call doctor if unpleasant adverse reactions occur.
- This drug masks common signs of shock and hypoglycemia.
- Food may increase the absorption of propranolol. Give consistently with meals.
- Compliance may be improved by administering this drug twice daily, or by sustained-release capsule. Check with doctor.
- Has also been used to treat aggression and rage, stage fright, recurrent GI bleeding, and menopausal symptoms.
- *Don't discontinue before surgery for pheochromocytoma.* Before any surgical procedure, notify anesthesiologist that patient is receiving propranolol.
- Double-check dose and route. I.V. doses are much smaller than P.O.
- Glucagon may be prescribed to reverse propranolol overdose.

verapamil hydrochloride
Calan, Calan SR, Cordilox Oral‡, Isoptin, Isoptin SR, Veradil‡

Pregnancy Risk Category: C

HOW SUPPLIED
Tablets: 40 mg, 80 mg, 120 mg
Tablets (sustained-release): 240 mg
Injection: 2.5 mg/ml

MECHANISM OF ACTION
Inhibits calcium ion influx across cardiac and smooth muscle cells, thus decreasing myocardial contractility and oxygen demand, and dilates coronary arteries and arterioles.

INDICATIONS & DOSAGE
Management of vasospastic (also called Prinzmetal's or variant) angina and classic chronic, stable angina pectoris—
Adults: starting dose is 80 mg P.O. t.i.d. or q.i.d. Dosage may be increased at weekly intervals. Some patients may require up to 480 mg daily.
Treatment of atrial arrhythmias—
Adults: 0.075 to 0.15 mg/kg (5 to 10 mg) I.V. push over 2 minutes with ECG and blood pressure monitoring. Repeat dose in 30 minutes if no response.
Children 1 to 15 years: 0.1 to 0.3 mg/kg as I.V. bolus over 2 minutes.
Children less than 1 year: 0.1 to 0.2 mg/kg as I.V. bolus over 2 minutes under continuous ECG monitoring.
Dose can be repeated in 30 minutes if no response.
Migraine headache prophylaxis—
Adults: 80 mg P.O. q.i.d.
Treatment of hypertension—
Adults: 240-mg sustained-release tablet once daily in the morning. If response is not adequate, may give an additional half tablet in the evening or one tablet q 12 hours. Alternatively, may give 80-mg immediate-release tablet t.i.d. or q.i.d.

ADVERSE REACTIONS
CNS: dizziness, headache, fatigue.
CV: *transient hypotension, CHF*, bradycardia, AV block, ventricular asystole, peripheral edema.
GI: *constipation*, nausea (primarily from oral form).
Hepatic: elevated liver enzymes.

INTERACTIONS
Carbamazepine, digitalis glycosides: verapamil may increase the serum levels of these drugs. Monitor patient for toxicity.
Lithium: verapamil may decrease serum lithium levels. Monitor patient closely.
Propranolol (and other beta blockers, including ophthalmic timolol), disopyramide: may cause heart failure. Use together cautiously.
Quinidine, antihypertensives: may result in hypotension. Monitor blood pressure.
Rifampin: may decrease oral bioavailability of verapamil. Monitor patient for lack of effect.

NURSING CONSIDERATIONS
• Contraindicated in advanced heart failure, AV block, severe left ventricular dysfunction, cardiogenic shock, sinus node disease, and severe hypotension.
• Use cautiously in elderly patients because duration of action may be prolonged. Administer I.V. doses over at least 3 minutes to minimize the risk of adverse reactions.
• Use cautiously in myocardial infarction followed by coronary occlusion, sick sinus syndrome, impaired AV conduction, or heart failure with atrial tachyarrhythmia; and in hepatic or renal disease.
• All patients receiving I.V. verapamil should be on a cardiac monitor. Monitor the R-R interval.
• Liver function tests should be done periodically.
• Patients with severely compromised cardiac function or those receiving beta blockers should receive lower doses of verapamil. Monitor these patients closely. Do not administer I.V. beta blockers at the same time as I.V. verapamil.
• Notify doctor if such signs of CHF as swelling of hands and feet or shortness of breath occur.
• If patient is kept on nitrate therapy while drug dosage of oral verapamil is being titrated, urge him to continue his compliance. Sublingual nitroglycerin, especially, may be taken as needed when anginal symptoms are acute.
• Taking extended-release tablets with food may decrease rate and extent of absorption, but allows smaller fluctuations of peak and trough blood levels.
• Preliminary studies show verapamil to be highly effective in the prophylaxis of migraine headache.

Italicized adverse reactions are common or life-threatening.
*Liquid form contains alcohol.   **May contain tartrazine.

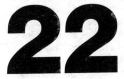

Antihypertensives

acebutolol
atenolol
betaxolol hydrochloride
captopril
carteolol
clonidine hydrochloride
deserpidine
diazoxide
diltiazem hydrochloride
(See Chapter 21, ANTIANGINALS.)
enalaprilat
enalapril maleate
guanabenz acetate
guanadrel sulfate
guanethidine sulfate
guanfacine hydrochloride
hydralazine hydrochloride
labetalol hydrochloride
lisinopril
mecamylamine hydrochloride
methyldopa
methyldopate hydrochloride
metoprolol tartrate
metyrosine
minoxidil
nadolol
(See Chapter 21, ANTIANGINALS.)
nitroprusside sodium
pargyline hydrochloride
penbutolol sulfate
phenoxybenzamine
hydrochloride
phentolamine mesylate
pindolol
prazosin hydrochloride
propranolol hydrochloride
(See Chapter 21, ANTIANGINALS.)
rauwolfia serpentina
rescinnamine
reserpine
terazocin hydrochloride

timolol maleate
trimethaphan camsylate
verapamil hydrochloride
(See Chapter 21, ANTIANGINALS.)

COMBINATION PRODUCTS

ALDOCLOR-150: chlorothiazide 150 mg and methyldopa 250 mg.
ALDOCLOR-250: chlorothiazide 250 mg and methyldopa 250 mg.
ALDORIL-15: hydrochlorothiazide 15 mg and methyldopa 250 mg.
ALDORIL-25: hydrochlorothiazide 25 mg and methyldopa 250 mg.
ALDORIL D30: hydrochlorothiazide 30 mg and methyldopa 500 mg.
ALDORIL D50: hydrochlorothiazide 50 mg and methyldopa 500 mg.
APRESAZIDE 25/25: hydrochlorothiazide 25 mg and hydralazine hydrochloride 25 mg.
APRESAZIDE 50/50: hydrochlorothiazide 50 mg and hydralazine hydrochloride 50 mg.
APRESAZIDE 100/50: hydrochlorothiazide 50 mg and hydralazine hydrochloride 100 mg.
APRESODEX: hydrochlorothiazide 15 mg and hydralazine hydrochloride 25 mg.
APRESOLINE-ESIDRIX: hydrochlorothiazide 15 mg and hydralazine hydrochloride 25 mg.
CAM-AP-ES: hydrochlorothiazide 15 mg, hydralazine hydrochloride 25 mg, and reserpine 0.1 mg.
CAPOZIDE 25/15: hydrochlorothiazide 15 mg and captopril 25 mg.
CAPOZIDE 25/25: hydrochlorothiazide 25 mg and captopril 25 mg.

CAPOZIDE 50/15: hydrochlorothiazide 15 mg and captopril 50 mg.

CAPOZIDE 50/25: hydrochlorothiazide 25 mg and captopril 50 mg.

CHERAPAS: hydrochlorothiazide 15 mg, hydralazine hydrochloride 25 mg, and reserpine 0.1 mg.

COMBIPRES 0.1: chlorthalidone 15 mg and clonidine hydrochloride 0.1 mg.

COMBIPRES 0.2: chlorthalidone 15 mg and clonidine hydrochloride 0.2 mg.

CORZIDE: nadolol 40 mg or 80 mg and bendroflumethiazide 5 mg.

DEMI-REGROTON: chlorthalidone 25 mg and reserpine 0.125 mg.

DIUPRES-250: chlorothiazide 250 mg and reserpine 0.125 mg.

DIUPRES-500: chlorothiazide 500 mg and reserpine 0.125 mg.

DIURESE-R: trichlormethiazide 4 mg and reserpine 0.1 mg.

DIURIGEN WITH RESERPINE: chlorothiazide 250 mg and reserpine 0.125 mg.

DIUTENSEN: methyclothiazide 2.5 mg and cryptenamine 2 mg (as tannate).

DIUTENSEN-R: methyclothiazide 2.5 mg and reserpine 0.1 mg.

ENDURONYL: methyclothiazide 5 mg and deserpidine 0.25 mg.

ENDURONYL-FORTE: methyclothiazide 5 mg and deserpidine 0.5 mg.

ESIMIL: hydrochlorothiazide 25 mg and guanethidine sulfate 10 mg.

EUTRON FILMTABS: methyclothiazide 5 mg and pargyline hydrochloride 25 mg.

EXNA-R TABLETS: benzthiazide 50 mg and reserpine 0.125 mg.

H.H.R.: hydrochlorothiazide 15 mg, hydralazine hydrochloride 25 mg, and reserpine 0.1 mg.

HYDROMOX-R: quinethazone 50 mg and reserpine 0.125 mg.

HYDROPINE: hydroflumethiazide 25 mg and reserpine 0.125 mg.

HYDROPINE HP: hydroflumethiazide 50 mg and reserpine 0.125 mg.

HYDROPRES-25: hydrochlorothiazide 25 mg and reserpine 0.125 mg.

HYDRO-RESERP: hydrochlorothiazide 25 or 50 mg and reserpine 0.125 mg.

HYDRO-SERP: hydrochlorothiazide 25 or 50 mg and reserpine 0.125 mg.

HYDROSERPINE: hydrochlorothiazide 25 or 50 mg and reserpine 0.125 mg.

HYDROTENSIN-25 TABLETS: hydrochlorothiazide 25 mg and reserpine 0.125 mg.

INDERIDE 40/25: propranolol hydrochloride 40 mg and hydrochlorothiazide 25 mg.

INDERIDE 80/25: propranolol hydrochloride 80 mg and hydrochlorothiazide 25 mg.

INDERIDE LA 80/50: propranolol hydrochloride 80 mg and hydrochlorothiazide 50 mg.

LOPRESSOR HCT 50/25: metoprolol tartrate 50 mg and hydrochlorothiazide 25 mg.

LOPRESSOR HCT 100/25: metoprolol tartrate 100 mg and hydrochlorothiazide 25 mg.

MAXZIDE: triamterene 75 mg and hydrochlorothiazide 50 mg.

METATENSIN TABLETS #2 or #4: trichlormethiazide 2 or 4 mg and reserpine 0.1 mg.

MINIZIDE 1: polythiazide 0.5 mg and prazosin hydrochloride 1 mg.

MINIZIDE 2: polythiazide 0.5 mg and prazosin hydrochloride 2 mg.

MINIZIDE 5: polythiazide 0.5 mg and prazosin hydrochloride 5 mg.

NAQUIVAL: trichlormethiazide 4 mg and reserpine 0.1 mg.

NATURETIN W/K 2.5 mg: bendroflumethiazide 2.5 mg and potassium chloride 500 mg.

NATURETIN W/K 5 mg: bendroflumethiazide 5 mg and potassium chloride 500 mg.

NORMOZIDE 100/25: labetalol hydrochloride 100 mg and hydrochlorothiazide 25 mg.

NORMOZIDE 200/25: labetalol hydrochloride 200 mg and hydrochlorothiazide 25 mg.

NORMOZIDE 300/25: labetalol hydro-

Italicized adverse reactions are common or life-threatening.
*Liquid form contains alcohol.   **May contain tartrazine.

chloride 300 mg and hydrochlorothiazide 25 mg.
ORETICYL 25: hydrochlorothiazide 25 mg and deserpidine 0.125 mg.
ORETICYL 50: hydrochlorothiazide 50 mg and deserpidine 0.125 mg.
ORETICYL FORTE: hydrochlorothiazide 25 mg and deserpidine 0.25 mg.
RAUZIDE**: bendroflumethiazide 4 mg and powdered rauwolfia serpentina 50 mg.
REGROTON: chlorthalidone 50 mg and reserpine 0.25 mg.
RENESE-R: polythiazide 2 mg and reserpine 0.25 mg.
REZIDE: hydrochlorothiazide 15 mg, hydralazine hydrochloride 25 mg, and reserpine 0.1 mg.
R-HCTZ-H: hydrochlorothiazide 15 mg, hydralazine hydrochloride 25 mg, and reserpine 0.1 mg.
SALUTENSIN: hydroflumethiazide 50 mg and reserpine 0.125 mg.
SALUTENSIN DEMI: hydroflumethiazide 25 mg and reserpine 0.125 mg.
SER-A-GEN: hydrochlorothiazide 15 mg, hydralazine hydrochloride 25 mg, and reserpine 0.1 mg.
SERALAZIDE: hydrochlorothiazide 15 mg, hydralazine hydrochloride 25 mg, and reserpine 0.1 mg.
SER-AP-ES: hydrochlorothiazide 15 mg, reserpine 0.1 mg, and hydralazine hydrochloride 25 mg.
SERPASIL-APRESOLINE #1**: reserpine 0.1 mg and hydralazine hydrochloride 25 mg.
SERPASIL-APRESOLINE #2: reserpine 0.2 mg and hydralazine hydrochloride 50 mg.
SERPASIL-ESIDRIX #1: hydrochlorothiazide 25 mg and reserpine 0.1 mg (called Serpasil-Esidrix 25 in Canada).
SERPASIL ESIDRIX #2: hydrochlorothiazide 50 mg and reserpine 0.1 mg.
SERPAZIDE: hydrochlorothiazide 15 mg, hydralazine hydrochloride 25 mg, and reserpine 0.1 mg.
TENORETIC 50: atenolol 50 mg and chlorthalidone 25 mg.

TENORETIC 100: atenolol 100 mg and chlorthalidone 25 mg.
TIMOLIDE 10/25: timolol maleate 10 mg and hydrochlorothiazide 25 mg.
TRI-HYDROSERPINE: hydrochlorothiazide 15 mg, hydralazine hydrochloride 25 mg, and reserpine 0.1 mg.
UNIPRES: hydrochlorothiazide 15 mg, reserpine 0.1 mg, and hydralazine hydrochloride 25 mg.
VASERETIC: enalapril maleate 10 mg and hydrochlorothiazide 25 mg.

acebutolol
Monitan†, Sectral
Pregnancy Risk Category: B

HOW SUPPLIED
Capsules: 200 mg, 400 mg

MECHANISM OF ACTION
A beta-selective blocking agent, acebutolol decreases myocardial contractility and decreases heart rate. It has mild intrinsic sympathomimetic activity.

INDICATIONS & DOSAGE
Treatment of hypertension—
Adults: 400 mg P.O. either as a single daily dosage or divided b.i.d. Patients may receive as much as 1,200 mg daily.
Ventricular arrhythmias—
Adults: 400 mg P.O. daily divided b.i.d. Dosage is then increased to provide an adequate clinical response. Usual dosage is 600 to 1,200 mg daily.

ADVERSE REACTIONS
CNS: *fatigue*, headache, dizziness, insomnia.
CV: chest pain, edema, bradycardia, CHF, *hypotension*.
GI: nausea, constipation, diarrhea, dyspepsia.
Metabolic: hypoglycemia without tachycardia.

Respiratory: dyspnea, broncho-
spasm.
Skin: rash.
Other: fever.

INTERACTIONS
Cardiac glycosides: excessive bradycardia and increased depressant effect
on myocardium. Use together cautiously.
Indomethacin: decreased antihypertensive effect. Monitor blood pressure
and adjust dosage.
Insulin, hypoglycemic drugs (oral):
can alter dosage requirements in previously stabilized diabetics. Observe
patient carefully.

NURSING CONSIDERATIONS
• Contraindicated in persistently severe bradycardia, second- and third-
degree heart block, overt cardiac failure, and cardiogenic shock.
• Use cautiously in patients with cardiac failure.
• Similar to metoprolol, acebutolol is
a cardioselective beta blocker. This
drug should be used with caution in
patients with bronchospastic diseases
such as asthma and emphysema.
• Dosage should be reduced in patients with decreased renal function.
• Elderly patients may require lower
acebutolol doses. For such patients,
dosage should not exceed 800 mg
daily.
• Always check patient's apical pulse
before giving this drug; if slower than
60 beats/minute, hold drug and call
doctor.
• Acebutolol may mask the signs of
hyperthyroidism and hyperglycemia,
and potentiate insulin-induced hypoglycemia.
• Before surgery, notify anesthesiologist if patient is receiving this drug.
• Do not discontinue abruptly; can
exacerbate angina and myocardial infarction.
• Teach patient about his disease and
therapy. Explain the importance of
taking this drug as prescribed, even
when he's feeling well. Tell patient
not to discontinue drug suddenly, but
to call the doctor if unpleasant adverse reactions occur.
• Instruct patient to check with doctor or pharmacist before taking OTC
medications.

atenolol
Noten‡, Tenormin

Pregnancy Risk Category: C

HOW SUPPLIED
Tablets: 50 mg, 100 mg
Injection: 5 mg/10 ml

MECHANISM OF ACTION
Blocks response to beta stimulation
and depresses renin secretion.

INDICATIONS & DOSAGE
Treatment of hypertension—
Adults: initially, 50 mg P.O. daily as
a single dose. Dosage may be increased to 100 mg once daily after 7
to 14 days. Dosages greater than 100
mg are unlikely to produce further
benefit. Dosage adjustment is necessary in patients with creatinine clearance below 35 ml/minute.
Angina pectoris—
Adults: 50 mg P.O. once daily. May
increase to 100 mg daily after 7 days
for optimal effect. May give as much
as 200 mg daily.
*To reduce cardiovascular mortality
and risk of reinfarction in patients
with acute myocardial infarction—*
Adults: 5 mg I.V. over 5 minutes, followed by another 5 mg I.V. 10 minutes later. After an additional 10 minutes, administer 50 mg P.O., followed
by 50 mg P.O. in 12 hours. Thereafter, give 100 mg P.O. daily (as a single dose or 50 mg b.i.d.) for at least 7
days.
*To reduce the incidence of supraven-
tricular tachycardia in patients undergoing coronary artery bypass—*

Italicized adverse reactions are common or life-threatening.
*Liquid form contains alcohol.   **May contain tartrazine.

Adults: 50 mg P.O. daily starting 3 days before surgery.

ADVERSE REACTIONS
CNS: fatigue, lethargy.
CV: *bradycardia, hypotension, congestive heart failure,* peripheral vascular disease.
GI: nausea, vomiting, diarrhea.
Respiratory: dyspnea, bronchospasm.
Skin: rash.
Other: fever.

INTERACTIONS
Antihypertensives: enhanced hypotensive effect. Use together cautiously.
Cardiac glycosides: excessive bradycardia and increased depressant effect on myocardium. Use together cautiously.
Indomethacin: decrease in antihypertensive effect. Monitor blood pressure and adjust dosage.
Insulin, hypoglycemic drugs (oral): can alter dosage requirements in previously stablilized diabetics. Observe patient carefully.

NURSING CONSIDERATIONS
• Contraindicated in sinus bradycardia and greater than first-degree conduction block, and cardiogenic shock.
• Use cautiously in cardiac failure.
• Similar to metoprolol, atenolol is a cardioselective beta blocker. Although atenolol can be used in patients with bronchospastic diseases such as asthma and emphysema, the drug should still be used cautiously in such patients—especially when 100 mg are given. Twice-daily dosing may help minimize this risk.
• Dosage should be reduced if patient has renal insufficiency. Patients with a creatinine clearance of 15 to 35 ml/mm/1.73 m^2 should receive a maximum of 50 mg daily; if creatinine clearance is <15 ml/mm/1.73 m^2, the maximum dosage is 50 mg every other day. Hemodialysis patients

should receive 50 mg after each dialysis session, but close supervision is mandatory because of the risk of marked decreases in blood pressure.
• I.V. doses may be mixed with 5% dextrose, sodium chloride injection, or dextrose and sodium chloride injection. The solution is stable for 48 hours after mixing.
• Once-a-day dosage encourages patient compliance. Counsel your patient to take the drug at a regular time every day. Drug can be dispensed in a 28-day calendar pack.
• Full antihypertensive effect may not appear for 1 to 2 weeks after initiating therapy.
• Always check patient's apical pulse before giving this drug; if slower than 60 beats/minute, hold drug and call doctor.
• Monitor blood pressure frequently.
• Don't discontinue abruptly; can exacerbate angina and myocardial infarction. Drug should be withdrawn gradually over a 2-week period.
• Teach patient about his disease and therapy. Explain the importance of taking this drug as prescribed, even when he's feeling well. Tell patient not to discontinue drug suddenly, but to call the doctor if unpleasant adverse reactions occur.
• Instruct patient to check with doctor or pharmacist before taking OTC medications.
• This drug masks common signs of shock and hypoglycemia. However, atenolol doesn't potentiate insulin-induced hypoglycemia or delay recovery of blood glucose to normal levels.
• Has been prescribed effectively in the treatment of angina pectoris and in patients with alcohol withdrawal syndrome.

betaxolol hydrochloride
Kerlone

Pregnancy Risk Category: C

HOW SUPPLIED
Tablets: 10 mg, 20 mg

MECHANISM OF ACTION
A beta$_1$-selective blocking agent that decreases blood pressure, probably by slowing heart rate and decreasing cardiac output.

INDICATIONS & DOSAGE
Management of hypertension (used alone or with other antihypertensives)—
Adults: initially, 10 mg P.O. once daily. After 7 to 14 days, full antihypertensive effect should be seen. If necessary, may double dosage to 20 mg P.O. once daily.

ADVERSE REACTIONS
CV: bradycardia, chest pain, hypotension, worsening of angina, peripheral vascular insufficiency, *CHF,* edema, syncope, postural hypotension, conduction disturbances.
CNS: dizziness, fatigue, headache, lethargy, anxiety.
GI: flatulence, constipation, nausea, diarrhea, dry mouth, vomiting, anorexia.
Respiratory: dyspnea, wheezing, bronchospasm.
Skin: rash.

INTERACTIONS
Calcium channel blocking agents: increased risk of hypotension, left ventricular failure, and AV conduction disturbances. I.V. calcium antagonists should be used with caution.
General anesthetics: increased hypotensive effects. Observe carefully for excessive hypotension or bradycardia, or orthostatic hypotension.
Lidocaine: beta blockers may increase the effects of lidocaine.

Reserpine, catecholamine-depleting drugs: may have an additive effect when administered with a beta blocker.

NURSING CONSIDERATIONS
• Contraindicated in patients with severe bradycardia, greater than first-degree heart block, cardiogenic shock, or uncontrolled CHF. It may be used cautiously in patients with CHF controlled by digitalis and diuretics because beta-adrenergic blocking agents do not block the inotropic effects of digitalis.
• Note that asymptomatic patients with a history of CHF may exhibit signs of cardiac decompensation with beta blocker therapy.
• Patients with bronchospastic disease (including asthma, chronic bronchitis, emphysema) should avoid beta blocker therapy because some beta$_2$ receptor antagonism may be associated with cardioselective agents such as betaxolol. However, some clinicians will use cardioselective beta blockers in such patients if the patients cannot tolerate other antihypertensives.
• Patients with unrecognized coronary artery disease may exhibit signs of angina pectoris upon withdrawal of the drug.
• Beta-blockade may inhibit glycogenolysis and the signs and symptoms of hypoglycemia (such as tachycardia and blood pressure changes).
• Beta blocking agents may mask tachycardia associated with hyperthyroidism. In patients with suspected thyrotoxicosis, beta blocker therapy should be withdrawn gradually to avoid thyroid storm.
• The anesthesiologist should be advised that the patient is receiving a beta blocking agent so that isoproterenol or dobutamine is made readily available for reversal of the cardiac effects of the drug.
• Withdrawal of beta blocker therapy

Italicized adverse reactions are common or life-threatening.
*Liquid form contains alcohol.   **May contain tartrazine.

before surgery is controversial. Some clinicians advocate withdrawal to prevent any impairment of cardiac responsiveness to reflex stimuli and decreased responsiveness to administration of catecholamines.

• Advise the patient to take the drug exactly as prescribed and not to discontinue the drug suddenly. Emphasize the importance of promptly reporting shortness of breath or difficulty breathing, unusually fast heartbeat, cough, or fatigue with exertion.

captopril
Capoten

Pregnancy Risk Category: C

HOW SUPPLIED
Tablets: 12.5 mg, 25 mg, 50 mg, 100 mg

MECHANISM OF ACTION
By inhibiting angiotensin-converting enzyme, prevents pulmonary conversion of angiotensin I to angiotensin II.

INDICATIONS & DOSAGE
Hypertension—
Adults: 25 mg P.O. b.i.d. or t.i.d. initially. If blood pressure isn't satisfactorily controlled in 1 to 2 weeks, dosage may be increased to 50 mg t.i.d. If not satisfactorily controlled after another 1 to 2 weeks, a diuretic should be added to regimen. If further blood pressure reduction is necessary, dosage may be raised to as high as 150 mg t.i.d. while continuing the diuretic. Maximum dosage is 450 mg daily. Daily dose may also be administered b.i.d.
Congestive heart failure—
Adults: 6.25 to 12.5 mg P.O. t.i.d. initially. May be gradually increased to 50 mg t.i.d. Maximum dosage is 450 mg daily.

ADVERSE REACTIONS
Blood: *leukopenia, agranulocytosis, pancytopenia.*
CNS: dizziness, fainting.
CV: *tachycardia, hypotension,* angina pectoris, CHF, pericarditis.
EENT: *loss of taste (dysgeusia).*
GI: anorexia.
GU: *proteinuria, nephrotic syndrome, membranous glomerulopathy, renal failure* (patients with preexisting renal disease or patients receiving high dosages), urinary frequency.
Metabolic: hyperkalemia.
Skin: *urticarial rash, maculopapular rash,* pruritus.
Other: fever, angioedema of face and extremities, transient increases in liver enzymes, persistent cough.

INTERACTIONS
Antacids: decreased captopril effect. Separate administration times.
Digitalis glycosides: may increase serum digoxin concentration by 15% to 30%.
NSAIDs: may reduce antihypertensive effect. Monitor blood pressure.
Potassium supplements: increased risk of hyperkalemia. Avoid these supplements unless hypokalemic blood levels are confirmed.

NURSING CONSIDERATIONS
• Use cautiously in impaired renal function or serious autoimmune disease (particularly systemic lupus erythematosus), or in patients who have been exposed to other drugs known to affect white cell counts or immune response.

• Proteinuria and nephrotic syndrome may occur in patients who are on captopril therapy. Those who develop persistent proteinuria or proteinuria that exceeds 1 g daily should have their captopril therapy reevaluated.

• Monitor patient's blood pressure and pulse rate frequently.

• Perform WBC and differential counts before starting treatment, ev-

ery 2 weeks for the first 3 months of therapy, and periodically thereafter.
• Advise patients to report any sign of infection (sore throat, fever).
• Although captopril can be used alone, its beneficial effects are increased when a thiazide diuretic is added.
• May cause dizziness or fainting, especially during initiation of therapy. Advise patient to avoid sudden postural changes.
• Teach patient about his disease and therapy. Explain the importance of taking this drug as prescribed, even when he's feeling well. Tell outpatient not to discontinue drug suddenly, but to call the doctor if unpleasant adverse reactions occur.
• Instruct patient to check with doctor or pharmacist before taking OTC medications.
• Elderly patients may be more sensitive to the drug's hypotensive effects.
• Should be taken 1 hour before meals since food in the GI tract may reduce absorption.
• Has been prescribed to treat rheumatoid arthritis.

---

carteolol
Cartrol

Pregnancy Risk Category: C

HOW SUPPLIED
Tablets: 2.5 mg, 5 mg

MECHANISM OF ACTION
A nonselective beta-adrenergic blocking agent with intrinsic sympathomimetic activity (ISA). Its antihypertensive effects are probably caused by decreased sympathetic outflow from the brain and decreased cardiac output. Carteolol does not have a consistent effect on renin output.

INDICATIONS & DOSAGE
Hypertension—
Adults: initially, 2.5 mg P.O. as a single daily dose. Gradually increase dosage as required to 5 mg or 10 mg daily as a single dose.

ADVERSE REACTIONS
CNS: weakness, lassitude, tiredness, fatigue, somnolence.
CV: conduction disturbances.
Other: *muscle cramps, asthenia.*

INTERACTIONS
Calcium channel blocking agents: increased risk of hypotension, left ventricular failure, and AV conduction disturbances. I.V. calcium antagonists should be used with caution.
General anesthetics: increased hypotensive effects. Observe carefully for excessive hypotension or bradycardia, or orthostatic hypotension.
Insulin, oral hypoglycemic agents: hypoglycemic response may be altered by beta blockers. Dosage adjustments may be necessary.
Reserpine, catecholamine-depleting drugs: may have an additive effect when administered with a beta blocker.

NURSING CONSIDERATIONS
• Contraindicated in patients with bronchial asthma, severe bradycardia, greater than first-degree heart block, cardiogenic shock, or uncontrolled CHF. It may be used cautiously in patients with CHF controlled by digitalis and diuretics because beta-adrenergic blocking agents do not block the inotropic effects of digitalis.
• Food may slow the rate, but not the extent, of carteolol absorption. Under normal circumstances, the patient may take the drug without regard to meals.
• Patients with substantial renal failure should receive the usual dose of carteolol at increased intervals. If creatinine clearance is >60 ml/minute, the drug is given at 24-hour intervals; if creatinine clearance is 20 to 60 ml/minute, the drug is given at 48-hour

---

Italicized adverse reactions are common or life-threatening.
*Liquid form contains alcohol.   **May contain tartrazine.

intervals; if creatinine clearance is <20 ml/minute, the drug is given at 72-hour intervals.
• Note that asymptomatic patients with a history of CHF may exhibit signs of cardiac decompensation with beta blocker therapy.
• Patients with unrecognized coronary artery disease may exhibit signs of angina pectoris upon withdrawal of the drug.
• Beta-blockade may inhibit glycogenolysis and the signs and symptoms of hypoglycemia (such as tachycardia and blood pressure changes). It may also attenuate insulin release.
• Beta blocking agents may mask tachycardia associated with hyperthyroidism. In patients with suspected thyrotoxicosis, beta blocker therapy should be withdrawn gradually to avoid thyroid storm.
• Withdrawal of beta blocker therapy before surgery is controversial. Some clinicians advocate withdrawal to prevent any impairment of cardiac responsiveness to reflex stimuli and decreased responsiveness to administration of catecholamines. However, the beta blocking effects of carteolol may persist for weeks, and discontinuing the drug before surgery may be impractical.
• The anesthesiologist should be advised that the patient is receiving a beta blocking agent so that isoproterenol or dobutamine is made readily available for reversal of the cardiac effects of the drug.
• Dosages that exceed 10 mg daily do not produce a greater response and may actually decrease response.
• Advise the patient to take the drug exactly as prescribed, and not to discontinue the drug suddenly. Emphasize the importance of reporting shortness of breath or difficulty breathing, unusually fast heartbeat, cough, or fatigue with exertion.

clonidine hydrochloride
Catapres, Catapres-TTS, Dixarit†‡

Pregnancy Risk Category: C

HOW SUPPLIED
Tablets: 0.025 mg†‡, 0.1 mg, 0.2 mg, 0.3 mg
Transdermal: TTS-1 (releases 0.1 mg/24 hours), TTS-2 (releases 0.2 mg/24 hours), TTS-3 (releases 0.3 mg/24 hours)

MECHANISM OF ACTION
Inhibits the central vasomotor centers, thereby decreasing sympathetic outflow.

INDICATIONS & DOSAGE
Essential, renal, and malignant hypertension—
Adults: initially, 0.1 mg P.O. b.i.d. Then increase by 0.1 to 0.2 mg daily on a weekly basis. Usual dosage range is 0.2 to 0.8 mg daily in divided doses; infrequently, dosages as high as 2.4 mg daily. No dosing recommendations for children.
Or, apply transdermal patch to a hairless area of intact skin on the upper arm or torso, once every 7 days.
Prophylactic treatment of migraine; treatment of menopausal flushing—
Adults: 0.025 mg P.O. b.i.d. If there has been no remission after 2 weeks, increase dosage to 0.050 mg b.i.d.
To suppress abstinence symptoms during narcotics withdrawal—
Adults: 0.1 mg P.O. t.i.d.

ADVERSE REACTIONS
CNS: *drowsiness,* dizziness, fatigue, sedation, nervousness, headache, vivid dreams.
CV: orthostatic hypotension, bradycardia, *severe rebound hypertension.*
EENT: *dry mouth.*
GI: *constipation.*
GU: urine retention, impotence.
Metabolic: transient glucose intolerance (after large doses).

---

†Available in Canada only. ‡Available in Australia only. ◊ Available OTC.

Skin: *pruritus, dermatitis* (from transdermal patch).

INTERACTIONS

CNS depressants: enhanced CNS depression. Use together cautiously.
Propranolol and other beta blockers: paradoxical hypertensive response. Monitor carefully.
Tricyclic antidepressants and MAO inhibitors: may decrease antihypertensive effect. Use together cautiously.

NURSING CONSIDERATIONS

• Use cautiously in patients with severe coronary insufficiency, diabetes, myocardial infarction, cerebral vascular disease, chronic renal failure, or history of depression, or in those taking other antihypertensives.
• Monitor blood pressure and pulse rate frequently. Dosage is usually adjusted to patient's blood pressure and tolerance.
• May be given to rapidly lower blood pressure in some hypertensive emergency situations.
• Discontinuing clonidine for surgery is not recommended.
• Reduce dosage gradually over 2 to 4 days. If discontinued abruptly, this drug may cause severe hypertension.
• In patients receiving both clonidine and a beta blocker, the beta blocker should be gradually withdrawn before clonidine to minimize adverse reactions.
• Teach patient about his disease and therapy. Explain the importance of taking this drug exactly as prescribed, even when he's feeling well. Tell outpatient not to discontinue this drug suddenly because this can cause severe rebound hypertension, but to call the doctor if unpleasant adverse reactions occur. Warn that this drug can cause drowsiness, but that tolerance to this side effect will develop.
• Instruct patient to check with doctor or pharmacist before taking OTC medications.

• Observe for tolerance to the drug's therapeutic effects that may require an increased dosage.
• Inform patient that orthostatic hypotension can be minimized by rising slowly and avoiding sudden position changes.
• Periodic eye examinations are recommended.
• Elderly patients may be more sensitive to hypotensive effects.
• Last dose should be taken immediately before retiring.
• Transdermal patch provides antihypertensive activity for up to 7 days. Available in three strengths: TTS-1 contains 2.5 mg; TTS-2 contains 5 mg; TTS contains 7.5 mg of clonidine.
• Transdermal patch usually adheres despite showering and other routine daily activities. An adhesive "overlay" is available to provide additional skin adherence if necessary. Instruct the patient to place the patch at a different site each week.
• Antihypertensive effects of transdermal clonidine may take 2 to 3 days to become apparent. Oral antihypertensive therapy may have to be continued in the interim.
• Remove patch before defibrillation to prevent arcing.
• Has been used investigationally for the treatment of dysmenorrhea. May also suppress craving for nicotine in nicotine addiction.

deserpidine

Harmonyl

Pregnancy Risk Category: C

HOW SUPPLIED

Tablets: 0.25 mg

MECHANISM OF ACTION

Acts peripherally, inhibiting norepinephrine release and depleting norepinephrine stores in adrenergic nerve endings.

Italicized adverse reactions are common or life-threatening.
*Liquid form contains alcohol.   **May contain tartrazine.

INDICATIONS & DOSAGE
Mild essential hypertension—
Adults: 0.25 mg P.O. once daily. No dosing recommendations for children.

ADVERSE REACTIONS
CNS: mental confusion, *depression, drowsiness, nervousness, paradoxical anxiety,* nightmares, *sedation, extrapyramidal symptoms.*
CV: bradycardia.
EENT: *dry mouth, nasal stuffiness,* glaucoma.
GI: *hypersecretion of gastric acid, nausea, vomiting,* GI bleeding.
Skin: pruritus, rash.
Other: *impotence, weight gain.*

INTERACTIONS
MAO inhibitors: may cause excitability and hypertension. Avoid if possible.

NURSING CONSIDERATIONS
• Contraindicated in mental depression. Use cautiously in severe cardiac or cerebrovascular disease, peptic ulcer, ulcerative colitis, gallstones, or mental depressive disorders; in patients undergoing surgery; and in patients taking other antihypertensives or anticonvulsants.
• Monitor patient's blood pressure and pulse rate frequently.
• Teach patient about his disease and therapy. Explain the importance of taking this drug as prescribed, even when he's feeling well. Tell outpatient not to discontinue this drug suddenly, but to call the doctor if unpleasant adverse reactions, such as mental depression, insomnia, or loss of appetite, occur. Warn that drug can cause drowsiness.
• Instruct patient to check with doctor or pharmacist before taking OTC medications.
• Advise patients to have periodic eye examinations.
• Watch patient closely for signs of mental depression. Warn him to no-

tify doctor promptly if he experiences nightmares.
• Tell patient to avoid alcohol and to follow prescribed diet.
• Dry mouth can be relieved with chewing gum, sour hard candy, or ice chips. Tell patient to contact doctor if relief is needed for nasal stuffiness.
• Give this drug with meals to increase absorption.
• Patient should weigh himself daily and notify doctor of any significant weight gain.

diazoxide
Hyperstat
Pregnancy Risk Category: C

HOW SUPPLIED
Injection: 300 mg/20 ml

MECHANISM OF ACTION
Directly relaxes arteriolar smooth muscle.

INDICATIONS & DOSAGE
Hypertensive crisis—
Adults and children: 1 to 3 mg/kg I.V. (up to a maximum of 150 mg) q 5 to 15 minutes until adequate response is seen. Repeat at intervals q 4 to 24 hours p.r.n.

ADVERSE REACTIONS
CNS: *headaches,* dizziness, lightheadedness, euphoria.
CV: *sodium and water retention, orthostatic hypotension,* sweating, flushing, warmth, angina, myocardial ischemia, arrhythmias, ECG changes.
GI: *nausea, vomiting,* abdominal discomfort.
Metabolic: *hyperglycemia,* hyperuricemia.
Local: inflammation and pain from extravasation.

INTERACTIONS
Hydralazine: may cause severe hypotension. Use together cautiously.

Thiazide diuretics: may increase the effects of diazoxide. Use together cautiously.

NURSING CONSIDERATIONS
• Use cautiously in patients with impaired cerebral or cardiac function, diabetes, or uremia, or in those taking other antihypertensives.
• Monitor blood pressure and ECG continuously. Patient should be supine or in Trendelenberg's position during and for 1 hour after infusion. Notify doctor immediately if severe hypotension develops. Keep norepinephrine available.
• Monitor patient's intake/output carefully. If fluid or sodium retention develops, doctor may want to order diuretics.
• Check patient's standing blood pressure before discontinuing close monitoring for hypotension.
• Take care to avoid extravasation.
• This drug may alter requirements for insulin, diet, or oral hypoglycemic drugs in previously controlled diabetics. Monitor blood glucose daily.
• Weigh patient daily. Notify doctor of any weight increase.
• Watch diabetics closely for signs of severe hyperglycemia or hyperosmolar nonketotic coma. Insulin may be needed.
• Check patient's uric acid levels frequently. Report abnormalities to doctor.
• Inform patient that orthostatic hypotension can be minimized by rising slowly and avoiding sudden position changes. Instruct patient to remain supine for 30 minutes after injection.
• Infusion of diazoxide has been shown to be as effective as a bolus in some patients.
• Protect I.V. solutions from light. Darkened I.V. solutions of diazoxide are subpotent and should not be used.

---

enalaprilat
Vasotec I.V.

enalapril maleate
Amprace‡, Renitec‡, Vasotec
Pregnancy Risk Category: C

HOW SUPPLIED
Tablets: 2.5 mg, 5 mg, 10 mg, 20 mg
Injection: 1.25 mg/ml in 2-ml vials

MECHANISM OF ACTION
By inhibiting angiotensin-converting enzyme, prevents pulmonary conversion of angiotensin I to angiotensin II.

INDICATIONS & DOSAGE
Treatment of hypertension—
Adults: initially, 5 mg P.O. once daily, then adjust according to response. Usual dosage range is 10 to 40 mg daily as a single dose or two divided doses. Alternatively, give by I.V. infusion 1.25 mg q 6 hours over 5 minutes.
To convert from I.V. therapy to oral therapy—
Adults: initially, 5 mg P.O. once a day. Adjust dosage to response.
To convert from oral therapy to I.V. therapy—
Adults: 1.25 mg I.V. over 5 minutes q 6 hours. Higher doses have not demonstrated greater efficacy.

ADVERSE REACTIONS
Blood: neutropenia, *agranulocytosis.*
CNS: *headache, dizziness, fatigue,* insomnia.
CV: *hypotension.*
GI: diarrhea, nausea.
GU: decreased renal function (patients with bilateral renal artery stenosis or CHF).
Skin: rash.
Other: persistent cough, *angioedema.*

Italicized adverse reactions are common or life-threatening.
*Liquid form contains alcohol.   **May contain tartrazine.

INTERACTIONS

Lithium: lithium toxicity can occur. Monitor lithium levels.

NSAIDs: may reduce antihypertensive effect. Monitor blood pressure.

Potassium supplements: increased risk of hyperkalemia. Avoid these supplements unless hypokalemic blood levels are confirmed.

NURSING CONSIDERATIONS

• Use cautiously in preexisting renal impairment or collagen vascular disease. Diabetic patients, patients with impaired renal function or CHF, and patients receiving drugs that can increase serum potassium may develop hyperkalemia. Monitor potassium intake and serum potassium level.

• If patient is taking a diuretic, it should be discontinued 2 to 3 days before beginning enalapril therapy. This will reduce the risk of hypotension. Then, if enalapril does not control blood pressure, diuretic therapy may be added.

• A response to I.V. enalaprilat is usually seen in 15 minutes, but peak effects may not be seen for up to 4 hours.

• Teach patient about his disease and therapy. Explain the importance of taking this drug as prescribed, even when he's feeling well. Tell outpatient not to discontinue drug suddenly, but to call the doctor if unpleasant adverse reactions occur.

• Instruct patient to check with doctor or pharmacist before taking OTC medications.

• Angioedema (including laryngeal edema) may occur, especially after the first enalapril dose. Advise patient to report any signs or symptoms such as swelling of face, eyes, lips, tongue, or breathing difficulty.

• Advise patient to report lightheadedness, especially during the first few days of therapy, when it's most likely to occur.

• Advise patient to report any sign of infection.

• Enalapril is similar to captopril, the other angiotensin-converting enzyme inhibitor, but has a longer duration of action. Many patients may get satisfactory therapeutic results by taking enalapril once daily.

guanabenz acetate
Wytensin

Pregnancy Risk Category: C

HOW SUPPLIED
Tablets: 4 mg, 8 mg

MECHANISM OF ACTION
Inhibits the central vasomotor centers, thereby decreasing sympathetic outflow.

INDICATIONS & DOSAGE
Treatment of hypertension—
Adults: initially, 4 mg P.O. b.i.d. Dosage may be increased in increments of 4 to 8 mg/day q 1 to 2 weeks. Maximum dosage is 32 mg b.i.d. To ensure adequate overnight blood pressure control, give last dose h.s.

ADVERSE REACTIONS
CNS: *drowsiness, sedation, dizziness, weakness,* headache, ataxia, depression.
CV: *severe rebound hypertension.*
EENT: *dry mouth.*
GU: sexual dysfunction.

INTERACTIONS
CNS depressants: may cause increased sedation. Use together cautiously.
Tricyclic antidepressants, MAO inhibitors: may decrease antihypertensive effect.

NURSING CONSIDERATIONS
• Use cautiously in vascular insufficiency, coronary insufficiency, recent myocardial infarction, cerebrovascu-

---

lar disease, or severe hepatic or renal failure.
• Don't stop guanabenz therapy abruptly. Rebound hypertension may occur.
• Advise patient to drive a car or operate machinery very cautiously until the CNS effects of the drug are known.
• Elderly patients may be more sensitive to hypotensive effects.
• Warn patient that his tolerance to alcohol or other CNS depressants may be diminished.
• Guanabenz can be used alone or in combination with a thiazide diuretic.
• Teach patient about his disease and therapy. Explain the importance of taking this drug as prescribed, even when he's feeling well. Tell outpatient not to discontinue drug suddenly, but to call the doctor if unpleasant adverse reactions occur.
• Instruct patient to check with doctor or pharmacist before taking OTC medications.
• To relieve dry mouth, tell patient to chew sugarless gum or dissolve ice chips in the mouth.
• Has been used investigationally as an adjunct in the treatment of opiate withdrawal (4 mg P.O. b.i.d.).

guanadrel sulfate
Hylorel

Pregnancy Risk Category: B

HOW SUPPLIED
Tablets: 10 mg, 25 mg

MECHANISM OF ACTION
Acts peripherally, inhibiting norepinephrine release and depleting norepinephrine stores in adrenergic nerve endings.

INDICATIONS & DOSAGE
Treatment of hypertension—
Adults: initially, 5 mg P.O. b.i.d. Dosage can be adjusted until blood pressure is controlled. Most patients require doses of 20 to 75 mg/day, usually given b.i.d.; however, tolerance to hypotensive effect may necessitate upward titration of dosage to 100 to 400 mg daily, given in three to four divided doses.

ADVERSE REACTIONS
CNS: *fatigue, dizziness,* drowsiness, faintness.
CV: *orthostatic hypotension,* edema.
GI: diarrhea.
Other: impotence, ejaculation disturbances.

INTERACTIONS
MAO inhibitors, ephedrine, norepinephrine, methylphenidate, tricyclic antidepressants, amphetamines, phenothiazines: may inhibit the antihypertensive effect of guanadrel. Adjust dose accordingly.

NURSING CONSIDERATIONS
• Contraindicated in known or suspected pheochromocytoma or frank CHF.
• Use cautiously in known peripheral vascular disease, asthma, and history of peptic ulcer disease.
• Guanadrel should be discontinued 48 to 72 hours before surgery to minimize the risk of vascular collapse during anesthesia.
• Don't give concurrently or within 1 week of therapy with an MAO inhibitor.
• Patient response varies widely with this drug and dosage must be individualized. Monitor both supine and standing blood pressure, especially during the period of dosage adjustment.
• Teach patient about his disease and therapy. Explain the importance of taking this drug as prescribed, even when he's feeling well. Tell patient not to discontinue this drug suddenly, but to call the doctor if unpleasant adverse reactions occur.

Italicized adverse reactions are common or life-threatening.
*Liquid form contains alcohol.   **May contain tartrazine.

- Instruct patient to check with doctor or pharmacist before taking OTC medications.
- Tell outpatient to avoid strenuous exercise, and warn that hot showers may cause hypotensive reaction.
- Inform patient that orthostatic hypotension can be minimized by rising slowly from a supine position and by avoiding sudden position changes.
- Elderly patients may be more sensitive to hypotensive effects.

---

guanethidine sulfate
Apo-Guanethidine†, Ismelin

Pregnancy Risk Category: C

HOW SUPPLIED
Tablets: 10 mg, 25 mg

MECHANISM OF ACTION
Acts peripherally, inhibiting norepinephrine release and depleting norepinephrine stores in adrenergic nerve endings.

INDICATIONS & DOSAGE
For moderate to severe hypertension; usually used in combination with other antihypertensives—
Adults: initially, 10 mg P.O. daily. Increase by 10 mg at weekly to monthly intervals, p.r.n. Usual dose is 25 to 50 mg daily. Some patients may require up to 300 mg.
Children: initially, 200 mcg/kg P.O. daily. Increase gradually q 1 to 3 weeks to maximum of 8 times initial dose.

ADVERSE REACTIONS
CNS: *dizziness, weakness, syncope.*
CV: *orthostatic hypotension, bradycardia,* CHF, arrhythmias.
EENT: *nasal stuffiness.*
GI: *diarrhea.*
Other: *edema, weight gain, inhibition of ejaculation.*

INTERACTIONS
Levodopa, alcohol: may increase hypotensive effect of guanethidine. Use together cautiously.
MAO inhibitors, ephedrine, norepinephrine, methylphenidate, tricyclic antidepressants, amphetamines, phenothiazines: may inhibit the antihypertensive effect of guanethidine. Adjust dose accordingly.

NURSING CONSIDERATIONS
- Contraindicated in pheochromocytoma. Use cautiously in severe cardiac disease, recent myocardial infarction, cerebrovascular disease, peptic ulcer, impaired renal function, or bronchial asthma, or in patients taking other antihypertensives.
- Full antihypertensive effect may not appear for 1 to 3 weeks.
- Discontinue drug 2 to 3 weeks before elective surgery to reduce the possibility of vascular collapse and cardiac arrest during anesthesia.
- Teach patient about his disease and therapy. Explain the importance of taking this drug as prescribed, even when he's feeling well. Tell patient not to discontinue this drug suddenly, but to call the doctor if unpleasant adverse reactions occur.
- Instruct patient to check with doctor or pharmacist before taking OTC medications.
- Tell outpatient to avoid strenuous exercise, and warn that hot showers may cause hypotensive reaction.
- A hot environment may also potentiate the hypotensive effects of guanethidine.
- Patient should receive instruction on low-sodium diet. Monitor for possible weight gain and edema.
- Inform patient that orthostatic hypotension can be minimized by rising slowly and avoiding sudden position changes. Dry mouth can be relieved with sugarless chewing gum, sour hard candy, or ice chips.

---

†Available in Canada only.   ‡Available in Australia only.   ◊ Available OTC.

- Elderly patients may be more sensitive to hypotensive effects.
- If patient develops diarrhea, doctor may prescribe atropine or paregoric.

guanfacine hydrochloride
Tenex

Pregnancy Risk Category: B

HOW SUPPLIED
Tablets: 1 mg

MECHANISM OF ACTION
Inhibits the central vasomotor center, thereby decreasing sympathetic outflow.

INDICATIONS & DOSAGE
Treatment of mild to moderate hypertension—
Adults: initially, 0.5 to 1 mg P.O. daily, h.s. Average dose is 1 to 3 mg daily.

ADVERSE REACTIONS
CNS: *drowsiness, dizziness,* fatigue, headache, insomnia.
CV: bradycardia, orthostatic hypotension, rebound hypertension.
EENT: dry mouth.
GI: *constipation,* diarrhea, nausea.
Skin: dermatitis, pruritus.

INTERACTIONS
None significant.

NURSING CONSIDERATIONS
- Use cautiously in severe coronary insufficiency, recent myocardial infarction, cerebrovascular disease, or chronic renal or hepatic insufficiency.
- Warn patients not to discontinue therapy abruptly. Rebound hypertension is less common than with similar drugs, such as clonidine, but may occur.
- Guanfacine reportedly has no adverse effect on blood lipids.
- May be used alone or with a diuretic.

- The incidence and severity of adverse reactions increase with higher dosages.
- Teach patient about his disease and therapy. Explain the importance of taking this drug as prescribed, even when he's feeling well. Tell outpatient not to discontinue drug suddenly, but to call the doctor if unpleasant adverse reactions occur.
- Instruct patient to check with doctor or pharmacist before taking OTC medications.
- Because guanfacine causes drowsiness, advise patient to avoid activities that require alertness until response to the drug is established.
- Guanfacine appears to be as effective as methyldopa and clonidine; long half-life permits once-daily dosing.

hydralazine hydrochloride
Alazine, Apresoline**, Novo-Hylazin†, Supres‡

Pregnancy Risk Category: C

HOW SUPPLIED
Tablets: 10 mg, 25 mg, 50 mg, 100 mg
Injection: 20 mg/ml

MECHANISM OF ACTION
Directly relaxes arteriolar smooth muscle.

INDICATIONS & DOSAGE
Essential hypertension (oral, alone or in combination with other antihypertensives); to reduce afterload in severe CHF (with nitrates); and severe essential hypertension (parenteral to lower blood pressure quickly)—
Adults: initially, 10 mg P.O. q.i.d.; gradually increased to 50 mg q.i.d. Maximum recommended dosage is 200 mg daily, but some patients may require 300 to 400 mg daily. Can be given b.i.d. for CHF.
*I.V.—*10 to 20 mg given slowly and

Italicized adverse reactions are common or life-threatening.
*Liquid form contains alcohol.   **May contain tartrazine.

repeated as necessary, generally q 4 to 6 hours. Switch to oral antihypertensives as soon as possible.
I.M.—20 to 40 mg repeated as necessary, generally q 4 to 6 hours. Switch to oral antihypertensives as soon as possible.
Children: initially, 0.75 mg/kg P.O. daily in four divided doses (25 mg/m² daily). May increase gradually to 10 times this dosage, if necessary.
I.V.—give slowly 1.7 to 3.5 mg/kg daily or 50 to 100 mg/m² daily in four to six divided doses.
I.M.—1.7 to 3.5 mg/kg daily or 50 to 100 mg/m² daily in four to six divided doses.

ADVERSE REACTIONS
Blood: neutropenia, leukopenia.
CNS: peripheral neuritis, *headache,* dizziness.
CV: orthostatic hypotension, *tachycardia,* arrhythmias, *angina, palpitations, sodium retention.*
GI: *nausea, vomiting, diarrhea, anorexia.*
Skin: rash.
Other: *lupus erythematosus-like syndrome (especially with high doses), weight gain.*

INTERACTIONS
Diazoxide: may cause severe hypotension. Use together cautiously.

NURSING CONSIDERATIONS
• Use cautiously in cardiac disease, CVA, or severe renal impairment, and in those taking other antihypertensives.
• Monitor patient's blood pressure, pulse rate, and body weight frequently. Some clinicians combine hydralazine therapy with diuretics and beta-adrenergic blocking agents to decrease sodium retention and tachycardia, and to prevent anginal attacks.
• Watch patient closely for signs of lupus erythematosus-like syndrome (sore throat, fever, muscle and joint aches, skin rash). Call doctor immediately if any of these develop.
• Teach patient about his disease and therapy. Explain the importance of taking this drug as prescribed, even when he's feeling well. Tell outpatient not to discontinue this drug suddenly, but to call the doctor if unpleasant adverse reactions occur.
• Instruct patient to check with doctor or pharmacist before taking OTC medications.
• Inform patient that orthostatic hypotension can be minimized by rising slowly and avoiding sudden position changes.
• Elderly patients may be more sensitive to hypotensive effects.
• Give this drug with meals to increase absorption.
• Compliance may be improved by administering this drug b.i.d. Check with doctor.
• CBC, LE cell preparation, and antinuclear antibody titer determinations should be done before therapy and periodically during long-term therapy.
• Has been prescribed during pregnancy for treatment of eclampsia. Administered I.V.

labetalol hydrochloride
Normodyne, Presolol‡, Trandate
Pregnancy Risk Category: C

HOW SUPPLIED
Tablets: 100 mg, 200 mg, 300 mg
Injection: 5 mg/ml

MECHANISM OF ACTION
Blocks response to alpha and beta stimulation and depresses renin secretion.

INDICATIONS & DOSAGE
Treatment of hypertension—
Adults: 100 mg P.O. b.i.d. with or without a diuretic. Dose may be increased to 200 mg b.i.d. after 2 days.

Further dose increases may be made q 1 to 3 days until optimum response is reached. Usual maintenance dosage is 200 to 400 mg b.i.d.

For severe hypertension and hypertensive emergencies—

Adults: Dilute 200 mg to 200 ml with dextrose 5% in water. Infuse at 2 mg/minute until satisfactory response is obtained. Then stop the infusion. May repeat q 6 to 8 hours.

Alternatively, administer by repeated I.V. injection: Initially, give 20 mg I.V. slowly over 2 minutes. May repeat injections of 40 to 80 mg q 10 minutes until maximum dose of 300 mg is reached.

ADVERSE REACTIONS
CNS: vivid dreams, fatigue, headache.
CV: *orthostatic hypotension and dizziness,* peripheral vascular disease, bradycardia.
EENT: nasal stuffiness.
Endocrine: hypoglycemia without tachycardia.
GI: nausea, vomiting, diarrhea.
GU: sexual dysfunction, urine retention.
Skin: rash.
Other: increased airway resistance, transient scalp tingling.

INTERACTIONS
Cimetidine: may enhance labetalol's effect. Give together cautiously.
Halothane: additive hypotensive effect.
Insulin, hypoglycemic drugs (oral): can alter dosage requirements in previously stabilized diabetics. Observe patient carefully.

NURSING CONSIDERATIONS
• Contraindicated in bronchial asthma.
• Use cautiously in CHF, hepatic failure, chronic bronchitis, emphysema, preexisting peripheral vascular disease, and pheochromocytoma.

• Monitor blood pressure frequently.
• Teach patient about his disease and therapy. Explain the importance of taking this drug as prescribed, even when he's feeling well. Tell outpatient not to discontinue this drug suddenly; abrupt discontinuation can exacerbate angina and myocardial infarction. Tell patient to call the doctor if unpleasant adverse reactions occur.
• Instruct patient to check with doctor or pharmacist before taking OTC medications.
• This drug masks common signs of shock and hypoglycemia.
• Labetalol is a beta-adrenergic blocker which also has unique alpha-adrenergic blocking effects.
• Unlike other beta blockers, labetalol does not decrease heart rate or cardiac output.
• Dizziness is the most troublesome adverse reaction and tends to occur in early stages of treatment, in patients also receiving diuretics, and in patients receiving higher dosages. Inform patient that this can be minimized by rising slowly and avoiding sudden position changes. Taking a dose at bedtime or taking smaller doses t.i.d. will also help minimize this adverse reaction. Discuss changes in medication schedule with doctor.
• Transient scalp tingling occurs occasionally at the beginning of labetalol therapy. This usually subsides quickly.
• When administered I.V. for hypertensive emergencies, labetalol produces a rapid, predictable fall in blood pressure within 5 to 10 minutes. Labetolol injection should be administered with a controlled infusion pump. Monitor blood pressure closely: q 5 minutes for 30 minutes, then q 30 minutes for 2 hours, then hourly for 6 hours. Patient should remain supine for 3 hours after infusion.

Italicized adverse reactions are common or life-threatening.
*Liquid form contains alcohol.   **May contain tartrazine.

lisinopril
Prinivil, Zestril

Pregnancy Risk Category: C

HOW SUPPLIED
Tablets: 5 mg, 10 mg, 20 mg

MECHANISM OF ACTION
Lisinopril inhibits angiotensin converting enzyme (ACE), preventing pulmonary conversion of angiotensin I to angiotensin II, a potent vasoconstrictor. This decreases peripheral arterial resistance and aldosterone secretion, thereby reducing sodium and water retention and blood pressure.

INDICATIONS & DOSAGE
Mild to severe hypertension—
Adults: initially, 10 mg P.O. daily. Most patients are well controlled on 20 to 40 mg daily as a single dose.

ADVERSE REACTIONS
Blood: neutropenia.
CNS: *dizziness, headache, fatigue,* depression, somnolence, paresthesia.
CV: hypotension, *orthostasis,* chest pain.
EENT: *nasal congestion.*
GI: *diarrhea,* nausea, dyspepsia, dysgeusia.
GU: impotence.
Metabolic: hyperkalemia.
Skin: rash.
Other: *upper respiratory symptoms, cough, muscle cramps, angiodema,* decreased libido.

INTERACTIONS
Diuretics: excessive hypotension.
Indomethacin: attenuated hypotensive effect.
Potassium-sparing diuretics, potassium supplements, potassium-containing salt substitutes: possible hyperkalemia.

NURSING CONSIDERATIONS
• Lower dosage is necessary in patients with impaired renal function.
• Lisinopril absorption is unaffected by food.
• Lisinopril attenuates potassium loss of thiazide diuretics. If patient is taking a diuretic, the diuretic should be discontinued 2 to 3 days before lisinopril therapy, or lisinopril dosage should be reduced to 5 mg once daily.
• If drug does not adequately control blood pressure, diuretics may be added.
• Teach patient about his disease and therapy. Explain the importance of taking this drug as prescribed, even when he's feeling well. Tell outpatient not to discontinue drug suddenly, but to call the doctor if unpleasant adverse reactions occur.
• Instruct patient to check with doctor or pharmacist before taking OTC medications.
• Review WBC and differential counts before treatment every 2 weeks for 3 months, and periodically thereafter.
• Beneficial effects of lisinopril may require several weeks of therapy.
• Tell patient to report light-headedness, especially in first few days of treatment, so dose can be adjusted; signs of infection such as sore throat or fever, because drugs may decrease WBC count; facial swelling or difficulty breathing, because drug may cause angioedema; and loss of taste, which may necessitate discontinuation of drug.
• Advise patient to avoid sudden postural changes to minimize orthostatic hypotension.

---

mecamylamine hydrochloride
Inversine

Pregnancy Risk Category: C

HOW SUPPLIED
Tablets: 2.5 mg

MECHANISM OF ACTION
A ganglionic blocker; competes with acetylcholine for ganglionic cholinergic receptors.

INDICATIONS & DOSAGE
For moderate to severe essential hypertension and uncomplicated malignant hypertension—
Adults: initially, 2.5 mg P.O. b.i.d. Increase by 2.5 mg daily q 2 days. Average daily dose is 25 mg given in three divided doses. No dosing recommendations for children.

ADVERSE REACTIONS
CNS: *paresthesias,* sedation, *fatigue, tremor, choreiform movements,* seizures, psychic changes, dizziness, *weakness, headaches.*
CV: *orthostatic hypotension.*
EENT: *dry mouth,* glossitis, dilated pupils, *blurred vision.*
GI: *anorexia, nausea, vomiting, constipation, adynamic ileus, diarrhea.*
GU: urine retention, impotence.
Other: decreased libido.

INTERACTIONS
Alcohol, bethanecol: excessive hypotension. Don't use together.
Sodium bicarbonate, acetazolamide: may increase effect of mecamylamine. Use together cautiously. Watch for increased hypotensive effects and toxicity.

NURSING CONSIDERATIONS
• Contraindicated in recent myocardial infarction, uremia, or chronic pyelonephritis. Use cautiously in lower urinary tract pathology, renal insufficiency, glaucoma, pyloric stenosis, coronary insufficiency, or in patients taking other antihypertensives. Mecamylamine is usually reserved for moderate to severe hypertension that is refractory to other drugs.
• Effects of this drug are increased by high environmental temperature, fever, stress, or severe illness.
• Don't withdraw this drug suddenly; rebound hypertension may occur.
• Frequently monitor patient's standing blood pressure.
• Give with meals for more gradual absorption. Schedule the administration consistently with meals. Don't restrict sodium intake.
• If patient develops constipation from this drug, the doctor may want him to take milk of magnesia. Instruct patient to avoid bulk laxatives.
• Teach the patient about his disease and therapy. Explain the importance of taking this drug as prescribed, even when he's feeling well. Tell outpatient to call the doctor if unpleasant adverse reactions develop. Warn him against discontinuing the drug suddenly because this may cause severe rebound hypertension.
• Instruct patient to check with doctor or pharmacist before taking OTC medications.
• Inform patient that orthostatic hypotension can be minimized by rising slowly and avoiding sudden position changes. Dry mouth can be relieved with sugarless chewing gum, sour hard candy, or ice chips.

Italicized adverse reactions are common or life-threatening.
*Liquid form contains alcohol.   **May contain tartrazine.

methyldopa
Aldomet, Aldomet M‡, Apo-
Methyldopa†, Dopamet†, Hydopa‡,
Novomedopa†

methyldopate
hydrochloride
Aldomet, Aldomet Ester Injection‡,

Pregnancy Risk Category: B

HOW SUPPLIED
methyldopa
Tablets: 125 mg, 250 mg, 500 mg
Oral suspension: 250 mg/5 ml
methyldopate hydrochloride
Injection: 250 mg/5 ml in 5-ml vials

MECHANISM OF ACTION
Inhibits the central vasomotor centers, thereby decreasing sympathetic outflow.

INDICATIONS & DOSAGE
For sustained mild to severe hypertension; should not be used for acute treatment of hypertensive emergencies—
Adults: initially, 250 mg P.O. b.i.d. to t.i.d. in first 48 hours. Then increase as needed q 2 days. May give entire daily dosage in the evening or h.s. Dosages may need adjustment if other antihypertensive drugs are added to or deleted from therapy. Maintenance dosage is 500 mg to 2 g daily in two to four divided doses. Maximum recommended daily dosage is 3 g.
I.V.—500 mg to 1 g q 6 hours, diluted in dextrose 5% in water, and administered over 30 to 60 minutes. Switch to oral antihypertensives as soon as possible.
Children: initially, 10 mg/kg P.O. daily in two to three divided doses; or 20 to 40 mg/kg I.V. daily in four divided doses. Increase dose daily until desired response occurs. Maximum daily dose is 65 mg/kg.

ADVERSE REACTIONS
Blood: *hemolytic anemia,* reversible granulocytopenia, thrombocytopenia.
CNS: *sedation,* headache, asthenia, weakness, dizziness, *decreased mental acuity,* involuntary choreoathetotic movements, psychic disturbances, depression, nightmares.
CV: bradycardia, *orthostatic hypotension,* aggravated angina, myocarditis, *edema, and weight gain.*
EENT: *dry mouth, nasal stuffiness.*
GI: diarrhea, pancreatitis.
Hepatic: *hepatic necrosis.*
Other: gynecomastia, lactation, skin rash, *drug-induced fever,* impotence.

INTERACTIONS
Levodopa: additive hypotensive effects; possible increased CNS adverse reactions.
Norepinephrine, phenothiazines, tricyclic antidepressants, amphetamines: possible hypertensive effects. Monitor carefully.

NURSING CONSIDERATIONS
• Use cautiously in patients receiving other antihypertensives or MAO inhibitors and in patients with impaired hepatic function. Monitor blood pressure and pulse rate frequently.
• Methyldopa is frequently used to treat hypertension in pregnant women, apparently without ill effects to the fetus if the patient is closely monitored. Some clinicians recommend that therapy not begin between 16 and 20 weeks' gestation, if possible.
• Observe for involuntary choreoathetoid movements. Report to doctor; he may discontinue drug.
• Observe patient for adverse reactions, particularly unexplained fever. Report adverse reactions to doctor.
• After dialysis, monitor patient for hypertension. Patient may need an extra dose of methyldopa.
• If patient has received this drug for several months, positive reaction to

direct Coombs' test indicates hemolytic anemia.

• If patient requires blood transfusion, make sure he gets direct and indirect Coombs' tests to avoid cross-matching problems.

• Monitor blood studies (CBC) before and during therapy. Monitor hepatic function periodically, especially during the first 6 to 12 weeks of therapy.

• Weigh patient daily. Notify doctor of any weight increase. Sodium and water retention may occur but can be relieved with diuretics.

• Teach patient about his disease and therapy. Explain the importance of taking this drug as prescribed, even when he's feeling well. Tell outpatient not to stop this drug suddenly, but to call the doctor if unpleasant adverse reactions occur. Check dosage schedule with doctor.

• Warn patient that this drug may impair ability to perform tasks that require mental alertness, particularly at start of therapy. Once-daily dosage given at bedtime will minimize daytime drowsiness.

• Instruct patient to check with doctor or pharmacist before taking OTC medications.

• Inform patient that orthostatic hypotension can be minimized by rising slowly and avoiding sudden position changes. Dry mouth can be relieved with sugarless chewing gum, sour hard candy, or ice chips.

• Tell patient that urine may turn dark in toilet bowls treated with bleach.

• Elderly patients are more likely to experience sedation and hypotension.

metoprolol tartrate
Apo-Metoprolol†, Betaloc†‡,
Betaloc Durules†, Lopresor†,
Lopresor SR†, Lopressor,
Novometoprol†

Pregnancy Risk Category: B

HOW SUPPLIED
Tablets: 50 mg, 100 mg
Tablets (sustained-release): 100 mg†,
200 mg†
Injection: 1 mg/ml in 5-ml ampules or refilled syringes

MECHANISM OF ACTION
Blocks cardiac beta receptors and depresses renin secretion.

INDICATIONS & DOSAGE
For hypertension; may be used alone or in combination with other antihypertensives—
Adults: 50 mg b.i.d. or 100 mg once daily P.O. initially. Up to 200 to 400 mg daily in two to three divided doses. No dosage recommendations for children.
Early intervention in acute myocardial infarction—
Adults: Three injections of 5-mg I.V. boluses q 2 minutes. Then, 15 minutes after last dose, administer 50 mg P.O. q 6 hours for 48 hours. Maintenance dosage is 100 mg P.O. b.i.d.

ADVERSE REACTIONS
CNS: fatigue, lethargy, dizziness.
CV: *bradycardia, hypotension, CHF,* peripheral vascular disease.
GI: nausea, vomiting, diarrhea.
Skin: rash.
Respiratory: dyspnea, bronchospasm.
Other: fever, arthralgias.

INTERACTIONS
Barbiturates, rifampin: increased metabolism of metoprolol. Monitor for decreased effect.
Cardiac glycosides: excessive brady-

Italicized adverse reactions are common or life-threatening.
*Liquid form contains alcohol.   **May contain tartrazine.

cardia and increased depressant effect on myocardium. Use together cautiously.

Chlorpromazine, cimetidine, verapamil: decreased hepatic clearance. Monitor for greater beta-blocking effect.

Indomethacin: decrease in antihypertensive effect. Monitor blood pressure and adjust dosage.

Insulin, hypoglycemic drugs (oral): can alter dosage requirements in previously stabilized diabetics. Observe patient carefully.

NURSING CONSIDERATIONS

• Use cautiously in heart failure, diabetes, respiratory or hepatic disease, or in patients taking other antihypertensives. Always check patient's apical pulse rate before giving this drug. If it's slower than 60 beats/minute, hold drug and call doctor immediately.

• Although most patients with asthma and bronchitis can take this drug without fear of worsening their condition, doses over 100 mg daily should be used cautiously.

• Monitor blood pressure frequently.

• Teach patient about his disease and therapy. Explain the importance of taking this drug as prescribed, even when he's feeling well. Tell outpatient not to discontinue this drug suddenly; abrupt discontinuation can exacerbate angina and myocardial infarction. Instruct patient to call the doctor if unpleasant adverse reactions occur.

• Instruct patient to check with doctor or pharmacist before taking OTC medications.

• This drug masks common signs of shock and hypoglycemia. However, metoprolol doesn't potentiate insulin-induced hypoglycemia or delay recovery of blood glucose to normal levels.

• Food may increase absorption of metoprolol. Give consistently with meals.

• Patient should have periodic eye examinations while taking drug.

metyrosine
Demser

Pregnancy Risk Category: C

HOW SUPPLIED
Capsules: 250 mg

MECHANISM OF ACTION
Inhibits the enzyme tyrosine hydroxylase, thus inhibiting endogenous catecholamine synthesis.

INDICATIONS & DOSAGE
Preoperative preparation of patients with pheochromocytoma; management of such patients when surgery is contraindicated; to control or prevent hypertension before or during pheochromocytomectomy—
Adults and children over 12 years: 250 mg P.O. q.i.d. May be increased by 250 to 500 mg q day to a maximum of 4 g daily in divided doses. When used for preoperative preparation, optimally effective dosage should be given for at least 5 to 7 days. In normotensive patients, doses are adjusted to produce a 50% reduction in urinary metanephrines and vanillylmandelic acid.

ADVERSE REACTIONS
CNS: *sedation,* extrapyramidal symptoms, such as speech difficulty and tremors, disorientation.
GI: *diarrhea,* nausea, vomiting, abdominal pain.
GU: *crystalluria,* hematuria.
Other: impotence, hypersensitivity.

INTERACTIONS
Phenothiazines and haloperidol: increased inhibition of catecholamine synthesis may result in extrapyramidal symptoms. Use cautiously.

---

†Available in Canada only.   ‡Available in Australia only.   ◊ Available OTC.

NURSING CONSIDERATIONS
• During surgery, monitor blood pressure and ECG continuously. If a serious arrhythmia occurs during anesthesia and surgery, treatment with a beta-blocking drug or lidocaine may be necessary.
• Warn patient that sedation almost always occurs in those treated with metyrosine. Sedation usually subsides after several days' treatment.
• Instruct patient to increase daily fluid intake to prevent crystalluria. Daily urine volume should be 2,000 ml or more.
• Insomnia may occur when metyrosine is stopped.
• If patient's hypertension is not adequately controlled by metyrosine, an alpha-adrenergic blocking agent, such as phenoxybenzamine, should be added to the regimen.

---

minoxidil
Loniten, Minodyl

Pregnancy Risk Category: C

HOW SUPPLIED
Tablets: 2.5 mg, 10 mg, 25 mg‡

MECHANISM OF ACTION
Produces direct arteriolar vasodilation.

INDICATIONS & DOSAGE
Treatment of severe hypertension—
Adults: 5 mg P.O. initially as a single dose. Effective dosage range is usually 10 to 40 mg daily. Maximum dosage is 100 mg daily.
Children under 12 years: 0.2 mg/kg as a single daily dose. Effective dosage range usually is 0.25 to 1 mg/kg daily. Maximum dosage is 50 mg.

ADVERSE REACTIONS
CV: *edema, tachycardia, pericardial effusion and tamponade, CHF,* ECG changes.

Skin: rash, *Stevens-Johnson syndrome*.
Other: *hypertrichosis* (elongation, thickening, and enhanced pigmentation of fine body hair), breast tenderness.

INTERACTIONS
Guanethidine: severe orthostatic hypotension. Advise patient to stand up slowly.

NURSING CONSIDERATIONS
• Contraindicated in pheochromocytoma. Patients with malignant hypertension should be hospitalized during initial therapy.
• A potent vasodilator: use only when other antihypertensives have failed.
• Instruct patient to take his own pulse. Patient should report an increase greater than 20 beats/minute to the doctor.
• Closely monitor blood pressure and pulse at beginning of therapy.
• Monitor intake/output and check for weight gain and edema. Tell outpatients to weigh themselves at least weekly and report substantial weight gain (more than 5 lb per week).
• Elderly patients may be more sensitive to hypotensive effects.
• About 8 out of 10 patients will experience hypertrichosis within 3 to 6 weeks of beginning treatment. Unwanted hair can be controlled with a depilatory or shaving. Assure patient that extra hair will disappear within 1 to 6 months of stopping minoxidil. Advise patient, however, not to discontinue drug without doctor's approval.
• Drug is usually prescribed with a beta-blocking drug to control tachycardia and a diuretic to counteract fluid retention. Make sure patient complies with total treatment regimen.
• Teach patient about his disease and therapy. Explain the importance of taking this drug as prescribed, even

---

Italicized adverse reactions are common or life-threatening.
*Liquid form contains alcohol.   **May contain tartrazine.

when he's feeling well. Tell outpatient not to discontinue drug suddenly, but to call the doctor if unpleasant adverse reactions occur.

• A patient package insert has been prepared by the manufacturer of minoxidil, describing in layman's terms the drug and its adverse reactions. Be sure your patient receives this insert and reads it thoroughly. Provide an oral explanation also.

• Instruct patient to check with doctor or pharmacist before taking OTC medications.

• Prescribed in various topical forms for treatment of some types of male pattern baldness.

• Minoxidil is removed by hemodialysis. Be sure to administer dose after dialysis.

---

nitroprusside sodium
Nipride, Nitropress

Pregnancy Risk Category: C

HOW SUPPLIED
Injection: 50 mg/vial in 2-ml, 5-ml vials

MECHANISM OF ACTION
Relaxes both arteriolar and venous smooth muscle.

INDICATIONS & DOSAGE
To lower blood pressure quickly in hypertensive emergencies; to control hypotension during anesthesia; to reduce preload and afterload in cardiac pump failure or cardiogenic shock; may be used with or without dopamine—
Adults: 50-mg vial diluted with 2 to 3 ml of dextrose 5% in water I.V. and then added to 250, 500, or 1,000 ml dextrose 5% in water. Infuse at 0.5 to 10 mcg/kg/minute. Average dose is 3 mcg/kg/minute. Maximum infusion rate is 10 mcg/kg/minute.

Patients taking other antihypertensive drugs along with nitroprusside

are very sensitive to this drug. Adjust dosage accordingly.

ADVERSE REACTIONS
The following adverse reactions usually indicate overdosage:
CNS: *headache, dizziness,* ataxia, loss of consciousness, coma, weak pulse, absent reflexes, widely dilated pupils, *restlessness, muscle twitching, diaphoresis.*
CV: distant heart sounds, palpitations, dyspnea, shallow breathing.
GI: *vomiting, nausea, abdominal pain.*
Metabolic: acidosis.
Skin: pink color.

INTERACTIONS
None significant.

NURSING CONSIDERATIONS
• Use cautiously in hypothyroidism or hepatic or renal disease, or in patients receiving other antihypertensives. Keep patient supine when initiating or titrating nitroprusside therapy.

• Because of light sensitivity, wrap I.V. solution in foil. It's not necessary to wrap the tubing in foil. Fresh solution should have faint brownish tint. Discard after 24 hours.

• Obtain baseline vital signs before giving this drug, and find out what parameters the doctor wants to achieve.

• Check blood pressure every 5 minutes at start of infusion and every 15 minutes thereafter. If severe hypotension occurs, turn off I.V. nitroprusside—effects of drug quickly reverse. Notify doctor. If possible, an arterial pressure line should be started. Regulate drug flow to specified level.

• Don't use bacteriostatic water for injection or sterile saline solution for reconstitution.

• Infuse with a continuous infusion pump.

• This drug is best run piggyback through a peripheral line with no

---

other medication. Don't adjust rate of main I.V. line while drug is running. Even small bolus of nitroprusside can cause severe hypotension.

• Excessive doses or rapid infusion (>15 mcg/kg/minute) of this drug can cause cyanide toxicity, so check serum thiocyanate levels every 72 hours. Thiocyanate levels of greater than 100 mcg/ml are associated with toxicity. Watch for signs of thiocyanate toxicity: profound hypotension, metabolic acidosis, dyspnea, headache, loss of consciousness, ataxia, vomiting. If these occur, discontinue drug immediately and notify doctor.

---

pargyline hydrochloride
Eutonyl

Pregnancy Risk Category: C

HOW SUPPLIED
Tablets (film-coated): 10 mg, 25 mg

MECHANISM OF ACTION
Inhibits the enzyme MAO.

INDICATIONS & DOSAGE
For moderate to severe hypertension, usually given in combination with other drugs—
Adults: initially, 25 to 50 mg P.O. once daily, if not receiving any other antihypertensive drugs. Then increase dosage by 10 mg daily at weekly intervals. Maximum daily dosage is 200 mg. Usual daily dosage for elderly patients or those who've had sympathectomy is 10 to 25 mg. When used in combination with other drugs, total daily dosage of pargyline should not exceed 25 mg. No dosage recommendations for children.

ADVERSE REACTIONS
CNS: *tremors,* convulsions, choreiform movements, psychic changes, *nightmares, hyperexcitability, sweating,* dizziness, fainting, drowsiness.

CV: palpitations, *orthostatic hypotension,* fluid retention.
EENT: *dry mouth,* optic damage.
GI: *nausea, vomiting, increased appetite, constipation.*
Other: impotence.

INTERACTIONS
Alcohol, barbiturates, and other sedatives; tranquilizers; narcotics; dextromethorphan; tricyclic antidepressants: unpredictable interactions. Should be used with caution and in reduced dosage.
Amphetamines, ephedrine, levodopa, metaraminol, methotrimeprazine, methylphenidate, phenylephrine, phenylpropanolamine, pseudoephedrine: enhanced pressor effects. Use together cautiously.

NURSING CONSIDERATIONS
• Contraindicated in advanced renal failure, pheochromocytoma, hyperthyroidism, or Parkinson's disease; in hyperactive and hyperexcitable patients. Use cautiously in patients who are receiving other antihypertensives or who have hepatic disease. Pargyline should not be used to treat malignant hypertension.
• Discontinue this drug at least 2 weeks before elective surgery.
• Hypotensive effects of this drug are increased by high environmental temperatures, fever, stress, or severe illness. If patient develops severe hypotension, counteract with ephedrine or phenylephrine.
• Monitor blood pressure and pulse rate frequently. Take blood pressure while patient is standing.
• Patient should have periodic eye examinations during therapy.
• If patient is scheduled for surgery and has been taking this drug, be sure narcotic dosages are reduced.
• This drug may require up to several weeks to reach optimal effect. Tolerance to its hypotensive actions may

---

Italicized adverse reactions are common or life-threatening.
*Liquid form contains alcohol.   **May contain tartrazine.

develop, and other drugs may be necessary.

• Advise patient to take drug in the morning to avoid insomnia.

• Warn patient not to take any other medications, including over-the-counter cold remedies, without first getting medical approval.

• This drug is an MAO inhibitor. Tell patient not to eat foods with high tyramine content: for example, aged cheese, chianti wine, sour cream, canned figs, raisins, chicken livers, yeast extract, and pickled herring.

• Teach patient about his disease and therapy. Explain the importance of taking this drug as prescribed, even when he's feeling well. Tell outpatient not to discontinue this drug suddenly, but to call the doctor if unpleasant adverse reactions occur.

• Instruct patient to check with doctor or pharmacist before taking OTC medications.

• Inform patient that orthostatic hypotension can be minimized by rising slowly and avoiding sudden position changes. Dry mouth can be relieved with sugarless chewing gum, sour hard candy, or ice chips.

---

penbutolol sulfate
Levatol

Pregnancy Risk Category: C

HOW SUPPLIED
Tablets: 20 mg

MECHANISM OF ACTION
Blocks both beta$_1$- and beta$_2$-adrenergic receptors.

INDICATIONS & DOSAGE
Treatment of mild to moderate hypertension—
Adults: 20 mg P.O. once daily. Usually given with other antihypertensive agents, such as thiazide diuretics.

ADVERSE REACTIONS
CNS: syncope, *dizziness,* vertigo, headache, fatigue, mental depression, paresthesias, hypoesthesia or hyperesthesia, lethargy, anxiety, nervousness, diminished concentration, sleep disturbances, nightmares, bizarre or frequent dreams, sedation, changes in behavior, reversible mental depression, catatonia, hallucinations, alteration of time perception, memory loss, emotional lability, light-headedness.
CV: *bradycardia,* chest pain, *CHF,* asymptomatic hypotension, peripheral ischemia, worsening of angina or arterial insufficiency, peripheral vascular insufficiency, claudication, edema, *pulmonary edema,* vasodilation, symptomatic postural hypotension, tachycardia, palpitations, conduction disturbances, first-degree and third-degree heart block, intensification of AV block.
EENT: dry mouth.
GI: gastric pain, flatulence, nausea, constipation, heartburn, vomiting, taste alteration.
GU: impotence, nocturia, urine retention.
Metabolic: hyperglycemia, hypoglycemia.
Respiratory: pharyngitis, laryngospasm, respiratory distress, shortness of breath.
Skin: pallor, flushing, rash.
Other: allergic reactions, eye discomfort, decreased libido.

INTERACTIONS
Clonidine: may cause paradoxical hypertension when combined with beta-adrenergic blocking agents. Also, beta blockers may enhance rebound hypertension when clonidine is withdrawn.
Insulin, oral hypoglycemic agents: beta-adrenergic blocking agents may alter the hypoglycemic response to these drugs. Monitor patient closely.
NSAIDs: possibly decreased antihypertensive effects.

Prazocin, terazocin: beta blockers may enhance the "first dose" orthostatic hypotension seen with these drugs.

Sympathomimetics, including isoproterenol, dopamine, dobutamine, or norepinephrine: decreased hypotensive response.

Theophylline: possibly decreased bronchodilator effect.

NURSING CONSIDERATIONS

• Contraindicated in patients allergic to penbutolol or other beta blockers. Also contraindicated in sinus bradycardia, cardiogenic shock, CHF, overt cardiac failure, and patients with greater than first-degree heart block. Beta-adrenergic blocking agents should be avoided in patients with pheochromocytoma unless alpha-adrenergic blocking agents are also used. They should also be avoided in patients with chronic airway disease, such as chronic bronchitis or emphysema.

• Administer cautiously to patients with a history of CHF controlled by digitalis glycosides and diuretics.

• Advise patients not to discontinue the drug abruptly, because sudden withdrawal of other beta blockers has precipitated angina and myocardial infarction. However, clinical experience has shown that withdrawal of beta blocker therapy in patients who have had a myocardial infarction does not present major problems.

• Administer with caution to patients with a history of bronchospastic disease. Teach patient the signs and symptoms of CHF (edema and pulmonary congestion). Advise them to contact the doctor if these symptoms occur.

• Always check patient's apical pulse before giving this drug. If you detect extremes in pulse rates, hold drug and call doctor immediately.

• Monitor blood pressure, ECG, and heart rate and rhythm frequently.

• Teach patient about his disease and therapy. Explain the importance taking this drug, even when he's feeling well. Tell patient to call doctor if unpleasant adverse reactions occur.

• Advise patient to check with his doctor or pharmacist before taking OTC medications.

---

phenoxybenzamine hydrochloride
Dibenyline‡, Dibenzyline
Pregnancy Risk Category: C

HOW SUPPLIED
Capsules: 10 mg

MECHANISM OF ACTION
An alpha-adrenergic blocker that noncompetitively blocks the effect of catecholamines on alpha-adrenergic receptors.

INDICATIONS & DOSAGE
To control hypertension and sweating secondary to pheochromocytoma; may be used in combination with propranolol to control excessive tachycardia—
Adults: initially, 10 mg P.O. daily. Increase by 10 mg daily q 4 days. Maintenance dosage is 20 to 60 mg daily.
Children: initially, 0.2 mg/kg or 6 mg/m^2 P.O. daily in a single dose. Maintenance dosage is 12 to 36 mg/m^2 daily as a single dose or in divided doses.
To control Raynaud's disease, frostbite, acrocyanosis—
Adults: initially, 10 mg P.O., then increase by 10 mg q 4 days to a maximum of 60 mg daily.

ADVERSE REACTIONS
CNS: lethargy, drowsiness.
CV: *orthostatic hypotension, tachycardia,* shock.
EENT: *nasal stuffiness, dry mouth, miosis.*
GI: vomiting, abdominal distress.

Italicized adverse reactions are common or life-threatening.
*Liquid form contains alcohol.   **May contain tartrazine.

Other: *impotence, inhibition of ejaculation.*

INTERACTIONS
Antihypertensives: excessive hypotension. Use together cautiously.

NURSING CONSIDERATIONS
• Use cautiously in cerebrovascular or coronary insufficiency, advanced renal disease, or respiratory disease.
• Watch patient closely for side effects, and call doctor promptly if they occur. If severe hypotension develops, patient may require norepinephrine to counteract effect.
• Nasal congestion, inhibition of ejaculation, and impotence usually decrease with continued therapy.
• Patient with tachycardia may require concurrent propranolol therapy.
• Monitor patient's heart rate and blood pressure frequently.
• This drug may take several weeks to achieve optimal effect.
• Monitor respiratory status carefully. This drug may aggravate symptoms of pneumonia and asthma.
• Teach patient about his disease and therapy. Explain the importance of taking this drug as prescribed, even when he's feeling well. Tell outpatient not to discontinue this drug suddenly, but to call the doctor if unpleasant adverse reactions occur.
• Instruct patient to check with doctor or pharmacist before taking OTC medications.
• Inform patient that orthostatic hypotension can be minimized by rising slowly and avoiding sudden position changes.
• Dry mouth can be relieved with sugarless chewing gum, sour hard candy, or ice chips. GI distress can be relieved by taking the drug in divided doses or with milk.
• Used investigationally to treat chronic urine retention.
• Small initial doses are increased gradually until desired effect is obtained. Patient should be observed after each dose for at least 4 days.

phentolamine mesylate
Regitine, Rogitine†

Pregnancy Risk Category: C

HOW SUPPLIED
Injection: 5 mg/ml in 1-ml vials, 10 mg/ml‡

MECHANISM OF ACTION
An alpha-adrenergic blocker that competitively blocks the effects of catecholamines on alpha-adrenergic receptors.

INDICATIONS & DOSAGE
To aid in diagnosis of pheochromocytoma; to control or prevent hypertension before or during pheochromocytomectomy—
Adults: I.V. diagnostic dose is 5 mg, with close monitoring of blood pressure.
  Before surgical removal of tumor, give 2 to 5 mg I.M. or I.V. During surgery, patient may need small I.V. doses (1 mg) or small I.M. doses (3 mg).
Children: I.V. diagnostic dose is 0.1 mg/kg or 3 mg/m^2 as single dose, with close monitoring of blood pressure.
  Before surgical removal of tumor, give 1 mg I.V. or 3 mg I.M. During surgery, patient may need small I.V. doses (1 mg).
To treat extravasation—
Adults and children: infiltrate area with 5 to 10 mg phentolamine in 10 ml normal saline solution. Must be done within 12 hours.

ADVERSE REACTIONS
CNS: *dizziness, weakness, flushing.*
CV: *hypotension,* shock, *arrhythmias,* palpitations, *tachycardia,* angina pectoris.
GI: *diarrhea,* abdominal pain, *nausea, vomiting,* hyperperistalsis.

Other: *nasal stuffiness*, hypoglycemia.

INTERACTIONS
Epinephrine: excessive hypotension. Don't use together.

NURSING CONSIDERATIONS
• Contraindicated in angina, coronary artery disease, and history of myocardial infarction. Use cautiously in gastritis or peptic ulcer and in patients receiving other antihypertensives.
• Don't administer epinephrine to treat phentolamine-induced hypotension. May cause additional fall in blood pressure ("epinephrine reversal"). Use norepinephrine instead.
• When this drug is given as a diagnostic test for pheochromocytoma, check patient's blood pressure first; check blood pressure frequently during administration.
• Test is positive for pheochromocytoma if I.V. test dose causes severe hypotension.
• Don't give sedatives or narcotics 24 hours before diagnostic test. Rauwolfia alkaloids should be withdrawn at least 4 weeks before such testing.
• Has been used experimentally, alone or with papaverine, to treat impotence. Patients are taught to self-administer this drug by intercavernosal injection.

pindolol
Barbloc‡, Visken

Pregnancy Risk Category: B

HOW SUPPLIED
Tablets: 5 mg, 10 mg, 15 mg‡

MECHANISM OF ACTION
Blocks response to beta stimulation.

INDICATIONS & DOSAGE
Treatment of hypertension—
Adults: initially, 5 mg P.O. b.i.d.

Dosage may be increased by 10 mg/ day q 2 to 3 weeks up to a maximum of 60 mg/day.

ADVERSE REACTIONS
CNS: *insomnia, fatigue, dizziness, nervousness,* vivid dreams, hallucinations, lethargy.
CV: *edema,* bradycardia, CHF, peripheral vascular disease, hypotension.
EENT: visual disturbances.
GI: *nausea,* vomiting, diarrhea.
Metabolic: hypoglycemia without tachycardia.
Skin: rash.
Other: *increased airway resistance, muscle pain, joint pain,* chest pain.

INTERACTIONS
Cardiac glycosides: excessive bradycardia and increased depressant effect on myocardium. Use together cautiously.
Epinephrine: severe vasoconstriction. Monitor blood pressure and observe patient carefully.
Indomethacin: decreased antihypertensive effect. Monitor blood pressure and adjust dosage.
Insulin, hypoglycemic drugs (oral): can alter requirements for these drugs in previously stabilized diabetics. Monitor for hypoglycemia.

NURSING CONSIDERATIONS
• Contraindicated in diabetes mellitus, asthma, allergic rhinitis; during ethyl ether anesthesia; in sinus bradycardia and heart block greater than first degree; in cardiogenic shock; in right ventricular failure secondary to pulmonary hypertension. Use with caution in CHF or respiratory disease, and in patients taking other antihypertensive drugs.
• Always check patient's apical pulse rate before giving this drug. If you detect extremes in pulse rates, hold medication and call doctor immediately.

Italicized adverse reactions are common or life-threatening.
*Liquid form contains alcohol.   **May contain tartrazine.

• Monitor blood pressure frequently. If patient develops severe hypotension, notify doctor. He may prescribe a vasopressor.

• Teach patient about his disease and therapy. Explain the importance of taking this drug as prescribed, even when he's feeling well. Tell outpatient not to discontinue this drug suddenly; abrupt discontinuation can exacerbate angina and myocardial infarction. Tell patient to call doctor if unpleasant adverse reactions occur.

• Instruct patient to check with doctor or pharmacist before taking OTC medications.

• This drug masks common signs of shock and hypoglycemia.

• Pindolol may be taken without any special regard for meals.

• Many patients respond favorably to a dose of 5 mg t.i.d.

• The first commercially available beta blocker with partial beta-*agonist* activity. In other words, pindolol also *stimulates* beta-adrenergic receptors as well as blocks them. Therefore, it decreases cardiac output less than other beta-adrenergic blockers.

• May be advantageous for patients who develop bradycardia with other beta blockers.

• Withdraw drug gradually (over 1 to 2 weeks) after long-term administration.

---

prazosin hydrochloride
Minipress

Pregnancy Risk Category: C

HOW SUPPLIED
Capsules: 1 mg, 2 mg, 5 mg

MECHANISM OF ACTION
Relaxes both arteriolar and venous smooth muscle probably by blocking postsynaptic alpha receptors.

INDICATIONS & DOSAGE
For mild to moderate hypertension; *used alone or in combination with a diuretic or other antihypertensive drugs; also used to decrease afterload in severe chronic congestive heart failure—*

Adults: P.O. test dose is 1 mg given before bedtime to prevent "first-dose syncope." Initial dose is 1 mg t.i.d. Increase dosage slowly. Maximum daily dosage is 20 mg. Maintenance dosage is 3 to 20 mg daily in three divided doses. A few patients have required dosages larger than this (up to 40 mg daily). If other antihypertensive drugs or diuretics are added to this drug, decrease prazosin dosage to 1 to 2 mg t.i.d. and retitrate.

ADVERSE REACTIONS
CNS: *dizziness,* headache, drowsiness, weakness, *"first-dose syncope,"* depression.
CV: orthostatic hypotension, *palpitations.*
EENT: blurred vision, dry mouth.
GI: vomiting, diarrhea, abdominal cramps, constipation, *nausea.*
GU: priapism, impotence.

INTERACTIONS
Propranolol and other beta blockers: syncope with loss of consciousness may occur more frequently. Advise patient to sit or lie down if he feels dizzy.

NURSING CONSIDERATIONS
• Use cautiously in patients receiving other antihypertensive drugs.

• Monitor patient's blood pressure and pulse rate frequently.

• If initial dose is greater than 1 mg, patient may develop severe syncope with loss of consciousness (first-dose syncope). Increase dosage slowly. Instruct patient to sit or lie down if he experiences dizziness.

• Elderly patients may be more sensitive to hypotensive effects.

• Teach patient about his disease and therapy. Explain the importance of

---

†Available in Canada only.   ‡Available in Australia only.   ◊ Available OTC.

taking this drug as prescribed, even when he's feeling well. Tell outpatient not to discontinue this drug suddenly, but to call the doctor if unpleasant adverse reactions occur.
• Instruct patient to check with doctor or pharmacist before taking OTC medications.
• Inform patient that orthostatic hypotension can be minimized by rising slowly and avoiding sudden position changes. Dry mouth can be relieved with sugarless chewing gum, sour hard candy, or ice chips.
• Compliance *may* be improved by giving this drug once a day. Check with doctor.
• Has been used to treat Raynaud's disease.

---

rauwolfia serpentina
Raudixin**, Rauverid, Wolfina

Pregnancy Risk Category: D

HOW SUPPLIED
Tablets: 50 mg, 100 mg

MECHANISM OF ACTION
Acts peripherally, inhibiting norepinephrine release and depleting norepinephrine stores in adrenergic nerve endings.

INDICATIONS & DOSAGE
Mild to moderate hypertension—
Adults: initially and for 1 to 3 weeks thereafter, 200 to 400 mg P.O. daily as a single dose or in two divided doses.
   Maintenance dosage is 50 to 300 mg daily. No dosing recommendations for children.

ADVERSE REACTIONS
CNS: mental confusion, *depression, drowsiness, nervousness, paradoxical anxiety,* nightmares, sedation, headache, extrapyramidal symptoms.
CV: orthostatic hypotension, bradycardia, syncope.

EENT: *dry mouth, nasal stuffiness,* glaucoma.
GI: *hypersecretion of gastric acid, nausea, vomiting,* GI bleeding.
Skin: pruritus, rash.
Other: impotence, weight gain.

INTERACTIONS
Digitalis glycosides: rauwolfia may predispose patients to digitalis-induced arrhythmias. Use together cautiously.
MAO inhibitors: may cause excitability and hypertension. Use together cautiously.

NURSING CONSIDERATIONS
• Contraindicated in depression. Use cautiously in severe cardiac or cerebrovascular disease, impaired renal function, peptic ulcer, ulcerative colitis, gallstones; in those undergoing surgery; in elderly or debilitated patients; and in those taking other antihypertensives or tricyclic antidepressants.
• Monitor patient's blood pressure and pulse rate frequently.
• Teach patient about his disease and therapy. Explain the importance of taking this drug as prescribed, even when he's feeling well. Tell outpatient not to discontinue this drug suddenly, but to call the doctor if unpleasant adverse reactions occur.
• Instruct patient to check with doctor or pharmacist before taking OTC medications.
• Warn that this drug can cause drowsiness. Patient should not drive or perform other activities that require alertness and good coordination until CNS effects are known.
• Watch patient closely for signs of mental depression. Warn him to notify doctor promptly if he experiences nightmares.
• Inform patient that orthostatic hypotension can be minimized by rising slowly and avoiding sudden position changes. Dry mouth can be relieved

---

Italicized adverse reactions are common or life-threatening.
*Liquid form contains alcohol.   **May contain tartrazine.

with sugarless chewing gum, sour hard candy, or ice chips. Tell patient to contact doctor if relief is needed for nasal stuffiness.
- Give this drug with meals.
- Patient should weigh himself daily and notify doctor of any weight gain.
- Effects of this drug may last for 10 days after it's discontinued.
- Advise patient to have periodic eye examinations.

---

rescinnamine
Moderil

Pregnancy Risk Category: D

HOW SUPPLIED
Tablets: 0.25 mg, 0.5 mg

MECHANISM OF ACTION
Acts peripherally, inhibiting norepinephrine release and depleting norepinephrine stores in adrenergic nerve endings.

INDICATIONS & DOSAGE
For mild to moderate hypertension; may be used alone or in combination with other antihypertensives—
Adults: initially, 0.5 mg P.O. b.i.d. Maintenance dosage is 0.25 to 0.5 mg daily. No dosing recommendations for children.

ADVERSE REACTIONS
CNS: mental confusion, *depression, drowsiness, nervousness, anxiety, nightmares,* sedation, parkinsonism.
CV: *orthostatic hypotension, bradycardia, syncope.*
EENT: *dry mouth, nasal stuffiness,* glaucoma.
GI: *hypersecretion of gastric acid, nausea, vomiting,* GI bleeding.
Skin: pruritus, rash.
Other: *impotence, weight gain.*

INTERACTIONS
MAO inhibitors: may cause excitabil-

ity and hypertension. Use together cautiously.

NURSING CONSIDERATIONS
- Contraindicated in depression. Use cautiously in severe cardiac or cerebrovascular disease, peptic ulcer, ulcerative colitis, gallstones, or in patients undergoing surgery; and in elderly or debilitated patients. Also use cautiously in patients taking other antihypertensives.
- Monitor patient's blood pressure and pulse rate frequently.
- Teach patient about his disease and therapy. Explain the importance of taking this drug as prescribed, even when he's feeling well. Tell outpatient not to discontinue this drug suddenly, but to call the doctor if unpleasant adverse reactions develop.
- Instruct patient to check with doctor or pharmacist before taking OTC medications.
- Warn that this drug can cause drowsiness. Patients should not drive or perform other tasks that require alertness and coordination until the adverse CNS effects of the drug are known.
- Watch patient closely for signs of mental depression. Warn him to notify doctor promptly if he experiences nightmares.
- Inform patient that orthostatic hypotension can be minimized by rising slowly and avoiding sudden position changes. Dry mouth can be relieved with sugarless chewing gum, sour hard candy, or ice chips. Tell patient to contact doctor if relief is needed for nasal stuffiness.
- Give this drug with meals.
- Patient should weigh himself daily and notify doctor of any weight gain.
- Effects of this drug may last for 10 days after it's discontinued.
- Advise patient to have periodic eye examinations.

---

reserpine
Novoreserpine†, Serpalan,
Serpasil*

Pregnancy Risk Category: C

HOW SUPPLIED
Tablets: 0.1 mg, 0.25 mg, 1 mg

MECHANISM OF ACTION
Acts peripherally, inhibiting norepinephrine release and depleting norepinephrine stores in adrenergic nerve endings.

INDICATIONS & DOSAGE
Mild to moderate essential hypertension—
Adults: 0.1 to 0.25 mg P.O. daily.
Children: 5 to 20 mcg/kg P.O. daily.

ADVERSE REACTIONS
CNS: mental confusion, *depression, drowsiness, nervousness, paradoxical anxiety, nightmares,* extrapyramidal symptoms, sedation.
CV: *orthostatic hypotension, bradycardia, syncope.*
EENT: *dry mouth, nasal stuffiness,* glaucoma.
GI: *hyperacidity, nausea, vomiting,* GI bleeding.
Skin: pruritus, rash.
Other: *impotence, weight gain.*

INTERACTIONS
MAO inhibitors: may cause excitability and hypertension. Use together cautiously.

NURSING CONSIDERATIONS
• Contraindicated in depression. Use cautiously in severe cardiac or cerebrovascular disease, history of seizures, peptic ulcer, ulcerative colitis, gallstones, or mental depressive disorders; in patients undergoing surgery; and in those taking other antihypertensive drugs.
• Monitor patient's blood pressure and pulse rate frequently.

• Teach patient about his disease and therapy. Explain the importance of taking this drug as prescribed, even when he's feeling well. Tell outpatient not to discontinue this drug suddenly, but to call doctor if unpleasant adverse reactions occur.
• Instruct patient to check with doctor or pharmacist before taking OTC medications.
• Warn patient that this drug can cause drowsiness. Tell him to avoid hazardous activities that require alertness and coordination until CNS effects of the drug are known.
• Warn female patient to notify doctor if she becomes pregnant.
• Watch patient closely for signs of mental depression. Warn him to notify doctor promptly if he experiences nightmares.
• Inform patient that orthostatic hypotension can be minimized by rising slowly and avoiding sudden position changes. Dry mouth can be relieved with sugarless chewing gum, sour hard candy, or ice chips. Tell patient to contact doctor if relief is needed for nasal stuffiness.
• Give this drug with meals.
• Patient should weigh himself daily and notify doctor of any weight gain.
• Effects of this drug may last for 10 days after it's discontinued.
• Advise patient to have periodic eye examinations.

terazocin hydrochloride
Hytrin

Pregnancy Risk Category: C

HOW SUPPLIED
Tablets: 1 mg, 2 mg, 5 mg

MECHANISM OF ACTION
Decreases blood pressure by vasodilation produced in response to blockade of alpha$_1$ adrenergic receptors.

Italicized adverse reactions are common or life-threatening.
*Liquid form contains alcohol.   **May contain tartrazine.

INDICATIONS & DOSAGE
Hypertension—
Adults: initial dose is 1 mg P.O. h.s., gradually increased according to patient response. Usual dosage range is 1 to 5 mg daily. Maximum recommended dosage is 20 mg/day.

ADVERSE REACTIONS
CNS: asthenia, *dizziness,* headache, nervousness, paresthesia, somnolence, decreased libido.
CV: *palpitations,* postural hypotension, tachycardia, *peripheral edema.*
EENT: *nasal congestion,* sinusitis, blurred vision.
GI: *nausea.*
Respiratory: dyspnea.
Other: back pain, muscle pain, weight gain, impotence.

INTERACTIONS
Antihypertensives: excessive hypotension. Use together cautiously.

NURSING CONSIDERATIONS
• Do not exceed initial dose of 1 mg.
• Instruct patient to avoid hazardous activities that require mental alertness (such as driving or operating heavy machinery) for 12 hours after the first dose.
• If terazocin is discontinued for several days, patient will need to be retitrated using initial dosing regimen (1 mg P.O. at bedtime).
• Teach patient about his disease and therapy. Explain the importance of taking this drug as prescribed, even when he's feeling well. Tell outpatient not to discontinue drug suddenly, but to call the doctor if unpleasant adverse reactions occur.
• Instruct patient to check with doctor or pharmacist before taking OTC medications.

timolol maleate
Apo-Timol†, Blocadren
Pregnancy Risk Category: C

HOW SUPPLIED
Tablets: 5 mg, 10 mg, 20 mg

MECHANISM OF ACTION
Blocks response to beta stimulation and depresses renin secretion.

INDICATIONS & DOSAGE
Hypertension—
Adults: initially 10 mg P.O. b.i.d. Usual daily maintenance dosage is 20 to 40 mg. Maximum daily dosage is 60 mg. Drug is used either alone or in combination with diuretics.
Myocardial infarction (long-term prophylaxis in patients who have survived acute phase)—
Adults: Recommended dosage for long-term prophylaxis in survivors of acute myocardial infarction is 10 mg P.O. b.i.d.

ADVERSE REACTIONS
CNS: fatigue, lethargy, vivid dreams.
CV: *bradycardia, hypotension, CHF,* peripheral vascular disease.
GI: nausea, vomiting, diarrhea.
Metabolic: hypoglycemia without tachycardia.
Respiratory: dyspnea, bronchospasm.
Skin: rash.
Other: *increased airway resistance,* fever.

INTERACTIONS
Cardiac glycosides: excessive bradycardia and increased depressant effect on myocardium. Use together cautiously.
Indomethacin: decrease in antihypertensive effect. Monitor blood pressure and adjust dosage.
Insulin, hypoglycemic drugs (oral): can alter requirements for these drugs

---

in previously stabilized diabetics. Monitor for hypoglycemia.

NURSING CONSIDERATIONS
• Contraindicated in diabetes mellitus, asthma, allergic rhinitis; during ethyl ether anesthesia; in sinus bradycardia and heart block greater than first degree; in cardiogenic shock; in right ventricular failure secondary to pulmonary hypertension. Use with caution in CHF, hepatic, renal, or respiratory disease, and in patients taking other antihypertensives.
• Always check patient's apical pulse rate before giving this drug. If you detect extremes in pulse rates, withhold medication and call the doctor immediately.
• Monitor blood pressure frequently.
• Teach patient about his disease and therapy. Explain the importance of taking drug as prescribed, even when he's feeling well. Tell patient not to discontinue drug suddenly: abrupt discontinuation can exacerbate angina and myocardial infarction. Tell patient to call doctor if unpleasant adverse reactions occur.
• Instruct patient to check with doctor or pharmacist before taking OTC medications.
• This drug masks common signs of shock and hypoglycemia.
• If patient is taking the drug for hypertension, warn him not to increase the dosage without first consulting his doctor. At least 7 days should intervene between increases in dosage.
• Do not discontinue therapy abruptly. Reduce dosage gradually over 1 to 2 weeks.
• Timolol is the first beta blocker approved for use in post-myocardial infarction patients. Like other beta blockers, it prolongs survival of myocardial infarction patients.

trimethaphan camsylate
Arfonad

Pregnancy Risk Category: C

HOW SUPPLIED
Injection: 50 mg/ml in 10-ml ampules, 250 mg/vial‡

MECHANISM OF ACTION
A ganglionic blocker that stabilizes postsynaptic membranes.

INDICATIONS & DOSAGE
To lower blood pressure quickly in hypertensive emergencies; for controlled hypotension during surgery—
Adults: 500 mg (10 ml) diluted in 500 ml dextrose 5% in water to yield concentration of 1 mg/ml I.V. Start I.V. drip at 1 to 2 mg/minute and titrate to achieve desired hypotensive response. Range is 0.3 mg to 6 mg/minute.

ADVERSE REACTIONS
CNS: dilated pupils, *extreme weakness.*
CV: *severe orthostatic hypotension, tachycardia.*
GI: anorexia, *nausea, vomiting, dry mouth.*
GU: urine retention.
Other: respiratory depression.

INTERACTIONS
Anesthetics, diuretics, procainamide: Increased hypotensive effect. Monitor patient closely.

NURSING CONSIDERATIONS
• Contraindicated in anemia, respiratory insufficiency. Use cautiously in arteriosclerosis; cardiac, hepatic, or renal disease; degenerative CNS disorders; Addison's disease; diabetes. Also use cautiously in patients receiving glucocorticoids or other antihypertensives.
• Monitor patient's blood pressure and vital signs continuously.

Italicized adverse reactions are common or life-threatening.
*Liquid form contains alcohol.   **May contain tartrazine.

• Patient should be supine during drug administration. May require elevation of the head of the bed for maximal effect to avoid cerebral anoxia. Do not elevate bed more than 30°.

• Watch closely for respiratory distress, especially if large doses are used. Large doses have caused apnea and respiratory arrest.

• If extreme hypotension occurs, discontinue drug and call doctor. Use phenylephrine or mephentermine to counteract hypotension.

• Patient should receive oxygen therapy during use of this agent.

• Use continuous infusion pump to administer this drug slowly and precisely.

• Discontinue drug before wound closure in surgery to allow blood pressure to return to normal.

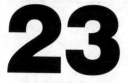

Vasodilators

amyl nitrite
cyclandelate
dipyridamole
ethaverine hydrochloride
isoxsuprine hydrochloride
nimodipine
nylidrin hydrochloride
papaverine hydrochloride
tolazoline hydrochloride

COMBINATION PRODUCTS
HYDERGINE: dihydroergocornine mesylate 0.167 mg, dihydroergocristine mesylate 0.167 mg, and dihydroergocryptine mesylate 0.167 mg.

---

amyl nitrite

Pregnancy Risk Category: C

HOW SUPPLIED
Ampules (crushable): 0.18 ml, 0.3 ml

MECHANISM OF ACTION
Reduces cardiac oxygen demand by decreasing left ventricular end-diastolic pressure (preload) and systemic vascular resistance (afterload). Also increases blood flow through the collateral coronary vessels. Converts hemoglobin to methemoglobin (which binds cyanide) to treat cyanide poisoning.

INDICATIONS & DOSAGE
Relief of angina pectoris; relief of renal or gallbladder colic—
Adults and children: 0.2 to 0.3 ml by inhalation (one glass ampule inhaler), p.r.n.
Antidote for cyanide poisoning—
0.2 or 0.3 ml by inhalation for 30 to 60 seconds q 5 minutes until conscious.

ADVERSE REACTIONS
Blood: methemoglobinemia.
CNS: *headache, sometimes with throbbing;* dizziness; weakness.
CV: *orthostatic hypotension, tachycardia,* flushing, palpitations, fainting.
GI: nausea, vomiting.
Skin: cutaneous vasodilation.
Other: hypersensitivity reactions.

INTERACTIONS
None significant.

NURSING CONSIDERATIONS
• Contraindicated in hypersensitivity to nitrites and during acute myocardial infarction. Use with caution in cerebral hemorrhage, hypotension, head injury, or glaucoma.
• Watch for orthostatic hypotension. Have patient sit down and avoid rapid position changes while inhaling drug.
• Extinguish all cigarettes before use, or ampule may ignite.
• Wrap ampule in cloth and crush. Hold near patient's nose and mouth so vapor is inhaled.
• Effective within 30 seconds but has a short duration of action (3 to 5 minutes).
• Keeping the head low, deep breathing, and movement of extremities may help relieve dizziness, syncope, or weakness from orthostatic hypotension.
• Drug is often abused. Claimed to

Italicized adverse reactions are common or life-threatening.
*Liquid form contains alcohol.   **May contain tartrazine.

have aphrodisiac benefits. Street name is "Amy."
• Seldom, if ever, used for treatment of angina because it is expensive, inconvenient, and frequently causes adverse reactions.
• Sometimes used to induce changes in heart murmurs. Patient inhales the drug until reflex tachycardia is induced, then discontinues.
• Store away from light.

cyclandelate
Cyclan, Cyclospasmol
Pregnancy Risk Category: C

HOW SUPPLIED
Tablets: 200 mg, 400 mg
Capsules: 200 mg, 400 mg

MECHANISM OF ACTION
Directly relaxes smooth muscle due to the inhibition of phosphodiesterase, resulting in increased concentrations of cyclic adenosine monophosphate.

INDICATIONS & DOSAGE
Adjunct in intermittent claudication, arteriosclerosis obliterans, vasospasm and muscular ischemia associated with thrombophlebitis, nocturnal leg cramps, Raynaud's phenomenon, selected cases of ischemic cerebral vascular disease—
Adults: initially, 1.2 to 1.6 g P.O. daily, in divided doses before meals and at bedtime. For maintenance, decrease dosage by 200 mg/day to the lowest effective level. Maintenance dosage is usually 400 to 800 mg daily in two to four divided doses.

ADVERSE REACTIONS
CNS: *headache, tingling of the extremities, dizziness.*
CV: *mild flushing, tachycardia.*
GI: pyrosis, eructation, nausea, heartburn.
Other: *sweating.*

INTERACTIONS
None significant.

NURSING CONSIDERATIONS
• Use with extreme caution in severe obliterative coronary artery or cerebrovascular disease, because circulation to these diseased areas may be compromised by vasodilatory effects of the drug elsewhere (coronary steal syndrome). Use with caution in glaucoma or hypotension.
• Give with food or antacids to lessen GI distress.
• Use in conjunction with, not as a substitute for, appropriate medical or surgical therapy for peripheral or cerebrovascular disease.
• Short-term therapy is of little benefit. Instruct patient to expect long-term treatment and to continue to take medication.
• Adverse reactions usually disappear after several weeks of therapy.

dipyridamole
Apo-Dipyridamole†, Persantin 100‡, Persantine**
Pregnancy Risk Category: C

HOW SUPPLIED
Tablets: 25 mg, 50 mg, 75 mg
Injection: 10 mg/2 ml†

MECHANISM OF ACTION
Inhibits platelet adhesion. Also inhibits the enzymes adenosine deaminase and phosphodiesterase.

INDICATIONS & DOSAGE
Inhibition of platelet adhesion in prosthetic heart valves, in combination with warfarin or aspirin—
Adults: 75 to 100 mg P.O. q.i.d.
Transient ischemic attack—
Adults: 400 to 800 mg P.O. daily in divided doses.
Acute coronary insufficiency‡—
Adults: 10 mg I.V. or I.M.

ADVERSE REACTIONS
CNS: *headache, dizziness,* weakness.
CV: flushing, fainting, *hypotension.*
GI: *nausea,* vomiting, diarrhea.
Skin: rash.

INTERACTIONS
None significant.

NURSING CONSIDERATIONS
• Use with caution in hypotension, and in patients receiving anticoagulant therapy.
• Observe for adverse reactions, especially with large doses. Monitor blood pressure.
• Administer 1 hour before meals. May administer with meals if patient develops GI distress.
• Watch for signs of bleeding, prolonged bleeding time (large doses, long-term).
• Dipyridamole should not be used alone for the prophylaxis of thromboembolism in postoperative prosthetic valve patients; it should be used with oral anticoagulants. Its value as part of an antithrombotic regimen is controversial and may not be significantly better than aspirin alone.

---

ethaverine hydrochloride
Ethaquin, Ethatab, Ethavex-100, Isovex

Pregnancy Risk Category: C

HOW SUPPLIED
Tablets: 100 mg
Capsules: 100 mg

MECHANISM OF ACTION
Directly relaxes smooth muscle due to the inhibition of phosphodiesterase, resulting in increased concentrations of cyclic adenosine monophosphate.

INDICATIONS & DOSAGE
Long-term treatment of peripheral and cerebrovascular insufficiency associated with arterial spasm; spastic conditions of GI and GU tracts—
Adults: 100 to 200 mg P.O. t.i.d.

ADVERSE REACTIONS
CNS: *headache,* drowsiness.
CV: *hypotension, flushing,* sweating, vertigo, cardiac depression, arrhythmias.
GI: *nausea, anorexia, abdominal distress, dry throat,* constipation, diarrhea.
Hepatic: jaundice, altered liver function tests.
Skin: rash.
Other: respiratory depression, malaise, lassitude.

INTERACTIONS
None significant.

NURSING CONSIDERATIONS
• Contraindicated in complete AV dissociation and severe hepatic disease. Use with caution in women who are pregnant or of childbearing age, and in glaucoma or pulmonary embolus; may precipitate arrhythmias.
• Withhold dose and call doctor if signs of hepatic hypersensitivity develop (GI symptoms, altered liver function tests, jaundice, and eosinophilia).
• The FDA has announced this drug may not be effective for disease states indicated.

---

isoxsuprine hydrochloride
Duvadilan‡, Vasodilan, Vasoprine

Pregnancy Risk Category: C

HOW SUPPLIED
Tablets: 10 mg, 20 mg

MECHANISM OF ACTION
Stimulates beta receptors and may also be a direct-acting peripheral vasodilator.

Italicized adverse reactions are common or life-threatening.
*Liquid form contains alcohol.   **May contain tartrazine.

INDICATIONS & DOSAGE
Adjunct for relief of symptoms associated with cerebrovascular insufficiency, peripheral vascular diseases (such as arteriosclerosis obliterans, thromboangiitis obliterans, Raynaud's disease)—
Adults: 10 to 20 mg P.O. t.i.d. or q.i.d.

ADVERSE REACTIONS
CV: tachycardia, hypotension.
GI: vomiting, abdominal distress, intestinal distention.
Skin: severe rash.

INTERACTIONS
None significant.

NURSING CONSIDERATIONS
• Contraindicated in immediate postpartum period and arterial bleeding. Use with caution in cardiovascular or cerebrovascular disease.
• Safe use in pregnancy and lactation not established, although drug has been used to inhibit contractions in premature labor.
• Isoxsuprine has also been used to minimize cramping in patients with severe primary dysmenorrhea.
• Discontinue if rash develops.
• Instruct patient to avoid sudden position changes to minimize the risk of orthostasis.

nimodipine
Nimotop

Pregnancy Risk Category: C

HOW SUPPLIED
Capsules: 30 mg

MECHANISM OF ACTION
Inhibits calcium ion influx across cardiac and smooth muscle cells, thus decreasing myocardial contractility and oxygen demand, and dilates coronary arteries and arterioles. Initially thought to relieve vasospasm in pa-

tients after subarachnoid hemorrhage, its mechanism of action is not fully known.

INDICATIONS & DOSAGE
Improvement of neurologic deficits in patients after subarachnoid hemorrhage from ruptured congenital aneurysms—
Adults: 60 mg P.O. q 4 hours for 21 days. Therapy should begin within 96 hours after subarachnoid hemorrhage.

ADVERSE REACTIONS
CNS: headaches.
CV: decreased blood pressure, flushing, edema.

INTERACTIONS
Antihypertensives: possible enhanced hypotensive effect.
Calcium channel blockers: possible enhanced cardiovascular effects.

NURSING CONSIDERATIONS
• There are no known contraindications to nimodipine therapy, and the drug was relatively well tolerated in clinical trials. Nimodipine should be reserved for patients who are in good neurologic condition post-ictus (for example, Hunt and Hess grades I to III).
• Patients with hepatic failure should receive lower doses. Begin therapy at 30 mg P.O. every 4 hours, with close monitoring of blood pressure and heart rate.
• Monitor blood pressure and heart rate in all patients, especially at the initiation of therapy.

nylidrin hydrochloride
Adrin, Arlidin, Arlidin Forte†, PMS Nylidrin†

Pregnancy Risk Category: C

HOW SUPPLIED
Tablets: 6 mg, 12 mg

MECHANISM OF ACTION
Stimulates beta receptors and may directly relax vascular smooth muscle.

INDICATIONS & DOSAGE
To increase blood supply in vasospastic disorders (arteriosclerosis obliterans, thromboangiitis obliterans, diabetic vascular disease, night leg cramps, Raynaud's phenomenon and disease, ischemic ulcer, frostbite, acrocyanosis, acroparesthesia, sequelae of thrombophlebitis) and in circulatory disturbances of the middle ear (primary cochlear ischemia, cochlear striae, vascular ischemia, macular or ampullar ischemia); other disturbances caused by labyrinth artery spasm or obstruction—
Adults: 3 to 12 mg P.O. t.i.d. or q.i.d.

ADVERSE REACTIONS
CNS: trembling, *nervousness,* weakness, *dizziness (not associated with labyrinth artery insufficiency).*
CV: *palpitations, hypotension,* flushing.
GI: nausea, vomiting.

INTERACTIONS
None significant.

NURSING CONSIDERATIONS
• Contraindicated in acute myocardial infarction, paroxysmal tachycardia, angina pectoris, or thyrotoxicosis. Use with caution in uncompensated heart disease or peptic ulcer.
• Advise patient to avoid tasks that require mental alertness (such as driving or operating heavy machinery) until CNS effects of the drug are known.
• Instruct patient to avoid sudden posture changes to minimize the risks of orthostasis.

papaverine hydrochloride
Cerespan, Genabid, Pavabid, Pavabid HP Capsulets, Pavabid Plateau Caps, Pavarine Spancaps, Pavasule, Pavatine, Pavatym, Paverolan Lanacaps

Pregnancy Risk Category: C

HOW SUPPLIED
Tablets: 30 mg, 60 mg, 100 mg, 150 mg, 200 mg, 300 mg
Tablets (timed-release): 200 mg
Capsules (timed-release): 150 mg
Injection: 30 mg/ml

MECHANISM OF ACTION
Directly relaxes smooth muscle from the inhibition of phosphodiesterase, resulting in increased concentrations of cyclic adenosine monophosphate.

INDICATIONS & DOSAGE
Relief of cerebral and peripheral ischemia associated with arterial spasm and myocardial ischemia; treatment of smooth muscle spasm (coronary occlusion, angina pectoris, sequelae of peripheral and pulmonary embolism, certain cerebral angiospastic states) and visceral spasms (biliary, ureteral, or GI colic)—
Adults: 60 to 300 mg P.O. 1 to 5 times daily, or 150- to 300-mg sustained-release preparations q 8 to 12 hours; 30 to 120 mg I.M. or I.V. q 3 hours, as indicated.

ADVERSE REACTIONS
CNS: *headache.*
CV: *increased heart rate, increased blood pressure* (with parenteral use), depressed AV and intraventricular conduction, hypotension, arrhythmias.
GI: constipation, *nausea.*
Other: *sweating, flushing,* malaise, hepatic damage, increased depth of respiration.

Italicized adverse reactions are common or life-threatening.
*Liquid form contains alcohol.   **May contain tartrazine.

INTERACTIONS
Levodopa: papaverine may interfere with the therapeutic effects of levodopa in patients with Parkinson's disease.

NURSING CONSIDERATIONS
• Contraindicated for I.V. use in patients with Parkinson's disease or complete AV block. Use with caution in glaucoma.
• Monitor blood pressure and heart rate and rhythm, especially in cardiac disease. Withhold dose and notify doctor immediately if changes occur.
• Not often used parenterally, except when immediate effect is desired.
• Give I.V. slowly (over 1 to 2 minutes) to avoid serious adverse reactions.
• Most effective when given early in the course of a disorder.
• Tell patient to take medication regularly; long-term therapy is required.
• Monitor for adverse hepatic reactions in patients receiving long-term therapy.
• Do not add lactated Ringer's injection to the injectable form; will precipitate.
• Advise patient to avoid tasks that require mental alertness (such as driving or operating heavy machinery) until CNS effects of the drug are known.
• Instruct patient to avoid sudden posture changes to minimize the risks of orthostatic hypotension.
• The FDA has announced this drug may not be effective for disease states indicated.
• Has been used experimentally, alone or with phenoxybenzamine, to treat impotence in males. Patients are taught to self-administer by intercavernosal injection.

tolazoline hydrochloride
Priscoline
Pregnancy Risk Category: C

HOW SUPPLIED
Injection: 25 mg/ml

MECHANISM OF ACTION
Direct-acting vasodilator. May have some alpha receptor blocking effects.

INDICATIONS & DOSAGE
Persistent pulmonary hypertension of the newborn—
Neonates: initially, 1 to 2 mg/kg I.V. over 10 minutes, followed by infusion of 1 to 2 mg/kg/hour.
Peripheral vasospastic disorders—
Adults: 10 to 50 mg I.M. or I.V. q.i.d.

ADVERSE REACTIONS
CV: *arrhythmias, anginal pain, hypertension, flushing,* transient postural vertigo, palpitations, *orthostatic hypotension.*
GI: *nausea, vomiting, diarrhea, epigastric discomfort, exacerbation of peptic ulcer.*
Local: burning at injection site.
Other: weakness, paradoxical response in seriously damaged limbs, increased pilomotor activity, tingling, chilliness, apprehension, pulmonary hemorrhage.

INTERACTIONS
Ethyl alcohol: possible disulfiram reaction from accumulation of acetaldehyde. Use together cautiously.
Vasopressors (epinephrine, norepinephrine): may cause a paradoxical fall in blood pressure.

NURSING CONSIDERATIONS
• Contraindicated in coronary artery disease or active peptic ulcer, or following CVA. Use with caution in patients with history of peptic ulcer dis-

---

ease, gastritis, or known or suspected mitral stenosis.

• Response to treatment of persistent pulmonary hypertension of the newborn should be evident within 30 minutes. There is little information regarding infusions lasting longer than 48 hours.

• Keep patient warm during parenteral administration to increase response.

• Patient should be supine during infusion.

• Appearance of flushing usually indicates maximum tolerable dose.

• Monitor vital signs. Watch especially for blood pressure changes and arrhythmias.

• Instruct patient to avoid sudden posture changes to minimize risks of orthostatic hypotension.

• Instruct patient to avoid alcohol; chills and flushing may occur.

• Warn patient against exposure to cold, which can aggravate tissue damage.

• Often used to distinguish between functional (vasospastic) and organic (obstructive) forms of peripheral vascular disease.

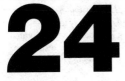

24

Antilipemics

cholestyramine
clofibrate
colestipol hydrochloride
dextrothyroxine sodium
gemfibrozil
lovastatin
niacin
 (See Chapter 92, VITAMINS AND MINERALS.)
probucol

COMBINATION PRODUCTS
None.

cholestyramine
Cholybar, Questran**

Pregnancy Risk Category: C

HOW SUPPLIED
Bar: 4 g
Powder: 378-g cans, 9-g single-dose
packets. Each scoop of powder or single-dose packet contains 4 g of cholestyramine resin.

MECHANISM OF ACTION
Combines with bile acid to form an insoluble compound that is excreted.

INDICATIONS & DOSAGE
*Primary hyperlipidemia, pruritus,
and diarrhea due to excess bile acid;
as adjunctive therapy for the reduction
of elevated serum cholesterol in patients with primary hypercholesterolemia; and to reduce the risks of atherosclerotic coronary artery disease
and myocardial infarction—*
Adults: 4 g before meals and h.s., not
to exceed 32 g daily. Each scoop or
packet of Questran contains 4 g cho-

lestyramine. Also available as Cholybar, a chewable candy bar (raspberry
or caramel flavored) containing 4 g
cholestyramine.
Children: 240 mg/kg daily P.O. in
three divided doses with beverage or
food. Safe dosage not established for
children under 6 years.

ADVERSE REACTIONS
GI: *constipation,* fecal impaction,
hemorrhoids, *abdominal discomfort,*
flatulence, *nausea,* vomiting, steatorrhea.
Skin: *rashes,* irritation of skin,
tongue, and perianal area.
Other: *vitamin A, D, and K deficiency from decreased absorption;* hyperchloremic acidosis with long-term
use or very high dosage.

INTERACTIONS
*Acetaminophen, coumarin anticoagulants, beta-adrenergic blocking
agents, corticosteroids, digitalis glycosides, fat soluble vitamins (A,D,E and
K), iron preparations, thiazide diuretics, thyroid hormone:* absorption may
be substantially decreased by cholestyramine. Separate administration
times by at least 2 hours.

NURSING CONSIDERATIONS
• Patients who are taking this drug to
reduce the risks of atherosclerotic
heart disease should be encouraged to
be aware of other cardiac disease risk
factors. Recommend weight control
and stop smoking programs.
• Monitor serum cholesterol and triglyceride levels regularly during cho-

---

†Available in Canada only.   ‡Available in Australia only.   ◇ Available OTC.

lestyramine therapy. Teach the patient about proper dietary management (restricting total fat and cholesterol intake), weight control, and exercise. Explain their importance in controlling elevated serum lipids.

• To mix powder, sprinkle powder on surface of preferred beverage or wet food. Let stand a few minutes, then stir to obtain uniform suspension.

• Mixing with carbonated beverages may result in excess foaming. Use large glass and mix slowly.

• Administer all other medications at least 1 hour before or 4 to 6 hours after cholestyramine to avoid blocking their absorption.

• Monitor bowel habits; treat constipation as needed. Encourage a diet high in fiber and fluids. If severe constipation develops, decrease dosage, add a stool softener, or discontinue drug.

• Monitor cardiac glycosides in patients receiving both medications concurrently. Should cholestyramine therapy be discontinued, cardiac glycoside toxicity may result unless dosage is adjusted.

• Watch for signs of folic acid and vitamin A, D, E, and K deficiency.

• May bind many drugs and cause decreased absorption. Check drug interaction list of individual drugs.

clofibrate
Arterioflexin‡, Atromid-S, Claripex†, Novofibrate†

Pregnancy Risk Category: C

HOW SUPPLIED
Capsules: 500 mg

MECHANISM OF ACTION
Seems to inhibit biosynthesis of cholesterol at an early stage, but the exact mechanism is unknown.

INDICATIONS & DOSAGE
Hyperlipidemia and xanthoma tubero-sum; Type III hyperlipidemia that does not respond adequately to diet—
Adults: 2 g P.O. daily in four divided doses. Some patients may respond to lower doses as assessed by serum lipid monitoring.

Should not be used in children.

ADVERSE REACTIONS
Blood: leukopenia.
CNS: fatigue, weakness.
CV: arrhythmias.
GI: *nausea, diarrhea, vomiting,* stomatitis, *dyspepsia,* flatulence.
GU: impotence and decreased libido, acute renal failure.
Hepatic: gallstones, *transient and reversible elevations of liver function tests.*
Skin: rashes, urticaria, pruritus, dry skin and hair.
Other: myalgias and arthralgias, resembling a flu-like syndrome; *weight gain; polyphagia;* fever, decreased libido.

INTERACTIONS
Furosemide, sulfonylureas: clofibrate may potentiate the clinical effect of these agents. Monitor patient closely.
Oral anticoagulants: clofibrate may potentiate the anticoagulant effects of warfarin or dicoumarol. Decreased anticoagulant dosage is necessary.
Oral contraceptives, rifampin: may antagonize clofibrate's lipid-lowering effect. Monitor serum lipids.
Probenecid: increased clofibrate effect. Monitor for toxicity.

NURSING CONSIDERATIONS
• Contraindicated in severe renal or hepatic disease.
• Warn patient to report flu-like symptoms to doctor immediately.
• Monitor renal and hepatic function, blood counts, and serum electrolyte and blood sugar levels. If liver function tests show steady rise, clofibrate should be discontinued.
• Should not be used indiscrimi-

Italicized adverse reactions are common or life-threatening.
*Liquid form contains alcohol.   **May contain tartrazine.

nately. May pose increased risk of gallstones, heart disease, and cancer.
• Monitor serum cholesterol and triglycerides regularly during clofibrate therapy.
• Teach patient about proper dietary management (restricting total fat and cholesterol intake), weight control, and exercise. Explain their importance in controlling elevated serum lipids.
• If significant lipid lowering is not ~~tionally to treat diabetes insipidus~~ at doses of 1.5 to 2 g daily.

---

colestipol hydrochloride
Colestid

Pregnancy Risk Category: C

HOW SUPPLIED
Granules: 500-g bottles, 5-g packets

MECHANISM OF ACTION
Combines with bile acid to form an insoluble compound that is excreted.

INDICATIONS & DOSAGE
Primary hypercholesterolemia and xanthomas—
Adults: 15 to 30 g P.O. daily in two to four divided doses.

ADVERSE REACTIONS
CNS: headache, dizziness.
GI: *constipation (common, may require decreasing the dosage),* fecal impaction, hemorrhoids, abdominal discomfort, flatulence, nausea, vomiting, steatorrhea.
Skin: rashes, irritation of skin, tongue, and perianal area.
Other: vitamin A, D, and K deficiency from decreased absorption; hyperchloremic acidosis with long-term use or very high dosage.

INTERACTIONS
Oral hypoglycemics: may antagonize response to colestipol. Monitor serum lipids.
Orally administered drugs: absorption may be decreased by colestipol. Separate administration times: other drugs should be taken at least 1 hour before or 4 hours after colestipol.

NURSING CONSIDERATIONS
• Administer all other medications at least 1 hour before or 4 to 6 hours after colestipol to avoid blocking their absorption.
• Monitor cardiac glycoside levels in patients receiving both medications concurrently. Should colestipol therapy be discontinued, cardiac glycoside toxicity may result unless dosage is adjusted.
• Watch for signs of vitamin A, D, and K deficiency.
• Lowering dosage, increasing dietary fiber, or adding stool softener may relieve constipation.
• May bind many drugs and cause decreased absorption. Check drug interaction list of individual drugs.
• Administer this drug in at least 3 oz (90 ml) of juice, milk, or water. After drinking this preparation, patient should swirl a small additional amount of liquid in the same glass and then drink it to ensure ingestion of the entire dose.
• Palatability may be enhanced if the next daily dose is mixed and refrigerated the previous evening.
• Teach patient about proper dietary management (restricting total fat and cholesterol intake), weight control, and exercise. Explain their importance in controlling elevated serum lipids.

---

dextrothyroxine sodium (d-thyroxine sodium)
Choloxin**

Pregnancy Risk Category: C

HOW SUPPLIED
Tablets: 1 mg, 2 mg, 4 mg, 6 mg

MECHANISM OF ACTION
Accelerates hepatic catabolism of cholesterol and increases bile secretion to lower cholesterol levels.

INDICATIONS & DOSAGE
Hyperlipidemia in euthyroid patients, especially when cholesterol and triglyceride levels are elevated—
Adults: initial dose 1 to 2 mg P.O. daily, increased by 1 to 2 mg daily at monthly intervals to a total of 4 to 8 mg daily.
Children: initial dose 0.05 mg/kg P.O. daily, increased by 0.05 mg/kg daily at monthly intervals to a total of 4 mg daily.

ADVERSE REACTIONS
CV: palpitations, angina pectoris, arrhythmias, ischemic myocardial changes on ECG, myocardial infarction.
EENT: visual disturbances, ptosis.
GI: nausea, vomiting, diarrhea, constipation, decreased appetite.
Metabolic: insomnia, weight loss, sweating, flushing, hyperthermia, hair loss, menstrual irregularities.

INTERACTIONS
Digitalis glycosides: dextrothyroxine may enhance clinical effect. Use together cautiously.
Oral anticoagulants: dextrothyroxine may potentiate the anticoagulant effect of warfarin or dicumarol.
Sympathomimetics: dextrothyroxine may precipitate arrhythmias or coronary insufficiency in patients with cardiac disease.

NURSING CONSIDERATIONS
• Contraindicated in hepatic or renal disease, or iodism. Patients with history of cardiac disease, including arrhythmias, hypertension, or angina pectoris, should receive very small doses.
• May increase need for insulin, diet therapy, or oral hypoglycemics in patients with diabetes.
• If the use of anticoagulants is considered, discon...
...observe patient for signs of hyperthyroidism, such as nervousness, insomnia, and weight loss. If these occur, dosage should be decreased or drug discontinued.
• Teach patient about proper dietary management (restricting total fat and cholesterol intake), weight control, and exercise. Explain their importance in controlling elevated serum lipids.

gemfibrozil
Lopid

Pregnancy Risk Category: B

HOW SUPPLIED
Tablets: 600 mg
Capsules: 300 mg

MECHANISM OF ACTION
Inhibits peripheral lipolysis and also reduces triglyceride synthesis in the liver.

INDICATIONS & DOSAGE
Treatment of type IV hyperlipidemia (hypertriglyceridemia) and severe hypercholesterolemia unresponsive to diet and other drugs—
Adults: 1,200 mg P.O. administered in two divided doses. Usual dosage range is 900 to 1,500 mg daily. If no beneficial effect is seen after 3 months of therapy, drug should be discontinued.

Italicized adverse reactions are common or life-threatening.
*Liquid form contains alcohol.   **May contain tartrazine.

ADVERSE REACTIONS
Blood: anemia, leukopenia.
CNS: blurred vision, headache, dizziness.
GI: *abdominal and epigastric pain, diarrhea, nausea,* vomiting, flatulence.
Hepatic: bile duct obstruction, elevated enzymes.
Skin: rash, dermatitis, pruritus.
Other: painful extremities.

INTERACTIONS
Oral anticoagulants: gemfibrozil may enhance the clinical effects of oral anticoagulants. Monitor patient closely.

NURSING CONSIDERATIONS
• Contraindicated in hepatic or severe renal dysfunction—including primary biliary cirrhosis—and preexisting gallbladder disease.
• CBC and liver function tests should be done periodically during the first 12 months of therapy.
• Gemfibrozil is very closely related to clofibrate both chemically and pharmacologically.
• Instruct patient to take drug half an hour before breakfast and dinner.
• Should not be used indiscriminately. May pose risk of gallstones, heart disease, and cancer.
• Observe bowel movements for evidence of steatorrhea or other signs of bile duct obstruction.
• Because of possible dizziness and blurred vision, patient should avoid driving or other hazardous activities until CNS effects of the drug are known.
• Teach patient about proper dietary management (restricting total fat and cholesterol intake), weight control, and exercise. Explain their importance in controlling elevated serum lipids.

lovastatin
Mevacor
Pregnancy Risk Category: X

HOW SUPPLIED
Tablets: 20 mg

MECHANISM OF ACTION
Lovastatin inhibits 3-hydroxy-3-methylglutaryl-coenzyme A (HMG-CoA) reductase. This enzyme is an early (and rate-limiting) step in the synthetic pathway of cholesterol.

INDICATIONS & DOSAGE
Reduction of low-density lipoprotein and total cholesterol levels in patients with primary hypercholesterolemia (types IIa and IIb)—
Adults: initially, 20 mg P.O. once daily with the evening meal. For patients with severely elevated cholesterol levels (for example, over 300 mg/dl), the initial dose should be 40 mg. The recommended range is 20 to 80 mg in single or divided doses.

ADVERSE REACTIONS
CNS: headache, dizziness.
EENT: blurred vision, dysgeusia.
GI: constipation, diarrhea, dyspepsia, flatus, abdominal pain or cramps, heartburn, nausea.
Metabolic: elevated serum transaminase levels, abnormal liver test results.
Skin: rash, pruritus.
Other: peripheral neuropathy, muscle cramps, myalgia, myositis, *rhabdomyolysis.*

INTERACTIONS
Cholestyramine, clofibrate: enhanced lipid-reducing effects.
Immunosuppressive agents, gemfibrozil: possible increased risk of polymyositis and rhabdomyolysis. Maximum recommended lovastatin dosage is 20 mg daily; monitor patient closely.

NURSING CONSIDERATIONS
• Initiate lovastatin only after diet and other nonpharmacologic therapies have proven ineffective. Patient should be on a standard cholesterol-lowering diet during therapy.
• Give lovastatin with the evening meal; absorption is enhanced and cholesterol biosynthesis is greater in the evening.
• Therapeutic response occurs in about 2 weeks, with maximum effects in 4 to 6 weeks. Effects of long-term use are unknown.
• Watch for signs of myositis.
• Liver function tests should be performed frequently at start of therapy and periodically thereafter.
• Store tablets at room temperature in a light-resistant container.
• Advise patient to restrict alcohol intake.
• Tell patient to advise doctor of any adverse reactions, particularly muscle aches and pains.
• Advise patient to have periodic eye examinations.
• Teach patient about proper dietary management (restricting total fat and cholesterol intake), weight control, and exercise. Explain their importance in controlling elevated serum lipids.

probucol
Lorelco, Lurselle ‡

Pregnancy Risk Category: B

HOW SUPPLIED
Tablets: 250 mg, 500 mg

MECHANISM OF ACTION
Inhibits cholesterol transport from the intestine and may also decrease cholesterol synthesis. Appears to be more effective in patients with mild cholesterol elevations than in those with severe hypercholesterolemia.

INDICATIONS & DOSAGE
Primary hypercholesterolemia—
Adults: 500 mg P.O. b.i.d. with morning and evening meals. Do not exceed 1 g/day.
　Not recommended for children.

ADVERSE REACTIONS
CV: prolonged QT interval, arrhythmias.
GI: *diarrhea, flatulence, abdominal pain, nausea, vomiting.*
Other: *hyperhidrosis,* fetid sweat, angioneurotic edema.

INTERACTIONS
Clofibrate: additive pharmacologic effects.
Tricyclic antidepressants, class Ia antiarrhythmics, phenothiazines, beta blockers, digitalis glycosides, calcium channel blocking agents: increased risk of arrhythmias.

NURSING CONSIDERATIONS
• Drug's effect is enhanced when taken with food.
• Contraindicated in patients with arrhythmias. Drug should be stopped in any patient whose ECG shows prolonged Q-T interval. Monitor ECG periodically.
• Teach patient about proper dietary management (restricting total fat and cholesterol intake), weight control, and exercise. Explain their importance in controlling elevated serum lipids.
• If female patient wishes to become pregnant, withdrawal of drug and effective contraception is recommended for 6 months due to the persistence of the drug in the body.

Italicized adverse reactions are common or life-threatening.
*Liquid form contains alcohol.　　**May contain tartrazine.

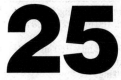

Nonnarcotic analgesics and antipyretics

Salicylates
aspirin
choline magnesium trisalicylate
choline salicylate
magnesium salicylate
salsalate
sodium salicylate
sodium thiosalicylate

Urinary tract analgesic
phenazopyridine hydrochloride

Miscellaneous
acetaminophen
diflunisal
methotrimeprazine
(See Chapter 28, SEDATIVE-HYPNOTICS.)

COMBINATION PRODUCTS
AMAPHEN: acetaminophen 325 mg, caffeine 40 mg, and butalbital 50 mg.
ANOQUAN: acetaminophen 325 mg, caffeine 40 mg, and butalbital 50 mg.
ARTHRALGEN: acetaminophen 250 mg and salicylamide 250 mg.
AXOTAL: aspirin 650 mg and butalbital 50 mg.
BC POWDER: aspirin 650 mg, salicylamide 195 mg, and caffeine 32 mg.
BC TABLETS: aspirin 325 mg, salicylamide 95 mg, and caffeine 16 mg.
BUTAL: aspirin 325 mg, caffeine 40 mg, and butalbital 50 mg.
CAMA, ARTHRITIS STRENGTH: aspirin 500 mg, magnesium oxide 150 mg, and aluminum hydroxide 150 mg.
COPE◊: aspirin 421 mg, caffeine 32 mg, magnesium hydroxide 50 mg, and aluminum hydroxide 25 mg.
DURADYNE◊: acetaminophen 180 mg, aspirin 230 mg, and caffeine 15 mg.

ESGIC: acetaminophen 325 mg, caffeine 40 mg, and butalbital 50 mg.
EXCEDRIN P.M.◊: acetaminophen 500 mg and diphenhydramine citrate 38 mg.
EXCEDRIN TABLETS◊: aspirin 250 mg, acetaminophen 250 mg, caffeine 65 mg.
FEMCAPS◊: acetaminophen 324 mg, caffeine 32 mg, ephedrine sulfate 8 mg, and atropine sulfate 0.0325 mg.
FIORICET: acetaminophen 325 mg, butalbital 50 mg, and caffeine 40 mg
FIORINAL: aspirin 325 mg, caffeine 40 mg, and butalbital 50 mg.
G-1: acetaminophen 500 mg, caffeine 40 mg, and butalbital 50 mg.
GEMNISYN◊: aspirin 325 mg and acetaminophen 325 mg.
ISOLLYL: aspirin 325 mg, caffeine 40 mg, and butalbital 50 mg.
MIDOL◊: aspirin 454 mg, caffeine 32.4 mg, and cinnemedrine hydrochloride 14.9 mg.
PAC NEW REVISED FORMULA◊: aspirin 400 mg and caffeine 32 mg.
PHRENILIN: acetaminophen 325 mg and butalbital 50 mg.
PHRENILIN FORTE: acetaminophen 650 mg and butalbital 50 mg.
SINUTAB◊: acetaminophen 325 mg, chlorpheniramine 2 mg, and pseudo-ephedrine hydrochloride 30 mg.
SINUTAB II MAXIMUM STRENGTH: acetaminophen 500 mg and pseudo-ephedrine hydrochloride 30 mg.
SYNALGOS◊: aspirin 356.4 mg and caffeine 30 mg.
TRIGESIC◊: acetaminophen 125 mg, aspirin 230 mg, and caffeine 30 mg.

†Available in Canada only. ‡Available in Australia only. ◊ Available OTC.

TRILISATE: choline salicylate 293 mg and magnesium salicylate 362 mg.
VANQUISH◇: aspirin 227 mg, acetaminophen 194 mg, caffeine 33 mg, aluminum hydroxide 25 mg, and magnesium hydroxide 50 mg.

acetaminophen (paracetamol)

Acephen◇, Aceta*◇, Ace-Tabs†◇, Acetaminophen Unicerts◇, Actamin◇, Actamin Extra◇, Anacin-3◇, Anacin-3 Maximum Strength◇, Anuphen◇, Apacet◇, Apacet Extra Strength◇, Apacet Oral Solution◇, APAP◇, Apo-Acetaminophen†◇, Atasol†◇, Atasol Forte†◇, Banesin◇, Campain†◇, Ceetamol‡, Children's Anacin-3◇, Children's Apacet◇, Children's Genapap◇, Children's Panadol◇, Children's Tylenol◇, Children's Ty-PAP◇, Children's Ty-Tabs◇, Dapa◇, Datril◇, Datril Extra Strength◇, Dolanex*◇, Dymadon‡, Exdol†◇, Exdol Strong†◇, Genapap◇, Genebs◇, Genebs Extra Strength◇, Gentabs◇, Halenol◇, Infant's Anacin-3◇, Infant's Apacet◇, Infant's Tylenol◇, Infant's Ty-PAP◇, Junior Disprol‡, Liquiprin◇, Meda Cap◇, Meda Tab◇, Myapap◇, Neopap◇, Oraphen-PD◇, Panadol◇, Panadol Junior Strength◇, Panamax‡, Panex◇, Paraphen†◇, Parmol‡, Pedric*◇, Phenaphen◇, Robigesic†◇, Rounox†◇, Suppap◇, Tapanol◇, Tapanol Extra Strength◇, Tempra◇, Tenol◇, Ty Caplets◇, Ty Caps◇, Tylenol*, Tylenol Extra Strength◇, Ty Tabs◇, Valadol*◇, Valorin◇

Pregnancy Risk Category: B

HOW SUPPLIED
Tablets: 160 mg◇, 325 mg◇, 500 mg◇, 650 mg◇
Tablets (chewable): 80 mg◇
Capsules: 325 mg◇, 500 mg◇
Oral solution: 100 mg/ml◇
Oral suspension: 120 mg/5 ml‡
Oral liquid: 160 mg/5 ml◇, 500 mg/15 ml◇
Elixir: 120 mg/5 ml◇, 160 mg/5 ml◇, 320 mg/5 ml◇
Wafers: 120 mg◇
Effervescent granules: 325 mg/capful◇
Suppositories: 120 mg◇, 125 mg◇, 135 mg◇, 650 mg◇

MECHANISM OF ACTION
Produces analgesia by blocking generation of pain impulses. This action is probably caused by inhibition of prostaglandin synthesis; it may also be caused by inhibition of the synthesis or action of other substances that sensitize pain receptors to mechanical or chemical stimulation. It relieves fever by central action in the hypothalamic heat-regulating center.

INDICATIONS & DOSAGE
Mild pain or fever—
Adults and children over 11 years: 325 to 650 mg P.O. or rectally q 4 hours; or 1 g P.O. q.i.d. p.r.n. Maximum dosage should not exceed 4 g daily. Dosage for long-term therapy should not exceed 2.6 g daily.
Children 11 years: 480 mg/dose.
Children 9 to 10 years: 400 mg/dose.
Children 6 to 8 years: 320 mg/dose.
Children 4 to 5 years: 240 mg/dose.
Children 2 to 3 years: 160 mg/dose.
Children 12 to 23 months: 120 mg/dose.
Children 4 to 11 months: 80 mg/dose.
Children up to 3 months: 40 mg/dose.

ADVERSE REACTIONS
Hepatic: *severe liver damage with toxic doses.*
Skin: rash, urticaria.

INTERACTIONS
Diflunisal: increases acetaminophen blood levels. Don't use together.

Italicized adverse reactions are common or life-threatening.
*Liquid form contains alcohol.   **May contain tartrazine.

Ethanol: increased risk of hepatic damage.

Warfarin: increased hypoprothrombinemic effect with chronic acetaminophen use.

NURSING CONSIDERATIONS
• Repeated use is contraindicated in anemia, or renal or hepatic disease.
• Has no significant anti-inflammatory effect.
• Warn patient that high doses or unsupervised chronic use can cause hepatic damage. Excessive ingestion of alcoholic beverages may increase the risk of hepatotoxicity.
• Should not be used for self-medication of marked fever (greater than 103.1° F. [39.5° C.]), fever persisting longer than 3 days, or recurrent fever unless directed by doctor.
• Many nonprescription products contain acetaminophen. Be aware of this when calculating total daily dosages.
• Recommend the liquid form for children and for all patients who have difficulty swallowing.

---

aspirin (acetylsalicylic acid)
Ancasal†◊, Arthrinol†◊, Artria SR◊, ASA◊, ASA Enseals◊, Aspergum◊, Aspro‡, Astrin†◊, Bayer Aspirin◊, Bex‡, Coryphen†◊, Easprin◊, Ecotrin◊, Empirin◊, Entrophen†◊, Measurin◊, Norwich Aspirin◊, Novasen†◊, Riphen-10†◊, Sal-Adult†◊, Sal-Infant†◊, Solprin‡, Supasa†◊, Triaphen-10†◊, Vincent's Powders‡, Winsprin Capsules‡, ZORprin◊

Pregnancy Risk Category: C (D in 3rd trimester)

HOW SUPPLIED
Tablets◊: 65 mg, 75 mg, 81 mg, 300 mg, 325 mg, 500 mg, 600 mg, 650 mg
Tablets (chewable): 81 mg◊

Tablets (enteric-coated): 325 mg◊, 500 mg◊, 650 mg◊, 975 mg
Tablets (extended-release): 800 mg
Tablets (timed-release): 650 mg◊
Capsules: 325 mg◊, 500 mg◊
Powder: 500 mg
Chewing gum: 227.5 mg◊
Suppositories: 60 to 120 mg◊

MECHANISM OF ACTION
• Produces analgesia by an ill-defined effect on the hypothalamus (central action) and by blocking generation of pain impulses (peripheral action). The peripheral action may involve inhibition of prostaglandin synthesis.
• Exerts its anti-inflammatory effect by inhibiting prostaglandin synthesis, may also inhibit the synthesis or action of other mediators of the inflammatory response.
• Relieves fever by acting on the hypothalamic heat-regulating center to produce peripheral vasodilation. This increases peripheral blood supply and promotes sweating, which leads to loss of heat and to cooling by evaporation.
• Also appears to impede clotting by blocking prostaglandin synthesis, which prevents formation of the platelet-aggregating substance thromboxane A_2.

INDICATIONS & DOSAGE
Adults:
Arthritis—2.6 to 5.4 g P.O. daily in divided doses.
Mild pain or fever—325 to 650 mg P.O. or rectally q 4 hours, p.r.n.
Thromboembolic disorders—325 to 650 mg P.O. daily or b.i.d.
Transient ischemic attacks in men—650 mg P.O. b.i.d. or 325 mg q.i.d.
To reduce the risk of heart attack in patients with previous myocardial infarction or unstable angina—325 mg P.O. once daily.
Children:
Arthritis—90 to 130 mg/kg P.O. daily

---

†Available in Canada only.   ‡Available in Australia only.   ◊Available OTC.

divided q 4 to 6 hours.
Fever—40 to 80 mg/kg P.O. or rectally daily divided q 6 hours, p.r.n.
Mild pain—65 to 100 mg/kg P.O. or rectally daily divided q 4 to 6 hours, p.r.n.

ADVERSE REACTIONS
Blood: *prolonged bleeding time*.
EENT: *tinnitus and hearing loss*.
GI: *nausea, vomiting, GI distress, occult bleeding*.
Hepatic: abnormal liver function studies, hepatitis.
Skin: *rash*, bruising.
Other: *hypersensitivity manifested by anaphylaxis and/or asthma*.

INTERACTIONS
Ammonium chloride (and other urine acidifiers): increased blood levels of aspirin products. Monitor for aspirin toxicity.
Antacids in high doses (and other urine alkalinizers): decreased levels of aspirin products. Monitor for decreased aspirin effect.
Corticosteroids: enhance salicylate elimination. Monitor for decreased salicylate effect.
Oral anticoagulants, heparin: increased risk of bleeding. Avoid using together if possible.
Oral hypoglycemic agents: increased hypoglycemic effect.

NURSING CONSIDERATIONS
• Contraindicated in GI ulcer, GI bleeding, patients with bleeding disorders, or aspirin hypersensitivity. Use cautiously in patients with hypoprothrombinemia, vitamin K deficiency, and in asthmatics with nasal polyps (may cause severe bronchospasm).
• Because of epidemiologic association with Reye's syndrome, the Centers for Disease Control recommends that children or teenagers with chicken pox or influenza-like illness should not be given salicylates.
• Febrile, dehydrated children can develop toxicity rapidly.
• Elderly patients may be more susceptible to aspirin's toxic effects.
• Give with food, milk, antacid, or large glass of water to reduce GI adverse reactions.
• Because of the many possible drug interactions involving aspirin, warn patients taking prescription drugs to check with doctor or pharmacist before taking OTC combinations containing aspirin.
• Therapeutic blood salicylate level in arthritis is 10 to 30 mg/100 ml. Tinnitus may occur at plasma levels of 30 mg/100 ml and above, but this is not a reliable indicator of toxicity, especially in very young and elderly patients.
• Concomitant use with alcohol, steroids or other NSAIDs may increase risk of GI bleeding.
• May cause an increase in serum levels of AST (SGOT), ALT (SGPT), alkaline phosphatase, and bilirubin.
• Keep out of reach of children—aspirin is one of the leading causes of poisoning in children. Encourage use of child-resistant containers in households with children.
• Advise patients receiving large doses of aspirin for an extended period of time to watch for petechiae, bleeding gums, and signs of GI bleeding, and to maintain adequate fluid intake. Obtain hemoglobin and prothrombin tests periodically.
• Enteric-coated products are slowly absorbed and are not suitable for acute effects. They do cause less GI bleeding and may be more suited for long-term therapy, such as arthritic therapy.
• There's no evidence that aspirin is effective in reducing the incidence of transient ischemic attacks in women.
• There is some evidence that aspirin may prevent sunburn and treat sun-

---

Italicized adverse reactions are common or life-threatening.
*Liquid form contains alcohol.   **May contain tartrazine.

burn pain by preventing cells from manufacturing prostaglandins.
• If possible, stop aspirin dosage 5 to 7 days before elective surgery.
• For patients with swallowing difficulties, aspirin can be crushed and combined with soft food or dissolved in liquid. After mixing it with a liquid, administer it immediately, because the drug doesn't stay in solution. Don't crush enteric-coated aspirin.

choline magnesium trisalicylate (choline salicylate and magnesium salicylate)
Trilisate

Pregnancy Risk Category: C

HOW SUPPLIED
Tablets: 500 mg, 750 mg, 1,000 mg of salicylate
Solution: 500 mg of salicylate/5 ml

MECHANISM OF ACTION
• Produces analgesia by an ill-defined effect on the hypothalamus (central action) and by blocking generation of pain impulses (peripheral action). The peripheral action may involve inhibition of prostaglandin synthesis.
• Exerts its anti-inflammatory effect by inhibiting prostaglandin synthesis.
• Relieves fever by acting on the hypothalamic heat-regulating center to produce peripheral vasodilation. This increases peripheral blood supply and promotes sweating, which leads to loss of heat and to cooling by evaporation.

INDICATIONS & DOSAGE
Arthritis, mild—
Adults: 1 to 2 teaspoonfuls or tablets P.O. b.i.d. Total daily dosage can also be given at one time (usually h.s.)
Rheumatoid arthritis and osteoarthritis—

Adults: initially, 3 g P.O. daily either as a single dose h.s. or b.i.d. Dosage is adjusted according to patient response. Dosage range is 1 to 4.5 g daily.
Juvenile rheumatoid arthritis—
Children (12 to 37 kg): 50 mg/kg/day P.O. in divided doses.
Children (more than 37 kg): 2,250 mg P.O. given in divided doses.
Mild to moderate pain and fever—
Adults: 2 to 3 g P.O. daily divided b.i.d.
Children (12 to 37 kg): 50 mg/kg/day P.O. in divided doses.

ADVERSE REACTIONS
EENT: tinnitus and hearing loss.
GI: GI distress.
Skin: rash.
Other: *hypersensitivity manifested by anaphylaxis (rare).*

INTERACTIONS
Alcohol, steroids, and other NSAIDs: enhanced risk of adverse GI effects.
Ammonium chloride (and other urine acidifiers): increased blood levels of salicylates. Monitor for salicylate toxicity.
Antacids in high doses (and other urine alkalinizers): decreased levels of salicylates. Monitor for decreased salicylate effect.
Corticosteroids: enhance salicylate elimination. Monitor for decreased salicylate effect.
Oral anticoagulants: increased risk of bleeding. Use together cautiously.

NURSING CONSIDERATIONS
• Use cautiously in chronic renal failure, peptic ulcer disease, gastritis, and in patients with a known allergy to salicylates.
• Each '500' tablet or teaspoonful is equal in salicylate content to 650 mg aspirin.
• Because of epidemiologic association with Reye's syndrome, the Centers for Disease Control recommends

---

†Available in Canada only.   ‡Available in Australia only.   ◊ Available OTC.

that children or teenagers with chicken pox or influenza-like illness should not be given salicylates.
• Causes less GI distress than aspirin. If antacid is needed, give it 2 hours after meals and give choline magnesium trisalicylate before meals.
• Tell patient to take tablets with food or a full glass of water. Solution may be mixed with fruit juice, but not antacids.
• Febrile, dehydrated children can develop toxicity rapidly.
• Therapeutic blood salicylate level in arthritis is 10 to 30 mg/100 ml. Tinnitus may occur at plasma levels of 30 mg/100 ml and above, but this is not a reliable indicator of toxicity, especially in very young and elderly patients.
• Obtain hemoglobin and prothrombin tests periodically in patients receiving large doses over an extended period of time.

choline salicylate
Arthropan, Teejel†*

Pregnancy Risk Category: C

HOW SUPPLIED
Liquid: 870 mg/5 ml◇
Gel: 87 mg/g†*

MECHANISM OF ACTION
• Produces analgesia by an ill-defined effect on the hypothalamus (central action) and by blocking generation of pain impulses (peripheral action). The peripheral action may involve inhibition of prostaglandin synthesis.
• Exerts its anti-inflammatory effect by inhibiting prostaglandin synthesis.
• Relieves fever by acting on the hypothalamic heat-regulating center to produce peripheral vasodilation. This increases peripheral blood supply and promotes sweating, which leads to loss of heat and to cooling by evaporation.

INDICATIONS & DOSAGE
Rheumatoid arthritis, osteoarthritis, minor pain or fever—
Adults and children over 12 years: 1 teaspoonful (870 mg choline salicylate) P.O. q 3 to 4 hours p.r.n. If tolerated and needed, dosage may be increased to 2 teaspoonfuls. Do not exceed 6 teaspoons daily.
Relief of pain from inflamed gums—
Adults and children over 2 years: apply 1 cm of gel to affected area q 3 to 4 hours and h.s., p.r.n.

ADVERSE REACTIONS
EENT: tinnitus and hearing loss.
GI: nausea, vomiting, GI distress.
Skin: rash.
Other: *hypersensitivity manifested by anaphylaxis (rare).*

INTERACTIONS
Alcohol, steroids, and other NSAIDs: enhanced risk of adverse GI reactions.
Ammonium chloride (and other urine acidifiers): increased blood levels of salicylates. Monitor for salicylate toxicity.
Antacids in high doses (and other urine alkalinizers): decreased levels of salicylates. Monitor for decreased salicylate effect.
Corticosteroids: enhance salicylate elimination. Monitor for decreased salicylate effect.

NURSING CONSIDERATIONS
• Use cautiously in chronic renal failure, peptic ulcer disease, gastritis, and in patients with a known allergy to salicylates.
• Because of epidemiologic association with Reye's syndrome, the Centers for Disease Control recommends that children or teenagers with chicken pox or influenza-like illness should not be given salicylates.
• Causes less GI distress than aspirin. If antacid is needed, give it 2 hours after meals and give choline salicylate before meals.

Italicized adverse reactions are common or life-threatening.
*Liquid form contains alcohol.   **May contain tartrazine.

- May mix drug with water, fruit juice, or carbonated drinks, but not antacids.
- Febrile, dehydrated children can develop toxicity rapidly.
- Therapeutic blood salicylate level in arthritis is 10 to 30 mg/100 ml. Tinnitus may occur at plasma levels of 30 mg/100 ml and above, but this is not a reliable indicator of toxicity, especially in very young and elderly patients.
- Obtain hemoglobin and prothrombin tests periodically in patients receiving large dosages over an extended period of time.

diflunisal
Dolobid

Pregnancy Risk Category: C

HOW SUPPLIED
Tablets: 250 mg, 500 mg

MECHANISM OF ACTION
Mechanism of action is unknown, but it is probably related to inhibition of prostaglandin synthesis.

INDICATIONS & DOSAGE
Mild to moderate pain and osteoarthritis—
Adults— 500 to 1,000 mg P.O. daily in two divided doses, usually q 12 hours. Maximum dosage 1,500 mg daily.
Adults over 65: Start with one-half the usual adult dose.

ADVERSE REACTIONS
CNS: *dizziness,* somnolence, insomnia, *headache,* fatigue.
EENT: *tinnitus, visual disturbances (rare).*
GI: *nausea, dyspepsia, gastrointestinal pain, diarrhea,* vomiting, constipation, flatulence.
Skin: *rash,* pruritus, sweating, dry mucous membranes, stomatitis.

INTERACTIONS
Aspirin, antacids: decreased diflunisal blood levels. Monitor for possible decreased therapeutic effect.
Oral anticoagulants, thrombolytic agents: diflunisal may enhance pharmacologic effects of these agents. Use together cautiously.
Sulindac: diflunisal decreases blood levels of sulindac's active metabolite. Monitor for decreased pharmacologic effect.

NURSING CONSIDERATIONS
- Contraindicated for patients in whom acute asthmatic attacks, urticaria, or rhinitis are precipitated by aspirin or other nonsteroidal anti-inflammatory drugs.
- Use cautiously in patients with active GI bleeding or history of peptic ulcer disease, renal impairment, liver disease, compromised cardiac function, or those taking anticoagulants.
- Similar to aspirin, diflunisal is a salicylic acid derivative but is metabolized differently and has less effect on platelet function.
- May be administered with water, milk, or meals.
- Avoid the use of diflunisal in children and teenagers with viral illnesses and flu because of possible association with Reye's syndrome.

magnesium salicylate
Extra-Strength Doan's◇, Magan◇, Mobidin◇, Original Doan's◇

Pregnancy Risk Category: C

HOW SUPPLIED
Tablets: 545 mg, 600 mg
Caplets: 325 mg◇, 500 mg◇

MECHANISM OF ACTION
- Produces analgesia by an ill-defined effect on the hypothalamus (central action) and by blocking generation of pain impulses (peripheral action). The peripheral action may in-

---

volve inhibition of prostaglandin synthesis.

• Exerts its anti-inflammatory effect by inhibiting prostaglandin synthesis.

• Relieves fever by acting on the hypothalamic heat-regulating center to produce peripheral vasodilation. This increases peripheral blood supply and promotes sweating, which leads to loss of heat and to cooling by evaporation.

INDICATIONS & DOSAGE
Arthritis—
Adults: 545 mg to 1.2 g P.O. t.i.d. or q.i.d. not to exceed 4.8 g daily.
Mild pain or fever—
Adults: 300 to 600 mg P.O. q 4 hours, not to exceed 3.5 g/24 hours.

ADVERSE REACTIONS
EENT: *tinnitus and hearing loss.*
GI: *nausea, vomiting, GI distress, occult bleeding.*
Hepatic: abnormal liver function studies, hepatitis.
Skin: *rash,* bruising.
Other: *hypersensitivity manifested by anaphylaxis and/or asthma.*

INTERACTIONS
Ammonium chloride (and other urine acidifiers): increased blood levels of salicylates. Monitor for salicylate toxicity.
Antacids in high doses (and other urine alkalinizers): decreased levels of salicylates. Monitor for decreased salicylate effect.
Corticosteroids: enhance salicylate elimination. Monitor for decreased salicylate effect.
Oral anticoagulants, heparin: increased risk of bleeding. Avoid using together if possible.

NURSING CONSIDERATIONS
• Contraindicated in severe chronic renal insufficiency because of risk of magnesium toxicity; GI ulcer; GI bleeding; or aspirin hypersensitivity.

Use cautiously in hypoprothrombinemia, vitamin K deficiency, and bleeding disorders.

• Because of epidemiologic association with Reye's syndrome, the Centers for Disease Control recommends that children or teenagers with chicken pox or influenza-like illness should not be given salicylates.

• Febrile, dehydrated children can develop toxicity rapidly.

• Give with food, milk, antacid, or large glass of water to reduce GI adverse reactions.

• Therapeutic blood salicylate level in arthritis is 10 to 30 mg/100 ml. Tinnitus may occur at plasma levels of 300 mg/100 ml and above, but this is not a reliable indicator of toxicity, expecially in very young and elderly patients.

• Concomitant use with alcohol, steroids, or other NSAIDs may increase risk of GI bleeding.

• May cause an increase in serum levels of AST (SGOT), ALT (SGPT), alkaline phosphatase, and bilirubin.

• Obtain hemoglobin and prothrombin tests periodically in patients receiving large doses over an extended period of time.

---

phenazopyridine hydrochloride
Azo-Standard◇, Baridium◇, Di-Azo◇, Eridium◇, Geridium◇, Phenazo†, Phenazodine◇, Pyrazodine◇, Pyridiate◇, Pyridin◇, Pyridium, Pyronium†, Urodine◇, Urogesic◇, Viridium◇

Pregnancy Risk Category: B

HOW SUPPLIED
Tablets: 100 mg◇, 200 mg

MECHANISM OF ACTION
Exerts local anesthetic action on urinary mucosa through unknown mechanism.

Italicized adverse reactions are common or life-threatening.
*Liquid form contains alcohol.   **May contain tartrazine.

INDICATIONS & DOSAGE
Pain with urinary tract irritation or infection—
Adults: 100 to 200 mg P.O. t.i.d.
Children: 100 mg P.O. t.i.d.

ADVERSE REACTIONS
CNS: headache, vertigo.
GI: nausea.
Skin: rash.

INTERACTIONS
None significant.

NURSING CONSIDERATIONS
• Contraindicated in renal and hepatic insufficiency.
• Colors urine red or orange. May stain fabrics.
• Taking the drug with meals may minimize GI distress.
• Use only as analgesic. Use with antibiotic to treat urinary tract infection.
• Drug may be stopped in 3 days if pain is relieved.
• May alter Clinistix or Tes-Tape results. Use Clinitest for accurate urine glucose test results.
• Stop drug if skin or sclera becomes yellow-tinged. May indicate accumulation caused by impaired renal excretion.

---

salsalate
Arthra-G, Disalcid, Mono-Gesic, Salflex, Salgesic, Salsitab

Pregnancy Risk Category: C

HOW SUPPLIED
Tablets: 500 mg, 750 mg
Capsules: 500 mg

MECHANISM OF ACTION
• The salicylic ester of salicylic acid, each molecule of salsalate is hydrolyzed to two molecules of salicylate in vivo.
• Produces analgesia by an ill-defined effect on the hypothalamus (central action) and by blocking generation of pain impulses (peripheral action). The peripheral action may involve inhibition of prostaglandin synthesis.
• Exerts its anti-inflammatory effect by inhibiting prostaglandin synthesis; may also inhibit the synthesis or action of other mediators of the inflammatory response.

INDICATIONS & DOSAGE
Arthritis—
Adults: 3 g P.O. daily, divided b.i.d. or t.i.d. Usual maintenance dose is 2 to 4 g daily.

ADVERSE REACTIONS
EENT: *tinnitus and hearing loss.*
GI: *nausea, vomiting, GI distress, occult bleeding.*
Hepatic: abnormal liver function studies, hepatitis.
Skin: *rash,* bruising.
Other: *hypersensitivity manifested by anaphylaxis and asthma.*

INTERACTIONS
Ammonium chloride (and other urine acidifiers): increased blood levels of salicylates. Monitor for salicylate toxicity.
Antacids in high doses (and other urine alkalinizers): decreased levels of salicylates. Monitor for decreased salicylate effect.
Corticosteroids: compete for binding sites. Monitor for decreased salicylate effect.
Oral anticoagulants: possible increased risk of bleeding. Avoid using together if possible.

NURSING CONSIDERATIONS
• Contraindicated in salsalate hypersensitivity. Use cautiously in GI bleeding, aspirin hypersensitivity, and renal insufficiency. Use cautiously in hypoprothrombinemia, vitamin K deficiency, and bleeding disorders.
• Because of epidemiologic association with Reye's syndrome, the Cen-

---

ters for Disease Control recommends that children or teenagers with chicken pox or influenza-like illness should not be given salicylates.
• Give with food, milk, antacid, or large glass of water to reduce possible GI adverse reactions.
• Therapeutic blood salicylate level in arthritis is 10 to 30 mg/100 ml. Tinnitus may occur at plasma levels of 30 mg/100 ml and above, but this is not a reliable indicator of toxicity, especially in very young and elderly patients.
• Concomitant use with alcohol, steroids, or other NSAIDs may increase risk of GI bleeding.
• May cause an increase in serum levels of AST (SGOT), ALT (SGPT), alkaline phosphatase, and bilirubin.
• Advise patients receiving large doses for extended period of time to watch for petechiae, bleeding gums, and signs of GI bleeding, and to maintain adequate fluid intake. Obtain hemoglobin and prothrombin tests periodically.

---

sodium salicylate
Uracel-5◊

Pregnancy Risk Category: C

HOW SUPPLIED
Tablets: 325 mg◊, 650 mg◊
Tablets (enteric-coated): 324 mg◊, 325 mg◊, 650 mg◊
Injection: 1 g/10 ml

MECHANISM OF ACTION
• Produces analgesia by an ill-defined effect on the hypothalamus (central action) and by blocking generation of pain impulses (peripheral action). The peripheral action may involve inhibition of prostaglandin synthesis.
• Exerts its anti-inflammatory effect by inhibiting prostaglandin synthesis; may also inhibit the synthesis or ac-

tion of other mediators of the inflammatory response.
• Relieves fever by acting on the hypothalamic heat-regulating center to produce peripheral vasodilation. This increases peripheral blood supply and promotes sweating, which leads to loss of heat and to cooling by evaporation.

INDICATIONS & DOSAGE
Minor pain or fever—
Adults: 325 to 650 mg P.O. q 4 to 6 hours, p.r.n., or 500 mg slow I.V. infusion over 4 to 8 hours. Maximum dosage is 1 g daily.
Arthritis—
Adults: 3.5 to 5.4 g P.O. daily in divided doses.

ADVERSE REACTIONS
EENT: *tinnitus, hearing loss.*
GI: *nausea, vomiting, GI distress, occult bleeding.*
Hepatic: abnormal liver function studies, hepatitis.
Skin: *rash,* bruising.
Local: thrombophlebitis (from I.V.).
Other: *hypersensitivity manifested by anaphylaxis and/or asthma.*

INTERACTIONS
Ammonium chloride (and other urine acidifiers): increased blood levels of salicylates. Monitor for salicylate toxicity.
Antacids in large doses (and other urine alkalinizers): decreased levels of salicylates. Monitor for decreased salicylate effect.
Corticosteroids: enhance salicylate elimination. Monitor for decreased salicylate effect.
Oral anticoagulants: increased risk of bleeding. Avoid using together if possible.

NURSING CONSIDERATIONS
• Contraindicated in GI ulcer, GI bleeding, or aspirin hypersensitivity. Use cautiously in hypoprothrombine-

---

Italicized adverse reactions are common or life-threatening.
*Liquid form contains alcohol.   **May contain tartrazine.

mia, vitamin K deficiency, bleeding disorders, and asthma with nasal polyps (may cause severe bronchospasm).
• Use cautiously in CHF and hypertension because of increased sodium load.
• Because of epidemiologic association with Reye's syndrome, the Centers for Disease Control recommends that children or teenagers with chicken pox or influenza-like illness should not be given salicylates.
• Febrile, dehydrated children can develop toxicity rapidly.
• Give with food, milk, antacid, or large glass of water to reduce GI adverse reactions.
• Therapeutic salicylate level in arthritis is 10 to 30 mg/100 ml. Tinnitus may occur at plasma levels of 30 mg/100 ml and above, but this is not a reliable indicator of toxicity, especially in very young and elderly patients.
• Concomitant use with alcohol, steroids, or other NSAIDs may increase risk of GI bleeding.
• May cause an increase in serum levels of AST (SGOT), ALT (SGPT), alkaline phosphatase, and bilirubin.
• Advise patients receiving large doses for extended period of time to watch for petechiae, bleeding gums, and signs of GI bleeding, and to maintain adequate fluid intake. Obtain hemoglobin and prothrombin tests periodically.

sodium thiosalicylate
Asproject, Rexolate, Tusal

Pregnancy Risk Category: C

HOW SUPPLIED
Injection: 50 mg/ml in 2-ml ampules or 30-ml vials.

MECHANISM OF ACTION
• Produces analgesia by an ill-defined effect on the hypothalamus (central action) and by blocking generation of pain impulses (peripheral action). The peripheral action may involve inhibition of prostaglandin synthesis.
• Relieves fever by acting on the hypothalamic heat-regulating center to produce peripheral vasodilation. This increases peripheral blood supply and promotes sweating, which leads to loss of heat and to cooling by evaporation.

INDICATIONS & DOSAGE
Mild pain—
Adults: 50 to 100 mg daily or every other day, I.M. or slow I.V.
Acute gout—
Adults: 100 mg I.M. or slow I.V. q 3 to 4 hours for 2 days; then 100 mg daily.
Rheumatic fever—
Adults: 100 to 150 mg I.M. or slowly I.V. q 4 to 6 hours for 3 days, followed by 100 mg b.i.d. until asymptomatic.

ADVERSE REACTIONS
EENT: *tinnitus and hearing loss.*
GI: *nausea, vomiting, GI distress, occult bleeding.*
Hepatic: abnormal liver function studies, hepatitis.
Skin: *rash,* bruising.
Other: *hypersensitivity manifested by anaphylaxis and/or asthma.*

INTERACTIONS
Ammonium chloride (and other urine acidifiers): increased blood levels of salicylates. Monitor for salicylate toxicity.
Antacids in large doses (and other urine alkalinizers): decreased levels of salicylates. Monitor for decreased salicylate effect.
Corticosteriods: enhance salicylate elimination. Monitor for decreased salicylate effects.
Oral anticoagulants, heparin: increased risk of bleeding. Avoid using together if possible.

NURSING CONSIDERATIONS
• Contraindicated in GI ulcer, GI bleeding, or aspirin sensitivity. Use cautiously in hypoprothrombinemia, vitamin K deficiency, bleeding disorders, and asthma with nasal polyps (may cause severe bronchospasm).
• Because of epidemiologic association with Reye's syndrome, the Centers for Disease Control recommends that children or teenagers with chicken pox or influenza-like illness should not be given salicylates.
• Tinnitus, headache, dizziness, confusion, fever, sweating, thirst, drowsiness, dim vision, hyperventilation, and tachycardia are signs of mild toxicity.
• May cause an increase in serum levels of AST (SGOT), ALT (SGPT), alkaline phosphatase, and bilirubin.
• I.M. route is preferred because of increased risk of complications associated with I.V. use.

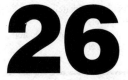

Nonsteroidal anti-inflammatory drugs

diclofenac sodium
fenoprofen calcium
flurbiprofen
ibuprofen
indomethacin
indomethacin sodium trihydrate
ketoprofen
ketorolac tromethamine
meclofenamate
mefenamic acid
naproxen
naproxen sodium
oxyphenbutazone
phenylbutazone
piroxicam
sulindac
tolmetin sodium

COMBINATION PRODUCTS
None.

---

diclofenac sodium
Voltaren, Voltaren SR†

Pregnancy Risk Category: B

HOW SUPPLIED
Tablets (enteric-coated): 25 mg, 50 mg, 75 mg
Tablets (slow-release): 100 mg†
Suppositories: 50 mg†, 100 mg†

MECHANISM OF ACTION
Produces anti-inflammatory, analgesic, and antipyretic effects, possibly through inhibition of prostaglandin synthesis.

INDICATIONS AND DOSAGE
Ankylosing spondylitis—
Adults: 25 mg P.O. q.i.d. and h.s.

Osteoarthritis—
Adults: 50 mg P.O. b.i.d. or t.i.d., or 75 mg P.O. b.i.d.
Rheumatoid arthritis—
Adults: 75 to 100 mg P.O. b.i.d., or 50 to 100 mg P.R. (where available) h.s. as a substitute for the last oral dose of the day. Do not exceed 150 mg daily.

ADVERSE REACTIONS
CNS: anxiety, depression, drowsiness, insomnia, irritability, *headache*.
CV: *CHF*, hypertension.
EENT: *tinnitus*, laryngeal edema, swelling of the lips and tongue.
GI: *abdominal pain or cramps, constipation, diarrhea, indigestion, nausea*, abdominal distention, flatulence, peptic ulceration, GI bleeding, melena, bloody diarrhea, appetite change, colitis.
GU: azotemia, proteinuria, acute renal failure, oliguria, interstitial nephritis, papillary necrosis, nephrotic syndrome, *fluid retention*.
Hepatic: elevated hepatic enzymes, jaundice, hepatitis, hepatotoxicity.
Respiratory: asthma.
Skin: rash, pruritus, urticaria, eczema, dermatitis, alopecia, photosensitivity, bullous eruption, *Stevens-Johnson syndrome (rare)*, allergic purpura.
Other: *anaphylaxis,* anaphylactoid reactions, angioedema.

INTERACTIONS
Anticoagulants (including warfarin): possible increased incidence of bleeding. Monitor patient closely.

Aspirin: concomitant use not recommended by manufacturer.

Cyclosporine, digoxin, lithium, methotrexate: diclofenac may reduce renal clearance of these drugs, and increase risk of toxicity. Monitor patient closely.

Diuretics: diclofenac may decrease the effectiveness of diuretics.

Insulin, oral hypoglycemic agents: diclofenac may alter requirements for hypoglycemic agents. Monitor patient closely.

Potassium-sparing diuretics: diclofenac may enhance potassium retention resulting in increased serum potassium levels.

NURSING CONSIDERATIONS
• Contraindicated in patients with hypersensitivity to diclofenac, aspirin, or other NSAIDs. Also contraindicated in patients with a history of asthma, urticaria, or other allergic reactions after taking these drugs.
• Use cautiously in patients with a history of peptic ulcer disease.
• Elevations of liver tests may occur during therapy. Measure serum transaminase, especially ALT (SGPT) periodically, in patients undergoing long-term therapy. The first serum transaminase measurement should be made no later than 8 weeks after initiation of therapy.
• Tell patient to take diclofenac with milk or meals to minimize G.I. distress.
• Peptic ulceration and GI bleeding have occurred in patients taking NSAIDs despite the absence of GI symptoms. Teach patient the signs and symptoms of GI bleeding, and tell him to contact the doctor if these symptoms appear.
• Teach patient the signs and symptoms of hepatotoxicity, including nausea, fatigue, lethargy, pruritus, jaundice, right upper quadrant tenderness, and flulike symptoms. Tell him to

contact doctor immediately if these symptoms appear.
• Tablets are enteric-coated. Do not crush, break, or chew.

---

fenoprofen calcium
Nalfon

Pregnancy Risk Category: B (D in 3rd trimester)

HOW SUPPLIED
Tablets: 600 mg
Capsules: 200 mg, 300 mg, 600 mg

MECHANISM OF ACTION
Produces anti-inflammatory, analgesic, and antipyretic effects, possibly through inhibition of prostaglandin synthesis.

INDICATIONS & DOSAGE
Rheumatoid arthritis and osteoarthritis—
Adults: 300 to 600 mg P.O. q.i.d. Maximum dosage is 3.2 g daily.
Mild to moderate pain—
Adults: 200 mg P.O. q 4 to 6 hours, p.r.n.

ADVERSE REACTIONS
Blood: prolonged bleeding time, anemia.
CNS: *headache, drowsiness, dizziness.*
CV: peripheral edema.
GI: *epigastric distress, nausea, vomiting, occult blood loss, peptic ulceration,* constipation, anorexia.
GU: reversible renal failure.
Hepatic: elevated enzymes.
Skin: *pruritus,* rash, urticaria.

INTERACTIONS
Aspirin: decreases fenoprofen half-life.
Oral anticoagulants, sulfonylureas: fenoprofen enhances pharmacologic effects of these drugs. Use together cautiously.

Italicized adverse reactions are common or life-threatening.
*Liquid form contains alcohol.   **May contain tartrazine.

NURSING CONSIDERATIONS

• Contraindicated in asthmatics with nasal polyps and in patients with hypersensitivity to aspirin. Use cautiously in elderly patients and patients with GI disorders, angioedema, cardiovascular disease, or hypersensitivity to other noncorticosteroid anti-inflammatory drugs.

• Use cautiously in patients with history of peptic ulcer disease.

• Serious GI toxicity can occur at any time in patients taking chronic NSAID therapy. Teach patient signs and symptoms of GI bleeding. Tell patient to report any signs or symptoms to doctor immediately.

• Concomitant use with aspirin, alcohol, or steroids may increase the risk of GI adverse reactions.

• Tell patient that full therapeutic effect for arthritis may be delayed for 2 to 4 weeks.

• Check renal, hepatic, and auditory function periodically in long-term therapy. Stop drug if abnormalities occur.

• Give dose 30 minutes before or 2 hours after meals. If GI adverse reactions occur, give with milk or meals.

• Prothrombin time may be prolonged in patients receiving coumarin-type anticoagulants. Fenoprofen decreases platelet aggregation and may prolong bleeding time.

---

flurbiprofen
Ansaid

Pregnancy Risk Category: B

HOW SUPPLIED
Tablets: 50 mg, 100 mg

MECHANISM OF ACTION
A NSAID, flurbiprofen interferes with prostaglandin synthesis.

INDICATIONS AND DOSAGE
Rheumatoid arthritis and osteoarthritis—

Adults: 200 to 300 mg P.O. daily, divided b.i.d. to q.i.d.

ADVERSE REACTIONS
CNS: *headache,* anxiety, insomnia, increased reflexes, tremors, amnesia, asthenia, drowsiness, malaise, depression, dizziness.
CV: *edema.*
EENT: rhinitis, tinnitus, visual changes.
GI: *dyspepsia, diarrhea, abdominal pain, nausea,* constipation, *GI bleeding,* flatulence, vomiting.
GU: *symptoms suggesting urinary tract infection.*
Hepatic: elevated liver enzymes.
Skin: rash.
Other: weight changes.

INTERACTIONS
Aspirin: decreased flurbiprofen levels. Concomitant use is not recommended.
Diuretics: possible decreased diuretic effect. Monitor patient closely.
Oral anticoagulants: increased bleeding tendencies. Monitor patient closely.

NURSING CONSIDERATIONS
• Contraindicated in patients with hypersensitivity including asthma or urticaria to aspirin or NSAIDs.

• Serious GI toxicity can occur at any time with patients taking chronic NSAID therapy. Teach patient the signs and symptoms of GI bleeding, and tell him to discontinue the drug and call the doctor if these symptoms appear.

• Elderly or debilitated patients and patients with impaired hepatic or renal function should be closely monitored and probably should receive lower doses. These patients may be at risk for renal toxicity. Periodically monitor renal function.

• Patients receiving long-term therapy should have periodic liver func-

---

tion studies, eye examinations, and hematocrit determinations.
- Tell patient to take drug with food, milk, or antacid if GI upset occurs.
- Advise patient to avoid hazardous activities that require mental alertness until the CNS effects of the drug are known.
- Tell patient to call doctor immediately if edema, substantial weight gain, black stools, skin rash, itching, or visual disturbances occur.

ibuprofen
Aches-N-Pain◇, Advil◇, Apo-Ibuprofen†, Amersol†, Cap-Profen◇, Brufen‡, Genpril◇, Haltran◇, Ibuprin◇, Inflam‡, Medipren Caplets◇, Medipren Tablets◇, Midol-200◇, Motrin, Motrin IB◇, Novoprofen†, Nuprin◇, Pamprin-IB◇, Rafen‡, Rufen, Trendar◇

Pregnancy Risk Category: B (D in 3rd trimester)

HOW SUPPLIED
Tablets: 200 mg◇, 300 mg, 400 mg, 600 mg, 800 mg
Caplets: 200 mg◇
Oral suspension: 100 mg/5 ml

MECHANISM OF ACTION
Produces anti-inflammatory, analgesic, and antipyretic effects, possibly through inhibition of prostaglandin synthesis.

INDICATIONS & DOSAGE
Mild to moderate pain, arthritis, primary dysmenorrhea, gout, postextraction dental pain—
Adults: 200 to 800 mg P.O. t.i.d. or q.i.d. not to exceed 3.2 g/day.

ADVERSE REACTIONS
Blood: prolonged bleeding time.
CNS: *headache, drowsiness, dizziness,* aseptic meningitis.
CV: *peripheral edema.*

EENT: visual disturbances, *tinnitus.*
GI: *epigastric distress, nausea, occult blood loss, peptic ulceration.*
GU: reversible renal failure.
Hepatic: elevated enzymes.
Skin: pruritus, rash, urticaria.
Other: bronchospasm, edema.

INTERACTIONS
Furosemide, thiazide diuretics: ibuprofen may decrease the effectiveness of diuretics.
Oral anticoagulants, lithium: ibuprofen may increase plasma levels or pharmacologic effects of these agents. Monitor for toxicity.

NURSING CONSIDERATIONS
- Contraindicated in asthmatics with nasal polyps. Use cautiously in GI disorders, angioedema, hypersensitivity to other noncorticosteroid anti-inflammatory drugs (including aspirin), hepatic or renal disease, cardiac decompensation, or known intrinsic coagulation defects.
- Use cautiously with history of peptic ulcer disease.
- Tell patient that full therapeutic effect for arthritis may be delayed for 2 to 4 weeks. Analgesic effect occurs at low dosage levels. However, anti-inflammatory effect does not occur at dosages below 400 mg q.i.d.
- Check renal and hepatic function periodically in long-term therapy. Stop drug if abnormalities occur.
- Serious GI toxicity can occur at any time in patients taking chronic NSAID therapy. Teach patient signs and symptoms of GI bleeding, and tell patient to report these to the doctor immediately.
- Give with meals or milk to reduce GI adverse reactions.
- Concomitant use with aspirin, alcohol, or steroids may increase the risk of GI adverse reactions.
- Available OTC in several brands (200 mg strength). Instruct patient not to exceed 1.2 g/day, or self-medicate

---

Italicized adverse reactions are common or life-threatening.
*Liquid form contains alcohol.   **May contain tartrazine.

for extended periods without consulting doctor.

indomethacin
Apo-Indomethacin†, Arthrexin‡, Indameth, Indocid†‡, Indocid SR†, Indocin, Indocin SR, Indomed, Novomethacin†, Rheumacin‡, Zendole

indomethacin sodium trihydrate
Apo-Indomethacin†, Indocid†, Indocin I.V., Indometh, Novomethacin

Pregnancy Risk Category: B (D in 3rd trimester)

HOW SUPPLIED
Capsules: 10 mg, 25 mg, 50 mg, 75 mg
Capsules (sustained-release): 75 mg
Oral suspension: 25 mg/5 ml
Injection: 1-mg vials
Suppositories: 50 mg

MECHANISM OF ACTION
Produces anti-inflammatory, analgesic, and antipyretic effects, possibly through inhibition of prostaglandin synthesis.

INDICATIONS & DOSAGE
Moderate to severe arthritis, ankylosing spondylitis—
Adults: 25 mg P.O. or rectally b.i.d. or t.i.d. with food or antacids; may increase dosage by 25 mg daily q 7 days up to 200 mg daily. Alternatively, sustained-release capsules (75 mg) may be given: 75 mg to start, in the morning or h.s., followed, if necessary, by 75 mg b.i.d.—
Acute gouty arthritis—
Adults: 50 mg P.O. t.i.d. Reduce dose as soon as possible, then stop. Sustained-release capsules shouldn't be used for this condition.
To close a hemodynamically signifi-cant patent ductus arteriosus in premature infants (I.V. form only)—
Neonates under 48 hours: 0.2 mg/kg I.V. followed by 2 doses of 0.1 mg/kg at 12- to 24-hour intervals.
Neonates 2 to 7 days: 0.2 mg/kg I.V. followed by 2 doses of 0.2 mg/kg at 12- to 24-hour intervals.
Over 7 days: 0.2 mg/kg I.V. followed by 2 doses of 0.25 mg/kg at 12- to 24-hour intervals.

ADVERSE REACTIONS
Oral form:
Blood: *hemolytic anemia, aplastic anemia, agranulocytosis,* leukopenia, *thrombocytopenic purpura,* iron deficiency anemia.
CNS: *headache, dizziness,* depression, drowsiness, confusion, peripheral neuropathy, seizures, psychic disturbances, syncope, *vertigo.*
CV: hypertension, *edema.*
EENT: *blurred vision, corneal and retinal damage,* hearing loss, tinnitus.
GI: *nausea, vomiting,* anorexia, *diarrhea, peptic ulceration, severe GI bleeding.*
GU: hematuria, hyperkalemia, acute renal failure.
Hepatic: elevated enzymes.
Skin: pruritus, urticaria, *Stevens-Johnson syndrome.*
Other: hypersensitivity (shocklike symptoms, rash, respiratory distress, angioedema).
I.V. form:
Blood: decreased platelet aggregation.
GI: *bleeding,* vomiting.
GU: *renal dysfunction.*
Metabolic: *hyponatremia, hyperkalemia,* hypoglycemia.

INTERACTIONS
Antihypertensive agents: reduced antihypertensive effect.
Aspirin: decreased blood levels of indomethacin.
Diflunisal, probenecid: decreases indomethacin excretion; watch for in-

creased incidence of indomethacin adverse reactions.
Lithium: increased plasma lithium levels. Monitor for toxicity.
Thiazide diuretics, furosemide: impaired response to both drugs. Avoid using together if possible.
Triamterene: possible nephrotoxicity. Don't use together.

NURSING CONSIDERATIONS
Oral form:
• Contraindicated in aspirin hypersensitivity and GI disorders. Use cautiously in epilepsy, parkinsonism, hepatic or renal disease, cardiovascular disease, infection, and history of mental illness, and in elderly patients.
• Severe headache may occur. Decrease dose if headache persists.
• Has an antipyretic effect.
• Tell patient to notify doctor immediately if any visual or hearing changes occur. Patients taking drug long-term should have regular eye examinations, hearing tests, CBC, and renal function tests to monitor for toxicity.
• Serious GI toxicity can occur at any time in patients taking chronic NSAID therapy. Teach patient signs and symptoms of GI bleeding, and tell patient to report these to the doctor immediately.
• Concomitant use with asprin, alcohol, or steroids may increase the risk of GI adverse reactions.
• CNS adverse reactions are more common and serious in elderly patients.
• Monitor for bleeding in patients receiving anticoagulants.
• Causes sodium retention; monitor for weight gain (especially in elderly patients) and increased blood pressure in patients with hypertension.
• Used as prophylaxis for gout when colchicine is not well tolerated.
• Due to high incidence of side effects when used chronically, indo-

methacin should not be used routinely as an analgesic or antipyretic.
I.V. form:
• Contraindicated in infants with untreated infection, active bleeding, coagulation defects or thrombocytopenia, necrotizing enterocolitis, or impaired renal function.
• Don't administer second or third scheduled dose if anuria or marked oliguria is evident.
• If ductus arteriosus reopens, a second course of one to three doses may be given. If ineffective, surgery may be necessary.
• Monitor carefully for bleeding and for reduced urine output. Stop drug and notify doctor if either occurs.

---

ketoprofen
Orudis, Orudis E†, Orudis SR†‡
Pregnancy Risk Category: B (D in 3rd trimester)

HOW SUPPLIED
Tablets (sustained-release): 200 mg†
Capsules: 25 mg, 50 mg, 75 mg
Suppositories: 100 mg†

MECHANISM OF ACTION
Produces anti-inflammatory, analgesic, and antipyretic effects, possibly through inhibition of prostaglandin synthesis.

INDICATIONS & DOSAGE
Rheumatoid arthritis and osteoarthritis—
Adults: 150 to 300 mg P.O. in three or four divided doses. Usual dosage is 75 mg t.i.d. Maximum dosage is 300 mg/day.
  Alternatively, may use suppository where available—
Adults: 100 mg P.R. b.i.d.; or 1 suppository h.s. (in conjunction with oral ketoprofen during the day).
Mild to moderate pain; dysmenorrhea—

Italicized adverse reactions are common or life-threatening.
*Liquid form contains alcohol.   **May contain tartrazine.

Adults: 25 to 50 mg P.O. q 6 to 8 hours p.r.n.

ADVERSE REACTIONS
Blood: prolonged bleeding time.
CNS: *headache,* dizziness, *CNS inhibition or excitation.*
EENT: tinnitus, visual disturbances.
GI: *nausea, abdominal pain, diarrhea, constipation, flatulence, peptic ulceration,* anorexia, vomiting, stomatitis.
GU: nephrotoxicity, *elevated BUN.*
Hepatic: elevated enzymes.
Skin: rash.

INTERACTIONS
Oral anticoagulants: increased risk of bleeding.
Probenecid, aspirin: decreased plasma levels of ketoprofen.

NURSING CONSIDERATIONS
• Contraindicated in patients who are hypersensitive to aspirin or other NSAIDs.
• Use cautiously in patients with history of peptic ulcer disease or renal dysfunction.
• Serious GI toxicity can occur at any time in patients taking chronic NSAID therapy. Teach patient signs and symptoms of GI bleeding, and tell patient to report these to the doctor immediately.
• Tell patient to report visual or auditory adverse reactions immediately.
• Concomitant use with aspirin, alcohol, or steroids may increase the risk of GI adverse reactions.
• Tell patient that full therapeutic effect may be delayed for 2 to 4 weeks.
• Check renal and hepatic function periodically during long-term therapy.
• Give dose 30 minutes before or 2 hours after meals. If GI adverse reactions occur, give with milk or meals.

ketorolac tromethamine
Toradol
Pregnancy Risk Category: B

HOW SUPPLIED
Injection: 15 mg, 30 mg, 60 mg

MECHANISM OF ACTION
An NSAID that acts by inhibiting the synthesis of prostaglandins.

INDICATIONS & DOSAGE
Short-term management of pain—
Adults: initially, give 30 or 60 mg I.M as a loading dose, followed by half of the loading dose (15 or 30 mg) q 6 hours on a regular schedule or p.r.n. Subsequent dosage should be based on patient response. If pain returns before 6 hours, dosage may be increased by as much as 50% (up to 60 mg); if pain relief continues for 8 to 12 hours, increase interval between doses to q 8 to 12 hours, or reduce dose. The recommended maximum dosage is 150 mg on the first day and 120 mg daily thereafter.

ADVERSE REACTIONS
CNS: *drowsiness,* dizziness, headache, sweating.
CV: edema.
GI: *nausea, dyspepsia, GI pain,* diarrhea.
Local: pain at the injection site.

INTERACTIONS
Lithium: NSAIDs increase lithium levels.
Methotrexate: NSAIDs decrease methotrexate clearance and increase its toxicity.
Salicylates, warfarin: ketorolac may increase the levels of free (unbound) salicylates or warfarin in the blood. Clinical significance is unknown.

NURSING CONSIDERATIONS
• Contraindicated in patients hypersensitive to ketorolac and in patients

---

with the complete or partial triad syndrome: nasal polyps, angioedema, and bronchospasm after use of aspirin or other NSAIDs.

• This drug is intended solely for short-term management of pain. The rate and severity of adverse reactions should be less than that observed in patients taking NSAIDs on a chronic basis.

• Because NSAIDs can cause fluid retention and edema, use ketorolac cautiously in patients with cardiac disease or hypertension.

• Carefully observe patients with coagulopathies and those who are taking anticoagulants. Ketorolac inhibits platelet aggregation and can prolong bleeding time. This effect will disappear within 48 hours of discontinuing the drug. It will not alter platelet count, partial thromboplastin time, or prothrombin time.

• GI ulceration, bleeding, and perforation can occur at any time, with or without warning, in any patient taking NSAIDs on a chronic basis. Teach patients the signs and symptoms of GI bleeding.

• Use with caution in patients with hepatic or renal impairment.

• Use lower initial doses in patients who are over 65 years or who weigh less than 110 lb (50 kg).

• Trace amounts of the drug have been detected in breast milk. Use with caution in breast-feeding women.

---

meclofenamate
Meclomen

Pregnancy Risk Category: B (D in 3rd trimester)

HOW SUPPLIED
Tablets: 50 mg, 100 mg
Capsules: 50 mg, 100 mg

MECHANISM OF ACTION
Produces anti-inflammatory, analgesic, and antipyretic effects, possibly through inhibition of prostaglandin synthesis.

INDICATIONS & DOSAGE
Rheumatoid arthritis and osteoarthritis—
Adults: 200 to 400 mg/day P.O. in three or four equally divided doses.
Mild to moderate pain—
Adults: 50 to 100 mg P.O. q 4 to 6 hours. Maximum dose is 400 mg/day.

ADVERSE REACTIONS
Blood: leukopenia, thrombocytopenia, *agranulocytosis, aplastic anemia.*
CNS: fatigue, malaise, insomnia, *dizziness,* nervousness, *headache.*
CV: edema.
EENT: blurred vision, eye irritation.
GI: *abdominal pain, flatulence, peptic ulceration,* nausea, vomiting, *diarrhea,* hemorrhage.
GU: dysuria, hematuria, nephrotoxicity.
Hepatic: hepatotoxicity.
Skin: rash, urticaria.

INTERACTIONS
Aspirin: decreased plasma levels of meclofenamate.
Oral anticoagulants: enhanced anticoagulant effect. Monitor for toxicity.

NURSING CONSIDERATIONS
• Contraindicated in GI ulceration or inflammation. Use cautiously in hepatic or renal disease, cardiovascular disease, blood dyscrasias, diabetes mellitus, and in asthmatics with nasal polyps.

• Use cautiously in history of peptic ulcer disease. Also use cautiously in elderly patients, who are more likely to experience adverse reactions.

• Serious GI toxicity can occur at any time in patients taking chronic NSAID therapy. Teach patient signs and symptoms of GI bleeding, and tell patient to report these to the doctor immediately.

Italicized adverse reactions are common or life-threatening.
*Liquid form contains alcohol.   **May contain tartrazine.

- Concomitant use with other NSAIDs, alcohol, or steroids may increase the risk of GI adverse reactions.
- Warn patient against activities that require alertness until CNS effects of drug are known.
- Stop drug if rash, visual disturbances, or diarrhea develops.
- Administer with food to minimize GI adverse reactions.
- Almost identical in chemical structure to mefenamic acid.
- False-positive reactions for urine bilirubin using the diazo tablet test have been reported.
- Patients taking drug long-term should receive periodic testing of CBC and renal and hepatic function.

mefenamic acid
Ponstan†, Ponstel

Pregnancy Risk Category: C

HOW SUPPLIED
Capsules: 250 mg

MECHANISM OF ACTION
Produces anti-inflammatory, analgesic, and antipyretic effects, possibly through inhibition of prostaglandin synthesis.

INDICATIONS & DOSAGE
Mild to moderate pain, dysmenorrhea—
Adults and children over 14 years: Initially 500 mg P.O., then 250 mg q 6 hours, p.r.n. Maximum therapy 1 week.

ADVERSE REACTIONS
Blood: leukopenia, thrombocytopenia, *agranulocytosis, aplastic anemia.*
CNS: *drowsiness, dizziness,* nervousness, headache.
CV: edema.
EENT: blurred vision, eye irritation.
GI: nausea, vomiting, *diarrhea, peptic ulceration,* hemorrhage.
GU: dysuria, hematuria, nephrotoxicity.
Hepatic: hepatotoxicity.
Skin: rash, urticaria.

INTERACTIONS
Oral anticoagulants, sulfonylureas, and other drugs that are highly protein bound: increased risk of toxicity.

NURSING CONSIDERATIONS
- Contraindicated in GI ulceration or inflammation. Use cautiously in hepatic or renal disease, cardiovascular disease, blood dyscrasias, diabetes mellitus, and in asthmatics with nasal polyps.
- Use cautiously in history of peptic ulcer disease.
- Serious GI toxicity can occur at any time in patients taking chronic NSAID therapy. Teach patient signs and symptoms of GI bleeding, and tell patient to report these to the doctor immediately.
- Concomitant use with aspirin, alcohol, or steroids may increase the risk of GI adverse reactions.
- Warn patient against hazardous activities that require alertness until CNS effects of the drug are known.
- Severe hemolytic anemia may occur with prolonged use. Monitor CBC periodically.
- Stop drug if rash, visual disturbances, or diarrhea develops.
- Should not be administered for more than 1 week at a time, because risk of toxicity increases.
- Administer with food to minimize GI adverse reactions.
- False-positive reactions for urine bilirubin using the diazo tablet test have been reported.

---

†Available in Canada only.   ‡Available in Australia only.   ◊ Available OTC.

naproxen
Apo-Naproxen†, Naprosyn, Naxen†‡, Novonaprox†

naproxen sodium
Anaprox, Anaprox DS, Naprogesic‡

Pregnancy Risk Category: B (D in 3rd trimester)

HOW SUPPLIED
naproxen
Tablets: 250 mg, 375 mg, 500 mg
Oral suspension: 125 mg/5 ml
Suppositories: 500 mg‡
naproxen sodium
Tablets (film-coated): 275 mg, 550 mg
   Note: 275 mg naproxen sodium = 250 mg naproxen

MECHANISM OF ACTION
Produces anti-inflammatory, analgesic, and antipyretic effects, possibly through inhibition of prostaglandin synthesis.

INDICATIONS & DOSAGE
Arthritis, primary dysmenorrhea (free base)—
Adults: 250 to 500 mg P.O. b.i.d.
   Alternatively, may use suppository where available—
Adults: 500 mg P.R. h.s. with oral naproxen during the day.
   Maximum dosage is 1,250 mg daily.
Mild to moderate pain and for treatment of primary dysmenorrhea (naproxen sodium)—
Adults: 2 tablets (275 mg each tablet) P.O. to start, followed by 275 mg q 6 to 8 hours as needed. Maximum daily dosage should not exceed 1,375 mg.

ADVERSE REACTIONS
Blood: prolonged bleeding time, *agranulocytosis,* neutropenia.
CNS: *headache,* drowsiness, *dizziness,* tinnitus.
CV: peripheral edema, dyspnea.
EENT: visual disturbances.
GI: *epigastric distress, occult blood loss, nausea, peptic ulceration.*
GU: nephrotoxicity.
Hepatic: elevated enzymes.
Skin: *pruritus, rash,* urticaria.

INTERACTIONS
Oral anticoagulants, sulfonylureas, and drugs that are highly protein bound: increased risk of toxicity.

NURSING CONSIDERATIONS
• Contraindicated in asthmatics with nasal polyps.
• Use cautiously in elderly patients and in patients with renal disease, cardiovascular disease, GI disorders, angioedema, and in those allergic to NSAIDs, including aspirin.
• Use cautiously in patients with history of peptic ulcer disease.
• Serious GI toxicity can occur at any time in patients taking chronic NSAID therapy. Teach patient signs and symptoms of GI bleeding, and tell patient to report these to the doctor immediately.
• Concomitant use with aspirin, alcohol, or steroids may increase the risk of GI adverse reactions.
• Monitor CBC and renal and hepatic function periodically during long-term therapy. Advise patient to have periodic eye examinations.
• Tell patient taking naproxen that full therapeutic effect may be delayed 2 to 4 weeks.
• Advise patient to take drug with food or milk to minimize GI upset.
• Warn patient against taking both naproxen and naproxen sodium at the same time because both circulate in the blood as the naproxen anion.
• Naproxen sodium is more rapidly absorbed.

Italicized adverse reactions are common or life-threatening.
*Liquid form contains alcohol.   **May contain tartrazine.

oxyphenbutazone

Pregnancy Risk Category: D

HOW SUPPLIED
Tablets: 100 mg

MECHANISM OF ACTION
Produces anti-inflammatory, analgesic, and antipyretic effects, possibly through inhibition of prostaglandin synthesis.

INDICATIONS & DOSAGE
Pain, inflammation in arthritis, bursitis, superficial venous thrombosis—
Adults: 100 to 200 mg P.O. with food or milk t.i.d. or q.i.d.
Acute gouty arthritis—
Adults: 400 mg initially as single dose, then 100 mg q 4 hours for 4 days or until relief is obtained.
Note: Do not continue therapy for longer than 1 week.

ADVERSE REACTIONS
Blood: *bone marrow suppression (fatal aplastic anemia, agranulocytosis, thrombocytopenia),* hemolytic anemia, leukopenia.
CNS: restlessness, confusion, lethargy.
CV: hypertension, pericarditis, myocarditis, *cardiac decompensation.*
EENT: optic neuritis, blurred vision, retinal hemorrhage or detachment, hearing loss.
GI: *nausea, vomiting, diarrhea, peptic ulceration, occult blood loss.*
GU: proteinuria, hematuria, glomerulonephritis, nephrotic syndrome, *renal failure.*
Hepatic: *hepatitis.*
Metabolic: toxic and nontoxic goiter, respiratory alkalosis, metabolic acidosis.
Skin: petechiae, pruritus, purpura, various dermatoses from rash to *toxic necrotizing epidermolysis.*

INTERACTIONS
Insulin, oral hypoglycemic agents: enhanced hypoglycemic effect. Monitor patient closely.
Oral anticoagulants: enhanced risk of bleeding. Monitor patient closely.
Phenytoin, lithium: increased plasma levels after oxyphenbutazone administration.

NURSING CONSIDERATIONS
• Contraindicated in children under 14 years and in patients with senility, GI ulcer, blood dyscrasias, and renal, hepatic, cardiac, and thyroid disease. Should not be used in patients receiving long-term anticoagulant therapy.
• Tell patient to stop drug and notify doctor immediately if fever, sore throat, mouth ulcers, GI discomfort, black or tarry stools, bleeding, bruising, rash, or weight gain occurs.
• Give with food, milk, or antacids.
• Complete physical examination and laboratory evaluation are recommended before therapy. Warn patient to remain under close medical supervision and to keep all doctor and laboratory appointments.
• Monitor CBC before therapy and after 3 days.
• Record patient's weight and intake/output daily. May cause sodium retention and edema.
• Response should be seen in 2 or 3 days. Stop drug if no response seen within 1 week.
• Patients over 60 years should not receive drug for longer than 1 week.
• Has antipyretic effect.

phenylbutazone

Apo-Phenylbutazone†, Azolid, Butazolidin, Butazone, Intrabutazone†, Novobutazone†

Pregnancy Risk Category: D

HOW SUPPLIED
Tablets: 100 mg
Capsules: 100 mg

MECHANISM OF ACTION
Produces anti-inflammatory, analgesic, and antipyretic effects, possibly through inhibition of prostaglandin synthesis.

INDICATIONS & DOSAGE
Pain, inflammation in arthritis, bursitis, acute superficial thrombophlebitis—
Adults: initially, 100 to 200 mg P.O. t.i.d. or q.i.d. Maximum dosage is 600 mg daily. When improvement is obtained, decrease dosage to 100 mg t.i.d. or q.i.d.
Acute, gouty arthritis—
Adults: 400 mg P.O. initially as single dose, then 100 mg q 4 hours for 4 days or until relief is obtained.
Note: Do not continue therapy for longer than 1 week.

ADVERSE REACTIONS
Blood: *bone marrow suppression (fatal aplastic anemia, agranulocytosis,* thrombocytopenia), hemolytic anemia, leukopenia.
CNS: agitation, confusion, lethargy.
CV: hypertension, edema, pericarditis, myocarditis, *cardiac decompensation.*
EENT: optic neuritis, blurred vision, retinal hemorrhage or detachment, hearing loss.
GI: *nausea, vomiting, diarrhea, peptic ulceration, occult blood loss.*
GU: proteinuria, hematuria, glomerulonephritis, nephrotic syndrome, *renal failure.*
Hepatic: *hepatitis.*
Metabolic: hyperglycemia, toxic and nontoxic goiter, respiratory alkalosis, metabolic acidosis.
Skin: petechiae, pruritus, purpura, various dermatoses from rash to *toxic necrotizing epidermolysis.*

INTERACTIONS
Cholestyramine: may alter phenylbutazone absorption. Give 1 hour before cholestyramine.

Insulin, oral hypoglycemics: enhanced hypoglycemic effect. Monitor patient closely.
Oral anticoagulants: enhanced risk of bleeding. Monitor patient closely.
Phenytoin, lithium: increased plasma levels after oxyphenbutazone administration.

NURSING CONSIDERATIONS
• Contraindicated in children under 14 years and in patients with senility, GI ulcer, blood dyscrasias, and renal, hepatic, cardiac, and thyroid disease. Should not be used in patients receiving long-term anticoagulant therapy.
• Warn patient to stop drug and notify doctor immediately if fever, sore throat, mouth ulcers, GI discomfort, black or tarry stools, bleeding, bruising, rash, or weight gain occurs.
• Give with food, milk, or antacids.
• Complete physical examination and laboratory evaluation are recommended before therapy. Patient should remain under close medical supervision and keep all doctor and laboratory appointments.
• Monitor CBC before therapy and after 3 days.
• Record patient's weight and intake/output daily. May cause sodium retention and edema.
• Response should be seen in 3 to 4 days. Stop drug if no response within 1 week.
• Patients over 60 years should not receive this drug for longer than 1 week.
• This drug has limited use because it produces severe adverse reactions in up to 45% of patients.

piroxicam
Apo-Piroxicam†, Feldene, Novopirocam†
Pregnancy Risk Category: C

HOW SUPPLIED
Capsules: 10 mg, 20 mg

Italicized adverse reactions are common or life-threatening.
*Liquid form contains alcohol.   **May contain tartrazine.

MECHANISM OF ACTION
Produces anti-inflammatory, analgesic, and antipyretic effects, possibly through inhibition of prostaglandin synthesis.

INDICATIONS & DOSAGE
Osteoarthritis and rheumatoid arthritis—
Adults: 20 mg P.O. once daily. If desired, the dose may be divided.

ADVERSE REACTIONS
Blood: prolonged bleeding time, anemia.
CNS: headache, drowsiness, dizziness.
CV: peripheral edema.
GI: *epigastric distress, nausea, occult blood loss, peptic ulceration, severe GI bleeding.*
GU: nephrotoxicity.
Hepatic: elevated enzymes.
Skin: pruritus, rash, urticaria, *photosensitivity.*

INTERACTIONS
Aspirin: decreased plasma levels of piroxicam.
Lithium: increased plasma lithium levels.
Oral anticoagulants: enhanced risk of bleeding. Monitor closely.
Oral hypoglycemic agents: enhanced hypoglycemic effects. Monitor patient closely.

NURSING CONSIDERATIONS
• Contraindicated in asthmatics with nasal polyps. Use cautiously in elderly patients and patients with angioedema, GI disorders, history of renal or peptic ulcer disease, cardiac disease, or hypersensitivity to other nonsteroidal anti-inflammatory drugs.
• Serious GI toxicity can occur at any time in patients taking chronic NSAID therapy. Teach patient signs and symptoms of GI bleeding, and tell him to report these immediately.

• Tell patient full therapeutic effect may be delayed for 2 to 4 weeks.
• Causes adverse skin reactions more often than other drugs in its class. Photosensitivity reactions are the most common.
• Check renal, hepatic, and auditory function periodically during prolonged therapy. Drug should be discontinued if abnormalities occur.
• If GI adverse reactions occur, give with milk or meals.
• The first NSAID approved by the FDA for once-daily administration. Has a longer half-life and, hence, a longer duration of action than other similar drugs.

sulindac
Clinoril

Pregnancy Risk Category: B (D in 3rd trimester)

HOW SUPPLIED
Tablets: 100 mg◊, 150 mg, 200 mg

MECHANISM OF ACTION
Produces anti-inflammatory, analgesic, and antipyretic effects, possibly through inhibition of prostaglandin synthesis.

INDICATIONS & DOSAGE
Osteoarthritis, rheumatoid arthritis, ankylosing spondylitis—
Adults: 150 mg P.O. b.i.d. initially; may increase to 200 mg P.O. b.i.d.
Acute subacromial bursitis or supraspinatus tendinitis, acute gouty arthritis—
Adults: 200 mg P.O. b.i.d. for 7 to 14 days. Dose may be reduced as symptoms subside.

ADVERSE REACTIONS
Blood: prolonged bleeding time, *aplastic anemia.*
CNS: dizziness, headache, nervousness.

EENT: tinnitus, transient visual disturbances.
GI: *epigastric distress, peptic ulceration, occult blood loss, nausea.*
Hepatic: elevated enzymes.
Skin: rash, pruritus.
Other: edema.

INTERACTIONS
None significant.

NURSING CONSIDERATIONS
• Contraindicated in acute asthmatics whose conditions are precipitated by aspirin or other nonsteroidal anti-inflammatory agents; in patients who have active ulcers and GI bleeding. Use cautiously in patients with a history of ulcers and GI bleeding, renal dysfunction, compromised cardiac function, hypertension; or in those receiving oral anticoagulants or oral hypoglycemic agents.
• To reduce GI adverse reactions, give with food, milk, or antacids.
• Serious GI toxicity can occur at any time in patients taking chronic NSAID therapy. Teach patient signs and symptoms of GI bleeding, and tell him to report these immediately.
• Patient should notify doctor and have complete visual examination if any visual disturbances occur.
• Tell patient to notify doctor immediately if prolonged bleeding occurs.
• Drug causes sodium retention, but is thought to have the least effect on the kidneys as compared to all other NSAIDs. Patient should report edema and have blood pressure checked periodically.

---

tolmetin sodium
Tolectin, Tolectin DS

Pregnancy Risk Category: B (D in 3rd trimester)

HOW SUPPLIED
Tablets: 200 mg
Capsules: 400 mg

MECHANISM OF ACTION
Produces anti-inflammatory, analgesic, and antipyretic effects, possibly through inhibition of prostaglandin synthesis.

INDICATIONS & DOSAGE
Rheumatoid arthritis, osteoarthritis, gout, dysmenorrhea, juvenile rheumatoid arthritis—
Adults: 400 mg P.O. t.i.d. or q.i.d. Maximum dosage is 2 g daily.
Children 2 years or older: 15 to 30 mg/kg P.O. daily in divided doses.

ADVERSE REACTIONS
Blood: prolonged bleeding time.
CNS: headache, dizziness, drowsiness.
GI: *epigastric distress, peptic ulceration, occult blood loss, nausea.*
GU: nephrotoxicity, pseudoproteinuria.
Skin: rash, urticaria, pruritus.
Other: sodium retention, edema.

INTERACTIONS
Oral anticoagulants: increased risk of bleeding. Monitor patient closely.

NURSING CONSIDERATIONS
• Contraindicated in asthmatics with nasal polyps. Use cautiously in cardiac and renal disease, GI bleeding, and history of peptic ulcer disease.
• Serious GI toxicity can occur at any time in patients taking chronic NSAID therapy. Teach patient signs and symptoms of GI bleeding, and tell him to report these immediately.
• Give with food, milk, or antacids to reduce GI adverse reactions.
• Tell patient therapeutic effect should begin within 1 week, but full effect may be delayed 2 to 4 weeks.
• Prolonged therapy requires periodic eye examinations and liver and renal function studies.
• Only NSAID reported to falsely elevate urinary protein, causing pseudoproteinuria.

Italicized adverse reactions are common or life-threatening.
*Liquid form contains alcohol.   **May contain tartrazine.

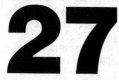

Narcotic and opioid analgesics

alfentanil hydrochloride
buprenorphine hydrochloride
butorphanol tartrate
codeine phosphate
codeine sulfate
fentanyl citrate
hydromorphone hydrochloride
levorphanol tartrate
meperidine hydrochloride
methadone hydrochloride
morphine hydrochloride
morphine sulfate
nalbuphine hydrochloride
oxycodone hydrochloride
oxycodone pectinate
oxymorphone hydrochloride
pentazocine hydrochloride
pentazocine hydrochloride and
   naloxone hydrochloride
pentazocine lactate
propoxyphene hydrochloride
propoxyphene napsylate
sufentanil citrate

COMBINATION PRODUCTS

AMACODONE: hydrocodone bitartrate 5 mg and acetaminophen 500 mg.

BANCAP HC: hydrocodone bitartrate 5 mg and acetaminophen 500 mg.

BUFF-A-COMP NO. 3: codeine phosphate 30 mg, aspirin 325 mg, caffeine 40 mg, and butalbital 50 mg.

DARVOCET-N 50: propoxyphene napsylate 50 mg and acetaminophen 325 mg.

DARVOCET-N 100: propoxyphene napsylate 100 mg and acetaminophen 650 mg.

DARVON COMPOUND: propoxyphene hydrochloride 32 mg, aspirin 389 mg, and caffeine 32.4 mg.

DARVON COMPOUND-65: propoxyphene hydrochloride 65 mg, aspirin 389 mg, and caffeine 32.4 mg.

DARVON-N WITH ASA: propoxyphene napsylate 100 mg and aspirin 325 mg.

DARVON WITH ASA: propoxyphene hydrochloride 65 mg and aspirin 325 mg.

DEMEROL APAP: meperidine hydrochloride 50 mg and acetaminophen 300 mg.

DOLACET: propoxyphene hydrochloride 65 mg and acetaminophen 650 mg.

DOLENE AP-65: propoxyphene hydrochloride 65 mg and acetaminophen 650 mg.

DOLENE COMPOUND-65: propoxyphene hydrochloride 65 mg, aspirin 389 mg, and caffeine 32.4 mg.

DOXAPHENE COMPOUND: propoxyphene hydrochloride 65 mg, aspirin 389 mg, and caffeine 32.4 mg.

DURADYNE DHC: hydrocodone bitartrate 5 mg and acetaminophen 500 mg.

EMPIRIN WITH CODEINE NO. 2: aspirin 325 mg and codeine phosphate 15 mg.

EMPIRIN WITH CODEINE NO. 3: aspirin 325 mg and codeine phosphate 30 mg.

EMPIRIN WITH CODEINE NO. 4: aspirin 325 mg and codeine phosphate 60 mg.

EMPRACET WITH CODEINE NO. 3: codeine phosphate 30 mg and acetaminophen 300 mg.

EMPRACET WITH CODEINE NO. 4: codeine phosphate 60 mg and acetaminophen 300 mg.

FIORINAL WITH CODEINE NO. 1: codeine phosphate 7.5 mg, aspirin 325 mg, caffeine 40 mg, and butalbital 50 mg.

FIORINAL WITH CODEINE NO. 2: codeine phosphate 15 mg, aspirin 325 mg, caffeine 40 mg, and butalbital 50 mg.

FIORINAL WITH CODEINE NO. 3: codeine phosphate 30 mg, aspirin 325 mg, caffeine 40 mg, and butalbital 50 mg.

HYCODAPHEN: hydrocodone bitartrate 5 mg and acetaminophen 500 mg.

INNOVAR (INJECTION): fentanyl (as the citrate) 0.05 mg and droperidol 2.5 mg per ml.

PANTOPON: hydrochlorides of opium alkaloids. 20 mg is therapeutically equivalent to 15 mg morphine.

PERCOCET: acetaminophen 325 mg and oxycodone hydrochloride 5 mg.

PERCODAN: oxycodone hydrochloride 4.5 mg, oxycodone terephthalate 0.38 mg, and aspirin 325 mg.

PERCODAN-DEMI: oxycodone hydrochloride 2.25 mg, oxycodone terephthalate 0.19 mg, and aspirin 325 mg.

PHENAPHEN-650 WITH CODEINE: codeine phosphate 30 mg and acetaminophen 650 mg.

PHENAPHEN WITH CODEINE NO. 3: codeine phosphate 30 mg and acetaminophen 325 mg.

PHENAPHEN WITH CODEINE NO. 4: codeine phosphate 60 mg and acetaminophen 325 mg.

PHRENILIN WITH CODEINE NO. 3: codeine phosphate 30 mg, acetaminophen 325 mg, and butalbital 50 mg.

PROVAL NO. 3: codeine phosphate 30 mg and acetaminophen 325 mg.

TALACEN: pentazocine hydrochloride 25 mg and acetaminophen 650 mg.

TALWIN COMPOUND: pentazocine hydrochloride 12.5 mg and aspirin 325 mg.

TYLENOL WITH CODEINE NO 1: acetaminophen 300 mg and codeine phosphate 7.5 mg.

TYLENOL WITH CODEINE NO. 2: acetaminophen 300 mg and codeine phosphate 15 mg.

TYLENOL WITH CODEINE NO. 3: acetaminophen 300 mg and codeine phosphate 30 mg.

TYLENOL WITH CODEINE NO. 4: acetaminophen 300 mg and codeine phosphate 60 mg.

TYLOX: acetaminophen 500 mg and oxycodone hydrochloride 5 mg.

VICODIN: hydrocodone bitartrate 5 mg and acetaminophen 500 mg.

WYGESIC: propoxyphene hydrochloride 65 mg and acetaminophen 650 mg.

ZYDONE: hydrocodone bitartrate 5 mg and acetaminophen 500 mg.

---

alfentanil hydrochloride
Alfenta
Controlled Substance Schedule II

Pregnancy Risk Category: B (D for prolonged use or use of high doses at term)

HOW SUPPLIED
Injection: 500 mcg/ml

MECHANISM OF ACTION
Binds with opiate receptors at many sites in the CNS (brain, brain stem, and spinal cord), altering both perception of and emotional response to pain through an unknown mechanism.

INDICATIONS & DOSAGE
Adjunct to general anesthetic—
Adults: initially, 8 to 50 mcg/kg I.V., then give increments of 3 to 15 mcg/kg I.V.
As a primary anesthetic—
Adults: initially, 130 to 245 mcg/kg I.V., then give 0.5 to 1.5 mcg/kg/minute I.V.

ADVERSE REACTIONS
CV: hypotension, hypertension, bradycardia, tachycardia.
GI: nausea, vomiting.

Italicized adverse reactions are common or life-threatening.
*Liquid form contains alcohol.   **May contain tartrazine.

Skin: itching.
Other: chest wall rigidity, intraoperative muscle movement, *respiratory depression*.

INTERACTIONS
Alcohol, CNS depressants: additive effects. Use together cautiously.

NURSING CONSIDERATIONS
• Use cautiously in patients with head injury, pulmonary disease, or decreased respiratory reserve.
• Should be administered only by persons specifically trained in the use of I.V. anesthetics.
• As a primary anesthetic, alfentanil may be prescribed for induction of anesthesia for general surgery requiring endotracheal intubation and medical ventilation.
• Discontinue infusion at least 10 to 15 minutes before the end of surgery.
• To administer small volumes of alfentanil accurately, use a tuberculin syringe.
• Keep narcotic antagonist (naloxone) and resuscitative equipment available when giving drug I.V.
• Dose should be reduced in elderly and debilitated patients.
• Monitor postoperative vital signs and bladder function periodically.

---

buprenorphine hydrochloride
Buprenex, Temgesic Injection‡
Controlled Substance Schedule V

Pregnancy Risk Category: C (D for prolonged use or use of high doses at term)

HOW SUPPLIED
Injection: 0.324 mg (equivalent to 0.3 mg base)/ml.

MECHANISM OF ACTION
Binds with opiate receptors at many sites in the CNS (brain, brain stem, and spinal cord), altering both perception of and emotional response to pain through an unknown mechanism.

INDICATIONS & DOSAGE
Moderate to severe pain—
Adults: 0.3 mg I.M. or slow I.V. q 6 hours, p.r.n. or around the clock. May administer up to 0.6 mg/dose if necessary.

ADVERSE REACTIONS
CNS: *dizziness, sedation, headache,* confusion, nervousness, euphoria.
CV: hypotension.
EENT: *miosis.*
GI: *nausea,* vomiting, constipation.
Skin: pruritus, *sweating.*
Other: *respiratory depression,* hypoventilation.

INTERACTIONS
Alcohol, CNS depressants: additive effects. Use together cautiously.
Narcotic analgesics: avoid concomitant use. Possible decreased analgesic effect.

NURSING CONSIDERATIONS
• Use cautiously in head injury and increased intracranial pressure, severe liver and kidney impairment, CNS depression, thyroid irregularities, and prostatic hypertrophy.
• Naloxone will not completely reverse the respiratory depression caused by buprenorphine overdose. Therefore, an overdose may necessitate mechanical ventilation. Larger than customary doses of naloxone (more than 0.4 mg) and doxapram may also be ordered.
• Psychological and physical addiction may occur.
• If dependence occurs, withdrawal symptoms may appear up to 14 days after drug is stopped.
• Possesses narcotic antagonist properties. May precipitate abstinence syndrome in narcotic-dependent patients.

---

†Available in Canada only.   ‡Available in Australia only.   ◊Available OTC.

• S.C. administration not recommended.

• Buprenorphine 0.3 mg is equal to 10 mg morphine and 75 mg meperidine in analgesic potency. Has longer duration of action than morphine or meperidine.

butorphanol tartrate
Stadol

Pregnancy Risk Category: B (D for prolonged use or use of high doses at term)

HOW SUPPLIED
Injection: 1 mg/ml, 2 mg/ml

MECHANISM OF ACTION
Binds with opiate receptors at many sites in the CNS (brain, brain stem, and spinal cord), altering both perception of and emotional response to pain through an unknown mechanism.

INDICATIONS & DOSAGE
Moderate to severe pain—
Adults: 1 to 4 mg I.M. q 3 to 4 hours, p.r.n. or around the clock; or 0.5 to 2 mg I.V. q 3 to 4 hours, p.r.n. or around the clock.

ADVERSE REACTIONS
CNS: *sedation, headache, vertigo, floating sensation,* lethargy, confusion, nervousness, unusual dreams, agitation, euphoria, hallucinations, flushing.
CV: palpitations, fluctuation in blood pressure.
EENT: diplopia, blurred vision.
GI: *nausea,* vomiting, dry mouth, constipation.
Skin: rash, hives, *clamminess, excessive sweating.*
Other: respiratory depression.

INTERACTIONS
Alcohol, CNS depressants: additive effects. Use together cautiously.
Narcotic analgesics: avoid concomi-

tant use. Possible decreased analgesic effect.

NURSING CONSIDERATIONS
• Contraindicated in narcotic addiction; may precipitate narcotic abstinence syndrome. Use cautiously in head injury, increased intracranial pressure, acute myocardial infarction, ventricular dysfunction, coronary insufficiency, respiratory disease or depression, and renal or hepatic dysfunction.
• Psychological and physical addiction may occur.
• Possesses narcotic antagonist properties. May precipitate abstinence syndrome in narcotic-dependent patients.
• Respiratory depression apparently does not increase with increased dosage.
• S.C. route not recommended.
• Also used as a preoperative medication, as the analgesic component of balanced anesthesia, and for relief of postpartum pain.

codeine phosphate
Paveral†

codeine sulfate
Controlled Substance Schedule II
Pregnancy Risk Category: C (D for prolonged use or use of high doses at term)

HOW SUPPLIED
phosphate
Oral solution: 15 mg/5 ml, 10 mg/ml†
Injection: 30 mg/ml, 60 mg/ml
sulfate
Tablets: 15 mg, 30 mg, 60 mg
Soluble tablets: 15 mg, 30 mg, 60 mg

MECHANISM OF ACTION
Binds with opiate receptors at many sites in the CNS (brain, brain stem, and spinal cord), altering both perception of and emotional response to

---

Italicized adverse reactions are common or life-threatening.
*Liquid form contains alcohol.   **May contain tartrazine.

pain through an unknown mechanism. Also supresses the cough reflex by direct action on the cough center in the medulla.

INDICATIONS & DOSAGE
Mild to moderate pain—
Adults: 15 to 60 mg P.O. or 15 to 60 mg (phosphate) S.C. or I.M. q 4 hours, p.r.n. or around the clock.
Children: 3 mg/kg P.O. daily divided q 4 hours, p.r.n. or around the clock.
Nonproductive cough—
Adults: 10 to 20 mg P.O. q 4 to 6 hours. Maximum dosage is 120 mg/24 hours.
Children 6 to 12 years: 5 to 10 mg P.O. q 4 to 6 hours. Maximum dosage is 60 mg/24 hours.
Children 2 to 6 years: 2.5 to 5 mg P.O. q 4 to 6 hours. Do not exceed 30 mg in 24 hours.

ADVERSE REACTIONS
CNS: *sedation, clouded sensorium, euphoria,* dizziness, seizures with large doses.
CV: *hypotension,* bradycardia.
GI: *nausea, vomiting, constipation, dry mouth,* ileus.
GU: *urine retention.*
Skin: pruritus, flushing.
Other: *respiratory depression,* physical dependence.

INTERACTIONS
Alcohol, CNS depressants: additive effects. Use together cautiously.

NURSING CONSIDERATIONS
• Use with extreme caution in head injury, increased intracranial pressure, increased cerebrospinal fluid pressure, hepatic or renal disease, hypothyroidism, Addison's disease, acute alcoholism, seizures, severe CNS depression, bronchial asthma, chronic obstructive pulmonary disease, respiratory depression, and shock; and in elderly or debilitated patients.

• Warn ambulatory patient to avoid activities that require alertness.
• Monitor respiratory and circulatory status and bowel function.
• For full analgesic effect, give before patient has intense pain.
• Codeine and aspirin or acetaminophen are often prescribed together to provide enhanced pain relief.
• Do not administer discolored injection solution.
• If used with general anesthetics, other narcotic analgesics, tranquilizers, sedatives, hypnotics, alcohol, tricyclic antidepressants, or MAO inhibitors, CNS depression is increased. Use together with extreme caution. Monitor patient response.
• An antitussive; don't use when cough is a valuable diagnostic sign or beneficial (as after thoracic surgery).
• Monitor cough type and frequency.
• Constipating effect makes codeine useful in the treatment of diarrhea.
• The abuse potential is much less than that of morphine.

---

fentanyl citrate
Sublimaze
Controlled Substance Schedule II

Pregnancy Risk Category: B (D for prolonged use or use of high doses at term)

HOW SUPPLIED
Injection: 50 mcg/ml

MECHANISM OF ACTION
Binds with opiate receptors at many sites in the CNS (brain, brain stem, and spinal cord), altering both perception of and emotional response to pain through an unknown mechanism.

INDICATIONS & DOSAGE
Adjunct to general anesthetic—
Adults: 0.05 to 0.1 mg I.V. repeated q 2 to 3 minutes, p.r.n. Dose should be reduced in elderly and high-risk patients.

Postoperatively—
Adults: 0.05 to 0.1 mg I.M. q 1 to 2 hours p.r.n.
Preoperatively—
Adults: 0.05 to 0.1 mg I.M. 30 to 60 minutes before surgery.
Children 2 to 12 years: 1.7 to 3.3 mcg/kg I.M.

ADVERSE REACTIONS
CNS: *sedation, somnolence, clouded sensorium, euphoria,* dizziness, seizures with large doses.
CV: *hypotension,* bradycardia.
GI: nausea, vomiting, *constipation,* ileus.
GU: *urine retention.*
Other: *respiratory depression,* muscle rigidity, physical dependence.

INTERACTIONS
Alcohol, CNS depressants: additive effects. Use together cautiously.

NURSING CONSIDERATIONS
• Contraindicated in patients who have received MAO inhibitors within 14 days and who have myasthenia gravis. Use cautiously in head injury, increased cerebrospinal fluid pressure, asthma, chronic obstructive pulmonary disease, respiratory depression, seizures, hepatic or renal disease, hypothyroidism, Addison's disease, alcoholism, increased intracranial pressure, CNS depression, and shock; and in elderly or debilitated patients.
• Keep narcotic antagonist (naloxone) and resuscitative equipment available when giving drug I.V.
• Monitor respirations of newborns exposed to drug during labor.
• Use as postoperative analgesic only in recovery room. Make sure another analgesic is ordered for later use.
• Often used with droperidol (Innovar) to produce neuroleptanalgesia.
• Monitor circulatory and respiratory status carefully.
• Respiratory depression, hypotension, profound sedation, and coma may result if used with other narcotic analgesics, general anesthetics, tranquilizers, alcohol, sedatives, hypnotics, tricyclic antidepressants, or MAO inhibitors. Fentanyl citrate dose should be reduced by one-fourth to one-third. Also give above drugs in reduced dosages.
• For better analgesic effect, give before patient has intense pain.
• When used postoperatively, encourage turning, coughing, and deep breathing to avoid atelectasis.
• Monitor bladder function in postoperative patients.
• Epidural injection or infusion has been used for postoperative analgesia, chronic pain management, or postpartum pain control.
• When administered by epidural injection, monitor the patient closely for respiratory depression. Immediately report a respiratory rate below 12.
• High doses can produce muscle rigidity. This effect can be reversed by administration of neuromuscular blocking agents.

hydromorphone hydrochloride
Dilaudid, Dilaudid HP
Controlled Substance Schedule II

Pregnancy Risk Category: B (D for prolonged use or use of high doses at term)

HOW SUPPLIED
Tablets: 1 mg, 2 mg, 3 mg, 4 mg
Injection: 1 mg/ml, 2 mg/ml, 3 mg/ml, 4 mg/ml, 10 mg/ml
Suppositories: 3 mg

MECHANISM OF ACTION
Binds with opiate receptors at many sites in the CNS (brain, brain stem, and spinal cord), altering both perception of and emotional response to pain through an unknown mechanism. Also suppresses the cough reflex by

---

Italicized adverse reactions are common or life-threatening.
*Liquid form contains alcohol.   **May contain tartrazine.

direct action on the cough center in the medulla.

INDICATIONS & DOSAGE
Moderate to severe pain—
Adults: 1 to 6 mg P.O. q 4 to 6 hours, p.r.n. or around the clock; or 2 to 4 mg I.M., S.C., or I.V. q 4 to 6 hours, p.r.n., or q 6 to 8 hours around the clock (I.V. dose should be given over 3 to 5 minutes); or 3 mg rectal suppository h.s., p.r.n., or q 6 to 8 hours around the clock.
Cough—
Adults: 1 mg P.O. q 3 to 4 hours p.r.n.
Children 6 to 12 years: 0.5 mg P.O. q 3 to 4 hours p.r.n.

ADVERSE REACTIONS
CNS: *sedation, somnolence, clouded sensorium,* dizziness, *euphoria,* seizures with large doses.
CV: *hypotension,* bradycardia.
GI: *nausea, vomiting, constipation,* ileus.
GU: *urine retention.*
Local: induration with repeated S.C. injections.
Other: *respiratory depression,* physical dependence.

INTERACTIONS
Alcohol, CNS depressants: additive effects. Use together cautiously.

NURSING CONSIDERATIONS
• Contraindicated in increased intracranial pressure and status asthmaticus. Use with extreme caution in patients with increased cerebrospinal fluid pressure, respiratory depression, hepatic or renal disease, hypothyroidism, shock, Addison's disease, acute alcoholism, seizures, head injury, severe CNS depression, brain tumor, bronchial asthma, and chronic obstructive pulmonary disease; and in elderly or debilitated patients.
• Warn ambulatory patient to avoid activities that require alertness.

• Monitor respiratory and circulatory status and bowel function.
• Keep narcotic antagonist (naloxone) available.
• Respiratory depression and hypotension can occur with I.V. administration. Give very slowly and monitor constantly. Keep recusitative equipment available.
• Rotate injection sites to avoid induration with S.C. injection.
• Commonly abused narcotic.
• If used with general anesthetics, other narcotic analgesics, tranquilizers, sedatives, hypnotics, alcohol, tricyclic antidepressants, or MAO inhibitors, CNS depression is increased. Hydromorphone dose should be reduced. Use together with extreme caution. Monitor patient response.
• Oral dosage form is particularly convenient for patients with chronic pain because tablets are available in 1 mg, 2 mg, 3 mg, and 4 mg. This enables these patients to titrate their own dose.
• For better analgesic effect, give before patient has intense pain.
• When used postoperatively, encourage turning, coughing, and deep breathing to avoid atelectasis.
• May worsen or mask gallbladder pain.
• Dilaudid HP, a highly concentrated form (10 mg/ml), may be administered in smaller volumes, preventing the discomfort associated with large-volume I.M. or S.C. injections.

---

levorphanol tartrate
Levo-Dromoran
Controlled Substance Schedule II

Pregnancy Risk Category: B (D for prolonged use or use of high doses at term)

HOW SUPPLIED
Tablets: 2 mg
Injection: 2 mg/ml

MECHANISM OF ACTION
Binds with opiate receptors at many sites in the CNS (brain, brain stem, and spinal cord), altering both perception of and emotional response to pain through an unknown mechanism.

INDICATIONS & DOSAGE
Moderate to severe pain—
Adults: 2 to 3 mg P.O. or S.C. q 6 to 8 hours, p.r.n. or around the clock.

ADVERSE REACTIONS
CNS: *sedation, somnolence, clouded sensorium,* dizziness, *euphoria,* seizures with large doses.
CV: *hypotension,* bradycardia.
GI: *nausea, vomiting, constipation,* ileus.
GU: urine retention.
Other: *respiratory depression,* physical dependence.

INTERACTIONS
Alcohol, CNS depressants: additive effects. Use together cautiously.

NURSING CONSIDERATIONS
• Contraindicated in acute alcoholism, bronchial asthma, increased intracranial pressure, respiratory depression, and anoxia. Use with extreme caution in hepatic or renal disease, hypothyroidism, Addison's disease, seizures, head injury, severe CNS depression, brain tumor, chronic obstructive pulmonary disease, and shock; and in elderly or debilitated patients.
• Warn ambulatory patient to avoid activities that require alertness.
• Monitor circulatory and respiratory status and bowel function.
• Warn patient drug has bitter taste.
• Protect from light.
• Keep narcotic antagonist (naloxone) available.
• If used with general anesthetics, other narcotic analgesics, tranquilizers, sedatives, hypnotics, alcohol, tricyclic antidepressants, or MAO inhibitors, CNS depression is increased. Reduce levorphanol dose. Use together with extreme caution. Monitor patient response.
• For better analgesic effect, give before patient has intense pain.
• When used postoperatively, encourage turning, coughing, and deep breathing to avoid atelectasis.

---

meperidine hydrochloride (pethidine hydrochloride)
Demerol
Controlled Substance Schedule II

Pregnancy Risk Category: B (D for prolonged use or use of high doses at term)

HOW SUPPLIED
Tablets: 50 mg, 100 mg
Syrup: 50 mg/ml
Injection: 10 mg/ml, 25 mg/ml, 50 mg/ml, 75 mg/ml, 100 mg/ml

MECHANISM OF ACTION
Binds with opiate receptors at many sites in the CNS (brain, brain stem, and spinal cord), altering both perception of and emotional response to pain through an unknown mechanism.

INDICATIONS & DOSAGE
Moderate to severe pain—
Adults: 50 to 150 mg P.O., I.M., or S.C. q 3 to 4 hours, p.r.n. or around the clock; or 15 to 35 mg/hour by continuous I.V. infusion.
Children: 1 to 1.8 mg/kg P.O., I.M., or S.C. q 4 to 6 hours. Maximum dosage is 100 mg q 4 hours, p.r.n. or around the clock.
Preoperatively—
Adults: 50 to 100 mg I.M. or S.C. 30 to 90 minutes before surgery.
Children: 1 to 2.2 mg/kg I.M. or S.C. 30 to 90 minutes before surgery.

ADVERSE REACTIONS
CNS: *sedation, somnolence, clouded sensorium, euphoria,* paradoxical ex-

---

Italicized adverse reactions are common or life-threatening.
*Liquid form contains alcohol.   **May contain tartrazine.

citement, tremors, dizziness, seizures with large doses.
CV: *hypotension,* bradycardia, tachycardia.
GI: *nausea, vomiting, constipation,* ileus.
GU: *urine retention.*
Local: pain at injection site, local tissue irritation and induration after S.C. injection; phlebitis after I.V. injection.
Other: *respiratory depression,* physical dependence, muscle twitching.

INTERACTIONS
Alcohol, CNS depressants: additive effects. Use together cautiously.
MAO inhibitors, barbiturates, isoniazid: increased CNS excitation or depression can be severe or fatal. Don't use together.
Phenytoin: decreased blood levels of meperidine. Monitor for decreased analgesia.

NURSING CONSIDERATIONS
• Contraindicated in patients who have received MAO inhibitors within 14 days. Use with extreme caution in patients with increased intracranial pressure, increased cerebrospinal fluid pressure, shock, CNS depression, head injury, asthma, chronic obstructive pulmonary disease, respiratory depression, supraventricular tachycardias, seizures, acute abdominal conditions, hepatic or renal disease, hypothyroidism, Addison's disease, urethral stricture, prostatic hypertrophy, and alcoholism; in children under 12 years; and in elderly or debilitated patients.
• May be used in some patients allergic to morphine.
• Meperidine and active metabolite normeperidine accumulate. Monitor for increased toxic effect, especially in patients with impaired renal function.
• Because meperidine toxicity often appears after several days of treat-

ment, this drug is not recommended for treatment of chronic pain.
• Meperidine may be given slow I.V., preferably as a diluted solution. S.C. injection is very painful.
• Keep narcotic antagonist (naloxone) available when giving this drug I.V.
• Warn ambulatory patient to avoid activities that require alertness.
• Monitor respirations of newborns exposed to drug during labor. Have resuscitation equipment and naloxone available.
• P.O. dose less than half as effective as parenteral dose. Give I.M. if possible. When changing from parenteral to P.O. route, dose should be increased.
• Syrup has local anesthetic effect. Give with full glass of water.
• Chemically incompatible with barbiturates. Don't mix together.
• Monitor respiratory and cardiovascular status carefully. Don't give if respirations are below 12/minute or if change in pupils is noted.
• Monitor bladder function in postoperative patients.
• Monitor bowel function. Patient may need a laxative or stool softener.
• Watch for withdrawal symptoms if stopped abruptly after long-term use.
• If used with other narcotic analgesics, general anesthetics, phenothiazines, sedatives, hypnotics, tricyclic antidepressants, or alcohol, respiratory depression, hypotension, profound sedation, or coma may occur. Reduce meperidine dose. Use together with extreme caution.
• For better analgesic effect, give before patient has intense pain. Initially, administration on a fixed schedule may result in better pain control with a smaller daily dose by reducing patient anxiety. Once good pain control has been achieved, adjust scheduling per individual requirements.
• Alternating a centrally active narcotic with a more peripherally active

nonnarcotic analgesic (aspirin, acetaminophen, or NSAID) may improve pain control while requiring lower narcotic doses.
• When used postoperatively, encourage turning, coughing, and deep breathing to avoid atelectasis.

methadone hydrochloride
Dolophine, Methadose, Physeptone‡
Controlled Substance Schedule II

Pregnancy Risk Category: B (D for prolonged use or use of high doses at term)

HOW SUPPLIED
Tablets: 5 mg, 10 mg
Dispersible tablets (for methadone maintenance therapy): 40 mg
Oral solution: 5 mg/5 ml, 10 mg/5 ml, 10 mg/ml (concentrate)
Injection: 10 mg/ml

MECHANISM OF ACTION
Binds with opiate receptors at many sites in the CNS (brain, brain stem, and spinal cord), altering both perception of and emotional response to pain through an unknown mechanism.

INDICATIONS & DOSAGE
Severe pain—
Adults: 2.5 to 10 mg P.O., I.M., or S.C. q 6 to 8 hours, p.r.n. or around the clock.
Narcotic abstinence syndrome—
Adults: 15 to 40 mg P.O. daily (highly individualized). Maintenance dosage is 20 to 120 mg P.O. daily. Adjust dose as needed. Daily dosages greater than 120 mg require special state and federal approval.

ADVERSE REACTIONS
CNS: *sedation, somnolence, clouded sensorium, euphoria,* dizziness, seizures with large doses.
CV: *hypotension,* bradycardia.

GI: *nausea, vomiting, constipation,* ileus.
GU: *urine retention.*
Local: pain at injection site, tissue irritation, induration following S.C. injection.
Other: *respiratory depression,* decreased libido, sweating, physical dependence.

INTERACTIONS
Alcohol, CNS depressants: additive effects. Use together cautiously.
Ammonium chloride and other urine acidifiers, phenytoin: may reduce methadone effect. Monitor for decreased pain control.
Rifampin: withdrawal symptoms; reduced blood levels of methadone. Use together cautiously.

NURSING CONSIDERATIONS
• Use with extreme caution in elderly or debilitated patients, or in patients with acute abdominal conditions, severe hepatic or renal impairment, hypothyroidism, Addison's disease, prostatic hypertrophy, urethral stricture, head injury, increased intracranial pressure, asthma, chronic obstructive pulmonary disease, respiratory depression, and CNS depression.
• When used as an adjunct in the treatment of narcotic addiction ("maintenance"), withdrawal will usually be delayed and mild.
• Safe use as maintenance drug in adolescent addicts not established.
• Once-daily dosage is adequate for maintenance. No advantage to divided doses.
• Oral liquid form legally required in maintenance programs. Completely dissolve tablets in 120 ml of orange juice or powdered citrus drink.
• Oral dose is half as potent as injected dose.
• Rotate injection sites.
• Has cumulative effect; marked sedation can occur after repeated doses.
• Monitor circulatory and respiratory

Italicized adverse reactions are common or life-threatening.
*Liquid form contains alcohol.   **May contain tartrazine.

status and bladder and bowel function. Patient may need laxatives or stool softeners.

• Warn ambulatory patient to avoid activities that require alertness.

• Regimented scheduling (around the clock) beneficial in severe, chronic pain. When used for severe, chronic pain, tolerance may develop with long-term use, requiring a higher dose to achieve the same degree of analgesia. This is *not* a sign of addiction.

• Patient treated for narcotic abstinence syndrome will usually require an additional analgesic if pain control is necessary.

• Use with general anesthetics, tranquilizers, sedatives, hypnotics, alcohol, tricyclic antidepressants, or MAO inhibitors may cause respiratory depression, hypotension, profound sedation, or coma. Use together with extreme caution. Monitor patient response.

• Liquid form available for patients who are unable to swallow tablets.

---

morphine hydrochloride
Morphitec†, M.O.S.†, M.O.S.-S.R.†

morphine sulfate
Astramorph, Astramorph P.F., Duramorph PF, Epimorph†, Morphine H.P.†, MS Contin, MSIR, RMS Uniserts, Roxanol, Roxanol SR, Statex†

Controlled Substance Schedule II

Pregnancy Risk Category: B (D for prolonged use or use of high doses at term)

HOW SUPPLIED
hydrochloride
Tablets: 10 mg†, 20 mg†, 40 mg†, 60 mg†
Oral solution†: 1 mg/ml, 5 mg/ml, 10 mg/ml, 20 mg/ml, 50 mg/ml
Syrup: 1 mg/ml†, 5 mg/ml†
Suppositories: 20 mg†, 30 mg†

sulfate
Tablets: 15 mg, 30 mg
Tablets (controlled-release): 30 mg, 60 mg
Soluble tablets: 10 mg, 15 mg, 30 mg
Oral solution: 10 mg/5 ml, 20 mg/5 ml, 20 mg/ml (concentrate)
Syrup: 1 mg/ml, 5 mg/ml
Injection (with preservative): 1 mg/ml, 2 mg/ml, 3 mg/ml, 4 mg/ml, 5 mg/ml, 8 mg/ml, 10 mg/ml, 15 mg/ml
Injection (without preservative): 500 mcg/ml, 1 mg/ml
Suppositories: 5 mg, 10 mg, 20 mg, 30 mg

MECHANISM OF ACTION
Binds with opiate receptors at many sites in the CNS (brain, brain stem, and spinal cord), altering both perception of and emotional response to pain through an unknown mechanism.

INDICATIONS & DOSAGE
Severe pain—
Adults: 4 to 15 mg S.C. or I.M.; or 30 to 60 mg P.O. or rectally q 4 hours, p.r.n. or around the clock. May be injected slow I.V. (over 4 to 5 minutes) diluted in 4 to 5 ml water for injection. May also administer controlled-release tablets q 8 to 12 hours. As an epidural injection, 5 mg via an epidural catheter q 24 hours.
Children: 0.1 to 0.2 mg/kg dose S.C. or I.M. q 4 hours. Maximum dosage is 15 mg.

In some situations, morphine may be administered by continuous I.V. infusion or by intraspinal and intrathecal injection.

ADVERSE REACTIONS
CNS: *sedation, somnolence, clouded sensorium, euphoria,* seizures with large doses, dizziness, *nightmares* (with long-acting oral forms).
CV: *hypotension,* bradycardia.
GI: *nausea, vomiting, constipation,* ileus.

---

†Available in Canada only.　　　　‡Available in Australia only.　　　　◇Available OTC.

GU: *urine retention.*
Other: *respiratory depression, physical dependence, pruritus and skin flushing (with epidural administration).*

INTERACTIONS
Alcohol, CNS depressants: additional effects. Use together cautiously.

NURSING CONSIDERATIONS
• Use with extreme caution in head injury, increased intracranial pressure, seizures, asthma, chronic obstructive pulmonary disease, alcoholism, prostatic hypertrophy, severe hepatic or renal disease, acute abdominal conditions, hypothyroidism, Addison's disease, increased cerebrospinal fluid pressure, urethral stricture, cardiac arrhythmias, reduced blood volume, and toxic psychosis; and in elderly or debilitated patients.
• Warn ambulatory patient to avoid activities that require alertness.
• Monitor circulatory and respiratory status and bladder and bowel function. Don't give if respirations are below 12/minute.
• Constipation often severe with maintenance. Make sure stool softener or other laxative is ordered.
• Drug of choice in relieving pain of myocardial infarction. May cause transient decrease in blood pressure.
• Keep narcotic antagonist (naloxone) and resuscitative equipment available.
• Respiratory depression, hypotension, profound sedation, or coma may occur if used with general anesthetics, tranquilizers, sedatives, hypnotics, alcohol, tricyclic antidepressants, or MAO inhibitors. Reduce morphine dose. Use together with extreme caution. Monitor patient response.
• Regimented scheduling (around the clock) beneficial in severe, chronic pain.
• When used postoperatively, encourage turning, coughing, and deep breathing to avoid atelectasis.
• Oral solutions of various concentrations are available, as well as an intensified oral solution (20 mg/ml). Be sure to note the strength you are administering.
• Do not crush or break controlled-release tablets.
• Sublingual administration may be ordered. Measure out oral solution with tuberculin syringe. Administer dose a few drops at a time to allow maximal sublingual absorption and to minimize swallowing.
• Rectal suppository available in 5-, 10-, and 20-mg dosages. Refrigeration is not necessary. Note that in some patients, rectal and oral absorption may not be equivalent.
• Preservative-free preparations now available for epidural and intrathecal administration. The popularity of the epidural route is increasing.
• When given epidurally, monitor closely for respiratory depression up to 24 hours after the injection. Check respiratory rate and depth every 30 to 60 minutes for 24 hours.
• May worsen or mask gallbladder pain.

nalbuphine hydrochloride
Nubain

Pregnancy Risk Category: B (D for prolonged use or use of high doses at term)

HOW SUPPLIED
Injection: 10 mg/ml, 20 mg/ml

MECHANISM OF ACTION
Binds with opiate receptors at many sites in the CNS (brain, brain stem, and spinal cord), altering both perception of and emotional response to pain through an unknown mechanism.

INDICATIONS & DOSAGE
Moderate to severe pain—
Adults: 10 to 20 mg S.C., I.M., or

I.V. q 3 to 6 hours, p.r.n. or around the clock. Maximum daily dosage is 160 mg.

ADVERSE REACTIONS
CNS: *headache, sedation,* dizziness, nervousness, depression, restlessness, crying, euphoria, hostility, unusual dreams, confusion, hallucinations, delusions.
GI: cramps, dyspepsia, bitter taste, *nausea, vomiting,* constipation.
GU: urinary urgency.
Skin: itching; burning; urticaria; *sweaty, clammy feeling.*
Other: *respiratory depression.*

INTERACTIONS
Alcohol, CNS depressants: additive effects. Use together cautiously.
Narcotic analgesics: avoid concomitant use. Possible decreased analgesic effect.

NURSING CONSIDERATIONS
• Contraindicated in emotional instability, history of drug abuse, head injury, or increased intracranial pressure. Use cautiously in hepatic and renal disease. These patients may overreact to customary doses.
• Causes respiratory depression, which at 10 mg is equal to the respiratory depression produced by 10 mg of morphine.
• Montior respirations of newborns exposed to the drug during labor.
• Respiratory depression can be reversed with naloxone. Keep recusitative equipment available, particulary when administering I.V.
• Psychological and physical dependence may occur.
• Monitor circulatory and respiratory status and bladder and bowel function. Don't give if respirations are below 12/minute.
• Constipation often severe with maintenance. Make sure stool softener or other laxative is ordered.
• Also acts as a narcotic antagonist;

may precipitate abstinence syndrome. When administering to patients who have chronically received opiates, administer 25% of the usual dose initially. Observe for signs of withdrawal.
• Warn patient to avoid hazardous activities that require alertness until CNS effects of the drug are known.

---

oxycodone hydrochloride
Endone‡, Roxicodone, Supeudol†
Controlled Substance Schedule II

oxycodone pectinate
Proladone‡

Pregnancy Risk Category: B (D for prolonged use or use of high doses at term)

HOW SUPPLIED
hydrochloride
Tablets: 5 mg
Oral solution: 5 mg/ml
Suppositories: 10 mg, 20 mg
pectinate
Suppositories: 30 mg‡

MECHANISM OF ACTION
Binds with opiate receptors at many sites in the CNS (brain, brain stem, and spinal cord), altering both perception of and emotional response to pain through an unknown mechanism.

INDICATIONS & DOSAGE
Moderate to severe pain—
Adults: available in combination with other drugs, such as aspirin (Codoxy, Percodan, Percodan-Demi) or acetaminophen (Percocet, Tylox). One to 2 tablets P.O. q 6 hours, p.r.n. or around the clock. Or 5 mg (5 ml) of oxycodone oral solution or tablets P.O. q 6 hours.
Adults: (Supeudol) 1 to 3 suppositories rectally daily, p.r.n. or around the clock.
Children: (Percodan-Demi) ¼ to ½

---

tablet P.O. q 6 hours, p.r.n. or around the clock.

ADVERSE REACTIONS
CNS: *sedation, somnolence, clouded sensorium, euphoria,* dizziness, seizures with large doses.
CV: *hypotension,* bradycardia.
GI: *nausea, vomiting, constipation,* ileus.
GU: *urine retention.*
Other: *respiratory depression,* physical dependence.

INTERACTIONS
Alcohol, CNS depressants: additive effects. Use together cautiously.
Anticoagulants: oxycodone hydrochloride products containing aspirin may increase anticoagulant effect. Monitor clotting times. Use together cautiously.

NURSING CONSIDERATIONS
• Use with extreme caution in head injury, increased intracranial pressure, increased cerebrospinal fluid pressure, seizures, asthma, chronic obstructive pulmonary disease, alcoholism, prostatic hypertrophy, severe hepatic or renal disease, acute abdominal conditions, urethral stricture, hypothyroidism, Addison's disease, cardiac arrhythmias, reduced blood volume, and toxic psychosis; and in elderly or debilitated patients.
• Don't give to children, except for Percodan-Demi and Percocet-Demi.
• Warn ambulatory patient to avoid activities that require alertness.
• Monitor circulatory and respiratory status and bladder and bowel function. Do not give if respirations are below 12/minute.
• Patient may require laxative or stool softener.
• For full analgesic effect, give before patient has intense pain.
• Give after meals or with milk.
• If used with general anesthetics, other narcotic analgesics, tranquilizers, sedatives, hypnotics, alcohol, tricyclic antidepressants, or MAO inhibitors, CNS depression is increased. Reduce oxycodone dose. Use together with extreme caution. Monitor patient's response.
• Single-agent oxycodone solution or tablets are especially good for patients who shouldn't take aspirin or acetaminophen.

---

oxymorphone hydrochloride
Numorphan
Controlled Substance Schedule II

Pregnancy Risk Category: B (D for prolonged use or use of high doses at term)

HOW SUPPLIED
Injection: 1 mg/ml, 1.5 mg/ml
Suppositories: 5 mg

MECHANISM OF ACTION
Binds with opiate receptors at many sites in the CNS (brain, brain stem, and spinal cord), altering both perception of and emotional response to pain through an unknown mechanism.

INDICATIONS & DOSAGE
Moderate to severe pain—
Adults: 1 to 1.5 mg I.M. or S.C. q 4 to 6 hours, p.r.n. or around the clock; or 0.5 mg I.V. q 4 to 6 hours, p.r.n. or around the clock; or 2.5 to 5 mg rectally q 4 to 6 hours, p.r.n. or around the clock.

ADVERSE REACTIONS
CNS: *sedation, somnolence, clouded sensorium, euphoria,* dizziness, seizures with large doses.
CV: *hypotension,* bradycardia.
GI: *nausea, vomiting, constipation,* ileus.
GU: *urine retention.*
Other: *respiratory depression,* physical dependence.

Italicized adverse reactions are common or life-threatening.
*Liquid form contains alcohol.   **May contain tartrazine.

INTERACTIONS
Alcohol, CNS depressants: additive effects. Use together cautiously.

NURSING CONSIDERATIONS
• Use with extreme caution in head injury, increased intracranial pressure, seizures, asthma, chronic obstructive pulmonary disease, alcoholism, increased cerebrospinal fluid pressure, acute abdominal conditions, prostatic hypertrophy, severe hepatic or renal disease, urethral stricture, CNS depression, respiratory depression, hypothyroidism, Addison's disease, cardiac arrhythmias, reduced blood volume, and toxic psychosis; and in elderly or debilitated patients.
• Warn ambulatory patient to avoid activities that require alertness.
• Monitor cardiovascular and respiratory status and bladder and bowel function. Don't give if respirations are below 12/minute.
• Patient may need laxative or stool softener.
• Well absorbed rectally. Alternative to narcotics with more limited dosage forms.
• Keep narcotic antagonist (naloxone) and resuscitative equipment available.
• If used with general anesthetics, tranquilizers, sedatives, hypnotics, alcohol, tricyclic antidepressants, or MAO inhibitors, CNS depression is increased. Reduce oxymorphone dose. Use together with extreme caution. Monitor patient's response.
• For better analgesic effect, give before patient has intense pain.
• When used postoperatively, encourage turning, coughing, and deep breathing to avoid atelectasis.
• Not intended for mild to moderate pain. May worsen gallbladder pain.

pentazocine hydrochloride
Fortral†‡, Talwin†

pentazocine hydrochloride and naloxone hydrochloride
Talwin Nx
Controlled Substance Schedule IV

pentazocine lactate
Fortral‡, Talwin
Controlled Substance Schedule IV

Pregnancy Risk Category: B (D for prolonged use or use of high doses at term)

HOW SUPPLIED
pentazocine hydrochloride
Tablets: 25 mg‡, 50 mg†‡
pentazocine hydrochloride and naloxone hydrochloride
Tablets: 50 mg pentazocine hydrochloride and 500 mcg naloxone hydrochloride
pentazocine lactate
Injection: 30 mg/ml

MECHANISM OF ACTION
Binds with opiate receptors at many sites in the CNS (brain, brain stem, and spinal cord), altering both perception of and emotional response to pain through an unknown mechanism.

INDICATIONS & DOSAGE
Moderate to severe pain—
Adults: 50 to 100 mg P.O. q 3 to 4 hours, p.r.n. or around the clock. Maximum oral dosage is 600 mg daily. Alternatively, may give 30 mg I.M., I.V., or S.C. q 3 to 4 hours, p.r.n. or around the clock. Maximum parenteral dosage is 360 mg daily. Single doses above 30 mg I.V. or 60 mg I.M. or S.C. not recommended.

ADVERSE REACTIONS
CNS: *sedation,* visual disturbances, *hallucinations,* drowsiness, *dizziness, light-headedness,* confusion, eu-

---

phoria, headache, *psychotomimetic effects.*
GI: *nausea, vomiting,* dry mouth, constipation.
GU: *urine retention.*
Local: induration, nodules, sloughing, and sclerosis of injection site.
Other: *respiratory depression,* physical and psychological dependence.

INTERACTIONS
Alcohol, CNS depressants: additive effects. Use together cautiously.
Narcotic analgesics: avoid concomitant use. Possible decreased analgesic effect.

NURSING CONSIDERATIONS
• Contraindicated in emotional instability, drug abuse, head injury, and increased intracranial pressure. Use cautiously in hepatic or renal disease.
• Tablets not well absorbed.
• Possesses narcotic antagonist properties. May precipitate abstinence syndrome in narcotic-dependent patients.
• Psychological and physical dependence may occur.
• Respiratory depression can be reversed with naloxone.
• Do not mix in same syringe with soluble barbiturates.
• Warn ambulatory patient to avoid activities that require alertness.
• Talwin Nx, the oral pentazocine available in the U.S., contains the narcotic antagonist naloxone. This prevents illicit I.V. use.

propoxyphene hydrochloride (dextropropoxyphene hydrochloride)
Darvon, Dolene, Doraphen, Doxaphene, Novopropoxyn†, Pro-Pox, Propoxycon, 642†

propoxyphene napsylate (dextropropoxyphene napsylate)
Darvocet-N, Darvon-N, Doloxene‡, Doloxene Co‡

Controlled Substance Schedule IV
Pregnancy Risk Category: C (D for prolonged use)

HOW SUPPLIED
hydrochloride
Capsules: 32 mg, 65 mg
napsylate
Tablets: 100 mg
Capsules: 50 mg, 100 mg
Oral suspension: 10 mg/ml

MECHANISM OF ACTION
Binds with opiate receptors at many sites in the CNS (brain, brain stem, and spinal cord), altering both perception of and emotional response to pain through an unknown mechanism.

INDICATIONS & DOSAGE
Mild to moderate pain—
Adults: 65 mg (hydrochloride) P.O. q 4 hours p.r.n.
Mild to moderate pain—
Adults: 100 mg (napsylate) P.O. q 4 hours p.r.n.

ADVERSE REACTIONS
CNS: *dizziness,* headache, sedation, euphoria, paradoxical excitement, insomnia.
GI: nausea, vomiting, constipation.
Other: psychological and physical dependence.

Italicized adverse reactions are common or life-threatening.
*Liquid form contains alcohol.   **May contain tartrazine.

INTERACTIONS
Alcohol, CNS depressants: additive effects. Use together cautiously.

NURSING CONSIDERATIONS
• Not to be prescribed for maintenance purposes in narcotic addiction.
• Warn ambulatory patient to avoid activities that require alertness until CNS effects of the drug are known.
• Warn patient not to exceed recommended dosage.
• Do not use caffeine or amphetamines to treat overdose; may cause fatal seizures. Use narcotic antagonist instead.
• May cause false decreases in urinary steroid excretion tests.
• 65 mg propoxyphene hydrochloride equals 100 mg propoxyphene napsylate.
• Can be considered a mild narcotic analgesic, but pain relief is equivalent to aspirin. Often used with aspirin or acetaminophen to maximize analgesia.
• Advise patient to limit alcohol intake when taking this drug.

---

sufentanil citrate
Sufenta
Controlled Substance Schedule II

Pregnancy Risk Category: C (D for prolonged use or use of high doses at term)

HOW SUPPLIED
Injection: 50 mcg/ml

MECHANISM OF ACTION
Binds with opiate receptors at many sites in the CNS (brain, brain stem, and spinal cord), altering both perception of and emotional response to pain through an unknown mechanism.

INDICATIONS & DOSAGE
Adjunct to general anesthetic—
Adults: 1 to 8 mcg/kg I.V. administered with nitrous oxide/oxygen.

As a primary anesthetic—
Adults: 8 to 30 mcg/kg I.V. administered with 100% oxygen and a muscle relaxant.

ADVERSE REACTIONS
CNS: chills.
CV: *hypotension,* hypertension, bradycardia, tachycardia.
GI: nausea, vomiting.
Skin: itching.
Other: *chest wall rigidity,* intraoperative muscle movement, *respiratory depression.*

INTERACTIONS
Alcohol, CNS depressants: additive effects. Use together cautiously.

NURSING CONSIDERATIONS
• Use cautiously in head injury, pulmonary disease, or decreased respiratory reserve.
• Should only be administered by persons specifically trained in the use of I.V. anesthetics.
• When used at doses of greater than 8 mcg/kg, postoperative mechanical ventilation and observation are essential because of extended postoperative respiratory depression.
• Keep narcotic antagonist (naloxone) and resuscitative equipment available when giving drug.
• Dose should be reduced in elderly and debilitated patients.
• Monitor postoperative vital signs frequently.
• Compared to fentanyl, sufentanil has a more rapid onset and shorter duration of action.
• High doses can produce muscle rigidity reversible by neuromuscular blocking agents.

---

† Available in Canada only.   ‡ Available in Australia only.   ◊ Available OTC.

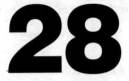

28

Sedative-hypnotics

amobarbital
amobarbital sodium
aprobarbital
butabarbital sodium
chloral hydrate
ethchlorvynol
ethinamate
flurazepam hydrochloride
glutethimide
methotrimeprazine
 hydrochloride
methyprylon
midazolam hydrochloride
paraldehyde
 (See Chapter 29, ANTICONVULSANTS.)
pentobarbital
pentobarbital sodium
phenobarbital sodium
 (See Chapter 29, ANTICONVULSANTS.)
quazepam
secobarbital sodium
talbutal
temazepam
triazolam

COMBINATION PRODUCTS
Barbiturates
TRI-BARBS CAPSULE: phenobarbital
32 mg, butabarbital sodium 32 mg,
and secobarbital sodium 32 mg.
TUINAL 50 MG PULVULES: amobarbital sodium 25 mg and secobarbital sodium 25 mg.
TUINAL 100 MG PULVULES: amobarbital sodium 50 mg and secobarbital sodium 50 mg.
TUINAL 200 MG PULVULES: amobarbital sodium 100 mg and secobarbital sodium 100 mg.

amobarbital
Amytal

amobarbital sodium
Amytal Sodium

Controlled Substance Schedule II
Pregnancy Risk Category: B

HOW SUPPLIED
amobarbital
Tablets: 30 mg, 50 mg, 100 mg
amobarbital sodium
Capsules: 65 mg, 200 mg
Powder for injection: 250 mg, 500 mg

MECHANISM OF ACTION
Probably interferes with transmission
of impulses from the thalamus to the
cortex of the brain. A barbiturate.

INDICATIONS & DOSAGE
Sedation—
Adults: usually 30 to 50 mg P.O.
b.i.d. or t.i.d. but may range from 15
to 120 mg b.i.d. to q.i.d.
Children: 3 to 6 mg/kg P.O. daily in
four equally divided doses.
Insomnia—
Adults: 65 to 200 mg P.O. or deep
I.M. h.s.; I.M. injection not to exceed
5 ml in any one site. Maximum dosage is 500 mg.
Children: 3 to 5 mg/kg deep I.M.
h.s.; I.M. injection not to exceed 5 ml
in any one site.
Preanesthetic sedation—
Adults and children: 200 mg P.O. or
I.M. 1 to 2 hours before surgery.
Manic reactions, as an adjunct in psychotherapy, anticonvulsant—

Italicized adverse reactions are common or life-threatening.
*Liquid form contains alcohol.   **May contain tartrazine.

Adults and children over 6 years: 65 to 500 mg slow I.V.; rate not to exceed 100 mg/minute. Maximum dosage is 1 g.
Children under 6 years: 3 to 5 mg/kg slow I.V. or I.M.

ADVERSE REACTIONS

CNS: *drowsiness, lethargy, hangover,* paradoxical excitement in elderly patients.
GI: nausea, vomiting.
Skin: rash, urticaria.
Local: pain, irritation, sterile abscess at injection site.
Other: *Stevens-Johnson syndrome,* angioedema, exacerbation of porphyria.

INTERACTIONS

Alcohol or other CNS depressants, including narcotic analgesics: excessive CNS and respiratory depression. Use together cautiously.
Griseofulvin: decreased absorption of griseofulvin.
MAO inhibitors: inhibit metabolism of barbiturates; may cause prolonged CNS depression. Reduce barbiturate dosage.
Oral anticoagulants, estrogens and oral contraceptives, doxycycline, corticosteroids: amobarbital may enhance the metabolism of these drugs. Monitor for decreased effect.
Rifampin: may decrease barbiturate levels. Monitor for decreased effect.

NURSING CONSIDERATIONS

• Contraindicated in uncontrolled severe pain, respiratory disease with dyspnea or obstruction, hypersensitivity to barbiturates, previous addiction to sedatives, or porphyria. Use with caution in hepatic or renal impairment.
• Elderly patients are more sensitive to the drug's adverse CNS effects. Assess mental status before and after initiating therapy.
• Use injection solution within 30 minutes after opening container to minimize deterioration. Don't use cloudy or precipitated solution. Don't shake solution; mix with sterile water only.
• Reserve I.V. injection for emergency treatment. Give under close supervision. Be prepared to give artificial respiration. Administer slowly I.V.; do not exceed 100 mg/minute.
• Administer I.M. injection deeply. Superficial injection may cause pain, sterile abscess, and sloughing.
• Because barbiturates potentiate narcotics, reduce dose when giving during labor. Excessive dose may cause respiratory depression in neonate.
• Remove cigarettes of patient receiving hypnotic dose.
• Supervise walking; raise bed rails, especially for elderly patients.
• Long-term high dosage may cause drug dependence and severe withdrawal symptoms. Withdraw barbiturates gradually.
• Prevent hoarding or self-overdosing by patients who are depressed, suicidal, or drug-dependent, or who have a history of drug abuse.
• Watch for signs of barbiturate toxicity: coma, pupillary constriction, cyanosis, clammy skin, and hypotension. Overdose can be fatal.
• Morning "hangover" common after hypnotic dose. Hypnotic doses suppress REM sleep. When drug is discontinued, patient may experience increased dreaming.
• Used in psychiatric settings as an "Amytal interview" to elicit information that patient can't or won't offer when fully conscious.

---

aprobarbital
Alurate*
Controlled Substance Schedule III
Pregnancy Risk Category: D

HOW SUPPLIED
Elixir: 40 mg/5 ml

MECHANISM OF ACTION
Probably interferes with transmission of impulses from the thalamus to the cortex of the brain. A barbiturate.

INDICATIONS & DOSAGE
Sedation—
Adults: 15 to 40 mg P.O. t.i.d. or q.i.d.; usual dose is 40 mg t.i.d.
Insomnia—
Adults: 40 to 160 mg P.O. h.s.

ADVERSE REACTIONS
CNS: *drowsiness, lethargy, hangover,* paradoxical excitement in elderly patients.
GI: nausea, vomiting.
Skin: rash, urticaria.
Other: *Stevens-Johnson syndrome,* angioedema, exacerbation of porphyria.

INTERACTIONS
Alcohol or other CNS depressants, including narcotic analgesics: excessive CNS and respiratory depression. Use together cautiously.
Griseofulvin: decreased absorption of griseofulvin.
MAO inhibitors: inhibit metabolism of barbiturates; may cause prolonged CNS depression. Reduce barbiturate dosage.
Oral anticoagulants, estrogens and oral contraceptives, doxycycline, corticosteroids: aprobarbital may enhance the metabolism of these drugs. Monitor for decreased effectiveness.
Rifampin: may decrease barbiturate levels. Monitor for decreased effect.

NURSING CONSIDERATIONS
• Contraindicated in uncontrolled severe pain, respiratory disease with dyspnea or obstruction, hypersensitivity to barbiturates, previous addiction to sedatives, or porphyria. Use with caution in hepatic or renal impairment and in elderly patients.
• Remove cigarettes of patient receiving hypnotic dose.
• Supervise walking; raise bed rails, especially for elderly patients.
• Long-term high dosage may cause drug dependence and severe withdrawal symptoms. Withdraw barbiturates gradually.
• Prevent hoarding or self-overdosing by patients who are depressed, suicidal, or drug-dependent, or who have a history of drug abuse.
• Watch for signs of barbiturate toxicity: coma, pupillary constriction, cyanosis, clammy skin, and hypotension. Overdose can be fatal.
• Morning "hangover" common after hypnotic dose.
• Hypnotic doses suppress REM sleep. When drug discontinued, patient may experience increased dreaming.
• Women who use oral contraceptives should consider alternate birth control methods when taking this drug because it may enhance contraceptive hormone metabolism and decrease its effect.

---

butabarbital sodium
Barbased*, Butalan*, Buticaps, Butisol* **, Day-Barb†, Sarisol No. 2* **
Controlled Substance Schedule III
Pregnancy Risk Category: D

HOW SUPPLIED
Tablets: 15 mg, 30 mg, 50 mg, 100 mg
Capsules: 15 mg, 30 mg
Elixir: 30 mg/5 ml, 33.3 mg/5 ml

MECHANISM OF ACTION
Probably interferes with transmission of impulses from the thalamus to the cortex of the brain. A barbiturate.

INDICATIONS & DOSAGE
Sedation—
Adults: 15 to 30 mg P.O. t.i.d. or q.i.d.

Italicized adverse reactions are common or life-threatening.
*Liquid form contains alcohol.   **May contain tartrazine.

Children: 6 mg/kg P.O. divided t.i.d. Dosage range 7.5 to 30 mg P.O. t.i.d.
Preoperatively—
Adults: 50 to 100 mg P.O. 60 to 90 minutes before surgery.
Insomnia—
Adults: 50 to 100 mg P.O. h.s.

ADVERSE REACTIONS
CNS: *drowsiness, lethargy, hangover,* paradoxical excitement in elderly patients.
GI: nausea, vomiting.
Skin: rash, urticaria.
Other: *Stevens-Johnson syndrome,* angioedema, exacerbation of porphyria.

INTERACTIONS
Alcohol or other CNS depressants, including narcotic analgesics: excessive CNS and respiratory depression. Use together cautiously.
Griseofulvin: decreased absorption of griseofulvin.
MAO inhibitors: inhibit the metabolism of barbiturates; may cause prolonged CNS depression. Reduce barbiturate dosage.
Oral anticoagulants, estrogens and oral contraceptives, doxycycline, corticosteroids: butabarbital may enhance the metabolism of these drugs. Monitor for decreased effect.
Rifampin: may decrease barbiturate levels. Monitor for decreased effect.

NURSING CONSIDERATIONS
• Contraindicated in uncontrolled severe pain, respiratory disease with dyspnea or obstruction, hypersensitivity to barbiturates, previous addiction to sedatives, or porphyria. Use with caution in hepatic or renal impairment.
• Elderly patients are more sensitive to the drug's adverse CNS reactions. Assess mental status before and after initiating therapy.
• Remove cigarettes of patient receiving hypnotic dose.

• Supervise walking; raise bed rails, especially for elderly patients.
• Long-term high dosage may cause drug dependence and severe withdrawal symptoms. Withdraw barbiturates gradually.
• Prevent hoarding or self-overdosing by patients who are depressed, suicidal, or drug-dependent, or who have a history of drug abuse.
• Butisol sodium elixir is sugar-free.
• Watch for signs of barbiturate toxicity: coma, pupillary constriction, cyanosis, clammy skin, and hypotension. Overdose can be fatal.
• Prolonged administration is not recommended: drug is not shown to be effective after 14 days. A drug-free interval of at least 1 week is advised.
• Morning "hangover" common after hypnotic dose.
• Hypnotic doses suppress REM sleep. When drug is discontinued, patient may experience increased dreaming.
• Women who use oral contraceptives should consider alternate birth control methods when taking this drug because it may enhance contraceptive hormone metabolism and decrease its effect.

---

chloral hydrate
Aquachloral Supprettes, Noctec, Novochlorhydrate†
Controlled Substance Schedule IV
Pregnancy Risk Category: C

HOW SUPPLIED
Capsules: 250 mg, 500 mg
Syrup: 250 mg/5 ml, 500 mg/5 ml
Suppositories: 325 mg, 500 mg, 648 mg

MECHANISM OF ACTION
Unknown. Sedative effects may be caused by its primary metabolite, trichloroethanol.

---

†Available in Canada only.   ‡Available in Australia only.   ◊Available OTC.

INDICATIONS & DOSAGE
Sedation—
Adults: 250 mg P.O. or rectally t.i.d. after meals.
Children: 8 mg/kg P.O. t.i.d. Maximum dosage is 500 mg t.i.d.
Insomnia—
Adults: 500 mg to 1 g P.O. or rectally 15 to 30 minutes before bedtime.
Children: 50 mg/kg P.O. single dose. Maximum dosage is 1 g.
Premedication for EEG—
Children: 25 mg/kg P.O. single dose. Maximum dosage is 1 g.

ADVERSE REACTIONS
Blood: eosinophilia.
CNS: *hangover, drowsiness,* nightmares, dizziness, ataxia, paradoxical excitement.
GI: *nausea,* vomiting, diarrhea, flatulence.
Skin: hypersensitivity reactions.

INTERACTIONS
Alcohol or other CNS depressants, including narcotic analgesics: excessive CNS depression or vasodilation reaction. Use together cautiously.
Furosemide I.V.: sweating, flushes, variable blood pressure, and uneasiness. Use together cautiously or use a different hypnotic drug.
Oral anticoagulants: increased risk of bleeding. Monitor patient closely.

NURSING CONSIDERATIONS
• Contraindicated in marked hepatic or renal impairment and hypersensitivity to chloral hydrate or triclofos. Oral administration contraindicated in gastric disorders. Use with caution in severe cardiac disease, mental depression, and suicidal tendencies.
• Dilute or administer with liquid to minimize unpleasant taste and stomach irritation. Administer after meals.
• Prevent hoarding or self-overdosing by patients who are depressed, suicidal, or drug-dependent, or who have a history of drug abuse.

• Remove cigarettes of patient receiving hypnotic dose.
• Supervise walking; raise bed rails, especially for elderly patients.
• Large dosage may raise BUN level.
• May interfere with fluorometric tests for urine catecholamines and Reddy, Jenkins, Thorn test for urine 17-hydroxycorticosteroids. Do not administer drug for 48 hours before fluorometric test.
• Aqueous solutions are incompatible with alkaline substances.
• Store in dark container; store suppositories in refrigerator.

---

ethchlorvynol
Placidyl**
Controlled Substance Schedule IV
Pregnancy Risk Category: C

HOW SUPPLIED
Capsules: 200 mg, 500 mg, 750 mg

MECHANISM OF ACTION
Unknown.

INDICATIONS & DOSAGE
Sedation—
Adults: 100 to 200 mg P.O. b.i.d. or t.i.d.
Insomnia—
Adults: 500 mg to 1 g P.O. h.s. May repeat 100 to 200 mg if awakened in early morning.

ADVERSE REACTIONS
Blood: thrombocytopenia.
CNS: facial numbness, drowsiness, fatigue, nightmares, dizziness, residual sedation, muscular weakness, syncope, ataxia.
CV: hypotension.
EENT: unpleasant aftertaste, blurred vision.
GI: distress, nausea, vomiting.
Skin: rashes, urticaria.

INTERACTIONS
Alcohol or other CNS depressants, in-

Italicized adverse reactions are common or life-threatening.
*Liquid form contains alcohol.   **May contain tartrazine.

cluding narcotic analgesics, tricyclic antidepressants, and MAO inhibitors: excessive CNS depression. Use together cautiously.
Oral anticoagulants: ethchlorvynol may enhance the metabolism of coumarin derivitives, decreasing their effectiveness. Monitor closely.

NURSING CONSIDERATIONS
• Contraindicated in uncontrolled pain and porphyria. Use cautiously in hepatic or renal impairment; in elderly or debilitated patients; in mental depression with suicidal tendencies; and if patient has previously overreacted to barbiturates or alcohol.
• Give with milk or food to minimize transient dizziness or ataxia caused by rapid absorption.
• May cause dependence and severe withdrawal symptoms. Withdraw gradually.
• Prevent hoarding or self-overdosing by patients who are depressed, suicidal, or drug-dependent, or who have a history of drug abuse. Overdosage very difficult to treat and has a high mortality.
• Watch for signs of toxicity, such as poor muscle coordination, confusion, hypothermia, speech or vision disturbances, tremors, and weakness.
• 750-mg strength contains tartrazine dye. May cause allergic reactions in susceptible patients.
• Remove cigarettes of patient receiving hypnotic dose.
• Supervise walking; raise bed rails, especially for elderly patients.
• Slight darkening of liquid from exposure to air and light doesn't affect safety or potency, but store in tight, light-resistant container to avoid possible deterioration.
• Drug is effective for short-term use only; treatment period should not exceed 1 week.

ethinamate
Valmid
Controlled Substance Schedule IV
Pregnancy Risk Category: C

HOW SUPPLIED
Capsules: 500 mg

MECHANISM OF ACTION
Unknown.

INDICATIONS & DOSAGE
Insomnia—
Adults: 500 mg to 1 g P.O. 20 minutes before bedtime. Starting dose should be 500 mg for elderly or debilitated patients.

ADVERSE REACTIONS
Blood: thrombocytic purpura.
GI: mild upset.
Skin: rashes.
Other: fever (allergic reaction).

INTERACTIONS
Alcohol, CNS depressants: increased CNS depression. Avoid concomitant use.

NURSING CONSIDERATIONS
• Contraindicated for uncontrolled pain. Use cautiously in mental depression, suicidal tendencies, or history of drug abuse.
• Not recommended for use in children under age 15; paradoxical excitement in children has been reported.
• Long-term use may cause dependence and severe withdrawal symptoms. Withdraw gradually.
• Prevent hoarding or self-overdosing by patients who are depressed, suicidal, or drug-dependent, or who have a history of drug abuse.
• Abrupt withdrawal may cause blood pressure and pulse rate changes, sweating, and hallucinations.
• Remove cigarettes of patient receiving dose.

---

†Available in Canada only.   ‡Available in Australia only.   ◊Available OTC.

• Supervise walking; raise bed rails, especially for elderly patients.
• In overdosage, treat CNS and respiratory depression same as barbiturate intoxication; ethinamate is dialyzable.
• May cause falsely elevated urine 17-ketosteroid (modified Zimmermann reaction) and 17-hydroxycorticosteroid levels (Porter-Silber test).
• Prolonged therapy not recommended; drug is not effective for more than 7 days.

flurazepam hydrochloride
Apo-Flurazepam†, Dalmane, Durapam, Novoflupam†, Sam-Pam†
Controlled Substance Schedule IV

Pregnancy Risk Category: D

HOW SUPPLIED
Capsules: 15 mg, 30 mg

MECHANISM OF ACTION
Acts on the limbic system, thalamus, and hypothalamus of the central nervous system to produce hypnotic effects. A benzodiazepine.

INDICATIONS & DOSAGE
Insomnia—
Adults: 15 to 30 mg P.O. h.s. May repeat dose once.
Adults over 65 years: 15 mg P.O. h.s.

ADVERSE REACTIONS
Blood: leukopenia, granulocytopenia.
CNS: *daytime sedation, dizziness, drowsiness, disturbed coordination,* lethargy, confusion, *headache*.
GI: nausea, vomiting, heartburn.
Metabolic: elevated liver enzymes.

INTERACTIONS
Alcohol or other CNS depressants, including narcotic analgesics: excessive CNS depression. Use together cautiously.

Cimetidine: increased sedation. Monitor carefully.

NURSING CONSIDERATIONS
• Use cautiously in impaired hepatic or renal function, mental depression, suicidal tendencies, or history of drug abuse.
• Elderly patients are more sensitive to the drug's adverse CNS reactions. Assess mental status before initiating therapy.
• Prevent hoarding or self-overdosing by patients who are depressed, suicidal, or drug-dependent, or who have a history of drug abuse.
• Remove cigarettes of patient receiving drug.
• Supervise walking; raise bed rails, especially for elderly patients.
• Dependence is possible with long-term use.
• More effective on second, third, and fourth nights of use because active metabolite accumulates. Encourage patient to continue drug if it doesn't work the first night.

glutethimide
Doriden, Doriglute
Controlled Substance Schedule III

Pregnancy Risk Category: C

HOW SUPPLIED
Tablets: 250 mg, 500 mg
Capsules: 500 mg

MECHANISM OF ACTION
Unknown.

INDICATIONS & DOSAGE
Insomnia—
Adults: 250 to 500 mg P.O. h.s. May be repeated, but not less than 4 hours before intended awakening. Total daily dosage should not exceed 1 g.

ADVERSE REACTIONS
CNS: *residual sedation, dizziness,*

Italicized adverse reactions are common or life-threatening.
*Liquid form contains alcohol.   **May contain tartrazine.

ataxia, paradoxical excitation, headache, vertigo.
EENT: dry mouth, blurred vision.
GI: irritation, nausea.
GU: bladder atony.
Skin: rash, urticaria.

INTERACTIONS

Alcohol or other CNS depressants, including narcotic analgesics: excessive CNS depression. Use together cautiously.
Oral anticoagulants: glutethimide enhances the metabolism of coumarin derivitives. Monitor for decreased effect.

NURSING CONSIDERATIONS

• Contraindicated in uncontrolled pain, severe renal impairment, or porphyria. Use cautiously in mental depression, suicidal tendencies, history of drug abuse, prostatic hypertrophy, stenosing peptic ulcer, pyloroduodenal or bladder-neck obstruction, narrow-angle glaucoma, and cardiac arrhythmias.
• Drug is effective for short-term use only.
• Remove cigarettes of patient receiving drug.
• Supervise walking; raise bed rails, especially for elderly patients.
• Prevent hoarding or self-overdosing by patients who are depressed, suicidal, or drug-dependent, or who have a history of drug abuse.
• Abrupt withdrawal may produce nausea, vomiting, nervousness, tremors, chills, fever, nightmares, insomnia, tachycardia, delirium, numbness of extremities, hallucinations, dysphagia, and seizures. Withdraw gradually.
• Monitor prothrombin times carefully when patient on glutethimide starts or ends anticoagulant therapy. Anticoagulant dose may need to be adjusted.
• Suppresses REM sleep, as do barbiturates. When drug is discontinued,

patient may experience increased dreaming.

---

methotrimeprazine hydrochloride (levomepromazine hydrochloride)

Levoprome, Nozinan†*

Pregnancy Risk Category: C

HOW SUPPLIED

Tablets: 2 mg†, 5 mg†, 25 mg†, 50 mg†
Oral solution: 40 mg/ml†
Drops: 40 mg/ml†
Injection: 20 mg/ml in 10-ml vials, 25 mg/ml†

MECHANISM OF ACTION

Acts on the limbic system, thalamus, and hypothalamus of the central nervous system to produce hypnotic effects. A phenothiazine.

INDICATIONS & DOSAGE

Postoperative analgesia—
Adults and children over 12 years: initially, 2.5 to 7.5 mg I.M. q 4 to 6 hours, then adjust dose.
Preanesthetic medication—
Adults and children over 12 years: 2 to 20 mg I.M. 45 minutes to 3 hours before surgery.
Sedation, analgesia—
Adults and children over 12 years: 10 to 20 mg deep I.M. q 4 to 6 hours as required; or 6 to 25 mg P.O. daily in three divided doses with meals. For severe pain, dosage may be increased to 50 to 75 mg daily in two or three divided doses with meals.
Adults over 65 years: 5 to 10 mg I.M. q 4 to 6 hours.
Psychosis—
Adults: 6 to 25 mg P.O. daily in three divided doses with meals. Dosage may be gradually increased as needed and tolerated to 50 to 75 mg P.O. daily in two or three divided doses.

ADVERSE REACTIONS
Blood: *agranulocytosis* and other dyscrasias after long-term high dosage.
CNS: *fainting, weakness, dizziness,* drowsiness, excessive sedation, amnesia, disorientation, euphoria, headache, slurred speech.
CV: *orthostatic hypotension,* palpitations.
EENT: dry mouth, nasal congestion.
GI: nausea, vomiting, abdominal discomfort.
GU: difficulty urinating.
Local: *pain, inflammation, swelling at injection site.*

INTERACTIONS
All antihypertensive agents: increased orthostatic hypotension. Don't use together.

NURSING CONSIDERATIONS
• Contraindicated in patients receiving concurrent antihypertensive drug therapy, including MAO inhibitors; also, in history of seizure disorders; hypersensitivity to phenothiazines; severe cardiac, hepatic, or renal disease; previous overdose of CNS depressant; or coma. Use with extreme caution in elderly or debilitated patients with cardiac disease or in any patient who may suffer serious consequences from a sudden drop in blood pressure. Because the injectable form contains sulfites, use with caution in asthmatic patients or in patients with sulfite sensitivity.
• Use low initial dose in susceptible patients; increase gradually while frequently checking pulse rate, blood pressure, and circulation.
• Expect drop in blood pressure 10 to 20 minutes after I.M. injection.
• Keep patient in bed or closely supervised for 6 to 12 hours after each of the first several injections because orthostatic hypotension may occur. If hypotension is severe, combat with phenylephrine, methoxamine, or levarterenol. Don't use epinephrine because it may worsen hypotension.
• Don't use for longer than 30 days except in terminal illness or when narcotics are contraindicated.
• In prolonged use, monitor liver function and blood studies periodically.
• Inject I.M. into large muscle masses. Rotate sites. Do not administer subcutaneously, as local irritation results. I.V. injection not recommended.
• May be mixed in same syringe with reduced dose of atropine and scopolamine. Do not mix with other drugs. Protect solution from light.
• If high oral doses (> 100 mg) are used, patient should be confined to bed for the first few days to prevent orthostatic hypotension.
• Rarely may cause neuroleptic malignant syndrome, with fever, leukocytosis, and dystonic reaction. Can be fatal if untreated.

---

methyprylon
Noludar
Controlled Substance Schedule III
Pregnancy Risk Category: B

HOW SUPPLIED
Tablets: 50 mg, 200 mg
Capsules: 300 mg

MECHANISM OF ACTION
Raises threshold of arousal centers in the brain stem.

INDICATIONS & DOSAGE
Insomnia—
Adults: 200 to 400 mg P.O. 15 minutes before bedtime.
Children over 3 months: 50 mg P.O. at bedtime, increased to 200 mg, if necessary. Maximum dosage is 400 mg daily.

Italicized adverse reactions are common or life-threatening.
*Liquid form contains alcohol.   **May contain tartrazine.

ADVERSE REACTIONS
Blood: thrombocytopenic purpura, neutropenia, *aplastic anemia*.
CNS: *morning drowsiness, dizziness,* headache, paradoxical excitation.
CV: hypotension.
GI: nausea, vomiting, diarrhea, esophagitis.
Skin: rash, pruritus.

INTERACTIONS
Alcohol or other CNS depressants, including narcotic analgesics: excessive CNS and respiratory depression. Use together cautiously.

NURSING CONSIDERATIONS
• Contraindicated in intermittent porphyria. Use cautiously in renal or hepatic impairment.
• Periodic blood counts are advisable during repeated or long-term use.
• May cause drug dependence and severe life-threatening withdrawal symptoms. Withdrawal should be gradual and closely monitored.
• Prevent hoarding or self-overdosing by patients who are depressed, suicidal, or drug-dependent, or who have a history of drug abuse.
• Remove cigarettes of patient receiving drug.
• Supervise walking; raise bed rails, especially for elderly patients.
• Value of this drug as a sedative has not been established.
• Overdosage symptoms include somnolence, confusion, constricted pupils, respiratory depression, hypotension, and coma. Hemodialysis is useful in severe intoxication.
• Suppresses REM sleep, as do barbiturates. When drug is discontinued, patient may experience increased dreaming.

midazolam hydrochloride
Versed
Controlled Substance Schedule IV
Pregnancy Risk Category: D

HOW SUPPLIED
Injection: 1 mg/ml, 5 mg/ml

MECHANISM OF ACTION
Depresses the CNS at the limbic and subcortical levels of the brain.

INDICATIONS & DOSAGE
Preoperative sedation (to induce sleepiness or drowsiness and relieve apprehension)—
Adults: 0.07 mg to 0.08 mg/kg I.M. approximately 1 hour before surgery. May be administered with atropine or scopolamine and reduced doses of narcotics.
Conscious sedation before short diagnostic or endoscopic procedures—
Adults: initially, 0.035 mg/kg slowly I.V. (not to exceed 2.5 mg). Dose is then titrated in small amounts to a total dosage of 0.1 mg/kg.
Induction of general anesthesia—
Adults: 0.3 to 0.35 mg/kg I.V. over 20 to 30 seconds. Additional increments of 25% of the initial dose may be needed to complete induction. Up to 0.6 mg/kg total dosage may be given.

ADVERSE REACTIONS
CNS: headache, oversedation, involuntary movements, combativeness.
CV: variations in blood pressure and pulse rate.
GI: nausea, vomiting, hiccups.
Local: pain and tenderness at injection site.
Other: *decreased respiratory rate, apnea.*

INTERACTIONS
CNS depressants: may increase the risk of apnea. Prepare to adjust drug dosage.

---

†Available in Canada only. ‡Available in Australia only. ◊ Available OTC.

NURSING CONSIDERATIONS
• Contraindicated in acute narrow-angle glaucoma. Don't give to patients in shock, coma, or acute alcohol intoxication. Use cautiously in CHF, COPD, or renal disease, and in elderly or debilitated patients.
• Before administering I.V. midazolam, have oxygen and resuscitative equipment available in case of severe respiratory depression. Excessive dosage or rapid infusion has been associated with respiratory arrest, particularly in elderly or debilitated patients.
• Monitor blood pressure during procedure, especially in patients who have also been premedicated with narcotics.
• Midazolam has a beneficial amnestic effect, which diminishes patient's recall of perioperative events. This drug offers advantages over diazepam, hydrozyzine, and barbiturates, which are also prescribed for similar indications.
• When injecting I.M., give deep into a large muscle mass.
• May be mixed in the same syringe with morphine sulfate, meperidine, atropine sulfate, or scopolamine.
• When administering I.V., take care to avoid extravasation.

---

pentobarbital
Nembutal* **

pentobarbital sodium
Nembutal Sodium*,
Novopentobarb†

Controlled Substance Schedule II
Pregnancy Risk Category: D

HOW SUPPLIED
pentobarbital
Elixir: 20 mg/5 ml
pentobarbital sodium
Capsules: 50 mg, 100 mg
Injection: 50 mg/ml
Suppositories: 30 mg, 60 mg, 120 mg, 200 mg

MECHANISM OF ACTION
Probably interferes with transmission of impulses from the thalamus to the cortex of the brain. A barbiturate.

INDICATIONS & DOSAGE
Sedation—
Adults: 20 to 40 mg P.O. b.i.d., t.i.d., or q.i.d.
Children: 6 mg/kg daily P.O. in divided doses.
Insomnia—
Adults: 100 to 200 mg P.O. h.s. or 150 to 200 mg deep I.M.; 100 mg initially, I.V., then additional doses up to 500 mg; 120 to 200 mg rectally.
Children: 3 to 5 mg/kg I.M. Maximum dosage is 100 mg. Rectal dosages are 2 months to 1 year, 30 mg; 1 to 4 years, 30 to 60 mg; 5 to 12 years, 60 mg; 12 to 14 years, 60 to 120 mg.
Preanesthetic medication—
Adults: 150 to 200 mg I.M. or P.O. in two divided doses.

ADVERSE REACTIONS
CNS: *drowsiness, lethargy, hangover,* paradoxical excitement in elderly patients.
GI: nausea, vomiting.
Skin: rash, urticaria.
Other: *Stevens-Johnson syndrome,* angioedema, exacerbation of porphyria.

INTERACTIONS
Alcohol or other CNS depressants, including narcotic analgesics: excessive CNS and respiratory depression. Use together cautiously.
Griseofulvin: decreased absorption of griseofulvin.
MAO inhibitors: inhibit metabolism of barbiturates; may cause prolonged CNS depression. Reduce barbiturate dosage.
Oral anticoagulants, estrogens and oral contraceptives, doxycycline, corticosteroids: pentobarbital may enhance the metabolism of these drugs. Monitor for decreased effect.

Italicized adverse reactions are common or life-threatening.
*Liquid form contains alcohol.   **May contain tartrazine.

Rifampin: may decrease barbiturate levels. Monitor for decreased effect.

NURSING CONSIDERATIONS
• Contraindicated in uncontrolled severe pain, respiratory disease with dyspnea or obstruction, hypersensitivity to barbiturates, previous addiction to sedatives, or porphyria. Use with caution in hepatic or renal impairment.
• Elderly patients are more sensitive to the drug's adverse CNS reactions. Assess mental status before initiating therapy.
• Use injection solution within 30 minutes after opening container to minimize deterioration. Don't use cloudy solution.
• Parenteral solution alkaline. Avoid extravasation; may cause tissue necrosis.
• I.V. injection should be reserved for emergency treatment and should be given under close supervision. Be prepared to give artificial respiration.
• Administer I.M. injection deeply. Superficial injection may cause pain, sterile abscess, and sloughing.
• Do not mix with other medications.
• Remove cigarettes of patient receiving hypnotic dose.
• Supervise walking; raise bed rails, especially for elderly patients.
• May cause drug dependence and severe withdrawal symptoms. Withdraw barbiturates gradually.
• Prevent hoarding or self-overdosing by patients who are depressed, suicidal, or drug-dependent, or who have a history of drug abuse.
• No analgesic effect. May cause restlessness or delirium in presence of pain.
• Watch for signs of barbiturate toxicity: coma, pupillary constriction, cyanosis, clammy skin, and hypotension. Overdose can be fatal.
• To ensure accurate dosage, don't divide suppositories.

• Morning "hangover" common after hypnotic dose.
• Hypnotic doses suppress REM sleep. When drug is discontinued, patient may experience increased dreaming.

---

quazepam
Doral
Controlled Substance Schedule IV
Pregnancy Risk Category: X

HOW SUPPLIED
Tablets: 7.5 mg, 15 mg

MECHANISM OF ACTION
Acts on the limbic system and thalamus of the CNS by binding to specific benzodiazepine receptors.

INDICATIONS & DOSAGE
Insomnia—
Adults: 15 mg P.O. h.s. Some patients may respond to lower doses. Decrease dosage in elderly patients to 7.5 mg P.O. h.s. after 2 days of therapy.

ADVERSE REACTIONS
CNS: *fatigue, dizziness, daytime drowsiness, headache.*

INTERACTIONS
Alcohol or other CNS depressants, including antihistamines, opiate analgesics, and other benzodiazepines: increased CNS depression.

NURSING CONSIDERATIONS
• Contraindicated in patients allergic to the drug or other benzodiazepines, in pregnant patients, and in patients with suspected or established sleep apnea.
• Warn the patient about the possible additive depressant effects that can occur with alcohol consumption. Additive effects can occur if alcohol is consumed on the day after the use of quazepam.

• Patients who receive prolonged therapy with benzodiazepines may experience withdrawal symptoms if the drug is suddenly withdrawn (possibly after 6 weeks of continuous therapy).
• Prevent hoarding or self-overdosing by patients who are depressed, suicidal, or known drug abusers.
• Supervise walking and use bed rails, especially for elderly patients. Warn patients to avoid activities that require alertness, such as driving a car, until the adverse CNS reactions of the drug are known.
• Warn patients not to increase the drug dosage on their own, and to inform the doctor if they feel that the drug is no longer effective.

---

secobarbital sodium
Novosecobarb†, Seconal Sodium
Controlled Substance Schedule II

Pregnancy Risk Category: D

HOW SUPPLIED
Tablets: 100 mg
Capsules: 50 mg, 100 mg
Injection: 50 mg/ml
Rectal injection: 50 mg/ml
Suppositories: 200 mg

MECHANISM OF ACTION
Probably interferes with transmission of impulses from the thalamus to the cortex of the brain. A barbiturate.

INDICATIONS & DOSAGE
Sedation, preoperatively—
Adults: 200 to 300 mg P.O. 1 to 2 hours before surgery.
Children: 50 to 100 mg P.O. or 4 to 5 mg/kg rectally 1 to 2 hours before surgery.
Insomnia—
Adults: 100 to 200 mg P.O. or I.M.
Children: 3 to 5 mg/kg I.M., not to exceed 100 mg, with no more than 5 ml injected in any one site or 4 to 5 mg/kg rectally.
Acute tetanus seizure—

Adults and children: 5.5 mg/kg I.M. or slow I.V., repeated q 3 to 4 hours, if needed; I.V. injection rate not to exceed 50 mg per 15 seconds.
Acute psychotic agitation—
Adults: 50 mg/minute I.V. up to 250 mg I.V. initially, additional doses given cautiously after 5 minutes if desired response is not obtained. Not to exceed 500 mg total.
Status epilepticus—
Adults and children: 250 to 350 mg I.M. or I.V.

ADVERSE REACTIONS
CNS: *drowsiness, lethargy, hangover,* paradoxical excitement in elderly patients.
GI: nausea, vomiting.
Skin: rash, urticaria.
Other: *Stevens-Johnson syndrome, angioedema, exacerbation of porphyria.*

INTERACTIONS
Alcohol or other CNS depressants, including narcotic analgesics: excessive CNS and respiratory depression. Use together cautiously.
Griseofulvin: decreased absorption of griseofulvin.
MAO inhibitors: inhibit metabolism of barbiturates; may cause prolonged CNS depression. Reduce barbiturate dosage.
Oral anticoagulants, estrogens and oral contraceptives, doxycycline, corticosteroids: secobarbital may enhance the metabolism of these drugs. Monitor for decreased effect.
Rifampin: may decrease barbiturate levels. Monitor for decreased effect.

NURSING CONSIDERATIONS
• Contraindicated in uncontrolled severe pain, respiratory disease with dyspnea or obstruction, hypersensitivity to barbiturates, previous addiction to sedatives, or porphyria. Use with caution in hepatic or renal impair-

---

Italicized adverse reactions are common or life-threatening.
*Liquid form contains alcohol.   **May contain tartrazine.

ment; also, in pregnant women with toxemia or history of bleeding.

• Elderly patients are more sensitive to the drug's adverse CNS reactions. Assess mental status before initiating therapy.

• Use injection solution within 30 minutes after opening container to minimize deterioration. Don't use cloudy solution.

• I.V. injection should be reserved for emergency treatment and should be given under close supervision. Be prepared to give artificial respiration.

• Give I.M. injection deeply. Superficial injection may cause pain, sterile abscess, and sloughing.

• Because barbiturates potentiate narcotics, reduce dose when giving during labor. Excessive dose may cause respiratory depression in neonate.

• Remove cigarettes of patient receiving hypnotic dose.

• Supervise walking; raise bed rails, especially for elderly patients.

• May cause drug dependence and severe withdrawal symptoms. Withdraw barbiturates gradually.

• Prevent hoarding or self-overdosing by patients who are depressed, suicidal, or drug-dependent, or who have a history of drug abuse.

• In renal insufficiency, use sterile drug reconstituted with sterile water for injection. Avoid commercial solution containing polyethylene glycol; it may irritate kidneys.

• Secobarbital in polyethylene glycol must be refrigerated.

• Secobarbital sodium injection not compatible with lactated Ringer's solution.

• Sterile secobarbital sodium compatible with Ringer's injection and normal saline solution. Don't mix with acidic solutions.

• To reconstitute, rotate ampule. Do not shake.

• Watch for signs of barbiturate toxicity: coma, pupillary construction,

cyanosis, clammy skin, and hypotension. Overdose can be fatal.

• Morning "hangover" common after hypnotic dose.

• Hypnotic doses suppress REM sleep. When drug is discontinued, patient may experience increased dreaming.

talbutal
Lotusate
Controlled Substance Schedule III
Pregnancy Risk Category: D

HOW SUPPLIED
Caplets: 120 mg

MECHANISM OF ACTION
Probably interferes with transmission of impulses from the thalamus to the cortex of the brain. A barbiturate.

INDICATIONS & DOSAGE
Insomnia—
Adults: 120 mg P.O. h.s.

ADVERSE REACTIONS
CNS: *drowsiness, lethargy, hangover, paradoxical excitement in elderly patients.*
GI: nausea, vomiting.
Skin: rash, urticaria.
Other: *Stevens-Johnson syndrome, angioedema, exacerbation of porphyria.*

INTERACTIONS
Alcohol or other CNS depressants, including narcotic analgesics: excessive CNS and respiratory depression. Use together cautiously.
Griseofulvin: decreased absorption of griseofulvin.
MAO inhibitors: inhibit the metabolism of barbiturates; may cause prolonged CNS depression. Reduce barbiturate dosage.
Oral anticoagulants, estrogens and oral contraceptives, doxycycline, corticosteroids: talbutal may enhance the

metabolism of these drugs. Monitor for decreased effect.
Rifampin: may decrease barbiturate levels. Monitor for decreased effect.

NURSING CONSIDERATIONS
• Contraindicated in uncontrolled severe pain, respiratory disease with dyspnea or obstruction, hypersensitivity to barbiturates, previous addiction to sedatives, or porphyria. Use with caution in hepatic or renal impairment.
• Remove cigarettes of patient receiving hypnotic dose.
• Supervise walking; raise bed rails, especially for elderly patients.
• May cause drug dependence and severe withdrawal symptoms. Withdraw barbiturates gradually.
• Prevent hoarding or self-overdosing by patients who are depressed, suicidal, or drug-dependent, or who have a history of drug abuse.
• Watch for signs of barbiturate toxicity: coma, pupillary constriction, cyanosis, clammy skin, and hypotension. Overdose can be fatal.
• Morning "hangover" common after hypnotic dose.
• Hypnotic doses suppress REM sleep. When drug is discontinued, patient may experience increased dreaming.
• Indicated only for short-term management of insomnia. Tolerance to hypnotic effects may develop after approximately 2 weeks.

---

temazepam
Restoril, Temaz
Controlled Substance Schedule IV
Pregnancy Risk Category: X

HOW SUPPLIED
Capsules: 15 mg, 30 mg

MECHANISM OF ACTION
Acts on the limbic system, thalamus, and hypothalamus of the central nervous system to produce hypnotic effects. A benzodiazepine.

INDICATIONS & DOSAGE
Insomnia—
Adults: 15 to 30 mg P.O. h.s.
Adults over 65 years: 15 mg P.O. h.s.

ADVERSE REACTIONS
CNS: *drowsiness, dizziness, lethargy,* disturbed coordination, daytime sedation, confusion.
GI: anorexia, diarrhea.

INTERACTIONS
Alcohol or CNS depressants, including narcotic analgesics: increased CNS depression. Use together cautiously.

NURSING CONSIDERATIONS
• Use cautiously in impaired hepatic or renal function, mental depression, suicidal tendencies, and history of drug abuse. Use caution and low end of dosage range for elderly or debilitated patients.
• Elderly patients are more sensitive to the drug's adverse CNS reactions. Assess mental status before initiating therapy.
• Prevent hoarding or self-overdosing by patients who are depressed, suicidal, or drug-dependent, or who have a history of drug abuse. Warn about increased alcohol effects and against hazardous activity requiring alertness or skill.
• Remove cigarettes of patient receiving drug.
• Supervise walking; raise bed rails, especially for elderly patients.
• May have less residual sedative effects ("hangover") the next day than flurazepam and diazepam. Relatively short-acting.
• May take as long as 2 to 2½ hours for onset of action.

Italicized adverse reactions are common or life-threatening.
*Liquid form contains alcohol.   **May contain tartrazine.

triazolam
Halcion
Controlled Substance Schedule IV
Pregnancy Risk Category: X

HOW SUPPLIED
Tablets: 0.125 mg, 0.25 mg

MECHANISM OF ACTION
Acts on the limbic system, thalamus, and hypothalamus of the central nervous system to produce hypnotic effects. A benzodiazepine.

INDICATIONS & DOSAGE
Insomnia—
Adults: 0.25 to 0.5 mg P.O. h.s.
Adults over 65: 0.125 mg P.O. h.s.; increase as needed to 0.25 mg P.O. H.S.

ADVERSE REACTIONS
CNS: *drowsiness, dizziness, headache,* rebound insomnia, amnesia, light-headedness, lack of coordination, mental confusion.
GI: nausea, vomiting.

INTERACTIONS
Alcohol or other CNS depressants, including narcotic analgesics: excessive CNS depression. Use together cautiously.
Cimetidine, erythromycin: may cause prolonged triazolam blood levels. Monitor for increased sedation.

NURSING CONSIDERATIONS
• Use cautiously in impaired hepatic or renal function, mental depression, suicidal tendencies, or history of drug abuse.
• Elderly patients are more sensitive to the drug's adverse CNS reactions. Assess mental status before initiating therapy.
• Prevent hoarding or self-overdosing by patients who are depressed, suicidal, or drug-dependent, or who have a history of drug abuse.
• Remove cigarettes of patient receiving drug.
• Supervise walking; raise bed rails, especially for elderly patients.
• Dependence is possible with long-term use.
• Triazolam is a benzodiazepine compound with similarities to flurazepam. However, it is very short-acting and therefore has less tendency to cause morning drowsiness.
• Faster acting than temazepam, another benzodiazepine derivative.
• Warn patient not to take more than the prescribed amount since overdosage can occur at a total daily dose of 2 mg (or four times the highest recommended amount).
• Tell patient that rebound insomnia may develop for one or two nights after stopping therapy.

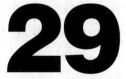

Anticonvulsants

COMBINATION PRODUCT
DILANTIN WITH PHENOBARBITAL:
phenytoin sodium 100 mg and phenobarbital 16 mg; phenytoin sodium 100
mg and phenobarbital 32 mg.

carbamazepine
Apo-Carbamazepine†, Epitol,
Mazepine†, Tegretol, Tegretol CR†,
Teril‡

Pregnancy Risk Category: C

HOW SUPPLIED
Tablets: 200 mg
Tablets (chewable): 100 mg
Oral suspension: 100 mg/5 ml

MECHANISM OF ACTION
Stabilizes neuronal membranes and
limits seizure activity by either increasing efflux or decreasing influx of
sodium ions across cell membranes in
the motor cortex during generation of
nerve impulses.

INDICATIONS & DOSAGE
*Generalized tonic-clonic (grand mal)
and complex-partial (psychomotor)
seizures, mixed seizure patterns—*
Adults and children over 12 years:
initially, 200 mg P.O. b.i.d. May increase by 200 mg P.O. daily, in divided doses at 6- to 8-hour intervals.
Adjust to minimum effective level
when control achieved.
Children under 12 years: 10 to 20
mg/kg P.O. daily in two to four divided doses.
Trigeminal neuralgia—
Adults: initially, 100 mg P.O. b.i.d.
with meals. Increase by 100 mg q 12
hours until pain is relieved. Don't exceed 1.2 g daily. Maintenance dose is
200 to 400 mg P.O. b.i.d.

ADVERSE REACTIONS

Blood: *aplastic anemia, agranulocytosis,* eosinophilia, leukocytosis, *thrombocytopenia.*

CNS: dizziness, *vertigo, drowsiness,* fatigue, *ataxia,* worsening of seizures.

CV: CHF, hypertension, hypotension, aggravation of coronary artery disease.

EENT: conjunctivitis, dry mouth and pharynx, blurred vision, diplopia, nystagmus.

GI: *nausea,* vomiting, abdominal pain, diarrhea, anorexia, *stomatitis,* glossitis.

GU: urinary frequency, urine retention, impotence, albuminuria, glycosuria, elevated BUN.

Hepatic: abnormal liver function tests, hepatitis.

Metabolic: water intoxication.

Skin: *rash,* urticaria, erythema multiforme, *Stevens-Johnson syndrome.*

Other: diaphoresis, fever, chills, pulmonary hypersensitivity.

INTERACTIONS

Phenytoin, primidone, phenobarbital, nicotinic acid: may decrease carbamazepine levels. Monitor for decreased effect.

Phenytoin, warfarin, doxycycline, theophylline, haloperidol: carbamazepine may decrease blood levels of these drugs. Monitor for decreased effect.

Propoxyphene, troleandomycin, erythromycin, isoniazid, verapamil: may increase carbamazepine blood levels. Use cautiously.

NURSING CONSIDERATIONS

• Contraindicated in bone marrow suppression, or hypersensitivity to carbamazepine or tricyclic antidepressants. Use cautiously in cardiac, renal, or hepatic damage and increased intraocular pressure.

• Warn patient to avoid activities that require alertness and good psychomotor coordination until CNS effects of the drug are known.

• May cause mild to moderate dizziness and drowsiness when first taken. Effect usually disappears within 3 to 4 days. Should be taken three times a day, when possible, to provide consistent blood levels.

• Observe for signs of anorexia or subtle appetite changes, which may indicate excessive blood levels.

• Never stop the drug suddenly when treating seizures or status epilepticus. Notify doctor immediately if side effects occur.

• Obtain CBC, platelet and reticulocyte counts, and serum iron levels weekly for first 3 months, then monthly. If bone marrow suppression develops, stop drug. Obtain urinalysis, BUN, and liver function tests every 3 months. Periodic eye examinations are recommended.

• Tell patient to notify doctor immediately if fever, sore throat, mouth ulcers, or easy bruising occurs.

• Therapeutic carbamazepine blood level is 3 to 9 mcg/ml.

• Monitor blood levels and effects closely. Ask patient when last dose of medication was taken to approximately evaluate blood levels.

• When used for trigeminal neuralgia, an attempt should be made every 3 months to decrease dosage or stop drug.

• Generally reserved for seizures unresponsive to other anticonvulsants.

• Adverse reactions may be minimized by increasing dosage gradually.

• An alternative to lithium in treatment of some affective disorders.

• Patient may take with food to minimize GI distress.

---

clonazepam
Klonopin, Rivotril
Controlled Substance Schedule IV
Pregnancy Risk Category: C

HOW SUPPLIED
Tablets: 0.5 mg, 1 mg, 2 mg
Drops: 2.5 mg/ml‡
Injection: 1 mg/ml‡

MECHANISM OF ACTION
Appears to act on the limbic system, thalamus, and hypothalamus to produce anticonvulsant effects. A benzodiazepine.

INDICATIONS & DOSAGE
Absence (petit mal) and atypical absence seizures; akinetic and myoclonic seizures—
Adults: initial dosage should not exceed 1.5 mg P.O. daily, in three divided doses. May be increased by 0.5 to 1 mg q 3 days until seizures are controlled. Maximum recommended daily dosage is 20 mg.
Children up to 10 years or 30 kg: 0.01 to 0.03 mg/kg P.O. daily (not to exceed 0.05 mg/kg daily), divided q 8 hours. Increase dosage by 0.25 to 0.5 mg q third day to a maximum maintenance dosage of 0.1 to 0.2 mg/kg daily.
Status epilepticus (where parenteral form is available)—
Adults: 1 mg by slow I.V. infusion.
Children: 0.5 mg by slow I.V. infusion.

ADVERSE REACTIONS
Blood: leukopenia, thrombocytopenia, eosinophilia.
CNS: *drowsiness, ataxia, behavioral disturbances (especially in children),* slurred speech, tremor, confusion.
EENT: *increased salivation,* diplopia, nystagmus, abnormal eye movements.
GI: constipation, gastritis, change in appetite, nausea, abnormal thirst, sore gums.
GU: dysuria, enuresis, nocturia, urinary retention.
Skin: rash.
Other: respiratory depression.

INTERACTIONS
Alcohol, CNS depressants: increased CNS depression. Monitor closely.

NURSING CONSIDERATIONS
• Contraindicated in hepatic disease; chlordiazepoxide, diazepam, or other benzodiazepine sensitivity; or acute narrow-angle glaucoma. Use with caution in chronic respiratory disease, impaired renal function, and open-angle glaucoma.
• Elderly patients are more sensitive to the drug's CNS effects.
• Warn patient to avoid activities that require alertness and good psychomotor coordination until CNS effects of the drug are known.
• Never withdraw drug suddenly. Call doctor at once if adverse reactions develop.
• Obtain periodic CBC and liver function tests.
• Monitor patient for oversedation.
• Withdrawal symptoms similar to those of barbiturates.

ethosuximide
Zarontin
Pregnancy Risk Category: C

HOW SUPPLIED
Capsules: 250 mg
Syrup: 250 mg/5 ml

MECHANISM OF ACTION
Increases seizure threshold. Reduces the paroxysmal spike-and-wave pattern of absence seizures by depressing nerve transmission in the motor cortex. A succinimide derivative.

Italicized adverse reactions are common or life-threatening.
*Liquid form contains alcohol.   **May contain tartrazine.

INDICATIONS & DOSAGE
Absence (petit mal) seizure—
Adults and children over 6 years:
initially, 250 mg P.O. b.i.d. May increase by 250 mg q 4 to 7 days up to 1.5 g daily.
Children 3 to 6 years: 250 mg P.O. daily or 125 mg P.O. b.i.d. May increase by 250 mg q 4 to 7 days up to 1.5 g daily.

ADVERSE REACTIONS
Blood: leukopenia, eosinophilia, *agranulocytosis,* pancytopenia, *aplastic anemia.*
CNS: *drowsiness,* headache, *fatigue, dizziness,* ataxia, irritability, hiccups, *euphoria, lethargy.*
EENT: myopia.
GI: *nausea, vomiting,* diarrhea, gum hypertrophy, weight loss, cramps, tongue swelling, *anorexia, epigastric and abdominal pain.*
GU: vaginal bleeding.
Skin: urticaria, pruritic and erythematous rashes, hirsutism.

INTERACTIONS
None significant.

NURSING CONSIDERATIONS
• Contraindicated in hypersensitivity to succinimide derivatives. Use cautiously in hepatic or renal disease.
• Never withdraw drug suddenly. Abrupt withdrawal may precipitate absence seizures. Call doctor immediately if adverse reactions develop.
• Warn patient to avoid activities that require alertness and good psychomotor coordination until CNS effects of the drug are known.
• Obtain CBC every 3 months.
• Therapeutic blood levels 40 to 80 mcg/ml.
• May increase frequency of generalized tonic-clonic seizures when used alone in patients who have mixed types of seizures.
• May cause positive direct Coombs' test.

• Currently the drug of choice for treating absence seizures.
• Patient may take with food to minimize GI distress.

---

ethotoin
Peganone
Pregnancy Risk Category: D

HOW SUPPLIED
Tablets: 250 mg, 500 mg

MECHANISM OF ACTION
Stabilizes neuronal membranes and limits seizure activity by either increasing efflux or decreasing influx of sodium ions across cell membranes in the motor cortex during generation of nerve impulses. Hydantoin derivative.

INDICATIONS & DOSAGE
Generalized tonic-clonic (grand mal) or complex-partial (psychomotor) seizures—
Adults: initially, 250 mg P.O. q.i.d. after meals. May increase slowly over several days to 3 g daily divided q.i.d.
Children: initially, 250 mg P.O. b.i.d. May increase up to 250 mg P.O. q.i.d.

ADVERSE REACTIONS
Blood: thrombocytopenia, leukopenia, *agranulocytosis,* pancytopenia, megaloblastic anemia.
CNS: fatigue, insomnia, dizziness, headache, numbness.
CV: chest pain.
EENT: diplopia, nystagmus.
GI: *nausea, vomiting, diarrhea,* gingival hyperplasia (rare).
Skin: rash.
Other: fever, lymphadenopathy.

INTERACTIONS
Alcohol, folic acid: monitor for decreased ethotoin activity.
Oral anticoagulants, antihistamines, chloramphenicol, cimetidine, diazepam, diazoxide, disulfiram, isoniazid,

phenylbutazone, salicylates, sulfa-methizole, valproate: monitor for increased ethotoin activity and toxicity. *Phenacemide:* paranoia. Use together cautiously.

NURSING CONSIDERATIONS
• Contraindicated in hydantoin hypersensitivity or hepatic or hematologic disorders. Use cautiously in patients receiving other hydantoin derivatives.
• Never withdraw drug suddenly. Call doctor at once if adverse reactions develop.
• Warn patient to avoid activities that require alertness and good psychomotor coordination until CNS effects of the drug are known.
• Obtain CBC and urinalysis when therapy starts and monthly thereafter. Periodically monitor liver function tests on long-term use.
• Give after meals. Schedule doses as evenly as possible over 24 hours.
• Discontinue drug if lymphadenopathy or lupus-like syndrome (fever, bruising, and sore throat) develops.
• Heavy use of alcohol may diminish benefits of drug.
• Hydantoin derivative of choice in young adults who are prone to gingival hyperplasia caused by phenytoin. Otherwise, infrequently used in the treatment of epilepsy.
• Ethotoin generally produces milder adverse reactions than phenytoin; however, the large doses required to maintain its therapeutic effect frequently cause GI distress.

---

magnesium sulfate
Pregnancy Risk Category: B

HOW SUPPLIED
Injection: 10% (0.8 mEq/ml), 12.5% (1 mEq/ml), 25% (2 mEq/ml), 50% (4 mEq/ml)

MECHANISM OF ACTION
May decrease acetylcholine released by nerve impulse, but its anticonvulsant mechanism is unknown.

INDICATIONS & DOSAGE
Hypomagnesemic seizures—
Adults: 1 to 2 g (as 10% solution) I.V. over 15 minutes, then 1 g I.M. q 4 to 6 hours, based on patient response and blood magnesium levels.
Seizures secondary to hypomagnesemia in acute nephritis—
Children: 0.2 ml/kg of 50% solution I.M. q 4 to 6 hours, p.r.n. or 100 mg/kg of 10% solution I.V. very slowly. Titrate dosage according to blood magnesium levels and seizure response.
Prevention or control of seizures in preeclampsia or eclampsia—
Women: initially, 4 g I.V. in 250 ml dextrose 5% in water and 4 g deep I.M. each buttock; then 4 g deep I.M. into alternate buttock q 4 hours, p.r.n. Alternatively, 4 g I.V. loading dose followed by 1 to 4 g hourly as an I.V. infusion.

ADVERSE REACTIONS
CNS: *sweating,* drowsiness, *depressed reflexes,* flaccid paralysis, hypothermia.
CV: *hypotension, flushing, circulatory collapse,* depressed cardiac function, *heart block.*
Other: *respiratory paralysis,* hypocalcemia.

INTERACTIONS
Neuromuscular blocking agents: may cause increased neuromuscular blockade. Use cautiously.

NURSING CONSIDERATIONS
• Use cautiously in impaired renal function, myocardial damage, and heart block, and in women in labor.
• Magnesium sulfate can decrease the frequency and force of uterine contractions.

• Keep I.V. calcium gluconate available to reverse magnesium intoxication; however, use cautiously in patients undergoing digitalization due to danger of arrhythmias.
• Monitor vital signs every 15 minutes when giving drug I.V.
• Watch for respiratory depression and signs of heart block. Respirations should be approximately 16/minute before each dose given.
• Monitor intake/output. Urine output should be 100 ml or more in 4-hour period before each dose.
• Check blood magnesium levels after repeated doses. Disappearance of knee-jerk and patellar reflexes is a sign of pending magnesium toxicity.
• Maximum infusion rate is 150 mg/minute. Rapid drip will induce uncomfortable feeling of heat.
• Especially when given I.V. to toxemic mothers within 24 hours before delivery, observe neonates for signs of magnesium toxicity, including neuromuscular or respiratory depression.
• Signs of hypermagnesemia begin to appear at blood levels of 4 mEq/liter.
• Has been used as a tocolytic agent (suppresses uterine contractions) to inhibit premature labor.

---

mephenytoin
Mesantoin

Pregnancy Risk Category: C

HOW SUPPLIED
Tablets: 100 mg

MECHANISM OF ACTION
Stabilizes neuronal membranes and limits seizure activity by either increasing efflux or decreasing influx of sodium ions across cell membranes in the motor cortex during generation of nerve impulses. Hydantoin derivative.

INDICATIONS & DOSAGE
Generalized tonic-clonic (grand mal)
or complex-partial (psychomotor) seizures—
Adults: 50 to 100 mg P.O. daily. May increase by 50 to 100 mg at weekly intervals up to 200 mg P.O. t.i.d.
Children: initially, 50 to 100 mg P.O. daily or 100 to 450 mg/m² P.O. daily in three divided doses. May increase slowly by 50 to 100 mg at weekly intervals up to 200 mg P.O. t.i.d., divided q 8 hours. Dosage must be adjusted individually.

ADVERSE REACTIONS
Blood: *leukopenia,* neutropenia, *agranulocytosis,* thrombocytopenia, pancytopenia, eosinophilia.
CNS: ataxia, *drowsiness,* fatigue, irritability, choreiform movements, depression, tremor, sleeplessness, dizziness (usually transient).
EENT: conjunctivitis, diplopia, nystagmus.
GI: gingival hyperplasia, nausea and vomiting (with prolonged use).
Skin: *rashes, exfoliative dermatitis.*
Other: hypertrichosis, edema, dysarthria, lymphadenopathy, polyarthropathy, pulmonary fibrosis, photosensitivity.

INTERACTIONS
Alcohol, folic acid: monitor for decreased mephenytoin activity.
Oral anticoagulants, antihistamines, chloramphenicol, cimetidine, diazepam, diazoxide, disulfiram, isoniazid, phenylbutazone, salicylates, sulfamethizole, valproate: monitor for increased mephenytoin activity and toxicity.

NURSING CONSIDERATIONS
• Contraindicated in hydantoin hypersensitivity. Use cautiously in patients receiving other hydantoin derivatives.
• Tell patient to notify doctor if fever, sore throat, bleeding, or rash occurs.
• Periodically monitor liver function studies with long-term use. Check

---

CBC and platelet count initially and every 2 weeks thereafter, up to 2 weeks after full dose is attained; then monthly for first year and every 3 months thereafter. Discontinue drug if neutrophil count becomes less than 1,600/mm³.
• Never withdraw drug suddenly. Call doctor if adverse reactions develop.
• Warn patient to avoid activities that require alertness and good psychomotor coordination until CNS effects of the drug are known.
• Therapeutic blood level of mephenytoin and its active metabolite is 25 to 40 mcg/ml.
• Heavy use of alcohol may diminish benefit of drug.
• Potentially life-threatening blood dyscrasias limit this drug's usefulness.

mephobarbital
Mebaral
Controlled Substance Schedule IV
Pregnancy Risk Category: D

HOW SUPPLIED
Tablets: 32 mg, 50 mg, 100 mg

MECHANISM OF ACTION
Depresses monosynaptic and polysynaptic transmission in the CNS and increases the threshold for seizure activity in the motor cortex. A barbiturate.

INDICATIONS & DOSAGE
Generalized tonic-clonic (grand mal) or absence (petit mal) seizures—
Adults: 400 to 600 mg P.O. daily or in divided doses.
Children: 6 to 12 mg/kg P.O. daily, divided q 6 to 8 hours (smaller doses are given initially and increased over 4 to 5 days as needed).

ADVERSE REACTIONS
Blood: megaloblastic anemia, *agranulocytosis,* thrombocytopenia.
CNS: *dizziness,* headache, *hangover,*

confusion, paradoxical excitation, exacerbation of existing pain, drowsiness.
CV: hypotension, bradycardia.
GI: nausea, vomiting, epigastric pain.
Skin: urticaria, morbilliform rash, blisters, purpura, erythema multiforme.
Other: allergic reactions (facial edema).

INTERACTIONS
Alcohol and other CNS depressants, including narcotic analgesics: excessive CNS depression. Use cautiously.
Griseofulvin: decreased absorption of griseofulvin.
MAO inhibitors: potentiated barbiturate effect. Monitor patient for increased CNS and respiratory depression.
Oral anticoagulants, estrogens and oral contraceptives, doxycycline, corticosteroids: mephobarbital may enhance the metabolism of these drugs. Monitor for decreased effect.
Rifampin: may decrease barbiturate levels. Monitor for decreased effect.

NURSING CONSIDERATIONS
• Contraindicated in barbiturate hypersensitivity, porphyria, or respiratory disease with dyspnea or obstruction. Use cautiously in hepatic, renal, cardiac, or respiratory function impairment; myasthenia gravis; and myxedema.
• Never withdraw drug suddenly. Call doctor at once if adverse reactions develop.
• Warn patient to avoid activities that require alertness and good psychomotor coordination until CNS effects of drug are known.
• Store in light-resistant container.
• In adults, give total or largest dose at night if seizures occur then.
• Three-quarters of drug is metabolized to phenobarbital; therapeutic

---

Italicized adverse reactions are common or life-threatening.
*Liquid form contains alcohol.   **May contain tartrazine.

blood levels as phenobarbital are 15 to 40 mcg/ml.
• Periodically monitor CBC, BUN, and creatinine.
• Women who use oral contraceptives should consider alternate birth control methods when receiving this drug because it may enhance contraceptive hormone metabolism and decrease its effectiveness.
• Suppresses REM sleep, as do other barbiturates. When drug is discontinued, patient may experience increased dreaming.

metharbital
Gemonil
Controlled Substance Schedule III
Pregnancy Risk Category: D

HOW SUPPLIED
Tablets: 100 mg

MECHANISM OF ACTION
Depresses monosynaptic and polysynaptic transmission in the CNS and increases the threshold for seizure activity in the motor cortex. A barbiturate.

INDICATIONS & DOSAGE
Generalized tonic-clonic (grand mal) or absence (petit mal) seizures; myoclonic or mixed seizures—
Adults: initially, 100 mg P.O. daily to t.i.d. May increase to 800 mg daily in divided doses.
Children: 5 to 15 mg/kg P.O. daily, divided t.i.d. May increase to 50 to 100 mg P.O. daily, b.i.d., or t.i.d.

ADVERSE REACTIONS
Blood: megaloblastic anemia, *agranulocytosis,* thrombocytopenia.
CNS: *dizziness,* irritability, *drowsiness,* headache, confusion, excitation.
CV: hypotension.
GI: nausea, vomiting, discomfort.
Skin: rash, urticaria, purpura, erythema multiforme.

INTERACTIONS
Alcohol and other CNS depressants, including narcotic analgesics: excessive CNS depression. Use cautiously.
Griseofulvin: decreased absorption of griseofulvin.
MAO inhibitors: potentiated barbiturate effect. Monitor patient for increased CNS and respiratory depression.
Oral anticoagulants, estrogens and oral contraceptives, doxycycline, corticosteroids: metharbital may enhance the metabolism of these drugs. Monitor for decreased effect.
Rifampin: may decrease barbiturate levels. Monitor for decreased effect.

NURSING CONSIDERATIONS
• Contraindicated in barbiturate hypersensitivity, manifest or latent porphyria, or respiratory disease with dyspnea or obstruction. Use cautiously in hepatic, cardiac, or renal impairment.
• Don't stop drug abruptly. Call doctor at once if adverse reactions develop.
• Warn patient to avoid activities that require alertness and good psychomotor coordination until CNS effects of the drug are known.
• Periodically monitor CBC, BUN, and creatinine.
• Women who use oral contraceptives should consider alternate birth control methods when receiving this drug because it may enhance contraceptive hormone metabolism and decrease its effectiveness.
• Seldom-used anticonvulsant. More sedative effects than phenobarbital.

methsuximide
Celontin
Pregnancy Risk Category: C

HOW SUPPLIED
Capsules: 150 mg, 300 mg

MECHANISM OF ACTION

Increases seizure threshold. Reduces the paroxysmal spike-and-wave pattern of absence seizures by depressing nerve transmission in the motor cortex. A succinimide derivative.

INDICATIONS & DOSAGE

Refractory absence (petit mal) seizures—

Adults and children: initially, 300 mg P.O. daily. May increase by 300 mg weekly. Maximum daily dosage is 1.2 g in divided doses.

ADVERSE REACTIONS

Blood: eosinophilia, leukopenia, monocytosis, pancytopenia.
CNS: *drowsiness, ataxia, dizziness,* irritability, nervousness, headache, insomnia, confusion, depression, aggressiveness.
EENT: blurred vision, photophobia, periorbital edema.
GI: *nausea, vomiting, anorexia,* diarrhea, weight loss, abdominal or epigastric pain.
Skin: urticaria, pruritic and erythematous rashes.

INTERACTIONS

None significant.

NURSING CONSIDERATIONS

• Contraindicated in hypersensitivity to succinimide derivatives. Use cautiously in hepatic or renal dysfunction.
• Never change or withdraw drug suddenly. Abrupt withdrawal may precipitate petit mal seizures. Call doctor immediately if adverse reactions develop.
• Warn patient to avoid activities that require alertness and good psychomotor coordination until CNS effects of the drug are known.
• Obtain CBC every 3 months; urinalysis and liver function tests every 6 months.

• Tell patient to call doctor promptly if lupus-like syndrome develops.
• May color urine pink or brown.
• Not as popular an anticonvulsant as ethosuximide.

paraldehyde

Paral
Controlled Substance Schedule IV
Pregnancy Risk Category: C

HOW SUPPLIED

Rectal or oral liquid: 1 g/ml
Injection: 5 ml‡

MECHANISM OF ACTION

Unknown.

INDICATIONS & DOSAGE

Refractory generalized tonic-clonic (grand mal) seizures, status epilepticus—
Adults: 5 to 10 ml I.M. (divide 10 ml dose into 2 injections); 0.2 to 0.4 ml/kg in 0.9% saline injection I.V.
Children: 0.15 ml/kg dose deep I.M. q 4 to 6 hours, p.r.n.; or 0.3 ml/kg rectally in olive oil q 4 to 6 hours; or 1 ml per year of age not to exceed 5 ml, repeated in 1 hour, p.r.n.; or dilute 5 ml in 95 ml 0.9% saline injection for I.V. infusion and titrate dose beginning at 5 ml/hour.
Sedation—
Adults: 4 to 10 ml P.O. or rectally; or 5 ml deep I.M. in upper outer quadrant of buttock. 3 to 5 ml I.V. (in emergency only).
Children: 0.15 ml/kg or 6 ml/m² P.O., rectally, or deep I.M.
Insomnia—
Adults: 10 to 30 ml P.O. or rectally; 10 ml I.M. or I.V.
Children: 0.3 ml/kg P.O., rectally, or deep I.M.
Alcohol withdrawal syndrome—
Adults: 5 to 10 ml P.O. or rectally; or 5 ml deep I.M. q 4 to 6 hours for the first 24 hours, not to exceed a total of 60 ml P.O. or 30 ml I.M.; then q 6

Italicized adverse reactions are common or life-threatening.
*Liquid form contains alcohol.   **May contain tartrazine.

hours on following days, not to exceed 40 ml P.O. or 20 ml I.M. per 24 hours.

Tetanus—

Adults: 4 to 5 ml I.V. (well diluted) or 12 ml (diluted 1:10) via gastric tube q 4 hours, p.r.n.; 5 to 10 ml I.M., p.r.n. to control seizures.

ADVERSE REACTIONS

CNS: confusion, tremor, weakness, irritability, dizziness.

CV: *I.V. administration may cause pulmonary edema or hemorrhage,* dilatation of right side of heart, *circulatory collapse.*

GI: irritation, *foul breath odor.*

GU: nephrosis with prolonged use.

Skin: *erythematous rash.*

Local: *pain,* sterile abscesses, sloughing of skin, fat necrosis, muscular irritation, nerve damage (if injection is near nerve trunk) at I.M. injection site.

Other: respiratory depression.

INTERACTIONS

Alcohol: increased CNS depression. Use with caution.

Disulfiram: increased paraldehyde and acetaldehyde blood levels; possible toxic disulfiram reaction. Use together cautiously.

NURSING CONSIDERATIONS

• Contraindicated in gastroenteritis with ulceration. Use cautiously in impaired hepatic function and asthma or other pulmonary disease.

• Use fresh supply. Don't expose to air. Don't use if liquid is brown or has a vinegary odor, or if container has been open longer than 24 hours.

• Watch closely for respiratory depression, especially in repeated doses.

• Dilute paraldehyde in olive oil or cottonseed oil 1:2 for rectal administration. Give as retention enema. May also use 200 ml normal saline solution to prepare enema.

• Keep patient's room well ventilated to remove exhaled paraldehyde.

• May cause drug dependence and severe withdrawal symptoms.

• Oral or rectal administration of decomposed paraldehyde may cause severe corrosion of stomach or rectum.

• Dilute oral dose with iced juice or milk to mask taste and odor and to reduce GI distress.

• Parenteral form may be difficult to obtain commercially in the United States. Check with pharmacy for availability.

• Paraldehyde is rarely given parenterally because of the availability of less toxic alternatives. I.V. administration is not advisable except in extreme emergencies.

• Drug reacts with plastic. Use glass syringe and bottle for parenteral dose. Prepare fresh I.V. solution every 4 hours. I.V. administration very hazardous.

• Give I.M. dose deeply, away from nerve trunks; massage injection site. Limit I.M. volume to a maximum of 5 ml at any one site.

---

paramethadione
Paradione* **

Pregnancy Risk Category: D

HOW SUPPLIED

Capsules: 150 mg, 300 mg

Oral solution: 300 mg/ml (65% alcohol) with dropper

MECHANISM OF ACTION

Raises the threshold for cortical seizures but does not modify seizure pattern. Decreases projection of focal activity and reduces both repetitive spinal-cord transmission and spike-and-wave patterns of absence (petit mal) seizures.

INDICATIONS & DOSAGE

Refractory absence (petit mal) seizures—

Adults: initially, 300 mg P.O. t.i.d. May increase by 300 mg weekly, up to 600 mg q.i.d., if needed.
Children over 6 years: 0.9 g P.O. daily in divided doses t.i.d. or q.i.d.
Children 2 to 6 years: 0.6 g P.O. daily in divided doses t.i.d. or q.i.d.
Children under 2 years: 0.3 g P.O. daily in divided doses b.i.d.

ADVERSE REACTIONS
Blood: neutropenia, leukopenia, eosinophilia, thrombocytopenia, pancytopenia, *agranulocytosis, hypoplastic and aplastic anemia.*
CNS: *drowsiness,* fatigue, vertigo, headache, paresthesias, irritability.
CV: hypertension, hypotension.
EENT: hemeralopia, photophobia, diplopia, epistaxis, retinal hemorrhage.
GI: nausea, vomiting, abdominal pain, weight loss, bleeding gums.
GU: albuminuria, vaginal bleeding.
Hepatic: abnormal liver function tests.
Skin: acneiform or morbilliform rash, *exfoliative dermatitis,* erythema multiforme, petechiae, alopecia.
Other: lymphadenopathy, lupus erythematosus.

INTERACTIONS
None significant.

NURSING CONSIDERATIONS
• Contraindicated in renal and hepatic dysfunction or severe blood dyscrasias. Use cautiously in retinal or optic nerve diseases.
• Never withdraw drug suddenly. Call doctor at once if adverse reactions develop.
• Discontinue drug if scotomata or signs of hepatitis, systemic lupus erythematosus, lymphadenopathy, skin rash, nephrosis, hair loss, or generalized tonic-clonic seizures appear.
• Tell patient to report sore throat, fever, malaise, bruises, petechiae, or epistaxis to doctor immediately. Advise patient to wear dark glasses if photosensitivity occurs. Warn him not to drive car or operate machinery until CNS effects of the drug are known.
• Obtain liver function studies and urinalysis before therapy; then monthly.
• Dilute oral solution with water before giving because it contains 65% alcohol.
• Give drug with food or milk to minimize GI upset.
• Monitor CBC. Discontinue drug if neutrophil count falls below 2,500/mm³.

---

phenacemide
Phenurone

Pregnancy Risk Category: D

HOW SUPPLIED
Tablets: 500 mg

MECHANISM OF ACTION
Stabilizes neuronal membranes and limits seizure activity by either increasing efflux or decreasing influx of sodium ions across cell membranes in the motor cortex during generation of nerve impulses. Hydantoin derivative.

INDICATIONS & DOSAGE
Refractory, complex-partial (psychomotor), generalized tonic-clonic (grand mal), absence (petit mal), and atypical absence seizures—
Adults: 500 mg P.O. t.i.d. May increase by 500 mg weekly up to 5 g daily, p.r.n.
Children 5 to 10 years: 250 mg P.O. t.i.d. May increase by 250 mg weekly, up to 1.5 g daily, p.r.n.

ADVERSE REACTIONS
Blood: *aplastic anemia, agranulocytosis,* leukopenia.
CNS: drowsiness, dizziness, insomnia, headaches, paresthesias, *depression, suicidal tendencies,* aggressiveness.

GI: anorexia, weight loss.
GU: nephritis with marked albumin-uria.
Hepatic: hepatitis, jaundice.
Skin: rashes.

INTERACTIONS
Anticonvulsants: enhanced risk of toxicity.
Ethotoin: paranoia. Use together cautiously.

NURSING CONSIDERATIONS
• Contraindicated in patients with preexisting personality disturbances or in patients achieving satisfactory seizure control with other anticonvulsants. Use with caution in patients with hepatic dysfunction or history of allergy, and when a hydantoin derivative is used concomitantly.
• Extremely toxic. Use drug only when other anticonvulsants are ineffective.
• Obtain liver function tests, CBCs, and urinalyses before and at monthly intervals during therapy.
• Tell patient to report sore throat or fever to doctor immediately.
• Warn patient to avoid activities that require alertness or good psychomotor coordination until CNS effects of the drug are known.
• Never withdraw drug suddenly. Call doctor at once if adverse reactions develop.
• Tell patient's family to watch for personality or psychological changes and report them to doctor at once.
• When phenacemide replaces another anticonvulsant, phenacemide dosage should be increased slowly while the dosage of the drug being discontinued is decreased slowly to maintain adequate seizure control.
• Notify doctor if patient develops jaundice or other signs of hepatitis, abnormal urinary findings, or WBC count below 4,000/mm³.

phenobarbital (phenobarbitone)
Barbita, Gardenal†, Luminal†, Solfoton

phenobarbital sodium (phenobarbitone sodium)
Luminal Sodium†
Controlled Substance Schedule IV
Pregnancy Risk Category: D

HOW SUPPLIED
Tablets: 8 mg, 15 mg, 16 mg, 30 mg, 32 mg, 60 mg, 65 mg, 100 mg
Capsules: 16 mg
Oral solution: 15 mg/5 ml, 20 mg/5 ml
Elixir: 20 mg/5 ml
Injection: 30 mg/ml, 60 mg/ml, 65 mg/ml, 130 mg/ml
Powder for injection: 120 mg/ampule

MECHANISM OF ACTION
Depresses monosynaptic and polysynaptic transmission in the CNS and increases the threshold for seizure activity in the motor cortex. As a sedative, probably interferes with transmission of impulses from the thalamus to the cortex of the brain. A barbiturate.

INDICATIONS & DOSAGE
All forms of epilepsy, febrile seizures in children—
Adults: 100 to 200 mg P.O. daily, divided t.i.d. or given as single dosage at bedtime.
Children: 4 to 6 mg/kg P.O. daily, usually divided q 12 hours. It can, however, be administered once daily.
Status epilepticus—
Adults: 10 mg/kg as I.V. infusion no faster than 50 mg/minute. May give up to 20 mg/kg total. Administer in acute care or emergency area only.
Children: 5 to 10 mg/kg I.V. May repeat q 10 to 15 minutes up to total of 20 mg/kg. I.V. injection rate should not exceed 50 mg/minute.

Sedation—
Adults: 30 to 120 mg P.O. daily in two or three divided doses.
Children: 6 mg/kg P.O. divided t.i.d.
Insomnia—
Adults: 100 to 320 mg P.O. or I.M.
Children: 3 to 6 mg/kg.
Preoperative sedation—
Adults: 100 to 200 mg I.M. 60 to 90 minutes before surgery.
Children: 16 to 100 mg I.M. 60 to 90 minutes before surgery.
Hyperbilirubinemia—
Neonates: 7 mg/kg daily P.O. from first to fifth day of life; or 5 mg/kg daily I.M. on first day, repeated P.O. on second to seventh days.
Chronic cholestasis—
Adults: 90 to 180 mg P.O. daily in two or three divided doses.
Children under 12 years: 3 to 12 mg/kg daily P.O. in two or three divided doses.

ADVERSE REACTIONS
CNS: *drowsiness, lethargy, hangover,* paradoxical excitement in elderly patients.
GI: nausea, vomiting.
Skin: rash, *Stevens-Johnson syndrome,* urticaria.
Local: pain, swelling, thrombophlebitis, necrosis, nerve injury.
Other: angioedema.

INTERACTIONS
Alcohol and other CNS depressants, including narcotic analgesics: excessive CNS depression. Use cautiously.
Diazepam: increased effects of both drugs. Use together cautiously.
Griseofulvin: decreased absorption of griseofulvin.
MAO inhibitors: potentiated barbiturate effect. Monitor for increased CNS and respiratory depression.
Oral anticoagulants, estrogens and oral contraceptives, doxycycline, corticosteroids: may enhance the metabolism of these drugs. Monitor for decreased effect.

Primidone: monitor for excessive phenobarbital blood levels.
Rifampin: may decrease barbiturate levels. Monitor for decreased effect.
Valproic acid: increased phenobarbital levels. Monitor for toxicity.

NURSING CONSIDERATIONS
• Contraindicated in barbiturate hypersensitivity, porphyria, hepatic dysfunction, respiratory disease with dyspnea or obstruction, nephritis, and in lactating women. Use cautiously in hyperthyroidism, diabetes mellitus, anemia, and in elderly or debilitated patients.
• Elderly patients are more sensitive to the drug's effects.
• I.V. injection should be reserved for emergency treatment and should be given slowly under close supervision. Monitor respirations closely.
• When administering I.V., do not give more than 60 mg/minute. Have recusitative equipment readily available.
• Give I.M. injection deeply. Superficial injection may cause pain, sterile abscess, and tissue sloughing.
• Do not use injectable solution if it contains a precipitate.
• Do not mix parenteral form with acidic solutions; precipitation may result.
• Watch for signs of barbiturate toxicity: coma, asthmatic breathing, cyanosis, clammy skin, and hypotension. Overdose can be fatal.
• Warn patient to avoid activities that require alertness and good psychomotor coordination until CNS effects of the drug are known.
• Don't stop drug abruptly. Call doctor immediately if adverse reactions develop.
• Full therapeutic effects not seen for 2 to 3 weeks, except when loading dose is used.
• Therapeutic blood levels are 15 to 40 mcg/ml.
• Make sure patient is aware that phe-

Italicized adverse reactions are common or life-threatening.
*Liquid form contains alcohol.   **May contain tartrazine.

nobarbital is available in different milligram strengths and sizes.

---

phensuximide
Milontin

Pregnancy Risk Category: D

HOW SUPPLIED
Capsules: 500 mg

MECHANISM OF ACTION
Increases seizure threshold. Reduces the paroxysmal spike-and-wave pattern of absence seizures by depressing nerve transmission in the motor cortex. A succinimide derivative.

INDICATIONS & DOSAGE
Absence (petit mal) seizures—
Adults and children: 500 mg to 1 g P.O. b.i.d. to t.i.d.

ADVERSE REACTIONS
Blood: transient leukopenia, pancytopenia, *agranulocytosis.*
CNS: muscular weakness, *drowsiness,* dizziness, ataxia, headache.
GI: nausea, vomiting, anorexia.
GU: urinary frequency, renal damage, hematuria.
Skin: pruritus, eruptions, erythema.
Other: lupus-like syndrome.

INTERACTIONS
None significant.

NURSING CONSIDERATIONS
• Contraindicated in hypersensitivity to succinimide derivatives. Use cautiously in patients with hepatic or renal disease.
• Never withdraw drug suddenly. Abrupt withdrawal may precipitate absence seizures. Call doctor immediately if adverse reactions develop.
• Warn patient to avoid hazardous activities that require alertness and good coordination until CNS effects of the drug are known.
• Obtain CBCs every 3 months; uri-

nalyses and liver function tests every 6 months.
• Tell patient to report lupus-like symptoms immediately.
• May color urine pink or red to reddish brown.
• Therapeutic blood level 40 to 80 mcg/ml.
• May increase incidence of generalized tonic-clonic seizures if used alone to treat patients with mixed seizure types.

---

phenytoin
Dilantin, Dilantin Infatabs, Dilantin-30 Pediatric, Dilantin-125

phenytoin sodium
Dilantin

phenytoin sodium (extended)
Dilantin Kapseals

phenytoin sodium (prompt)
Diphenylan

Pregnancy Risk Category: D

HOW SUPPLIED
phenytoin
Tablets (chewable): 50 mg
Oral suspension: 30 mg/5 ml, 125 mg/5 ml
phenytoin sodium
Capsules: 30 mg (27.6-mg base), 100 mg (92-mg base)
Injection: 50 mg/ml (46-mg base)
phenytoin sodium (extended)
Capsules: 30 mg (27.6-mg base), 100 mg (92-mg base)
phenytoin sodium (prompt)
Capsules: 30 mg (27.6-mg base), 100 mg (92 mg-base)

MECHANISM OF ACTION
Stabilizes neuronal membranes and limits seizure activity by either increasing efflux or decreasing influx of sodium ions across cell membranes in the motor cortex during generation of

---

nerve impulses. Produces antiarrhythmic effect by normalizing sodium influx to Purkinje's fibers when used to treat digitalis-induced arrhythmias. A hydantoin derivative.

INDICATIONS & DOSAGE
Generalized tonic-clonic (grand mal) seizures, status epilepticus, nonepileptic seizures (post-head trauma, Reye's syndrome)—
Adults: loading dose is 900 mg to 1.5 g I.V. at 50 mg/minute or P.O. divided t.i.d., then start maintenance dosage of 300 mg P.O. daily (extended only) or divided t.i.d. (extended or prompt).
Children: loading dose is 15 mg/kg I.V. at 50 mg/minute or P.O. divided q 8 to 12 hours, then start maintenance dosage of 5 to 7 mg/kg P.O. or I.V. daily, divided q 12 hours.
If patient has not received phenytoin previously or has no detectable blood level, use loading dose—
Adults: 900 mg to 1.5 g I.V. divided into t.i.d. at 50 mg/minute. Do not exceed 500 mg each dose.
Children: 15 mg/kg I.V. at 50 mg/minute.
If patient has been receiving phenytoin but has missed one or more doses and has subtherapeutic levels—
Adults: 100 to 300 mg I.V. at 50 mg/minute.
Children: 5 to 7 mg/kg I.V. at 50 mg/minute. May repeat lower dose in 30 minutes if needed.
Neuritic pain (migraine, trigeminal neuralgia, Bell's palsy)—
Adults: 200 to 400 mg P.O. daily.
Ventricular arrhythmias unresponsive to lidocaine or procainamide; supraventricular and ventricular arrhythmias induced by cardiac glycosides—
Adults: loading dose is 1 g P.O. divided over first 24 hours, followed by 500 mg daily for 2 days, then maintenance dose of 300 mg P.O. daily; 250 mg I.V. over 5 minutes until arrhythmias subside, adverse reactions de-

velop, or 1 g has been given. Infusion rate should never exceed 50 mg/minute (slow I.V. push).
Alternate method: 100 mg I.V. q 15 minutes until adverse reactions develop, arrhythmias are controlled, or 1 g has been given. May also administer entire loading dose of 1 g I.V. slowly at 25 mg/minute. Can be diluted in normal saline solution. I.M. dose not recommended because of pain and erratic absorption.
Children: 3 to 8 mg/kg P.O. or slow I.V. daily or 250 mg/m² daily given as single dose or in two divided doses.

ADVERSE REACTIONS
Blood: thrombocytopenia, leukopenia, *agranulocytosis,* pancytopenia, macrocytosis, megaloblastic anemia.
CNS: *ataxia, slurred speech, confusion,* dizziness, insomnia, nervousness, twitching, headache.
CV: hypotension, *ventricular fibrillation.*
EENT: *nystagmus, diplopia,* blurred vision.
GI: *nausea, vomiting, gingival hyperplasia (especially children).*
Hepatic: toxic hepatitis.
Skin: scarlatiniform or morbilliform rash; bullous, *exfoliative,* or purpuric *dermatitis; Stevens-Johnson syndrome;* lupus erythematosus; *hirsutism; toxic epidermal necrolysis;* photosensitivity.
Local: pain, necrosis, and inflammation at injection site; purple glove syndrome.
Other: periarteritis nodosa, lymphadenopathy, hyperglycemia, osteomalacia, hypertrichosis.

INTERACTIONS
Alcohol, dexamethasone, folic acid: monitor for decreased phenytoin activity.
Oral anticoagulants, antihistamines, amiodarone, chloramphenicol, cimetidine, cycloserine, diazepam, diazoxide, disulfiram, influenza vaccine,

---

Italicized adverse reactions are common or life-threatening.
*Liquid form contains alcohol.   **May contain tartrazine.

isoniazid, phenylbutazone, salicylates, sulfamethizole, valproate: monitor for increased phenytoin activity and toxicity.
Oral tube feedings with Osmolite or Isocal: may interfere with absorption of oral phenytoin. Schedule feedings as far as possible from drug administration.

NURSING CONSIDERATIONS

• Contraindicated in phenacemide or hydantoin hypersensitivity, bradycardia, SA and AV block, or Stokes-Adams syndrome. Use cautiously in hepatic or renal dysfunction, hypotension, myocardial insufficiency, and respiratory depression; in elderly or debilitated patients; and in patients receiving other hydantoin derivatives.
• Elderly patients tend to metabolize phenytoin slowly. Therefore, they may require lower dosages.
• Phenytoin requirements usually increase during pregnancy. Monitor serum levels closely.
• Don't withdraw drug suddenly. Call doctor at once if adverse reactions develop.
• Warn patient to avoid activities that require alertness and good psychomotor coordination until CNS effects of the drug are known.
• Don't mix drug with dextrose 5% in water because it will precipitate. Clear I.V. tubing first with normal saline solution. Never use cloudy solution. May mix with normal saline solution if necessary and give as an infusion. Administer infusion over 30 to 60 minutes, when possible. Infusion must begin within 1 hour after preparation and should run through an in-line filter. Discard 4 hours after preparation. Preferably, administer slowly (50 mg/minute) as an I.V. bolus.
• Do not give I.M. unless dosage adjustments are made. Drug may precipitate at injection site, cause pain, and be erratically absorbed.
• Obtain CBC and serum calcium lev-

els every 6 months, and periodically monitor hepatic function. Doctor may order folic acid and vitamin B_{12} if megaloblastic anemia is evident.
• Drug may color urine pink, red, or reddish-brown.
• Tell patient to carry identification stating that he's taking phenytoin.
• Stress importance of good oral hygiene and regular dental examinations. Gingivectomy may be necessary periodically.
• Drug should be stopped if rash appears. If rash is scarlet or measles-like, drug may be resumed after rash clears. If rash reappears, therapy should be stopped. If rash is exfoliative, purpuric, or bullous, don't resume drug.
• Use only clear solution for injection. Slight yellow color acceptable. Don't refrigerate.
• Avoid administering I.V. push phenytoin injections into veins in the back of the hand. Inject into larger veins to avoid discoloration known as purple glove syndrome.
• Divided doses given with or after meals may decrease GI adverse reactions.
• Shake suspension well before each dose. Use solid forms (tablets or capsules) if possible.
• Therapeutic phenytoin blood level is 10 to 20 mcg/ml.
• Heavy use of alcohol may diminish benefits of drug.
• Phenytoin levels may be decreased in mononucleosis. Monitor for increased seizure activity.
• Dilantin brand and Bolar generic capsules are the only oral forms that can be given once daily. Toxic levels may result if any other brand is given once daily. Dilantin brand tablets and oral suspension should not be taken once daily.
• Advise patient not to change brands or dosage forms once stabilized on therapy.

• Suspension available as 30 mg/5 ml or 125 mg/5 ml. Read label carefully.
• The drug was formerly known as diphenylhydantoin.

---

primidone
Apo-Primidone†, Myidone, Mysoline, Sertan†
Pregnancy Risk Category: D

HOW SUPPLIED
Tablets: 50 mg, 250 mg
Oral suspension: 250 mg/5 ml

MECHANISM OF ACTION
Unknown, but some activity may be caused by phenobarbital, which is an active metabolite.

INDICATIONS & DOSAGE
Generalized tonic-clonic (grand mal) seizures, complex-partial (psychomotor) seizures—
Adults and children over 8 years: 250 mg P.O. daily. Increase by 250 mg weekly, up to maximum of 2 g daily, divided q.i.d.
Children under 8 years: 125 mg P.O. daily. Increase by 125 mg weekly, up to maximum of 1 g daily, divided q.i.d.

ADVERSE REACTIONS
Blood: leukopenia, eosinophilia.
CNS: *drowsiness, ataxia,* emotional disturbances, vertigo, hyperirritability, fatigue.
EENT: *diplopia,* nystagmus, edema of the eyelids.
GI: anorexia, *nausea, vomiting.*
GU: impotence, polyuria.
Skin: morbilliform rash, alopecia.
Other: edema, thirst.

INTERACTIONS
Carbamezepine: increased primidone levels. Observe for toxicity.
Phenytoin: stimulated conversion of primidone to phenobarbital. Observe for increased phenobarbital effect.

NURSING CONSIDERATIONS
• Contraindicated in phenobarbital hypersensitivity or porphyria.
• Don't withdraw drug suddenly. Call doctor at once if adverse reactions develop.
• Warn patient to avoid hazardous activities that require alertness and good psychomotor coordination until CNS effects of the drug are known. Full therapeutic response may take 2 weeks or more.
• Therapeutic blood level of primidone is 5 to 12 mcg/ml. Therapeutic blood level of phenobarbital is 15 to 40 mcg/ml.
• CBC and routine blood chemistry should be done every 6 months.
• Partially converted to phenobarbital; use cautiously with phenobarbital.
• Shake liquid suspension well.

---

trimethadione
Tridione
Pregnancy Risk Category: D

HOW SUPPLIED
Capsules: 150 mg, 300 mg
Oral solution: 40 mg/ml

MECHANISM OF ACTION
Raises the threshold for cortical seizure but does not modify seizure pattern. Decreases projection of focal activity and reduces both repetitive spinal-cord transmission and spike-and-wave patterns of absence (petit mal) seizures. An oxazolidinedione derivative.

INDICATIONS & DOSAGE
Refractory absence (petit mal) seizures—
Adults and children over 13 years: initially, 300 mg P.O. t.i.d. May increase by 300 mg weekly up to 600 mg P.O. q.i.d.
Children: 13 mg/kg P.O. t.i.d. or 335 mg/m^2 P.O. t.i.d.; alternatively,

---

Italicized adverse reactions are common or life-threatening.
*Liquid form contains alcohol.   **May contain tartrazine.

Children under 2 years: 100 mg
P.O. t.i.d.
Children 2 to 6 years: 200 mg P.O.
t.i.d.
Children 6 to 13 years: 300 mg P.O.
t.i.d.

ADVERSE REACTIONS
Blood: neutropenia, leukopenia, eosinophilia, thrombocytopenia, pancytopenia, *agranulocytosis, hypoplastic
and aplastic anemia.*
CNS: *drowsiness,* fatigue, *malaise,*
insomnia, dizziness, headache, paresthesias, irritability.
CV: hypertension, hypotension.
EENT: *hemeralopia,* diplopia, photophobia, epistaxis, retinal hemorrhage.
GI: nausea, vomiting, anorexia, abdominal pain, bleeding gums.
GU: nephrosis, albuminuria, vaginal
bleeding.
Hepatic: abnormal liver function
tests.
Skin: acneiform and morbilliform
rash, *exfoliative dermatitis,* erythema
multiforme, petechiae, alopecia.
Other: lymphadenopathy, systemic
lupus-like syndrome, myasthenia-like
syndrome.

INTERACTIONS
None significant.

NURSING CONSIDERATIONS
• Contraindicated in paramethadione
and trimethadione hypersensitivity,
severe blood dyscrasias, or hepatic
dysfunction. Use with extreme caution in retinal and optic nerve diseases.
• Don't withdraw drug suddenly.
Abrupt withdrawal may precipitate
absence seizures. Call doctor immediately if adverse reactions develop.
• Check CBC, hepatic function, and
urinalysis before starting therapy and
monthly thereafter. Drug should be
stopped if neutrophil count falls below 2,500/mm³.

• Watch for impending toxicity; may
precipitate tonic-clonic seizure.
• Warn patient to report skin rash, alopecia, sore throat, fever, bruises, or
epistaxis to doctor immediately.
• Warn patient to avoid activities requiring alertness and good psychomotor coordination until CNS effects of
the drug are known.
• Suggest sunglasses if vision blurs in
bright light. Notify doctor.
• If scotomata or rash develops, drug
should be discontinued.
• May increase risk of tonic-clonic
seizures if used alone to treat patients
who have mixed types of seizures.
• Has been largely replaced by succinimide derivatives.

---

valproate sodium
Depakene Syrup, Epilim‡, Myproic
Acid Syrup

valproic acid
Dalpro, Depa, Depakene, Myproic
Acid

divalproex sodium
Depakote, Epival†, Valcote‡

Pregnancy Risk Category: D

HOW SUPPLIED
valproate sodium
Syrup: 250 mg/ml‡
valproic acid
Tablets (enteric-coated): 200 mg‡,
500 mg‡
Crushable tablets: 100 mg‡
Capsules: 250 mg
Syrup: 200 mg/5 ml‡
divalproex sodium
Tablets (enteric-coated): 125 mg, 250
mg, 500 mg

MECHANISM OF ACTION
Increases brain levels of gamma-ami-
nobutyric acid, which transmits in-
hibitory nerve impulses in the CNS.

INDICATIONS & DOSAGE
Simple and complex absence seizures (including petit mal), mixed seizure types (including absence seizures), investigationally in major motor (grand mal, tonic-clonic) seizures—
Adults and children: initially, 15 mg/kg P.O. daily divided b.i.d. or t.i.d.; then may increase by 5 to 10 mg/kg daily at weekly intervals up to maximum of 60 mg/kg daily, divided b.i.d. or t.i.d.

ADVERSE REACTIONS
Because drug usually used in combination with other anticonvulsants, adverse reactions reported may not be caused by valproic acid alone.
Blood: *inhibited platelet aggregation, thrombocytopenia, increased bleeding time.*
CNS: *sedation,* emotional upset, depression, psychosis, aggression, hyperactivity, behavioral deterioration, muscle weakness, tremor.
EENT: stomatitis.
GI: *nausea, vomiting,* indigestion, diarrhea, abdominal cramps, constipation, increased appetite and weight gain, *anorexia,* pancreatitis. (*Note:* lower incidence of GI effects with divalproex.)
Hepatic: *elevated enzymes, toxic hepatitis.*
Metabolic: *elevated serum ammonia.*
Other: alopecia.

INTERACTIONS
Antacids, aspirin: May cause valproic acid toxicity. Use together cautiously and monitor blood levels.
Phenobarbital: increased phenobarbital levels.
Phenytoin: increased or decreased phenytoin levels.

NURSING CONSIDERATIONS
• Contraindicated in hepatic dysfunction. Use cautiously in children under 2 years; in children with congenital metabolic disorders or mental retardation; in patients with organic brain disease; and those taking multiple anticonvulsants.
• Tell patient not to disontinue the drug suddenly. Call doctor at once if adverse reactions develop.
• Obtain liver function studies, platelet counts, and prothrombin time before starting drug and every month thereafter, especially during the first 6 months of therapy.
• Serious or fatal hepatotoxicity may follow nonspecific symptoms, such as malaise, fever, and lethargy.
• Warn patient to avoid activities that require alertness and good psychomotor coordination until CNS effects of the drug are known.
• May give drug with food or milk to reduce GI adverse reactions. Advise against chewing capsules; causes irritation of mouth and throat.
• May need to reduce dosage if tremors occur.
• May produce false-positive test results for ketones in urine.
• Available as tasty red syrup. Keep out of reach of children.
• Syrup is more rapidly absorbed. Peak effect within 15 minutes.
• Syrup shouldn't be mixed with carbonated beverages; may be irritating to mouth and throat.
• Don't administer syrup to patients who need sodium restriction. Check with doctor.
• Valproic acid has been used investigationally to prevent recurrent febrile seizures in children.

Italicized adverse reactions are common or life-threatening.
*Liquid form contains alcohol.   **May contain tartrazine.

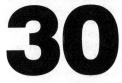

Antidepressants

Monoamine oxidase inhibitors
isocarboxazid
phenelzine sulfate
tranylcypromine sulfate

Tricyclic antidepressants
amitriptyline hydrochloride
amoxapine
clomipramine hydrochloride
desipramine hydrochloride
doxepin hydrochloride
imipramine hydrochloride
imipramine pamoate
maprotiline hydrochloride
nortriptyline hydrochloride
protriptyline hydrochloride
trimipramine maleate

Miscellaneous
bupropion hydrochloride
fluoxetine hydrochloride
trazodone hydrochloride

COMBINATION PRODUCTS
ETRAFON 2-10: perphenazine 2 mg and amitriptyline hydrochloride 10 mg.
ETRAFON: perphenazine 2 mg and amitriptyline hydrochloride 25 mg.
ETRAFON-A: perphenazine 4 mg and amitriptyline hydrochloride 10 mg.
ETRAFON-FORTE: perphenazine 4 mg and amitriptyline hydrochloride 25 mg.
LIMBITROL 5-12.5: chlordiazepoxide 5 mg and amitriptyline hydrochloride 12.5 mg.
LIMBITROL 10-25: chlordiazepoxide 10 mg and amitriptyline hydrochloride 25 mg.
TRIAVIL 2-10, TRIAVIL 4-10, TRIAVIL 2-25, TRIAVIL 4-25 are products identical to the Etrafon products listed above. Triavil is also available as TRIAVIL 4-50 (perphenazine 4 mg and amitriptyline hydrochloride 50 mg).

---

amitriptyline hydrochloride
Amitril, Apo-Amitriptylene†, Elavil, Emitrip, Endep, Enovil, Laroxyl‡, Levate†, Meravil†, Novo-Triptyn†
Pregnancy Risk Category: D

HOW SUPPLIED
Tablets: 10 mg, 25 mg, 50 mg, 75 mg, 100 mg, 150 mg
Injection: 10 mg/ml

MECHANISM OF ACTION
Increases the amount of norepinephrine or serotonin, or both, in the CNS by blocking their reuptake by the presynaptic neurons. This action allows these neurotransmitters to accumulate.

INDICATIONS & DOSAGE
Treatment of depression—
Adults: 50 to 100 mg P.O. h.s., increasing to 200 mg daily; maximum dosage is 300 mg daily if needed; or 20 to 30 mg I.M. q.i.d. Alternatively, the entire dosage can be given at bedtime.
Elderly patients and adolescents: 30 mg P.O. daily in divided doses. May be increased to 150 mg.

ADVERSE REACTIONS
CNS: *drowsiness, dizziness,* excita-

---

tion, tremors, weakness, confusion, headache, nervousness.
CV: *orthostatic hypotension, tachycardia, ECG changes,* hypertension.
EENT: *blurred vision,* tinnitus, mydriasis.
GI: *dry mouth, constipation,* nausea, vomiting, anorexia, paralytic ileus.
GU: *urine retention.*
Skin: rash, urticaria.
Other: *sweating,* allergy.
After abrupt withdrawal of long-term therapy: nausea, headache, malaise. (Does not indicate addiction.)

INTERACTIONS
Barbiturates: decrease tricyclic antidepressant (TCA) blood levels. Monitor for decreased antidepressant effect.
Cimetidine, methylphenidate: increases TCA blood levels. Monitor for enhanced antidepressant effect.
Epinephrine, norepinephrine: increase hypertensive effect. Use with caution.
MAO inhibitors: may cause severe excitation, hyperpyrexia, or seizures, usually with high dosage. Use together cautiously.

NURSING CONSIDERATIONS
• Contraindicated during acute recovery phase of myocardial infarction, in patients with history of seizure disorders, and in prostatic hypertrophy. Use with caution in patients who are suicide risks; in patients with urine retention, narrow-angle glaucoma, increased intraocular pressure, cardiovascular disease, impaired hepatic function, or hyperthyroidism; and in patients receiving thyroid medications, electroshock therapy, or elective surgery.
• Reduce dosage in elderly or debilitated persons and adolescents.
• Do not withdraw drug abruptly.
• If psychotic signs increase, dosage should be reduced. Record mood

changes. Watch for suicidal tendencies. Allow minimum supply of tablets to lessen suicide risk.
• Check for urine retention and constipation. Increase fluids to lessen constipation. Suggest stool softener or high-fiber diet, if needed.
• Warn patient to avoid activities that require alertness and good psychomotor coordination until CNS effects of the drug are known. Drowsiness and dizziness usually subside after first few weeks.
• Has strong anticholinergic effects; one of the most sedating tricyclic antidepressants. Avoid combining with alcohol or other depressants.
• Expect delay of 2 weeks or more before noticeable effect. Full effect may take 4 weeks or more.
• Dry mouth may be relieved with sugarless hard candy or gum. Saliva substitutes may be necessary.
• Advise the patient not to take any other drugs (prescription or OTC) without first consulting the doctor.
• Whenever possible, patient should take full dose at bedtime. Warn the patient about the possibility of morning orthostatic hypotension.
• Has been used to treat intractable hiccups, chronic severe pain, and patients with eating disorders (bulimia or anorexia nervosa).

amoxapine
Asendin

Pregnancy Risk Category: C

HOW SUPPLIED
Tablets: 25 mg, 50 mg, 100 mg, 150 mg

MECHANISM OF ACTION
Increases the amount of norepinephrine or serotonin, or both, in the CNS by blocking their reuptake by the presynaptic neurons. This action allows these neurotransmitters to accumulate.

Italicized adverse reactions are common or life-threatening.
*Liquid form contains alcohol.   **May contain tartrazine.

INDICATIONS & DOSAGE

Treatment of depression—
Adults: initial dose 50 mg P.O. t.i.d. May increase to 100 mg t.i.d. on third day of treatment. Increases above 300 mg daily should be made only if 300 mg daily has been ineffective during a trial period of at least 2 weeks. When effective dosage is established, entire dosage (not exceeding 300 mg) may be given at bedtime. Maximum dosage is 600 mg in hospitalized patients.

ADVERSE REACTIONS

CNS: *drowsiness, dizziness,* excitation, tremors, weakness, confusion, headache, nervousness, *tardive dyskinesia* (especially in elderly women).
CV: *orthostatic hypotension, tachycardia, ECG changes,* hypertension.
EENT: *blurred vision,* tinnitus, mydriasis.
GI: *dry mouth, constipation,* nausea, vomiting, anorexia, paralytic ileus.
GU: *urine retention, acute renal failure.*
Skin: rash, urticaria.
Other: *sweating,* weight gain and craving for sweets, allergy.
After abrupt withdrawal of long-term therapy: nausea, headache, malaise. (Does not indicate addiction.)

INTERACTIONS

Barbiturates: decrease tricyclic antidepressant (TCA) blood levels. Monitor for decreased antidepressant effect.
Cimetidine: may increase amoxapine serum levels. Monitor for increased adverse effects.
Epinephrine, norepinephrine: increase hypertensive effect. Use with caution.
MAO inhibitors: may cause severe excitation, hyperpyrexia, or seizures, usually with high dose. Use together cautiously.
Methylphenidate: increases TCA blood levels. Monitor for enhanced antidepressant effect.

NURSING CONSIDERATIONS

• Contraindicated in acute recovery phase of myocardial infarction, in patients with history of seizure disorders, and in prostatic hypertrophy. Use with caution in patients who are suicide risks; in urine retention, narrow-angle glaucoma, increased intraocular pressure, cardiovascular disease, impaired hepatic function, or hyperthyroidism; and in patients receiving thyroid medications, electroshock therapy, or elective surgery.
• Monitor for signs and symptoms of tardive dyskinesia, especially in elderly women.
• Reduce dosage in elderly or debilitated persons and adolescents.
• Do not withdraw drug abruptly.
• If psychotic signs increase, reduce dosage. Record mood changes. Watch for suicidal tendencies. Allow minimum supply of tablets to lessen suicide risk.
• Expect delay of 2 weeks or more before noticeable effect. Full effect may take 4 weeks or more.
• Check for urine retention and constipation. Increase fluids to lessen constipation. Suggest stool softener, if needed.
• Warn patient to avoid activities that require alertness and good psychomotor coordination until CNS effects of the drug are known. Drowsiness and dizziness usually subside after first few weeks.
• Dry mouth may be relieved with sugarless hard candy or gum. Saliva substitutes may be necessary.
• Whenever possible, patient should take full dose at bedtime.

bupropion hydrochloride
Wellbutrin

Pregnancy Risk Category: B

HOW SUPPLIED
Tablets: 75 mg, 100 mg

MECHANISM OF ACTION
Unknown. Bupropion does not inhibit monoamine oxidase and is a weak inhibitor of norepinephrine, dopamine, and serotonin reuptake.

INDICATIONS & DOSAGE
Treatment of depression—
Adults: initially, 100 mg P.O. b.i.d. If necessary, dosage is increased after 3 days to the usual dose of 100 mg P.O. t.i.d. If there is no response after several weeks of therapy, dosage may be increased to 150 mg t.i.d.

ADVERSE REACTIONS
CNS: *headache,* akathisia, *seizures, agitation,* anxiety, *confusion,* decreased libido, delusions, euphoria, hostility, impaired sleep quality, insomnia, sedation, sensory disturbance, tremor.
CV: cardiac arrhythmias, hypertension, hypotension, palpitations, syncope, tachycardia.
GI: appetite increase, constipation, dyspepsia, nausea, vomiting, dry mouth.
GU: impotence, menstrual complaints, urinary frequency.
Skin: pruritus, rash, cutaneous temperature disturbance.
Other: arthritis, fever and chills, excessive sweating, auditory disturbance, gustatory disturbance, blurred vision.

INTERACTIONS
Levodopa, phenothiazines, MAO inhibitors, or tricyclic antidepressants; or recent and rapid withdrawal of benzodiazepines: increased risk of adverse reactions, including seizures.

NURSING CONSIDERATIONS
• Contraindicated in patients who are allergic to the drug; patients who have taken MAO inhibitors within the previous 14 days; and patients with seizure disorders. About 0.4% of patients treated at doses up to 450 mg/day may experience seizures. If dosage is increased to 600 mg/day, the incidence of seizures increases about tenfold. Bupropion is also contraindicated in patients with a history of bulimia or anorexia nervosa because studies have revealed a higher incidence of seizures in these patients. Studies have also shown that patients who experience seizures often have predisposing factors, including history of head trauma; history of prior seizure; or CNS tumors; or they may be taking a drug that lowers the seizure threshold.
• Animal data suggest that bupropion may induce drug metabolizing enzymes, decreasing the effectiveness of other drugs taken concomitantly.
• Many patients experience a period of increased restlessness, especially at initiation of therapy. This may include agitation, insomnia, and anxiety. In clinical studies, some patients required sedative/hypnotic agents; about 2% had to discontinue the drug.
• Antidepressants can cause manic episodes during the depressed phase in patients with bipolar manic depression.
• Clinical trials revealed that 28% of the patients experienced a 5 lb or greater weight loss. This drug effect should be considered if weight loss is a major factor in the patient's depressive illness.
• Patients should be advised to take the drug regularly as scheduled, and to take each day's dosage in three divided doses to minimize the risk of seizures.
• Patients should be advised to avoid alcohol use, since it may contribute to the development of seizures.

Italicized adverse reactions are common or life-threatening.
*Liquid form contains alcohol.   **May contain tartrazine.

• Advise the patient to avoid hazardous activities that require alertness, including operating heavy machinery or driving a car, until the CNS effects of the drug are known.
• Patients should not take any other medications, including OTC medications, without first checking with their doctors.

---

clomipramine hydrochloride
Anafranil

Pregnancy Risk Category: C

HOW SUPPLIED
Capsules: 25 mg, 50 mg, 75 mg

MECHANISM OF ACTION
Mechanism is unknown; selectively inhibits reuptake of serotonin.

INDICATIONS & DOSAGE
Treatment of obsessive-compulsive disorder—
Adults: initially, 25 mg P.O. daily in divided doses with meals, gradually increasing to 100 mg daily during first 2 weeks. Maximum dosage, 250 mg/day in divided doses with meals. After titration, total daily dose may be given h.s.
Children and adolescents: initially, 25 mg P.O. daily, gradually increased to daily maximum of 3 mg/kg or 100 mg P.O., whichever is smaller; given in divided doses with meals during first 2 weeks. Maximum daily dosage is 3 mg/kg or 200 mg, whichever is smaller; may be given h.s. afer titration.
  Maintenance dosage in children, adolescents, and adults is the lowest effective dose h.s. Periodic reassessment and adjustment are necessary.

ADVERSE REACTIONS
CNS: *somnolence, tremor, dizziness,* headache, insomnia, *libido change,* *nervousness, myoclonus, increased appetite, fatigue.*
CV: postural hypotension, palpitations, tachycardia.
EENT: otitis media (children), *abnormal vision,* pharyngitis, rhinitis.
GI: *dry mouth, constipation, nausea, dyspepsia,* diarrhea, *anorexia,* abdominal pain, *nausea.*
GU: *micturition disorder,* urinary tract infection, dysmenorrhea, *ejaculation failure,* impotence.
Skin: *increased sweating,* rash, pruritus.
Other: myalgia.

INTERACTIONS
Barbiturates: decrease tricyclic antidepressant (TCA) blood levels. Monitor for decreased antidepressant effect.
Epinephrine, norepinephrine: increase hypertensive effect. Use with caution.
MAO inhibitors: hyperpyretic crisis, seizures, coma, death may result. Alcohol, barbiturates, other CNS depressants: exaggerated response.
Methylphenidate: increases TCA blood levels. Monitor for enhanced antidepressant effect.

NURSING CONSIDERATIONS
• Contraindicated during acute recovery period after myocardial infarction. Use with caution in patients with history of seizure disorder, in brain damage of varying etiology; in patients who are receiving other seizure threshold–lowering drugs; in patients at risk for suicide; in patients who are hyperthyroid or are receiving thyroid medication; in urine retention, narrow-angle glaucoma, increased intraocular pressure, cardiovascular disease, impaired hepatic function; and in patients with tumors of the adrenal medulla, or who are receiving electroshock therapy or electric surgery.
• Monitor for urine retention and constipation. Increase fluids to lessen

---

constipation. Suggest stool softener or high-fiber diet as needed.
• Warn patients to avoid hazardous activities requiring alertness and good psychomotor coordination, especially during titration. Daytime sedation, dizziness may occur.
• Avoid combining with other depressants or alcohol.
• Dry mouth may be relieved with sugarless candy or gum. Saliva substitutes may also be used.
• Total daily dose may be taken at bedtime after titration. During titration, dose may be divided and given with meals to minimize GI effects.
• Do not withdraw drug abruptly.

desipramine hydrochloride
Norpramin**, Pertofran‡, Pertofrane
Pregnancy Risk Category: C

HOW SUPPLIED
Tablets: 10 mg, 25 mg, 50 mg, 75 mg, 100 mg, 150 mg
Capsules: 25 mg, 50 mg

MECHANISM OF ACTION
Increases the amount of norepinephrine or serotonin, or both, in the CNS by blocking their reuptake by the presynaptic neurons. This action allows these neurotransmitters to accumulate.

INDICATIONS & DOSAGE
Treatment of depression—
Adults: 75 to 150 mg P.O. daily in divided doses, increasing to maximum of 300 mg daily. Alternatively, the entire dosage can be given at bedtime.
Elderly and adolescents: 25 to 50 mg P.O. daily, increasing gradually to maximum of 100 mg daily.

ADVERSE REACTIONS
CNS: *drowsiness, dizziness,* excitation, tremors, weakness, confusion, headache, nervousness.
CV: *orthostatic hypotension, tachycardia, ECG changes,* hypertension.
EENT: *blurred vision,* tinnitus, mydriasis.
GI: *dry mouth, constipation,* nausea, vomiting, anorexia, paralytic ileus.
GU: *urine retention.*
Skin: rash, urticaria.
Other: *sweating,* allergy.
After abrupt withdrawal of long-term therapy: nausea, headache, malaise. (Does not indicate addiction.)

INTERACTIONS
Barbiturates: decrease tricyclic antidepressant (TCA) blood levels. Monitor for decreased antidepressant effect.
Cimetidine: may increase desipramine serum levels. Monitor for increased adverse reactions.
Epinephrine, norepinephrine: increase hypertensive effect. Use with caution.
MAO inhibitors: may cause severe excitation, hyperpyrexia, or seizures, usually with high dose. Use together cautiously.
Methylphenidate: increases TCA blood levels. Monitor for enhanced antidepressant effect.

NURSING CONSIDERATIONS
• Contraindicated during acute recovery phase of myocardial infarction, in patients with history of seizure disorders, and in prostatic hypertrophy. Use with caution in cardiovascular disease, urine retention, narrow-angle glaucoma, thyroid disease, blood dyscrasias, or impaired hepatic function; in patients who are suicide risks; and in those receiving electroshock therapy, thyroid medication, or elective surgery.
• Reduce dosage in elderly or debilitated persons and adolescents.
• Do not withdraw drug abruptly.
• Orthostatic hypotension not as se-

Italicized adverse reactions are common or life-threatening.
*Liquid form contains alcohol.   **May contain tartrazine.

vere with this drug compared to other tricyclic antidepressants.

• If psychotic signs increase, dosage should be decreased. Record mood changes. Watch for suicidal tendencies. To lessen suicide risk, allow minimum supply of tablets.

• Check for urine retention and constipation. Increase fluids to lessen constipation. Suggest stool softener, if needed.

• Warn patient to avoid activities that require alertness and good psychomotor coordination until CNS effects of the drug are known. Drowsiness and dizziness usually subside after a few weeks.

• Dry mouth may be relieved with sugarless hard candy or gum. Saliva substitutes may be necessary.

• Drug has low potential for anticholinergic effects, is a metabolite of imipramine, and produces less sedation than amitriptyline or doxepin. Orthostatic hypotension is usually not a problem. Alcohol may antagonize effects of desipramine.

• Because it produces less tachycardia and other anticholinergic effects compared with other tricyclics, desipramine is often prescribed for cardiac patients.

• Expect delay of 2 weeks or more before noticeable effect. Full effect may take 4 weeks or more.

• Advise patient not to take any other drugs (prescription or OTC) without first consulting the doctor.

• Whenever possible, patient should take full dose at bedtime.

---

doxepin hydrochloride
Adapin**, Deptran‡, Sinequan, Triadapin†

Pregnancy Risk Category: C

HOW SUPPLIED
Tablets: 10 mg, 25 mg, 50 mg, 75 mg, 100 mg, 150 mg
Capsules: 10 mg‡, 25 mg‡

Oral concentrate: 10 mg/ml

MECHANISM OF ACTION
Increases the amount of norepinephrine or serotonin, or both, in the CNS by blocking their reuptake by the presynaptic neurons. This action allows these neurotransmitters to accumulate.

INDICATIONS & DOSAGE
Treatment of depression—
Adults: initially, 50 to 75 mg P.O. daily in divided doses, to maximum of 300 mg daily. Alternatively, entire dosage may be given at bedtime.

ADVERSE REACTIONS
CNS: *drowsiness, dizziness,* excitation, tremors, weakness, confusion, headache, nervousness.
CV: *orthostatic hypotension, tachycardia, ECG changes,* hypertension.
EENT: *blurred vision,* tinnitus, glossitis, mydriasis.
GI: *dry mouth, constipation,* nausea, vomiting, anorexia, paralytic ileus.
GU: *urine retention.*
Skin: rash, urticaria.
Other: *sweating,* allergy.
After abrupt withdrawal of long-term therapy: nausea, headache, malaise. (Does not indicate addiction.)

INTERACTIONS
Barbiturates: decrease tricyclic depressant (TCA) blood levels. Monitor for decreased antidepressant effect.
Cimetidine: may increase doxepin serum levels. Monitor for increased adverse reactions.
MAO inhibitors: may cause severe excitation, hyperpyrexia, or seizures, usually with high dose. Use together cautiously.
Methylphenidate: increases TCA blood levels. Monitor for enhanced antidepressant effect.

NURSING CONSIDERATIONS

• Contraindicated in urine retention, narrow-angle glaucoma, or prostatic hypertrophy. Use with caution in suicide risks.

• Reduce dose in elderly or debilitated patients, adolescents, and those receiving other medications (especially anticholinergics).

• Dilute oral concentrate with 120 ml water, milk, or juice (orange, grapefruit, tomato, prune, or pineapple). Incompatible with carbonated beverages.

• If psychotic symptoms increase, dosage should be decreased. Record mood changes. Watch for suicidal tendencies.

• Check for urine retention and constipation. Increase fluids to lessen constipation. Suggest stool softener, if needed.

• Warn patient to avoid activities that require alertness and good psychomotor coordination until CNS effects of the drug are known. Drowsiness and dizziness usually subside after a few weeks.

• Expect delay of 2 weeks or more before noticeable effect. Full effect may take 4 weeks or more.

• Dry mouth may be relieved with sugarless hard candy or gum. Saliva substitutes may be necessary.

• Has strong anticholinergic effects; one of the most sedating tricyclic antidepressants. Avoid combining with alcohol or other depressants.

• Advise patient not to take any other drugs (OTC or prescription) without first consulting the doctor.

• Liquid formulation available.

• Whenever possible, patient should take full dose at bedtime. Warn patient about the possibility of morning orthostatic hypotension.

• Especially well tolerated by elderly patients.

• May be useful for chronic, severe neurogenic pain.

---

fluoxetine hydrochloride
Prozac

Pregnancy Risk Category: B

HOW SUPPLIED
Pulvules: 20 mg.

MECHANISM OF ACTION
Inhibits the CNS neuronal uptake of serotonin.

INDICATIONS & DOSAGE
Short-term management of depressive illness—
Adults: initially, 20 mg P.O. in the morning; dosage increased according to patient response. May be given b.i.d. in the morning and at noon. Maximum dosage is 80 mg/day.

ADVERSE REACTIONS
CNS: *nervousness, anxiety, insomnia, headache, drowsiness, tremor, dizziness,* abnormal dreams.
CV: palpitations, flushing, bradycardia, arrhythmias.
EENT: flu-like syndrome, nasal congestion, upper respiratory infection, pharyngitis, cough sinusitis, visual disturbances, tinnitus, respiratory distress.
GI: *nausea, diarrhea, dry mouth, anorexia, dyspepsia,* constipation, abdominal pain, vomiting, taste change, flatulence, increased appetite.
GU: sexual dysfunction, urine retention.
Other: muscle pain, *weight loss, rash, pruritus, urticaria, asthenia,* edema, lymphadenopathy.

INTERACTIONS
Diazepam: half-life may be prolonged. Drugs highly bound to plasma proteins (warfarin, digitoxin) can cause displacement of drug and potential toxic effects.
Tryptophan: agitation, GI distress, and restlessness.

Italicized adverse reactions are common or life-threatening.
*Liquid form contains alcohol.   **May contain tartrazine.

NURSING CONSIDERATIONS
• Because this drug commonly causes nervousness and insomnia, patient should avoid taking this drug in the afternoon to prevent sleep disturbances.
• May cause dizziness or drowsiness in some patients. Warn patient to avoid driving or other hazardous activities that require alertness until CNS effects of the drug are known.
• Elderly or debilitated patients and patients with renal or hepatic dysfunction may require lower dosages or less frequent dosing.
• Fluoxetine and its active metabolite have a long elimination half-life. Clinical effects of dosage changes may not be evident for weeks; full antidepressant effects may not appear for 4 or more weeks of treatment.

---

imipramine hydrochloride
Apo-Imipramine†, Imiprin‡, Impril†, Janimine**, Novo-Pramine†, Tripramine, Tofranil**

imipramine pamoate
Tofranil-PM**

Pregnancy Risk Category: D

HOW SUPPLIED
Tablets: 10 mg, 25 mg, 50 mg
Injection: 12.5 mg/ml

MECHANISM OF ACTION
Increases the amount of norepinephrine or serotonin, or both, in the CNS by blocking their reuptake by the presynaptic neurons. This action allows these neurotransmitters to accumulate.

INDICATIONS & DOSAGE
Treatment of depression—
Adults: 75 to 100 mg P.O. or I.M. daily in divided doses, with 25- to 50-mg increments up to 200 mg. Maximum dosage is 300 mg daily. Alternatively, the entire dosage may be given at bedtime. (I.M. route rarely used.)
Childhood enuresis—
Children 6 years and older: 25 mg P.O. 1 hour before bedtime. If no response within 1 week, increase to 50 mg if the child is under 12 years; increase to 75 mg for children 12 years and over. In either case, do not exceed 2.5 mg/kg/day.

ADVERSE REACTIONS
CNS: *drowsiness, dizziness,* excitation, tremors, weakness, confusion, headache, nervousness.
CV: *orthostatic hypotension, tachycardia, ECG changes,* hypertension.
EENT: *blurred vision,* tinnitus, mydriasis.
GI: *dry mouth, constipation,* nausea, vomiting, anorexia, paralytic ileus.
GU: *urine retention.*
Skin: rash, urticaria.
Other: *sweating,* allergy.
After abrupt withdrawal of long-term therapy: nausea, headache, malaise. (Does not indicate addiction.)

INTERACTIONS
Barbiturates: decrease tricyclic antidepressant (TCA) blood levels. Monitor for decreased antidepressant effect.
Cimetidine: may increase imipramine serum levels. Monitor for increased adverse reactions.
Epinephrine, norepinephrine: increase hypertensive effect. Use with caution.
MAO inhibitors: may cause severe excitation, hyperpyrexia, or seizures, usually with high dose. Use together cautiously.
Methylphenidate: increases TCA blood levels. Monitor for enhanced antidepressant effect.

NURSING CONSIDERATIONS
• Contraindicated during acute recovery phase of myocardial infarction, in

---

prostatic hypertrophy, and in patients with history of seizure disorders. Use with extreme caution in cardiovascular disease, urine retention, narrow-angle glaucoma or increased intraocular pressure, thyroid disease, blood dyscrasias, or impaired hepatic function; in patients who are suicide risks; and in those receiving electroshock therapy, thyroid medication, or elective surgery.

• Reduce dosage in elderly or debilitated persons, adolescents, and patients with aggravated psychotic symptoms.

• Do not withdraw drug abruptly.

• If psychotic signs increase, dosage should be reduced. Record mood changes. Watch for suicidal tendencies. To lessen suicide risk, allow minimum supply of tablets.

• Check for urine retention and constipation. Increase fluids to lessen constipation. Suggest stool softener, if needed.

• Warn patient to avoid activities that require alertness and good psychomotor coordination until CNS effects of the drug are known. Drowsiness and dizziness usually subside after a few weeks.

• Expect delay of 2 weeks or more before noticeable effect. Full effect may take 4 weeks or more.

• Dry mouth may be relieved with sugarless hard candy or gum. Saliva substitutes may be necessary.

• Avoid combining with alcohol or other depressants.

• Advise patient not to take any other drugs (prescription or OTC) without first consulting the doctor.

• Imipramine has a high potential for inducing orthostatic hypotension. Whenever possible, patient should take full dose at bedtime. Warn patient about the possibility of morning orthostatic hypotension.

• May be useful for chronic, severe neurogenic pain.

• When treating enuresis, it may be more effective to divide dosage and administer the first dose earlier in the day (such as late afternoon) if the child is an "early night" bedwetter.

• To prevent relapse in children receiving the drug for enuresis, withdraw dosage gradually.

---

isocarboxazid
Marplan

Pregnancy Risk Category: C

HOW SUPPLIED
Tablets: 10 mg

MECHANISM OF ACTION
Promotes accumulation of neurotransmitters by inhibiting MAO.

INDICATIONS & DOSAGE
Treatment of depression—
Adults: 30 mg P.O. daily in divided doses. Reduce to 10 to 20 mg daily when condition improves. Not recommended for children under 16 years.

ADVERSE REACTIONS
CNS: *dizziness,* vertigo, weakness, headache, overactivity, hyperreflexia, tremors, muscle twitching, mania, *insomnia,* confusion, memory impairment, fatigue.
CV: *orthostatic hypotension,* arrhythmias, paradoxical hypertension.
EENT: blurred vision.
GI: dry mouth, *anorexia,* nausea, diarrhea, constipation.
Skin: rash.
Other: peripheral edema, sweating, weight changes, altered libido.

INTERACTIONS
Alcohol, barbiturates, and other sedatives; narcotics; dextromethorphan; tricyclic antidepressants: unpredictable interaction. Use with caution and in reduced dosage.
Amphetamines, ephedrine, levodopa, meperidine, metaraminol, methotrimeprazine, methylphenidate, phenyl-

---

Italicized adverse reactions are common or life-threatening.
*Liquid form contains alcohol.   **May contain tartrazine.

ephrine, phenylpropanolamine: pressor effects of these drugs are enhanced by isocarboxazid. Use together very cautiously.

Insulin, oral hypoglycemic agents: isocarboxazid may alter requirements for antidiabetic medications.

NURSING CONSIDERATIONS
• Contraindicated in elderly or debilitated patients; and in severe hepatic or renal impairment, CHF, pheochromocytoma; hypertensive, cardiovascular, or cerebrovascular disease; severe or frequent headaches. Also contraindicated with foods containing tryptophan or tyramine. Also during therapy with other MAO inhibitors (including pargyline hydrochloride, phenelzine sulfate, tranylcypromine sulfate) or within 10 days of such therapy; within 10 days of elective surgery requiring general anesthetic, cocaine, or local anesthetic containing sympathomimetic vasoconstrictors. Use cautiously with other psychotropic drugs or with spinal anesthetic; in hyperactive, agitated, or schizophrenic patients; in suicide risks; and in patients with diabetes or epilepsy.
• Avoid combining with alcohol or other depressant.
• Use only when tricyclic antidepressant or electroshock therapy is ineffective or contraindicated.
• If patient develops symptoms of overdosage (palpitations, frequent headaches, or severe orthostatic hypotension), hold dose and notify doctor.
• Watch for suicidal tendencies.
• Dosage is usually reduced to maintenance level as soon as possible.
• Do not withdraw drug abruptly.
• Weigh patient biweekly; check for edema and urine retention.
• Warn patient to avoid foods high in tyramine or tryptophan (aged cheese, Chianti wine, beer, avocados, chicken livers, chocolate, bananas, soy sauce, meat tenderizers, salami, bologna);

large amounts of caffeine; and self-medication with OTC cold, hay fever, or diet preparations.
• Incidence of orthostatic hypotension is high. Supervise walking. Tell patient to get out of bed slowly, sitting up first for 1 minute.
• Have phentolamine (Regitine) available to counteract severe hypertension.
• Continue precautions 10 days after stopping drug because it has long-lasting effects.
• Expect delay of 2 weeks or more before noticeable effect. Full effect may take 4 weeks or more.
• Obtain baseline blood pressure readings, CBC, and liver function tests before beginning therapy, and continue to monitor throughout treatment.

---

maprotiline hydrochloride
Ludiomil

Pregnancy Risk Category: B

HOW SUPPLIED
Tablets: 25 mg, 50 mg, 75 mg

MECHANISM OF ACTION
Increases the amount of norepinephrine or serotonin, or both, in the CNS by blocking their reuptake by the presynaptic neurons. This action allows these neurotransmitters to accumulate.

INDICATIONS & DOSAGE
Treatment of depression—
Adults: initial dose of 75 mg P.O. daily for patients with mild to moderate depression. The dosage may be increased as required to a dose of 150 mg daily. Maximum dosage is 225 mg in patients who are not hospitalized. More severely depressed, hospitalized patients may receive up to 300 mg daily.

ADVERSE REACTIONS
CNS: *drowsiness, dizziness,* excitation, *seizures,* tremors, weakness, confusion, headache, nervousness.
CV: orthostatic hypotension, tachycardia, *ECG changes,* hypertension.
EENT: *blurred vision,* tinnitus, mydriasis.
GI: *dry mouth, constipation,* nausea, vomiting, anorexia, paralytic ileus.
GU: *urine retention.*
Skin: rash, urticaria.
Other: *sweating,* allergy.
After abrupt withdrawal of long-term therapy: nausea, headache, malaise. (Does not indicate addiction.)

INTERACTIONS
Barbiturates: decrease maprotiline blood levels. Monitor for decreased antidepressant effect.
Cimetidine: may increase maprotiline serum levels. Monitor for increased adverse reactions.
Epinephrine, norepinephrine: increase hypertensive effect. Use with caution.
MAO inhibitors: may cause severe excitation, hyperpyrexia, or seizures, usually with high dose. Use together cautiously.
Methylphenidate: increases maprotiline blood levels. Monitor for enhanced antidepressant effect.

NURSING CONSIDERATIONS
• Contraindicated during acute recovery phase of myocardial infarction and in prostatic hypertrophy. Use with caution in CV disease, urine retention, narrow-angle glaucoma, thyroid disease or medication, blood dyscrasias, and impaired hepatic functon; in patients with a history of seizures; in patients who are suicide risks; and in those receiving electroshock therapy or elective surgery.
• Reduce dosage in elderly or debilitated persons and adolescents.
• Do not withdraw drug abruptly.

• If psychotic signs increase, reduce dosage. Record mood changes. Watch for suicidal tendencies. To lessen suicide risk, allow minimum supply of tablets.
• Check for urine retention and constipation. Increase fluids to lessen constipation. Suggest stool softener, if needed.
• Warn patient to avoid activities that require alertness and good psychomotor coordination until CNS effects of the drug are known. Drowsiness and dizziness usually subside after a few weeks.
• Dry mouth may be relieved with sugarless hard candy or gum, but maprolitine usually has a low potential for inducing anticholinergic effects. Saliva substitutes may be necessary.
• Whenever possible, patient should take full dose at bedtime.
• The first "tetracyclic" antidepressant.

---

nortriptyline hydrochloride
Aventyl*, Pamelor*
Pregnancy Risk Category: D

HOW SUPPLIED
Capsules: 10 mg, 25 mg, 75 mg
Oral solution: 10 mg/5ml (4% alcohol)

MECHANISM OF ACTION
Increases the amount of norepinephrine or serotonin, or both, in the CNS by blocking their reuptake by the presynaptic neurons. This action allows these neurotransmitters to accumulate.

INDICATIONS & DOSAGE
Treatment of depression—
Adults: 25 mg P.O. t.i.d. or q.i.d., gradually increasing to maximum of 150 mg daily. Alternatively, entire dose may be given at bedtime.

Italicized adverse reactions are common or life-threatening.
*Liquid form contains alcohol. **May contain tartrazine.

ADVERSE REACTIONS

CNS: *drowsiness, dizziness,* excitation, seizures, tremors, weakness, confusion, headache, nervousness.
CV: *tachycardia, ECG changes,* hypertension.
EENT: *blurred vision,* tinnitus, mydriasis.
GI: *dry mouth, constipation,* nausea, vomiting, anorexia, paralytic ileus.
GU: *urine retention.*
Skin: rash, urticaria.
Other: *sweating,* allergy.
After abrupt withdrawal of long-term therapy: nausea, headache, malaise. (Does not indicate addiction.)

INTERACTIONS

Barbiturates: decrease tricyclic depressant (TCA) blood levels. Monitor for decreased antidepressant effect.
Cimetidine: may increase nortriptyline serum levels. Monitor for increased adverse reactions.
Epinephrine, norepinephrine: increase hypertensive effect. Use with caution.
MAO inhibitors: may cause severe excitation, hyperpyrexia, or seizures, usually with high dose. Use together cautiously.
Methylphenidate: increases TCA blood levels. Monitor for enhanced antidepressant effect.

NURSING CONSIDERATIONS

• Contraindicated during acute recovery phase of myocardial infarction, in prostatic hypertrophy, and in patients with history of seizure disorders. Use with caution in CV disease, urine retention, glaucoma, thyroid disease, impaired hepatic function, or blood dyscrasias; in patients who are suicide risks; or in those receiving electroshock therapy, thyroid medication, or elective surgery.
• Reduce dosage in elderly or debilitated persons and adolescents.
• Do not withdraw drug abruptly.

• If psychotic signs increase, dosage should be reduced. Record mood changes. Watch for suicidal tendencies. To lessen suicide risk, allow minimum tablet supply.
• Check for urine retention and constipation. Increase fluids to lessen constipation. Suggest stool softener, if needed.
• Warn patient to avoid activities that require alertness and good psychomotor coordination until CNS effects of the drug are known. Drowsiness and dizziness usually subside after a few weeks.
• Expect delay of 2 weeks or more before noticeable effect. Full effect may take 4 weeks or more.
• Dry mouth may be relieved with sugarless hard candy or gum. Saliva substitutes may be necessary.
• Drug is tricyclic antidepressant, similar in anticholinergic effects to other cyclics. Has low potential for orthostatic hypotension. Avoid combining with alcohol or other depressants.
• Advise patient not to use other drugs (prescription or OTC) without first consulting the doctor.
• Liquid formulation available.
• Whenever possible, patient should take full dose at bedtime.

phenelzine sulfate
Nardil

Pregnancy Risk Category: C

HOW SUPPLIED
Tablets: 15 mg

MECHANISM OF ACTION
Promotes accumulation of neurotransmitters by inhibiting MAO.

INDICATIONS & DOSAGE
Treatment of depression—
Adults: 45 mg P.O. daily in divided doses, increasing rapidly to 60 mg daily. Then dosage can usually be re-

duced to 15 mg daily. Maximum is 90 mg daily.

ADVERSE REACTIONS
CNS: *dizziness,* vertigo, headache, overactivity, hyperreflexia, tremors, muscle twitching, mania, jitters, *insomnia,* confusion, memory impairment, drowsiness, weakness, fatigue.
CV: paradoxical hypertension, *orthostatic hypotension,* arrhythmias.
GI: dry mouth, *anorexia,* nausea, constipation.
Other: peripheral edema, sweating, weight changes.

INTERACTIONS
Alcohol, barbiturates, and other sedatives; narcotics; dextromethorphan; tricyclic antidepressants: unpredictable interaction. Use with caution and in reduced dosage.
Amphetamines, ephedrine, levodopa, meperidine, metaraminol, methotrimeprazine, methylphenidate, phenylephrine, phenylpropanolamine: enhance pressor effects. Use together cautiously.
Insulin, oral hypoglycemic agents: phenelzine may alter requirements for antidiabetic medications.

NURSING CONSIDERATIONS
• Contraindicated in elderly or debilitated patients, and in hepatic impairment, CHF, pheochromocytoma, hypertension, cardiovascular or cerebrovascular disease, or severe or frequent headaches. Also contraindicated with foods containing tryptophan (broad beans) or tyramine; during therapy with other MAO inhibitors (including pargyline HCl, isocarboxazid, tranylcypromine sulfate) or within 10 days of such therapy; within 10 days of elective surgery requiring general anesthetic, cocaine, or local anesthetic containing sympathomimetic vasoconstrictors; and in hyperactive, agitated, or schizophrenic patients. Use cautiously with antihypertensive

drugs containing thiazide diuretics or with spinal anesthetic; and in patients with suicide risk or diabetes.
• Avoid combining with alcohol or other depressant.
• Use only when tricyclic antidepressant or electroshock therapy is ineffective or contraindicated.
• If patient develops symptoms of overdose (severe hypotension, palpitations, or frequent headaches), hold dose and notify doctor.
• Watch for suicidal tendencies.
• Dosage is usually reduced to maintenance level as soon as possible.
• Store drug in tight container, away from heat and light.
• Have phentolamine (Regitine) available to counteract severe hypertension.
• Warn patient to avoid foods high in tyramine or tryptophan (aged cheese, Chianti wine, beer, avocados, chicken livers, chocolate, bananas, soy sauce, meat tenderizers, salami, bologna) and self-medication with OTC cold, hay fever, or diet preparations.
• Incidence of orthostatic hypotension is high. Supervise walking. Tell patient to get out of bed slowly, sitting up first for 1 minute.
• Continue precautions 10 days after stopping drug because it has long-lasting effects.
• Expect delay of 2 weeks or more before noticeable effect. Full effect may take 4 weeks or more.
• Obtain baseline blood pressure readings, CBC, and liver function tests before therapy, and continue to monitor throughout treatment.

---

protriptyline hydrochloride
Triptil†, Vivactil

Pregnancy Risk Category: C

HOW SUPPLIED
Tablets: 5 mg, 10 mg

MECHANISM OF ACTION

Increases the amount of norepinephrine or serotonin, or both, in the CNS by blocking their reuptake by the presynaptic neurons. This action allows these neurotransmitters to accumulate.

INDICATIONS & DOSAGE

Treatment of depression—
Adults: 15 to 40 mg P.O. daily in divided doses, increasing gradually to maximum of 60 mg daily.

ADVERSE REACTIONS

CNS: excitation, seizures, tremors, weakness, confusion, headache, nervousness.
CV: *orthostatic hypotension, tachycardia, ECG changes,* hypertension.
EENT: *blurred vision,* tinnitus, mydriasis.
GI: *dry mouth, constipation,* nausea, vomiting, anorexia, paralytic ileus.
GU: *urine retention.*
Skin: rash, urticaria.
Other: *sweating,* allergy.
After abrupt withdrawal of long-term therapy: nausea, headache, malaise. (Does not indicate addiction.)

INTERACTIONS

Barbiturates: decrease tricyclic antidepressant (TCA) blood levels. Monitor for decreased antidepressant effect.
Epinephrine, norepinephrine: increase hypertensive effect. Use with caution.
Cimetidine: may increase protriptyline serum levels. Monitor for increased adverse reactions.
MAO inhibitors: may cause severe excitation, hyperpyrexia, or seizures, and death, usually with high dose. Use together cautiously.
Methylphenidate: increases TCA blood levels. Monitor for enhanced antidepressant effect.

NURSING CONSIDERATIONS

• Contraindicated during acute recovery phase of myocardial infarction, in prostatic hypertrophy, and in patients with history of seizure disorders. Use with caution in elderly patients and in CV disease, urine retention, increased intraocular tension, thyroid disease, or blood dyscrasias; in suicide risks; and in those receiving electroshock therapy, thyroid medication, or elective surgery.
• Protriptyline has low potential for producing orthostatic hypotension, and is the least sedating of the tricyclic antidepressants. It may even have amphetamine-like effects. Avoid late-day dosing to prevent insomnia.
• Reduce dosage in elderly or debilitated patients and adolescents.
• Do not withdraw drug abruptly.
• Watch for increased psychotic signs, anxiety, agitation, or CV reactions; dosage should be reduced if they occur. Record mood changes. Watch for suicidal tendencies. To lessen suicide risk, allow minimum supply of tablets.
• Check for urine retention and constipation. Increase fluids to lessen constipation. Suggest stool softener, if needed.
• Protriptylene has high anticholinergic effects. Dry mouth may be relieved with sugarless hard candy or gum. Saliva substitutes may be necessary.
• Expect delay of 2 weeks or more before noticeable effect. Full effect may take 4 weeks or more.
• Advise patient not to use other drugs (prescription or OTC) without first consulting the doctor. Avoid combining with alcohol or other depressants.
• Used investigationally to treat obstructive sleep apnea.

---

†Available in Canada only.　　　‡Available in Australia only.　　　◊ Available OTC.

tranylcypromine sulfate
Parnate

Pregnancy Risk Category: C

HOW SUPPLIED
Tablets: 10 mg

MECHANISM OF ACTION
Promotes accumulation of neurotransmitters by inhibiting MAO.

INDICATIONS & DOSAGE
Treatment of depression—
Adults: 10 mg P.O. b.i.d. Increase to maximum of 30 mg daily, if necessary, after 2 weeks. Not recommended for children under 16 years.

ADVERSE REACTIONS
CNS: *dizziness,* vertigo, headache, overactivity, hyperreflexia, tremors, muscle twitching, mania, jitters, confusion, memory impairment, fatigue.
CV: *orthostatic hypotension,* arrhythmias, paradoxical hypertension.
EENT: blurred vision.
GI: dry mouth, *anorexia,* nausea, diarrhea, constipation, abdominal pain.
GU: impotence.
Skin: rash.
Other: peripheral edema, sweating, weight changes, chills, altered libido.

INTERACTIONS
Alcohol, barbiturates, and other sedatives; narcotics; dextromethorphan; tricyclic antidepressants: use with caution and in reduced dosage.
Amphetamines, ephedrine, levodopa, meperidine, metaraminol, methotrimeprazine, methylphenidate, phenylephrine, phenylpropanolamine: pressor effects of these drugs are enhanced by tranylcypromine. Use together cautiously.
Insulin, oral hypoglycemic agents: tranylcypromine may alter requirements of antidiabetic medications.

NURSING CONSIDERATIONS
• Contraindicated in severe hepatic or renal impairment; CHF; pheochromocytoma, hypertension, or cardiovascular or cerebrovascular disease; severe or frequent headaches; in patients taking antihypertensive drugs or diuretics; in elderly or debilitated patients; in patients for whom close supervision is not possible; and in hyperactive, agitated, or schizophrenic patients. Also contraindicated with foods containing tryptophan or tyramine. Also contraindicated during therapy with other MAO inhibitors (including pargyline, phenelzine sulfate, isocarboxazid) or within 7 days of such therapy; within 7 days of elective surgery requiring general anesthetic, cocaine, or local anesthetic containing sympathomimetic vasoconstrictors. Use cautiously with antiparkinsonian drugs, spinal anesthetics; in renal disease, diabetes, epilepsy, hyperthyroidism; and in suicide risks.
• MAO inhibitor most often reported to cause hypertensive crisis with high-tyramine ingestion.
• Avoid combining with alcohol or other depressants.
• Use only when tricyclic antidepressant or electroshock therapy is ineffective or contraindicated.
• If patient develops symptoms of overdose (palpitations, severe hypotension, or frequent headaches), hold dose and notify doctor.
• Watch for suicidal tendencies.
• Dosage is usually reduced to maintenance level as soon as possible.
• Do not withdraw drug abruptly.
• Have phentolamine (Regitine) available to counteract severe hypertension.
• Warn patient to avoid foods high in tyramine or tryptophan (aged cheese, Chianti wine, beer, avocados, chicken livers, chocolate, bananas, soy sauce, meat tenderizers, salami, bologna)

Italicized adverse reactions are common or life-threatening.
*Liquid form contains alcohol.   **May contain tartrazine.

and self-medication with OTC cold, hay fever, or reducing preparations.
• Tell patient to get out of bed slowly, sitting up for 1 minute.
• Continue precautions for 7 days after stopping drug; effects last that long.
• Expect delay of 2 weeks or more before noticeable effect. Full effect may take 4 weeks or more.
• Obtain baseline blood pressure readings, CBC, and liver function tests before beginning therapy, and continue to monitor throughout treatment.

trazodone hydrochloride
Desyrel, Trazon, Trialodine
Pregnancy Risk Category: C

HOW SUPPLIED
Tablets: 50 mg, 100 mg, 150 mg

MECHANISM OF ACTION
Inhibits serotonin uptake in the brain.

INDICATIONS & DOSAGE
Treatment of depression—
Adults: initial dosage is 150 mg P.O. daily in divided doses, which can be increased by 50 mg daily q 3 to 4 days. Average dosage ranges from 150 mg to 400 mg daily. Maximum dosage is 600 mg.

ADVERSE REACTIONS
CNS: *drowsiness, dizziness,* nervousness, fatigue, confusion, tremors, weakness.
CV: orthostatic hypotension, tachycardia.
EENT: blurred vision, tinnitus.
GI: dry mouth, constipation, nausea, vomiting, anorexia.
GU: urine retention, priapism possibly leading to impotence.
Skin: rash, urticaria.
Other: sweating.

INTERACTIONS
Alcohol, CNS depressants: enhanced CNS depression.
Antihypertensives: added hypotensive effect of trazodone. Dose of antihypertensive drug may have to be decreased.
Digoxin, phenytoin: trazodone may increase serum levels of these drugs. Monitor for toxicity.
MAO inhibitors: No clinical experience. Use together very cautiously.

NURSING CONSIDERATIONS
• Should not be used during initial recovery phase of myocardial infarction. Avoid concurrent administration with electroshock therapy. Drug may be discontinued before surgery.
• Use cautiously with preexisting cardiac disease.
• Priapism is a potential problem in men taking trazodone. Be sure to note if patient complains of prolonged and painful erections. May need surgical intervention.
• Watch for suicidal tendencies and record mood changes. Allow minimum amount of tablets to lessen suicide risk.
• Warn patient to avoid activities that require alertness and good psychomotor coordination until CNS effects of the drug are known. Drowsiness and dizziness usually subside after the first few weeks.
• Administer after meals or a light snack for optimal absorption and to decrease incidence of dizziness.
• Not chemically related to tricyclic antidepressants or MAO inhibitors.
• Anticholinergic and adverse cardiac effects are minimal.
• Expect delay of 2 weeks or more before noticeable effect. Full effect may take 4 weeks or more.

trimipramine maleate
Apo-Trimip†, Surmontil

Pregnancy Risk Category: C

HOW SUPPLIED
Tablets: 25 mg‡
Capsules: 25 mg, 50 mg, 100 mg

MECHANISM OF ACTION
Increases the amount of norepinephrine or serotonin, or both, in the CNS by blocking their reuptake by the presynaptic neurons. This action allows these neurotransmitters to accumulate.

INDICATIONS & DOSAGE
Treatment of depression—
Adults: 75 mg P.O. daily in divided doses, increased to 200 mg daily. Dosages over 300 mg daily not recommended.
Enuresis—
Children over 6 years: initial dosage 25 mg P.O. 1 hour before bedtime; if no response, increase dosage to 50 mg in children under 12 years, and to 75 mg in children over 12 years.

ADVERSE REACTIONS
CNS: *drowsiness, dizziness,* excitation, seizures, tremors, weakness, confusion, headache, nervousness.
CV: *orthostatic hypotension, tachycardia, ECG changes,* hypertension.
EENT: *blurred vision,* tinnitus, mydriasis.
GI: *dry mouth, constipation,* nausea, vomiting, anorexia, paralytic ileus.
GU: *urine retention.*
Skin: rash, urticaria.
Other: *sweating,* allergy.
After abrupt withdrawal of long-term therapy: nausea, headache, malaise. (Does not indicate addiction.)

INTERACTIONS
Barbiturates: decrease tricyclic antidepressant (TCA) blood levels. Monitor for decreased antidepressant effect.
Cimetidine: may increase trimipramine serum levels. Monitor for increased adverse reactions.
Epinephrine, norepinephrine: increase hypertensive effect. Use with caution.
MAO inhibitors: may cause severe excitation, hyperpyrexia, or seizures, usually with high dose. Use together cautiously.
Methylphenidate: increases TCA blood levels. Monitor for enhanced antidepressant effects.

NURSING CONSIDERATIONS
• Contraindicated during acute recovery phase of myocardial infarction, in prostatic hypertrophy, and in patients with history of seizure disorders. Use with extreme caution in CV disease, urine retention, narrow-angle glaucoma or increased intraocular pressure, thyroid disease, blood dyscrasias, or impaired hepatic function. Also contraindicated in patients who are suicide risks and in those receiving electroshock therapy, thyroid medicaton, or elective surgery.
• Reduce dosage in elderly or debilitated persons and adolescents.
• Do not withdraw drug abruptly.
• Watch for increased psychotic signs; dosage should be reduced if they occur. Record mood changes. Watch for suicidal tendencies. Allow only minimum supply of tablets to lessen suicide risk.
• Check for urine retention and constipation. Increase fluids to lessen constipation. Suggest stool softener, if necessary.
• Warn patient to avoid activities that require alertness and good psychomotor coordination until CNS effects of the drug are known. Drowsiness and dizziness usually subside after a few weeks.
• Don't combine with alcohol or other depressants.

Italicized adverse reactions are common or life-threatening.
*Liquid form contains alcohol.   **May contain tartrazine.

- Expect delay of 2 weeks or more before noticeable effect. Full effect may take 4 weeks or more.
- Dry mouth may be relieved with sugarless hard candy or gum. Saliva substitutes may be necessary.
- Effectiveness in enuresis may decrease over time. Similar in anticholinergic effects to other tricyclic antidepressants.
- Advise patient not to use other drugs (prescription or OTC) without first consulting the doctor.
- Trimipramine has high sedative effect. Whenever possible, patient should take full dose at bedtime. Warn patient about possible morning orthostatic hypotension.

31

Antianxiety agents

alprazolam
buspirone hydrochloride
chlordiazepoxide
chlordiazepoxide hydrochloride
clorazepate dipotassium
diazepam
halazepam
hydroxyzine hydrochloride
hydroxyzine pamoate
lorazepam
meprobamate
oxazepam
prazepam

COMBINATION PRODUCTS
DEPROL**: meprobamate 400 mg and benactyzine hydrochloride 1 mg.
EQUAGESIC: meprobamate 200 mg and aspirin 325 mg.
LIBRAX CAPSULES: chlordiazepoxide hydrochloride 5 mg and clidinium bromide 2.5 mg.
LIMBITROL 5-12.5: chlordiazepoxide 5 mg and amitriptyline hydrochloride 12.5 mg.
LIMBITROL 10-25: chlordiazepoxide 10 mg and amitriptyline hydrochloride 25 mg.
MENRIUM 5-2: chlordiazepoxide 5 mg and esterified estrogens 0.2 mg.
MENRIUM 5-4: chlordiazepoxide 5 mg and esterified estrogens 0.4 mg.
MENRIUM 10-4: chlordiazepoxide 10 mg and esterified estrogens 0.4 mg.
MILPREM-200: meprobamate 200 mg and conjugated estrogens 0.45 mg.
MILPREM-400: meprobamate 400 mg and conjugated estrogens 0.45 mg.
PMB 200: meprobamate 200 mg and conjugated estrogens 0.45 mg.
PMB 400: meprobamate 400 mg and conjugated estrogens 0.45 mg.

alprazolam
Xanax
Controlled Substance Schedule IV
Pregnancy Risk Category: D

HOW SUPPLIED
Tablets: 0.25 mg, 0.5 mg, 1 mg

MECHANISM OF ACTION
Depresses the CNS at the limbic and subcortical levels of the brain.

INDICATIONS & DOSAGE
Anxiety and tension—
Adults: usual starting dose is 0.25 to 0.5 mg P.O. t.i.d. Maximum total daily dosage is 4 mg in divided doses. In elderly or debilitated patients, usual starting dose is 0.25 mg b.i.d. or t.i.d.

ADVERSE REACTIONS
CNS: *drowsiness, light-headedness,* headache, confusion, hostility.
CV: transient hypotension, tachycardia.
EENT: dry mouth.
GI: nausea, vomiting, constipation, discomfort.

INTERACTIONS
Alcohol, other CNS depressants: increased CNS depression. Avoid concomitant use.
Cimetidine: increased sedation. Monitor carefully.
Tricyclic antidepressants: increased

Italicized adverse reactions are common or life-threatening.
*Liquid form contains alcohol.   **May contain tartrazine.

plasma levels of tricyclic antidepressants.

NURSING CONSIDERATIONS
• Contraindicated in acute narrow-angle glaucoma, psychoses, or anxiety-free psychiatric disorders.
• Reduce dosage in elderly or debilitated patients because they may be more susceptible to the adverse CNS effects of the drug.
• Do not withdraw drug abruptly. Abuse or addiction is possible. Withdrawal symptoms may occur.
• Warn patient not to combine drug with alcohol or other depressants, and also to avoid activities that require alertness and psychomotor coordination until CNS effects of the drug are known.
• Caution patient against giving medication to others.
• Drug should not be prescribed for everyday stress.
• Drug is not for long-term use (more than 4 months).
• Warn patient not to discontinue drug without doctor's approval.
• Alprazolam is the first of a new type of benzodiazepine, known as a triazolo-benzodiazepine. It's more rapidly metabolized and excreted than most of the other drugs in the benzodiazepine class and has a lower incidence of lethargy than other drugs of this class.
• May also be effective for treatment of depression.

---

buspirone hydrochloride
BuSpar

Pregnancy Risk Category: B

HOW SUPPLIED
Tablets: 5 mg, 10 mg

MECHANISM OF ACTION
Unknown. However, the drug may inhibit neuronal firing and reduce 5-HT turnover in cortical, amygdaloid, and septohippocampal tissue.

INDICATIONS & DOSAGE
Management of anxiety disorders; short-term relief of anxiety—
Adults: initially, 5 mg P.O. t.i.d. Dosage may be increased at 3-day intervals. Usual maintenance dosage is 20 to 30 mg daily in divided doses.

ADVERSE REACTIONS
CNS: *dizziness, drowsiness,* nervousness, insomnia, headache.
GI: nausea, dry mouth, diarrhea.
Other: fatigue.

INTERACTIONS
Alcohol, other CNS depressants: increased CNS depression. Avoid concomitant use.
MAO inhibitors: may elevate blood pressure.

NURSING CONSIDERATIONS
• Although buspirone is less sedating than other anxiolytics and does not produce any serious functional impairment, CNS effects in an individual patient may be unpredictable. Therefore, warn patients to avoid hazardous activities that require alertness and neuromuscular coordination until CNS effects of the drug are known.
• Unlike the benzodiazepines, buspirone is not an effective anticonvulsant or skeletal muscle relaxant. Its use is limited to the treatment of anxiety.
• Advise patient to take the drug with food.
• Before initiating buspirone therapy in patients already being treated with benzodiazepines, warn them against stopping the benzodiazepine abruptly. Abrupt discontinuation may cause a benzodiazepine withdrawal reaction.
• Signs of improvement with buspirone are usually evident within 7 to 10 days; optimal results are achieved after 3 to 4 weeks of therapy.
• This drug has shown no potential

---

for abuse and has not been classified as a controlled substance. However, it is not recommended for use to relieve everyday stress.

---

chlordiazepoxide
Libritabs

chlordiazepoxide hydrochloride
Apo-Chlordiazepoxide†, Librium, Lipoxide, Medilium†, Mitran, Novopoxide†, Reposans, Sereen, Solium†

Controlled Substance Schedule IV
Pregnancy Risk Category: D

HOW SUPPLIED
chlordiazepoxide
Tablets: 5 mg, 10 mg, 25 mg
chlordiazepoxide hydrochloride
Capsules: 5 mg, 10 mg, 25 mg
Powder for injection: 100 mg/ampule

MECHANISM OF ACTION
Depresses the CNS at the limbic and subcortical levels of the brain.

INDICATIONS & DOSAGE
Mild to moderate anxiety and tension—
Adults: 5 to 10 mg P.O. t.i.d. or q.i.d.
Children over 6 years: 5 mg P.O. b.i.d. to q.i.d. Maximum dosage is 10 mg P.O. b.i.d. to t.i.d.
Severe anxiety and tension—
Adults: 20 to 25 mg P.O. t.i.d. or q.i.d.
Withdrawal symptoms of acute alcoholism—
Adults: 50 to 100 mg P.O., I.M., or I.V. Maximum dosage is 300 mg daily.
Preoperative apprehension and anxiety—
Adults: 5 to 10 mg P.O. t.i.d. or q.i.d. on day preceding surgery; or 50 to 100 mg I.M. 1 hour before surgery.

Note: Parenteral form not recommended in children under 12 years.

ADVERSE REACTIONS
CNS: *drowsiness, lethargy, hangover,* fainting.
CV: transient hypotension.
GI: nausea, vomiting, abdominal discomfort.
Local: *pain at injection site.*

INTERACTIONS
Alcohol, other CNS depressants: increased CNS depression. Avoid concomitant use.
Cimetidine: increased sedation. Monitor carefully.

NURSING CONSIDERATIONS
• Use with caution in mental depression, psychiatric disturbances, blood dyscrasias, porphyria, hepatic or renal disease, or in those undergoing anticoagulant therapy.
• Dosage should be reduced in elderly or debilitated patients.
• Possibility of abuse and addiction. Do not withdraw drug abruptly; withdrawal symptoms may occur.
• Warn patient to avoid activities that require alertness and good psychomotor coordination until CNS effects of the drug are known.
• Warn patient not to combine drug with alcohol or other depressants.
• Although package recommends I.M. use only, this drug may be given I.V.
• Injectable form (as hydrochloride) comes as two ampules—diluent and powdered drug. Read directions carefully. For I.M., add 2 ml of diluent to powder and agitate gently until clear. Use immediately. I.M. form may be erratically absorbed.
• For I.V., use 5 ml of saline injection or sterile water for injection as diluent; do not give packaged diluent I.V. Give slowly over 1 minute.
• Keep powder away from light and

Italicized adverse reactions are common or life-threatening.
*Liquid form contains alcohol. **May contain tartrazine.

store in the refrigerator; mix just before use; discard remainder.
• Do not mix injectable form with any other parenteral drug.
• Caution patient against giving medication to others.
• Drug should not be prescribed regularly for everyday stress.

clorazepate dipotassium
Gen-Xene, Novoclopate†,
Tranxene, Tranxene-SD, Tranxene-T-Tab
Controlled Substance Schedule IV
Pregnancy Risk Category: C

HOW SUPPLIED
Tablets: 3.75 mg, 7.5 mg, 11.25 mg, 15 mg, 22.5 mg
Capsules: 3.75 mg, 7.5 mg, 15 mg

MECHANISM OF ACTION
Depresses the CNS at the limbic and subcortical levels of the brain. As an anticonvulsant, suppresses the spread of seizure activity produced by epileptogenic foci in the cortex, thalamus, and limbic structures.

INDICATIONS & DOSAGE
Acute alcohol withdrawal—
Adults: Day 1—30 mg P.O. initially, followed by 30 to 60 mg P.O. in divided doses; Day 2—45 to 90 mg P.O. in divided doses; Day 3—22.5 to 45 mg P.O. in divided doses; Day 4—15 to 30 mg P.O. in divided doses; gradually reduce daily dosage to 7.5 to 15 mg.
Anxiety—
Adults: 15 to 60 mg P.O. daily.
As an adjunct in epilepsy—
Adults and children over 12 years: Maximum recommended initial dosage is 7.5 mg P.O. t.i.d. Dosage increases should be no greater than 7.5 mg/week. Maximum daily dosage should not exceed 90 mg daily.
Children between 9 and 12 years: Maximum recommended initial dosage is 7.5 mg P.O. b.i.d. Dosage increases should be no greater than 7.5 mg/week. Maximum daily dosage should not exceed 60 mg/day.

ADVERSE REACTIONS
CNS: *drowsiness, lethargy, hangover, fainting.*
CV: transient hypotension.
GI: nausea, vomiting, abdominal discomfort.

INTERACTIONS
Alcohol, other CNS depressants: increased CNS depression. Avoid concomitant use.
Cimetidine: increased sedation. Monitor carefully.

NURSING CONSIDERATIONS
• Contraindicated in acute narrow-angle glaucoma, depressive neuroses, psychotic reactions, and in children under 18 years. Use with caution when hepatic or renal damage is present.
• Dosage should be reduced in elderly or debilitated patients.
• Possibility of abuse and addiction exists. Do not withdraw drug abruptly; withdrawal symptoms may occur.
• Warn patient to avoid activities requiring alertness and good psychomotor coordination until CNS effects of the drug are known.
• Warn patient not to combine drug with alcohol or other depressants.
• Suggest sugarless chewing gum or hard candy to relieve dry mouth.
• Caution patient against giving medication to others.
• Drug should not be prescribed regularly for everyday stress.

---

†Available in Canada only.　　‡Available in Australia only.　　◊Available OTC.

diazepam
Apo-Diazepam†, Diazemuls†,
Diazepam Intensol, E-Pam†,
Meval†, Novodipam†, Q-Pam,
Rival†, Valium, Valrelease,
Vasepam, Vivol†, Zetran
Controlled Substance Schedule IV

Pregnancy Risk Category: D

HOW SUPPLIED
Tablets: 2 mg, 5 mg, 10 mg
Capsules (extended-release): 15 mg
Oral solution: 5 mg/5 ml, 5 mg/ml
Injection: 5 mg/ml
Sterile emulsion for injection: 5 mg/
ml†

MECHANISM OF ACTION
Depresses the CNS at the limbic and
subcortical levels of the brain. As an
anticonvulsant, suppresses the spread
of seizure activity produced by epileptogenic foci in the cortex, thalamus, and limbic structures.

INDICATIONS & DOSAGE
*Tension, anxiety, adjunct in seizure
disorders or skeletal muscle spasm—*
Adults: 2 to 10 mg P.O. t.i.d. or
q.i.d. Or, 15 to 30 mg of extended-release capsule once daily.
Children over 6 months: 1 to 2.5 mg
P.O. t.i.d. or q.i.d.
*Tension, anxiety, muscle spasm, endo-
scopic procedures, seizures—*
Adults: 5 to 10 mg I.V. initially, up to
30 mg in 1 hour or possibly more for
cardioversion or status epilepticus,
depending on response.
Children 5 years and older: 1 mg
I.V. or I.M. slowly q 2 to 5 minutes to
maximum of 10 mg. Repeat q 2 to 4
hours.
Children 30 days to 5 years: 0.2 to
0.5 mg I.V. or I.M. slowly q 2 to 5
minutes to maximum of 5 mg. Repeat
q 2 to 4 hours.
Tetanic muscle spasms—
Children over 5 years: 5 to 10 mg
I.M. or I.V. q 3 to 4 hours, p.r.n.

Infants over 30 days: 1 to 2 mg I.M.
or I.V. q 3 to 4 hours, p.r.n.
Status epilepticus—
Adults: 5 to 20 mg slow I.V. push 2 to
5 mg/minute; may repeat q 5 to 10
minutes up to maximum total dose of
60 mg. Use 2 to 5 mg in elderly or debilitated patients. May repeat therapy
in 20 to 30 minutes with caution if
seizures recur.
Children: 0.1 to 0.3 mg/kg slow I.V.
push (1 mg/minute over 3 minutes).
May repeat q 15 minutes for 2 doses.
Maximum single dose in children under 5 years is 5 mg; in children over 5
years, 10 mg.

ADVERSE REACTIONS
CNS: *drowsiness, lethargy, hangover,
ataxia,* fainting, slurred speech,
tremor.
CV: transient hypotension, bradycar-
dia, *cardiovascular collapse*.
EENT: diplopia, blurred vision, nys-
tagmus.
GI: nausea, vomiting, abdominal dis-
comfort.
Skin: rash, urticaria.
Local: desquamation, *pain, phlebitis
at injection site*.
Other: respiratory depression.

INTERACTIONS
Alcohol, other CNS depressants: increased CNS depression. Avoid concomitant use.
Cimetidine: increased sedation. Monitor carefully.
Phenobarbital: increased effects of
both drugs. Use together cautiously.

NURSING CONSIDERATIONS
• Contraindicated in shock, coma,
acute alcohol intoxication, acute
narrow-angle glaucoma, psychoses,
myasthenia gravis; in oral form for
children under 6 months. Use with
caution in blood dyscrasias, hepatic or
renal damage, depression, open-angle
glaucoma; in elderly and debilitated

Italicized adverse reactions are common or life-threatening.
*Liquid form contains alcohol.   **May contain tartrazine.

patients; and in those with limited pulmonary reserve.

• Dosage should be reduced in elderly or debilitated patients because they may be more susceptible to the adverse CNS effects of the drug.

• Possibility of abuse and addiction exists. Do not withdraw drug abruptly; withdrawal symptoms may occur.

• Monitor CBC and hepatic function during long-term use.

• Warn patient to avoid activities that require alertness and good psychomotor coordination until CNS effects of the drug are known.

• Warn patient not to combine drug with alcohol or other depressants.

• Do not mix injectable form with other drugs because diazepam is incompatible with most drugs.

• There is considerable controversy about the use of diluted diazepam solutions for continuous I.V. infusion because of its low aqueous solubility. Under certain conditions, it may be compatible with sodium chloride 0.9% or Ringer's lactate injection, but the solution may not be stable. Consult hospital pharmacy for further information.

• Avoid extravasation. Do not inject into small veins.

• Watch daily for phlebitis at injection site.

• Give I.V. slowly, at rate not exceeding 5 mg per minute. When injecting I.V., best to administer directly into the vein. If this is not possible, inject slowly through the infusion tubing as close as possible to the vein insertion site.

• Monitor respirations every 5 to 15 minutes and before each repeated I.V. dose. Have emergency resuscitative equipment and oxygen at bedside. Note that naloxone does not reverse the respiratory depression produced by diazepam.

• I.V. route is more reliable; I.M. administration is not recommended because absorption is variable and injection is painful (because the solution is highly alkaline).

• Drug of choice (I.V. form) for status epilepticus.

• Seizures may recur within 20 to 30 minutes of initial control, because of redistribution of the drug.

• Continuous infusions of 1 to 10 mg hourly have been used to prevent seizure recurrence.

• Do not store diazepam in plastic syringes.

• Caution patient against giving medication to others.

• Drug should not be prescribed regularly for everyday stress.

halazepam
Paxipam
Controlled Substance Schedule IV
Pregnancy Risk Category: D

HOW SUPPLIED
Tablets: 20 mg, 40 mg

MECHANISM OF ACTION
Depresses the CNS at the limbic and subcortical levels of the brain.

INDICATIONS & DOSAGE
Relief of anxiety and tension—
Adults: Usual dose is 20 to 40 mg P.O. t.i.d. or q.i.d. Optimal daily dosage is generally 80 to 160 mg. Daily dosages up to 600 mg have been given. In elderly or debilitated patients, initial dosage is 20 mg once or twice daily.

ADVERSE REACTIONS
CNS: *drowsiness, lethargy, hangover,* fainting.
CV: transient hypotension.
EENT: dry mouth.
GI: nausea and vomiting, discomfort.

INTERACTIONS
Alcohol, other CNS depressants: in-

---

creased CNS depression. Avoid concomitant use.
Cimetidine: possible increased sedation. Monitor carefully.

NURSING CONSIDERATIONS
• Contraindicated in acute narrow-angle glaucoma, psychoses, or anxiety-free psychiatric disorders. Use with caution in hepatorenal impairment.
• Reduce dosage in elderly or debilitated patients.
• Do not withdraw drug abruptly.
• Abuse and addiction are possible. Withdrawal symptoms may occur.
• Warn patient not to combine drug with alcohol or other depressants, and to avoid activities that require alertness and psychomotor coordination until CNS effects of the drug are known.
• Caution patient against giving medication to others.
• Drug should not be prescribed for everyday stress.
• Halazepam is not for long-term use (more than 4 months).

---

hydroxyzine hydrochloride (hydroxyzine embonate)
Anxanil, Apo-Hydroxyzine†, Atarax*, Atozine, Durrax, E-Vista, Hydroxacen, Hyzine-50, Multipax†, Novohydroxyzin†, Quiess, Vistacon, Vistaject, Vistaquel, Vistaril, Vistazine

hydroxyzine pamoate
Hy-Pam, Vamate, Vistaril
Pregnancy Risk Category: C

HOW SUPPLIED
hydrochloride
Tablets: 10 mg, 25 mg, 50 mg, 100 mg
Capsules: 10 mg†‡, 25 mg†‡, 50 mg†‡
Syrup: 10 mg/5 ml
Injection: 25 mg/ml, 50 mg/ml

pamoate
Capsules: 25 mg, 50 mg, 100 mg
Oral suspension: 25 mg/5 ml

MECHANISM OF ACTION
A piperazine antihistamine. Depresses the CNS at the limbic and subcortical levels of the brain.

INDICATIONS & DOSAGE
Anxiety and tension—
Adults: 25 to 100 mg P.O. t.i.d. or q.i.d.
Anxiety, tension, hyperkinesia—
Children 6 years and over: 50 to 100 mg P.O. daily in divided doses.
Children under 6 years: 50 mg P.O. daily in divided doses.
Preoperative and postoperative adjunctive therapy—
Adults: 25 to 100 mg I.M. q 4 to 6 hours.
Children: 1.1 mg/kg I.M. q 4 to 6 hours.
Rashes, pruritus—
Adults: 25 mg P.O. t..i.d. or q.i.d.
Children 6 years and over: 50 to 100 mg P.O. daily in divided doses.
Children under 6 years: 50 mg P.O. daily in divided doses.

ADVERSE REACTIONS
CNS: *drowsiness,* involuntary motor activity.
GI: *dry mouth.*
Local: marked discomfort at site of I.M. injection.

INTERACTIONS
Alcohol, other CNS depressants: increased CNS depression. Avoid concomitant use.

NURSING CONSIDERATIONS
• Contraindicated in shock or comatose states.
• Dosage should be reduced in elderly or debilitated patients.
• Warn patient to avoid activities that require alertness and good psychomo-

---

Italicized adverse reactions are common or life-threatening.
*Liquid form contains alcohol.   **May contain tartrazine.

tor coordination until CNS effects of the drug are known.
- Warn patient not to combine drug with alcohol or other depressants.
- Observe for excessive sedation due to potentiation with other CNS drugs.
- Used perioperatively as an antiemetic and anxiolytic. Its sedative and antihistamine properties make it especially useful to treat pruritus that prevents sleep.
- Used in psychogenically induced allergic conditions, such as chronic urticaria and pruritus.
- Parenteral form (hydroxyzine hydrocholoride) for I.M. use only, never I.V. Z-track injection is preferred.
- Aspirate injection carefully to prevent inadvertent intravascular injection. Inject deep into a large muscle.
- Suggest sugarless hard candy or gum to relieve dry mouth.

lorazepam
Alzapam, Apo-Lorazepam†, Ativan, Loraz, Novolorazem†
Controlled Substance Schedule IV
Pregnancy Risk Category: D

HOW SUPPLIED
Tablets: 0.5 mg, 1 mg, 2 mg
Tablets (sublingual): 1 mg†, 2 mg†
Injection: 2 mg/ml, 4 mg/ml

MECHANISM OF ACTION
Depresses the CNS at the limbic and subcortical levels of the brain.

INDICATIONS & DOSAGE
Anxiety, tension, agitation, irritability, especially in anxiety neuroses or organic (especially GI or CV) disorders—
Adults: 2 to 6 mg P.O. daily in divided doses. Maximum dosage is 10 mg daily.
Insomnia—
Adults: 2 to 4 mg P.O. h.s.
Premedication before operative procedure—

Adults: 0.05 mg/kg I.M. or I.V., not to exceed 4 mg.

ADVERSE REACTIONS
CNS: *drowsiness, lethargy, hangover, fainting.*
CV: transient hypotension.
GI: dry mouth, abdominal discomfort.

INTERACTIONS
Alcohol, other CNS depressants: increased CNS depression. Avoid concomitant use.

NURSING CONSIDERATIONS
- Contraindicated in acute narrowangle glaucoma, psychoses, or mental depression. Use with caution in organic brain syndrome, myasthenia gravis, and renal or hepatic impairment.
- Dosage should be reduced in elderly or debilitated patients. Preoperative I.V. dose should not exceed 2 mg in patients over 50.
- Possibility of abuse and addiction exists with long-term use. Do not withdraw drug abruptly: withdrawal symptoms may occur.
- When administering I.M., inject deep into muscle mass. Don't dilute.
- When administering I.V., dilute with an equal volume of sterile water for injection, sodium chloride injection, or dextrose 5% injection.
- Used as a preoperative premedication before surgery, lorazepam provides substantial preoperative amnesia.
- Warn patient to avoid activities that require alertness or good psychomotor coordination until CNS effects of the drug are known.
- Warn patient not to combine drug with alcohol or other depressants.
- Caution patient against giving medication to others.
- Drug should not be prescribed regularly for everyday stress.
- Fewer cumulative effects than other

---

†Available in Canada only.   ‡Available in Australia only.   ◊ Available OTC.

benzodiazepines, due to short half-life.
• Store parenteral form in refrigerator to prolong shelf life.

---

meprobamate
Apo-Meprobamate†, Equanil**, Meditran, Meprospan, Miltown, Neuramate, Novo-Mepro†, Sedabamate, Tranmep
Controlled Substance Schedule IV

Pregnancy Risk Category: D

HOW SUPPLIED
Tablets: 200 mg, 400 mg, 600 mg
Capsules: 200 mg, 400 mg
Capsules (sustained-release): 200 mg, 400 mg

MECHANISM OF ACTION
Depresses the CNS at the limbic and subcortical levels of the brain.

INDICATIONS & DOSAGE
Anxiety and tension—
Adults: 1.2 to 1.6 g P.O. in three or four equally divided doses. Maximum dosage is 2.4 g daily.
Children 6 to 12 years: 100 to 200 mg P.O. b.i.d. or t.i.d. Not recommended for children under 6 years.

ADVERSE REACTIONS
Blood: *thrombocytopenia, leukopenia,* eosinophilia.
CNS: *drowsiness,* ataxia, dizziness, slurred speech, headache, vertigo.
CV: palpitation, tachycardia, hypotension.
GI: anorexia, nausea, vomiting, diarrhea, stomatitis.
Skin: pruritus, urticaria, erythematous maculopapular rash.

INTERACTIONS
Alcohol, other CNS depressants: increased CNS depression. Avoid concomitant use.

NURSING CONSIDERATIONS
• Contraindicated in patients with hypersensitivity to meprobamate, carisoprodol, mebutamate, tybamate, carbromal; and in renal insufficiency or porphyria. Use with caution in impaired hepatic or renal function and in patients with suicidal tendencies.
• Dosage should be reduced in elderly or debilitated patients.
• Possibility of abuse and addiction exists with long-term use. Meprobamate should not be used for everyday stress. Withdraw drug gradually (over 2 weeks) or withdrawal symptoms may occur, including severe generalized tonic-clonic seizures.
• Warn patient to avoid activities that require alertness or good psychomotor coordination until CNS effects of the drug are known.
• Warn patient not to combine drug with alcohol or other depressants.
• Give drug with meals to reduce GI distress.
• Therapeutic blood levels 0.5 to 2 mg/100 ml; levels above 20 mg/100 ml may cause coma and death.
• Periodic evaluation of CBC and liver function tests are indicated in patients receiving high doses.

---

oxazepam
Apo-Oxazepam†, Novoxapam†, Ox-Pam†, Serax**, Zapex†
Controlled Substance Schedule IV

Pregnancy Risk Category: C

HOW SUPPLIED
Tablets: 10 mg, 15 mg, 30 mg
Capsules: 10 mg, 15 mg, 30 mg

MECHANISM OF ACTION
Depresses the CNS at the limbic and subcortical levels of the brain.

INDICATIONS & DOSAGE
Alcohol withdrawal—
Adults: 15 to 30 mg P.O. t.i.d. or q.i.d.

Severe anxiety—
Adults: 15 to 30 mg P.O. t.i.d. or q.i.d.
Tension, mild to moderate anxiety—
Adults: 10 to 15 mg P.O. t.i.d. or q.i.d.

ADVERSE REACTIONS
Blood: *leukopenia*(rare).
CNS: *drowsiness, lethargy, hangover,* fainting.
CV: transient hypotension.
GI: nausea, vomiting, abdominal discomfort.
Metabolic: hepatic dysfunction.

INTERACTIONS
Alcohol, other CNS depressants: increased CNS depression. Avoid concomitant use.

NURSING CONSIDERATIONS
• Contraindicated in psychoses. Use cautiously in patients with history of convulsive disorders, drug allergies, blood dyscrasias, renal disease, and depression.
• Dose should be reduced in elderly or debilitated patients.
• Possibility of abuse and addiction exists. Don't stop drug abruptly; withdrawal symptoms may occur.
• Warn patient to avoid activities that require alertness or good psychomotor coordination until CNS effects of the drug are known.
• Warn patient not to combine drug with alcohol or other depressants.
• Fewer cumulative effects than many other benzodiazepines due to short half-life.
• Caution patient against giving medication to others.
• Monitor CBC and hepatic function periodically in patients on long-term therapy.
• Meprobamate should not be prescribed for everyday stress.

prazepam
Centrax
Controlled Substance Schedule IV
Pregnancy Risk Category: C

HOW SUPPLIED
Tablets: 10 mg
Capsules: 5 mg, 10 mg, 20 mg

MECHANISM OF ACTION
Depresses the CNS at the limbic and subcortical levels of the brain.

INDICATIONS & DOSAGE
Anxiety—
Adults: 30 mg P.O. in divided doses. Range 20 to 60 mg daily. May be administered as single daily dose at bedtime. Start with 20 mg.

ADVERSE REACTIONS
CNS: *drowsiness, lethargy, hangover,* dizziness, ataxia, fainting.
CV: transient hypotension.
GI: dry mouth, nausea, vomiting, abdominal discomfort.
Skin: rash.

INTERACTIONS
Alcohol, other CNS depressants: increased CNS depression. Avoid concomitant use.
Cimetidine: increased sedation. Monitor carefully.

NURSING CONSIDERATIONS
• Contraindicated in acute narrow-angle glaucoma, psychoses, or anxiety-free psychiatric disorders. Use with caution in renal or hepatic impairment.
• Dosage should be reduced in elderly or debilitated patients.
• Possibility of abuse and addiction exists. Don't stop drug abruptly: withdrawal symptoms may occur.
• Warn patient to avoid activities that require alertness and good psychomotor coordination until CNS effects of the drug are known.

● Warn patient not to combine drug with alcohol or other depressants.
● Caution patient against giving medication to others.
● Prazepam should not be prescribed for everyday stress.

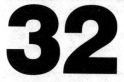

32

Antipsychotics

acetophenazine maleate
chlorpromazine hydrochloride
chlorprothixene
clozapine
fluphenazine decanoate
fluphenazine enanthate
fluphenazine hydrochloride
haloperidol
haloperidol decanoate
haloperidol lactate
loxapine hydrochloride
loxapine succinate
mesoridazine besylate
molindone hydrochloride
perphenazine
pimozide
prochlorperazine
   (See Chapter 48, ANTIEMETICS.)
promazine hydrochloride
thioridazine hydrochloride
thiothixene
thiothixene hydrochloride
trifluoperazine hydrochloride
triflupromazine hydrochloride

COMBINATION PRODUCTS
ETRAFON 2-10: perphenazine 2 mg and amitriptyline hydrochloride 10 mg.
ETRAFON-A: perphenazine 2 mg and amitriptyline hydrochloride 25 mg.
ETRAFON-FORTE: perphenazine 4 mg and amitriptyline hydrochloride 25 mg.
TRIAVIL 2-10, TRIAVIL 4-10, TRIAVIL 2-25 are identical to Etrafon products above; TRIAVIL 4-50: perphenazine 4 mg and amitriptyline hydrochloride 50 mg.

---

acetophenazine maleate
Tindal
Pregnancy Risk Category: C

HOW SUPPLIED
Tablets: 20 mg

MECHANISM OF ACTION
Blocks postsynaptic dopamine receptors in the brain. A piperazine phenothiazine.

INDICATIONS & DOSAGE
Psychotic disorders—
Adults: initially, 20 mg P.O. t.i.d. or q.i.d. Daily dosage ranges from 40 to 80 mg in outpatients, or 80 to 120 mg in hospitalized patients, but in severe psychotic states up to 600 mg daily has been safely administered. Smallest effective dosage should be used at all times.

ADVERSE REACTIONS
Blood: transient leukopenia, *agranulocytosis.*
CNS: *extrapyramidal reactions (high incidence), tardive dyskinesia,* sedation (low incidence), pseudoparkinsonism, EEG changes, dizziness.
CV: *orthostatic hypotension,* tachycardia, ECG changes.
EENT: ocular changes, *blurred vision.*
GI: *dry mouth, constipation.*
GU: *urine retention,* dark urine, menstrual irregularities, gynecomastia, inhibited ejaculation.
Hepatic: cholestatic jaundice, abnormal liver function tests.

Metabolic: hyperprolactinemia.
Skin: *mild photosensitivity,* dermal allergic reactions.
Other: weight gain; increased appetite; rarely, *neuroleptic malignant syndrome* (fever, tachycardia, tachypnea, profuse diaphoresis).
After abrupt withdrawal of long-term therapy: gastritis, nausea, vomiting, dizziness, tremors, feeling of warmth or cold, sweating, tachycardia, headache, insomnia.

INTERACTIONS
Alcohol, other CNS depressants: increased CNS depression. Avoid concomitant use.
Antacids: inhibit absorption of oral phenothiazines. Separate antacid and phenothiazine doses by at least 2 hours.
Barbiturates: may decrease phenothiazine effect. Observe patient.

NURSING CONSIDERATIONS
• Contraindicated in CNS depression, bone marrow suppression, subcortical damage, and coma; also with use of spinal or epidural anesthetic, or adrenergic blocking agents. Use cautiously with other CNS depressants, anticholinergics; in elderly or debilitated patients; and in hepatic disease, arteriosclerosis or cardiovascular disease (may cause sudden drop in blood pressure), exposure to extreme heat or cold (including antipyretic therapy), respiratory disorders, hypocalcemia, seizure disorders (may lower seizure threshold), severe reactions to insulin or electroshock therapy, suspected brain tumor or intestinal obstruction, glaucoma, or prostatic hypertrophy.
• Tardive dyskinesia may occur after prolonged use. It may not appear until months or years later and may disappear spontaneously or persist for life despite discontinuation of drug.
• Acute dystonic reactions may be treated with I.V. diphenhydramine.
• Neuroleptic malignant syndrome is rare, but frequently fatal. It is not necessarily related to length of drug use or type of neuroleptic, but over 60% of affected patients are men. Watch for symptoms.
• Hold dose and notify doctor if patient develops symptoms of blood dyscrasias (fever, sore throat, infection, cellulitis, weakness), persistent (longer than a few hours) extrapyramidal reactions, or any such reaction during pregnancy.
• Dose of 20 mg is therapeutic equivalent of 100 mg chlorpromazine.
• Monitor therapy by weekly bilirubin tests during first month; periodic blood tests (CBC and liver function); and ophthalmic tests (long-term use).
• Have patient report urine retention or constipation.
• Tell patient to use sunscreening agents and protective clothing to avoid photosensitivity reactions.
• Warn against activities requiring alertness or good psychomotor coordination until CNS effects of the drug are known.
• Obtain baseline measures of blood pressure before starting therapy and monitor routinely. Watch for orthostatic hypotension. Advise patient to get up slowly.
• Dry mouth may be relieved with sugarless gum, sour hard candy, or rinsing with mouthwash.
• Do not withdraw drug abruptly unless required by severe adverse reactions.
• Patient on maintenance may take medication at bedtime to facilitate sleep and decrease sedation during daytime.

Italicized adverse reactions are common or life-threatening.
*Liquid form contains alcohol.   **May contain tartrazine.

chlorpromazine hydrochloride

Chlorpromanyl†, Largactil†‡, Novo-Chlorpromazine†, Protran‡, Thorazine, Thor-Pram

Pregnancy Risk Category: C

HOW SUPPLIED

Tablets: 10 mg, 25 mg, 50 mg, 100 mg, 200 mg
Capsules (sustained-release): 30 mg, 75 mg, 150 mg, 200 mg, 300 mg
Oral concentrate: 30 mg/ml, 100 mg/ml
Syrup: 10 mg/5ml
Injection: 25 mg/ml
Suppositories: 25 mg, 100 mg

MECHANISM OF ACTION

Blocks postsynaptic dopamine receptors in the brain. As an antiemetic, inhibits the medullary chemoreceptor trigger zone. Aliphatic phenothiazine.

INDICATIONS & DOSAGE

Intractable hiccups—
Adults: 25 to 50 mg P.O. or I.M. t.i.d. or q.i.d.
Mild alcohol withdrawal, acute intermittent porphyria, and tetanus—
Adults: 25 to 50 mg I.M. t.i.d. or q.i.d.
Psychosis—
Adults: 500 mg P.O. daily in divided doses, increasing gradually to 2 g; or 25 to 50 mg I.M. q 1 to 4 hours, p.r.n.
Children: 0.25 mg/kg P.O. q 4 to 6 hours; or 0.25 mg/kg I.M. q 6 to 8 hours; or 0.5 mg/kg rectally q 6 to 8 hours. Maximum dose is 40 mg in children under 5 years, and 75 mg in children 5 to 12 years.
Nausea and vomiting—
Adults: 10 to 225 mg P.O. or I.M. q 4 to 6 hours, p.r.n.; or 50 to 100 mg rectally q 6 to 8 hours, p.r.n.
Children: 0.25 mg/kg P.O. q 4 to 6 hours; or 0.25 mg/kg I.M. q 6 to 8 hours; or 0.5 mg/kg rectally q 6 to 8 hours.

ADVERSE REACTIONS

Blood: transient leukopenia, *agranulocytosis.*
CNS: *extrapyramidal reactions (moderate incidence), sedation (high incidence), tardive dyskinesia,* pseudoparkinsonism, EEG changes, dizziness.
CV: *orthostatic hypotension,* tachycardia, ECG changes.
EENT: ocular changes, *blurred vision.*
GI: *dry mouth, constipation.*
GU: *urine retention,* dark urine, menstrual irregularities, gynecomastia, inhibited ejaculation.
Hepatic: cholestatic jaundice, abnormal liver function tests.
Metabolic: hyperprolactinemia.
Skin: *mild photosensitivity,* dermal allergic reactions.
Local: *pain on I.M. injection,* sterile abscess.
Other: weight gain; increased appetite; rarely, *neuroleptic malignant syndrome* (fever, tachycardia, tachypnea, profuse diaphoresis).
After abrupt withdrawal of long-term therapy: gastritis, nausea, vomiting, dizziness, tremors, feeling of warmth or cold, sweating, tachycardia, headache, insomnia.

INTERACTIONS

Alcohol, other CNS depressants: increased CNS depression. Avoid concomitant use.
Antacids: inhibit absorption of oral phenothiazines. Separate antacid and phenothiazine doses by at least 2 hours.
Anticholinergics (including antidepressant and antiparkinsonian agents): increased anticholinergic activity, aggravated parkinsonian symptoms. Use with caution.
Barbiturates, lithium: may decrease phenothiazine effect. Observe patient.
Centrally acting antihypertensive

---

agents: decreased antihypertensive effect.

Lithium: possible decreased response to chlorpromazine. Observe patient.

Oral anticoagulants: decreased anticoagulant effect.

Propranolol: increased levels of both propranolol and chlorpromazine.

NURSING CONSIDERATIONS

• Contraindicated in CNS depression, bone marrow suppresion, subcortical damage, Reye's syndrome, and coma; also contraindicated with use of spinal or epidural anesthetic, or adrenergic blocking agents. Use cautiously with other CNS depressants, anticholinergics; in elderly or debilitated patients; in hepatic disease, arteriosclerosis or CV disease (may cause sudden drop in blood pressure), exposure to extreme heat or cold (including antipyretic therapy), respiratory disorders, hypocalcemia, seizure disorders (may lower seizure threshold), severe reactions to insulin or electroshock therapy, suspected brain tumor or intestinal obstruction, glaucoma, or prostatic hypertrophy; and in acutely ill or dehydrated children. Use parenteral form cautiously in asthmatics and in patients allergic to sulfites.

• Tardive dyskinesia may occur after prolonged use. It may not appear until months or years later and may disappear spontaneously or persist for life despite discontinuation of drug.

• Neuroleptic malignant syndrome is rare, but frequently fatal. It is not necessarily related to length of drug use or type of neuroleptic, but over 60% of affected patients are men. Watch for symptoms.

• Acute dystonic reactions may be treated with I.V. diphenhydramine.

• Hold dose and notify doctor if patient develops jaundice, symptoms of blood dyscrasias (fever, sore throat, infection, cellulitis, weakness), persistent (longer than a few hours) extrapyramidal reactions, or any such reaction in pregnancy or in children.

• Monitor therapy by weekly bilirubin tests during first month; periodic blood tests (CBC and liver function); and ophthalmic tests (long-term use).

• Have patient report urine retention or constipation.

• Tell patient to use sunscreening agents and protective clothing to avoid photosensitivity reactions. Chlorpromazine causes higher incidence of photosensitivity than any other drug in its class.

• Warn against activities that require alertness or good psychomotor coordination until CNS effects of the drug are known. Drowsiness and dizziness usually subside after first few weeks.

• Obtain baseline measures of blood pressure before starting therapy and monitor regularly. Watch for orthostatic hypotension, especially with parenteral administration. Monitor blood pressure before and after I.M. administration. Keep patient supine for 1 hour afterward. Advise patient to get up slowly.

• Give deep I.M. only in upper outer quadrant of buttocks. Massage slowly afterward to prevent sterile abscess. Injection stings.

• Liquid (oral) and parenteral forms of drug can cause contact dermatitis. If susceptible, wear gloves when preparing solutions of this drug, and prevent any contact with skin and clothing.

• Protect liquid concentrate from light. Dilute with fruit juice, milk, or semisolid food just before administration.

• Slight yellowing of injection or concentrate is common; does not affect potency. Discard markedly discolored solutions.

• Do not withdraw drug abruptly unless required by severe adverse reactions.

• Dry mouth may be relieved by sug-

Italicized adverse reactions are common or life-threatening.
*Liquid form contains alcohol.   **May contain tartrazine.

arless gum, sour hard candy, or rinsing with mouthwash.
• Also available as a rectal suppository.

chlorprothixene
Taractan**, Tarasan†

Pregnancy Risk Category: C

HOW SUPPLIED
Tablets: 10 mg, 25 mg, 50 mg, 100 mg
Oral concentrate: 100 mg/5 ml (fruit)
Injection: 12.5 mg/ml

MECHANISM OF ACTION
Blocks postsynaptic dopamine receptors in the brain. A thioxanthene.

INDICATIONS & DOSAGE
Psychotic disorders—
Adults: initially, 10 mg P.O. t.i.d. or q.i.d. Increase gradually to maximum of 600 mg daily.
Children over 6 years: 10 to 25 mg P.O. t.i.d. or q.i.d.
Agitation of severe neurosis, depression, schizophrenia—
Adults: 25 to 50 mg P.O. or I.M. t.i.d. or q.i.d. Increase as needed up to maximum of 600 mg.

ADVERSE REACTIONS
Blood: transient leukopenia, *agranulocytosis.*
CNS: extrapyramidal reactions (low incidence), tardive dyskinesia, *sedation,* pseudoparkinsonism, EEG changes, dizziness.
CV: *orthostatic hypotension,* tachycardia, ECG changes.
EENT: ocular changes, *blurred vision.*
GI: *dry mouth, constipation.*
GU: *urine retention,* dark urine, menstrual irregularities, gynecomastia, inhibited ejaculation.
Hepatic: cholestatic jaundice, abnormal liver function tests.
Metabolic: hyperprolactinemia.

Skin: *mild photosensitivity,* dermal allergic reactions.
Local: pain on I.M. injection, sterile abscess.
Other: weight gain; increased appetite; rarely, *neuroleptic malignant syndrome* (fever, tachycardia, tachypnea, profuse diaphoresis).
After abrupt withdrawal of long-term therapy: gastritis, nausea, vomiting, dizziness, tremors, feeling of warmth or cold, sweating, tachycardia, headache, insomnia.

INTERACTIONS
Alcohol, other CNS depressants: increased CNS depression. Avoid concomitant use.
Anticholinergics: potentiated central anticholinergic effects.
Centrally acting antihypertensives: decreased antihypertensive effect.

NURSING CONSIDERATIONS
• Contraindicated in coma, CNS depression, bone marrow suppression, circulatory collapse, CHF, cardiac decompensation, coronary artery or cerebrovascular disorders, subcortical damage; with use of spinal or epidural anesthetic, or adrenergic blocking agents. Use cautiously with other CNS depressants, anticholinergics; in elderly or debilitated patients; in hepatic or renal disease, arteriosclerosis or CV disease (may cause sudden drop in blood pressure), exposure to extreme heat or cold (including antipyretic therapy), respiratory disorders, hypocalcemia, seizure disorders (may lower seizure threshold), severe reactions to insulin or electroshock therapy, suspected brain tumor or intestinal obstruction, glaucoma, or prostatic hypertrophy; and in acutely ill or dehydrated children.
• Tardive dyskinesia may occur after prolonged use. It may not appear until months or years later and may disappear spontaneously or persist for life despite discontinuation of drug.

• Neuroleptic malignant syndrome is rare, but frequently fatal. It is not necessarily related to length of drug use or type of neuroleptic, but over 60% of affected patients are men. Watch for symptoms.

• Acute dystonic reactions may be treated with I.V. diphenhydramine.

• Hold dose and notify doctor if patient develops symptoms of blood dyscrasias (fever, sore throat, infection, cellulitis, weakness), jaundice, persistent (longer than a few hours) extrapyramidal reactions, or any such reactions in children.

• Monitor therapy by weekly bilirubin tests during first month; periodic blood tests (CBC and liver function) before and during therapy; and ophthalmic tests (long-term therapy).

• Have patient report urine retention or constipation.

• Tell patient to use sunscreening agents and protective clothing to avoid photosensitivity reactions.

• Warn against activities that require alertness or good psychomotor coordination until CNS effects of the drug are known. Drowsiness and dizziness usually subside after first few weeks.

• Obtain baseline measures of blood pressure before starting therapy and monitor regularly. Watch for orthostatic hypotension, especially with parenteral administration, since adrenergic blockage is high. Keep patient in a supine position for 1 hour afterward. Advise patient to change positions slowly.

• Give deep I.M. only in upper outer quadrant of buttocks or midlateral thigh. Massage slowly afterward to prevent sterile abscess. Injection stings.

• Dilute liquid concentrate with fruit juice, milk, or semisolid food just before administration.

• Protect medication from light. Slight yellowing of injection or concentrate is common; does not affect potency. Discard markedly discolored solutions.

• Do not withdraw drug abruptly unless required by severe adverse reactions.

• Prevent contact dermatitis by keeping drug off patient's skin and clothes. Wear gloves when preparing liquid forms of the drug.

• Dry mouth may be relieved by sugarless gum, sour hard candy, or rinsing with mouthwash.

• Dose of 100 mg is the therapeutic equivalent of 100 mg chlorpromazine.

clozapine
Clozaril
Pregnancy Risk Category: B

HOW SUPPLIED
Available only through a special Patient Management System
Tablets: 25 mg, 100 mg

MECHANISM OF ACTION
Binds to dopamine receptors (both D-1 and D-2) within the limbic system of the CNS. It also may interfere with adrenergic, cholinergic, histaminergic, and serotoninergic receptors.

INDICATIONS & DOSAGE
Treatment of schizophrenia in severely ill patients unresponsive to other therapies—
Adults: initially, 25 mg P.O. q.i.d. or b.i.d., titrated upward at 25 to 50 mg daily (if tolerated) to a daily dosage of 300 to 450 mg daily by the end of 2 weeks. Individual dosage is based on clinical response, patient tolerance, and adverse reactions. Subsequent dosage should not be increased more than once or twice weekly, and should not exceed 100 mg. Many patients respond to doses of 300 to 600 mg daily, but some may require as much as 900 mg daily. Do not exceed 900 mg/day.

Italicized adverse reactions are common or life-threatening.
*Liquid form contains alcohol.   **May contain tartrazine.

ADVERSE REACTIONS
Blood: *leukopenia, granulocytopenia, agranulocytosis.*
CNS: *drowsiness, sedation, seizures, dizziness,* syncope, vertigo, headache, tremor, disturbed sleep or nightmares, restlessness, hypokinesia or akinesia, agitation, rigidity, akathisia, confusion, fatigue, insomnia, hyperkinesia, weakness, lethargy, ataxia, slurred speech, depression, myoclonia, anxiety.
CV: *tachycardia, hypotension,* hypertension, chest pain, ECG changes.
GI: *constipation,* nausea, vomiting, *salivation, dry mouth.*
GU: urinary abnormalities, incontinence, abnormal ejaculation, urinary frequency or urgency, urine retention.
Other: fever, muscle pain or spasm, muscle weakness, weight gain, rash.

INTERACTIONS
Anticholinergics: may potentiate the anticholinergic effects of clozapine.
Antihypertensives: hypotensive effects may be potentiated by clozapine.
Bone marrow suppressant drugs: potentially increased bone marrow toxicity.
CNS-active drugs: possible additive effects. Use together cautiously.
Warfarin, digoxin, and other highly protein bound drugs: increased serum levels of these drugs may occur. Monitor closely for adverse reactions.

NURSING CONSIDERATIONS
• Contraindicated in patients with a history of clozapine-induced agranulocytosis or severe granulocytopenia; in patients with a WBC count below 3,500/mm³; and in patients with severe CNS depression or coma. It is also contraindicated in patients who are taking other drugs that suppress bone marrow function and in patients with myelosuppressive disorders.
• Because clozapine has potent anticholinergic effects, use cautiously in patients with prostatic hypertrophy or glaucoma.
• Seizures may occur, especially in patients receiving high doses of the drug. Patients should avoid hazardous activities that require alertness and good coordination, such as driving, swimming, or climbing, while taking the drug.
• Clozapine therapy carries a significant risk of agranulocytosis (early trials estimate the incidence at 1.3%). If possible, patients should receive at least two trials of a standard antipsychotic drug therapy before clozapine therapy is initiated. Baseline WBC and differential counts are required before therapy; WBC counts must be monitored weekly and for at least 4 weeks after clozapine therapy is discontinued.
• Clozapine is available only through a special Clozaril Patient Management System that ensures weekly testing of WBC counts. Blood tests are performed once a week, and no more than a 1-week supply of drug is distributed.
• If WBC count drops below 3,500/mm³ after initiating therapy or exhibits a substantial drop from baseline, monitor patient closely for signs of infection. If WBC count is 3,000 to 3,500/mm³ and granulocyte count is above 1,500/mm³, perform twice weekly WBC and differential counts. If WBC count drops below 3,000/mm³ and granulocyte count drops below 1,500/mm³, therapy should be interrupted and the patient monitored for signs of infection. Therapy may be cautiously restarted if WBC count returns above 3,000/mm³ and granulocyte count returns above 1,500/mm³, but twice weekly monitoring of WBC and differential counts should occur until the WBC count exceeds 3,500/mm³.
• If the WBC count drops below 2,000/mm³ and granulocyte count drops below 1,000/mm³, the patient

may require protective isolation. If the patient develops infection, prepare cultures according to policy and administer antibiotics, as ordered. Some clinicians may perform bone marrow aspiration to assess bone marrow function. In such patients, future clozapine therapy is contraindicated.

• If clozapine therapy must be discontinued, the drug is usually withdrawn gradually (over a 1- to 2-week period). However, changes in the patient's medical condition (including the development of leukopenia) may require abrupt discontinuation of the drug. Monitor closely for the recurrence of psychotic symptoms.

• If therapy is reinstated in patients withdrawn from the drug, the usual guidelines for dosage build-up should be followed. However, reexposure of the patient to this drug may increase the severity and risk of adverse reactions. If therapy was terminated for WBC counts below 2,000/mm³ or granulocyte counts below 1,000/mm³, the drug should not be continued.

• Patients should be warned about the risk of agranulocytosis. They should know that the drug is available only through a special monitoring program that will require weekly blood tests to monitor for agranulocytosis. Advise the patient to report flu-like symptoms, fever, sore throat, lethargy, malaise, or other signs of infection.

• Some patients experience transient fevers (temperature >100.4° F., or 38° C.), especially in the first 3 weeks of therapy. Monitor patients closely.

• Advise patients to check with the doctor before taking any OTC drugs or alcohol.

• Recommend ice chips or sugarless candy or gum to help relieve dry mouth.

• Patients should rise slowly to avoid orthostatic hypotension.

fluphenazine decanoate
Modecate Decanoate†‡, Prolixin Decanoate

fluphenazine enanthate
Moditen Enanthate†, Prolixin Enanthate

fluphenazine hydrochloride
Anatensol‡*, Apo-Fluphenazine†, Moditen HCl†, Moditen HCl-HP†, Permitil* **, Prolixin* **

Pregnancy Risk Category: C

HOW SUPPLIED
decanoate
Depot injection: 25 mg/ml
enanthate
Depot injection: 25 mg/ml
hydrochloride
Tablets: 1 mg, 2.5 mg, 5 mg, 10 mg
Oral concentrate: 5 mg/ml (contains 14% alcohol)
Elixir: 2.5 mg/5 ml (with 14% alcohol)
I.M. injection: 2.5 mg/ml

MECHANISM OF ACTION
Blocks postsynaptic dopamine receptors in the brain. A piperazine phenothiazine.

INDICATIONS & DOSAGE
Psychotic disorders—
Adults: initially, 0.5 to 10 mg (fluphenazine hydrochloride) P.O. daily in divided doses q 6 to 8 hours; may increase cautiously to 20 mg. Higher doses (50 to 100 mg) have been given. Maintenance dosage is 1 to 5 mg P.O. daily. I.M. doses are ⅓ to ½ oral doses. Lower dosages for geriatric patients (1 to 2.5 mg daily).
Children: 0.25 to 3.5 mg fluphenazine hydrochloride P.O. daily in divided doses q 4 to 6 hours; or ⅓ to ½ of oral dose I.M.; maximum dosage is 10 mg daily.
Adults and children over 12 years: 12.5 to 25 mg of long-acting esters

---

Italicized adverse reactions are common or life-threatening.
*Liquid form contains alcohol.   **May contain tartrazine.

(fluphenazine decanoate and enanthate) I.M. or S.C. q 1 to 6 weeks. Maintenance dosage is 25 to 100 mg, p.r.n.

ADVERSE REACTIONS
Blood: transient leukopenia, *agranulocytosis.*
CNS: *extrapyramidal reactions (high incidence), tardive dyskinesia,* sedation (low incidence), pseudoparkinsonism, EEG changes, dizziness.
CV: *orthostatic hypotension,* tachycardia, ECG changes.
EENT: ocular changes, *blurred vision.*
GI: *dry mouth, constipation.*
GU: *urine retention,* dark urine, menstrual irregularities, gynecomastia, inhibited ejaculation.
Hepatic: cholestatic jaundice, abnormal liver function tests.
Metabolic: hyperprolactinemia.
Skin: *mild photosensitivity,* dermal allergic reactions.
Other: weight gain; increased appetite; rarely, *neuroleptic malignant syndrome* (fever, tachycardia, tachypnea, profuse diaphoresis).
After abrupt withdrawal of long-term therapy: gastritis, nausea, vomiting, dizziness, tremors, feeling of warmth or cold, sweating, tachycardia, headache, insomnia.

INTERACTIONS
Alcohol, other CNS depressants: increased CNS depression. Avoid concomitant use.
Antacids: inhibit absorption of oral phenothiazines. Separate antacid and phenothiazine doses by at least 2 hours.
Barbiturates, lithium: may decrease phenothiazine effect. Observe patient.
Centrally acting antihypertensives: decreased antihypertensive effect.

NURSING CONSIDERATIONS
• Contraindicated in coma, CNS depression, bone marrow suppression or other blood dyscrasia, subcortical damage, hepatic damage, renal insufficiency; and with use of spinal or epidural anesthetic, or adrenergic blocking agents. Use cautiously with other CNS depressants, anticholinergics; in elderly or debilitated patients; in acutely ill or dehydrated children; and in hepatic disease, pheochromocytoma, arteriosclerotic, cerebrovascular, or CV disease (may cause sudden drop in blood pressure), peptic ulcer, exposure to extreme heat or cold (including antipyretic therapy), respiratory disorders, hypocalcemia, seizure disorders (may lower seizure threshold), severe reactions to insulin or electroshock therapy, suspected brain tumor or intestinal obstruction, glaucoma, or prostatic hypertrophy. Use parenteral form cautiously in asthmatic patients and patients allergic to sulfites.
• For long-acting forms (decanoate and enanthate), which are oil preparations, use a dry needle of at least 21 gauge. Allow 24 to 96 hours for onset of action. Note and report adverse reactions in patients taking the long-acting drug forms.
• Tardive dyskinesia may occur after prolonged use. It may not appear until months or years later and may disappear spontaneously or persist for life despite discontinuation of drug.
• Neuroleptic malignant syndrome is rare, but frequently fatal. It is not necessarily related to length of drug use or type of neuroleptic, but over 60% of affected patients are men. Watch for symptoms.
• Acute dystonic reactions may be treated with I.V. diphenhydramine.
• Hold dose and notify doctor if patient develops symptoms of blood dyscrasias (fever, sore throat, infection, cellulitis, weakness), persistent (longer than a few hours) extrapyramidal reactions, or any such reactions in pregnancy or in children.

---

†Available in Canada only.   ‡Available in Australia only.   ◊ Available OTC.

• Monitor therapy by weekly bilirubin tests during first month; periodic blood tests (CBC and liver function); periodic renal function and ophthalmic tests (long-term use).

• Have patient report urine retention or constipation.

• Tell patient to use sunscreening agents and protective clothing to avoid photosensitivity reactions.

• Warn against activities that require alertness and good psychomotor coordination until CNS effects of the drug are known. Drowsiness and dizziness usually subside after first few weeks.

• Decanoate and enanthate may be given subcutaneously.

• Liquid (oral) and parenteral forms can cause contact dermatitis. If susceptible, wear gloves when preparing solutions of this drug, and prevent any contact with skin and clothing.

• Dilute liquid concentrate with water, fruit juice, milk, or semisolid food just before administration.

• Protect medication from light. Slight yellowing of injection or concentrate is common; does not affect potency. Discard markedly discolored solutions.

• Dry mouth may be relieved by sugarless gum, sour hard candy, or rinsing with mouthwash.

• Do not withdraw drug abruptly unless required by severe adverse reactions.

• Dose of 2 mg is therapeutic equivalent of 100 mg chlorpromazine.

• Note that Prolixin Concentrate and Permitil Concentrate are 10 times more concentrated than Prolixin Elixir (5 mg/ml vs. 0.5 mg/ml).

haloperidol
Apo-Haloperidol†, Haldol**, Halperon, Novoperidol†, Peridol†, Serenace‡

haloperidol decanoate
Haldol Decanoate, Haldol LA†

haloperidol lactate
Haldol

Pregnancy Risk Category: C

HOW SUPPLIED
haloperidol
Tablets: 0.5 mg, 1 mg, 2 mg, 5 mg, 10 mg, 20 mg
haloperidol decanoate
Injection: 50 mg/ml
haloperidol lactate
Oral concentrate: 2 mg/ml
Injection: 5 mg/ml

MECHANISM OF ACTION
Blocks postsynaptic dopamine receptors in the brain. A butyrophenone.

INDICATIONS & DOSAGE
Psychotic disorders—
Adults: dosage varies for each patient. Initial range is 0.5 to 5 mg P.O. b.i.d. or t.i.d.; or 2 to 5 mg I.M. q 4 to 8 hours, increasing rapidly if necessary for prompt control. Maximum dosage is 100 mg P.O. daily. Doses over 100 mg have been used for patients with severely resistant conditions.
Chronic psychotic patients who require prolonged therapy—
Adults: 50 to 100 mg I.M. haloperidol decanoate q 4 weeks.
Control of tics, vocal utterances in Gilles de la Tourette's syndrome—
Adults: 0.5 to 5 mg P.O. b.i.d. or t.i.d., increasing p.r.n.

ADVERSE REACTIONS
Blood: transient leukopenia and leukocytosis.
CNS: *high incidence of severe extra-*

Italicized adverse reactions are common or life-threatening.
*Liquid form contains alcohol.   **May contain tartrazine.

pyramidal reactions, tardive dyskinesia, low incidence of sedation.
CV: low incidence of cardiovascular effects with therapeutic dosages.
EENT: blurred vision, dry mouth.
GU: urine retention, menstrual irregularities, gynecomastia.
Skin: rash.
Other: rarely, neuroleptic malignant syndrome (fever, tachycardia, tachypnea, profuse diaphoresis).

INTERACTIONS
Alcohol, other CNS depressants: increased CNS depression. Avoid concomitant use.
Lithium: lethargy and confusion with high doses. Observe patient.
Methyldopa: possible symptoms of dementia. Observe patient.

NURSING CONSIDERATIONS
• Contraindicated in parkinsonism, coma, or CNS depression. Use with caution in elderly and debilitated patients; in severe CV disorders, allergies, glaucoma, urine retention; and in conjunction with anticonvulsant, anticoagulant, antiparkinsonian, or lithium medications.
• Tardive dyskinesia may occur after prolonged use. It may not appear until months or years later and may disappear spontaneously or persist for life despite discontinuation of drug.
• Neuroleptic malignant syndrome is rare, but frequently fatal. It is not necessarily related to length of drug use or type of neuroleptic, but over 60% of affected patients are men. Watch for symptoms.
• Acute dystonic reactions may be treated with I.V. diphenhydramine.
• Elderly patients usually require lower initial doses and a more gradual dosage titration.
• Haloperidol is the least sedating of the antipsychotic agents. However, warn patient against activities that require alertness and good psychomotor coordination until CNS effects of the drug are known. Drowsiness and dizziness usually subside after a few weeks.
• Protect medication from light. Slight yellowing of injection or concentrate is common; does not affect potency. Discard markedly discolored solutions.
• Do not withdraw drug abruptly unless required by severe adverse reactions.
• Dry mouth may be relieved by sugarless gum, sour hard candy, and rinsing with mouthwash.
• Dose of 2 mg is therapeutic equivalent of 100 mg chlorpromazine.
• Especially useful for agitation associated with senile dementia.
• When changing from tablets to decanoate injection, patient should receive 10 to 15 times the oral dose once a month (maximum 100 mg).
• Don't administer the decanoate form I.V.

loxapine hydrochloride
Loxapac†, Loxitane C, Loxitane I.M.

loxapine succinate
Loxapac†, Loxitane
Pregnancy Risk Category: C

HOW SUPPLIED
Capsules: 5 mg, 10 mg, 25 mg, 50 mg
Oral concentrate: 25 mg/ml
Injection: 50 mg/ml

MECHANISM OF ACTION
Blocks postsynaptic dopamine receptors in the brain. A dibenzoxazepine.

INDICATIONS & DOSAGE
Psychotic disorders—
Adults: 10 mg P.O. or I.M. b.i.d. to q.i.d., rapidly increasing to 60 to 100 mg P.O. daily for most patients; dosage varies from patient to patient.

ADVERSE REACTIONS
Blood: transient leukopenia.
CNS: *extrapyramidal reactions (moderate incidence), sedation (moderate incidence),* tardive dyskinesia, pseudoparkinsonism, EEG changes, dizziness.
CV: *orthostatic hypotension,* tachycardia, ECG changes.
EENT: *blurred vision.*
GI: *dry mouth, constipation.*
GU: *urine retention,* dark urine, menstrual irregularities, gynecomastia.
Skin: *mild photosensitivity,* dermal allergic reactions.
Other: weight gain; increased appetite; rarely, *neuroleptic malignant syndrome* (fever, tachycardia, tachypnea, profuse diaphoresis).

INTERACTIONS
Alcohol, other CNS depressants: increased CNS depression. Avoid concomitant use.

NURSING CONSIDERATIONS
• Contraindicated in coma, severe CNS depression, or drug-induced depressed states. Use with caution in epilepsy, CV disorders, glaucoma, urine retention, suspected intestinal obstruction or brain tumor, and renal damage.
• Tardive dyskinesia may occur after prolonged use. It may not appear until months or years later and may disappear spontaneously or persist for life despite discontinuation of drug.
• Neuroleptic malignant syndrome is rare, but frequently fatal. It is not necessarily related to length of drug use or type of neuroleptic, but over 60% of affected patients are men. Watch for symptoms.
• Acute dystonic reactions may be treated with I.V. diphenhydramine.
• Warn against activities that require alertness and good psychomotor coordination until CNS effects of the drug are known. Drowsiness and dizziness usually subside after first few weeks.

• Obtain baseline measures of blood pressure before starting therapy and monitor regularly. Advise patient to get up slowly to avoid orthostatic hypotension.
• Dilute liquid concentrate with orange or grapefruit juice just before giving.
• Dry mouth may be relieved by sugarless gum, sour hard candy, or rinsing with mouthwash.
• Periodic eye examinations are recommended.
• Tricyclic dibenzoxazepine; the only dibenzoxazepine derivative.
• Dose of 10 mg is therapeutic equivalent of 100 mg chlorpromazine.

mesoridazine besylate
Serentil* **
Pregnancy Risk Category: C

HOW SUPPLIED
Tablets: 10 mg, 25 mg, 50 mg, 100 mg
Oral concentrate: 25 mg/ml (0.6% alcohol)
Injection: 25 mg/ml

MECHANISM OF ACTION
Blocks postsynaptic dopamine receptors in the brain. It is a piperidine phenothiazine and the major sulfoxide metabolite of thioridazine.

INDICATIONS & DOSAGE
Alcoholism—
Adults and children over 12 years: 25 mg P.O. b.i.d. up to maximum of 200 mg daily.
Behavioral problems associated with chronic brain syndrome—
Adults and children over 12 years: 25 mg P.O. t.i.d. up to maximum of 300 mg daily.
Psychoneurotic manifestations (anxiety)—
Adults and children over 12 years: 10 mg P.O. t.i.d. up to maximum of 150 mg daily.

Schizophrenia—
Adults and children over 12 years:
initially, 50 mg P.O. t.i.d. or 25 mg
I.M. repeated in 30 to 60 minutes,
p.r.n.

ADVERSE REACTIONS

Blood: transient leukopenia, *agranulocytosis.*
CNS: extrapyramidal reactions (low incidence), *tardive dyskinesia, sedation (high incidence),* EEG changes, dizziness.
CV: *orthostatic hypotension,* tachycardia, ECG changes.
EENT: *ocular changes, blurred vision,* pigmentary retinopathy.
GI: *dry mouth, constipation.*
GU: *urine retention,* dark urine, menstrual irregularities, gynecomastia, inhibited ejaculation.
Hepatic: cholestatic jaundice, abnormal liver function tests.
Metabolic: hyperprolactinemia.
Skin: *mild photosensitivity,* dermal allergic reactions.
Local: pain at I.M. injection site, sterile abscess.
Other: weight gain; increased appetite; rarely, *neuroleptic malignant syndrome* (fever, tachycardia, tachypnea, profuse diaphoresis).
After abrupt withdrawal of long-term therapy: gastritis, nausea, vomiting, dizziness, tremors, feeling of warmth or cold, sweating, tachycardia, headache, insomnia.

INTERACTIONS

Alcohol, other CNS depressants: increased CNS depression. Avoid concomitant use.
Antacids: inhibit absorption of oral phenothiazines. Separate antacid and phenothiazine doses by at least 2 hours.
Barbiturates: may decrease phenothiazine effect. Observe patient.

NURSING CONSIDERATIONS

• Contraindicated in coma, CNS depression, bone marrow suppression, subcortical damage, and with use of spinal or epidural anesthetic or adrenergic blocking agents. Use cautiously with other CNS depressants, anticholinergics; in elderly or debilitated patients; in acutely ill or dehydrated children; and in hepatic disease, arteriosclerosis or CV disease (may cause sudden drop in blood pressure), exposure to extreme heat or cold (including antipyretic therapy), respiratory disorders, hypocalcemia, seizure disorders, severe reactions to insulin or electroshock therapy, suspected brain tumor or intestinal obstruction, glaucoma, and prostatic hypertrophy.
• Tardive dyskinesia may occur after prolonged use. It may not appear until months or years later and may disappear spontaneously or persist for life despite discontinuation of drug.
• Neuroleptic malignant syndrome is rare, but frequently fatal. It is not necessarily related to length of drug use or type of neuroleptic, but over 60% of affected patients are men. Watch for symptoms.
• Acute dystonic reactions may be treated with I.V. diphenhydramine.
• Hold dose and notify doctor if patient develops jaundice, symptoms of blood dyscrasias (fever, sore throat, infection, cellulitis, weakness), persistent (longer than a few hours) extrapyramidal reactions, or any such reactions in pregnancy or in children.
• Monitor therapy by weekly bilirubin tests during first month; periodic blood tests (CBC and liver function); and ophthalmic tests (long-term use).
• Have patient report urine retention or constipation.
• Tell patient to use sunscreening agents and protective clothing to avoid photosensitivity reactions.
• Warn against activities that require alertness and good psychomotor coordination until CNS effects of the drug are known. Drowsiness and dizziness usually subside after a few weeks.

• Obtain baseline measures of blood pressure before starting therapy and monitor regularly. Watch for orthostatic hypotension, especially with parenteral administration. Advise patient to change positions slowly.

• Give deep I.M. only in upper outer quadrant of buttocks. Massage slowly afterward to prevent sterile abscess. Injection may sting.

• Protect medication from light. Slight yellowing of injection or concentrate is common; does not affect potency. Discard markedly discolored solutions.

• Liquid (oral) and parenteral forms may cause contact dermatitis. If susceptible, wear gloves when preparing solutions of this drug, and prevent contact with skin and clothing.

• Dry mouth may be relieved with sugarless gum, sour hard candy, or rinsing with mouthwash.

• Do not withdraw drug abruptly unless required by severe adverse reactions.

• Dose of 50 mg is therapeutic equivalent of 100 mg chlorpromazine.

---

molindone hydrochloride
Moban

Pregnancy Risk Category: C

HOW SUPPLIED
Tablets: 5 mg, 10 mg, 25 mg, 50 mg, 100 mg
Oral solution: 20 mg/ml

MECHANISM OF ACTION
Blocks postsynaptic dopamine receptors in the brain. A dihydroindolone.

INDICATIONS & DOSAGE
Psychotic disorders—
Adults: 50 to 75 mg P.O. daily, increasing to maximum of 225 mg daily. Doses up to 400 mg may be required.

ADVERSE REACTIONS
Blood: transient leukopenia.
CNS: *extrapyramidal reactions (moderate incidence), tardive dyskinesia, sedation (moderate incidence),* pseudoparkinsonism, EEG changes, dizziness.
CV: *orthostatic hypotension,* tachycardia, ECG changes.
EENT: *blurred vision.*
GI: *dry mouth, constipation.*
GU: *urine retention,* dark urine, menstrual irregularities, gynecomastia, inhibited ejaculation.
Hepatic: cholestatic jaundice, abnormal liver function tests.
Metabolic: hyperprolactinemia.
Skin: *mild photosensitivity,* dermal allergic reactions.
Other: rarely, *neuroleptic malignant syndrome* (fever, tachycardia, tachypnea, profuse diaphoresis).

INTERACTIONS
Alcohol, other CNS depressants: increased CNS depression. Avoid concomitant use.

NURSING CONSIDERATIONS
• Contraindicated in coma or severe CNS depression. Use with caution when increased physical activity would be harmful, as this agent increases activity; in seizures (may lower seizure threshold), suicide risk, suspected brain tumor, or intestinal obstruction.

• Tardive dyskinesia may occur after prolonged use. It may not appear until months or years later and may disappear spontaneously or persist for life despite discontinuation of drug.

• Neuroleptic malignant syndrome is rare, but frequently fatal. It is not necessarily related to length of drug use or type of neuroleptic, but over 60% of affected patients are men. Watch for symptoms.

• Acute dystonic reactions may be treated with I.V. diphenhydramine.

• Warn against activities that require

Italicized adverse reactions are common or life-threatening.
*Liquid form contains alcohol.   **May contain tartrazine.

alertness or good psychomotor coordination until CNS effects of the drug are known. Drowsiness and dizziness usually subside after first few weeks.
• Dry mouth may be relieved with sugarless gum, sour hard candy, or rinsing with mouthwash.
• Drug is the only dihydroindolone derivative.
• Dose of 20 mg is therapeutic equivalent of 100 mg chlorpromazine.
• May be administered in a single daily dose.

---

perphenazine
Apo-Perphenazine†, Phenazine†, Trilafon

Pregnancy Risk Category: C

HOW SUPPLIED
Tablets: 2 mg, 4 mg, 8 mg, 16 mg
Repetabs (sustained-release): 8 mg
Oral concentrate: 16 mg/5ml
Injection: 5 mg/ml

MECHANISM OF ACTION
Blocks postsynaptic dopamine receptors in the brain. As an antiemetic, inhibits the medullary chemoreceptor trigger zone.

INDICATIONS & DOSAGE
Hospitalized psychiatric patients—
Adults: initially, 8 to 16 mg P.O. b.i.d., t.i.d., or q.i.d., increasing to 64 mg daily.
Children over 12 years: 6 to 12 mg P.O. daily in divided doses.
Mental disturbances, acute alcoholism, nausea, vomiting, hiccups—
Adults and children over 12 years: 5 to 10 mg I.M., p.r.n. Maximum 15 mg daily in ambulatory patients, 30 mg daily in hospitalized patients.

ADVERSE REACTIONS
Blood: transient leukopenia, *agranulocytosis.*
CNS: *extrapyramidal reactions (high incidence), tardive dyskinesia,* seda-

tion (low incidence), pseudoparkinsonism, EEG changes, dizziness.
CV: *orthostatic hypotension,* tachycardia, ECG changes.
EENT: ocular changes, *blurred vision.*
GI: *dry mouth, constipation.*
GU: *urine retention,* dark urine, menstrual irregularities, gynecomastia, inhibited ejaculation.
Hepatic: cholestatic jaundice, abnormal liver function tests.
Metabolic: hyperprolactinemia.
Skin: *mild photosensitivity,* dermal allergic reactions.
Local: pain at I.M. injection site, sterile abscess.
Other: weight gain; increased appetite; rarely, *neuroleptic malignant syndrome* (fever, tachycardia, tachypnea, profuse diaphoresis).
After abrupt withdrawal of long-term therapy: gastritis, nausea, vomiting, dizziness, tremors, feeling of warmth or cold, sweating, tachycardia, headache, insomnia.

INTERACTIONS
Alcohol, other CNS depressants: increased CNS depression. Avoid concomitant use.
Antacids: inhibit absorption of oral phenothiazines. Separate antacid and phenothiazine doses by at least 2 hours.
Barbiturates: may decrease phenothiazine effect. Observe patient.

NURSING CONSIDERATIONS
• Contraindicated in coma, CNS depression, bone marrow suppression, subcortical damage, use of spinal or epidural anesthetic or adrenergic blocking agents. Use cautiously with other CNS depressants, anticholinergics; in elderly or debilitated patients; in acutely ill or dehydrated children; and in hepatic disease, arteriosclerosis or CV disease (may cause sudden drop in blood pressure), exposure to extreme heat or cold (including anti-

---

pyretic therapy), respiratory disorders, hypocalcemia, seizure disorders (may lower seizure threshold), severe reactions to insulin or electroshock therapy, suspected brain tumor or intestinal obstruction, glaucoma, prostatic hypertrophy.

• Tardive dyskinesia may occur after prolonged use. It may not appear until months or years later and may disappear spontaneously or persist for life despite discontinuation of drug.

• Neuroleptic malignant syndrome is rare, but frequently fatal. It is not necessarily related to length of drug use or type of neuroleptic, but over 60% of affected patients are men. Watch for symptoms.

• Acute dystonic reactions may be treated with I.V. diphenhydramine.

• Hold dose and notify doctor if patient develops jaundice, symptoms of blood dyscrasias (fever, sore throat, infection, cellulitis, weakness), persistent (longer than a few hours) extrapyramidal reactions, or any such reactions in pregnancy or in children.

• Monitor therapy by weekly bilirubin tests during first month; periodic blood tests (CBC and liver function); and ophthalmic tests (long-term use).

• Have patient report urine retention or constipation.

• Tell patient to use sunscreening agents and protective clothing to avoid photosensitivity reactions.

• Warn against activities that require alertness or good psychomotor coordination until CNS effects of the drug are known. Drowsiness and dizziness usually subside after a few weeks.

• Obtain baseline measures of blood pressure before starting therapy and monitor regularly. Watch for orthostatic hypotension, especially with parenteral administration. Keep patient supine for 1 hour afterward. Advise patient to change positions slowly.

• Give deep I.M. only in upper outer quadrant of buttocks. Massage slowly afterward to prevent sterile abscess. Injection may sting.

• Do not withdraw drug abruptly unless required by severe adverse reactions.

• Protect drug from light. Slight yellowing of injection or concentrate is common; does not affect potency. Discard markedly discolored solutions.

• Prevent contact dermatitis by keeping drug off patient's skin and clothes. Wear gloves when preparing liquid forms of the drug.

• Dilute liquid concentrate with fruit juice, milk, carbonated beverage, or semisolid food just before giving. Exceptions: Oral concentrate causes turbidity or precipitation in colas, black coffee, grape or apple juice, or tea. Do not mix with these liquids.

• Dry mouth may be relieved with sugarless gum, sour hard candy, or rinsing with mouthwash.

• Dose of 8 mg is therapeutic equivalent of 100 mg chlorpromazine.

---

pimozide
Orap

Pregnancy Risk Category: C

HOW SUPPLIED
Tablets: 2 mg

MECHANISM OF ACTION
Blocks dopaminergic receptors.

INDICATIONS & DOSAGE
Suppression of severe motor and phonic tics in patients with Tourette's disorder—
Adults and children over 12 years: initially, 1 to 2 mg P.O. daily in divided doses. Then, increase dosage every other day. Maintenance dosage ranges from 7 to 16 mg daily.

ADVERSE REACTIONS
CNS: *parkinsonian-like symptoms,* other extrapyramidal symptoms (dys-

---

Italicized adverse reactions are common or life-threatening.
*Liquid form contains alcohol.   **May contain tartrazine.

tonia, akathisia, hyperreflexia, opisthotonus, oculogyric crisis), *tardive dyskinesia, sedation.*
CV: *ECG changes (prolonged Q-T interval),* hypotension.
EENT: visual disturbances.
GI: *dry mouth, constipation.*
GU: impotence.
Other: rarely, *neuroleptic malignant syndrome* (fever, tachycardia, tacypnea, profuse diaphoresis), muscle tightness.

INTERACTIONS

Alcohol, other CNS depressants: increased CNS depression.
Phenothiazines, tricyclic antidepressants, antiarrhythmics: increased incidence of ECG abnormalities.

NURSING CONSIDERATIONS

• Contraindicated in congenital long Q-T syndrome or history of cardiac arrhythmias, severe toxic CNS depression, or in coma. Use cautiously in hepatic or renal dysfunction, glaucoma, and prostatic hypertrophy.
• Tardive dyskinesia may occur after prolonged use. It may not appear until months or years later and may disappear spontaneously or persist for life despite discontinuation of drug.
• Neuroleptic malignant syndrome is rare, but frequently fatal. It is not necessarily related to length of drug use or type of neuroleptic, but over 60% of affected patients are men. Watch for symptoms.
• Acute dystonic reactions may be treated with I.V. diphenhydramine.
• Pimozide is not recommended for treatment of simple tics except those associated with Tourette's disorder. Don't use in drug-induced motor and phonic tics.
• Avoid concurrent administration of other drugs that prolong the Q-T interval, such as antiarrhythmic agents.
• Perform an ECG before treatment begins and periodically thereafter. Monitor for prolonged Q-T interval.

• Monitor patients who are also taking anticonvulsants for increased seizure activity. Pimozide may lower the seizure threshold.
• Because pimozide may cause serious adverse effects, the patient and his family should be thoroughly informed before deciding whether he should take the drug. Pimozide is indicated only in patients who have failed to respond satisfactorily to standard treatment.
• Warn patient not to stop taking drug abruptly and not to exceed prescribed dose.
• Tell patient to use sugarless hard candy, gum, and liquids, as needed, to relieve dry mouth.

promazine hydrochloride
Sparine**

Pregnancy Risk Category: C

HOW SUPPLIED
Tablets: 25 mg, 50 mg, 100 mg
Syrup: 10 mg/5 ml
Injection: 25 mg/ml, 50 mg/ml

MECHANISM OF ACTION
Blocks postsynaptic dopamine receptors in the brain. An aliphatic phenothiazine.

INDICATIONS & DOSAGE
Psychosis—
Adults: 10 to 200 mg P.O. or I.M. q 4 to 6 hours, up to 1 g daily. I.V. dose in concentrations no greater than 25 mg/ml for acutely agitated patients. Initial dose is 50 to 150 mg; repeat within 5 to 10 minutes if necessary.
Children over 12 years: 10 to 25 mg P.O. or I.M. q 4 to 6 hours.

ADVERSE REACTIONS
Blood: transient leukopenia, *agranulocytosis.*
CNS: *extrapyramidal reactions (moderate incidence), tardive dyskinesia,*

---

sedation (high incidence), pseudoparkinsonism, EEG changes, dizziness.
CV: *orthostatic hypotension,* tachycardia, ECG changes.
EENT: ocular changes, *blurred vision.*
GI: *dry mouth, constipation.*
GU: *urine retention,* dark urine, menstrual irregularities, gynecomastia, inhibited ejaculation.
Hepatic: cholestatic jaundice, abnormal liver function tests.
Metabolic: hyperprolactinemia.
Skin: *mild photosensitivity,* dermal allergic reactions.
Local: pain at I.M. injection site, sterile abscess.
Other: weight gain; increased appetite; rarely, *neuroleptic malignant syndrome* (fever, tachycardia, tachypnea, profuse diaphoresis).
After abrupt withdrawal of long-term therapy: gastritis, nausea, vomiting, dizziness, tremors, feeling of warmth or cold, sweating, tachycardia, headache, insomnia.

INTERACTIONS
Alcohol, other CNS depressants: increased CNS depression. Avoid concomitant use.
Antacids: inhibit absorption of oral phenothiazines. Separate antacid and phenothiazine doses by at least 2 hours.
Anticholinergics (including antidepressant and antiparkinsonian agents): increased anticholinergic activity, aggravated parkinsonian symptoms. Use with caution.
Barbiturates, lithium: may decrease phenothiazine effect. Observe patient.
Centrally acting antihypertensives: decreased antihypertensive effect.
Oral anticoagulants: decreased effectiveness.
Propranolol: increased serum levels of propranolol and promazine.

NURSING CONSIDERATIONS
• Contraindicated in coma, CNS depression, bone marrow suppression, subcortical damage, and with use of spinal or epidural anesthetic or adrenergic blocking agents. Use cautiously with other CNS depressants, anticholinergics; in elderly or debilitated patients; in hepatic disease, arteriosclerosis or CV disease (may cause sudden drop in blood pressure), exposure to extreme heat or cold (including antipyretic therapy), respiratory disorders, hypocalcemia, seizure disorders (may lower seizure threshold), severe reactions to insulin or electroshock therapy, suspected brain tumor or intestinal obstruction, glaucoma, prostatic hypertrophy; and in acutely ill or dehydrated children.
• Tardive dyskinesia may occur after prolonged use. It may not appear until months or years later and may disappear spontaneously or persist for life despite discontinuation of drug.
• Neuroleptic malignant syndrome is rare, but frequently fatal. It is not necessarily related to length of drug use or type of neuroleptic, but over 60% of affected patients are men. Watch for symptoms.
• Acute dystonic reactions may be treated with I.V. diphenhydramine.
• Hold dose and notify doctor if patient develops jaundice, symptoms of blood dyscrasias (fever, sore throat, infection, cellulitis, weakness), persistent (longer than a few hours) extrapyramidal reactions, or such reactions during pregnancy or in children.
• Monitor therapy by weekly bilirubin tests during first month; periodic blood tests (CBC and liver function); and ophthalmic tests (long-term use).
• Have patient report urine retention or constipation.
• Tell patient to use sunscreening agents and protective clothing to avoid photosensitivity reactions.
• Warn against activities that require alertness or good psychomotor coor-

---

Italicized adverse reactions are common or life-threatening.
*Liquid form contains alcohol.   **May contain tartrazine.

dination until CNS effects of the drug are known. Drowsiness and dizziness usually subside after a few weeks.
• Monitor blood pressure with patient lying and standing before starting therapy, and routinely throughout course of treatment.
• Watch for orthostatic hypotension, especially with parenteral administration. Keep patient supine for 1 hour afterward. Advise patient to change positions slowly.
• Give deep I.M. only in upper outer quadrant of buttocks. Massage slowly afterward to prevent sterile abscess. Injection may sting.
• Protect drug from light. Slight yellowing of injection or concentrate is common; does not affect potency. Discard markedly discolored solutions.
• Prevent contact dermatitis by keeping drug off patient's skin and clothes. Wear gloves when preparing liquid forms of the drug.
• Dilute liquid concentrate with fruit juice, milk, semisolid food, or chocolate-flavored drinks just before giving. For best taste, use at least 10 ml diluent per 25 mg drug.
• Do not withdraw drug abruptly unless required by severe adverse reactions.
• Dry mouth may be relieved with sugarless gum, sour hard candy, or rinsing with mouthwash.

thioridazine hydrochloride
Aldazine‡, Apo-Thioridazine†, Mellaril*, Mellaril-S, Novoridazine†, PMS Thioridazine†

Pregnancy Risk Category: C

HOW SUPPLIED
Tablets: 10 mg, 15 mg, 25 mg, 50 mg, 100 mg, 200 mg
Oral suspension: 25 mg/5 ml, 100 mg/5 ml
Oral concentrate: 30 mg/ml, 100 mg/ml (3% to 4.2% alcohol)
Syrup: 10 mg/5 ml

MECHANISM OF ACTION
Blocks postsynaptic dopamine receptors in the brain. A piperidine phenothiazine.

INDICATIONS & DOSAGE
Psychosis—
Adults: initially, 25 to 100 mg P.O. t.i.d., with gradual increments up to 800 mg daily in divided doses, if needed. Dosage varies.
Adults over 65 years: initial dose, 25 mg P.O. t.i.d.
Depressive neurosis, alcohol withdrawal, dementia in geriatric patients, behavioral problems in children—
Adults: initially, 25 mg P.O. t.i.d. Maintenance dosage is 20 to 200 mg daily.
Children over 2 years: 0.5 to 3 mg/ kg P.O. daily in divided doses.

ADVERSE REACTIONS
Blood: transient leukopenia, *agranulocytosis.*
CNS: extrapyramidal reactions (low incidence), *tardive dyskinesia, sedation (high incidence),* EEG changes, dizziness.
CV: *orthostatic hypotension,* tachycardia, ECG changes.
EENT: *ocular changes, blurred vision,* pigmentary retinopathy.
GI: *dry mouth, constipation.*
GU: *urine retention,* dark urine, menstrual irregularities, gynecomastia, inhibited ejaculation.
Hepatic: cholestatic jaundice.
Metabolic: hyperprolactinemia.
Skin: *mild photosensitivity,* dermal allergic reactions.
Other: weight gain; increased appetite; rarely, *neuroleptic malignant syndrome* (fever, tachycardia, tachypnea, profuse diaphoresis).
After abrupt withdrawal of long-term therapy: gastritis, nausea, vomiting, dizziness, tremors, feeling of

---

warmth or cold, sweating, tachycardia, headache, insomnia.

INTERACTIONS

Alcohol, other CNS depressants: increased CNS depression. Avoid concomitant use.

Antacids: inhibit absorption of oral phenothiazines. Separate antacid and phenothiazine doses by at least 2 hours.

Barbiturates, lithium: may decrease phenothiazine effect. Observe patient.

Centrally acting antihypertensives: decreased antihypertensive effect.

NURSING CONSIDERATIONS

• Contraindicated in coma, CNS depression, bone marrow suppression, hypertensive or hypotensive cardiac disease, subcortical damage, and with use of spinal or epidural anesthetic or adrenergic blocking agents. Use cautiously with other CNS depressants, anticholinergics; in elderly or debilitated patients; in hepatic disease, arteriosclerosis or CV disease (may cause sudden drop in blood pressure), exposure to extreme heat or cold (including antipyretic therapy), respiratory disorders, hypocalcemia, seizure disorders, severe reactions to insulin or electroshock therapy, suspected brain tumor or intestinal obstruction, glaucoma, or prostatic hypertrophy; and in acutely ill or dehydrated children.

• Tardive dyskinesia may occur after prolonged use. It may not appear until months or years later and may disappear spontaneously or persist for life despite discontinuation of drug.

• Neuroleptic malignant syndrome is rare, but frequently fatal. It is not necessarily related to length of drug use or type of neuroleptic, but over 60% of affected patients are men. Watch for symptoms.

• Acute dystonic reactions may be treated with I.V. diphenhydramine.

• Hold dose and notify doctor if patient develops jaundice, symptoms of blood dyscrasias (fever, sore throat, infection, cellulitis, weakness), persistent (longer than a few hours) extrapyramidal reactions, or such reactions during pregnancy or in children.

• Monitor therapy by weekly bilirubin tests during first month; periodic blood tests (CBC and liver function); and ophthalmic tests (long-term therapy).

• Have patient report urine retention or constipation.

• Watch for blurred vision, dry mouth; high incidence of anticholinergic effects.

• Tell patient to use sunscreening agents and protective clothing to avoid photosensitivity reactions.

• Warn against activities that require alertness or good psychomotor coordination until CNS effects of the drug are known. Drowsiness and dizziness usually subside after a few weeks.

• Watch for orthostatic hypotension, especially with parenteral administration. Advise patient to change positions slowly.

• Prevent contact dermatitis by keeping drug off patient's skin and clothes. Wear gloves when preparing liquid forms of the drug.

• Caution: Note different concentrations of liquid formulations.

• Not available in injectable form. Mesoridazine is prescribed when parenteral use of a thioridazine-like drug is desirable.

• Dilute liquid concentrate with water or fruit juice just before giving. Avoid contact with skin because contact dermatitis has been reported.

• Be sure to shake suspension well before using.

• Do not withdraw abruptly unless required by severe adverse reactions.

• Dry mouth may be relieved with sugarless gum, sour hard candy, or rinsing with mouthwash.

- Dose of 100 mg is the therapeutic equivalent of 100 mg chlorpromazine.
- Dosage above 800 mg may be associated with ocular toxicity (pigmentary retinopathy).

thiothixene
Navane

thiothixene hydrochloride
Navane*

Pregnancy Risk Category: C

HOW SUPPLIED
thiothixene
Capsules: 1 mg, 2 mg, 5 mg, 10 mg, 20 mg
thiothixene hydrochloride
Oral concentrate: 5 mg/ml (7% alcohol)
Injection: 2 mg, 5 mg/ml

MECHANISM OF ACTION
Blocks postsynaptic dopamine receptors in the brain. A thioxanthene.

INDICATIONS & DOSAGE
Acute agitation—
Adults: 4 mg I.M. b.i.d. to q.i.d. Maximum dosage is 30 mg daily I.M. Change to P.O. as soon as possible.
Mild to moderate psychosis—
Adults: initially, 2 mg P.O. t.i.d. May increase gradually to 15 mg daily.
Severe psychosis—
Adults: initially, 5 mg P.O. b.i.d. May increase gradually to 15 to 30 mg daily. Maximum recommended daily dose is 60 mg. Not recommended in children under 12 years.

ADVERSE REACTIONS
Blood: transient leukopenia, *agranulocytosis.*
CNS: *extrapyramidal reactions (high incidence), tardive dyskinesia,* sedation (low incidence), pseudoparkinsonism, EEG changes, dizziness.
CV: *orthostatic hypotension,* tachycardia, ECG changes.

EENT: ocular changes, *blurred vision.*
GI: *dry mouth, constipation.*
GU: *urine retention,* dark urine, menstrual irregularities, gynecomastia, inhibited ejaculation.
Hepatic: cholestatic jaundice.
Metabolic: hyperprolactinemia.
Skin: *mild photosensitivity,* dermal allergic reactions.
Local: pain at I.M. injection site, sterile abscess.
Other: weight gain; increased appetite; rarely, *neuroleptic malignant syndrome* (fever, tachycardia, tachypnea, profuse diaphoresis).
After abrupt withdrawal of long-term therapy: gastritis, nausea, vomiting, dizziness, tremors, feeling of warmth or cold, sweating, tachycardia, headache, insomnia.

INTERACTIONS
Alcohol, other CNS depressants: increased CNS depression. Avoid concomitant use.

NURSING CONSIDERATIONS
- Contraindicated in convulsive seizures, circulatory collapse, coma, CNS depression, blood dyscrasias, bone marrow suppression, alcohol withdrawal, akathisia or restlessness, subcortical damage, and with use of spinal or epidural anesthetic or adrenergic blocking agents. Use cautiously with other CNS depressants, anticholinergics; in elderly or debilitated patients; and in hepatic disease, arteriosclerosis or CV disease (may cause sudden drop in blood pressure), exposure to extreme heat or cold (including antipyretic therapy) or undue sunlight, respiratory disorders, hypocalcemia, severe reactions to insulin or electroshock therapy, suspected brain tumor or intestinal obstruction, glaucoma, and prostatic hypertrophy.
- Tardive dyskinesia may occur after prolonged use. It may not appear until months or years later and may disap-

pear spontaneously or persist for life despite discontinuation of drug.
• Neuroleptic malignant syndrome is rare, but frequently fatal. It is not necessarily related to length of drug use or type of neuroleptic, but over 60% of affected patients are men. Watch for symptoms.
• Acute dystonic reactions may be treated with I.V. diphenhydramine.
• Hold dose and notify doctor if patient develops jaundice, symptoms of blood dyscrasias (fever, sore throat, infection, cellulitis, weakness), persistent (longer than a few hours) extrapyramidal reactions, or any such reactions during pregnancy.
• Monitor therapy by weekly bilirubin tests during first month; periodic blood tests (CBC and liver function); and ophthalmic tests (long-term use).
• Have patient report urine retention or constipation.
• Tell patient to use sunscreening agents and protective clothing to avoid photosensitivity reactions.
• Warn against activities that require alertness or good psychomotor coordination until CNS effects of the drug are known. Drowsiness and dizziness usually subside after a few weeks.
• Watch for orthostatic hypotension, especially with parenteral administration. Keep patient in a supine position for 1 hour afterward. Advise patient to change positions slowly.
• Give I.M. only in upper outer quadrant of buttocks or midlateral thigh. Massage slowly afterward to prevent sterile abscess. Injection may sting.
• I.M. form must be stored in refrigerator.
• Slight yellowing of injection or concentrate is common; does not affect potency. Discard markedly discolored solutions.
• Prevent contact dermatitis by keeping drug off patient's skin and clothes. Wear gloves when preparing liquid forms of the drug.
• Dilute liquid concentrate with fruit juice, milk, or semisolid food just before giving.
• Do not withdraw abruptly unless required by severe adverse reactions.
• Dry mouth may be relieved with sugarless gum, sour hard candy, or rinsing with mouthwash.
• Dose of 4 mg is therapeutic equivalent of 100 mg chlorpromazine.

trifluoperazine hydrochloride
Apo-Trifluoperazine†, Calmazine‡, Novo-Flurazine†, Solazine†, Stelazine, Suprazine, Terfluzine†

Pregnancy Risk Category: C

HOW SUPPLIED
Tablets (regular and film-coated): 1 mg, 2 mg, 5 mg, 10 mg
Oral concentrate: 10 mg/ml
Injection: 2 mg/ml

MECHANISM OF ACTION
Blocks postsynaptic dopamine receptors in the brain. A piperazine phenothiazine.

INDICATIONS & DOSAGE
Anxiety states—
Adults: 1 to 2 mg P.O. b.i.d.
Schizophrenia and other psychotic disorders—
Adults: *outpatients*—1 to 2 mg P.O. b.i.d., up to 4 mg daily; *hospitalized*—2 to 5 mg P.O. b.i.d.; may gradually increase to 40 mg daily. 1 to 2 mg I.M. q 4 to 6 hours, p.r.n.
Children 6 to 12 years (hospitalized or under close supervision): 1 mg P.O. daily or b.i.d.; may increase gradually to 15 mg daily.

ADVERSE REACTIONS
Blood: transient leukopenia, *agranulocytosis.*
CNS: *extrapyramidal reactions (high incidence), tardive dyskinesia,* sedation (low incidence), pseudoparkinsonism, EEG changes, dizziness.

Italicized adverse reactions are common or life-threatening.
*Liquid form contains alcohol. 　　**May contain tartrazine.

CV: *orthostatic hypotension*, tachycardia, ECG changes.
EENT: ocular changes, *blurred vision*.
GI: *dry mouth, constipation*.
GU: *urine retention*, dark urine, menstrual irregularities, gynecomastia, inhibited ejaculation.
Hepatic: cholestatic jaundice.
Metabolic: hyperprolactinemia.
Skin: *mild photosensitivity*, dermal allergic reactions.
Local: pain at I.M. injection site, sterile abscess.
Other: weight gain; increased appetite; rarely, *neuroleptic malignant syndrome* (fever, tachycardia, tachypnea, profuse diaphoresis).
After abrupt withdrawal of long-term therapy: gastritis, nausea, vomiting, dizziness, tremors, feeling of warmth or cold, sweating, tachycardia, headache, insomnia.

INTERACTIONS

Alcohol, other CNS depressants: increased CNS depression. Avoid concomitant use.
Antacids: inhibit absorption of oral phenothiazines. Separate antacid and phenothiazine doses by at least 2 hours.
Barbiturates, lithium: may decrease phenothiazine effect. Observe patient.
Centrally acting antihypertensives: decreased antihypertensive effect.

NURSING CONSIDERATIONS

• Contraindicated in coma, CNS depression, bone marrow suppression, subcortical damage, and with use of spinal or epidural anesthetic or adrenergic blocking agents. Use cautiously with other CNS depressants, anticholinergics; in elderly or debilitated patients; in hepatic disease, arteriosclerosis or CV disease (may cause drop in blood pressure), exposure to extreme heat or cold (including antipyretic therapy), respiratory disorders, hypocalcemia, seizure disorders, severe reactions to insulin or electroshock therapy, suspected brain tumor or intestinal obstruction, glaucoma, or prostatic hypertrophy; and in acutely ill or dehydrated children.

• Tardive dyskinesia may occur after prolonged use. It may not appear until months or years later and may disappear spontaneously or persist for life despite discontinuation of drug.

• Neuroleptic malignant syndrome is rare, but frequently fatal. It is not necessarily related to length of drug use or type of neuroleptic, but over 60% of affected patients are men. Watch for symptoms.

• Acute dystonic reactions may be treated with I.V. diphenhydramine.

• Hold dose and notify doctor if patient develops jaundice, symptoms of blood dyscrasias (fever, sore throat, infection, cellulitis, weakness), persistent (longer than a few hours) extrapyramidal reactions, or any such reactions during pregnancy or in children.

• Monitor therapy by weekly bilirubin tests during first month; periodic blood tests (CBC and liver function); and ophthalmic tests (long-term use).

• Have patient report urine retention or constipation.

• Tell patient to use sunscreening agents and protective clothing to avoid photosensitivity reactions.

• Warn against activities that require alertness or good psychomotor coordination until CNS effects of the drug are known. Drowsiness and dizziness usually subside after a few weeks.

• Watch for orthostatic hypotension, especially with parenteral administration. Keep patient supine for 1 hour afterward. Advise patient to change positions slowly.

• Give deep I.M. only in upper outer quadrant of buttocks. Massage slowly afterward to prevent sterile abscess. Injection may sting.

• Protect drug from light. Slight yellowing of injection or concentrate is common; does not affect potency. Discard markedly discolored solutions.

• Prevent contact dermatitis by keeping drug off patient's skin and clothes. Wear gloves when preparing liquid forms of the drug.

• Dilute liquid concentrate with 60 ml tomato or fruit juice, carbonated beverages, coffee, tea, milk, water, or semisolid food just before giving.

• Do not withdraw abruptly unless required by severe adverse reactions.

• Dry mouth may be relieved with sugarless gum, sour hard candy, or rinsing with mouthwash.

• Drug is a prototype piperazine phenothiazine.

• Dose of 5 mg is therapeutic equivalent of 100 mg chlorpromazine.

---

triflupromazine hydrochloride
Vesprin

Pregnancy Risk Category: C

HOW SUPPLIED
Injection: 10 mg, 20 mg/ml

MECHANISM OF ACTION
Blocks postsynaptic dopamine receptors in the brain. An aliphatic phenothiazine.

INDICATIONS & DOSAGE
Acute, severe agitation—
Adults: 60 to 150 mg I.M. in two or three divided doses.
Children over 2½ years: 0.2 to 0.25 mg/kg I.M. in divided doses. Maximum dosage is 10 mg daily.
Nausea and vomiting—
Adults: 1 to 3 mg I.V. daily; or 5 to 15 mg I.M. daily up to maximum of 60 mg daily.
Children: 0.2 mg/kg I.M. up to maximum of 10 mg daily.

ADVERSE REACTIONS
Blood: transient leukopenia, *agranulocytosis.*
CNS: *extrapyramidal reactions (moderate incidence), tardive dyskinesia, sedation (high incidence),* pseudoparkinsonism, EEG changes, dizziness.
CV: *orthostatic hypotension,* tachycardia, ECG changes.
EENT: ocular changes, *blurred vision.*
GI: *dry mouth, constipation.*
GU: *urine retention,* dark urine, menstrual irregularities, gynecomastia, inhibited ejaculation.
Hepatic: cholestatic jaundice.
Metabolic: hyperprolactinemia.
Skin: *mild photosensitivity,* dermal allergic reactions.
Local: pain at I.M. injection site, sterile abscess.
Other: weight gain; increased appetite; rarely, *neuroleptic malignant syndrome (fever, tachycardia, tachypnea, profuse diaphoresis).*
After abrupt withdrawal of long-term therapy: gastritis, nausea, vomiting, dizziness, tremors, feeling of warmth or cold, sweating, tachycardia, headache, insomnia.

INTERACTIONS
Alcohol, other CNS depressants: increased CNS depression. Avoid concomitant use.
Anticholinergics (including antidepressant and antiparkinsonian agents): increased anticholinergic activity, aggravated parkinsonian symptoms. Use with caution.
Barbiturates, lithium: may decrease phenothiazine effect. Observe patient.
Centrally acting antihypertensives: decreased antihypertensive effect.

NURSING CONSIDERATIONS
• Contraindicated in coma, CNS depression, blood dyscrasias, bone marrow suppression, subcortical brain damage, and with use of spinal or epi-

---

Italicized adverse reactions are common or life-threatening.
*Liquid form contains alcohol.   **May contain tartrazine.

dural anesthetic or adrenergic blocking agents. Use cautiously with other CNS depressants, anticholinergics; in elderly or debilitated patients; in hepatic disease, arteriosclerosis or CV disease (may cause sudden drop in blood pressure), exposure to extreme heat or cold (including antipyretic therapy), respiratory disorders, pheochromocytoma, hypocalcemia, seizure disorders, severe reactions to insulin or electroshock therapy, suspected brain tumor or intestinal obstruction, glaucoma, prostatic hypertrophy; and in acutely ill or dehydrated children.

• Tardive dyskinesia may occur after prolonged use. It may not appear until months or years later and may disappear spontaneously or persist for life despite discontinuation of drug.

• Neuroleptic malignant syndrome is rare, but frequently fatal. It is not necessarily related to length of drug use or type of neuroleptic, but over 60% of affected patients are men. Watch for symptoms.

• Acute dystonic reactions may be treated with I.V. diphenhydramine.

• Hold dose and notify doctor if patient develops jaundice, symptoms of blood dyscrasias (fever, sore throat, infection, cellulitis, weakness), persistent (longer than a few hours) extrapyramidal reactions, or any such reactions during pregnancy or in children.

• Monitor therapy by weekly bilirubin tests during first month; periodic blood tests (CBC and liver function); and ophthalmic tests in long-term use.

• Have patient report urine retention or constipation.

• Tell patient to use sunscreening agents and protective clothing to avoid photosensitivity reactions.

• Warn against activities that require alertness or good psychomotor coordination until CNS effects of the drug are known. Drowsiness and dizziness usually subside after a few weeks.

• Watch for orthostatic hypotension, especially with parenteral administration. Keep patient supine for 1 hour afterward. Advise patient to change itions slowly.

• Give I.M. only in upper outer quadrant of buttocks. Massage slowly afterward to prevent sterile abscess. Injection may sting.

• Protect drug from light. Slight yellowing of injection or concentrate is common; does not affect potency. Discard markedly discolored solutions.

• Prevent contact dermatitis by avoiding contact with skin.

• Do not withdraw abruptly unless required by severe adverse reactions.

• Dry mouth may be relieved with sugarless gum, sour hard candy, or rinsing with mouthwash.

• Dose of 25 mg is therapeutic equivalent of 100 mg chlorpromazine.

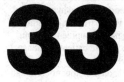

Miscellaneous psychotherapeutics

lithium carbonate
lithium citrate

COMBINATION PRODUCTS
None.

---

lithium carbonate
Camcolit‡, Carbolith†, Duralith†,
Eskalith, Eskalith CR, Lithane**,
Lithicarb‡, Lithizine†, Lithobid,
Lithonate, Lithotabs, Priadel‡

lithium citrate
Cibalith-S*

Pregnancy Risk Category: D

HOW SUPPLIED
Tablets: 250 mg‡, 300 mg (300 mg =
8.12 mEq lithium)
Tablets (sustained-release): 300 mg,
400 mg‡, 450 mg
Capsules: 300 mg
Syrup (sugarless): 300 mg/5 ml (0.3%
alcohol)

MECHANISM OF ACTION
Alters chemical transmitters in the
CNS, possibly by interfering with
ionic pump mechanisms in brain
cells. Its exact mechanism of action in
mania, however, is unknown.

INDICATIONS & DOSAGE
Prevention or control of mania—
Adults: 300 to 600 mg P.O. up to
q.i.d., increasing on the basis of
blood levels to achieve optimal dosage. Recommended therapeutic lithium blood levels: 1 to 1.5 mEq/liter
for acute mania; 0.6 to 1.2 mEq/liter

for maintenance therapy; and 2 mEq/
liter as maximum.
Note: 5 ml lithium citrate (liquid)
contains 8 mEq lithium equal to 300
mg lithium carbonate.

ADVERSE REACTIONS
Blood: *leukocytosis of 14,000 to
18,000 (reversible).*
CNS: tremors, drowsiness, headache,
confusion, restlessness, dizziness,
psychomotor retardation, stupor, lethargy, coma, blackouts, epileptiform
seizures, EEG changes, worsened organic brain syndrome, impaired
speech, ataxia, muscle weakness, incoordination, hyperexcitability.
CV: *reversible ECG changes,* arrhythmias, hypotension, peripheral
circulatory collapse, allergic vasculitis, ankle and wrist edema.
EENT: tinnitus, impaired vision.
GI: nausea, vomiting, anorexia, diarrhea, dry mouth, *thirst,* metallic
taste.
GU: *polyuria,* glycosuria, incontinence, renal toxicity with long-term
use.
Metabolic: transient hyperglycemia,
goiter, hypothyroidism (lowered T_3,
T_4, and protein-bound iodine, but elevated ^{131}I uptake), hyponatremia.
Skin: pruritus, rash, diminished or
lost sensation, drying and thinning of
hair.

INTERACTIONS
*Aminophylline, sodium bicarbonate,
and sodium chloride:* ingestion of
these salts increases lithium excre-

Italicized adverse reactions are common or life-threatening.
*Liquid form contains alcohol.   **May contain tartrazine.

tion. Avoid salt loads and monitor lithium levels.

Carbamazepine, probenecid, indomethacin, methyldopa and piroxicam: increased effect of lithium. Monitor for lithium toxicity.

Diuretics: increased reabsorption of lithium by kidneys, with possible toxic effect. Use with extreme caution, and monitor lithium and electrolyte levels (especially sodium).

Haloperidol and thioridazine: encephalopathic syndrome (lethargy, tremors, extrapyramidal symptoms). Watch for syndrome, and stop drug if it occurs.

Thyroid hormones: lithium may induce hypothyroidism.

NURSING CONSIDERATIONS

• Contraindicated if therapy cannot be closely monitored. Use with caution with haloperidol, other antipsychotics, neuromuscular blocking agents, and diuretics; in elderly or debilitated persons; and in thyroid disease, epilepsy, renal or cardiovascular disease, brain damage, severe debilitation or dehydration, and sodium depletion.

• Monitor baseline ECG, thyroid, and renal studies, and electrolyte levels. Monitor lithium blood levels 8 to 12 hours after first dose, usually before morning dose, two or three times weekly first month, then weekly to monthly on maintenance.

• Determination of lithium blood concentration is crucial to the safe use of the drug. Shouldn't be used in patients who can't have regular lithium blood level checks.

• Explain to patient that lithium has a narrow therapeutic margin of safety. A blood level that is even slightly too high can be dangerous.

• When blood levels of lithium are below 1.5 mEq/liter, adverse reactions usually remain mild.

• Check fluid intake/output, especially when surgery is scheduled.

• Warn patient and family to watch for signs of toxicity (diarrhea, vomiting, drowsiness, muscular weakness, ataxia) and to expect transient nausea, polyuria, thirst, and discomfort during first few days. Patient should withhold one dose and call doctor if toxic symptoms appear, but not stop drug abruptly.

• Expect lag of 1 to 3 weeks before drug's beneficial effects are noticed.

• Weigh patient daily; check for signs of edema or sudden weight gain.

• Adjust fluid and salt ingestion to compensate if excessive loss occurs through protracted sweating or diarrhea. Under normal conditions, patients should have fluid intake of 2,500 to 3,000 ml daily and a balanced diet with adequate salt intake.

• Have outpatient follow-up of thyroid and renal functions every 6 to 12 months. Palpate thyroid to check for enlargement.

• Patient should carry identification/instruction card (available from pharmacy) with toxicity and emergency information.

• Warn ambulatory patient to avoid activities that require alertness and good psychomotor coordination until CNS effects of the drug are known.

• Administer with plenty of water, and after meals to minimize GI upset.

• Check urine for specific gravity and report level below 1.005, which may indicate diabetes insipidus syndrome.

• May alter glucose tolerance in diabetics. Monitor blood glucose closely.

• Tell patient not to switch brands of lithium or to take other drugs (prescription or OTC) without doctor's guidance.

• Investigationally used to increase white cells in patients undergoing cancer chemotherapy.

• Also used investigationally for treatment of cluster headaches, aggression, organic brain syndrome, and tardive dyskinesia. Has been used to treat SIADH.

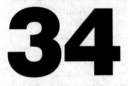

Cerebral stimulants

amphetamine sulfate
benzphetamine hydrochloride
caffeine
dextroamphetamine sulfate
diethylpropion hydrochloride
fenfluramine hydrochloride
mazindol
methamphetamine hydrochloride
methylphenidate hydrochloride
pemoline
phendimetrazine tartrate
phenmetrazine hydrochloride
phentermine hydrochloride

COMBINATION PRODUCTS
BIPHETAMINE 12½: dextroamphetamine 6.25 mg and amphetamine
6.25 mg.
BIPHETAMINE 20: dextroamphetamine
10 mg and amphetamine 10 mg.

amphetamine sulfate
Controlled Substance Schedule II
Pregnancy Risk Category: C

HOW SUPPLIED
Tablets: 5 mg, 10 mg
Capsules: 5 mg, 10 mg

MECHANISM OF ACTION
Main site of activity appears to be the
cerebral cortex and the reticular activating system. Promotes nerve impulse transmission by releasing stored
norepinephrine from nerve terminals
in the brain. In children with hyperkinesia, amphetamines have a paradoxical calming effect.

INDICATIONS & DOSAGE
*Attention deficit disorder with hyper-
activity (ADDH)—*
Children 6 years and older: 5 mg
P.O. daily, with 5-mg increments
weekly, p.r.n.
Children 3 to 5 years: 2.5 mg P.O.
daily, with 2.5-mg increments
weekly, p.r.n.
Narcolepsy—
Adults: 5 to 60 mg P.O. daily in divided doses.
Children over 12 years: 10 mg P.O.
daily, with 10-mg increments weekly,
p.r.n.
Children 6 to 12 years: 5 mg P.O.
daily, with 5-mg increments weekly,
p.r.n.
*Short-term adjunct in exogenous obe-
sity—*
Adults: single 10- or 15-mg long-acting capsule daily, or 2 if needed, up to
30 mg daily; or 5 to 30 mg daily in divided doses 30 to 60 minutes before
meals. Not recommended for children
under 12 years.

ADVERSE REACTIONS
CNS: *restlessness,* tremor, *hyperactivity, talkativeness, insomnia,* irritability, dizziness, headache, chills, overstimulation, dysphoria.
CV: *tachycardia, palpitations,* hypertension, hypotension.
GI: nausea, vomiting, cramps, dry
mouth, diarrhea, constipation, metallic taste, anorexia, weight loss.
Other: urticaria, impotence, altered
libido.

Italicized adverse reactions are common or life-threatening.
*Liquid form contains alcohol.   **May contain tartrazine.

INTERACTIONS

Ammonium chloride, ascorbic acid: observe for decreased amphetamine effect.

Antacids, sodium bicarbonate, acetazolamide: increased renal reabsorption. Monitor for enhanced effect.

MAO inhibitors: severe hypertension; possible hypertensive crisis. Don't use together.

Phenothiazines, haloperidol: observe for decreased amphetamine effect.

NURSING CONSIDERATIONS

• Contraindicated in symptomatic CV diseases, hyperthyroidism, nephritis, angina pectoris, moderate to severe hypertension, parkinsonism due to arteriosclerosis, certain types of glaucoma, advanced arteriosclerosis, in agitated states, or patients with history of drug abuse. Use with caution in diabetes mellitus and in elderly, debilitated, or hyperexcitable patients.

• Use cautiously in children with Tourette's disorder.

• Psychic dependence or habituation may occur, especially in patients with history of drug addiction. Avoid prolonged administration. When used long-term, lower dosage gradually to prevent acute rebound depression.

• Not recommended for first-line treatment of obesity. Use as an anorexigenic agent is prohibited in some states.

• When used for obesity, make sure patient is also on a weight-reduction program. Give drug 30 to 60 minutes before meals. Monitor dietary intake. Do calorie counts, if necessary.

• Fatigue may result as drug effects wear off. Patient will need more rest.

• Tell patient to avoid drinks containing caffeine, which increase the effects of amphetamines and related amines.

• Have patient report signs of excessive stimulation.

• Urine acidification enhances renal excretion; urine alkalinization enhances renal reabsorption and recycling.

• When tolerance to anorexigenic effect develops, dosage should not be increased, but drug discontinued.

• Should not be used to combat fatigue.

• Warn patient to avoid activities that require alertness or good psychomotor coordination until CNS effects of the drug are known.

• May alter daily insulin needs in patients with diabetes. Monitor blood and urine sugars.

• Use as analeptic is usually discouraged, since CNS stimulation superimposed on CNS depression can lead to neuronal instability and seizures.

• May reverse beneficial effect of antihypertensives. Monitor blood pressure.

• Give at least 6 hours before bedtime to avoid sleep interference.

---

benzphetamine hydrochloride
Didrex**
Controlled Substance Schedule III
Pregnancy Risk Category: X

HOW SUPPLIED
Tablets: 25 mg, 50 mg

MECHANISM OF ACTION
Main site of activity appears to be the cerebral cortex and the reticular activating system. Promotes nerve impulse transmission by releasing stored norepinephrine from nerve terminals in the brain.

INDICATIONS & DOSAGE
Short-term adjunct in exogenous obesity—
Adults: 25 to 50 mg P.O. daily, b.i.d., or t.i.d.

ADVERSE REACTIONS
CNS: *restlessness,* tremor, *hyperactiv-*

---

†Available in Canada only.   ‡Available in Australia only.   ◊ Available OTC.

ity, talkativeness, insomnia, irritability, dizziness, headache, chills, overstimulation, dysphoria.
CV: *tachycardia, palpitations,* hypertension, hypotension.
GI: nausea, vomiting, cramps, dry mouth, diarrhea, constipation, metallic taste, anorexia, weight loss.
Skin: urticaria.
Other: impotence, altered libido.

INTERACTIONS
MAO inhibitors: severe hypertension; possible hypertensive crisis. Don't use together.
Antacids, sodium bicarbonate, acetazolamide: increased renal reabsorption. Monitor for enhanced effects.
Ammonium chloride, ascorbic acid: observe for decreased benzphetamine effects.
Phenothiazines, haloperidol: observe for decreased benzphetamine effects.

NURSING CONSIDERATIONS
• Contraindicated in symptomatic CV diseases, hyperthyroidism, nephritis, angina pectoris, moderate to severe hypertension, parkinsonism due to arteriosclerosis, certain types of glaucoma, advanced arteriosclerosis, agitated states, or patients with history of drug abuse. Use with caution in diabetes mellitus and in elderly, debilitated, or hyperexcitable patients.
• Psychic dependence or habituation may occur, especially in patients with history of drug addiction. Avoid prolonged administration. When used long-term, lower dosage gradually to prevent acute rebound depression.
• Use in conjunction with weight-reduction program. Monitor dietary intake. Do calorie counts, if necessary. Give 30 to 60 minutes before meals.
• Fatigue may result as drug effects wear off. Patient will need more rest.
• Tell patient to avoid drinks containing caffeine, which increase the effects of amphetamines and related amines.
• Have patient report signs of excessive stimulation.
• Urine acidification enhances renal excretion; urine alkalinization enhances renal reabsorption and recycling.
• When tolerance to anorexigenic effect develops, dosage should not be increased, but drug discontinued.
• Warn patient to avoid activities that require alertness or good psychomotor coordination until CNS effects of the drug are known.
• May alter daily insulin needs in patients with diabetes. Monitor blood and urine sugars.
• Give at least 6 hours before bedtime to avoid sleep interference.

caffeine
Caffedrine◇, Dexitac◇, No Doz◇, Quick Pep◇, Tirend◇, Vivarin◇
Pregnancy Risk Category: B

HOW SUPPLIED
Tablets: 100 mg◇, 150 mg◇, 200 mg◇
Capsules (timed-release): 200 mg◇, 250 mg◇
Injection: caffeine (125 mg/ml) with sodium benzoate (125 mg/ml)

MECHANISM OF ACTION
Inhibits phosphodiesterase, the enzyme that degrades cyclic adenosine monophosphate.

INDICATIONS & DOSAGE
CNS stimulant—
Adults: 100 to 200 mg anhydrous caffeine P.O.
Neonatal apnea—
Neonates: 5 to 10 mg/kg P.O., I.M., or I.V. as a loading dose, then 2.5 to 5 mg. P.O., I.M., or I.V. daily, according to patient tolerance and serum caffeine levels (therapeutic range is 5 to 20 mcg/ml).

ADVERSE REACTIONS
CNS: *stimulation, insomnia,* restlessness, nervousness, mild delirium, headache, excitement, agitation, muscle tremors, twitches.
CV: *tachycardia.*
GI: nausea, vomiting.
GU: *diuresis.*
Skin: hyperesthesia.

INTERACTIONS
Theophylline, beta-adrenergic agonists: Excessive CNS stimulation.

NURSING CONSIDERATIONS
• Contraindicated in gastric or duodenal ulcer, arrhythmias, or postmyocardial infarction.
• Caffeine-containing beverages should be restricted in patients who experience palpitations.
• Tolerance or psychological dependence may develop.
• Be alert for signs of overdose: GI pain, mild delirium, insomnia, diuresis, dehydration, and fever. Treat with short-acting barbiturates, gastric emesis, or lavage.
• Single dose should not exceed 1 g.
• Caffeine content in cola beverages, 17 to 55 mg/180 ml; tea, 40 to 100 mg/180 ml; instant coffee, 60 to 180 mg/180 ml; brewed coffee, 100 to 150 mg/180 ml; decaffeinated coffee, 1 to 6 mg/180 ml.
• Caffeine does not reverse alcohol intoxication or CNS depressant effects of alcohol. Overvigorous therapy with caffeine may aggravate depression in an already depressed patient.
• Sudden discontinuation of caffeine may cause headache and irritability.
• Caffeine is included in many OTC analgesic preparations. There's conflicting evidence regarding whether it increases pain relief.
• Treatment of neonatal apnea is an unlabeled indication. Solution may have to be made in pharmacy because most commercially available parenteral caffeine injections contain sodium benzoate, a preservative that may cause kernicterus in neonates.

dextroamphetamine sulfate
Dexedrine* **, Ferndex, Oxydess II, Robese, Spancap #1
Controlled Substance Schedule II
Pregnancy Risk Category: C

HOW SUPPLIED
Tablets: 5 mg, 10 mg
Capsules (sustained-release): 5 mg, 10 mg, 15 mg
Elixir: 5 mg/5 ml

MECHANISM OF ACTION
Main site of activity appears to be the cerebral cortex and the reticular activating system. Promotes nerve impulse transmission by releasing stored norepinephrine from nerve terminals in the brain. In children with hyperkinesia, amphetamines have a paradoxical calming effect.

INDICATIONS & DOSAGE
Narcolepsy—
Adults: 5 to 60 mg P.O. daily in divided doses.
Children over 12 years: 10 mg P.O. daily, with 10-mg increments weekly, p.r.n.
Children 6 to 12 years: 5 mg P.O. daily, with 5-mg increments weekly, p.r.n.
Short-term adjunct in exogenous obesity—
Adults: single 10- to 15-mg long-acting capsule, up to 30 mg daily; or in divided doses, 5 to 10 mg half hour before meals.
Attention deficit disorders with hyperactivity (ADDH)—
Children 6 years and older: 5 mg P.O. once daily or b.i.d., with 5-mg increments weekly, p.r.n.
Children 3 to 5 years: 2.5 mg P.O. daily, with 2.5-mg increments weekly, p.r.n.

ADVERSE REACTIONS
CNS: *restlessness,* tremor, *hyperactivity, talkativeness, insomnia,* irritability, dizziness, headache, chills, overstimulation, dysphoria.
CV: *tachycardia, palpitations,* hypertension, hypotension.
GI: nausea, vomiting, cramps, dry mouth, diarrhea, constipation, metallic taste, anorexia, weight loss.
Skin: urticaria.
Other: impotence, altered libido.

INTERACTIONS
Ammonium chloride, ascorbic acid: observe for decreased amphetamine effects.
Antacids, sodium bicarbonate, acetazolamide: increased renal reabsorption. Monitor for enhanced amphetamine effects.
MAO inhibitors: severe hypertension; possible hypertensive crisis. Don't use together.
Phenothiazines, haloperidol: observe for decreased amphetamine effects.

NURSING CONSIDERATIONS
• Contraindicated in hyperthyroidism, nephritis, severe hypertension, angina pectoris or other severe CV disease, some types of glaucoma, or history of drug abuse. Use with caution in diabetes mellitus and in elderly, debilitated, or hyperexcitable patients.
• Use cautiously in children with Tourette's disorder.
• Psychic dependence or habituation may occur, especially in patients with history of drug addiction. Avoid prolonged administration. When used long-term, lower dosage gradually to prevent acute rebound depression.
• Not recommended for first-line treatment of obesity. Use as an anorexigenic agent is prohibited in some states.
• When used for obesity, be sure patient is also on a weight-reduction program. Give 30 to 60 minutes before meals. Avoid giving within 6 hours of bedtime.
• Fatigue may result as drug effects wear off. Patient will need more rest.
• Tell patient to avoid drinks containing caffeine, which increase the effects of amphetamines and related amines.
• Have patient report signs of excessive stimulation.
• Urine acidification enhances renal excretion; urine alkalinization enhances renal reabsorption and recycling.
• When tolerance to anorexigenic effect develops, dosage should not be increased, but drug discontinued.
• Should not be used to prevent fatigue.
• Warn patient to avoid activities that require alertness or good psychomotor coordination until CNS effects of the drug are known.
• May alter daily insulin needs in patients with diabetes. Monitor blood and urine sugars.
• Use as analeptic is usually discouraged, since CNS stimulation superimposed on CNS depression can lead to neuronal instability and seizures.
• Give at least 6 hours before bedtime to avoid sleep interference.

---

diethylpropion hydrochloride
Nobesine†, Propion†, Tenuate, Tenuate Dospan, Tepanil, Tepanil Ten-Tab
Controlled Substance Schedule IV
Pregnancy Risk Category: B

HOW SUPPLIED
Tablets: 25 mg
Tablets (controlled-release): 75 mg

MECHANISM OF ACTION
Main site of activity appears to be the cerebral cortex and the reticular activating system. Promotes nerve impulse transmission by releasing stored

---

Italicized adverse reactions are common or life-threatening.
*Liquid form contains alcohol.   **May contain tartrazine.

norepinephrine from nerve terminals in the brain.

INDICATIONS & DOSAGE
Short-term adjunct in exogenous obesity—
Adults: 25 mg P.O. before meals, t.i.d.; or 75 mg controlled-release tablet P.O. in mid-morning.

ADVERSE REACTIONS
CNS: headache, *nervousness,* dizziness.
CV: *tachycardia, palpitations,* rise in blood pressure.
EENT: blurred vision.
GI: nausea, abdominal cramps, dry mouth, diarrhea, constipation.
Skin: urticaria.
Other: impotence, altered libido, menstrual changes.

INTERACTIONS
MAO inhibitors: hypertension; possible hypertensive crisis. Don't use together.

NURSING CONSIDERATIONS
• Contraindicated in hyperthyroidism, hypertension, angina pectoris, severe CV disease, glaucoma, or history of drug abuse. Use with caution in epilepsy, diabetes mellitus, and hyperexcitability states. May alter insulin requirements. Monitor blood and urine sugars.
• When tolerance to anorexigenic effect develops, dosage should not be increased, but drug discontinued.
• Habituation or psychic dependence may occur.
• Be sure patient is also on a weight-reduction program.
• Can be used to stop nighttime eating. Rarely causes insomnia.
• Fatigue may result as drug effects wear off. Patient will need more rest.
• Tell patient to avoid drinks containing caffeine, which increase the effects of amphetamines and related amines.

• Have patient report signs of excessive stimulation.
• Urine acidification enhances renal excretion; urine alkalinization enhances renal reabsorption and recycling.
• Use as analeptic is usually discouraged, since CNS stimulation superimposed on CNS depression can lead to neuronal instability and seizures.
• Give at least 6 hours before bedtime to avoid sleep interference.

---

fenfluramine hydrochloride
Ponderal†, Ponderal Pacaps†, Ponderax‡, Ponderax Pacaps‡, Pondimin, Pondimin Extentabs
Controlled Substance Schedule IV

Pregnancy Risk Category: C

HOW SUPPLIED
Tablets: 20 mg, 40 mg
Capsules (sustained-release): 60 mg†‡

MECHANISM OF ACTION
Stimulates ventromedial nucleus of the hypothalamus. May also affect serotonin metabolism.

INDICATIONS & DOSAGE
Short-term adjunct in exogenous obesity—
Adults: initially, 20 mg P.O. t.i.d. before meals. Maximum dosage is 40 mg t.i.d. Adjust dosage according to patient's response.

ADVERSE REACTIONS
CNS: *drowsiness,* dizziness, incoordination, headache, euphoria or depression, anxiety, *insomnia,* weakness, fatigue, agitation.
CV: *palpitations,* hypotension, hypertension, chest pain.
EENT: eye irritation, blurred vision.
GI: *diarrhea, dry mouth,* nausea, vomiting, abdominal pain, constipation.

---

†Available in Canada only.　　‡Available in Australia only.　　◊ Available OTC.

GU: dysuria, increased urinary frequency, impotence.
Skin: rashes, urticaria, burning sensation.
Other: sweating, chills, fever, increased libido.

INTERACTIONS
Alcohol, CNS depressants: enhanced CNS depression.
Centrally acting antihypertensives: decreased antihypertensive effect.
MAO inhibitors: severe hypertension; possible hypertensive crisis. Don't use together.

NURSING CONSIDERATIONS
• Contraindicated in glaucoma, hypersensitivity to sympathomimetic amines, symptomatic cardiovascular disease, alcoholism, or history of drug abuse. Use with caution in hypertension, history of mental depression, and diabetes mellitus.
• Because of possible hypoglycemia, patients with diabetes may have altered insulin or sulfonylurea requirements. Monitor blood and urine sugars.
• Differs pharmacologically from amphetamines in that it produces CNS depression more often than stimulation.
• Have patient report signs of excessive sedation, depression, or excessive stimulation. Closely monitor blood pressure.
• Be sure patient is on a weight-reduction program.
• Tolerance or dependence may occur. Avoid prolonged administration.
• Fenfluramine should not be discontinued abruptly; may precipitate an acute depressive reaction.
• Has been proven effective for treating autistic children.

mazindol
Mazanor, Sanorex
Controlled Substance Schedule IV
Pregnancy Risk Category: C

HOW SUPPLIED
Tablets: 1 mg, 2 mg

MECHANISM OF ACTION
Inhibits neuronal uptake of norepinephrine and dopamine.

INDICATIONS & DOSAGE
Short-term adjunct in exogenous obesity—
Adults: 1 mg P.O. t.i.d. 1 hour before meals, or 2 mg daily 1 hour before lunch. Use lowest effective dosage.

ADVERSE REACTIONS
CNS: *nervousness, restlessness, dizziness, insomnia,* dysphoria, headache, depression, drowsiness, weakness, tremor.
CV: *palpitations, tachycardia.*
GI: dry mouth, nausea, constipation, diarrhea, unpleasant taste.
GU: difficulty initiating micturition, impotence.
Skin: rash, clamminess, pallor.
Other: shivering, excessive sweating, altered libido.

INTERACTIONS
Centrally acting antihypertensives: decreased antihypertensive effect.
MAO inhibitors: severe hypertension; possible hypertensive crisis. Don't use together.

NURSING CONSIDERATIONS
• Contraindicated in glaucoma, CV disease including arrhythmias, agitated states, or history of drug abuse. Use with caution in diabetes mellitus, hypertension, and hyperexcitability states.
• Warn patient to avoid activities that require alertness or good psychomo-

---

Italicized adverse reactions are common or life-threatening.
*Liquid form contains alcohol.   **May contain tartrazine.

tor coordination until CNS effects of the drug are known.
• Fatigue may result as drug effects wear off. Patient will need more rest.
• Tell patient to avoid drinks containing caffeine, which increase the effects of amphetamines and related amines.
• Have patient report signs of excessive stimulation.
• Tolerance or dependence may develop. Avoid prolonged use.
• Be sure patient is also on a weight-reduction program.
• May alter insulin needs in patients with diabetes. Monitor blood and urine sugars.
• Give at least 6 hours before bedtime to avoid sleep interference.

---

methamphetamine hydrochloride
Desoxyn, Desoxyn Gradumet
Controlled Substance Schedule II
Pregnancy Risk Category: C

HOW SUPPLIED
Tablets: 5 mg, 10 mg
Tablets (long-acting): 5 mg, 10 mg, 15 mg

MECHANISM OF ACTION
Main site of activity appears to be the cerebral cortex and the reticular activating system. Promotes nerve impulse transmission by releasing stored norepinephrine from nerve terminals in the brain. In children with hyperkinesia, amphetamines have a paradoxical calming effect.

INDICATIONS & DOSAGE
Attention deficit disorder with hyperactivity (ADDH)—
Children 6 years and older: 2.5 to 5 mg P.O. once daily or b.i.d., with 5-mg increments weekly, p.r.n. Usual effective dosage is 20 to 25 mg daily.
Short-term adjunct in exogenous obesity—

Adults: 2.5 to 5 mg P.O. once to t.i.d. 30 minutes before meals; or 1 long-acting 5- to 15-mg tablet daily before breakfast.

ADVERSE REACTIONS
CNS: *nervousness, insomnia,* irritability, *talkativeness,* dizziness, headache, hyperexcitability, tremor.
CV: hypertension, hypotension, *tachycardia, palpitations,* cardiac arrhythmias.
EENT: blurred vision, mydriasis.
GI: nausea, vomiting, abdominal cramps, diarrhea, constipation, dry mouth, anorexia, metallic taste.
Skin: urticaria.
Other: impotence, altered libido.

INTERACTIONS
Ammonium chloride, ascorbic acid: observe for decreased amphetamine effects.
Antacids, sodium bicarbonate, acetazolamide: increased renal reabsorption. Monitor for enhanced effects.
MAO inhibitors: severe hypertension; possible hypertensive crisis. Don't use together.
Phenothiazines, haloperidol: observe for decreased amphetamine effects.

NURSING CONSIDERATIONS
• Contraindicated in hypertension, hyperthyroidism, nephritis, angina pectoris or other severe CV disease, glaucoma, parkinsonism due to arteriosclerosis, agitated states, or history of drug abuse. Use with caution in diabetes mellitus; and in patients who are elderly, debilitated, asthenic, psychopathic, or who have a history of suicidal or homicidal tendencies.
• Use cautiously in children with Tourette's disorder.
• Warn that potential for abuse is high. Should not be used to prevent fatigue.
• May alter insulin needs in patients with diabetes. Monitor blood and urine sugars.

• Not recommended for first-line treatment of obesity. Use as an anorexigenic agent is prohibited in some states.
• When used for obesity, be sure patient is on a weight-reduction program.
• Tell patient to avoid drinks containing caffeine, which increase the effects of amphetamines and related amines.
• Have patient report signs of excessive stimulation.
• Urine acidification enhances renal excretion; urine alkalinization enhances renal reabsorption and recycling.
• When tolerance to anorexigenic effect develops, dosage should not be increased, but drug discontinued.
• Warn patient to avoid activities that require alertness or good psychomotor coordination until CNS effects of the drug are known.
• Give at least 6 hours before bedtime to avoid sleep interference.

---

methylphenidate hydrochloride
Ritalin, Ritalin SR
Controlled Substance Schedule II
Pregnancy Risk Category: C

HOW SUPPLIED
Tablets: 5 mg, 10 mg, 20 mg
Tablets (sustained-release): 20 mg

MECHANISM OF ACTION
Main site of activity appears to be the cerebral cortex and the reticular activating system. Promotes nerve impulse transmission by releasing stored norepinephrine from nerve terminals in the brain. In children with hyperkinesia, amphetamines have a paradoxical calming effect.

INDICATIONS & DOSAGE
Attention deficit disorder with hyperactivity (ADDH)—

Children 6 years and older: initial dose 5 to 10 mg P.O. daily before breakfast and lunch, with 5- to 10-mg increments weekly as needed, up to 60 mg daily.
Narcolepsy—
Adults: 10 mg P.O. b.i.d. or t.i.d. half hour before meals. Dosage varies with patient needs. Dosage range is 5 to 50 mg daily.

ADVERSE REACTIONS
Blood: thrombocytopenia.
CNS: *nervousness, insomnia,* dizziness, headache, akathisia, dyskinesia, *Tourette's disorder.*
CV: *palpitations,* angina, *tachycardia,* changes in blood pressure and pulse rate.
EENT: difficulty with accommodation and blurring of vision.
GI: nausea, dry throat, abdominal pain, anorexia, weight loss.
Skin: rash, urticaria, *exfoliative dermatitis,* erythema multiforme, thrombocytopenic purpura.
Other: growth suppression.

INTERACTIONS
Anticonvulsants, tricyclic antidepressants, oral anticoagulants: methylphenidate may increase plasma levels of these drugs and enhance their pharmacologic effects.
Centrally acting antihypertensives: decreased antihypertensive effect.
MAO inhibitors: severe hypertension; possible hypertensive crisis. Don't use together.

NURSING CONSIDERATIONS
• Contraindicated in symptomatic cardiac disease; hyperthyroidism; moderate to severe hypertension; angina pectoris; advanced arteriosclerosis; severe depression of either endogenous or exogenous form; glaucoma; parkinsonism; history of drug abuse or dependency; or history of marked anxiety, tension, or agitation. Use with caution in elderly, debilitated, or

---

Italicized adverse reactions are common or life-threatening.
*Liquid form contains alcohol.   **May contain tartrazine.

hyperexcitable patients, and those with history of CV disease, diabetes, or seizures.
• May precipitate Tourette's disorder in children. Monitor especially at start of therapy.
• Closely monitor blood pressure. Observe for signs of excessive stimulation.
• Should not be used to prevent fatigue.
• Observe for interactions, as treatment of other disease states may be affected. May alter daily insulin needs in patients with diabetes. Monitor blood and urine sugars. May decrease seizure threshold in patients with seizure disorders.
• Drug of choice for ADDH. Usually stopped after puberty.
• Periodic CBC, differential, and platelet counts advised with long-term use.
• Tolerance, psychic dependence, or habituation may develop, especially in patients with history of drug addiction. High abuse potential. Avoid prolonged administration. When used long-term, lower dosage gradually to prevent acute rebound depression.
• Fatigue may result as drug effects wear off. Patient will need more rest.
• Tell patient to avoid drinks containing caffeine, which increase the effects of amphetamines and related amines.
• Warn patient to avoid activities that require alertness or good psychomotor coordination until CNS effects of the drug are known.
• Monitor height and weight in children on prolonged therapy because drug has been associated with growth suppression. Recent evidence suggests it may delay "growth spurt," but children will attain normal height when drug is discontinued.
• Now available in a sustained-release form (duration, 6 to 8 hours). Warn patient against chewing these tablets.
• Give at least 6 hours before bedtime to prevent insomnia. Administer after meals to reduce appetite-suppressive effects.

pemoline
Cylert, Cylert Chewable
Controlled Substance Schedule IV
Pregnancy Risk Category: B

HOW SUPPLIED
Tablets: 18.75 mg, 37.5 mg, 75 mg
Tablets (chewable and containing povidine): 37.5 mg

MECHANISM OF ACTION
Main site of activity appears to be the cerebral cortex and the reticular activating system. Promotes nerve impulse transmission by releasing stored norepinephrine from nerve terminals in the brain.

INDICATIONS & DOSAGE
Attention deficit disorder with hyperactivity (ADDH)—
Children 6 years and older: initially, 37.5 mg P.O. given in the morning. Daily dose can be raised by 18.75 mg weekly. Effective dosage range is 56.25 to 75 mg daily; maximum dosage is 112.5 mg daily.

ADVERSE REACTIONS
CNS: *insomnia,* malaise, irritability, fatigue, mild depression, dizziness, headache, drowsiness, hallucinations, nervousness (large doses), seizures, *Tourette's disorder,* psychosis.
CV: *tachycardia (large doses).*
GI: anorexia, abdominal pain, nausea, diarrhea.
Hepatic: elevated liver enzymes.
Skin: rash.

INTERACTIONS
Insulin, oral hypoglycemics: pemoline may alter requirements of antidiabetic agents.

NURSING CONSIDERATIONS
• Contraindicated in patients with hepatic dysfunction, and in children under 6 years. Use with caution in patients with impaired renal function or a history of Tourette's disorder. Drug may accumulate.
• May precipitate Tourette's disorder in children. Monitor especially at start of therapy.
• Closely monitor patients on long-term therapy for possible blood or hepatic function abnormalities and for growth suppression.
• Structurally dissimilar to amphetamines or methylphenidate. However, may produce similar adverse reactions, including lowered seizure threshold. Also, has a greater potential for drug abuse and dependence than previously thought.
• Therapeutic effects may not be evident for up to 3 to 4 weeks.
• Give at least 6 hours before bedtime to avoid sleep interference.

---

phendimetrazine tartrate
Adipost, Adphen, Anorex, Bacarate, Bontril PDM, Bontril Slow Release, Dyrexan OD, Melfiat, Metra, Obalan, Obeval, Phenazine-35, Phenzine, Plegine, Prelu-2, Slyn-LL, Sprx-105, Statobex**, Trimtabs, Trimstat, Wehless, Weightrol, X-Trozine, X-Trozine LA
Controlled Substance Schedule IV

Pregnancy Risk Category: C

HOW SUPPLIED
Tablets: 35 mg
Capsules: 35 mg
Capsules (sustained-release): 105 mg

MECHANISM OF ACTION
Main site of activity appears to be the cerebral cortex and the reticular activating system. Promotes nerve impulse transmission by releasing stored norepinephrine from nerve terminals in the brain.

INDICATIONS & DOSAGE
Short-term adjunct in exogenous obesity—
Adults: 35 mg P.O. b.i.d. to t.i.d. 1 hour before meals. Maximum dosage is 70 mg t.i.d. Use lowest effective dosage. Adjust dose to individual response.

ADVERSE REACTIONS
CNS: *nervousness,* dizziness, *insomnia,* tremor, headache.
CV: *tachycardia, palpitations,* rise in blood pressure.
EENT: blurred vision
GI: dry mouth, nausea, abdominal cramps, diarrhea, constipation.
GU: dysuria.

INTERACTIONS
Ammonium chloride, ascorbic acid: observe for decreased phendimetrazine effects.
Antacids, sodium bicarbonate, acetazolamide: increased renal reabsorption. Monitor for enhanced effects.
MAO inhibitors: severe hypertension; possible hypertensive crisis. Don't use together.
Phenothiazines, haloperidol: observe for decreased effect.

NURSING CONSIDERATIONS
• Contraindicated in hyperthyroidism, hypertension, angina pectoris or other severe CV disease, or glaucoma. Use with caution in hyperexcitability states or with history of drug addiction.
• Warn patient to avoid activities that require alertness or good psychomotor coordination until CNS effects of the drug are known.
• Be sure patient is following weight-reduction program.
• Tolerance or dependence can develop. Not advised for prolonged use.
• Fatigue may result as drug effects wear off. Patient will need more rest.
• Tell patient to avoid drinks containing caffeine, which increase the ef-

---

Italicized adverse reactions are common or life-threatening.
*Liquid form contains alcohol.   **May contain tartrazine.

fects of amphetamines and related amines.
• Have patient report signs of excessive stimulation.
• Urine acidification enhances renal excretion; urine alkalinization enhances renal reabsorption and recycling.
• May alter daily insulin needs in patients with diabetes. Monitor blood urine sugars.
• Give at least 6 hours before bedtime to avoid sleep interference.

phenmetrazine hydrochloride
Preludin**
Controlled Substance Schedule II

Pregnancy Risk Category: C

HOW SUPPLIED
Tablets: 25 mg
Tablets (sustained-release): 75 mg

MECHANISM OF ACTION
Main site of activity appears to be the cerebral cortex and the reticular activating system. Promotes nerve impulse transmission by releasing stored norepinephrine from nerve terminals in the brain.

INDICATIONS & DOSAGE
Short-term adjunct in exogenous obesity—
Adults: 25 mg P.O. b.i.d. or t.i.d. 1 hour before meals, up to 75 mg daily; or single 50- to 75-mg extended-release tablet daily in midmorning.

ADVERSE REACTIONS
CNS: *nervousness,* dizziness, *insomnia,* headache.
CV: *tachycardia, palpitations,* increased blood pressure.
EENT: blurred vision.
GI: dry mouth, nausea, abdominal cramps, constipation.
Skin: urticaria.
Other: altered libido, impotence.

INTERACTIONS
Ammonium chloride, ascorbic acid: observe for decreased phenmetrazine effects.
Antacids, sodium bicarbonate, acetazolamide: increased renal reabsorption. Monitor for enhanced effects.
MAO inhibitors: severe hypertension; possible hypertensive crisis. Don't use together.
Phenothiazines, haloperidol: observe for decreased effect.

NURSING CONSIDERATIONS
• Contraindicated in patients with hyperthyroidism, hypertension, angina pectoris or other CV disease, glaucoma, or history of drug addiction. Use with caution in hyperexcitability states.
• Tolerance or dependence may develop. High abuse potential. Not advised for prolonged use.
• Be sure patient is also following weight-reduction program.
• Fatigue may result as drug effects wear off. Patient will need more rest.
• Tell patient to avoid drinks containing caffeine, which increase the effects of amphetamines and related amines.
• Have patient report signs of excessive stimulation.
• Urine acidification enhances renal excretion; urine alkalinization enhances renal reabsorption and recycling.

phentermine hydrochloride
Adipex-P, Dapex, Duromine‡, Fastin, Ionamin, Obe-Nix, Obephen, Obermine, Obestin, Oby-Trim, Parmine, Phentrol, Span R/D, Teramine, Unifast
Controlled Substance Schedule IV

Pregnancy Risk Category: C

HOW SUPPLIED
Tablets and capsules: 8 mg, 15 mg, 18.75 mg, 30 mg, 37.5 mg

---

†Available in Canada only.　　‡Available in Australia only.　　◊Available OTC.

Capsules (resin complex, sustained-release): 15 mg, 30 mg

MECHANISM OF ACTION
Main site of activity appears to be the cerebral cortex and the reticular activating system. Promotes nerve impulse transmission by releasing stored norepinephrine from nerve terminals in the brain.

INDICATIONS & DOSAGE
Short-term adjunct in exogenous obesity—
Adults: 8 mg P.O. t.i.d. half hour before meals; or 15 to 30 mg daily before breakfast (resin complex).

ADVERSE REACTIONS
CNS: *nervousness,* dizziness, *insomnia.*
CV: *palpitations, tachycardia,* increased blood pressure.
GI: dry mouth, unpleasant taste, nausea, constipation, diarrhea.
Skin: urticaria.
Other: altered libido, impotence.

INTERACTIONS
Ammonium chloride, ascorbic acid: observe for decreased phentermine effects.
Antacids, sodium bicarbonate, acetazolamide: increased renal reabsorption. Monitor for enhanced effects.
MAO inhibitors: severe hypertension; possible hypertensive crisis. Don't use together.
Phenothiazines, haloperidol: observe for decreased effects.

NURSING CONSIDERATIONS
• Contraindicated in hyperthyroidism, hypertension, angina pectoris or other severe CV disease, or glaucoma. Use with caution in hyperexcitability states or history of drug addiction.
• Tolerance or dependence may develop. Avoid prolonged administration.
• Use with weight-reduction program. Give 30 minutes before meals.
• Fatigue may result as drug effects wear off. Patient will need more rest.
• Tell patient to avoid drinks containing caffeine, which increase the effects of amphetamines and related amines.
• Have patient report signs of excessive stimulation.
• Urine acidification enhances renal excretion; urine alkalinization enhances renal reabsorption and recycling.
• Give at least 6 hours before bedtime to avoid sleep interference.

Italicized adverse reactions are common or life-threatening.
*Liquid form contains alcohol.   **May contain tartrazine.

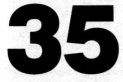

Cholinergics (parasympathomimetics)

ambenonium chloride
bethanechol chloride
edrophonium chloride
neostigmine bromide
neostigmine methylsulfate
physostigmine salicylate
  (eserine)
pyridostigmine bromide

COMBINATION PRODUCTS
None.

---

ambenonium chloride
Mytelase

Pregnancy Risk Category: C

HOW SUPPLIED
Tablets: 10 mg

MECHANISM OF ACTION
Inhibits the destruction of acetylcholine released from the parasympathetic and somatic efferent nerves. Acetylcholine accumulates, promoting increased stimulation of the receptor.

INDICATIONS & DOSAGE
Symptomatic treatment of myasthenia gravis in patients who cannot take neostigmine bromide or pyridostigmine bromide—
Adults: dosage must be individualized for each patient, but usually ranges from 5 to 25 mg P.O. t.i.d. to q.i.d. Starting dose usually is 5 mg P.O. t.i.d. to q.i.d. Increase gradually and adjust at 1- to 2-day intervals to avoid drug accumulation and overdosage. Usual dosage range is 15 to 100 mg daily, but some patients may require as much as 75 mg two to four times a day.

ADVERSE REACTIONS
CNS: headache, dizziness, muscle weakness, incoordination, seizures, mental confusion, jitters, sweating.
CV: bradycardia, hypotension.
EENT: miosis, blurred vision.
GI: *nausea, vomiting, diarrhea, abdominal cramps,* increased salivation.
GU: urinary frequency, incontinence.
Other: bronchospasm, *muscle cramps,* bronchoconstriction, increased bronchial secretions, *respiratory paralysis.*

INTERACTIONS
Atropine, corticosteroids, magnesium, procainamide, quinidine: may impair drug effect. Observe for lack of drug effect.

NURSING CONSIDERATIONS
• Contraindicated in mechanical obstruction of intestine or urinary tract, bradycardia, or hypotension.
• Use with extreme caution in bronchial asthma.
• Use cautiously in epilepsy, recent coronary occlusion, vagotonia, hyperthyroidism, cardiac arrhythmias, and peptic ulcer.
• Avoid large dose in patients with decreased GI motility or megacolon.
• Discontinue all other cholinergics before administering this drug.
• Watch patient very closely for adverse reactions, particularly if total dosage is greater than 200 mg daily.

Adverse reactions may indicate drug toxicity. Notify doctor immediately if they develop.

• Monitor and document vital signs frequently, being especially careful to check respirations. Always have atropine injection readily available and be prepared to give atropine 0.5 mg subcutaneously or slow I.V. push as ordered, and provide respiratory support as needed.

• Administer each dose exactly as ordered, on time. Amount and frequency of dosage should vary with patient's activity level. The doctor will probably order larger doses to be given when patient is fatigued, for example, in the afternoon and at mealtime.

• If muscle weakness is severe, doctor must determine if this is caused by drug toxicity or exacerbation of myasthenia gravis. A test dose of edrophonium I.V. will aggravate drug-induced weakness but will temporarily relieve weakness that results from the disease.

• Weakness occurring 30 to 60 minutes after taking dose is a warning sign of drug toxicity. Notify doctor immediately.

• Observe and record the patient's variations in muscle strength. Show him how to do it himself.

• When given for myasthenia gravis, explain to patient that this drug will relieve symptoms of ptosis, double vision, difficulty in chewing and swallowing, and trunk and limb weakness. Stress the importance of taking this drug exactly as ordered. Explain to patient and his family that he may have to take this drug for the rest of his life. Teach them about the disease and the drug's effect on symptoms.

• Patient may develop resistance to drug.

• Seek approval when indicated for hospitalized patient to have bedside supply of tablets to take himself. Patients with long-standing disease often insist on this.

• Give with milk or food to produce fewer muscarinic adverse reactions.

• Advise patient to wear identification tag indicating he has myasthenia gravis.

---

bethanechol chloride
Duvoid, Urabeth, Urecholine, Urocarb Liquid‡, Urocarb Tablets‡

Pregnancy Risk Category: C

HOW SUPPLIED
Tablets: 5 mg, 10 mg, 25 mg, 50 mg
Liquid: 1 mg/5 ml‡
Injection: 5 mg/ml

MECHANISM OF ACTION
Binds to cholinergic (muscarinic) receptors, mimicking the action of acetylcholine.

INDICATIONS & DOSAGE
Acute postoperative and postpartum nonobstructive (functional) urine retention, neurogenic atony of urinary bladder with retention, abdominal distention, megacolon, or reflux esophagitis caused by low esophageal sphincter pressure—
Adults: 10 to 30 mg P.O. b.i.d. to q.i.d. Or, 2.5 to 10 mg S.C. Never give I.M. or I.V. When used for urine retention, some patients may require 50 to 100 mg P.O. per dose. Use such doses with extreme caution.

Test dose is 2.5 mg S.C. repeated at 15- to 30-minute intervals to total of 4 doses to determine the minimal effective dose; then use minimal effective dose q 6 to 8 hours. All doses must be adjusted individually.

ADVERSE REACTIONS
Dose-related:
CNS: headache, malaise.
CV: bradycardia, hypotension, *cardiac arrest,* reflex tachycardia.
EENT: lacrimation, miosis.

Italicized adverse reactions are common or life-threatening.
*Liquid form contains alcohol.   **May contain tartrazine.

GI: *abdominal cramps, diarrhea,* salivation, nausea, vomiting, belching, borborygmus, esophageal spasms.
GU: urinary urgency.
Skin: flushing, sweating.
Other: bronchoconstriction, increased bronchial secretions.

INTERACTIONS
Atropine, anticholinergic agents, procainamide, quinidine: may reverse cholinergic effects. Observe for lack of drug effect.

NURSING CONSIDERATIONS
• Contraindicated in patients with uncertain strength or integrity of bladder wall; when increased muscular activity of GI or urinary tract is harmful; in mechanical obstructions of GI or urinary tract; in hyperthyroidism, peptic ulcer, latent or active bronchial asthma, cardiac or coronary artery disease, vagotonia, epilepsy, Parkinson's disease, bradycardia, chronic obstructive pulmonary disease, hypotension. Use cautiously in hypertension, vasomotor instability, peritonitis, and other acute inflammatory conditions of GI tract.
• *Never* give I.M. or I.V.; could cause circulatory collapse, hypotension, severe abdominal cramping, bloody diarrhea, shock, or cardiac arrest.
• Should stop all other cholinergics before giving this drug.
• Watch closely for adverse reactions that may indicate drug toxicity, especially with S.C. administration.
• Monitor vital signs frequently, being especially careful to check respirations. Always have atropine injection readily available and be prepared to give atropine 0.5 mg subcutaneously or slow I.V. push as ordered, and provide respiratory support if needed.
• If used to treat urine retention, make sure bedpan is readily available. Monitor intake/output.
• When used to prevent abdominal

distention and GI distress, the doctor may also order a rectal tube inserted to help passage of gas.
• Poor and variable oral absorption requires larger oral doses. Oral and S.C. doses are *not* interchangeable.
• Drug usually effective 5 to 15 minutes after injection and 30 to 90 minutes after oral use.
• Give on empty stomach; if taken after meals, may cause nausea and vomiting.

edrophonium chloride
Enlon, Reversol, Tensilon
Pregnancy Risk Category: C

HOW SUPPLIED
Injection: 10 mg/ml in 1-ml ampules or 10-ml vials

MECHANISM OF ACTION
Inhibits the destruction of acetylcholine released from the parasympathetic and somatic efferent nerves. Acetylcholine accumulates, promoting increased stimulation of the receptor. Edrophonium has a very short duration of action.

INDICATIONS & DOSAGE
As a curare antagonist (to reverse neuromuscular blocking action)—
Adults: 10 mg I.V. given over 30 to 45 seconds. Dose may be repeated as necessary to 40 mg maximum dosage. Larger dosages may potentiate rather than antagonize effect of curare.
Diagnostic aid in myasthenia gravis (Tensilon test)—
Adults: 1 to 2 mg I.V. within 15 to 30 seconds, then 8 mg if no response (increase in muscular strength).
Children over 34 kg: 2 mg I.V. If no response within 45 seconds, give 1 mg q 45 seconds to maximum of 10 mg.
Children up to 34 kg: 1 mg I.V. If no response within 45 seconds, give 1

mg q 45 seconds to maximum of 5 mg.
Infants: 0.5 mg I.V.
To differentiate myasthenic crisis from cholinergic crisis—
Adults: 1 mg I.V. If no response in 1 minute, repeat dose once. Increased muscular strength confirms myasthenic crisis; no increase or exaggerated weakness confirms cholinergic crisis.
Paroxysmal supraventricular tachycardia—
Adults: 5 to 10 mg I.V. given over 1 minute or less.
Children: 2 mg I.V. Administer slowly.

ADVERSE REACTIONS
CNS: seizures, weakness, dysphagia, respiratory paralysis, sweating.
CV: hypotension, bradycardia, AV block.
EENT: excessive lacrimation, diplopia, miosis.
GI: nausea, vomiting, *diarrhea, abdominal cramps,* excessive salivation.
GU: urinary frequency.
Other: increased bronchial secretions, bronchospasm, muscle cramps, muscle fasciculation.

INTERACTIONS
Digitalis glycosides: may increase the heart's sensitivity to edrophonium. Use together cautiously.
Procainamide, quinidine: may reverse cholinergic effects. Observe for lack of drug effect.

NURSING CONSIDERATIONS
• Contraindicated in mechanical obstruction of intestine or urinary tract, bradycardia, or hypotension. Use cautiously in hyperthyroidism, cardiac disease, peptic ulcer, and bronchial asthma.
• Should stop all other cholinergics before giving this drug.
• Watch closely for adverse reactions; may indicate toxicity.

• Monitor vital signs frequently, being especially careful to check respirations. Always have atropine injection readily available and be prepared to give atropine 0.5 mg subcutaneously or slow I.V. push as ordered, and provide respiratory support as needed.
• When giving drug to differentiate myasthenic crisis from cholinergic crisis, observe patient's muscle strength closely.
• Edrophonium not effective against muscle relaxation induced by decamethonium bromide and succinylcholine chloride.
• This cholinergic has the most rapid onset but shortest duration; therefore, not used for treatment of myasthenia gravis.
• For easier parenteral administration, use a tuberculin syringe with an I.V. needle.
• I.M. route may be used in children because of difficulty with I.V. route: for children under 34 kg, inject 2 mg I.M.; children over 34 kg, 5 mg I.M. Expect same reactions as with I.V. test, but these appear after 2- to 10-minute delay.
• Continuous I.V. infusions have been used to control atrial tachycardia or supraventricular tachycardia associated with Wolff-Parkinson-White syndrome that is unresponsive to digitalis glycosides.

neostigmine bromide
Prostigmin Bromide

neostigmine methylsulfate
Prostigmin
Pregnancy Risk Category: C

HOW SUPPLIED
Tablets: 15 mg
Injection: 0.25 mg/ml, 0.5 mg/ml, 1 mg/ml

MECHANISM OF ACTION
Inhibits the destruction of acetylcholine released from the parasympathetic and somatic efferent nerves. Acetylcholine accumulates, promoting increased stimulation of the receptor.

INDICATIONS & DOSAGE
Antidote for nondepolarizing neuromuscular blocking agents—
Adults: 0.5 to 2 mg I.V. slowly. Repeat p.r.n. to a total of 5 mg. Give 0.6 to 1.2 mg atropine sulfate I.V. before antidote dose.
Postoperative abdominal distention and bladder atony—
Adults: 0.5 to 1 mg I.M. or S.C. q 4 to 6 hours.
Postoperative ileus—
Adults: 0.25 to 1 mg I.M. or S.C. q 4 to 6 hours.
Diagnosis of myasthenia gravis—
Adults: 0.022 mg/kg I.M. 30 minutes after 0.011 mg of atropine sulfate.
Treatment of myasthenia gravis—
Adults: 15 to 30 mg P.O. t.i.d. (range is 15 to 375 mg daily); or 0.5 to 2 mg I.M. or I.V. q 1 to 3 hours. Dosage must be individualized, depending on response and tolerance of adverse reactions. Therapy may be required day and night.
Children: 7.5 to 15 mg P.O. t.i.d. to q.i.d.
Note: 1:1,000 solution of injectable solution contains 1 mg/ml; 1:2,000 solution contains 0.5 mg/ml.

ADVERSE REACTIONS
CNS: dizziness, muscle weakness, mental confusion, jitters, sweating, respiratory depression.
CV: bradycardia, hypotension.
EENT: miosis.
GI: *nausea, vomiting, diarrhea, abdominal cramps,* excessive salivation.
GU: urinary frequency.
Skin: rash (bromide).
Other: bronchospasm, *muscle cramps,* muscle fasciculations, bronchoconstriction.

INTERACTIONS
Atropine, anticholinergic agents, procainamide, aminoglycosides, quinidine: may reverse cholinergic effect on muscle. Observe for lack of drug effect.

NURSING CONSIDERATIONS
• Contraindicated in hypersensitivity to cholinergics or to bromide, mechanical obstruction of the intestine or urinary tract, bradycardia, or hypotension. Use with extreme caution in bronchial asthma. Use cautiously in epilepsy, recent coronary occlusion, peritonitis, vagotonia, hyperthyroidism, cardiac arrhythmias, and peptic ulcer.
• Should stop all other cholinergics before giving this drug.
• Monitor vital signs frequently, being especially careful to check respirations. Have atropine injection readily available and be prepared to give as ordered, and provide respiratory support as needed.
• Difficult to judge optimum dosage. Monitor and document patient's response after each dose. Observe closely for improvement in strength, vision, and ptosis 45 to 60 minutes after each dose. Show patient how to observe and record variations in muscle strength.
• When using for myasthenia gravis, explain that this drug will relieve ptosis, double vision, difficulty in chewing and swallowing, trunk and limb weakness. Stress importance of taking drug exactly as ordered. Explain that drug may have to be taken for life.
• In myasthenia gravis, schedule the largest dose before periods of fatigue. For example, if patient has dysphagia, schedule dose 30 minutes before each meal.
• When used to prevent abdominal distention and GI distress, the doctor

---

may order a rectal tube inserted to help passage of gas.
• Patients sometimes develop a resistance to neostigmine.
• If muscle weakness is severe, doctor determines if it is caused by drug-induced toxicity or exacerbation of myasthenia gravis. Test dose of edrophonium I.V. will aggravate drug-induced weakness but will temporarily relieve weakness caused by disease.
• Hospitalized patient with long-standing myasthenia may request bedside supply of tablets. This will enable patient to take each dose precisely as ordered. Seek approval for self-medication program according to hospital policy, but continue to oversee medication regimen.
• GI adverse reactions may be reduced by taking drug with milk or food.
• Advise patient to wear an identification tag indicating that he has myasthenia gravis.
• I.M. neostigmine may be used instead of edrophonium to diagnose myasthenia gravis. May be preferable to edrophonium when limb weakness is the only symptom.

physostigmine salicylate (eserine)
Antilirium

Pregnancy Risk Category: C

HOW SUPPLIED
Injection: 1 mg/ml

MECHANISM OF ACTION
Inhibits the destruction of acetylcholine released from the parasympathetic and somatic efferent nerves. Acetylcholine accumulates, promoting increased stimulation of the receptor.

INDICATIONS & DOSAGE
To reverse the CNS toxicity associated with tricyclic antidepressant and anticholinergic poisoning—
Adults: 0.5 to 2 mg I.M. or I.V. (1 mg/minute I.V.) repeated as necessary if life-threatening signs recur (coma, seizures, arrhythmias).

ADVERSE REACTIONS
CNS: seizures, hallucinations, muscular twitching, muscle weakness, ataxia, *restlessness, excitability, sweating.*
CV: irregular pulse, palpitations.
EENT: miosis.
GI: nausea, vomiting, epigastric pain, *diarrhea, excessive salivation.*
Other: bronchospasm, bronchial constriction, dyspnea.

INTERACTIONS
Atropine, anticholinergic agents, procainamide, quinidine: may reverse cholinergic effects. Observe for lack of drug effect.

NURSING CONSIDERATIONS
• Use cautiously in preexisting conditions: mechanical obstruction of intestine or urogenital tract, bronchial asthma, gangrene, diabetes, cardiovascular disease, vagotonia, bradycardia, hypotension, epilepsy, Parkinson's disease, hyperthyroidism, and peptic ulcer.
• Watch closely for adverse reactions, particularly CNS disturbances. Use side rails if patient becomes restless or hallucinates. Adverse reactions may indicate drug toxicity.
• Monitor vital signs frequently, being especially careful to check respirations. Position patient to make breathing easier. Always have atropine injection readily available and be prepared to give atropine 0.5 mg subcutaneously or slow I.V. push as ordered, and provide respiratory support as needed. Best administered in presence of doctor.
• Use only clear solution. Darkening may indicate loss of potency.

Italicized adverse reactions are common or life-threatening.
*Liquid form contains alcohol.   **May contain tartrazine.

- Give I.V. at controlled rate; use slow, direct injection at no more than 1 mg/minute.
- Only cholinergic that crosses blood-brain barrier; therefore the only one useful for treating CNS effects of anticholinergic or tricyclic antidepressant toxicity.
- Effectiveness often immediate and dramatic but may be transient and may require repeat dose.
- Is used investigationally to improve cognitive function in patients with Alzheimer's disease. Investigators have used 0.5 mg P.O. q 2 hours, increasing to 2 to 2.5 mg P.O. q 2 hours, 6 or 7 times a day. Maximum dose is 16 mg/day.

---

pyridostigmine bromide
Mestinon*, Mestinon Supraspan†, Mestinon Timespan, Regonol

Pregnancy Risk Category: C

HOW SUPPLIED
Tablets: 60 mg
Tablets (timed-release): 180 mg
Syrup: 60 mg/5 ml
Injection: 5 mg/ml in 2-ml ampules or 5-ml vials

MECHANISM OF ACTION
Inhibits the destruction of acetylcholine released from the parasympathetic and somatic efferent nerves. Acetylcholine accumulates, promoting increased stimulation of the receptor.

INDICATIONS & DOSAGE
Antidote for nondepolarizing neuromuscular blocking agents—
Adults: 10 to 20 mg I.V. preceded by atropine sulfate 0.6 to 1.2 mg I.V.
Myasthenia gravis—
Adults: 60 to 120 mg P.O. q 3 or 4 hours. Usual dosage is 600 mg daily but higher dosage may be needed (up to 1,500 mg daily). Give ⅟₃₀ of oral dose I.M. or I.V. Dosage must be ad-

justed for each patient, depending on response and tolerance of adverse reactions. Alternatively, may give 180 to 540 mg timed-release tablets (1 to 3 tablets) b.i.d., with at least 6 hours between doses.

ADVERSE REACTIONS
CNS: headache (with high doses), weakness, sweating, seizures.
CV: bradycardia, hypotension.
EENT: miosis.
GI: abdominal cramps, nausea, vomiting, diarrhea, excessive salivation.
Skin: rash.
Local: thrombophlebitis.
Other: bronchospasm, bronchoconstriction, increased bronchial secretions, muscle cramps, muscle fasciculations.

INTERACTIONS
Atropine, anticholinergic agents, procainamide, quinidine: may reverse cholinergic effects. Observe for lack of drug effect.

NURSING CONSIDERATIONS
- Contraindicated in mechanical obstruction of intestine or urinary tract, bradycardia, or hypotension. Use with extreme caution in bronchial asthma. Use cautiously in epilepsy, recent coronary occlusion, vagotonia, hyperthyroidism, cardiac arrhythmias, and peptic ulcer. Avoid large doses in decreased GI motility.
- Difficult to judge optimum dosage. Monitor and document patient's response after each dose.
- Should stop all other cholinergics before giving this drug.
- Monitor vital signs frequently, being especially careful to check respirations. Position patient to make breathing easier. Have atropine injection readily available and be prepared to give as ordered, and provide respiratory support as needed.
- If muscle weakness is severe, doctor determines if it is caused by drug-

induced toxicity or exacerbation of myasthenia gravis. Test dose of edrophonium I.V. will aggravate drug-induced weakness but will temporarily relieve weakness caused by disease.
• When using for myasthenia gravis, stress importance of taking drug exactly as ordered, on time, in evenly spaced doses. If doctor has ordered extended-release tablets, explain how these work. Patient must take them at the same time each day, at least 6 hours apart. Explain that he may have to take this drug for life.
• Has longest duration of the cholinergics used for myasthenia gravis.
• Used by the oral route in the treatment of senility associated with Alzheimer's disease.
• Don't crush the timed-release (Timespan or Supraspan) tablets.
• Available as a syrup for patients who have difficulty swallowing. Syrup is very sweet; give over ice chips if patient can't tolerate flavor.
• Store tablets in a tightly capped bottle, away from moisture.

Italicized adverse reactions are common or life-threatening.
*Liquid form contains alcohol.   **May contain tartrazine.

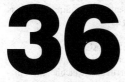

Cholinergic blockers (parasympatholytics)

atropine sulfate
  (See Chapter 20, ANTIARRHYTHMICS.)
benztropine mesylate
biperiden hydrochloride
biperiden lactate
glycopyrrolate
procyclidine hydrochloride
scopolamine butylbromide
scopolamine hydrobromide
trihexyphenidyl hydrochloride

COMBINATION PRODUCTS
Cholinergic blocking agents are available in tablets and capsules, combined with varying amounts of sedatives.

---

benztropine mesylate
Apo-Benztropine†, Bensylate†, Cogentin, PMS Benztropine†

Pregnancy Risk Category: C

HOW SUPPLIED
Tablets: 0.5 mg, 1 mg, 2 mg
Injection: 1 mg/ml in 2-ml ampules

MECHANISM OF ACTION
Blocks central cholinergic receptors, helping to balance cholinergic activity in the basal ganglia.

INDICATIONS & DOSAGE
Acute dystonic reaction—
Adults: 1 to 2 mg I.V. or I.M. followed by 1 to 2 mg P.O. b.i.d. to prevent recurrence.
Parkinsonism—
Adults: 0.5 to 6 mg P.O. daily. Initial dose is 0.5 mg to 1 mg. Increase 0.5 mg q 5 to 6 days. Adjust dosage to meet individual requirements. Usual dose is 1 to 2 mg per day.

ADVERSE REACTIONS
CNS: disorientation, restlessness, irritability, incoherence, hallucinations, headache, sedation, depression, muscular weakness.
CV: palpitations, tachycardia, paradoxical bradycardia.
EENT: dilated pupils, blurred vision, photophobia, difficulty swallowing.
GI: *constipation, dry mouth,* nausea, vomiting, epigastric distress.
GU: urinary hesitancy, urine retention.
Skin: warming, dry, flushing.
  Some adverse reactions may be due to pending atropine-like toxicity and are dose related.

INTERACTIONS
Amantadine, phenothiazines, tricyclic antidepressants: additive anticholinergic adverse reactions, such as confusion and hallucinations. Reduce dosage before administering amantadine.

NURSING CONSIDERATIONS
• Contraindicated in narrow-angle glaucoma. Use cautiously in prostatic hypertrophy, tendency to tachycardia, and in elderly or debilitated patients; produces atropine-like adverse reactions and may aggravate tardive dyskinesia.
• Monitor vital signs carefully. Watch closely for adverse reactions, especially in elderly or debilitated patients. Call doctor promptly.

• Never discontinue this drug abruptly. Dosage must be reduced gradually.

• Warn patient to avoid activities that require alertness until CNS effects of the drug are known. If patient is to receive single daily dose, give at bedtime.

• Explain that drug may take 2 to 3 days to exert full effect.

• Advise patient to report signs of urinary hesitancy or urine retention.

• Watch for intermittent constipation, distention, abdominal pain; may be onset of paralytic ileus.

• Relieve dry mouth with cool drinks, ice chips, sugarless gum or hard candy.

• To help prevent GI distress, administer after meals.

• Advise patient to limit activities during hot weather because drug-induced anhydrosis may result in hyperthermia.

---

biperiden hydrochloride
Akineton

biperiden lactate
Akineton Lactate

Pregnancy Risk Category: C

HOW SUPPLIED
Tablets: 2 mg
Injection: 5 mg/ml in 1-ml ampules

MECHANISM OF ACTION
Blocks central cholinergic receptors, helping to balance cholinergic activity in the basal ganglia.

INDICATIONS & DOSAGE
Extrapyramidal disorders—
Adults: 2 to 6 mg P.O. daily, b.i.d., or t.i.d., depending on severity. Usual dose is 2 mg daily, or 2 mg I.M. or I.V. q half hour, not to exceed 4 doses or 8 mg total daily.
Parkinsonism—
Adults: 2 mg P.O. t.i.d. to q.i.d.

Some patients may require as much as 16 mg per day.

ADVERSE REACTIONS
CNS: disorientation, euphoria, restlessness, irritability, incoherence, dizziness, increased tremor.
CV: transient postural hypotension (with parenteral use).
EENT: blurred vision.
GI: *constipation, dry mouth,* nausea, vomiting, epigastric distress.
GU: urinary hesitancy, urine retention.

Adverse reactions are dose-related and may resemble atropine toxicity.

INTERACTIONS
Phenothiazines, tricyclic antidepressants: excessive CNS anticholinergic effects.

NURSING CONSIDERATIONS
• Use with caution in prostatism, cardiac arrhythmias, narrow-angle glaucoma, and epilepsy.

• Monitor vital signs carefully. Watch closely for adverse reactions, especially in elderly or debilitated patients. Call doctor promptly.

• Give oral doses with or after meals to decrease GI adverse reactions.

• When giving parenterally, keep patient in a supine position. Parenteral administration may cause transient postural hypotension and coordination disturbances.

• I.V. injections should be made very slowly.

• Because of possible dizziness, help patient when he gets out of bed.

• Tolerance may develop, requiring increased dosage.

• In severe parkinsonism, tremors may increase as spasticity is relieved.

• Warn patient to avoid activities that require alertness until CNS effects of the drug are known.

• Advise patient to report signs of urinary hesitancy or urine retention.

• Relieve dry mouth with cool drinks,

Italicized adverse reactions are common or life-threatening.
*Liquid form contains alcohol.   **May contain tartrazine.

ice chips, sugarless gum, or hard candy.

glycopyrrolate
Robinul, Robinul Forte

Pregnancy Risk Category: B

HOW SUPPLIED
Tablets: 1 mg, 2 mg
Injection: 0.2 mg/ml

MECHANISM OF ACTION
Inhibits cholinergic (muscarinic) actions of acetylcholine on autonomic effectors innervated by postganglionic cholinergic nerves.

INDICATIONS & DOSAGE
To reverse neuromuscular blockade—
Adults: 0.2 mg I.V. for each 1 mg neostigmine or 5 mg of pyridostigmine. May be given I.V. without dilution or may be added to dextrose injection and given by infusion.
Preoperatively to diminish secretions and block cardiac vagal reflexes—
Adults: 0.002 mg/lb of body weight I.M. 30 to 60 minutes before anesthesia.
Adjunctive therapy in peptic ulcers and other GI disorders—
Adults: 1 to 2 mg P.O. t.i.d. or 0.1 mg I.M. t.i.d. or q.i.d. Dosage must be individualized. Maximum P.O. dose is 8 mg/day.

ADVERSE REACTIONS
CNS: disorientation, irritability, incoherence, weakness, nervousness, drowsiness, dizziness, headache.
CV: palpitations, tachycardia, paradoxical bradycardia.
EENT: *dilated pupils, blurred vision,* photophobia, increased intraocular pressure, difficulty swallowing.
GI: *constipation, dry mouth,* nausea, vomiting, epigastric distress.
GU: *urinary hesitancy, urine retention,* impotence.
Skin: urticaria, decreased sweating or anhidrosis, other dermal manifestations.
Local: burning at injection site.
Other: bronchial plugging, fever.

INTERACTIONS
None significant.

NURSING CONSIDERATIONS
• Contraindicated in narrow-angle glaucoma, obstructive uropathy, obstructive disease of the GI tract, myasthenia gravis, paralytic ileus, intestinal atony, unstable cardiovascular status in acute hemorrhage, or toxic megacolon. Use with caution in patients with autonomic neuropathy, hyperthyroidism, coronary artery disease, cardiac arrhythmias, CHF, hypertension, hiatal hernia associated with reflux esophagitis, hepatic or renal disease, and ulcerative colitis; and in patients over 40 years because of increased incidence of glaucoma. Use with caution in hot or humid environments. Drug-induced heatstroke possible.
• Check all dosages carefully. Even slight overdose could lead to toxicity.
• Don't mix with I.V. solution containing sodium bicarbonate or alkaline solutions with a pH >6.
• Monitor vital signs carefully. Watch closely for adverse reactions, especially in elderly or debilitated patients. Call doctor promptly.
• Advise patient to report signs of urinary hesitancy or urine retention.
• Warn patient to avoid activities that require alertness until CNS effects of the drug are known.
• Administer 30 minutes to 1 hour before meals.
• Administer smaller doses to elderly patients.

procyclidine hydrochloride
Kemadrin, PMS Procyclidine†,
Procyclid†

Pregnancy Risk Category: C

HOW SUPPLIED
Tablets: 5 mg

MECHANISM OF ACTION
Blocks central cholinergic receptors,
helping to balance cholinergic activity
in the basal ganglia.

INDICATIONS & DOSAGE
Parkinsonism, muscle rigidity—
Adults: initially, 2 to 2.5 mg P.O.
t.i.d., after meals. Increase gradually
as needed. Usual dosage range is 20 to
30 mg/day, but some patients may require up to 60 mg daily.
 Also used to relieve extrapyramidal
dysfunction that accompanies treatment with phenothiazines and rauwolfia derivatives. Also controls excessive salivation from neuroleptic medications.

ADVERSE REACTIONS
CNS: light-headedness, giddiness.
EENT: blurred vision, mydriasis.
GI: *constipation, dry mouth,* nausea,
vomiting, epigastric distress.
Skin: rash.
Other: muscle weakness.

INTERACTIONS
None significant.

NURSING CONSIDERATIONS
• Contraindicated in narrow-angle
glaucoma. Use cautiously in tachycardia, hypotension, urine retention, and
prostatic hypertrophy.
• Watch closely for mental confusion,
disorientation, agitation, hallucinations, and psychotic symptoms, especially in the elderly. Call doctor
promptly if these occur.
• In severe parkinsonism, tremors
may increase as spasticity is relieved.

• Give after meals to minimize GI
distress.
• Warn patient to avoid activities that
require alertness until CNS effects of
the drug are known.
• Relieve dry mouth with cool drinks,
ice chips, sugarless gum, or hard
candy.

scopolamine butylbromide (hyoscine butylbromide)
Buscospan†‡

scopolamine hydrobromide (hyoscine hydrobromide)
Pregnancy Risk Category: C

HOW SUPPLIED
Capsules: 0.25 mg
Injection: 0.3, 0.4, 0.5, 0.6, and 1
mg/ml in 1-ml vials and ampules;
0.86 mg/ml in 0.5-ml ampules

MECHANISM OF ACTION
Inhibits muscarinic actions of acetylcholine on autonomic effectors innervated by postganglionic cholinergic
neurons.

INDICATIONS & DOSAGE
*Postencephalitic parkinsonism and
other spastic states—*
Adults: 0.5 to 1 mg P.O. t.i.d. to
q.i.d.; 0.3 to 0.6 mg S.C., I.M., or
I.V. (with suitable dilution) t.i.d. to
q.i.d.
Children: 0.006 mg/kg P.O. or S.C.
t.i.d. to q.i.d.; or 0.2 mg/m².
*Preoperatively to reduce secretions
and block cardiac vagal reflexes—*
Adults: 0.4 to 0.6 mg S.C. 30 to 60
minutes before induction of anesthesia.

ADVERSE REACTIONS
CNS: disorientation, restlessness, irritability, dizziness, drowsiness, headache.
CV: palpitations, tachycardia, paradoxical bradycardia.

EENT: dilated pupils, blurred vision, photophobia, increased intraocular pressure, difficulty swallowing.
GI: *constipation, dry mouth, nausea, vomiting, epigastric distress.*
GU: urinary hesitancy, urine retention.
Skin: rash, flushing, dryness.
Other: bronchial plugging, fever, depressed respirations.

Adverse reactions may be caused by pending atropine-like toxicity and are dose related. Individual tolerance varies greatly.

INTERACTIONS
Alcohol, CNS depressants: increased CNS depression.
Centrally acting anticholinergics (tricyclic antidepressants, phenothiazines): increased CNS adverse reactions.
Digoxin: increased digoxin levels.

NURSING CONSIDERATIONS
• Contraindicated in narrow-angle glaucoma, obstructive uropathy, obstructive disease of the GI tract, asthma, chronic pulmonary disease, myasthenia gravis, paralytic ileus, intestinal atony, unstable cardiovascular status in acute hemorrhage, or toxic megacolon. Use with caution in patients with autonomic neuropathy, hyperthyroidism, coronary artery disease, cardiac arrhythmias, CHF, hypertension, hiatal hernia associated with reflux esophagitis, hepatic or renal disease, ulcerative colitis; in patients over 40 years because of the increased incidence of glaucoma; and in children under 6 years. Use with caution in hot or humid environments. Drug-induced heatstroke possible.
• Some patients become temporarily excited or disoriented. Symptoms disappear when sedative effect is complete. Raise side rails as a precaution.
• In therapeutic doses, scopolamine may produce amnesia, drowsiness, and euphoria. These effects are desir-

able when used as an adjunct to anesthesia. May need to reorient patient.
• Warn patient to avoid activities requiring alertness until CNS effects of the drug are known.
• Advise patient to report signs of urinary hesitancy or urine retention.
• Tolerance may develop when given over a long period of time.
• Many of the adverse reactions (such as dry mouth, constipation) are an expected extension of the drug's pharmacologic activity.
• To determine m^2 for dosage calculation in children, use a nomogram.

---

trihexyphenidyl hydrochloride
Aparkane†, Apo-Trihex†, Artane*, Artane Sequels, Novohexidyl†, Trihexane, Trihexy-2, Trihexy-5
Pregnancy Risk Category: C

HOW SUPPLIED
Tablets: 2 mg, 5 mg
Capsules (sustained-release): 5 mg
Elixir: 2 mg/5 ml

MECHANISM OF ACTION
Blocks central cholinergic receptors, helping to balance cholinergic activity in the basal ganglia.

INDICATIONS & DOSAGE
Drug-induced parkinsonism—
Adults: 1 mg P.O. 1st day, 2 mg 2nd day, then increases by 2 mg q 3 to 5 days until total of 6 to 10 mg is given daily. Usually given t.i.d. with meals and, if needed, q.i.d. (last dose should be before bedtime) or may switch to extended-release form b.i.d. Postencephalitic parkinsonism may require 12 to 15 mg total daily dosage.

ADVERSE REACTIONS
CNS: nervousness, dizziness, headache, restlessness, agitation, hallucinations, euphoria, delusion, amnesia.

CV: tachycardia.
EENT: blurred vision, mydriasis, increased intraocular pressure.
GI: constipation, *dry mouth, nausea.*
GU: urinary hesitancy, urine retention.
   Adverse reactions are dose-related.

INTERACTIONS
Amantadine: additive anticholinergic adverse reactions, such as confusion and hallucinations. Reduce dosage before administering amantadine.

NURSING CONSIDERATIONS
• Use cautiously in patients with narrow-angle glaucoma; cardiac, hepatic, or renal disorders; hypertension; obstructive disease of the GI and GU tracts; possible prostatic hypertrophy; patients over 60 years; and those with arteriosclerosis or history of drug hypersensitivities. Adverse reactions are usually mild and transient.
• Warn patient to avoid activities that require alertness until CNS effects of the drug are known.
• Causes nausea if given before meals.
• Relieve dry mouth with cool drinks, ice chips, sugarless gum, or hard candy.
• Patient may develop a tolerance to this drug, so dosage may need to be gradually increased.
• Advise patient to report signs of urinary hesitancy or urine retention.
• Gonioscopic evaluation and close monitoring of intraocular pressure is advised, especially in patients over 40 years.

37

Adrenergics (sympathomimetics)

dobutamine hydrochloride
dopamine hydrochloride
mephentermine sulfate
metaraminol bitartrate
norepinephrine injection
phenylephrine hydrochloride
pseudoephedrine hydrochloride
pseudoephedrine sulfate

COMBINATION PRODUCTS
ENTEX: phenylephrine hydrochloride
5 mg, phenylpropanolamine hydrochloride 45 mg, guaifenesin 400 mg.
ENTEX LIQUID: phenylephrine hydrochloride 5 mg/5 ml, phenylpropanolamine hydrochloride 20 mg/5 ml, guaifenesin 100 mg/5 ml (alcohol 5%).

---

dobutamine hydrochloride
Dobutrex

Pregnancy Risk Category: C

HOW SUPPLIED
Injection: 12.5 mg/ml in 20-ml vials
(parenteral)

MECHANISM OF ACTION
Directly stimulates beta$_1$ receptors of
the heart to increase myocardial contractility and stroke volume, resulting
in increased cardiac output.

INDICATIONS & DOSAGE
Refractory heart failure and as ad-
junct in cardiac surgery—
Adults: 2.5 to 10 mcg/kg/minute as
an I.V. infusion. Rarely, infusion rates
up to 40 mcg/kg/minute may be
needed.

ADVERSE REACTIONS
CNS: headache.
CV: *increased heart rate, hyperten-*
sion, premature ventricular contrac-
tions, angina, nonspecific chest pain.
GI: nausea, vomiting.
Other: shortness of breath.

INTERACTIONS
Beta blockers: may antagonize dobutamine effects. Do not use together.
General anesthetics: greater incidence
of ventricular arrhythmias.

NURSING CONSIDERATIONS
• Contraindicated in idiopathic hypertrophic subaortic stenosis.
• A unique agent. Increases contractility of failing heart without inducing
marked tachycardia, except at high
doses.
• Hypovolemia should be corrected
with plasma volume expanders before
initiating therapy with dobutamine.
• Dobutamine is chemical modification of isoproterenol.
• Often used with nitroprusside for
additive effects.
• ECG, blood pressure, pulmonary
wedge pressure, and cardiac output
should be monitored continuously.
Also monitor urine output.
• Incompatible with alkaline solutions. Do not mix with sodium bicarbonate injection.
• Infusions of up to 72 hours produce
no more adverse effects than shorter
infusions.
• Oxidation of drug may slightly discolor admixtures containing dobut-

amine. This does not indicate a significant loss of potency.
• I.V. solutions remain stable for 24 hours.

dopamine hydrochloride
Intropin, Revimine†‡

Pregnancy Risk Category: C

HOW SUPPLIED
Injection: 40 mg/ml, 80 mg/ml, 160 mg/ml parenteral concentrate for injection for I.V. infusion; 0.8 mg/ml (200 or 400 mg) in dextrose 5%; 1.6 mg/ml (400 or 800 mg) in dextrose 5%, 3.2 mg/ml (800 mg) in dextrose 5% parenteral injection for I.V. infusion.

MECHANISM OF ACTION
Stimulates dopaminergic, beta-adrenergic, and alpha-adrenergic receptors of the sympathetic nervous system.

INDICATIONS & DOSAGE
To treat shock and correct hemodynamic imbalances; to improve perfusion to vital organs; to increase cardiac output; to correct hypotension; to treat acute renal failure—
Adults: 2 to 5 mcg/kg/minute I.V. infusion, up to 50 mcg/kg/minute. Titrate the dosage to the desired hemodynamic and/or renal response.

ADVERSE REACTIONS
CNS: headache.
CV: ectopic beats, tachycardia, anginal pain, palpitations, *hypotension.* Less frequently, bradycardia, widening of QRS complex, conduction disturbances, vasoconstriction.
GI: nausea, vomiting.
Local: necrosis and tissue sloughing with extravasation.
Other: piloerection, dyspnea.

INTERACTIONS
Beta blockers: may antagonize dopamine's effects.

Ergot alkaloids: extreme elevations in blood pressure. Don't use together.
MAO inhibitors: may cause hypertensive crisis. Avoid if possible.
Phenytoin: may lower blood pressure of dopamine-stabilized patients. Monitor carefully.

NURSING CONSIDERATIONS
• Contraindicated in uncorrected tachyarrhythmias, pheochromocytoma, or ventricular fibrillation. Use cautiously in patients with occlusive vascular disease, cold injuries, diabetic endarteritis, and arterial embolism; also, in pregnant patients and those taking MAO inhibitors.
• Not a substitute for blood or fluid volume deficit. Volume deficit should be replaced before vasopressors are administered.
• Use large vein, as in the antecubital fossa, to minimize risk of extravasation. Watch site carefully for signs of extravasation. If it occurs, stop infusion immediately and call doctor. He may want to counteract effect by infiltrating the area with 5 to 10 mg phentolamine and 10 to 15 ml normal saline solution.
• Monitor blood pressure, cardiac output, pulse rate, urine output, and extremity color and temperature often during infusion. Titrate infusion rate according to findings, using doctor's guidelines. Use a continuous infusion pump to regulate flow rate.
• Observe patient closely for adverse effects. If adverse effects develop, dosage may need to be adjusted or discontinued.
• If a disproportionate rise in the diastolic pressure (a marked decrease in pulse pressure) is observed in patients receiving dopamine, decrease infusion rate and observe carefully for further evidence of predominant vasoconstrictor activity, unless such an effect is desired.
• Patient response depends upon dosage and pharmacologic effect. Doses

---

Italicized adverse reactions are common or life-threatening.
*Liquid form contains alcohol.   **May contain tartrazine.

of 0.5 to 2 mcg/kg/minute predominately stimulate dopamine receptors, and produce vasodilation. Doses of 2 to 10 mcg/kg/minute stimulate beta-adrenergic receptors. Higher doses also stimulate alpha-adrenergic receptors.

• Most patients satisfactorily maintained on less than 20 mcg/kg/minute.
• If doses exceed 50 mcg/kg/minute, check urine output often. If urine flow decreases without hypotension, consider reducing dose.
• If drug is stopped, watch closely for sudden drop in blood pressure.
• Don't mix with alkaline solutions. Use dextrose 5% in water, normal saline solution, or combination of dextrose 5% in water and saline solution. Mix just before use.
• Dopamine solutions deteriorate after 24 hours. Discard at that time or earlier if solution is discolored.
• Do not mix other drugs in I.V. container with dopamine.
• Do not give alkaline drugs (e.g., sodium bicarbonate, phenytoin sodium) through I.V. line containing dopamine.
• Acidosis decreases effectiveness of dopamine.

---

mephentermine sulfate
Wyamine

Pregnancy Risk Category: C

HOW SUPPLIED
Injection: 15 mg/ml, 30 mg/ml

MECHANISM OF ACTION
Indirectly stimulates beta- and alpha-adrenergic receptors by releasing norepinephrine.

INDICATIONS & DOSAGE
Hypotension following spinal anesthesia—
Adults: 30 to 45 mg I.V. in a single injection, then 30 mg I.V. repeated p.r.n. Maintenance of blood pressure:

continuous I.V. infusion of 0.1% solution of mephentermine in dextrose 5% in water.
Children: 0.4 mg/kg I.M. or I.V.
Hypotension following spinal anesthesia during obstetric procedures—
Adults: initially 15 mg I.V. p.r.n.
Prevention of hypotension during spinal anesthesia—
Adults: 30 to 45 mg I.M. 10 to 20 minutes before anesthesia.

ADVERSE REACTIONS
CNS: euphoria, nervousness, anxiety, tremor, incoherence, drowsiness, seizures.
CV: *arrhythmias, marked elevation of blood pressure (with large doses).*

INTERACTIONS
Antihypertensives, nitrates: decreased effects of these adrenergic blocking agents.
Beta-adrenergic blocking agents, rauwolfia alkaloids: mutual inhibition of therapeutic effects.
CNS stimulants, mazindol, methylphenidate, sympathomimetics: increased CNS stimulation.
Digitalis glycosides, levodopa, inhalation anesthetics: increased risk of cardiac arrhythmias.
Ergot alkaloids, oxytocin: enhanced vasoconstriction.
MAO inhibitors: may cause severe hypertension (hypertensive crisis) or arrhythmias. Don't use together.
Thyroid hormones: enhanced risk of coronary insufficiency.
Tricyclic antidepressants, maprotiline: decreased pressure of mephentermine.

NURSING CONSIDERATIONS
• Contraindicated in concealed hemorrhage or hypotension from hemorrhage, except in emergencies; also in patients receiving phenothiazines, or who have received MAO inhibitors within 2 weeks. Use cautiously in arteriosclerosis, cardiovascular disease,

---

hyperthyroidism, hypertension, chronic illness.
• Not a substitute for blood or fluid volume deficit. If deficit exists, it should be replaced before vasopressors are administered.
• During infusion, check blood pressure every 2 minutes until stabilized; then every 10 to 15 minutes.
• Observe patient closely for adverse effects. If adverse effects develop, dosage may need to be adjusted or discontinued.
• Monitor blood pressure until stable, even after stopping drug.
• I.M. route may be used since drug is not irritating to tissue.
• I.V. drug is not irritating to tissue, and extravasation is not dangerous. To prepare 0.1% I.V. solution; add 16.6 ml mephentermine (30 mg/ml) to 500 ml dextrose 5% in water.
• Can be given I.V. undiluted.
• Don't mix with I.V. hydralazine or epinephrine because they are physically incompatable with mephentermine.
• May increase uterine contractions during third trimester of pregnancy.
• Hypercapnia, hypoxia, acidosis may reduce effectiveness or increase adverse effects. Identify and correct before and during administration.

---

metaraminol bitartrate
Aramine

Pregnancy Risk Category: D

HOW SUPPLIED
Injection: 10 mg/ml

MECHANISM OF ACTION
Predominantly stimulates alpha-adrenergic receptors within the sympathetic nervous system.

INDICATIONS & DOSAGE
Prevention of hypotension—
Adults: 2 to 10 mg I.M. or S.C.
Severe shock—

Adults: 0.5 to 5 mg direct I.V. followed by I.V. infusion.
Treatment of hypotension caused by shock—
Adults: 15 to 100 mg in 500 ml normal saline solution or dextrose 5% in water I.V. infusion. Adjust rate to maintain blood pressure.
All indications—
Children: 0.01 mg/kg as single I.V. injection; 1 mg/25 ml dextrose 5% in water as I.V. infusion. Adjust rate to maintain blood pressure in normal range. 0.1 mg/kg I.M. as single dose, p.r.n. Allow at least 10 minutes to elapse before increasing dose because maximum effect is not immediately apparent.

ADVERSE REACTIONS
CNS: apprehension, restlessness, dizziness, headache, tremor, weakness; with excessive use, seizures.
CV: hypertension; hypotension; precordial pain; palpitations; arrhythmias, including sinus or ventricular tachycardia; bradycardia; premature supraventricular contractions; atrioventricular dissociation.
GI: nausea, vomiting.
GU: decreased urine output.
Metabolic: hyperglycemia.
Skin: flushing, pallor, sweating.
Local: abscess, necrosis, and sloughing upon extravasation.
Other: *metabolic acidosis in hypovolemia, increased body temperature, respiratory distress.*

INTERACTIONS
General anesthetics: increased risk of adverse cardiac effects. Monitor closely.
MAO inhibitors: may cause severe hypertension (hypertensive crisis). Don't use together.

NURSING CONSIDERATIONS
• Contraindicated in peripheral or mesenteric thrombosis, pulmonary edema, hypercarbia, or acidosis; also

---

Italicized adverse reactions are common or life-threatening.
*Liquid form contains alcohol.   **May contain tartrazine.

during anesthesia with cyclopropane and halogenated hydrocarbon anesthetics. Use cautiously in hypertension, thyroid disease, diabetes, cirrhosis, malaria, or sulfite sensitivity, and those receiving digitalis.

• Not a substitute for blood or fluid volume deficit. Volume deficit should be replaced before vasopressors are administered.

• Keep solution in light-resistant container, away from heat.

• Use large veins, as in the antecubital fossa, to minimize risk of extravasation. Watch infusion site carefully for signs of extravasation. If it occurs, stop infusion immediately and call doctor.

• During infusion, check blood pressure every 5 minutes until stabilized; then every 15 minutes. Check pulse rates, urine output, and color and temperature of extremities. Titrate infusion rate according to findings, using doctor's guidelines.

• Use a continuous infusion pump to regulate infusion flow rate.

• Observe patient closely for adverse effects. If adverse effects develop, dosage may need to be adjusted or discontinued.

• For I.V. therapy, use a piggyback setup so I.V. can continue if this drug is stopped.

• Blood pressure should be raised to slightly less than the patient's normal level. Be careful to avoid excessive blood pressure response. Rapidly induced hypertensive response can cause acute pulmonary edema, arrhythmias, and cardiac arrest.

• Because of prolonged action, a cumulative effect is possible. With an excessive vasopressor response, elevated blood pressure may persist after the drug is stopped.

• Urine output may decrease initially, then increase as blood pressure reaches normal level. Report persistent decreased urine output.

• When discontinuing therapy with this drug, slow infusion rate gradually. Continue monitoring vital signs, watching for possible severe drop in blood pressure. Keep equipment nearby to start drug again, if necessary. Pressor therapy should not be reinstated until the systolic blood pressure falls below 70 to 80 mm Hg.

• Keep emergency drugs on hand to reverse effects of metaraminol: atropine for reflex bradycardia; phentolamine to decrease vasopressor effects; and propranolol for arrhythmias.

• Closely monitor patients with diabetes. Adjustment in insulin dose may be needed.

• Metaraminol should not be mixed with other drugs.

norepinephrine injection (levarterenol bitartrate)
Levophed

Pregnancy Risk Category: D

HOW SUPPLIED
Injection: 1 mg/ml

MECHANISM OF ACTION
Stimulates alpha- and beta-adrenergic receptors within the sympathetic nervous system.

INDICATIONS & DOSAGE
To restore blood pressure in acute hypotensive states—
Adults: initially, 8 to 12 mcg/minute I.V. infusion, then adjust to maintain normal blood pressure. Average maintenance dosage is 2 to 4 mcg/minute.

ADVERSE REACTIONS
CNS: *headache,* anxiety, weakness, dizziness, tremor, restlessness, insomnia.
CV: bradycardia, severe hypertension, marked increase in peripheral resistance, decreased cardiac output, arrhythmias, *ventricular tachycardia, fibrillation,* bigeminal rhythm, atrio-

---

ventricular dissociation, precordial pain.
GU: *decreased urine output.*
Metabolic: *metabolic acidosis,* hyperglycemia, increased glycogenolysis.
Local: irritation with extravasation.
Other: fever, respiratory difficulty.

INTERACTIONS
Alpha-adrenergic blocking agents: may antagonize drug effects.
MAO inhibitors: increased risk of hypertensive crisis.
Tricyclic antidepressants: when given with sympathomimetics, may cause severe hypertension (hypertensive crisis). Don't give together.

NURSING CONSIDERATIONS
• Contraindicated in mesenteric or peripheral vascular thrombosis, pregnancy, profound hypoxia, hypercarbia, hypotension from blood volume deficits; and during cyclopropane and halothane anesthesia. Use cautiously in hypertension, hyperthyroidism, severe cardiac disease, and sulfite sensitivity. Use with extreme caution in patients receiving MAO inhibitors or tricyclic antidepressants.
• Not a substitute for blood or fluid volume deficit. Volume deficit should be replaced before vasopressors are administered.
• Norepinephrine solutions deteriorate after 24 hours.
• Use large vein, as in the antecubital fossa, to minimize risk of extravasation. Check site frequently for signs of extravasation. If it occurs, stop infusion immediately and call doctor. He may counteract effect by infiltrating area with 5 to 10 mg phentolamine and 10 to 15 ml normal saline solution. Also check for blanching along course of infused vein; may progress to superficial sloughing.
• During infusion, check blood pressure every 2 minutes until stabilized; then every 5 minutes. Also check pulse rates, urine output, and color and temperature of extremities. Titrate infusion rate according to findings, using doctor's guidelines. In previously hypertensive patients, blood pressure should be raised no more than 40 mm Hg below preexisting systolic pressure.
• Never leave patient unattended during infusion.
• Use a continuous infusion pump to regulate infusion flow rate.
• For I.V. therapy, use a piggyback setup so I.V. can continue if norepinephrine is stopped.
• Report decreased urine output to doctor immediately.
• If prolonged I.V. therapy is necessary, change injection site frequently.
• When stopping drug, slow infusion rate gradually. Monitor vital signs, even after drug is stopped. Watch for severe drop in blood pressure.
• Keep emergency drugs on hand to reverse effects of norepinephrine: atropine for reflex bradycardia; phentolamine for increased vasopressor effects; and propranolol for arrhythmias.
• Administer in dextrose 5% in water and saline solution; saline solution alone is not recommended.

---

phenylephrine hydrochloride
Neo-Synephrine
Pregnancy Risk Category: C

HOW SUPPLIED
Injection: 10 mg/ml

MECHANISM OF ACTION
Predominantly stimulates alpha-adrenergic receptors in the sympathetic nervous system.

INDICATIONS & DOSAGE
Hypotensive emergencies during spinal anesthesia—

Italicized adverse reactions are common or life-threatening.
*Liquid form contains alcohol.   **May contain tartrazine.

Adults: initially, 0.2 mg I.V., then subsequent doses of 0.1 to 0.2 mg.
Maintenance of blood pressure during spinal or inhalation anesthesia—
Adults: 2 to 3 mg S.C. or I.M. 3 or 4 minutes before anesthesia.
Children: 0.04 mg to 0.088 mg/kg S.C. or I.M.
Mild to moderate hypotension—
Adults: 2 to 5 mg S.C. or I.M.; 0.1 to 0.5 mg I.V. Not to be repeated more often than 10 to 15 minutes.
Paroxysmal supraventricular tachycardia—
Adults: initially, 0.5 mg rapid I.V.; subsequent doses should not exceed the preceding dose by more than 0.1 to 0.2 mg and should not exceed 1 mg.
Prolongation of spinal anesthesia—
Adults: 2 to 5 mg added to anesthetic solution.
Severe hypotension and shock (including drug-induced)—
Adults: 10 mg in 500 ml dextrose 5% in water. Start 100 to 180 drops per minute I.V. infusion, then 40 to 60 drops per minute. Adjust to patient response.
Vasoconstrictor for regional anesthesia—
Adults: 1 mg phenylephrine added to 20 ml local anesthetic.

ADVERSE REACTIONS
CNS: *headache, restlessness, light-headedness, weakness.*
CV: palpitations, bradycardia, arrhythmias, hypertension, anginal pain.
EENT: blurred vision.
Skin: goose bumps, feeling of coolness.
Local: tissue sloughing with extravasation.
Other: tachyphylaxis may occur with continued use.

INTERACTIONS
MAO inhibitors: may cause severe hypertension (hypertensive crisis). Don't use together.
Oxytocics, tricyclic antidepressants: increased pressor response. Observe patient.

NURSING CONSIDERATIONS
• Contraindicated in narrow-angle glaucoma, hypotension, ventricular tachycardia, severe coronary disease, or cardiovascular disease (including myocardial infarction), and in patients who are taking MAO inhibitors or tricyclic antidepressants. Use with extreme caution in patients with heart disease, hyperthyroidism, diabetes, severe atherosclerosis, bradycardia, partial heart block, myocardial disease, sulfite sensitivity, and in elderly patients.
• Longer acting than ephedrine and epinephrine.
• Causes little or no CNS stimulation.
• Monitor blood pressure frequently. Avoid excessive rise in blood pressure. Maintain blood pressure at slightly below the patient's normal level. In previously normotensive patients, maintain systolic blood pressure at 80 to 100 mm Hg; in previously hypertensive patients, maintain systolic blood pressure at 30 to 40 mm Hg below their usual level.
• May reverse severe increase in blood pressure with phentolamine.
• With I.V. infusions, avoid abrupt withdrawal. Monitor blood pressure throughout. Reverse therapy if blood pressure falls too rapidly.

---

†Available in Canada only.   ‡Available in Australia only.   ◊ Available OTC.

pseudoephedrine hydrochloride

Cenafed◇, Children's Sudafed Liquid◇, Decofed◇, Dorcol Children's Decongestant◇, Eltor†◇, Genaphed◇, Halofed◇, NeoFed◇, Robidrine◇, Ornex Cold†◇, Pediacare Infant's Oral Decongestant Drops◇, Pseudofrin†◇, Pseudogest◇, Sinufed◇, Sudafed◇, Sudafed 12-Hour◇, Sudrin◇, Sufedrin◇

pseudoephedrine sulfate

Afrinol Repetabs

Pregnancy Risk Category: C

HOW SUPPLIED
Tablets: 30 mg◇, 60 mg◇
Tablets (extended-release): 120 mg◇
Oral solution: 15 mg/5 ml◇, 30 mg/5 ml◇, 7.5 mg/0.8 ml◇

MECHANISM OF ACTION
Stimulates alpha-adrenergic receptors in the respiratory tract, producing vasoconstriction.

INDICATIONS & DOSAGE
Nasal and eustachian tube decongestant—
Adults: 60 mg P.O. q 4 hours. Maximum dosage is 240 mg daily.
Children 6 to 12 years: 30 mg P.O. q 4 hours. Maximum dosage is 120 mg daily.
Children 2 to 6 years: 15 mg P.O. q 4 hours. Maximum dosage is 60 mg/day.
Extended-release tablets:
Adults and children over 12 years: 60 to 120 mg P.O. q 12 hours. This form is contraindicated for children under 12 years.
Relief of nasal congestion—
Adults: 120 mg q 12 hours.

ADVERSE REACTIONS
CNS: *anxiety,* transient stimulation, tremors, dizziness, headache, insomnia, *nervousness.*
CV: arrhythmias, *palpitations,* tachycardia.
EENT: dry mouth.
GI: anorexia, nausea, vomiting.
GU: difficulty in urinating.
Skin: pallor.

INTERACTIONS
Antihypertensives: hypotensive effect may be attenuated.
MAO inhibitors: may cause severe hypertension (hypertensive crisis). Don't use together.

NURSING CONSIDERATIONS
• Contraindicated in severe hypertension or severe coronary artery disease; in patients receiving MAO inhibitors; and in breast-feeding women. Use cautiously in hypertension, cardiac disease, diabetes, glaucoma, hyperthyroidism, and prostatic hypertrophy.
• Elderly patients are more sensitive to the drug's effects.
• Tell patient to stop drug if he becomes unusually restless and to notify doctor promptly.
• Warn against using OTC products containing other sympathomimetic amines.
• Tell patient not to take drug within 2 hours of bedtime because it can cause insomnia.
• Tell patient to relieve dry mouth with sugarless gum or sour hard candy.

Italicized adverse reactions are common or life-threatening.
*Liquid form contains alcohol.   **May contain tartrazine.

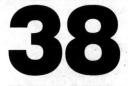

Adrenergic blockers (sympatholytics)

**dihydroergotamine mesylate
ergotamine tartrate
methysergide maleate
phenoxybenzamine
hydrochloride**
(See Chapter 22, ANTIHYPERTENSIVES.)
propranolol hydrochloride
(See Chapter 21, ANTIANGINALS.)

COMBINATION PRODUCTS
CAFERGOT: ergotamine tartrate 1 mg
and caffeine 100 mg.
CAFERGOT SUPPOSITORIES: ergotamine tartrate 2 mg and caffeine 100
mg.
ERGOCAFF: ergotamine tartrate 1 mg
and caffeine 100 mg.
MIGRAL: ergotamine tartrate 1 mg,
caffeine 50 mg, and cyclizine hydrochloride 25 mg.
WIGRAINE: ergotamine tartrate 1 mg,
caffeine 100 mg, levorotatory belladonna alkaloids 0.1 mg, and phenace-
tin 130 mg.
WIGRAINE SUPPOSITORIES: ergotamine tartrate 2 mg, caffeine 100 mg,
and tartaric acid 21.5 mg.

---

dihydroergotamine mesylate
D.H.E. 45, Dihydergot‡

Pregnancy Risk Category: X

HOW SUPPLIED
Injection: 1 mg/ml

MECHANISM OF ACTION
Inhibits the effects of epinephrine,
norepinephrine, and other sympathomimetic amines. Also has antiserotonin effects.

INDICATIONS & DOSAGE
Vascular or migraine headache—
Adults: 1 mg I.M. or I.V. May repeat
q 1 to 2 hours, p.r.n., up to total of 3
mg per attack. Maximum weekly dosage is 6 mg.

ADVERSE REACTIONS
CV: numbness and tingling in fingers
and toes, transient tachycardia or bradycardia, precordial distress and
pain, increased arterial pressure.
GI: nausea, vomiting.
Skin: itching.
Other: weakness in legs, muscle
pains in extremities, localized edema.

INTERACTIONS
Propranolol and other beta blockers:
blocked natural pathway for vasodilation in patients receiving ergot alkaloids and thus could result in excessive vasoconstriction. Watch closely if
drugs are used together.

NURSING CONSIDERATIONS
• Contraindicated in pregnancy and
in peripheral and occlusive vascular
disease, coronary artery disease, hypertension, hepatic or renal dysfunction, sepsis.
• Avoid prolonged administration;
don't exceed recommended dosage.
• Tell patient to report any feeling of
coldness in extremities or tingling of
fingers and toes from vasoconstriction. Severe vasoconstriction may result in tissue damage.

• Most effective when used at first sign of migraine or soon after onset. Provide a quiet, low-light environment to help patient relax.
• Help patient evaluate underlying causes of stress.
• Protect ampules from heat and light. Discard if solution is discolored.
• Best results are obtained by adjusting the dose in order to determine the most effective, minimal dose.
• Ergotamine rebound, or an increase in frequency and duration of headache, may occur when the drug is stopped.
• For short-term use only.

---

ergotamine tartrate
Ergomar, Ergostat, Gynergen†, Medihaler-Ergotamine

Pregnancy Risk Category: X

HOW SUPPLIED
Tablets (sublingual): 2 mg
Aerosal inhaler: 360 mcg/metered spray
Suppositories: 2 mg

MECHANISM OF ACTION
Inhibits the effects of epinephrine, norepinephrine, and other sympathomimetic amines. Also has antiserotonin effects.

INDICATIONS & DOSAGE
Vascular or migraine headache—
Adults: initially, 2 mg P.O. or S.L., then 1 to 2 mg P.O. q hour or S.L. q ½ hour, to maximum of 6 mg daily and 10 mg weekly. Alternatively, use aerosol inhaler: 1 spray (360 mcg) initially, repeated every 5 minutes p.r.n. to a maximum of 6 sprays (2.16 mg) per 24 hours or 15 sprays (5.4 mg) per week.

Patient may also use rectal suppositories. Initially, 2 mg rectally at the onset of the attack, repeated in 1 hour p.r.n. Maximum dose is 2 suppositories per attack or 5 suppositories per week.

ADVERSE REACTIONS
CV: numbness and tingling in fingers and toes, *transient tachycardia or bradycardia,* precordial distress and pain, increased arterial pressure, angina pectoris.
GI: nausea, vomiting, diarrhea, abdominal cramps.
Skin: itching.
Other: weakness in legs, muscle pains in extremities, localized edema.

INTERACTIONS
Propranolol and other beta blockers: blocked natural pathway for vasodilation in patients receiving ergot alkaloids and thus could result in excessive vasoconstriction. Watch closely if drugs are used together.

NURSING CONSIDERATIONS
• Contraindicated in pregnancy and in peripheral and occlusive vascular diseases, coronary artery disease, hypertension, hepatic or renal dysfunction, sepsis.
• Avoid prolonged administration; don't exceed recommended dosage.
• Most effective when used during prodromal stage of headache or as soon as possible after onset.
• Provide a quiet, low-light environment to help patient relax.
• Help patient evaluate underlying causes of physical or emotional stress, which may precipitate attacks.
• Prolonged exposure to cold weather should be avoided whenever possible. Cold may increase many of the adverse reactions.
• Instruct patient on long-term therapy to check for and report feeling of coldness in extremities or tingling of fingers and toes due to vasoconstriction. Severe vasoconstriction may result in tissue damage.
• Store drug in light-resistant container.

Italicized adverse reactions are common or life-threatening.
*Liquid form contains alcohol.   **May contain tartrazine.

- Sublingual tablet is preferred during early stage of attack because of its rapid absorption.
- Warn patient not to increase dosage without first consulting the doctor.
- Obtain an accurate dietary history from patient to determine if a relationship exists between certain foods and onset of headache.
- Ergotamine rebound, or an increase in frequency and duration of headache, may occur if the drug is stopped.
- Instruct patient how to use the inhaler correctly.

methysergide maleate
Deseril‡, Sansert**

Pregnancy Risk Category: C

HOW SUPPLIED
Tablets: 1 mg‡, 2 mg

MECHANISM OF ACTION
Specifically blocks serotonin (a neurotransmitter).

INDICATIONS & DOSAGE
Prevention of frequent, severe, uncontrollable, or disabling migraine or vascular headache—
Adults: 4 to 8 mg P.O. daily with meals.
To control diarrhea caused by carcinoid disease—
Adults: initially, 2 mg P.O. t.i.d., increased p.r.n. to 4 to 16 mg t.i.d.

ADVERSE REACTIONS
Blood: neutropenia, eosinophilia.
CNS: insomnia, drowsiness, *euphoria, vertigo*, ataxia, *light-headedness*, hyperesthesia, weakness, *hallucinations or feelings of dissociation*.
CV: *fibrotic thickening of cardiac valves and aorta, inferior vena cava, and common iliac branches (retroperitoneal fibrosis);* vasoconstriction, causing chest pain, abdominal pain, vascular insufficiency of lower limbs;

cold, numb, painful extremities with or without paresthesias and diminished or absent pulses; postural hypotension; tachycardia; peripheral edema; murmurs; bruits.
EENT: nasal stuffiness.
GI: nausea, vomiting, diarrhea, constipation, epigastric pain.
Skin: hair loss, dermatitis, sweating, flushing, rash.
Other: *retroperitoneal fibrosis,* causing general malaise, fatigue, weight gain, backache, low-grade fever, urinary obstruction; *pulmonary fibrosis,* causing dyspnea, tightness and pain in chest, pleural friction rubs and effusion, arthralgia, myalgia.

INTERACTIONS
None significant.

NURSING CONSIDERATIONS
- Contraindicated in severe hypertension, arteriosclerosis, peripheral vascular insufficiency, renal or hepatic disease, severe coronary artery diseases, thromboembolic disorders, phlebitis or cellulitis of lower limbs, fibrotic processes, valvular heart disease; and in debilitated patients. Use cautiously in peptic ulcers or suspected coronary artery disease. ECG and cardiac status evaluation advisable before giving to patients over 40 years.
- GI effects may be prevented by gradual introduction of medication and by administering with meals.
- Obtain laboratory studies of cardiac and renal function, blood count, and sedimentation rate before and during therapy.
- Drug may be gradually withdrawn every 6 months; then restart after at least 3 or 4 weeks.
- Tell patient not to stop drug abruptly; may cause rebound headaches. Stop gradually over 2 to 3 weeks.
- Patient should keep daily weight record and report unusually rapid

weight gain. Teach him to check for peripheral edema. Explain and suggest low-salt diet if necessary.
• Give drug for 3 weeks before evaluating effectiveness.
• Tell patient to report to doctor promptly if he experiences cold, numb, or painful hands and feet; leg cramps when walking; pelvic, chest, or flank pain.
• Not for treatment of migraine or vascular headache in progress or for treatment of tension (muscle contraction) headaches.
• Indicated only for patients who are unresponsive to other drugs and who can be kept under close medical supervision.

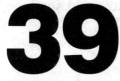

Skeletal muscle relaxants

baclofen
carisoprodol
chlorphenesin carbamate
chlorzoxazone
cyclobenzaprine
dantrolene sodium
methocarbamol
orphenadrine citrate

COMBINATION PRODUCTS
BLANEX: chlorzoxazone 250 mg and acetaminophen 300 mg.
CHLOROFON-F: chlorzoxazone 250 mg and acetaminophen 300 mg.
CHLORZONE FORTE: chlorzoxazone 250 mg and acetaminophen 300 mg.
LOBAC: chlorzoxazone 250 mg and acetaminophen 300 mg.
MUS-LAX: chlorzoxazone 250 mg and acetaminophen 300 mg.
NORGESIC: orphenadrine citrate 25 mg, aspirin 385 mg, and caffeine 30 mg.
NORGESIC FORTE: orphenadrine citrate 50 mg, aspirin 770 mg, and caffeine 60 mg.
PARACET FORTE: chlorzoxazone 250 mg and acetaminophen 300 mg.
POLYFLEX: chlorzoxazone 250 mg and acetaminophen 300 mg.
ROBAXISAL: methocarbamol 400 mg and aspirin 325 mg.
SKELEX: chlorzoxazone 250 mg and acetaminophen 300 mg.
SOMA COMPOUND: carisoprodol 200 mg and aspirin 325 mg.
SOMA COMPOUND WITH CODEINE: carisoprodol 200 mg, aspirin 325 mg, caffeine 32 mg, and codeine phosphate 16 mg.

ZOXAPHEN: chlorzoxazone 250 mg and acetaminophen 300 mg.

---

baclofen
Lioresal, Lioresal DS

Pregnancy Risk Category: C

HOW SUPPLIED
Tablets: 10 mg, 20 mg, 25 mg‡

MECHANISM OF ACTION
Reduces transmission of impulses from the spinal cord to skeletal muscle.

INDICATIONS & DOSAGE
Spasticity in multiple sclerosis, spinal cord injury—
Adults: initially, 5 mg P.O. t.i.d. for 3 days, 10 mg t.i.d. for 3 days, 15 mg t.i.d. for 3 days, 20 mg t.i.d. for 3 days. Increase according to response up to maximum of 80 mg daily.

ADVERSE REACTIONS
CNS: *drowsiness, dizziness,* headache, *weakness, fatigue,* confusion, insomnia, dysarthria, *seizures.*
CV: hypotension.
EENT: nasal congestion, blurred vision.
GI: *nausea,* constipation.
GU: urinary frequency.
Hepatic: increased AST (SGOT) and alkaline phosphatase.
Metabolic: hyperglycemia.
Skin: rash, pruritus.
Other: ankle edema, excessive perspiration, weight gain.

INTERACTIONS
Alcohol, CNS depressants: increased CNS depression.

NURSING CONSIDERATIONS
• Use cautiously in impaired renal function, stroke (minimal benefit, poor tolerance), epilepsy, and when spasticity is used to maintain motor function.
• Give with meals or milk to prevent GI distress.
• Amount of relief determines if dosage (and drowsiness) can be reduced.
• Tell patient to avoid activities that require alertness until CNS effects of the drug are known. Drowsiness is usually transient.
• Watch for increased incidence of seizures in epileptics.
• Watch for sensitivity reactions, such as fever, skin eruptions, and respiratory distress.
• Advise patient to follow doctor's orders regarding rest and physical therapy.
• Do not withdraw abruptly unless required by severe adverse reactions; may precipitate hallucinations or rebound spasticity.
• Overdosage treatment is supportive only; do not induce emesis or use a respiratory stimulant in obtunded patients.
• Used investigationally for treatment of unstable bladder.

---

carisoprodol
Rela, Sodol, Soma, Soprodol, Soridol

Pregnancy Risk Category: C

HOW SUPPLIED
Tablets: 350 mg

MECHANISM OF ACTION
Reduces transmission of impulses from the spinal cord to skeletal muscle.

INDICATIONS & DOSAGE
As an adjunct in acute, painful musculoskeletal conditions—
Adults and children over 12 years: 350 mg P.O. t.i.d. and h.s.
  Not recommended for children under 12 years.

ADVERSE REACTIONS
CNS: *drowsiness, dizziness,* vertigo, ataxia, tremor, agitation, irritability, headache, depressive reactions, insomnia.
CV: orthostatic hypotension, tachycardia, facial flushing.
GI: nausea, vomiting, hiccups, increased bowel activity, epigastric distress.
Skin: rash, *erythema multiforme,* pruritus.
Other: asthmatic episodes, fever, angioneurotic edema, *anaphylaxis.*

INTERACTIONS
Alcohol, CNS depressants: increased CNS depression.

NURSING CONSIDERATIONS
• Contraindicated in hypersensitivity to related compounds (e.g., meprobamate, tybamate) or intermittent porphyria. Use with caution in impaired hepatic or renal function.
• Watch for idiosyncratic reactions after first to fourth dose (weakness, ataxia, visual and speech difficulties, fever, skin eruptions, and mental changes) or severe reactions, including bronchospasm, hypotension, and anaphylactic shock. Withhold dose and notify doctor immediately of any unusual reactions.
• Record amount of relief to determine whether dosage can be reduced.
• Warn patient to avoid activities that require alertness until CNS effects of the drug are known. Drowsiness is transient.
• Avoid combining with alcohol or other depressants.
• Advise patient to follow doctor's or-

Italicized adverse reactions are common or life-threatening.
*Liquid form contains alcohol.   **May contain tartrazine.

ders regarding rest and physical therapy.
• Do not stop drug abruptly, mild withdrawal effects, such as insomnia, headache, nausea, and abdominal cramps, may result.

chlorphenesin carbamate
Maolate**

Pregnancy Risk Category: C

HOW SUPPLIED
Tablets: 400 mg

MECHANISM OF ACTION
Reduces transmission of impulses from the spinal cord to skeletal muscle.

INDICATIONS & DOSAGE
As an adjunct in short-term, acute, painful musculoskeletal conditions—
Adults: initial dose is 800 mg P.O. t.i.d. Maintenance dose is 400 mg P.O. q.i.d. for maximum of 8 weeks.

ADVERSE REACTIONS
Blood: thrombocytopenia, leukopenia, *agranulocytosis.*
CNS: *drowsiness, dizziness,* confusion, headache, weakness. Dose-related adverse reactions include paradoxical stimulation, agitation, insomnia, nervousness, headache.
GI: *nausea, GI distress.*
Other: *anaphylaxis.*

INTERACTIONS
Alcohol and CNS depressants: increased CNS depression.

NURSING CONSIDERATIONS
• Use cautiously in hepatic disease or impaired renal function, and in patients hypersensitive to aspirin.
• Safe use for periods over 8 weeks not established.
• Take with meals or milk to prevent GI distress.
• Amount of relief determines if dosage (and drowsiness) can be reduced.

• Watch for sensitivity reactions, such as fever, skin eruptions, and respiratory distress. Withhold dose and notify doctor of unusual reactions.
• Monitor CBC and platelet studies in patients on long-term therapy. Watch for unusual bleeding and infections that may indicate blood dyscrasia.
• Tell patient to avoid activities that require mental alertness (such as driving or operating heavy machinery) until adverse CNS effects of the drug are known.

chlorzoxazone
Paraflex, Parafon Forte DSC, Strifon Forte DSC

Pregnancy Risk Category: C

HOW SUPPLIED
Tablets: 250 mg
Caplets: 500 mg

MECHANISM OF ACTION
Reduces transmission of impulses from the spinal cord to skeletal muscle.

INDICATIONS & DOSAGE
As an adjunct in acute, painful musculoskeletal conditions—
Adults: 250 to 750 mg P.O. t.i.d. or q.i.d.
Children: 20 mg/kg P.O. daily in divided doses t.i.d. or q.i.d.

ADVERSE REACTIONS
Blood: anemia, granulocytopenia.
CNS: *drowsiness, dizziness, lightheadedness,* malaise, headache, overstimulation.
GI: anorexia, nausea, vomiting, heartburn, abdominal distress, constipation, diarrhea.
GU: urine discoloration (orange or purple-red).
Hepatic: hepatic dysfunction.
Skin: urticaria, redness, itching, petechiae, bruising.

---

†Available in Canada only.   ‡Available in Australia only.   ◊Available OTC.

INTERACTIONS
Alcohol and CNS depressants: increased CNS depression.

NURSING CONSIDERATIONS
• Contraindicated in impaired hepatic function. Use cautiously in history of drug allergies.
• Amount of relief determines if dosage (and drowsiness) can be reduced.
• Watch for signs of hepatic dysfunction. Withhold dose and notify doctor.
• Warn patient to avoid activities that require alertness until CNS effects of the drug are known. Drowsiness is usually mild and transient.
• Avoid combining with alcohol or other depressants.
• Tell patient that the drug may discolor urine orange or purple-red.
• Advise patient to follow doctor's orders regarding rest and physical therapy.
• Give with meals or milk to prevent GI distress.

---

cyclobenzaprine
Flexeril

Pregnancy Risk Category: B

HOW SUPPLIED
Tablets: 10 mg

MECHANISM OF ACTION
Reduces transmission of impulses from the spinal cord to skeletal muscle.

INDICATIONS & DOSAGE
Short-term treatment of muscle spasm—
Adults: 10 mg P.O. t.i.d. for 7 days. Maximum dosage is 60 mg daily for 2 to 3 weeks.

ADVERSE REACTIONS
CNS: *drowsiness,* euphoria, weakness, headache, insomnia, nightmares, paresthesias, dizziness, depression, visual disturbances, precipitation of seizures.

CV: tachycardia.
EENT: blurred vision, dry mouth.
GI: abdominal pain, dyspepsia, peculiar taste, constipation.
GU: urine retention.
Skin: rash, urticaria, pruritus.
Other: in high doses, watch for adverse reactions like those of other tricyclic drugs (e.g., amitriptyline, imipramine).

INTERACTIONS
None significant.

NURSING CONSIDERATIONS
• Contraindicated in patients who have received MAO inhibitors within 14 days; during acute recovery phase of myocardial infarction; in heart block, arrhythmias, conduction disturbances, or CHF. Use cautiously in urine retention, narrow-angle glaucoma, increased intraocular pressure, cardiovascular disease, impaired hepatic function, and seizures; and in elderly or debilitated patients.
• Withdrawal symptoms (nausea, headache, and malaise) may occur if drug is stopped abruptly after long-term use.
• Watch for symptoms of overdose, including possible cardiotoxicity. Notify doctor immediately and have physostigmine available.
• Advise patient to report urinary hesitancy or urine retention. If constipation is a problem, increase fluid intake and get an order for a stool softener.
• Warn patient to avoid activities that require alertness until CNS effects of the drug are known. Drowsiness and dizziness usually subside after 2 weeks.
• Avoid combining alcohol or other depressants with cyclobenzaprine.
• Tell patient that dry mouth may be relieved with sugarless candy or gum.

Italicized adverse reactions are common or life-threatening.
*Liquid form contains alcohol.   **May contain tartrazine.

dantrolene sodium
Dantrium, Dantrium I.V.

Pregnancy Risk Category: C

HOW SUPPLIED
Capsules: 25 mg, 50 mg, 100 mg
Injection: 20 mg/vial

MECHANISM OF ACTION
Acts directly on skeletal muscle to interfere with intracellular calcium
movement.

INDICATIONS & DOSAGE
Spasticity and sequelae secondary to
severe chronic disorders (multiple
sclerosis, cerebral palsy, spinal cord
injury, stroke)—
Adults: 25 mg P.O. daily. Increase
gradually in increments of 25 mg at 4-
to 7-day intervals, up to 100 mg b.i.d.
to q.i.d., to maximum of 400 mg
daily.
Children: 1 mg/kg daily P.O. b.i.d.
to q.i.d. Increase gradually as needed
by 1 mg/kg daily to maximum of 100
mg q.i.d.
Management of malignant hyperther-
mia—
Adults and children: 1 mg/kg I.V.
initially; may repeat dose up to cumulative dose of 10 mg/kg.
Prevention or attenuation of malignant
hyperthermia in susceptible patients
who require surgery—
Adults: 4 to 8 mg/kg P.O. daily given
in three to four divided doses for 1 to
2 days before procedure. Administer
final dose 3 to 4 hours before procedure.
Prevention of recurrence of malignant
hyperthermia—
Adults: 4 to 8 mg/kg/day P.O. given
in four divided doses for up to 3 days
following hyperthermic crisis.

ADVERSE REACTIONS
CNS: *muscle weakness, drowsiness,*
dizziness, light-headedness, malaise,
headache, confusion, nervousness, insomnia, exacerbation of precipitation
of seizures.
CV: tachycardia, blood pressure
changes.
EENT: excessive tearing, visual disturbances.
GI: anorexia, constipation, cramping,
dysphagia, metallic taste, *severe diar-*
rhea.
GU: urinary frequency, incontinence,
nocturia, dysuria, crystalluria, difficulty achieving erection.
Hepatic: *hepatitis.*
Skin: eczematous eruption, pruritus,
urticaria, photosensitivity.
Other: abnormal hair growth, drool-
ing, sweating, pleural effusion, myalgia, chills, fever.

INTERACTIONS
Alcohol, CNS depressants: increased
CNS depression. Monitor for decreased alertness.
Verapamil (I.V.): may result in cardiovascular collapse. Stop drug before
administering I.V. dantrolene.

NURSING CONSIDERATIONS
The following are considerations for
the P.O. form only:
• Contraindicated when spasticity is
used to maintain motor function; in
spasms in rheumatic disorders; and in
lactation. Use with caution in severely
impaired cardiac or pulmonary function or preexisting hepatic disease; in
women; and in patients over 35 years.
• Safety and efficacy in long-term use
not established; value may be determined by therapeutic trial. Do not
give more than 45 days if no benefits
are obtained.
• Give with meals or milk to prevent
GI distress.
• Prepare oral suspension for single
dose by dissolving capsule contents in
juice or other suitable liquid. For multiple doses, use acid vehicle, such as
citric acid in USP syrup; refrigerate.
Use within several days.

• Amount of relief determines if dosage (and drowsiness) can be reduced.
• Liver function tests should be performed at the beginning of therapy.
• Watch for hepatitis (fever and jaundice), severe diarrhea, severe weakness, or sensitivity reactions (fever and skin eruptions). Withhold dose and notify doctor.
• Warn patient to avoid driving and other hazardous activities until CNS effects of the drug are known. Adverse reactions should subside after 4 days.
• Tell patient to avoid combining with alcohol or other depressants; to avoid photosensitivity reactions by using sunscreening agents and protective clothing; to report abdominal discomfort or GI problems immediately; and to follow doctor's orders regarding rest and physical therapy.
The following are considerations for the I.V. form only:
• Administer as soon as malignant hyperthermia reaction is recognized.
• Reconstitute each vial by adding 60 ml of sterile water for injection and shaking vial until clear. Don't use a diluent that contains a bacteriostatic agent.
• Protect contents from light and use within 6 hours.
• Be careful to avoid extravasation.
• Has been used to treat neuroleptic malignant syndrome.

---

methocarbamol
Delaxin, Marbaxin-750, Robaxin, Robomol-500, Robomol-750

Pregnancy Risk Category: C

HOW SUPPLIED
Tablets: 500 mg, 750 mg
Injection: 100 mg/ml

MECHANISM OF ACTION
Reduces transmission of impulses from the spinal cord to skeletal muscle.

INDICATIONS & DOSAGE
As an adjunct in acute, painful musculoskeletal conditions—
Adults: 1.5 g P.O. for 2 to 3 days, then 1 g P.O. q.i.d., or not more than 500 ml (5 ml) I.M. into each gluteal region. May repeat q 8 hours. Or 1 to 3 g daily (10 to 30 ml) I.V. directly into vein at 3 ml/minute, or 10 ml may be added to no more than 250 ml of dextrose 5% in water or normal saline solution. Maximum dosage is 3 g daily.
Supportive therapy in tetanus management—
Adults: 1 to 2 g into tubing of running I.V. or 1 to 3 g in infusion bottle q 6 hours.
Children: 15 mg/kg I.V. q 6 hours.

ADVERSE REACTIONS
Blood: hemolysis, increased hemoglobin (I.V. only).
CNS: drowsiness, dizziness, light-headedness, headache, syncope, mild muscular incoordination (I.M. or I.V. only), seizures (I.V. only).
CV: hypotension, bradycardia (I.M. or I.V. only).
GI: nausea, anorexia, GI upset, metallic taste.
GU: hematuria (I.V. only), discoloration of urine.
Skin: urticaria, pruritus, rash.
Local: thrombophlebitis, extravasation (I.V. only).
Other: fever, flushing, *anaphylactic reactions* (I.M. or I.V. only).

INTERACTIONS
Alcohol and CNS depressants: increased CNS depression.

NURSING CONSIDERATIONS
• Contraindicated in impaired renal function (injectable form), myasthenia gravis, epilepsy (injectable form); in children under 12 years (except in tetanus); and in patients receiving anticholinesterase agents.
• I.V. irritates veins, may cause phle-

Italicized adverse reactions are common or life-threatening.
*Liquid form contains alcohol.   **May contain tartrazine.

bitis, aggravate seizures, and may cause fainting if injected rapidly.
• Give I.V. slowly. Maximum rate 300 mg (3 ml)/minute. Give I.M. deeply, only in upper outer quadrant of buttocks, with maximum of 5 ml in each buttock, and inject slowly. Do not give subcutaneously.
• In tetanus management, use methocarbamol with tetanus antitoxin, penicillin, tracheotomy, and aggressive supportive care. Long course of I.V. methocarbamol required.
• Watch for sensitivity reactions, such as fever and skin eruptions.
• Warn patient to avoid activities that require alertness until CNS effects of the drug are known. Drowsiness subsides.
• Avoid combining with alcohol or other depressants.
• Advise patient to follow doctor's orders regarding rest and physical therapy.
• Tell patient urine may turn green, black, or brown.
• Give with meals or milk to prevent GI distress.
• Watch for orthostatic hypotension, especially with parenteral administration. Keep patient supine for 15 minutes afterward, and supervise ambulation. Advise patient to get up slowly.
• Have epinephrine, antihistamines, and corticosteroids available.
• Prepare liquid by crushing tablets into water or saline solution. Give through nasogastric tube.
• Obtain CBC periodically during prolonged therapy.
• May interfere with urine tests for 5-hydroxyindoleacetic acid (5-HIAA) and vanillylmandelic acid (VMA).

---

orphenadrine citrate
Banflex, Flexoject, Flexon, K-Flex, Marflex, Myolin, Neocyten, Noradex, Norflex, O-Flex, Orflagen, Orphenate

Pregnancy Risk Category: C

HOW SUPPLIED
Tablets: 100 mg
Tablets (sustained-release): 100 mg
Injection: 30 mg/ml

MECHANISM OF ACTION
Reduces transmission of impulses from the spinal cord to skeletal muscle.

INDICATIONS & DOSAGE
Adjunctive treatment in painful, acute musculoskeletal conditions—
Adults: 100 mg P.O. b.i.d., or 60 mg I.V. or I.M. q 12 hours, p.r.n. For maintenance, switch to oral therapy beginning 12 hours after last parenteral dose.

ADVERSE REACTIONS
Blood: *aplastic anemia.*
CNS: disorientation, restlessness, irritability, weakness, *drowsiness,* headache, dizziness.
CV: palpitations, tachycardia.
EENT: dilated pupils, blurred vision, difficulty swallowing.
GI: constipation, *dry mouth,* nausea, vomiting, paralytic ileus, epigastric distress.
GU: urinary hesitancy or urine retention.

INTERACTIONS
Alcohol, other CNS depressants: increased CNS depression.

NURSING CONSIDERATIONS
• Contraindicated in narrow-angle glaucoma; prostatic hypertrophy; pyloric, duodenal, or bladder-neck obstruction; myasthenia gravis; tachycardia; severe hepatic or renal disease; or ulcerative colitis. Use cau-

tiously in elderly or debilitated patients with cardiac disease, arrhythmias, sulfite sensitivity, and those exposed to high temperatures.
• Check all dosages carefully. Even a slight overdose can lead to toxicity. Early signs are excessive dry mouth, dilated pupils, blurred vision, skin flushing, and fever.
• Monitor vital signs carefully.
• With I.V. administration, inject the drug over a period of approximately 5 minutes while patient is supine. Wait 5 to 10 minutes and then help patient to sit up.
• When given I.V., may cause paradoxical initial bradycardia. Usually disappears in 2 minutes.
• Have patient report urinary hesitancy and urine retention. Orphenadrine is an anticholinergic. Have patient void before taking the drug.
• Relieve dry mouth with cool drinks, sugarless gum, or hard candy.
• Monitor CBC and urinalysis in patients receiving drug over extended periods.
• Advise patients to avoid hazardous tasks (such as driving or operating heavy machinery) until CNS effects of the drug are known.

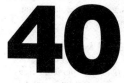

Neuromuscular blockers

atracurium besylate
gallamine triethiodide
hexafluorenium bromide
metocurine iodide
pancuronium bromide
succinylcholine chloride
tubocurarine chloride
vecuronium bromide

COMBINATION PRODUCTS
None.

---

atracurium besylate
Tracrium

Pregnancy Risk Category: C

HOW SUPPLIED
Injection: 10 mg/ml

MECHANISM OF ACTION
Prevents acetylcholine from binding to the receptors on the muscle end plate, thus blocking depolarization. Nondepolarizing agent.

INDICATIONS & DOSAGE
Adjunct to general anesthesia, to facilitate endotracheal intubation and to provide skeletal muscle relaxation during surgery or mechanical ventilation—
Dose depends on anesthetic used, individual needs, and response. Doses are representative and must be adjusted.
Adults and children over 2 years:
0.4 to 0.5 mg/kg by I.V. bolus. Maintenance dose of 0.08 to 0.10 mg/kg within 20 to 45 minutes of initial dose should be administered during pro-

longed surgical procedures. Maintenance doses may be administered q 12 to 25 minutes in patients receiving balanced anesthesia. For prolonged procedures, a constant infusion of 5 to 9 mcg/kg/minute may be used.
Children 1 month to 2 years: initial dose, 0.3 to 0.4 mg/kg. Frequent maintenance doses may be needed.

ADVERSE REACTIONS
CV: bradycardia.
Skin: skin flush, erythema, pruritus, urticaria.
Other: *prolonged dose-related apnea, wheezing, increased bronchial secretions.*

INTERACTIONS
Aminoglycoside antibiotics (including amikacin, gentamicin, kanamycin, neomycin, streptomycin); polymyxin antibiotics (polymyxin B sulfate, colistin); clindamycin; quinidine; general anesthetics such as halothane, enflurane, and isoflurane: potentiated neuromuscular blockade, leading to increased skeletal muscle relaxation and possible respiratory paralysis. Use cautiously during surgical and postoperative periods.
Lithium, narcotic analgesics: potentiated neuromuscular blockade, leading to increased skeletal muscle relaxation and possible respiratory paralysis. Use with extreme caution and reduce dose of atracurium.

NURSING CONSIDERATIONS
• Use cautiously in cardiovascular disease, severe electrolyte disorders,

---

bronchogenic carcinoma, and neuromuscular diseases.

• Atracurium should only be used by personnel experienced in airway management.

• Keep airway clear. Have emergency respiratory support equipment (endotracheal equipment, ventilator, oxygen, atropine, edrophonium, neostigmine, and epinephrine) on hand.

• Prior administration of succinylcholine does not prolong duration of action, but it quickens onset and may deepen neuromuscular blockade.

• Atracurium facilitates intubation within 2 to 2½ minutes. The duration of effect is 20 to 35 minutes.

• Once spontaneous recovery starts, atracurium-induced neuromuscular blockade may be reversed with an anticholinesterase agent (such as neostigmine or edrophonium). Usually administered together with an anticholinergic drug (such as atropine or glycopyrrolate).

• Don't administer by I.M. injection.

• Don't mix with alkaline solutions such as barbiturates (precipitate may form).

• Monitor respirations closely until patient is fully recovered from neuromuscular blockade, as evidenced by tests of muscle strength (hand grip, head lift, and ability to cough).

• Atracurium has a longer duration of action than succinylcholine and a shorter duration of action than *d*-tubocurarine or pancuronium.

---

gallamine triethiodide
Flaxedil

Pregnancy Risk Category: C

HOW SUPPLIED
Injection: 20 mg/ml

MECHANISM OF ACTION
Prevents acetylcholine from binding to the receptors on the muscle end plate, thus blocking depolarization. Nondepolarizing agent.

INDICATIONS & DOSAGE
Adjunct to anesthesia to induce skeletal muscle relaxation; facilitate intubation, reduction of fractures and dislocations; lessen muscle contractions in pharmacologically or electrically induced seizures; assist with mechanical ventilation—
Dosage depends on anesthetic used, individual needs, and response. Dosages are representative and must be adjusted.
Adults and children over 1 month: initially, 1 mg/kg I.V. to maximum of 100 mg, regardless of patient's weight; then 0.5 mg to 1 mg/kg q 30 to 40 minutes.
Children under 1 month but over 5 kg (11 lb): initially, 0.25 to 0.75 mg/kg I.V., then may give additional doses of 0.1 to 0.5 mg/kg q 30 to 40 minutes.

ADVERSE REACTIONS
CV: tachycardia.
Other: *respiratory paralysis, dose-related prolonged apnea,* residual muscle weakness, increased oropharyngeal secretions, allergic or idiosyncratic hypersensitivity reactions.

INTERACTIONS
Aminoglycoside antibiotics (amikacin, gentamicin, kanamycin, neomycin, streptomycin); polymyxin antibiotics (polymyxin B sulfate, colistin); clindamycin; quinidine; general anesthetics (such as halothane, enflurane, isoflurane: potentiated neuromuscular blockade, leading to increased skeletal muscle relaxation and possible respiratory paralysis. Use cautiously during surgical and postoperative periods.
Narcotic analgesics, I.V. diazepam: potentiated neuromuscular blockade, leading to increased skeletal muscle relaxation and possible respiratory pa-

---

Italicized adverse reactions are common or life-threatening.
*Liquid form contains alcohol.   **May contain tartrazine.

ralysis. Use with extreme caution, and reduce dose of gallamine.

NURSING CONSIDERATIONS
• Contraindicated in patients with hypersensitivity to iodides, impaired renal function, myasthenia gravis; patients in shock; and patients in whom tachycardia may be hazardous. Use cautiously in elderly or debilitated patients; in hepatic or pulmonary impairment, respiratory depression, myasthenic syndrome of lung cancer or bronchogenic carcinoma, dehydration, thyroid disorders, collagen diseases, porphyria, and electrolyte disturbances; in patients sensitive to sulfites; and in patients undergoing cesarean section.
• Gallamine should only be used by personnel experienced in airway management.
• Keep airway clear. Have emergency respiratory support equipment (endotracheal equipment, ventilator, oxygen, atropine, edrophonium, neostigmine, and epinephrine) on hand.
• Monitor baseline electrolyte determinations (electrolyte imbalance can potentiate neuromuscular effects).
• Take vital signs every 15 minutes, especially for developing tachycardia. Notify doctor immediately of significant changes.
• Measure intake and output (renal dysfunction prolongs duration of action, since drug is unchanged before excretion).
• Monitor respirations closely until patient is fully recovered from neuromuscular blockade, as evidenced by tests of muscle strength (hand grip, head lift, and ability to cough).
• Determine whether patient has iodide allergy.
• Protect drug from light or excessive heat; use only fresh solutions.
• Do not mix solution with meperidine HCl or barbiturate solutions.
• Give I.V. slowly (over 30 to 90 seconds).

• May be preferred in patients who have bradycardia.
• Once spontaneous recovery starts, gallamine-induced neuromuscular blockade may be reversed with an anticholinesterase agent (such as neostigmine or edrophonium). Usually administered together with an anticholinergic drug (such as atropine or glycopyrrollate).

hexafluorenium bromide
Mylaxen

Pregnancy Risk Category: C

HOW SUPPLIED
Injection: 20 mg/ml

MECHANISM OF ACTION
Inhibits the enzymatic breakdown of succinylcholine, prolonging its duration.

INDICATIONS & DOSAGE
Adjunct for use with succinylcholine to prolong neuromuscular blockade and reduce muscular fasciculations—
Adults and children: use in ratio of 2 mg:1 mg succinylcholine and administer by I.V. push. Maximum dosage is hexafluorenium bromide 10 to 36 mg; should not be administered more frequently than q 15 to 30 minutes.

ADVERSE REACTIONS
CV: hypotension, hypertension, tachycardia, bradycardia, arrhythmias, *cardiac arrest.*
EENT: increased intraocular pressure, salivation.
Other: increased bronchial tone, *bronchospasm, apnea, prolonged neuromuscular blockade,* hyperthermia.

INTERACTIONS
None reported for this drug alone; always used with succinylcholine. See succinylcholine.

NURSING CONSIDERATIONS

• Contraindicated in hypersensitivity to bromides, in bronchial asthma. Use cautiously in elderly or debilitated patient; in renal, hepatic, or pulmonary impairment, respiratory depression, myasthenia gravis, myasthenic syndrome of lung cancer or bronchogenic carcinoma, dehydration, thyroid disorders, collagen diseases, porphyria, electrolyte disturbances, and glaucoma; and during ocular surgery and (in large doses) cesarean section.

• Monitor baseline electrolyte determinations (electrolyte imbalance potentiates neuromuscular effects) and vital signs (watch respirations closely).

• Keep airway clear. Have emergency respiratory support equipment (endotracheal equipment, ventilator, oxygen, atropine, edrophonium, neostigmine, and epinephrine) on hand.

• Reassure patient that postoperative stiffness is normal and will soon subside.

• Use only fresh solutions.

• Give only under direct supervision of doctor.

---

metocurine iodide
Metubine

Pregnancy Risk Category: C

HOW SUPPLIED
Injection: 2mg/ml

MECHANISM OF ACTION
Prevents acetylcholine from binding to the receptors on the muscle end plate, thus blocking depolarization. Nondepolarizing agent.

INDICATIONS & DOSAGE
Adjunct to anesthesia to induce skeletal muscle relaxation; facilitate intubation, reduction of fractures and dislocations—
Dosage depends on anesthetic used, individual needs, and response. Dosages are representative and must be adjusted. Administer as sustained injection over 30 to 60 seconds.
Adults: given cyclopropane: 2 to 4 mg I.V. (2.68 mg average).
Given ether: 1.5 to 3 mg I.V. (2.1 mg average).
Given nitrous oxide: 4 to 7 mg I.V. (4.79 mg average). Supplemental injections of 0.5 to 1 mg in 25 to 90 minutes, repeated p.r.n.
Lessen muscle contractions in pharmacologically or electrically induced seizures—
Adults: 1.75 to 5.5 mg I.V.

ADVERSE REACTIONS
CV: hypotension secondary to histamine release, ganglionic blockade in rapid dose or overdose.
Other: *dose-related prolonged apnea,* residual muscle weakness, increased oropharyngeal secretions, allergic or idiosyncratic hypersensitivity reactions, *bronchospasm.*

INTERACTIONS
Aminoglycoside antibiotics (including amikacin, gentamicin, kanamycin, neomycin, streptomycin); polymyxin antibiotics (polymyxin B sulfate, colistin); clindamycin; quinidine; general anesthetics (such as halothane, enflurane, isoflurane), furosemide, thiazide diuretics, and beta-adrenergic blocking agents: potentiated neuromuscular blockade, leading to increased skeletal muscle relaxation and possible respiratory paralysis. Use cautiously during surgical and postoperative periods.
Narcotic analgesics: potentiated neuromuscular blockade, leading to increased skeletal muscle relaxation and possible respiratory paralysis. Use with extreme caution, and reduce dose of metocurine iodide.

NURSING CONSIDERATIONS
• Contraindicated in patients with hypersensitivity to iodides; and in whom

---

histamine release is a hazard (asthmatic or atopic patients). Use cautiously in elderly or debilitated patients; and in renal, hepatic, or pulmonary impairment, respiratory depression, myasthenia gravis, myasthenic syndrome of lung cancer or bronchogenic carcinoma, dehydration, thyroid disorders, collagen diseases, porphyria, electrolyte disturbances, hyperthermia, and (in large doses) cesarean section.
• Metocurine should only be used by personnel experienced in airway management.
• Keep airway clear. Have emergency respiratory support equipment (endotracheal equipment, ventilator, oxygen, atropine, edrophonium, epinephrine, and neostigmine) on hand.
• Once spontaneous recovery starts, metocurine-induced neuromuscular blockade may be reversed with an anticholinesterase agent (such as neostigmine or edrophonium). Usually administered together with an anticholinergic drug (such as atropine or glycopyrollate).
• Dose of 1 mg is the therapeutic equivalent of 3 mg *d*-tubocurarine chloride.
• Monitor baseline electrolyte determinations (electrolyte imbalance, especially potassium, calcium, and magnesium, can potentiate neuromuscular effects) and vital signs, especially respiration.
• Measure intake and output (renal dysfunction prolongs duration of action, since drug is mainly unchanged before excretion).
• Monitor respirations closely until patient is fully recovered from neuromuscular blockade, as evidenced by tests of muscle strength (hand grip, head lift, and ability to cough).
• Determine whether patient has iodide allergy.
• Store solution away from heat, sunlight; do not mix with barbiturates (precipitate will form). Use fresh solutions only.

---

pancuronium bromide
Pavulon

Pregnancy Risk Category: C

HOW SUPPLIED
Injection: 1 mg/ml, 2 mg/ml

MECHANISM OF ACTION
Prevents acetylcholine from binding to the receptors on the muscle end plate, thus blocking depolarization. Nondepolarizing agent.

INDICATIONS & DOSAGE
Adjunct to anesthesia to induce skeletal muscle relaxation; facilitate intubation; lessen muscle contractions in pharmacologically or electrically induced seizures; assist with mechanical ventilation—
Dosage depends on anesthetic used, individual needs, and response. Dosages are representative and must be adjusted.
Adults: initially, 0.04 to 0.1 mg/kg I.V.; then 0.01 mg/kg q 30 to 60 minutes.
Children over 10 years: initially, 0.04 to 0.1 mg/kg I.V., then ⅕ initial dose q 30 to 60 minutes.

ADVERSE REACTIONS
CV: tachycardia, increased blood pressure.
Skin: transient rashes.
Local: burning sensation.
Other: excessive sweating and salivation, *prolonged dose-related apnea*, wheezing, residual muscle weakness, allergic or idiosyncratic hypersensitivity reactions.

INTERACTIONS
Aminoglycoside antibiotics (including amikacin, gentamicin, kanamycin, neomycin, streptomycin); polymyxin antibiotics (polymyxin B sulfate, colis-

---

tin); clindamycin; quinidine; general anesthetics (such as halothane, enflurane, isoflurane): potentiated neuromuscular blockade, leading to increased skeletal muscle relaxation and possible respiratory paralysis. Use cautiously during surgical and postoperative periods.

Lithium, narcotic analgesics: potentiated neuromuscular blockade, leading to increased skeletal muscle relaxation and possible respiratory paralysis. Use with extreme caution, and reduce dose of pancuronium.

NURSING CONSIDERATIONS
• Contraindicated in hypersensitivity to bromides; preexisting tachycardia; and in patients for whom even a minor increase in heart rate is undesirable. Use cautiously in elderly or debilitated patients; renal, hepatic, or pulmonary impairment; respiratory depression; myasthenia gravis; myasthenic syndrome of lung cancer or bronchogenic carcinoma; dehydration; thyroid disorders; collagen diseases; porphyria; electrolyte disturbances; hyperthermia; toxemic states; and (in large doses) cesarean section.
• Pancuronium should only be used by personnel experienced in airway management.
• Have emergency respiratory support equipment (endotracheal equipment, ventilator, oxygen, atropine, edrophonium, epinephrine, and neostigmine) on hand.
• Causes no histamine release or hypotension.
• Dose of 1 mg is the approximate therapeutic equivalent of 5 mg *d*-tubocurarine chloride.
• Monitor baseline electrolyte determinations (electrolyte imbalance can potentiate neuromuscular effects) and vital signs (watch respiration and heart rate closely).
• Measure intake and output (renal dysfunction may prolong duration of

action, since 25% of the drug is unchanged before excretion).
• Monitor respirations closely until patient is fully recovered from neuromuscular blockade, as evidenced by tests of muscle strength (hand grip, head lift, and ability to cough).
• Allow succinylcholine effects to subside before giving pancuronium.
• Store in refrigerator. Do not store in plastic containers or syringes, although plastic syringes may be used for administration.
• Do not mix with barbiturate solutions (precipitate will form); use only fresh solutions.
• Once spontaneous recovery starts, pancuronium-induced neuromuscular blockade may be reversed with an anticholinesterase agent (such as neostigmine or edrophonium). Usually administered together with an anticholinergic drug (such as atropine or glycopyrollate).

---

succinylcholine chloride (suxamethonium chloride)
Anectine, Anectine Flo-Pack, Quelicin, Scoline‡, Sucostrin

Pregnancy Risk Category: C

HOW SUPPLIED
Injection: 20 mg/ml, 50 mg/ml, 100 mg/ml; 100 mg/vial, 500 mg/vial, 1 g/vial

MECHANISM OF ACTION
Prolongs depolarization of the muscle end plate. Depolarizing agent.

INDICATIONS & DOSAGE
Adjunct to anesthesia to induce skeletal muscle relaxation; facilitate intubation and assist with mechanical ventilation or orthopedic manipulations (drug of choice); lessen muscle contractions in pharmacologically or electrically induced seizures—
Dosage depends on anesthetic used, individual needs, and response. Dos-

ages are representative and must be adjusted.

Adults: 25 to 75 mg I.V., then 2.5 mg/minute, p.r.n., or 2.5 mg/kg I.M. up to maximum of 150 mg I.M. in deltoid muscle.

Children: 1 to 2 mg/kg I.M. or I.V. Maximum I.M. dosage is 150 mg. (Children may be less sensitive to succinylcholine than adults.)

ADVERSE REACTIONS

CV: bradycardia, tachycardia, hypertension, hypotension, arrhythmias.
EENT: increased intraocular pressure.
Other: *prolonged respiratory depression, apnea, malignant hyperthermia,* muscle fasciculation, *postoperative muscle pain,* myoglobinemia, excessive salivation, allergic or idiosyncratic hypersensitivity reactions.

INTERACTIONS

Aminoglycoside antibiotics (including amikacin, gentamicin, kanamycin, neomycin, streptomycin); polymyxin antibiotics (polymyxin B sulfate, colistin); cholinesterase inhibitors such as neostigmine, pyridostigmine, edrophonium, physostigmine, or echothiophate; general anesthetics (such as halothane, enflurane, isoflurane): potentiated neuromuscular blockade, leading to increased skeletal muscle relaxation and possible respiratory paralysis. Use cautiously during surgical and postoperative periods.
Cardiac glycosides: possible cardiac arrhythmias. Use together cautiously.
Magnesium sulfate (parenterally): potentiated neuromuscular blockade, increased skeletal muscle relaxation, and possible respiratory paralysis. Use with caution, preferably with reduced doses.
MAO inhibitors, lithium, cyclophosphamide: prolonged apnea. Use with caution.
Narcotic analgesics, methotrimeprazine: potentiated neuromuscular

blockade, leading to increased skeletal muscle relaxation and possible respiratory paralysis. Use with extreme caution.

NURSING CONSIDERATIONS

• Contraindicated in abnormally low plasma pseudocholinesterase. Use with caution in patients with personal or family history of malignant hypertension or hyperthermia; elderly or debilitated patients; hepatic, renal, or pulmonary impairment; and in respiratory depression, severe burns or trauma, electrolyte imbalances, quinidine or digitalis therapy, hyperkalemia, paraplegia, spinal neuraxis injury, degenerative or dystrophic neuromuscular disease, myasthenia gravis, myasthenic syndrome of lung cancer or bronchogenic carcinoma, dehydration, thyroid disorders, collagen diseases, porphyria, fractures, muscle spasms, glaucoma, eye surgery or penetrating eye wounds, pheochromocytoma, and (in large doses) cesarean section.
• Succinylcholine should only be used by personnel experienced in airway management.
• Keep airway clear. Have emergency respiratory support equipment (endotracheal equipment, ventilator, oxygen, atropine, and epinephrine) on hand.
• Unlike nondepolarizing agents, neostigmine or edrophonium may worsen neuromuscular blockade. Don't use reversing agents.
• Drug of choice for short procedures (less than 3 minutes) and for orthopedic manipulations; use caution in fractures or dislocations.
• Duration of action prolonged to 20 minutes by continuous I.V. infusion or single-dose administration, along with hexafluorenium bromide.
• Repeated or continuous infusions of succinylcholine alone not advised; may cause reduced response or prolonged muscle relaxation and apnea.

• Monitor baseline electrolyte determinations and vital signs (check respiration every 5 to 10 minutes during infusion).
• Reassure patient that postoperative stiffness is normal and will soon subside.
• Store injectable form in refrigerator. Store powder form at room temperature, tightly closed. Use immediately after reconstitution. Do not mix with alkaline solutions (thiopental, sodium bicarbonate, barbiturates).
• Give test dose (10 mg I.M. or I.V.) after patient has been anesthetized. Normal response (no respiratory depression or transient depression for up to 5 minutes) indicates drug may be given. Do not give if patient develops respiratory paralysis sufficient to permit endotracheal intubation. (Recovery within 30 to 60 minutes.)
• Monitor respirations closely until patient is fully recovered from neuromuscular blockade, as evidenced by tests of muscle strength (hand grip, head lift, and ability to cough).
• If given I.M., give deep I.M., preferably high into the deltoid muscle.

---

tubocurarine chloride
Tubarine†

Pregnancy Risk Category: C

HOW SUPPLIED
Injection: 3 mg (20 units)/ml; 10 mg/ml‡

MECHANISM OF ACTION
Prevents acetylcholine from binding to the receptors on the muscle end plate, thus blocking depolarization. Nondepolarizing agent.

INDICATIONS & DOSAGE
Adjunct to anesthesia to induce skeletal muscle relaxation; facilitate intubation, orthopedic manipulations—
Dosage depends on anesthetic used, individual needs, and response. Dos-

ages listed are representative and must be adjusted.
Adults: 1 unit/kg or 0.15 mg/kg I.V. slowly over 60 to 90 seconds. Average, initially, 40 to 60 units I.V. May give 20 to 30 units in 3 to 5 minutes. For longer procedures, give 20 units, p.r.n.
Children: 1 unit/kg or 0.15 mg/kg.
Assist with mechanical ventilation—
Adults and children: initially, 0.0165 mg/kg I.V. (average 1 mg or 7 units), then adjust subsequent doses to patient's response.
Lessen muscle contractions in pharmacologically or electrically induced seizures—
Adults and children: 1 unit/kg or 0.15 mg/kg slowly over 60 to 90 seconds. Initial dose is 20 units (3 mg) less than calculated dose.

ADVERSE REACTIONS
CV: hypotension, circulatory depression.
Other: profound and prolonged muscle relaxation, *respiratory depression to the point of apnea,* hypersensitivity, idiosyncrasy, residual muscle weakness, increased salivation, *bronchospasm.*

INTERACTIONS
Aminoglycoside antibiotics (including amikacin, gentamicin, kanamycin, neomycin, streptomycin); polymyxin antibiotics (polymyxin B sulfate, colistin); general anesthetics (such as halothane, enflurane, isoflurane): potentiated neuromuscular blockade, leading to increased skeletal muscle relaxation and possible respiratory paralysis. Use cautiously during surgical and postoperative periods.
Quinidine: prolonged neuromuscular blockade. Use together with caution. Monitor closely.
Thiazide diuretics, furosemide, ethacrynic acid, amphotericin B, propranolol, methotrimeprazine, narcotic analgesics: potentiated neuromuscular

---

Italicized adverse reactions are common or life-threatening.
*Liquid form contains alcohol.   **May contain tartrazine.

blockade, leading to increased respiratory paralysis. Use with extreme caution during surgical and postoperative periods.

NURSING CONSIDERATIONS
• Contraindicated in patients for whom histamine release is a hazard (asthmatics). Use cautiously in elderly or debilitated patients; in hepatic or pulmonary impairment, respiratory depression, myasthenia gravis, myasthenic syndrome of lung cancer or bronchogenic carcinoma, dehydration, thyroid disorders, collagen diseases, porphyria, electrolyte disturbances, fractures, muscle spasms, and (in large doses) cesarean section.
• Tubocurarine should only be used by personnel experienced in airway management.
• Keep airway clear. Have emergency respiratory support equipment (endotracheal equipment, ventilator, oxygen, atropine, edrophonium, epinephrine, and neostigmine) on hand.
• Allow succinylcholine effects to subside before giving tubocurarine.
• Monitor baseline electrolyte determinations (electrolyte imbalance can potentiate neuromuscular effects).
• Monitor respirations closely until patient is fully recovered from neuromuscular blockade, as evidenced by tests of muscle strength (hand grip, head lift, and ability to cough).
• Check vital signs every 15 minutes. Notify doctor at once of changes.
• Measure intake and output (renal dysfunction prolongs duration of action, since much of drug is unchanged before excretion).
• Do not mix with barbiturates (precipitate will form). Use only fresh solutions and discard if discolored.
• Give I.V. slowly (60 to 90 seconds); give deep I.M. in deltoid muscle.
• Once spontaneous recovery starts, tubocurarine-induced neuromuscular blockade may be reversed with an anticholinesterase agent (such as neostigmine or edrophonium). Usually administered together with an anticholinergic drug (such as atropine or glycopyrollate).

vecuronium bromide
Norcuron

Pregnancy Risk Category: C

HOW SUPPLIED
Injection: 10 mg/vial

MECHANISM OF ACTION
Prevents acetylcholine from binding to the receptors on the muscle end plate, thus blocking depolarization. Nondepolarizing agent.

INDICATIONS & DOSAGE
Adjunct to general anesthesia, to facilitate endotracheal intubation and to provide skeletal muscle relaxation during surgery or mechanical ventilation—
Dosage depends on anesthetic used, individual needs, and response. Dosages are representative and must be adjusted.
Adults and children over 9 years:
Initially, 0.08 to 0.10 mg/kg I.V. bolus. Maintenance doses of 0.010 to 0.015 mg/kg within 25 to 40 minutes of initial dose should be administered during prolonged surgical procedures. Maintenance doses may be given q 12 to 15 minutes in patients receiving balanced anesthesia.
Children under 10 years may require a slightly higher initial dose and may also require supplementation slightly more often than adults.

ADVERSE REACTIONS
CV: transient increases in heart rate.
Local: redness, itching, induration.
Other: *prolonged dose-related apnea.*

INTERACTIONS
Aminoglycoside antibiotics (including

amikacin, gentamicin, kanamycin, neomycin, streptomycin); polymyxin antibiotics (polymyxin B sulfate, colistin); clindamycin; quinidine; general anesthetics (such as halothane, enflurane, isoflurane): potentiated neuromuscular blockade, leading to increased skeletal muscle relaxation and possible respiratory paralysis. Use cautiously during surgical and postoperative periods.
Narcotic analgesics: potentiated neuromuscular blockade, leading to increased skeletal muscle relaxation and possible respiratory paralysis. Use with extreme caution, and reduce dose of vecuronium.

NURSING CONSIDERATIONS
• Contraindicated in hypersensitivity to bromides. Use cautiously in altered circulation time from cardiovascular disease, old age, and edematous states; in hepatic disease; in severe obesity; in bronchogenic carcinoma; and in neuromuscular disease.
• Vecuronium should only be used by personnel experienced in airway management.
• Keep airway clear. Have emergency respiratory support equipment (endotracheal equipment, ventilator, oxygen, atropine, edrophonium, epinephrine, and neostigmine) on hand.
• Unlike other nondepolarizing neuromuscular blockers, vecuronium has no effect on cardiovascular system. Also, the drug causes no histamine release and therefore no histamine-related hypersensitivity reactions, such as bronchospasm, hypotension, or tachycardia.
• The drug is well tolerated in renal failure.
• Prior administration of succinylcholine may enhance the neuromuscular blocking effect and duration of action.
• Vecuronium provides conditions for intubation within 2½ to 3 minutes.

The duration of effect is 25 to 40 minutes.
• Once spontaneous recovery starts, vecuronium-induced neuromuscular blockade may be reversed with an anticholinesterase agent (such as neostigmine or edrophonium). Usually administered together with an anticholinergic drug (such as atropine or glycopyrrolate).
• Monitor respirations closely until patient is fully recovered from neuromuscular blockade, as evidenced by tests of muscle strength (hand grip, head lift, and ability to cough).
• Store reconstituted solution in refrigerator. Discard after 24 hours.

Italicized adverse reactions are common or life-threatening.
*Liquid form contains alcohol.   **May contain tartrazine.

41

Antihistamines

astemizole
azatadine maleate
brompheniramine maleate
carbinoxamine maleate
chlorpheniramine maleate
clemastine fumarate
cyproheptadine hydrochloride
dexchlorpheniramine maleate
diphenhydramine hydrochloride
methdilazine hydrochloride
promethazine hydrochloride
terfenadine
trimeprazine tartrate
tripelennamine citrate
tripelennamine hydrochloride
triprolidine hydrochloride

COMBINATION PRODUCTS

ALLEREST TABLETS◇: phenylpropanolamine hydrochloride 18.7 mg and chlorpheniramine maleate 2 mg.

ALLERGESIC: phenylpropanolamine hydrochloride 18.7 mg and chlorpheniramine maleate 2 mg.

BROMFED-AT: brompheniramine maleate 2 mg, dextromethorphan hydrobromide 10 mg, and pseudoephedrine hydrochloride 30 mg/5 ml.

CHLOR-TRIMETON DECONGESTANT◇: chlorpheniramine maleate 4 mg and pseudoephedrine sulfate 60 mg.

CHLOR-TRIMETON DECONGESTANT REPETABS◇: chlorpheniramine maleate 8 mg and pseudoephedrine sulfate 120 mg.

CODIMAL DH*: hydrocodone bitartrate 1.66 mg, phenylephrine hydrochloride 5 mg, pyrilamine maleate 8.33 mg, potassium guaiacolsulfonate 83.3 mg, sodium citrate 216 mg, and citric acid 50 mg.

CONDRIN-LA: phenylpropanolamine hydrochloride 75 mg and chlorpheniramine maleate 12 mg.

CONTAC CAPSULES◇: phenylpropanolamine 75 mg and chlorpheniramine maleate 8 mg.

CONTAC 12-HOUR CAPLETS◇: phenylpropanolamine 75 mg and chlorpheniramine maleate 12 mg.

CORICIDIN TABLETS◇: chlorpheniramine maleate 2 mg and aspirin 325 mg.

DECONADE: phenylpropanolamine hydrochloride 75 mg and chlorpheniramine maleate 12 mg.

DECONAMINE: pseudoephedrine hydrochloride 60 mg and chlorpheniramine maleate 4 mg.

DIMETAPP EXTENTABS: brompheniramine maleate 12 mg, and phenylpropanolamine hydrochloride 75 mg.

DISOPHROL CHRONOTABS◇: dexbrompheniramine maleate 6 mg and pseudoephedrine sulfate 120 mg.

DRIXORAL◇: dexbrompheniramine maleate 6 mg and pseudoephedrine sulfate 120 mg.

DRIZE: phenylpropanolamine hydrochloride 75 mg and chlorpheniramine maleate 12 mg.

FEDAHIST: pseudoephedrine hydrochloride 60 mg and chlorpheniramine maleate 4 mg.

HISTABID DURACAPS: phenylpropanolamine 75 mg and chlorpheniramine maleate 8 mg.

HISTASPAN-D: chlorpheniramine maleate 8 mg, phenylephrine hydrochloride 20 mg, and methscopolamine nitrate 2.5 mg.

NALDECON: phenylephrine hydrochloride 10 mg, phenylpropanolamine hydrochloride 40 mg, phenyltoloxamine citrate 15 mg, and chlorpheniramine maleate 5 mg.

NEOTEP-GRANUCAPS: chlorpheniramine maleate 9 mg and phenylephrine hydrochloride 21 mg.

NOLAMINE: chlorpheniramine maleate 4 mg, phenindamine tartrate 24 mg, and phenylpropanolamine hydrochloride 50 mg.

NOVAFED A: pseudoephedrine hydrochloride 120 mg and chlorpheniramine maleate 8 mg.

NOVAHISTINE ELIXIR◊*: phenylephrine 5 mg, chlorpheniramine maleate 2 mg, and alcohol 5%/5 ml.

ORAHIST: phenylpropanolamine hydrochloride 75 mg and chlorpheniramine maleate 12 mg.

ORNADE SPANSULES: phenylpropanolamine hydrochloride 75 mg and chlorpheniramine maleate 12 mg.

RHINEX D-LAY: acetaminophen 300 mg, salicylamide 300 mg, phenylpropanolamine hydrochloride 60 mg, and chlorpheniramine maleate 4 mg.

RONDEC: carbinoxamine maleate 4 mg and pseudoephedrine hydrochloride 60 mg.

SUDAFED PLUS◊: pseudoephedrine HCl 60 mg and chlorpheniramine maleate 4 mg.

TRIAMINIC-12: phenylpropanolamine HCl 75 mg and chlorpheniramine maleate 12 mg.

TRIAMINIC TABLETS: phenylpropanolamine hydrochloride 50 mg, pheniramine maleate 25 mg, and pyrilamine maleate 25 mg.

TRINALIN REPETABS: azatadine maleate 1 mg and pseudoephedrine sulfate 120 mg.

---

astemizole
Hismanal

Pregnancy Risk Category: C

HOW SUPPLIED
Tablets: 10 mg

Suspension: 2mg/ml‡

MECHANISM OF ACTION
Blocks the effects of histamine at H_1 receptors. Astemizole is a nonsedating antihistamine because its chemical structure prevents entry into the CNS.

INDICATIONS AND DOSAGE
Relief of symptoms associated with chronic idiopathic urticaria and seasonal allergic rhinitis—
Adults and children over 12 years: 10 mg P.O. daily. A loading dose may be given in order to achieve steady-state plasma levels quickly. Begin therapy at 30 mg on the first day, followed by 20 mg on the second day, and 10 mg daily thereafter.

ADVERSE REACTIONS
CNS: headache, nervousness, dizziness, drowsiness.
EENT: dry mouth, pharyngitis, conjunctivitis.
GI: nausea, diarrhea, abdominal pain, increased appetite.
Other: arthralgia, weight gain.

INTERACTIONS
None significant.

NURSING CONSIDERATIONS
• Contraindicated in patients with hypersensitivity to astemizole.
• Instruct patient to take this drug on an empty stomach at least 2 hours after a meal and to avoid eating for at least 1 hour after dosing.
• Because of its potential for anticholinergic effects, use cautiously in patients with lower respiratory diseases (including asthma) because drying effects can increase the risk of bronchial mucous plug formation.
• Warn patient to stop taking drug 4 days before allergy skin tests to preserve accuracy of tests.
• Use with caution in patients with

---

hepatic or renal disease. Astemizole is not believed to be dialysable.

azatadine maleate
Optimine, Zadine‡

Pregnancy Risk Category: B

HOW SUPPLIED
Tablets: 1 mg
Syrup: 0.5 mg/5 ml‡

MECHANISM OF ACTION
Competes with histamine for H_1-receptor sites on effector cells. Prevents but does not reverse histamine-mediated responses.

INDICATIONS & DOSAGE
Rhinitis, allergy symptoms, chronic urticaria—
Adults: 1 to 2 mg P.O. b.i.d. Maximum dosage is 4 mg daily.
　Not intended for children under 12 years.

ADVERSE REACTIONS
Blood: thrombocytopenia.
CNS: (especially in elderly patients) *drowsiness, dizziness,* vertigo, disturbed coordination.
CV: hypotension, palpitations.
GI: anorexia, nausea, vomiting, *dry mouth and throat,* epigastric distress.
GU: urine retention.
Skin: urticaria, rash.
Other: thick bronchial secretions.

INTERACTIONS
CNS depressants: increased sedation. Use together cautiously.

NURSING CONSIDERATIONS
• Contraindicated in acute asthmatic attacks. Use cautiously in elderly patients and in increased intraocular pressure, hyperthyroidism, cardiovascular or renal disease, hypertension, bronchial asthma, urine retention, prostatic hypertrophy, bladder-neck obstruction, and stenosing peptic ulcers.
• Warn patient against drinking alcoholic beverages during therapy and against activities that require alertness until CNS response to drug is determined.
• Reduce GI distress by giving with food or milk.
• Coffee or tea may reduce drowsiness. Sugarless gum or sour hard candy, or ice chips may relieve dry mouth.
• If tolerance develops, another antihistamine may be substituted.
• Warn patient to stop taking drug 4 days before allergy skin tests to preserve accuracy of tests.
• Monitor blood counts during long-term therapy; watch for signs of blood dyscrasias.

brompheniramine maleate
Brombay◊, Bromphen*◊, Chlorphed◊, Codimal-A, Conjec-B◊, Cophene-B, Dehist, Diamine TD, Dimetane*◊, Dimetane Extentabs◊, Dimetane-Ten◊, Histaject Modified, Nasahist B, ND-Stat Revised, Oraminic II, Sinusol-B, Veltane

Pregnancy Risk Category: C

HOW SUPPLIED
Tablets: 4 mg◊
Tablets (timed-release): 8 mg◊, 12 mg◊
Elixir: 2 mg/5 ml◊
Injection: 10 mg/ml◊

MECHANISM OF ACTION
Competes with histamine for H_1-receptor sites on effector cells. Prevents but does not reverse histamine-mediated responses.

INDICATIONS & DOSAGE
Rhinitis, allergy symptoms—
Adults: 4 to 8 mg P.O. t.i.d. or q.i.d.; or (timed-release) 8 to 12 mg P.O.

b.i.d. or t.i.d.; or 5 to 20 mg q 6 to 12 hours I.M., I.V., or S.C. Maximum dosage is 40 mg daily.

Children over 6 years: 2 to 4 mg P.O. t.i.d. or q.i.d.; or (timed-release) 8 to 12 mg q 12 hours; or 0.5 mg/kg I.M., I.V., or S.C. daily divided t.i.d. or q.i.d.

Children under 6 years: 0.5 mg/kg P.O., I.M., I.V., or S.C. daily divided t.i.d. or q.i.d.

Note: Children under 12 years should use only as directed by a doctor.

ADVERSE REACTIONS
Blood: thrombocytopenia, *agranulocytosis.*
CNS: (especially in elderly patients) dizziness, tremors, irritability, insomnia, *drowsiness, stimulation.*
CV: hypotension, palpitations.
GI: anorexia, nausea, vomiting, *dry mouth and throat.*
GU: urine retention.
Skin: urticaria, rash.
After parenteral administration: local reaction, sweating, syncope.

INTERACTIONS
CNS depressants: increased sedation. Use together cautiously.

NURSING CONSIDERATIONS
• Contraindicated in acute asthmatic attacks. Use cautiously in elderly patients, breast-feeding women, and in increased intraocular pressure, hyperthyroidism, cardiovascular or renal disease, hypertension, bronchial asthma, urine retention, prostatic hypertrophy, bladder-neck obstruction, and stenosing peptic ulcers.
• Warn patient against drinking alcoholic beverages during therapy and against activities that require alertness until adverse CNS effects are known.
• Reduce GI distress by giving with food or milk.

• Causes less drowsiness than some other antihistamines.
• Coffee or tea may reduce drowsiness. Sugarless gum or sour hard candy, or ice chips may relieve dry mouth.
• If tolerance develops, another antihistamine may be substituted.
• Warn patient to stop taking drug 4 days before allergy skin tests to preserve accuracy of tests.
• Injectable form containing 10 mg/ml can be given diluted or undiluted very slowly I.V. The 100 mg/ml injection should not be given I.V.
• Monitor blood count during long-term therapy; observe for signs of blood dyscrasias.

---

carbinoxamine maleate
Clistin*

Pregnancy Risk Category: C

HOW SUPPLIED
Tablets: 4 mg

MECHANISM OF ACTION
Competes with histamine for H_1-receptor sites on effector cells. Prevents but does not reverse histamine-mediated responses.

INDICATIONS & DOSAGE
Rhinitis, allergy symptoms—
Adults: 4 to 8 mg P.O. t.i.d. or q.i.d.
Children over 6 years: 4 to 6 mg P.O. t.i.d. or q.i.d.
Children 3 to 6 years: 2 to 4 mg P.O. t.i.d. or q.i.d.
Children 1 to 3 years: 2 mg P.O. t.i.d. or q.i.d.

Note: Children under 12 years should use only as directed by a doctor.

ADVERSE REACTIONS
CNS: (especially in elderly patients) *drowsiness, dizziness, stimulation.*
GI: anorexia, nausea, vomiting, *dry mouth.*

Italicized adverse reactions are common or life-threatening.
*Liquid form contains alcohol.   **May contain tartrazine.

GU: urine retention.

INTERACTIONS
CNS depressants: increased sedation. Use together cautiously.

NURSING CONSIDERATIONS
• Contraindicated in acute asthmatic attacks. Use cautiously in elderly patients, and in increased intraocular pressure, hyperthyroidism, cardiovascular or renal disease, hypertension, bronchial asthma, urine retention, prostatic hypertrophy, bladder-neck obstruction, and stenosing peptic ulcers.
• Warn patient against drinking alcoholic beverages during therapy and against driving or other activities that require alertness until CNS response to drug is determined.
• Reduce GI distress by giving with food or milk.
• Coffee or tea may reduce drowsiness. Sugarless gum or sour hard candy, or ice chips may relieve dry mouth.
• If tolerance develops, another antihistamine may be substituted.
• Warn patient to stop taking drug 4 days before allergy skin tests to preserve accuracy of tests.

---

chlorpheniramine maleate
Aller-Chlor*◊, Allergex‡, Chlo-Amine◊, Chlor-100◊, Chlorate◊, Chlor-Niramine◊, Chlor-Pro, Chlor-Pro 10, Chlorspan-12, Chlortab-4, Chlortab-8, Chlor-Trimeton*◊, Chlor-Trimeton Repetabs◊, Chlor-Tripolon†◊, Genallerate◊, Novopheniram‡◊, Pfeiffer's Allergy◊, Phenetron*, Piriton‡, Pyranistan◊, Telachlor, Teldrin◊, Trymegen◊

Pregnancy Risk Category: B

HOW SUPPLIED
Tablets: 4 mg◊
Tablets (chewable): 2 mg◊

Tablets (timed-release): 8 mg◊, 12 mg◊
Capsules (timed-release): 8 mg◊, 12 mg◊
Syrup: 2 mg/5 ml◊
Injection: 10 mg/ml, 100 mg/ml

MECHANISM OF ACTION
Competes with histamine for H_1-receptor sites on effector cells. Prevents but does not reverse histamine-mediated responses.

INDICATIONS & DOSAGE
Rhinitis, allergy symptoms—
Adults: 4 mg P.O. q 4 to 6 hours, not to exceed 24 mg/day; or (timed-release) 8 mg P.O. every 12 hours; or 5 to 40 mg I.M., I.V., or S.C. daily. Give I.V. injection over 1 minute.
Children 6 to 12 years: 2 mg P.O. q 4 to 6 hours, not to exceed 12 mg/day. Alternatively, may give 8 mg (timed-release) at bedtime.
Children 2 to 6 years: 1 mg P.O. q 4 to 6 hours.
Note: Children under 12 years should use only as directed by a doctor.

ADVERSE REACTIONS
CNS: *stimulation,* sedation, *drowsiness* (especially in elderly patients), excitability (in children).
CV: hypotension, palpitations.
GI: epigastric distress, *dry mouth.*
GU: urine retention.
Skin: rash, urticaria.
Other: thick bronchial secretions.
After parenteral administration: local stinging, burning sensation, pallor, weak pulse, transient hypotension.

INTERACTIONS
CNS depressants: increased sedation. Use together cautiously.

NURSING CONSIDERATIONS
• Contraindicated in acute asthmatic attacks. Use cautiously in elderly patients, and in increased intraocular

---

pressure, hyperthyroidism, cardiovascular or renal disease, hypertension, bronchial asthma, urine retention, prostatic hypertrophy, bladder-neck obstruction and stenosing peptic ulcers.

• Warn patient against drinking alcoholic beverages and using other CNS depressants during therapy and against driving or other activities that require alertness until CNS response to drug is determined.

• Available as nonprescription item for self-medication by adults. However, use on children under 12 years is not recommended without doctor's supervision.

• Coffee or tea may reduce drowsiness. Sugarless gum or sour hard candy, or ice chips may relieve dry mouth.

• If tolerance develops, another antihistamine may be substituted.

• Warn patient to stop taking drug 4 days before allergy skin tests to preserve accuracy of tests.

• Only injectable forms *without* preservatives can be given I.V. Give *slowly*.

• If symptoms occur during or after parenteral dose, discontinue drug. Notify doctor.

---

clemastine fumarate
Tavist*, Tavist-1

Pregnancy Risk Category: C

HOW SUPPLIED
Tablets: 1.34 mg, 2.68 mg
Syrup: 0.67 mg/5 ml (equivalent to 0.5 mg base/5 ml)

MECHANISM OF ACTION
Competes with histamine for H_1-receptor sites on effector cells. Prevents but does not reverse histamine-mediated responses.

INDICATIONS & DOSAGE
Rhinitis, allergy symptoms—

Adults: 1.34 to 2.68 mg P.O. b.i.d. or t.i.d. Maximum recommended daily dosage is 8.04 mg.
Children 6 to 12 years: 0.67 mg P.O. b.i.d. Maximum dosage is 4.02 mg/day.
Allergic skin manifestation of urticaria and angioedema—
Adults: 2.68 mg P.O. up to t.i.d. maximum.
Children 6 to 12 years: 1.34 mg P.O. b.i.d. Maximum dosage is 4.02 mg/day.
Note: Children under 12 years should use only as directed by a doctor.

ADVERSE REACTIONS
Blood: hemolytic anemia, thrombocytopenia, *agranulocytosis.*
CNS: (especially in elderly patients) *sedation, drowsiness.*
CV: hypotension, palpitations, tachycardia.
GI: epigastric distress, anorexia, nausea, vomiting, constipation, *dry mouth.*
GU: urine retention.
Skin: rash, urticaria.
Other: thick bronchial secretions.

INTERACTIONS
CNS depressants: increased sedation. Use together cautiously.

NURSING CONSIDERATIONS
• Contraindicated in acute asthmatic attacks. Use cautiously in elderly patients, and in increased intraocular pressure, hyperthyroidism, cardiovascular or renal disease, hypertension, bronchial asthma, urine retention, prostatic hypertrophy, bladder-neck obstruction, and stenosing peptic ulcers.

• Warn patient against drinking alcoholic beverages during therapy and against driving or other activities that require alertness until CNS response to drug is determined.

• Coffee or tea may reduce drowsi-

Italicized adverse reactions are common or life-threatening.
*Liquid form contains alcohol.   **May contain tartrazine.

ness. Sugarless gum or sour hard candy, or ice chips may relieve dry mouth.
• If tolerance develops, another antihistamine may be substituted.
• Warn patient to stop taking drug 4 days before allergy skin tests to preserve accuracy of tests.
• Monitor blood counts during long-term therapy; observe for signs of blood dyscrasias.

---

cyproheptadine hydrochloride
Periactin*

Pregnancy Risk Category: B

HOW SUPPLIED
Tablets: 4 mg
Syrup: 2 mg/5 ml

MECHANISM OF ACTION
Competes with histamine for H_1-receptor sites on effector cells. Prevents but does not reverse histamine-mediated responses.

INDICATIONS & DOSAGE
Allergy symptoms, pruritus—
Adults: 4 mg P.O. t.i.d. or q.i.d. Maximum dosage is 0.5 mg/kg daily.
Children 7 to 14 years: 4 mg P.O. b.i.d. or t.i.d. Maximum dosage is 16 mg daily.
Children 2 to 6 years: 2 mg P.O. b.i.d. or t.i.d. Maximum dosage is 12 mg daily.
Note: Children under 14 years should use only as directed by a doctor.

ADVERSE REACTIONS
CNS: (especially in elderly patients) *drowsiness,* dizziness, headache, fatigue.
GI: nausea, vomiting, epigastric distress, *dry mouth.*
GU: urine retention.
Skin: rash.
Other: weight gain.

INTERACTIONS
CNS depressants: increased sedation. Use together cautiously.

NURSING CONSIDERATIONS
• Contraindicated in acute asthmatic attacks. Use cautiously in elderly patients, and in increased intraocular pressure, hyperthyroidism, cardiovascular or renal disease, hypertension, bronchial asthma, urine retention, prostatic hypertrophy, bladder-neck obstruction, and stenosing peptic ulcers.
• Warn patient against drinking alcoholic beverages during therapy and against driving or other activities that require alertness until CNS response to drug is determined.
• Reduce GI distress by giving with food or milk.
• Coffee or tea may reduce drowsiness. Sugarless gum or sour hard candy, or ice chips may relieve dry mouth.
• If tolerance develops, another antihistamine may be substituted.
• Warn patient to stop taking drug 4 days before allergy skin tests to preserve accuracy of tests.
• Used experimentally to stimulate appetite and increase weight gain in children.

---

dexchlorpheniramine maleate
Dexchlor, Poladex TD, Polaramine*, Polaramine Repetabs, Polargen

Pregnancy Risk Category: B

HOW SUPPLIED
Tablets: 2 mg
Tablets (timed-release): 4 mg, 6 mg
Syrup: 2 mg/5 ml

MECHANISM OF ACTION
Competes with histamine for H_1-receptor sites on effector cells. Prevents but does not reverse histamine-mediated responses.

INDICATIONS & DOSAGE

Rhinitis, allergy symptoms, contact dermatitis, pruritus—

Adults: 2 mg P.O. q 4 to 6 hours, not to exceed 12 mg/day; or (timed-release) 4 to 6 mg b.i.d. or t.i.d.

Children 6 to 12 years: 1 mg P.O. q 4 to 6 hours, not to exceed 6 mg/day; or 4 mg (timed-release tablet) at bedtime.

Children 2 to 6 years: 0.5 mg P.O. q 4 to 6 hours, not to exceed 3 mg/day.

Note: Children under 6 years should use only as directed by a doctor. Do not use timed-release tablets for children younger than 6 years.

ADVERSE REACTIONS

CNS: (especially in elderly patients) *drowsiness,* dizziness, *stimulation.*
GI: nausea, *dry mouth.*
GU: polyuria, dysuria, urine retention.

INTERACTIONS

CNS depressants: increased sedation. Use together cautiously.

NURSING CONSIDERATIONS

• Contraindicated in acute asthmatic attacks. Use cautiously in elderly patients, and with increased intraocular pressure, hyperthyroidism, cardiovascular or renal disease, hypertension, bronchial asthma, urine retention, prostatic hypertrophy, bladder-neck obstruction, and stenosing peptic ulcers.

• Warn patient against drinking alcoholic beverages during therapy and against driving or other activities that require alertness until CNS response to drug is determined.

• Available as nonprescription item for self-medication by adults. However, use in children under 6 years is not recommended without doctor's supervision.

• Causes less drowsiness than some other antihistamines.

• Coffee or tea may reduce drowsiness. Sugarless gum or sour hard candy, or ice chips may relieve dry mouth.

• If tolerance develops, another antihistamine may be substituted.

• Warn patient to stop taking drug 4 days before allergy skin tests to preserve accuracy of tests.

diphenhydramine hydrochloride

Allerdryl†◇, AllerMax◇, Beldin*◇, Belix◇, Bena-D, Bena-D 50◇, Benadryl*◇, Benadryl Complete Allergy◇, Benahist 10, Benahist 50, Ben-Allergen-50, Benaphen◇, Benoject-10, Benoject-50, Benylin Cough*◇, Benylin Dietetic†, Benylin Expectorant†, Benylin Pediatric†, Bydramine Cough◇, Compoz Diahist◇, Dihydrex, Diphenacen-50, Diphenadryl◇, Diphen Cough*◇, Diphenhist◇, Dormarex 2◇, Fenylhist◇, Fynex◇, Hydramine*, Hydramyn, Hydril◇, Hyrexin-50, Insomnal†, Nervine Nighttime Sleep-Aid◇, Noradryl, Nordryl, Nytol with DPH◇, Sleep-Eze 3◇, Sominex◇, Sominex Liquid◇, Tusstat*◇, Twilite◇, Valdrene*◇, Wehdryl

Pregnancy Risk Category: B

HOW SUPPLIED

Tablets: 25 mg◇, 50 mg◇
Capsules: 25 mg◇, 50 mg◇
Elixir: 12.5 mg/5 ml (14% alcohol)◇
Syrup: 12.5 mg/5 ml◇, 13.3 mg/5 ml (5% alcohol)◇
Injection: 10 mg/ml, 50 mg/ml

MECHANISM OF ACTION

Competes with histamine for H_1-receptor sites on effector cells. Prevents but does not reverse histamine-mediated responses, particularly histamine's effects on the smooth muscle of the bronchial tubes, GI tract, uterus, and blood vessels. Structurally related to local anesthetics, diphenhy-

---

Italicized adverse reactions are common or life-threatening.
*Liquid form contains alcohol.   **May contain tartrazine.

dramine provides local anesthesia by preventing initiation and transmission of nerve impulses. Also suppresses the cough reflex by a direct effect in the medulla of the brain.

INDICATIONS & DOSAGE

Rhinitis, allergy symptoms, nighttime sedation, motion sickness, antiparkinsonism—
Adults: 25 to 50 mg P.O. t.i.d. or q.i.d.; or 10 to 50 mg deep I.M. or I.V. Maximum dosage is 400 mg daily.
Children under 12 years: 5 mg/kg daily P.O., deep I.M., or I.V. divided q.i.d. Maximum dosage is 300 mg daily.
Sedation—
Adults: 25 to 50 mg P.O., or deep I.M., p.r.n.
As a nighttime sleep aid—
Adults: 50 mg P.O. at bedtime.
Nonproductive cough—
Adults: 25 mg P.O. q 4 hours (not to exceed 100 mg daily).
Children 6 to 12 years: 12.5 mg P.O. q 4 hours (not to exceed 50 mg daily).
Children 2 to 6 years: 6.25 mg P.O. q 4 hours (not to exceed 25 mg daily).
   Note: Children under 12 years should use only as directed by a doctor.

ADVERSE REACTIONS

CNS: (especially in elderly patients) *drowsiness,* confusion, insomnia, headache, vertigo.
CV: palpitations.
EENT: diplopia, nasal stuffiness.
GI: *nausea,* vomiting, diarrhea, *dry mouth,* constipation.
GU: dysuria, urine retention.
Skin: urticaria, photosensitivity.

INTERACTIONS

CNS depressants: increased sedation. Use together cautiously.

NURSING CONSIDERATIONS

• Contraindicated in acute asthmatic attacks. Use cautiously in narrow-angle glaucoma, prostatic hypertrophy, pyloroduodenal and bladder-neck obstruction, and stenosing peptic ulcers; in newborns; and in asthmatic, hypertensive, or cardiac patients.
• Alternate injection sites to prevent irritation. Administer deep I.M. into large muscle.
• Warn patient against drinking alcoholic beverages during therapy and against driving or other hazardous activities until CNS response to drug is determined.
• Reduce GI distress by giving with food or milk.
• Coffee or tea may reduce drowsiness. Sugarless gum or sour hard candy, or ice chips may relieve dry mouth.
• If tolerance develops, another antihistamine may be substituted.
• For use to prevent motion sickness, instruct patient to take 30 minutes before travel.
• Warn patient to stop taking drug 4 days before allergy skin tests to preserve accuracy of tests.
• Used with epinephrine in anaphylaxis.
• One of most sedating antihistamines; often used as a hypnotic.
• Warn patient of possible photosensitivity. Advise use of a sunscreen.

---

methdilazine hydrochloride
Dilosyn†, Tacaryl*

Pregnancy Risk Category: C

HOW SUPPLIED
Tablets: 8 mg
Tablets (chewable): 3.6 mg methdilazine (equal to 4 mg methdilazine hydrochloride)
Syrup: 4 mg/5 ml

MECHANISM OF ACTION
Competes with histamine for H_1-receptor sites on effector cells. Pre-

vents but does not reverse histamine-mediated responses.

INDICATIONS & DOSAGE
Allergic rhinitis; pruritus—
Adults: 8 mg P.O. b.i.d. to q.i.d. or (chewable tablets) 7.2 mg P.O. b.i.d. to q.i.d.
Children over 3 years: 4 mg P.O. b.i.d. to q.i.d. or (chewable tablets) 3.6 mg P.O. b.i.d. to q.i.d.

ADVERSE REACTIONS
CNS: (especially in elderly patients) *drowsiness,* dizziness, headache.
GI: nausea, *dry mouth and throat.*
GU: urine retention.
Hepatic: cholestatic jaundice.
Skin: rash.

INTERACTIONS
CNS depressants: increased sedation. Use together cautiously.
Phenothiazines: increased effects. Don't use together.

NURSING CONSIDERATIONS
• Contraindicated in acute asthmatic attacks. Use cautiously in elderly or debilitated patients; acutely ill or dehydrated children; in patients with a history of seizures; and in pulmonary, hepatic, or cardiovascular disease, asthma, hypertension, prostatic hypertrophy, bladder-neck obstruction, CNS depression, and stenosing peptic ulcers.
• Warn patient against drinking alcoholic beverages during therapy and against driving or other activities that require alertness until CNS response to drug is determined.
• Reduce GI distress by giving with food or milk.
• Coffee or tea may reduce drowsiness. Sugarless gum or sour hard candy, or ice chips may relieve dry mouth.
• If tolerance develops, another antihistamine may be substituted.
• Available as chewable tablet for children. Instruct child to chew completely and swallow promptly; may cause local anesthetic effect in mouth, which increases the risk of choking.
• Warn patient to stop taking drug 4 days before allergy skin tests to preserve accuracy of tests.

promethazine hydrochloride
Anergan 25, Anergan 50, Histanil†, K-Phen, Mallergan, Pentazine, Phenameth, Phenazine 25, Phenazine 50, Phencen-50, Phenergan*, Phenergan-Fortis*, Phenergan-Plain*, Phenoject-50, PMS-Promethazine†, Pro-50, Prometh-25, Prometh-50, Promethegan, Prothazine‡, Prothazine-25, Prothazine-50, Prothazine Plain, Remsed, V-Gan-25, V-Gan-50

Pregnancy Risk Category: C

HOW SUPPLIED
Tablets: 12.5 mg, 25 mg, 50 mg
Syrup: 5 mg/5 ml‡, 6.25 mg/5 ml, 10 mg/5 ml, 25 mg/5 ml
Injection: 25 mg/ml, 50 mg/ml
Suppositories: 12.5 mg, 25 mg, 50 mg

MECHANISM OF ACTION
Competes with histamine for H_1-receptor sites on effector cells. Prevents but does not reverse histamine-mediated responses.

INDICATIONS & DOSAGE
Motion sickness—
Adults: 25 mg P.O. b.i.d.
Children: 1 mg/kg P.O., I.M., or rectally b.i.d.
Nausea—
Adults: 12.5 to 25 mg P.O., I.M., or rectally q 4 to 6 hours, p.r.n.
Children: 1 mg/kg I.M. or rectally q 4 to 6 hours, p.r.n.
Rhinitis, allergy symptoms—

Adults: 12.5 mg P.O. q.i.d.; or 25 mg P.O. at bedtime.
Children: 6.25 to 12.5 mg P.O. t.i.d. or 25 mg P.O. or rectally at bedtime.
Sedation—
Adults: 25 to 50 mg P.O. or I.M. at bedtime or p.r.n.
Children: 12.5 to 25 mg P.O., I.M., or rectally at bedtime.
Routine preoperative or postoperative sedation or as an adjunct to analgesics—
Adults: 25 to 50 mg I.M., I.V., or P.O.
Children: 12.5 to 25 mg I.M., I.V., or P.O.

ADVERSE REACTIONS
Blood: leukopenia, *agranulocytosis.*
CNS: (especially in elderly patients) *sedation,* confusion, restlessness, tremors, *drowsiness.*
CV: hypotension.
EENT: transient myopia, nasal congestion.
GI: anorexia, nausea, vomiting, constipation, *dry mouth.*
GU: urine retention.
Other: photosensitivity.

INTERACTIONS
CNS depressants: increased sedation. Use together cautiously.
Phenothiazines: increased effects. Don't give together.

NURSING CONSIDERATIONS
• Contraindicated in increased intraocular pressure, intestinal obstruction, prostatic hypertrophy, bladderneck obstruction, epilepsy, bone-marrow depression, coma, CNS depression, stenosing peptic ulcers, and in newborns and acutely ill or dehydrated children. Use cautiously in pulmonary, hepatic, or cardiovascular disease; asthma; hypertension; bone-marrow depression; elderly or debilitated patients; and in patients with a history of seizures.
• Warn patient against drinking alcoholic beverages during therapy and against driving or other activities that require alertness until CNS response to drug is determined.
• Reduce GI distress by giving with food or milk.
• Coffee or tea may reduce drowsiness. Sugarless gum or sour hard candy, or ice chips may relieve dry mouth.
• Warn patient to stop taking drug 4 days before allergy skin tests to preserve accuracy of tests.
• Pronounced sedative effect limits use in many ambulatory patients.
• May cause false-positive immunologic urine pregnancy test (Gravindex). Also may interfere with blood grouping in ABO system.
• When treating motion sickness, tell patient to take first dose 30 to 60 minutes before travel. On succeeding days of travel, he should take dose upon arising and with evening meal.
• Inject deep I.M. into large muscle mass. Don't administer S.C. Rotate injection sites.
• May be administered I.V., but don't give in a concentration greater than 25 mg/ml, nor at a rate exceeding 25 mg/minute. Shield I.V. infusion from direct light.
• Used as an adjunct to analgesics (usually to increase sedation), but promethazine has no analgesic activity.
• May be safely mixed with meperidine (Demerol) in the same syringe.
• Warn patient about possible photosensitivity and precautions to avoid it.

---

terfenadine
Seldane, Teldane‡
Pregnancy Risk Category: C

HOW SUPPLIED
Tablets: 60 mg

MECHANISM OF ACTION
Competes with histamine for H_1-

receptor sites on effector cells. Prevents but does not reverse histamine-mediated responses.

INDICATIONS & DOSAGE
Rhinitis, allergy symptoms—
Adults and children over 12 years: 60 mg P.O. b.i.d.
Children 6 to 12 years: 30 to 60 mg P.O. b.i.d.
Children 3 to 5 years: 15 mg P.O. b.i.d.

ADVERSE REACTIONS
CNS: fatigue, dizziness, *headache,* sedation.
GI: abdominal distress, nausea.
EENT: dry throat and mouth, nasal stuffiness.

INTERACTIONS
None significant.

NURSING CONSIDERATIONS
• May cause a mild anticholinergic drying effect in patients with lower airway disease, such as asthma. Keep patients well hydrated.
• Instruct patients not to exceed prescribed dose.
• Relief of symptoms begins within 1 hour.
• Terfenadine is a butyrophenone-derivative antihistamine. Significant lack of adverse reactions also makes it unique.
• Does not cause the degree of drowsiness and sedation associated with other antihistamines because drug does not cross blood-brain barrier; its anticholinergic and antiserotonin effects are mild.
• Tablets must be broken for children's dosages.

trimeprazine tartrate
Panectyl†, Temaril*
Pregnancy Risk Category: C

HOW SUPPLIED
Tablets: 2.5 mg
Spansule capsules (sustained-release): 5 mg
Syrup: 2.5 mg/5 ml (5.7% alcohol)

MECHANISM OF ACTION
Competes with histamine for H_1-receptor sites on effector cells. Prevents but does not reverse histamine-mediated responses.

INDICATIONS & DOSAGE
Pruritus—
Adults: 2.5 mg P.O. q.i.d.; or (timed-release) 5 mg P.O. b.i.d.
Children 3 to 12 years: 2.5 mg P.O. at bedtime or t.i.d., p.r.n.
Children 6 months to 3 years: 1.25 mg P.O. at bedtime or t.i.d., p.r.n.
Note: Children under 12 years should use only as directed by a doctor.

ADVERSE REACTIONS
Blood: *agranulocytosis,* leukopenia.
CNS: (especially in elderly patients) drowsiness, dizziness, confusion, headache, restlessness, tremors, irritability, insomnia; (in children) paradoxical excitation.
CV: hypotension, palpitations, tachycardia.
GI: anorexia, nausea, vomiting, *dry mouth and throat.*
GU: urinary frequency, urine retention.
Skin: urticaria, rash, *photosensitivity.*

INTERACTIONS
CNS depressants: increased sedation. Use together cautiously.
Phenothiazines: increased effects. Don't use together.

Italicized adverse reactions are common or life-threatening.
*Liquid form contains alcohol.   **May contain tartrazine.

NURSING CONSIDERATIONS
• Contraindicated in acute asthmatic attacks. Use cautiously in pulmonary, hepatic, or cardiovascular disease; asthma; hypertension; narrow-angle glaucoma; intestinal obstruction; prostatic hypertrophy; bladder-neck obstruction; epilepsy; bone-marrow depression; coma; CNS depression; stenosing peptic ulcers; in elderly or debilitated patients; and in acutely ill or dehydrated children.
• Warn patient against drinking alcoholic beverages during therapy and against driving or other activities that require alertness until CNS response to drug is determined.
• Reduce GI distress by giving with food or milk.
• Coffee or tea may reduce drowsiness. Sugarless gum or sour hard candy, or ice chips may relieve dry mouth.
• Warn patient to stop taking drug 4 days before allergy skin tests to preserve accuracy of tests.
• Monitor blood counts during long-term therapy.
• Warn patient about risk of photosensitivity. Recommend use of a sunscreen. If photosensitivity occurs, tell patient to stop taking the drug and call the doctor.

---

tripelennamine citrate
PBZ*

tripelennamine hydrochloride
PBZ*, PBZ-SR, Pelamine, Pyribenzamine

Pregnancy Risk Category: B

HOW SUPPLIED
citrate
Elixir: 37.5 mg/5 ml (equivalent to 25 mg/5 ml tripelennamine hydrochloride)
hydrochloride
Tablets: 25 mg, 50 mg

Tablets (sustained-release): 100 mg.

MECHANISM OF ACTION
Competes with histamine for H_1-receptor sites on effector cells. Prevents but does not reverse histamine-mediated responses.

INDICATIONS & DOSAGE
Rhinitis, allergy symptoms—
Adults: 25 to 50 mg P.O. q 4 to 6 hours; or (timed-release) 100 mg b.i.d. or t.i.d. Maximum dosage is 600 mg daily.
Children: 5 mg/kg P.O. daily in four to six divided doses. Maximum dosage is 300 mg daily.

ADVERSE REACTIONS
CNS: (especially in elderly patients) *drowsiness,* dizziness, confusion, restlessness, tremors, irritability, insomnia.
CV: palpitations.
GI: anorexia, diarrhea or constipation, *nausea, vomiting, dry mouth.*
GU: urinary frequency, urine retention.
Skin: urticaria, rash.
Other: thick bronchial secretions.

INTERACTIONS
CNS depressants: increased sedation. Use together cautiously.

NURSING CONSIDERATIONS
• Contraindicated in acute asthmatic attacks. Use cautiously in elderly patients, and in increased intraocular pressure, hyperthyroidism, cardiovascular or renal disease, hypertension, bronchial asthma, urine retention, prostatic hypertrophy, bladder-neck obstruction, and stenosing peptic ulcers.
• Warn patient against drinking alcoholic beverages during therapy and against driving or other activities that require alertness until CNS response to drug is determined.

• Reduce GI distress by giving with food or milk.
• Coffee or tea may reduce drowsiness. Sugarless gum or sour hard candy, or ice chips may relieve dry mouth.
• If tolerance develops, another antihistamine may be substituted.
• Warn patient to stop taking drug 4 days before allergy skin tests to preserve accuracy of tests.

---

triprolidine hydrochloride
Actidil*◇, Myidyl
Pregnancy Risk Category: C

HOW SUPPLIED
Tablets: 2.5 mg◇
Syrup: 1.25 mg/5 ml◇

MECHANISM OF ACTION
Competes with histamine for H_1-receptor sites on effector cells. Prevents but does not reverse histamine-mediated responses.

INDICATIONS & DOSAGE
Colds and allergy symptoms—
Adults: 2.5 mg P.O. q 4 to 6 hours. Maximum dosage is 10 mg/day.
Children over 6 years: 1.25 mg P.O. q 4 to 6 hours. Maximum dosage is 5 mg/day.
Children 4 to 6 years: 0.9 mg P.O. q 4 to 6 hours. Maximum dosage is 3.75 mg/day.
Children 2 to 4 years: 0.6 mg P.O. q 4 to 6 hours. Maximum dosage is 2.5 mg/day.
Children 4 months to 2 years: 0.3 mg P.O. q 4 to 6 hours. Maximum dosage is 1.25 mg/day.
   Note: Children under 12 years should use only as directed by a doctor.

ADVERSE REACTIONS
CNS: (especially in elderly patients) *drowsiness,* dizziness, confusion, restlessness, insomnia, *stimulation.*

GI: anorexia, diarrhea or constipation, nausea, vomiting, *dry mouth.*
GU: urinary frequency, urine retention.
Skin: urticaria, rash.

INTERACTIONS
CNS depressants: increased sedation.

NURSING CONSIDERATIONS
• Contraindicated in acute asthma attacks. Use cautiously in elderly patients, and in increased intraocular pressure, hyperthyroidism, cardiovascular or renal disease, hypertension, diabetes mellitus, bronchial asthma, urine retention, prostatic hypertrophy, bladder-neck obstruction, and stenosing peptic ulcers.
• Warn patient against drinking alcoholic beverages during therapy and against driving or other activities that require alertness until CNS response to drug is determined.
• Reduce GI distress by giving with food or milk.
• Coffee or tea may reduce drowsiness. Sugarless gum or sour hard candy, or ice chips may relieve dry mouth.
• Warn patient to stop taking drug 4 days before allergy skin tests to preserve accuracy of tests.

Italicized adverse reactions are common or life-threatening.
*Liquid form contains alcohol.   **May contain tartrazine.

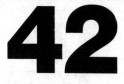

Bronchodilators

*Adrenergics
(sympathomimetics)*
albuterol
albuterol sulfate
bitolterol mesylate
ephedrine hydrochloride
ephedrine sulfate
epinephrine
epinephrine bitartrate
epinephrine hydrochloride
**ethylnorepinephrine
hydrochloride**
isoetharine hydrochloride
isoetharine mesylate
isoproterenol
isoproterenol hydrochloride
isoproterenol sulfate
metaproterenol sulfate
pirbuterol
terbutaline sulfate

Anticholinergics
atropine sulfate
(See Chapter 20, ANTIARRHYTHMICS.)
ipratropium bromide

Methylxanthines and derivatives
aminophylline
dyphylline
oxtriphylline
theophylline
theophylline sodium glycinate

COMBINATION PRODUCTS
Inhalants
DUO-MEDIHALER: isoproterenol hydrochloride 0.16 mg and phenylephrine bitartrate 0.24 mg per dose.
Oral bronchodilators
BRONCHIAL CAPSULES: 150 mg theophylline and 90 mg guaifenesin.

BRONCHOBID DURACAPS: theophylline 260 mg and ephedrine hydrochloride 35 mg.
BRONDECON TABLETS: 200 mg oxtriphylline and 100 mg guaifenesin.
DILOR-G TABLETS: 200 mg dyphylline and 200 mg guaifenesin.
DYFLEX-G TABLETS: 200 mg dyphylline and 200 mg guaifenesin.
DYLINE-GG TABLETS: 200 mg dyphylline and 200 mg guaifenesin.
ENTEX LA: phenylpropanolamine hydrochloride 75 mg and guaifenesin 400 mg.
GLYCERYL-T CAPSULES: 150 mg theophylline and 90 mg guaifenesin.
LANOPHYLLIN-GG CAPSULES: 150 mg theophylline and 90 mg guaifenesin.
MARAX*: theophylline 130 mg, ephedrine sulfate 25 mg, and hydroxyzine hydrochloride 10 mg.
NEOTHYLLINE-GG TABLETS: 200 mg dyphylline and 200 mg guaifenesin.
QUADRINAL: theophylline calcium salicylate 65 mg, ephedrine hydrochloride 24 mg, potassium iodide 320 mg, and phenobarbital 24 mg.
QUIBRON CAPSULES: 150 mg theophylline and 90 mg guaifenesin.
QUIBRON PLUS*: theophylline 150 mg, ephedrine hydrochloride 25 mg, guaifenesin 100 mg, and butabarbital 20 mg.
TEDRAL◇: theophylline 130 mg, ephedrine hydrochloride 24 mg, and phenobarbital 8 mg.
TEDRAL SA: theophylline 180 mg, ephedrine hydrochloride 48 mg, and phenobarbital 25 mg.
THALFED◇: theophylline 120 mg,

---

†Available in Canada only.　　　‡Available in Australia only.　　　◇ Available OTC.

ephedrine hydrochloride 25 mg, and phenobarbital 8 mg.

Decongestants

ACTIFED◊: pseudoephedrine hydrochloride 60 mg and triprolidine hydrochloride 2.5 mg.

CONGESPRIN◊: phenylephrine hydrochloride 1.25 mg and aspirin 81 mg.

DRISTAN◊: phenylephrine hydrochloride 5 mg, chlorpheniramine maleate 2 mg, aspirin 325 mg, and caffeine 16.2 mg.

HISTASPAN-PLUS: phenylephrine hydrochloride 20 mg and chlorpheniramine maleate 8 mg.

NALDECON: phenylpropanolamine hydrochloride 40 mg, phenylephrine hydrochloride 10 mg, chlorpheniramine maleate 5 mg, and phenyltoloxamine citrate 15 mg.

ORNEX◊: phenylpropanolamine hydrochloride 18 mg and acetaminophen 325 mg.

PHENERGAN-D: pseudoephedrine hydrochloride 60 mg and promethazine hydrochloride 6.25 mg.

TRIAMINIC◊: phenylpropanolamine hydrochloride 50 mg, pyrilamine maleate 25 mg, and pheniramine maleate 25 mg.

---

albuterol (salbutamol)
Proventil, Respolin‡

albuterol sulfate (salbutamol sulphate)
Proventil, Proventil Repetabs, Respolin Inhaler‡, Respolin Inhaler Solution‡, Ventolin Obstetric Injection‡

Pregnancy Risk Category: C

HOW SUPPLIED
albuterol
Aerosol inhaler: 90 mcg/metered spray, 100 mcg/metered spray‡
albuterol sulfate
Tablets (extended-release): 4 mg
Syrup: 2 mg/5 ml

Aqueous solution (for respirator): 5 mg/ml‡
Injection: 1 mg/ml‡

MECHANISM OF ACTION
Relaxes bronchial and uterine smooth muscle by acting on beta$_2$-adrenergic receptors.

INDICATIONS & DOSAGE
Prevention and treatment of bronchospasm in patients with reversible obstructive airway disease—
Adults and children over 13 years: 1 to 2 inhalations q 4 to 6 hours. More frequent administration or a greater number of inhalations is not recommended.
   Usual dosage range is 10 to 50 mcg/ minute.
Oral tablets—2 to 4 mg t.i.d. or q.i.d. Maximum dosage is 8 mg q.i.d.
Extended-release tablets—4 to 8 mg q 12 hours. Maximum dosage is 16 mg b.i.d.
Children 6 to 13 years: 2 mg (1 teaspoonful) P.O. t.i.d. or q.i.d.
Children 2 to 5 years: 0.1 mg/kg P.O. t.i.d., not to exceed 2 mg (1 teaspoonful) t.i.d.
Adults over 65 years: 2 mg P.O. t.i.d. or q.i.d.
To prevent exercise-induced asthma—
Adults: 2 inhalations 15 minutes before exercise.
Prevention of premature labor‡—
Adults: initially, 10 mcg/minute by continuous I.V. infusion (use an infusion pump). Dosage should be increased in 10-minute intervals until the desired response is achieved.

ADVERSE REACTIONS
CNS: *tremor, nervousness,* dizziness, insomnia, headache.
CV: tachycardia, palpitations, hypertension.
EENT: drying and irritation of nose and throat (with inhaled form).
GI: heartburn, nausea, vomiting.

Italicized adverse reactions are common or life-threatening.
*Liquid form contains alcohol.   **May contain tartrazine.

Other: muscle cramps.

INTERACTIONS
MAO inhibitors, tricyclic antidepressants: increased adverse cardiovascular effects.
Propranolol and other beta blockers: mutual antagonism. Monitor patient carefully.

NURSING CONSIDERATIONS
• Use cautiously in cardiovascular disorders, including coronary insufficiency and hypertension; in hyperthyroidism or diabetes mellitus; and in patients who are unusually responsive to adrenergics.
• Warn patient about the possibility of paradoxical bronchospasm. If this occurs, the drug should be discontinued immediately.
• Patients may use tablets and aerosol concomitantly. Monitor closely for toxicity.
• Albuterol reportedly produces less cardiac stimulation than other sympathomimetics, especially isoproterenol.
• Elderly patients usually require a lower dosage.
• May be prescribed for use 15 minutes before exercise to prevent exercise-induced bronchospasm.
• Teach patient how to administer metered dose correctly. Have him shake container; exhale through nose; administer aerosol while inhaling deeply on mouthpiece of inhaler; and hold breath for a few seconds, then exhale slowly. Tell him to allow 2 minutes between inhalations and not to use more than the prescribed amount.
• When used to prevent premature labor, monitor maternal heart rate closely. It should not exceed 140 beats/minute.
• After uterine contractions have ceased, the drip rate of the drug should be maintained for 1 hour, then gradually tapered at 50% increments

in six hourly intervals. Infusions should not continue for more than 48 hours. If therapy needs to continue over 48 hours, the doctor may prescribe 4 to 8 mg P.O. q.i.d.
• I.V. form (where available) may be used to prepare infusion using sodium chloride injection, glucose injection, or sodium chloride and glucose injection. The drug should never be administered without dilution. Do not mix with any other medication. Discard unused dilution after 24 hours.
• Pleasant-tasting syrup may be taken by children as young as age 2. Contains no alcohol or sugar.
• Store drug in light-resistant container.

---

aminophylline (theophylline ethylenediamine)
Aminophyllin, Cardophyllin‡, Corophyllin†, Phyllocontin, Somophyllin-DF
Pregnancy Risk Category: C

HOW SUPPLIED
Tablets: 100 mg, 200 mg
Tablets (controlled-release): 225 mg
Oral liquid: 105 mg/5 ml
Injection: 250 mg/10 ml, 500 mg/20 ml, 500 mg/2 ml, 100 mg/100 ml in 0.45% sodium chloride, 200 mg/100 ml in 0.45% sodium chloride
Rectal solution: 300 mg/5 ml
Rectal suppositories: 250 mg, 500 mg

MECHANISM OF ACTION
Inhibits phosphodiesterase, the enzyme that degrades cyclic AMP. Results in relaxation of smooth muscle of the bronchial airways and pulmonary blood vessels.

INDICATIONS & DOSAGE
Symptomatic relief of bronchospasm—
Patients not currently receiving theophylline who require rapid relief of symptoms: loading dose is 6 mg/kg

---

(equivalent to 4.7 mg/kg anhydrous theophylline) I.V. slowly (less than or equal to 25 mg/kg minute), then maintenance infusion.

Adults (nonsmokers): 0.7 mg/kg/hour for 12 hours; then 0.5 mg/kg/hour.

Otherwise healthy adult smokers: 1 mg/kg/hour for 12 hours; then 0.18 mg/kg/hour.

Older patients and adults with cor pulmonale: 0.6 mg/kg/hour for 12 hours; then 0.3 mg/kg/hour.

Adults with CHF or liver disease: 0.5 mg/kg/hour for 12 hours; then 0.1 to 0.2 mg/kg/hour.

Children 9 to 16 years: 1 mg/kg/hour for 12 hours; then 0.8 mg/kg/hour.

Children 6 months to 9 years: 1.2 mg/kg/hour for 12 hours; then 1 mg/kg/hour.

Patients currently receiving theophylline: aminophylline infusions of 0.63 mg/kg (0.5 mg/kg anhydrous theophylline) will increase plasma levels of theophylline by 1 mcg/ml. Some clinicians recommend a dose of 3.1 mg/kg (2.5 mg/kg anhydrous theophylline) if no obvious signs of theophylline toxicity are present.

Chronic bronchial asthma—
Adults: 600 to 1,600 mg P.O. daily divided t.i.d. or q.i.d.
Children: 12 mg/kg P.O. daily divided t.i.d. or q.i.d.

ADVERSE REACTIONS
CNS: *restlessness, dizziness,* headache, *insomnia,* light-headedness, *seizures,* muscle twitching.
CV: *palpitations, sinus tachycardia,* extrasystoles, flushing, marked hypotension, increase in respiratory rate.
GI: *nausea, vomiting, anorexia,* bitter aftertaste, dyspepsia, heavy feeling in stomach, diarrhea.
Skin: urticaria.
Local: *rectal suppositories may cause irritation.*

INTERACTIONS
Alkali-sensitive drugs: reduced activity. Do not add to I.V. fluids containing aminophylline.
Barbiturates, phenytoin, rifampin: enhanced metabolism and decreased theophylline blood levels. Monitor for decreased aminophylline effect.
Beta-adrenergic blockers: antagonism. Propranolol and nadolol, especially, may cause bronchospasm in sensitive patients. Use together cautiously.
Influenza virus vaccine, oral contraceptives, troleandomycin, erythromycin, cimetidine: decreased hepatic clearance of theophylline; elevated theophylline levels. Monitor for signs of toxicity.

NURSING CONSIDERATIONS
• Contraindicated in hypersensitivity to xanthine compounds (caffeine, theobromine) and in preexisting cardiac arrhythmias, especially tachyarrhythmias. Use cautiously in young children; in elderly patients with CHF or other cardiac or circulatory impairment, cor pulmonale, or hepatic disease; in active peptic ulcer, because drug may increase volume and acidity of gastric secretions; and in hyperthyroidism or diabetes mellitus.
• Individuals metabolize xanthines at different rates. Adjust dosage by monitoring response, tolerance, pulmonary function, and serum theophylline levels. Theophylline concentrations should range from 10 to 20 mcg/ml; toxicity has been reported with levels above 20 mcg/ml.
• Plasma clearance may be decreased in patients with CHF, hepatic dysfunction, or pulmonary edema. Smokers show accelerated clearance. Dosage adjustments are necessary.
• I.V. drug administration can cause burning; dilute with 5% dextrose in water solution.
• Monitor vital signs; measure and record intake/output. Expected clinical effects include improvement in quality of pulse and respiration.

Italicized adverse reactions are common or life-threatening.
*Liquid form contains alcohol.   **May contain tartrazine.

- Warn elderly patient of dizziness, a common adverse reaction at start of therapy.
- GI symptoms may be relieved by taking oral drug with full glass of water at meals, although food in stomach delays absorption. Enteric-coated tablets may also delay and impair absorption. No evidence that antacids reduce GI adverse reactions.
- Suppositories are slowly and erratically absorbed; retention enemas may be absorbed more rapidly. Rectally administered preparations can be given if patient cannot take drug orally. Schedule after evacuation, if possible; may be retained better if given before meal. Advise patient to remain recumbent 15 to 20 minutes after insertion.
- Question patient closely about other drugs used. Warn him that OTC remedies may contain ephedrine in combination with theophylline salts; excessive CNS stimulation may result. Tell him to check with doctor or pharmacist before taking *any* other medications.
- Before giving loading dose, check that patient has not had recent theophylline therapy.
- Supply instructions for home care and dosage schedule. Some patients may require an around-the-clock dosage schedule.
- Warn patients with allergies that exposure to allergens may exacerbate bronchospasm.

---

bitolterol mesylate
Tornalate

Pregnancy Risk Category: C

HOW SUPPLIED
Aerosol inhaler: 370 mcg/metered spray

MECHANISM OF ACTION
Relaxes bronchial smooth muscle by acting on beta$_2$-adrenergic receptors.

INDICATIONS & DOSAGE
To prevent and treat bronchial asthma and bronchospasm—
Adults and children over 12 years: to treat bronchospasm, two inhalations at an interval of at least 1 to 3 minutes followed by a third inhalation, if needed. To prevent bronchospasm, the usual dose is two inhalations q 8 hours. In either case, dose should never exceed three inhalations q 6 hours or two inhalations q 4 hours.

ADVERSE REACTIONS
CNS: *tremors,* nervousness, headache, dizziness, light-headedness.
CV: palpitations, chest discomfort, tachycardia.
EENT: throat irritation, cough.
GI: nausea.
Other: dyspnea, *hypersensitivity.*

INTERACTIONS
None significant.

NURSING CONSIDERATIONS
- Use cautiously in ischemic heart disease or hypertension, hyperthyroidism, diabetes mellitus, cardiac arrhythmias, and seizure disorders.
- Monitor blood pressure regularly.
- Advise patients not to exceed recommended dosages. Too frequent use may cause tachycardia.
- Remind patients that beneficial effects last for up to 8 hours, longer than most other similar bronchodilators.
- Has rapid onset of action (about 3 to 4 minutes). Peak effect occurs in 30 to 60 minutes.
- Show patient how to use inhaler correctly.

---

dyphylline
Brophylline, Dilin, Dilor*, Dyflex,
Dylline*, Emfabid, Lufyllin*,
Protophylline†

Pregnancy Risk Category: C

HOW SUPPLIED
Tablets: 200 mg, 400 mg
Elixir: 100 mg/15 ml, 160 mg/15 ml
Injection: 250 mg/ml

MECHANISM OF ACTION
Inhibits phosphodiesterase, the enzyme that degrades cyclic adenosine monophosphate. Results in relaxation of smooth muscle of the bronchial airways and pulmonary blood vessels.

INDICATIONS & DOSAGE
For relief of acute and chronic bronchial asthma and reversible bronchospasm associated with chronic bronchitis and emphysema—
Adults: 15 mg/kg P.O. q 6 hours.
I.M. route is rarely used, but patients may receive 250 to 500 mg I.M. injected slowly at 6-hour intervals. Dosage should be decreased in renal insufficiency.

ADVERSE REACTIONS
CNS: *restlessness, dizziness,* headache, *insomnia,* light-headedness, *seizures,* muscle twitching.
CV: *palpitations, sinus tachycardia,* extrasystoles, flushing, marked hypotension, increase in respiratory rate.
GI: *nausea, vomiting, anorexia,* bitter aftertaste, dyspepsia, heavy feeling in stomach.
Skin: urticaria.

INTERACTIONS
Barbiturates, phenytoin, rifampin: enhanced metabolism and decreased theophylline blood levels. Monitor for decreased theophylline effect.
Beta-adrenergic blockers: antagonism. Propanolol and nadolol, especially, may cause bronchospasm in sensitive patients. Use together cautiously.
Influenza virus vaccine, oral contraceptives, troleandomycin, erythromycin, cimetidine: decreased hepatic clearance of theophylline; elevated theophylline levels. Monitor for signs of toxicity.

NURSING CONSIDERATIONS
• Contraindicated in hypersensitivity to xanthine compounds (caffeine, theobromine); preexisting cardiac arrhythmias, especially tachycardias. Use cautiously in young children; in elderly patients with CHF, any impaired cardiac or circulatory function, cor pulmonale, renal or hepatic disease; and in peptic ulcer, hyperthyroidism, or diabetes mellitus.
• Do not administer I.V.
• Dyphylline is metabolized faster than theophylline; dosage intervals may have to be decreased to ensure continual therapeutic effect. Higher daily dosages may be needed.
• Monitor vital signs; measure and record intake/output. Expected clinical effects include improvement in quality of pulse and respiration.
• Warn elderly patient of dizziness, a common adverse reaction at start of therapy.
• Gastric irritation may be relieved by taking oral drug after meals; there is no evidence that antacids reduce this adverse reaction. May produce less gastric discomfort than theophylline.
• Discard injectable dyphylline if precipitate is present. Protect from light.
• Question patient closely about other drugs used. Warn him that OTC remedies may contain ephedrine in combination with theophylline salts; excessive CNS stimulation may result. Tell him to check with doctor or pharmacist before taking *any* other medications.

Italicized adverse reactions are common or life-threatening.
*Liquid form contains alcohol.   **May contain tartrazine.

- Supply instructions for home care and dosage schedule.

---

ephedrine hydrochloride
Fedrine†

ephedrine sulfate
Ephed II

Pregnancy Risk Category: C

HOW SUPPLIED
Tablets: 30 mg‡
Capsules: 25 mg, 50 mg
Capsules (extended-release): 15 mg, 30 mg, 60 mg
Oral solution: 11 mg/5 ml, 20 mg/5 ml
Injection: 5 mg/ml, 20 mg/ml, 25 mg/ml, 50 mg/ml (parenteral)

MECHANISM OF ACTION
Both a direct- and indirect-acting sympathomimetic that stimulates alpha- and beta-adrenergic receptors.

INDICATIONS & DOSAGE
To correct hypotensive states; to support ventricular rate in Adams-Stokes syndrome—
Adults: 25 to 50 mg I.M. or S.C., or 10 to 25 mg I.V. p.r.n. to maximum of 150 mg/24 hours.
Children: 3 mg/kg S.C. or I.V. daily, in four to six divided doses.
Bronchodilator or nasal decongestant—
Adults: 12.5 to 50 mg P.O. b.i.d., t.i.d., or q.i.d. Maximum dosage is 400 mg daily in six to eight divided doses.
Children: 2 to 3 mg/kg P.O. daily in four to six divided doses.

ADVERSE REACTIONS
CNS: *insomnia, nervousness,* dizziness, headache, muscle weakness, sweating, euphoria, confusion, delirium.
CV: *palpitations,* tachycardia, hypertension.

EENT: dryness of nose and throat.
GI: nausea, vomiting, anorexia.
GU: urine retention, painful urination due to visceral sphincter spasm.

INTERACTIONS
Alpha-adrenergic blocking agents: unopposed beta-adrenergic effects, resulting in hypotension.
Antihypertensives: decreased effects.
Beta-adrenergic blocking agents: unopposed alpha-adrenergic effects, resulting in hypertension.
Digitalis glycosides, general anesthetics (halogenated hydrocarbons): increased risk of ventricular arrhythmias.
Ergot alkaloids: enhanced vasoconstrictor activity.
Guanadrel, guanethidine: enhanced pressor effects of ephedrine.
Levodopa: enhanced risk of ventricular arrhythmias.
MAO inhibitors and tricyclic antidepressants: when given with sympathomimetics, may cause severe hypertension (hypertensive crisis).
Methyldopa: may inhibit effects of ephedrine. Use together cautiously.

NURSING CONSIDERATIONS
- Contraindicated in porphyria, severe coronary artery disease, cardiac arrhythmias, narrow-angle glaucoma, or psychoneurosis; and in patients on MAO-inhibitor therapy. Use with caution in elderly patients and those with hypertension, hyperthyroidism, nervous or excitable states, cardiovascular disease, and prostatic hypertrophy.
- Not a substitute for blood or fluid volume deficit. Volume deficit should be replaced before vasopressors are administered.
- Give I.V. injection slowly.
- Hypoxia, hypercapnia, and acidosis, which may reduce effectiveness or increase the incidence of adverse reactions, must be identified and corrected before or during ephedrine administration.

- Effectiveness decreases after 2 to 3 weeks. Then increased dosage may be needed. Tolerance develops, but drug is not known to cause addiction.
- To prevent insomnia, avoid giving within 2 hours before bedtime.
- Warn patient not to take OTC drugs that contain ephedrine without informing doctor.

---

epinephrine
Adrenalin◊, Bronkaid Mist◊, Bronkaid Mistometer†, Dysne-Inhal†, Primatene Mist Solution◊

epinephrine bitartrate
AsthmaHaler◊, Broniten Mist◊, Bronkaid Mist Suspension◊, Medihaler-Epi◊, Primatene Mist Suspension◊

epinephrine hydrochloride
Adrenalin Chloride◊, Epi-Pen, Epi-Pen Jr., Sus-Phrine

Pregnancy Risk Category: C

HOW SUPPLIED
Aerosol inhaler: 160 mcg◊, 200 mcg◊, 250 mcg/metered spray◊
Nebulizer inhaler: 1% (1:100)†◊, 1.25%†◊, 2.25%†◊
Injection: 0.01 mg/ml (1:100,000), 0.1 mg/ml (1:10,000), 0.5 mg/ml (1:2,000), 1 mg/ml (1:1,000) parenteral; 5 mg/ml (1:200) parenteral suspension

MECHANISM OF ACTION
Stimulates alpha- and beta-adrenergic receptors within the sympathetic nervous system.

INDICATIONS & DOSAGE
Bronchospasm, hypersensitivity reactions, anaphylaxis—
Adults: 0.1 to 0.5 ml of 1:1,000 S.C. or I.M. Repeat q 10 to 15 minutes, p.r.n. Or 0.1 to 0.25 ml 1:1,000 I.V.
Children: 0.01 ml (10 mcg) of 1:1,000/kg S.C. Repeat q 20 minutes to 4 hours, p.r.n.; 0.005 ml/kg of 1:200 (Sus-Phrine). Repeat q 8 to 12 hours, p.r.n.
Hemostasis—
Adults: 1:50,000 to 1:1,000, applied topically.
Acute asthmatic attacks (inhalation)—
Adults and children: 1 or 2 inhalations of 1:100 or 2.25% racemic, every 1 to 5 minutes until relief is obtained; 0.2 mg/dose usual content.
To prolong local anesthetic effect—
Adults and children: 0.2 to 0.4 ml of 1:1,000 intraspinal; 1:500,000 to 1:50,000 local mixed with local anesthetic.
To restore cardiac rhythm in cardiac arrest—
Adults: 0.5 to 1 mg I.V. or into endotracheal tube. May be given intracardiac if no I.V. route or intratracheal route available. Some clinicians advocate higher dose (up to 5 mg), especially in patients who don't respond to usual I.V dose. Following initial I.V. administration, may be infused I.V. at a rate of 1 to 4 mcg/minute.
Children: 10 mcg/kg I.V. or 5 to 10 mcg (0.05 to 0.1 ml of 1:10,000)/kg intracardiac.
    Note: 1 mg = 1 ml of 1:1,000 or 10 ml of 1:10,000.

ADVERSE REACTIONS
CNS: *nervousness,* tremor, euphoria, anxiety, coldness of extremities, vertigo, *headache,* sweating, disorientation, agitation. In patients with Parkinson's disease, the drug increases rigidity and tremor.
CV: *palpitations;* widened pulse pressure; hypertension; *tachycardia; ventricular fibrillation; CVA;* anginal pain; ECG changes, including a decrease in the T wave amplitude.
Metabolic: *hyperglycemia,* glycosuria.
Other: pulmonary edema, dyspnea, *pallor.*

Italicized adverse reactions are common or life-threatening.
*Liquid form contains alcohol.   **May contain tartrazine.

INTERACTIONS

Alpha-adrenergic blocking agents: hypotension due to unopposed beta-adrenergic effects.

Beta blockers, such as propranolol: vasoconstriction and reflex bradycardia. Monitor patient carefully.

Digitalis glycosides, general anesthetics (halogenated hydrocarbons): increased risk of ventricular arrhythmias.

Doxapram, mazindol, methylphenidate: enhanced CNS stimulation or pressor effects.

Ergot alkaloids: enhanced vasoconstrictor activity.

Guanadrel, guanethidine: enhanced pressor effects of epinephrine.

Levodopa: enhanced risk of cardiac arrhythmias.

MAO inhibitors: increased risk of hypertensive crisis.

Tricyclic antidepressants, antihistamines, thyroid hormones: when given with sympathomimetics, may cause severe adverse cardiac effects. Avoid giving together.

NURSING CONSIDERATIONS

• Contraindicated in narrow-angle glaucoma, shock (other than anaphylactic shock), organic brain damage, cardiac dilatation, or coronary insufficiency. Also contraindicated during general anesthesia with halogenated hydrocarbons or cyclopropane and in labor (may delay second stage). Use with extreme caution in long-standing bronchial asthma and emphysema who have developed degenerative heart disease. Use with caution in elderly patients, and those with hyperthyroidism, angina, hypertension, psychoneurosis, and diabetes.

• Don't mix with alkaline solutions. Use dextrose 5% in water, normal saline solution, or a combination of dextrose 5% in water and saline solution. Mix just before use.

• When administered I.V., monitor blood pressure, heart rate, and ECG when therapy is initiated and frequently thereafter.

• Epinephrine is rapidly destroyed by oxidizing agents, such as iodine, chromates, nitrates, nitrites, oxygen, and salts of easily reducible metals (such as iron).

• Epinephrine solutions deteriorate after 24 hours. Discard after that time or before if solution is discolored or contains precipitate. Keep solution in light-resistant container, and don't remove before use.

• Massage site after injection to counteract possible vasoconstriction. Repeated local injection can cause necrosis at site from vasoconstriction.

• Avoid I.M. administration of oil injection into buttocks. Gas gangrene may occur because epinephrine reduces oxygen tension of the tissues, encouraging the growth of contaminating organisms.

• In the event of a sharp blood pressure rise, rapid-acting vasodilators, such as nitrites or alpha-adrenergic blocking agents, can be given to counteract the marked pressor effect of large doses of epinephrine.

• Observe patient closely for adverse reactions. If adverse reactions develop, dosage may need to be adjusted or discontinued.

• If patient has acute hypersensitivity reactions, it may be necessary to instruct him to self-inject epinephrine at home.

• Drug of choice in emergency treatment of acute anaphylactic reactions.

---

ethylnorepinephrine hydrochloride

Bronkephrine

Pregnancy Risk Category: C

HOW SUPPLIED

Injection: 2 mg/ml

MECHANISM OF ACTION
Relaxes bronchial smooth muscle by acting on beta-adrenergic receptors.

INDICATIONS & DOSAGE
To relieve bronchospasm caused by asthma—
Adults: 0.6 to 2 mg S.C. or I.M.
Children: 0.2 to 1 mg S.C. or I.M.

ADVERSE REACTIONS
CNS: *headache*, dizziness.
CV: changes in blood pressure, *elevation in pulse rate*, palpitations.
GI: nausea.

INTERACTIONS
Beta blockers: mutual inhibition of clinical effects.
CNS stimulants, xanthine derivatives: enhanced CNS stimulation.
Digitalis glycosides, levodopa, inhalation anesthetics: increased risk of cardiac arrhythmias.
Nitrates, antihypertensives: decreased effects of these agents.
Rauwolfia alkaloids, sympathomimetics: enhanced effects.
Thyroid hormones: increased risk of coronary insufficiency.

NURSING CONSIDERATIONS
• Use with caution in cardiovascular disease or history of stroke.
• Safer than epinephrine for use in hypertensive or severely ill patients in whom significant pressor effects are undesirable.
• Valuable when used in children because of low incidence of adverse reactions; may be useful in diabetic asthmatics due to low glycogenolytic activity.
• Choose anatomic injection site carefully to avoid inadvertent intraneural or intravascular injection.

ipratropium bromide
Atrovent

Pregnancy Risk Category: B

HOW SUPPLIED
Inhaler: each metered dose supplies 18 mcg
Solution (for nebulizer): 0.025% (250 mcg/ml)‡

MECHANISM OF ACTION
Inhibits vagally mediated reflexes by antagonizing acetylcholine. An anticholinergic.

INDICATIONS & DOSAGE
Maintenance treatment of bronchospasm associated with chronic obstructive pulmonary disease—
Adults: 2 inhalations (26 mcg) q.i.d. Additional inhalations may be needed. However, total inhalations should not exceed 12 in 24 hours.

ADVERSE REACTIONS
CNS: nervousness, dizziness, headache.
CV: palpitations.
EENT: cough, blurred vision.
GI: nausea, GI distress, dry mouth.
Skin: rash.

INTERACTIONS
None significant.

NURSING CONSIDERATIONS
• Use cautiously in patients with narrow-angle glaucoma, prostatic hypertrophy, and bladder-neck obstruction.
• Warn patient that this drug is not effective in the treatment of acute episodes of bronchospasm where rapid response is required.
• Teach patient to use the inhaler correctly, as follows: Enclose mouthpiece with lips and hold the base of the canister vertically. Exhale deeply, then inhale slowly through the mouth and, at the same time, firmly press once on

---

Italicized adverse reactions are common or life-threatening.
*Liquid form contains alcohol.   **May contain tartrazine.

the up-ended canister base. Hold your breath for a few seconds. Remove mouthpiece and exhale slowly. Wait 15 seconds, then repeat inhalation.
• Tell patient to avoid accidentally spraying into eyes. Temporary blurring of vision may result.
• Ipratropium is the first anticholinergic bronchodilator available as an aerosol. Works by a different mechanism from either the adrenergics or theophylline compounds.

isoetharine hydrochloride
Arm-a-Med Isoetharine, Beta-2, Bisorine, Bronkosol, Dey-Dose Isoetharine, Dey-Dose Isoetharine S/F, Dey-Lute Isoetharine, Dispos-a-Med Isoetharine

isoetharine mesylate
Bronkometer

Pregnancy Risk Category: C

HOW SUPPLIED
Aerosol inhaler: 340 mcg/metered spray
Nebulizer inhaler: 0.062%, 0.08%, 0.1%, 0.125%, 0.14%, 0.167%, 0.17%, 0.2%, 0.25%, 0.5%, 1% solution

MECHANISM OF ACTION
Relaxes bronchial smooth muscle by acting on beta$_2$-adrenergic receptors.

INDICATIONS & DOSAGE
Bronchial asthma and reversible bronchospasm that may occur with bronchitis and emphysema—
Adults: (hydrochloride) administered by hand nebulizer, oxygen aerosolization, or IPPB.

Method	Dose	Dilution
Hand	3 to 7 inhalations	undiluted
Oxygen aerosolization	0.5 ml	1:3 with saline
IPPB	0.5 ml	1:3 with saline

Adults: (mesylate) 1 to 2 inhalations. Occasionally, more may be required.

ADVERSE REACTIONS
CNS: *tremor, headache,* dizziness, excitement.
CV: *palpitations,* increased heart rate.
GI: nausea, vomiting.

INTERACTIONS
Propranolol and other beta blockers: blocked bronchodilating effect of isoetharine. Monitor patient carefully if used together.

NURSING CONSIDERATIONS
• Use cautiously in hyperthyroidism, hypertension, or coronary disease, and in patients with sensitivity to sympathomimetics.
• Excessive use can lead to decreased effectiveness.
• Monitor for severe paradoxical bronchoconstriction after excessive use. Discontinue immediately if bronchoconstriction occurs.
• Although isoetharine has minimal effects on the heart, use cautiously in patients receiving general anesthetics that sensitize the myocardium to sympathomimetic drugs.
• Instruct patient in the use of aerosol and mouthpiece.
• Due to oxidation of drug when diluted with water, pink sputum mimicking hemoptysis may occur after inhaling isoetharine solution. Tell patient not to be concerned.

isoproterenol
Aerolone, Dey-Dose Isoproterenol,
Dispos-a-Med Isoproterenol,
Isuprel, Vapo-Iso

isoproterenol hydrochloride
Isuprel, Isuprel Mistometer,
Norisodrine Aerotrol

isoproterenol sulfate
Medihaler-Iso

Pregnancy Risk Category: C

HOW SUPPLIED
isoproterenol
Nebulizer inhaler: 0.25%, 0.5%, and
1%
isoproterenol hydrochloride
Tablets (sublingual): 10 mg, 15 mg
Aerosol inhaler: 120 mcg or 131 mcg/
metered spray
Injection: 200 mcg/ml
isoproterenol sulfate
Aerosol inhaler: 80 mcg/metered
spray

MECHANISM OF ACTION
Relaxes bronchial smooth muscle by
acting on $beta_2$-adrenergic receptors.
As a cardiac stimulant, acts on $beta_1$-
adrenergic receptors in the heart.

INDICATIONS & DOSAGE
Bronchial asthma and reversible bron-
chospasm—
Adults: 10 to 20 mg (hydrochloride)
S.L. q 6 to 8 hours.
Children: 5 to 10 mg (hydrochloride)
S.L. q 6 to 8 hours. Not recommended
for children under 6 years.
Bronchospasm—
Adults and children: (sulfate) acute
dyspneic episodes: 1 inhalation initially. May repeat if needed after 2 to
5 minutes.
    Maintenance dosage is 1 to 2 inha-
lations q.i.d. to 6 times daily. May repeat once more 10 minutes after second dose. Not more than 3 doses

should be administered for each attack.
Heart block and ventricular arrhyth-
mias—
Adults: (hydrochloride) initially,
0.02 to 0.06 mg I.V. Subsequent
doses 0.01 to 0.2 mg I.V. or 5 mcg/
minute I.V.; or 0.2 mg I.M. initially,
then 0.02 to 1 mg, p.r.n.
Children: (hydrochloride) may give
half of initial adult dose.
Shock—
Adults and children: (hydrochloride)
0.5 to 5 mcg/ minute by continuous
I.V. infusion. Usual concentration is 1
mg (5 ml) in 500 ml dextrose 5% in
water. Adjust rate according to heart
rate, central venous pressure, blood
pressure, and urine flow.

ADVERSE REACTIONS
CNS: *headache,* mild tremor, weakness, dizziness, nervousness, insomnia.
CV: *palpitations, tachycardia, an-*
ginal pain; blood pressure may rise
and then fall.
GI: nausea, vomiting.
Metabolic: hyperglycemia.
Other: sweating, flushing of face,
bronchial edema and inflammation.

INTERACTIONS
Epinephrine: increased risk of arrhythmias.
Propranolol and other beta blockers:
blocked bronchodilating effect of isoproterenol. Monitor patient carefully
if used together.

NURSING CONSIDERATIONS
• Contraindicated in tachycardia
caused by digitalis intoxication and in
preexisting arrhythmias, especially
tachycardia, because chronotropic effect on the heart may aggravate such
disorders. Contraindicated in recent
myocardial infarction. Use cautiously
in coronary insufficiency, diabetes, or
hyperthyroidism.
• Not a substitute for blood or fluid

Italicized adverse reactions are common or life-threatening.
*Liquid form contains alcohol.   **May contain tartrazine.

volume deficit. Volume deficit should be replaced before vasopressors are administered.

• If heart rate exceeds 110 beats/minute, it may be advisable to decrease infusion rate or temporarily stop infusion. Doses sufficient to increase the heart rate to more than 130 beats/minute may induce ventricular arrhythmias.

• If precordial distress or anginal pain occurs, stop drug immediately.

• When administering I.V. isoproterenol for shock, closely monitor blood pressure, central venous pressure, ECG, arterial blood gas measurements, and urine output. Carefully adjust infusion rate according to these measurements.

• Oral and sublingual tablets are poorly and erratically absorbed.

• Teach patient how to take sublingual tablet properly. Tell him to hold tablet under tongue until it dissolves and is absorbed and not to swallow saliva until that time. Prolonged use of sublingual tablets can cause tooth decay. Instruct patient to rinse mouth with water between doses. Will also help prevent dryness of oropharynx.

• If possible, don't give at bedtime because it interrupts sleep patterns.

• This drug may cause a slight rise in systolic blood pressure and a slight to marked drop in diastolic blood pressure.

• Use a continuous infusion pump to regulate infusion flow rate.

• Observe patient closely for adverse reactions. Dosage may need to be adjusted or discontinued.

• Tell patient to discontinue the drug if it causes an increase in airway resistance.

• Teach patient to perform oral inhalation correctly. Give the following instructions for using a metered-dose nebulizer:

—Clear nasal passages and throat.
—Breathe out, expelling as much air from lungs as possible.
—Place mouthpiece well into mouth as dose from nebulizer is released, and inhale deeply.
—Hold breath for several seconds, remove mouthpiece, and exhale slowly.

• Instructions for metered powder nebulizer are the same, except that deep inhalation is not necessary.

• Patient may develop a tolerance to this drug. Warn against overuse.

• Warn patient using oral inhalant that drug may turn sputum and saliva pink.

• May aggravate ventilation perfusion abnormalities; even while ease of breathing is improved, arterial oxygen tension may fall paradoxically.

• If ordered via inhalation with oxygen, be sure oxygen concentration will not suppress respiratory drive.

• Discard inhalation solution if it is discolored or contains precipitate.

---

metaproterenol sulfate
Alupent, Arm-A-Med
Metaproterenol, Dey-Dose
Metaproterenol, Dey-Med
Metaproterenol, Metaprel

Pregnancy Risk Category: C

HOW SUPPLIED
Tablets: 10 mg, 20 mg
Solution: 10 mg/5 ml
Aerosol inhaler: 0.65 mg/metered spray
Nebulizer inhaler: 0.6%, 5% solution

MECHANISM OF ACTION
Relaxes bronchial smooth muscle by acting on beta$_2$-adrenergic receptors.

INDICATIONS & DOSAGE
Acute episodes of bronchial asthma—
Adults and children. 2 to 3 inhalations. Should not repeat inhalations more often than q 3 to 4 hours. Should not exceed 12 inhalations daily.
Bronchial asthma and reversible bronchospasm—

Adults: 20 mg P.O. q 6 to 8 hours.
Children over 9 years or over 27 kg:
20 mg P.O. q 6 to 8 hours (0.4 mg to
0.9 mg/kg/dose t.i.d.).
**Children 6 to 9 years or less than 27
kg:** 10 mg P.O. q 6 to 8 hours (0.4 mg
to 0.9 mg/kg/dose t.i.d.).
Not recommended for children under 6 years.

ADVERSE REACTIONS
CNS: nervousness, weakness, drowsiness, tremor.
CV: tachycardia, hypertension, palpitations; *with excessive use, cardiac arrest*.
GI: vomiting, nausea, bad taste in
mouth.
Other: paradoxical bronchiolar constriction with excessive use.

INTERACTIONS
Propranolol and other beta blockers:
blocked bronchodilating effect of metaproterenol. Monitor patient carefully if used together.

NURSING CONSIDERATIONS
• Contraindicated in tachycardia and
arrhythmias associated with tachycardia. Use with caution in hypertension,
coronary artery disease, hyperthyroidism, and diabetes.
• Safe use of inhalant in children under 12 years not established.
• Teach patient how to administer
metered dose correctly. Instructions:
shake container; exhale through nose;
administer aerosol while inhaling
deeply on mouthpiece of inhaler; and
hold breath for a few seconds, then
exhale slowly. Allow 2 minutes between inhalations. Store drug in light-
resistant container.
• Metaproterenol inhalations should
precede steroid inhalations (when
prescribed) by 10 to 15 minutes to
maximize therapy.
• Warn patient about the possibility
of paradoxical bronchospasm. If this

occurs, the drug should be discontinued immediately.
• Patients may use tablets and aerosol
concomitantly. Monitor closely for
toxicity.
• Metaproterenol reportedly produces less cardiac stimulation than
other sympathomimetics, especially
isoproterenol.
• Inhalant solution can be administered by IPPB diluted in saline solution or via a hand nebulizer at full
strength.
• Tell patient to notify doctor if no response is derived from dosage. Warn
against changing dose without calling
doctor.

---

oxtriphylline (choline theophyllinate)
Choledyl*
Pregnancy Risk Category: C

HOW SUPPLIED
Tablets: 100 mg, 200 mg
Tablets (sustained-release): 400 mg,
600 mg
Elixir: 100 mg/5 ml
Syrup: 50 mg/5 ml

MECHANISM OF ACTION
Inhibits phosphodiesterase, the enzyme that degrades cyclic adenosine
monophosphate. Results in relaxation
of smooth muscle of the bronchial airways and pulmonary blood vessels.

INDICATIONS & DOSAGE
*To relieve acute bronchial asthma and
reversible bronchospasm associated
with chronic bronchitis and emphysema—*
Adults and children over 12 years:
200 mg P.O. q 6 hours; or 400 to 600
mg sustained-release form P.O. q 12
hours, then adjust dosage based upon
serum theophylline levels.
Children 2 to 12 years: 4 mg/kg P.O.
q 6 hours. Adjust as needed to main-

Italicized adverse reactions are common or life-threatening.
*Liquid form contains alcohol.   **May contain tartrazine.

tain therapeutic levels of theophylline (10 to 20 mcg/ml).

ADVERSE REACTIONS
CNS: *restlessness, dizziness,* headache, *insomnia,* light-headedness, *seizures,* muscle twitching.
CV: *palpitations, sinus tachycardia,* extrasystoles, flushing, marked hypotension, increase in respiratory rate.
GI: *nausea, vomiting, anorexia,* bitter aftertaste, dyspepsia, heavy feeling in stomach.
Skin: urticaria.

INTERACTIONS
Barbiturates, phenytoin, rifampin: enhanced metabolism and decreased theophylline blood levels. Monitor for decreased effect.
Beta-adrenergic blockers: antagonism. Propranolol and nadolol, especially, may cause bronchospasms in sensitive patients. Use together cautiously.
Erythromycin, troleandomycin, cimetidine, influenza virus vaccine, oral contraceptives: decreased hepatic clearance of theophylline; increased plasma level. Monitor for signs of toxicity.

NURSING CONSIDERATIONS
• Contraindicated in hypersensitivity to xanthines (caffeine, theobromine); preexisting cardiac arrhythmias, especially tachyarrhythmias.
• Tell patient to report GI distress, palpitations, irritability, restlessness, nervousness, or insomnia; may indicate excessive CNS stimulation.
• Administer drug after meals and at bedtime.
• Store at 15° to 30° C. (59° to 86° F.). Protect elixir from light and tablets from moisture.
• Equivalent to 64% anhydrous theophylline.
• Monitor therapy carefully.
• Combination products that contain ephedrine are not recommended; excessive CNS stimulation may result (nervousness, tremors, akathisia).

---

pirbuterol
Maxair

Pregnancy Risk Category: C

HOW SUPPLIED
Inhaler: 0.2 mg/metered dose

MECHANISM OF ACTION
Relaxes bronchial smooth muscle by acting on beta$_2$-adrenergic receptors.

INDICATIONS AND DOSAGE
Prevention and reversal of bronchospasm, asthma—
Adults: 1 or 2 inhalations (0.2 to 0.4 mg) repeated q 4 to 6 hours. Not to exceed 12 inhalations daily.

ADVERSE REACTIONS
CNS: tremors, nervousness, dizziness, insomnia, headache.
CV: tachycardia, palpitations, increased blood pressure.
EENT: drying or irritation of throat.

INTERACTIONS
Propranolol and other beta-adrenergic blocking agents: decreased bronchodilating effects.

NURSING CONSIDERATIONS
• Contraindicated in hypersensitivity to pirbuterol or other adrenergics, and in patients with digitalis toxicity or cardiac arrhythmias associated with tachycardia.
• Tell patient to call the doctor if he experiences increased bronchospasm after using the drug.
• Teach patient how to administer metered dose correctly. Have him shake container; exhale through nose; administer aerosol while inhaling deeply on mouthpiece of inhaler; and hold breath for a few seconds, then exhale slowly. Tell him to allow 2 minutes between inhalations and to

---

† Available in Canada only.   ‡ Available in Australia only.   ◊ Available OTC.

wait at least 5 minutes before using his steroid inhalant (if he's taking concomitant corticosteroid inhalants).
• Advise patient to seek medical attention if a previously effective dosage does not control symptoms because this may signify a worsening of the disease.

---

terbutaline sulfate
Brethaire, Brethine, Bricanyl
Pregnancy Risk Category: B

HOW SUPPLIED
Tablets: 2.5 mg, 5 mg
Aerosol inhaler: 200 mcg/metered spray
Injection: 1 mg/ml

MECHANISM OF ACTION
Relaxes bronchial smooth muscle by acting on beta$_2$-adrenergic receptors. Also relaxes uterine muscle.

INDICATIONS & DOSAGE
Relief of bronchospasm in patients with reversible obstructive airway disease—
Adults and children over 11 years: 2 inhalations separated by a 60-second interval, repeated q 4 to 6 hours. May also administer 2.5 to 5 mg P.O. q 8 hours or 0.25 mg S.C.
Treatment of premature labor—
Women: 0.01 mg/minute by I.V. infusion. Increase by 0.005 mg q 10 minutes up to 0.025 mg/minute or until contractions cease. Or, give 0.25 mg S.C. hourly until contractions cease. Maintenance dosage is 5 mg P.O. q 4 hours for 48 hours, then 5 mg q 6 hours.

ADVERSE REACTIONS
CNS: *nervousness, tremors, headache,* drowsiness, sweating.
CV: palpitations, increased heart rate.

EENT: drying and irritation of nose and throat (with inhaled form).
GI: vomiting, nausea.

INTERACTIONS
MAO inhibitors: when given with sympathomimetics, may cause severe hypertension (hypertensive crisis). Don't use together.
Propranolol and other beta blockers: blocked bronchodilating effects of terbutaline.

NURSING CONSIDERATIONS
• Use cautiously in patients with diabetes, hypertension, hyperthyroidism, severe cardiac disease, and cardiac arrhythmias.
• Protect injection from light. Do not use if discolored.
• Make sure patient and his family understand why drug is necessary.
• Give S.C. injections in lateral deltoid area.
• Tolerance may develop with prolonged use.
• Warn patient about the possibility of paradoxical bronchospasm. If this occurs, the drug should be discontinued immediately.
• Patient may use tablets and aerosol concomitantly. Monitor closely for toxicity.
• Teach patient how to administer metered dose correctly. Have him shake container; exhale through nose; administer aerosol while inhaling deeply on mouthpiece of inhaler; and hold breath for a few seconds, then exhale slowly.
• Although not approved by the FDA for treatment of preterm labor, it is considered very effective and is used in many hospitals. Monitor neonates for hypoglycemia.

Italicized adverse reactions are common or life-threatening.
*Liquid form contains alcohol.   **May contain tartrazine.

theophylline

Immediate-release liquids:
Accurbron*, Aerolate, Aquaphyllin, Asmalix*, Bronkodyl*, Elixicon, Elixomin*, Elixophyllin*, Lanophyllin*, Lixolin, Slo-Phyllin, Theolair, Theon*, Theophyl*
Immediate-release tablets and capsules: Bronkodyl, Elixophyllin, Nuelin‡, Slo-Phyllin, Somophyllin-T
Timed-release tablets: Constant-T, Duraphyl, Quibron-T/SR, Respbid, Sustaire, Theo-Dur, Theolair-SR, Theo-Time, Uniphyl
Timed-release capsules: Aerolate, Bronkodyl S-R, Elixophyllin SR, Lodrane, Nuelin-SR‡, Slo-bid Gyrocaps, Slo-Phyllin, Somophyllin-CRT, Theo-24, Theobid Duracaps, Theobid Jr., Theochron, Theo-Dur Sprinkle, Theophyl-SR, Theospan SR, Theovent Long-acting

theophylline sodium glycinate

Acet-Am†, Synophylate

Pregnancy Risk Category: C

HOW SUPPLIED
theophylline
Tablets: 100 mg, 125 mg, 200 mg, 225 mg, 250 mg, 300 mg
Tablets (chewable): 100 mg
Tablets (extended-release): 100 mg, 200 mg, 250 mg, 300 mg, 400 mg, 500 mg
Capsules: 50 mg, 100 mg, 200 mg, 250 mg
Capsules (extended-release): 50 mg, 60 mg, 65 mg, 75 mg, 100 mg, 125 mg, 130 mg, 200 mg, 250 mg, 260 mg, 300 mg
Elixir: 27 mg/5 ml, 50 mg/5 ml
Oral solution: 27 mg/5 ml, 53 mg/5 ml
Oral suspension: 100 mg/5 ml
Syrup: 27 mg/5 ml, 50 mg/5 ml
Dextrose 5% injection: 200 mg in 50 ml or 100 ml; 400 mg in 100 ml, 250 ml, 500 ml, or 1,000 ml; 800 mg in 500 ml or 1,000 ml
theophylline sodium glycinate
Elixir: 110 mg/5 ml (equivalent to 55 mg anhydrous theophylline/5 ml)

MECHANISM OF ACTION
Inhibits phosphodiesterase, the enzyme that degrades cyclic adenosine monophosphate. Results in relaxation of smooth muscle of the bronchial airways and pulmonary blood vessels.

INDICATIONS & DOSAGE
Prophylaxis and symptomatic relief of bronchial asthma, bronchospasm of chronic bronchitis and emphysema—
Adults: 6 mg/kg P.O. followed by 2 to 3 mg/kg q 4 hours for 2 doses. Maintenance dosage is 1 to 3 mg/kg q 8 to 12 hours.
Children 9 to 16 years: 6 mg/kg P.O. followed by 3 mg/kg q 4 hours for 3 doses. Maintenance dosage is 3 mg/kg q 6 hours.
Children 6 months to 9 years: 6 mg/kg P.O. followed by 4 mg/kg q 4 hours for 3 doses. Maintenance dosage is 4 mg/kg q 6 hours.
　　Most oral timed-release forms are given q 8 to 12 hours. Several products, however, may be given q 24 hours.
Symptomatic relief of bronchial asthma, pulmonary emphysema, and chronic bronchitis—
Adults: 330 to 660 mg (sodium glycinate) P.O. q 6 to 8 hours, after meals.
Children over 12 years: 220 to 330 mg (sodium glycinate) P.O. q 6 to 8 hours.
Children 6 to 12 years: 330 mg (sodium glycinate) P.O. q 6 to 8 hours.
Children 3 to 6 years: 110 to 165 mg (sodium glycinate) P.O. q 6 to 8 hours.
Children 1 to 3 years: 55 to 110 mg (sodium glycinate) P.O. q 6 to 8 hours.

Parenteral theophylline for patients not currently receiving theophylline—
Loading dose: 4.7 mg/kg I.V. slowly; then maintenance infusion.
Adults (nonsmokers): 0.55 mg/kg/ hour for 12 hours, then 0.39 mg/kg/ hour.
Otherwise-healthy adult smokers: 0.79 mg/kg/hour for 12 hours; then 0.63 mg/kg/hour.
Older adults with cor pulmonale: 0.47 mg/kg/hour for 12 hours; then 0.24 mg/kg/hour.
Adults with CHF or liver disease: 0.38 mg/kg/hour for 12 hours; then 0.08 to 0.16 mg/kg/hour.
Children 9 to 16 years: 0.79 mg/kg/ hour for 12 hours; then 0.63 mg/kg/ hour.
Children 6 months to 9 years: 0.95 mg/kg/hour for 12 hours; then 0.79 mg/kg/hour.

Switch to oral theophylline as soon as patient shows adequate improvement.
Sympotmatic relief of bronchospasm in patients currently receiving theophylline—
Adults and children: each 0.5 mg/kg I.V. or P.O. (loading dose) will increase plasma levels by 1 mcg/ml. Ideally, dose is based upon current theophylline level. In emergency situations, some clinicians recommend a 2.5 mg/kg P.O. dose of rapidly absorbed form if no obvious signs of theophylline toxicity are present.

ADVERSE REACTIONS
CNS: *restlessness, dizziness,* headache, *insomnia,* light-headedness, *seizures,* muscle twitching.
CV: *palpitations, sinus tachycardia,* extrasystoles, flushing, marked hypotension, increase in respiratory rate.
GI: *nausea, vomiting, anorexia,* bitter aftertaste, dyspepsia, heavy feeling in stomach, diarrhea.
Skin: urticaria.

INTERACTIONS
Barbiturates, phenytoin, rifampin: enhanced metabolism and decreased theophylline blood levels. Monitor for decreased effect.
Beta-adrenergic blockers: antagonism. Propranolol and nadolol, especially, may cause bronchospasms in sensitive patients. Use together cautiously.
Erythromycin, troleandomycin, cimetidine, influenza virus vaccine, oral contraceptives: decreased hepatic clearance of theophylline; increased plasma levels. Monitor for signs of toxicity.

NURSING CONSIDERATIONS
• Contraindicated in hypersensitivity to xanthine compounds (caffeine, theobromine); preexisting cardiac arrhythmias, especially tachyarrhythmias. Use cautiously in young children; in elderly patients with CHF or other circulatory impairment, cor pulmonale, renal or hepatic disease; and in peptic ulcer, hyperthyroidism, or diabetes mellitus.
• Individuals metabolize xanthines at different rates; determine dosage by monitoring response, tolerance, pulmonary function, and serum theophylline levels. Serum theophylline concentrations should range from 10 to 20 mcg/ml; toxicity has been reported with levels above 20 mcg/ml.
• Monitor vital signs; measure and record intake/output. Expected clinical effects include improvement in quality of pulse and respiration.
• Warn elderly patients of dizziness, a common adverse reaction at start of therapy.
• GI symptoms may be relieved by taking oral drug with full glass of water after meals, although food in stomach delays absorption.
• Question patient closely about other drugs used. Warn him that OTC remedies may contain ephedrine in combination with theophylline salts; ex-

---

Italicized adverse reactions are common or life-threatening.
*Liquid form contains alcohol. **May contain tartrazine.

cessive CNS stimulation may result. Tell him to check with doctor or pharmacist before taking *any* other medications.
• Supply instructions for home care and dosage schedule.
• Daily dosage may need to be decreased in patients with CHF or hepatic disease, or in elderly patients, since metabolism and excretion may be decreased. Monitor carefully, using blood levels, observation, examination, and patient interview. Give drug around the clock, using sustained-release product at bedtime.
• Drug dosage may need to be increased in cigarette smokers and in habitual marijuana smokers because smoking causes the drug to be metabolized faster.
• Be careful not to confuse sustained-release dosage forms with standard-release dosage forms.
• Warn patient not to dissolve, crush, or chew slow-release products. Small children unable to swallow these can ingest (without chewing) the contents of bead-filled capsules sprinkled over soft food.
• Warn patients to take the drug regularly, as directed. Patients tend to want to take extra "breathing pills."
• Patients taking Theo-24 brand of theophylline should take it on an empty stomach because food accelerates the drug's absorption.

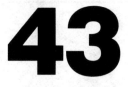

Expectorants and antitussives

Expectorants
acetylcysteine
ammonium chloride
(See Chapter 62, ACIDIFIER AND ALKALINIZERS.)
guaifenesin
iodinated glycerol
potassium iodide
terpin hydrate

Antitussives
benzonatate
codeine phosphate
(See Chapter 27, NARCOTIC AND OPIOID ANALGESICS.)
codeine sulfate
(See Chapter 27, NARCOTIC AND OPIOID ANALGESICS.)
dextromethorphan hydrobromide
diphenhydramine hydrochloride
(See Chapter 41, ANTIHISTAMINES.)
hydromorphone hydrochloride
(See Chapter 27, NARCOTIC AND OPIOID ANALGESICS.)

COMBINATION PRODUCTS
Preparations are available in the following combinations:
• expectorants with decongestants or antihistamines, or both
• antitussives with decongestants or antihistamines, or both
• expectorants and antitussives
• expectorants and antitussives with decongestants or antihistamines, or both.

acetylcysteine
Airbron†, Mucomyst, Mucosol, Parvolex†‡

Pregnancy Risk Category: B

HOW SUPPLIED
Solution: 10%, 20%
Injection: 200 mg/ml†‡*

MECHANISM OF ACTION
Increases production of respiratory tract fluids to help liquefy and reduce the viscosity of thick, tenacious secretions. Also restores liver stores of glutathione in the treatment of acetaminophen toxicity.

INDICATIONS & DOSAGE
Pneumonia, bronchitis, tuberculosis, cystic fibrosis, emphysema, atelectasis (adjunct), complications of thoracic surgery and CV surgery—
Adults and children: 1 to 2 ml 10% to 20% solution by direct instillation into trachea as often as every hour; or 3 to 5 ml 20% solution, or 6 to 10 ml 10% solution, by mouthpiece t.i.d. or q.i.d.
Acetaminophen toxicity—
140 mg/kg initially P.O., followed by 70 mg/kg q 4 hours for 17 doses (a total of 1,330 mg/kg).

ADVERSE REACTIONS
EENT: *rhinorrhea, hemoptysis.*
GI: *stomatitis, nausea.*
Other: *bronchospasm (especially in asthmatics).*

Italicized adverse reactions are common or life-threatening.
*Liquid form contains alcohol.   **May contain tartrazine.

INTERACTIONS
Activated charcoal: don't use together in treating acetaminophen toxicity. Limits acetylcysteine's effectiveness.

NURSING CONSIDERATIONS
• Use cautiously in asthma or severe respiratory insufficiency and in elderly or debilitated patients.
• Classified as a mucolytic.
• Use plastic, glass, stainless steel, or another nonreactive metal when administering by nebulization. Hand bulb nebulizers not recommended because output is too small and particle size too large.
• After opening, store in refrigerator; use within 96 hours.
• Incompatible with oxytetracycline, tetracycline, erythromycin lactobionate, amphotericin B, ampicillin, iodized oil, chymotrypsin, trypsin, and hydrogen peroxide. Administer separately.
• Monitor cough type and frequency. For maximum effect, instruct patient to clear his airway by coughing before aerosol administration.
• Dilute oral doses with cola, fruit juice, or water before administering.

benzonatate
Tessalon

Pregnancy Risk Category: C

HOW SUPPLIED
Capsules: 100 mg

MECHANISM OF ACTION
Suppresses the cough reflex by direct action on the cough center in the medulla (brain). Also has local anesthetic action.

INDICATIONS & DOSAGE
Nonproductive cough—
Adults and children over 10 years: 100 mg P.O. t.i.d.; up to 600 mg daily.

Children under 10 years: 8 mg/kg P.O. in 3 to 6 divided doses.

ADVERSE REACTIONS
CNS: dizziness, drowsiness, headache.
EENT: nasal congestion, sensation of burning in eyes.
GI: nausea, constipation.
Skin: rash.
Other: chills.

INTERACTIONS
None significant.

NURSING CONSIDERATIONS
• Patient should not chew capsules or leave in mouth to dissolve; local anesthesia will result. If capsules dissolve in mouth, CNS stimulation may cause restlessness, tremors, and possibly seizures.
• A nonnarcotic cough suppressant; don't use when cough is valuable as diagnostic sign or is beneficial (as after thoracic surgery).
• Monitor cough type and frequency.
• Use with percussion and chest vibration.
• Maintain fluid intake to help liquefy sputum.

dextromethorphan hydrobromide
Balminil D.M.◊, Benylin DM◊, Broncho-Grippol-DM†, Congespirin for Children◊, Cremacoat 1◊, Delsym◊, DM Cough*◊, Hold◊, Koffex†, Mediquell◊, Neo-DM†, Pediacare 1◊, Pertussin 8 Hour Cough Formula◊, Robidex†, Sedatuss†, St. Joseph for Children◊, Sucrets Cough Control Formula◊. More commonly available in combination products such as Contac Cough and Sore Throat Formula◊, Contact Cough Formula◊, Contac Jr.

Children's Cold Medicine◇, Contac Nighttime Cold Medicine◇, Contac Severe Cold Formula Caplets◇, Novahistine DMX Liquid, Phenergan with Dextromethorphan*, Robitussin-DM*◇, Rondec-DM*◇, Triaminicol Multi-Symptom Cold◇, Trind-DM Liquid*◇, Tussi-Organidin-DM Liquid*

Pregnancy Risk Category: C

HOW SUPPLIED
Chewable pieces: 15 mg◇
Liquid (sustained-action): 30 mg/5 ml◇
Lozenges: 5 mg◇
Syrup: 5 mg/5 ml◇, 7.5 mg/5 ml◇, 10 mg/5 ml◇, 15 mg/5 ml◇

MECHANISM OF ACTION
Suppresses the cough reflex by direct action on the cough center in the medulla (brain).

INDICATIONS & DOSAGE
Nonproductive cough—
Adults: 10 to 20 mg P.O. q 4 hours, or 30 mg q 6 to 8 hours. Or the controlled-release liquid twice daily (60 mg b.i.d.). Maximum 120 mg daily.
Children 6 to 12 years: 5 to 10 mg P.O. q 4 hours, or 15 mg q 6 to 8 hours. Or the controlled-release liquid twice daily (30 mg b.i.d.). Maximum 60 mg daily.
Children 2 to 6 years: 2.5 to 5 mg P.O. q 4 hours, or 7.5 mg q 6 to 8 hours. Maximum 30 mg daily.

ADVERSE REACTIONS
CNS: drowsiness, dizziness.
GI: nausea.

INTERACTIONS
MAO inhibitors: hypotension, coma, hyperpyrexia, and death have occurred. Do not use together.

NURSING CONSIDERATIONS
• Contraindicated in patients currently taking or within 2 weeks of discontinuing MAO inhibitors.
• Produces no analgesia or addiction and little or no CNS depression.
• An antitussive; don't use when cough is valuable diagnostic sign or beneficial (as after thoracic surgery).
• Use with percussion and chest vibration.
• Monitor cough type and frequency.
• Dose of 15 to 30 mg dextromethorphan is equivalent to 8 to 15 mg codeine as an antitussive.

guaifenesin (glyceryl guaiacolate)
Anti-Tuss*◇, Balminil Expectorant†, Baytussin◇, Breonesin◇, Colrex Expectorant*◇, Cremacoat 2◇, Gee-Gee◇, GG-CEN*◇, Glyate*◇, Glycotuss◇, Glytuss◇, Guiatuss*◇, Halotussin◇, Humibid L.A.◇, Hytuss◇, Hytuss-2X◇, Malotuss◇, Naldecon Senior EX◇, Neo-Spec†, Nortussin◇, Resyl†, Robafen◇, Robitussin*◇, S-T Expectorant◇

Pregnancy Risk Category: C

HOW SUPPLIED
Tablets: 100 mg◇, 200 mg◇
Capsules: 200 mg◇
Syrup: 67 mg/5 ml◇, 100 mg/5 ml◇

MECHANISM OF ACTION
Increases production of respiratory tract fluids to help liquefy and reduce the viscosity of thick, tenacious secretions.

INDICATIONS & DOSAGE
As expectorant—
Adults: 100 to 400 mg P.O. q 4 hours. Maximum 2,400 mg daily.
Children 6 to 12 years: 100 to 200 mg P.O. q 4 hours. Maximum 600 mg daily.
Children 2 to 5 years: 50 to 100 mg P.O. q 4 hours. Maximum 300 mg daily.

Italicized adverse reactions are common or life-threatening.
*Liquid form contains alcohol.   **May contain tartrazine.

ADVERSE REACTIONS
CNS: drowsiness.
GI: vomiting and nausea occur with large doses.

INTERACTIONS
Heparin: increased risk of bleeding. Use together cautiously.

NURSING CONSIDERATIONS
• May interfere with certain laboratory tests for 5-hydroxyindoleacetic acid and vanillylmandelic acid.
• Liquefies thick, tenacious sputum; maintain fluid intake. Advise patient to take with a glass of water whenever possible.
• Monitor cough type and frequency.
• Encourage deep-breathing exercises.
• Although a popular expectorant, its efficacy has not been established.

---

iodinated glycerol
Iophen Elixir*, Myodine*, Organidin*, R-Ger Elixir*

Pregnancy Risk Category: X

HOW SUPPLIED
Tablets: 30 mg
Elixir: 60 mg/5 ml
Solution: 50 mg/ml

MECHANISM OF ACTION
Increases production of respiratory tract fluids to help liquefy and reduce the viscosity of thick, tenacious secretions.

INDICATIONS & DOSAGE
Bronchial asthma, bronchitis, emphysema (adjunct)—
Adults: 60 mg P.O. q.i.d. (tablets), or 20 drops (solution) P.O. q.i.d. with fluids, or 5 ml (elixir) P.O. q.i.d.
Children: up to half adult dose based on child's weight.

ADVERSE REACTIONS
After long-term use:

GI: *nausea,* gastrointestinal distress.
Skin: *eruptions.*
Other: acute parotitis, thyroid enlargement, hypothyroidism.

INTERACTIONS
None significant.

NURSING CONSIDERATIONS
• Contraindicated in hypothyroidism, iodine sensitivity, and during pregnancy and lactation.
• Skin rash or other hypersensitivity reaction may require stopping drug.
• May liquefy thick, tenacious sputum; maintain fluid intake.
• Monitor cough type and frequency.
• Encourage deep-breathing exercises.
• Efficacy has not been established.

---

potassium iodide
Pregnancy Risk Category: D

HOW SUPPLIED
Tablets (enteric-coated): 300 mg
Oral solution: 500 mg/15 ml
Saturated solution (SSKI): 1 g/ml
Strong iodine solution (Lugol's solution): iodine 50 mg/ml and potassium iodide 100 mg/ml
Syrup: 325 mg/5 ml

MECHANISM OF ACTION
Increases production of respiratory tract fluids to help liquefy and reduce the viscosity of thick secretions.

INDICATIONS & DOSAGE
As expectorant, chronic bronchitis, chronic pulmonary emphysema, bronchial asthma—
Adults: 0.3 to 0.6 ml P.O. q 4 to 6 hours.
Children: 0.25 to 0.5 ml P.O. of saturated solution (1 g/ml) b.i.d. to q.i.d.
Nuclear radiation protection—
Adults and children: 0.13 ml P.O. of SSKI immediately before or after ini-

---

tial exposure will block 90% of radioactive iodine. Same dose given 3 to 4 hours after exposure will provide 50% block. Should be administered for up to 10 days under medical supervision.
Infants under 1 year: ½ adult dose.

ADVERSE REACTIONS
GI: *nausea,* vomiting, *epigastric pain,* metallic taste.
Metabolic: goiter, hyperthyroid adenoma, hypothyroidism (with excessive use), collagen disease-like syndrome.
Skin: rash.
Other: drug fever.
Prolonged use: chronic iodine poisoning, soreness of mouth, coryza, sneezing, swelling of eyelids.

INTERACTIONS
Lithium carbonate: may cause hypothyroidism. Don't use together.

NURSING CONSIDERATIONS
• Contraindicated in iodine hypersensitivity, tuberculosis, hyperkalemia, acute bronchitis, hyperthyroidism.
• Maintain adequate fluid intake.
• Has strong, salty, metallic taste. Dilute with milk, fruit juice, or broth to reduce GI distress and disguise taste.
• Sudden withdrawal may precipitate thyroid storm.
• If skin rash appears, discontinue use. Contact doctor.

---

terpin hydrate*
Pregnancy Risk Category: C

HOW SUPPLIED
Elixir: 85 mg/5 ml (43% alcohol)

MECHANISM OF ACTION
Increases production of respiratory tract fluids to help liquefy and reduce the viscosity of thick secretions.

INDICATIONS & DOSAGE
Excessive bronchial secretions—

Adults: 5 to 10 ml P.O. of elixir q 4 to 6 hours.

ADVERSE REACTIONS
GI: nausea, vomiting.

INTERACTIONS
None significant.

NURSING CONSIDERATIONS
• Contraindicated in peptic ulcer or severe diabetes mellitus.
• Don't give in large doses; *high alcoholic content of elixir* (86 proof).
• Monitor cough type and frequency.

Italicized adverse reactions are common or life-threatening.
*Liquid form contains alcohol.   **May contain tartrazine.

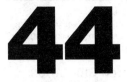

Antacids, adsorbents, and antiflatulents

aluminum carbonate
aluminum hydroxide
aluminum phosphate
calcium carbonate
dihydroxyaluminum sodium
  carbonate
magaldrate
magnesium oxide
magnesium hydroxide
  (See Chapter 47, LAXATIVES.)
simethicone
sodium bicarbonate
  (See Chapter 62, ACIDIFIER AND
  ALKALINIZERS.)

COMBINATION PRODUCTS

ALKA-SELTZER, MEDI-SELTZER◇: sodium bicarbonate 1,916 mg, aspirin 325 mg, and citric acid 1,000 mg.
ALKA-SELTZER WITHOUT ASPIRIN◇: sodium bicarbonate 958 mg, citric acid 832 mg, and potassium bicarbonate 312 mg.
ALUDROX SUSPENSION◇: aluminum hydroxide 307 mg, magnesium hydroxide 103 mg.
CAMALOX TABLETS◇: aluminum hydroxide 225 mg, magnesium hydroxide 200 mg, and calcium carbonate 250 mg.
DELCID SUSPENSION◇: aluminum hydroxide 600 mg, magnesium hydroxide 665 mg.
DI-GEL LIQUID◇: aluminum hydroxide 200 mg, magnesium hydroxide 200 mg, simethicone 20 mg.
GAVISCON◇: aluminum hydroxide 31.7 mg, magnesium carbonate 137 mg.
GELUSIL◇: aluminum hydroxide 200 mg, magnesium hydroxide 200 mg, simethicone 25 mg.
GELUSIL-II◇: aluminum hydroxide 400 mg, magnesium hydroxide 400 mg, simethicone 30 mg.
GELUSIL-M◇: aluminum hydroxide 300 mg, magnesium hydroxide 200 mg, simethicone 25 mg.
EXTRA STRENGTH MAALOX TABLETS◇: aluminum hydroxide 400 mg and magnesium hydroxide 400 mg.
MAALOX NO. 1◇: aluminum hydroxide 200 mg and magnesium hydroxide 200 mg.
MAALOX PLUS TABLETS◇: aluminum hydroxide 200 mg, magnesium hydroxide 200 mg, simethicone 25 mg.
MAALOX TC TABLETS◇: aluminum hydroxide 600 mg, magnesium hydroxide 300 mg.
MAGNATRIL◇: aluminum hydroxide 260 mg, magnesium hydroxide 130 mg, and magnesium trisilicate 455 mg.
MYLANTA TABLETS◇: aluminum hydroxide 200 mg, magnesium hydroxide 200 mg, simethicone 20 mg.
MYLANTA-II TABLETS◇: aluminum hydroxide 400 mg, magnesium hydroxide 400 mg, simethicone 40 mg.
RIOPAN PLUS CHEW TABLETS◇: magaldrate 540 mg, simethicone 20 mg.
RIOPAN PLUS SUSPENSION◇: magaldrate 540 mg and simethicone 20 mg/5 ml.
SILAIN-GEL◇: aluminum hydroxide 282 mg, magnesium hydroxide 285 mg, simethicone 25 mg per 5 ml.
TITRALAC LIQUID◇: calcium carbonate 1,000 mg in glycine.

TITRALAC TABLETS◇: calcium carbonate 420 mg, glycine 150 mg.
UNIVOL†◇: aluminum hydroxide and magnesium carbonate co-dried gel 300 mg and magnesium hydroxide 100 mg.
WINGEL◇: aluminum hydroxide 180 mg, magnesium hydroxide 160 mg.

---

aluminum carbonate
Basaljel◇

Pregnancy Risk Category: C

HOW SUPPLIED
Tablets or capsules: aluminum hydroxide equivalent 500 mg◇
Oral suspension: aluminum hydroxide equivalent 400 mg/5 ml◇, 1 g/5 ml◇

MECHANISM OF ACTION
Reduces total acid load in the GI tract and elevates gastric pH to reduce pepsin activity. Also strengthens the gastric mucosal barrier and increases esophageal sphincter tone. An antacid.

INDICATIONS & DOSAGE
As antacid—
Adults: suspension: 5 to 10 ml P.O., p.r.n. Extra-strength suspension: 2.5 to 5 ml, p.r.n. Tablets: 1 to 2, p.r.n. Capsules: 1 to 2, p.r.n.
To prevent formation of urinary phosphate stones (with low-phosphate diet)—
Adults: suspension: 15 to 30 ml suspension in water or juice P.O. 1 hour after meals and h.s.; 5 to 15 ml extra-strength suspension in water or juice 1 hour after meals and h.s.; 2 to 6 tablets or capsules 1 hour after meals and h.s.

ADVERSE REACTIONS
GI: anorexia, *constipation*, intestinal obstruction.
Metabolic: hypophosphatemia.

INTERACTIONS
Ciprofloxacin, quinolone antibiotics, tetracyclines: decreased antibiotic effect. Separate administration times.

NURSING CONSIDERATIONS
• Use cautiously in elderly patients, especially those with decreased GI motility (those receiving antidiarrheals, antispasmodics, or anticholinergics), dehydration, fluid restriction, chronic renal disease, and suspected intestinal obstruction.
• Record amount and consistency of stools. Manage constipation with laxatives or stool softeners; alternate with magnesium-containing antacids (if patient does not have renal disease).
• Shake suspension well; give with small amount of water or fruit juice to ensure passage to stomach. When administering through nasogastric tube, be sure tube is placed correctly and is patent; follow antacid with water to clear tube.
• Watch long-term high-dose use in patient on restricted sodium intake.
• Warn patient not to take aluminum carbonate indiscriminately and not to switch antacids without doctor's advice.
• Because it contains aluminum, it is used in renal failure to help control hyperphosphatemia. Binds phosphate in GI tract.
• Monitor serum phosphate.
• Watch for symptoms of hypophosphatemia with prolonged use (anorexia, malaise, muscle weakness); can also lead to resorption of calcium and bone demineralization.
• May cause enteric-coated drugs to be released prematurely in stomach. Separate doses by 1 hour.
• Basaljel liquid contains no sugar.

---

aluminum hydroxide
ALternaGEL◇, Alu-Cap◇, Alu-Tab◇,
Amphojel◇, Amphotabs‡,
Dialume◇, Nephrox◇

Pregnancy Risk Category: C

HOW SUPPLIED
Tablets: 300 mg◇, 600 mg◇
Capsules: 475 mg◇, 500 mg◇
Oral suspension◇: 320 mg/5 ml◇, 600 mg/5 ml◇

MECHANISM OF ACTION
Reduces total acid load in the GI tract and elevates gastric pH to reduce pepsin activity. Also strengthens the gastric mucosal barrier and increases esophageal sphincter tone. An antacid.

INDICATIONS & DOSAGE
Antacid—
Adults: 600 mg P.O. (5 to 10 ml of most products) 1 hour after meals and h.s.; 300- or 600-mg tablet, chewed before swallowing, taken with milk or water 5 to 6 times daily after meals and h.s.
Hyperphosphatemia in renal failure—
Adults: 500 mg to 2 g P.O. b.i.d. to q.i.d.

ADVERSE REACTIONS
GI: anorexia, *constipation*, intestinal obstruction.
Metabolic: hypophosphatemia.

INTERACTIONS
Ciprofloxacin, quinolone antibiotics, tetracyclines: decreased antibiotic effect. Separate administration times.

NURSING CONSIDERATIONS
• Use cautiously in elderly patients, especially those with decreased GI motility (those receiving antidiarrheals, antispasmodics, or anticholinergics), dehydration, fluid restriction, chronic renal disease, and suspected intestinal obstruction.
• Record amount and consistency of stools. Manage constipation with laxatives or stool softeners; alternate with magnesium-containing antacids (if patient does not have renal disease).
• Shake suspension well; give with small amount of milk or water to assure passage to stomach. When administering through nasogastric tube, make sure tube is placed correctly and is patent. After instilling antacid, flush tube with water.
• Watch long-term high-dose use in patient on restricted sodium intake.
• Warn patient not to take aluminum hydroxide indiscriminately or switch antacids without doctor's advice.
• Because it contains aluminum, it is used in renal failure to help control hyperphosphatemia. Binds phosphate in the GI tract.
• Monitor serum phosphate.
• Watch for symptoms of hypophosphatemia with prolonged use (anorexia, malaise, and muscle weakness); can also lead to resorption of calcium and bone demineralization.
• May cause enteric-coated drugs to be released prematurely in stomach. Separate doses by 1 hour.

aluminum phosphate
Phosphaljel◇

Pregnancy Risk Category: C

HOW SUPPLIED
Oral suspension: 233 mg/5 ml◇

MECHANISM OF ACTION
Reduces total acid load in the GI tract and elevates gastric pH to reduce pepsin activity. Also strengthens the gastric mucosal barrier and increases esophageal sphincter tone. An antacid.

INDICATIONS & DOSAGE
Antacid—

---

†Available in Canada only.   ‡Available in Australia only.   ◇ Available OTC.

Adults: 15 to 30 ml undiluted P.O. q 2 hours between meals and h.s.

ADVERSE REACTIONS
GI: *constipation,* intestinal obstruction.

INTERACTIONS
Ciprofloxacin, quinolone antibiotics, tetracyclines: decreased antibiotic effect. Separate administration times.

NURSING CONSIDERATIONS
• Use cautiously in elderly patients, especially those with decreased GI motility (those receiving antidiarrheals, antispasmodics, or anticholinergics), dehydration, fluid restriction, chronic renal disease, and suspected intestinal obstruction.
• Record amount and consistency of stools. Manage constipation with laxatives or stool softeners; alternate with magnesium-containing antacids (if patient does not have renal disease).
• Shake well; give alone or with small amount of milk or water. When administering through nasogastric tube, make sure tube is placed correctly and is patent; after instilling, flush tube with water to facilitate passage to stomach and maintain tube patency.
• Watch long-term high-dose use in patient on restricted sodium intake.
• Warn patient not to take aluminum phosphate indiscriminately and not to switch antacids without doctor's advice.
• This drug is a very weak antacid.
• Can reverse hypophosphatemia induced by aluminum hydroxide.
• May cause enteric-coated drugs to be released prematurely in stomach. Separate doses by 1 hour.
• Phosphaljel contains no sugar.

calcium carbonate
Alka-Mints◊, Amitone◊, Calcilac◊, Calcimax‡, Calglycine◊, Cal-Sup‡, Chooz◊, Dicarbosil◊, Effercal-600‡, Equilet◊, Genalac◊, Glycate◊, Gustalac◊, Mallamint◊, Pama No. 1◊, Rolaids Calcium Rich◊, Titracid◊, Titralac◊, Tums◊, Tums E-X◊, Tums Liquid Extra Strength◊

Pregnancy Risk Category: C

HOW SUPPLIED
Calcium carbonate contains 40% calcium; 20 mEq calcium/g.
Tablets: 350 mg, 420 mg, 500 mg, 650 mg, 750 mg, 850 mg, 1,250 mg‡
Oral suspension: 1 g/5 ml
Effervescent powder: 1,500 mg (600 g elemental calcium)/5 g

MECHANISM OF ACTION
Reduces total acid load in the GI tract and elevates gastric pH to reduce pepsin activity. Also strengthens the gastric mucosal barrier and increases esophageal sphincter tone. An antacid.

INDICATIONS & DOSAGE
Antacid—
Adults: 1-g tablet, P.O. 4 to 6 times daily, chewed well and taken with water; or 1 g of suspension (5 ml of most products), 1 hour after meals and h.s.

ADVERSE REACTIONS
GI: *constipation,* gastric distention, flatulence, rebound hyperacidity, *nausea.*
Metabolic: *hypercalcemia, hypophosphatemia;* if taken with milk—milk-alkali syndrome.

INTERACTIONS
Ciprofloxacin, quinolone antibiotics, tetracyclines: decreased antibiotic effect. Separate administration times.

Italicized adverse reactions are common or life-threatening.
*Liquid form contains alcohol.   **May contain tartrazine.

NURSING CONSIDERATIONS
• Contraindicated in severe renal disease. Use cautiously in elderly patients, especially those with decreased GI motility (those receiving antidiarrheals, antispasmodics, or anticholinergics), dehydration, fluid restriction, chronic renal disease, and suspected intestinal obstruction.
• Do not administer with milk or other foods high in vitamin D. Can cause milk-alkali syndrome (headache, confusion, distaste for food, nausea, vomiting, hypercalcemia, hypercalciuria, calcinosis, and hypophosphatemia).
• Record amount and consistency of stools. Manage constipation with laxatives or stool softeners.
• Watch for symptoms of hypercalcemia (nausea, vomiting, headache, mental confusion, and anorexia).
• Monitor serum calcium, especially in mild renal impairment.
• Warn patient not to take calcium carbonate indiscriminately and not to switch antacids without doctor's advice.
• May cause enteric-coated tablets to be released prematurely in stomach. Separate doses by 1 hour.

dihydroxyaluminum sodium carbonate
Rolaids◊

Pregnancy Risk Category: C

HOW SUPPLIED
Tablets: 334 mg◊

MECHANISM OF ACTION
Reduces total acid load in the GI tract and elevates gastric pH to reduce pepsin activity. Also strengthens the gastric mucosal barrier and increases esophageal sphincter tone. An antacid.

INDICATIONS & DOSAGE
Antacid—

Adults: chew 1 to 2 tablets (334 to 668 mg), p.r.n.

ADVERSE REACTIONS
GI: anorexia, *constipation,* intestinal obstruction.

INTERACTIONS
Ciprofloxacin, quinolone antibiotics, tetracyclines: decreased antibiotic effect. Separate administration times.

NURSING CONSIDERATIONS
• Use cautiously in elderly patients, especially those with decreased GI motility (those receiving antidiarrheals, antispasmodics, or anticholinergics), dehydration, fluid restriction, chronic renal disease, and suspected intestinal obstruction.
• Has high sodium content and may increase sodium and water retention.
• Record amount and consistency of stools. Manage constipation with laxatives or stool softeners; alternate with magnesium-containing antacids (if patient does not have renal disease).
• Watch long-term high-dose use in patient on restricted sodium intake.
• Warn patient not to take dihydroxyaluminum sodium carbonate indiscriminately.
• May cause enteric-coated drugs to be released prematurely in stomach. Separate doses by 1 hour.

magaldrate (aluminum-magnesium complex)
Antiflux†, Lowsium◊, Riopan◊
Pregnancy Risk Category: C

HOW SUPPLIED
Tablets: 480 mg◊
Tablets (chewable): 480 mg◊
Oral suspension: 540 mg/5 ml◊, 1,080 mg/5 ml◊

MECHANISM OF ACTION
Reduces total acid load in the GI tract

and elevates gastric pH to reduce pepsin activity. Also strengthens the gastric mucosal barrier and increases esophageal sphincter tone. An antacid.

INDICATIONS & DOSAGE
Antacid—
Adults: suspension: 540 to 1,080 mg (5 to 10 ml) P.O. between meals and h.s. with water. Tablet: 480 to 960 mg (1 to 2 tablets) P.O. with water between meals and h.s. Chewable tablet: 480 to 960 mg (1 to 2 tablets) P.O. chewed before swallowing, between meals and h.s.

ADVERSE REACTIONS
GI: mild constipation or diarrhea.

INTERACTIONS
Ciprofloxacin, quinolone antibiotics, tetracyclines: decreased antibiotic effect. Separate administration times.

NURSING CONSIDERATIONS
• Contraindicated in severe renal disease. Use cautiously in elderly patients, especially those with decreased GI motility (those receiving antidiarrheals, antispasmodics, or anticholinergics), dehydration, fluid restriction, and mild renal impairment.
• Record amount and consistency of stools.
• Shake suspension well; give with a little water to ensure passage to stomach. When giving through nasogastric tube, be sure tube is placed properly and is patent. After instilling, flush tube with water to ensure passage to stomach and maintain tube patency.
• Monitor serum magnesium in patients with mild renal impairment. Symptomatic hypermagnesemia usually occurs only in severe renal failure.
• Not usually used in renal failure (although it contains aluminum) to help control hypophosphatemia, because it

contains magnesium, which may accumulate in renal failure.
• Good for patient on restricted sodium intake; very low sodium content.
• Warn patient not to take magaldrate indiscriminately and not to switch antacids without doctor's advice.
• May cause enteric-coated drugs to be released prematurely in stomach. Separate doses by 1 hour.
• Riopan, Riopan Plus liquid, and Riopan Swallow Tablet contain no sugar. Chewable tablets contain sugar.

---

magnesium oxide
Mag-Ox 400◊, Maox◊, Par-Mag◊, Uro-Mag◊

Pregnancy Risk Category: C

HOW SUPPLIED
Tablets: 400 mg◊, 420 mg◊
Capsules: 140 mg◊
Oral suspension: 7.75%◊

MECHANISM OF ACTION
Reduces total acid load in the GI tract and elevates gastric pH to reduce pepsin activity. Also strengthens the gastric mucosal barrier and increases esophageal spincter tone. An antacid.

INDICATIONS & DOSAGE
Antacid—
Adults: 140 mg P.O. with water or milk after meals and h.s.
Laxative—
Adults: 4 g P.O. with water or milk, usually h.s.
Oral replacement therapy in mild hypomagnesemia—
Adults: 400 mg to 840 mg P.O. daily. Monitor serum magnesium response.

ADVERSE REACTIONS
GI: *diarrhea,* nausea, abdominal pain.
Metabolic: hypermagnesemia.

Italicized adverse reactions are common or life-threatening.
*Liquid form contains alcohol.   **May contain tartrazine.

INTERACTIONS
Ciprofloxacin, quinolone antibiotics, tetracyclines: decreased antibiotic effect. Separate administration times.

NURSING CONSIDERATIONS
• Contraindicated in severe renal disease. Use cautiously in elderly patients, and in mild renal impairment.
• With prolonged use and some degree of renal impairment, watch for symptoms of hypermagnesemia (hypotension, nausea, vomiting, depressed reflexes, respiratory depression, and coma). Monitor serum magnesium.
• When used as laxative, do not give other oral drugs 1 to 2 hours before or after.
• If diarrhea occurs on antacid doses, suggest alternate preparation.
• Warn patient not to take magnesium oxide indiscriminately and not to switch antacid without doctor's advice.
• May cause enteric-coated drugs to be released prematurely in stomach. Separate doses by 1 hour.

simethicone
Extra Strength Gas-X◇, Gas-X◇, Mylicon-80◇, Mylicon-125◇, Ovol-40†, Ovol-80†, Phazyme◇, Phazyme 55◇, Phazyme 95◇, Phazyme 125◇, Silain◇

Pregnancy Risk Category: C

HOW SUPPLIED
Tablets◇: 40 mg, 50 mg, 60 mg, 80 mg, 95 mg, 125 mg
Capsules: 40 mg/0.6 ml◇

MECHANISM OF ACTION
By its defoaming action, disperses or prevents formation of mucus-surrounded gas pockets in the GI tract.

INDICATIONS & DOSAGE
Flatulence, functional gastric bloating—

Adults and children over 12 years: 40 to 125 mg after each meal and h.s.

ADVERSE REACTIONS
GI: expulsion of excessive liberated gas as belching, rectal flatus.

INTERACTIONS
None significant.

NURSING CONSIDERATIONS
• Warn patient not to take simethicone indiscriminately.
• Tell patient to chew tablet before swallowing.

---

†Available in Canada only.   ‡Available in Australia only.   ◇Available OTC.

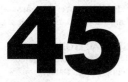

Digestants

chenodiol
monooctanoin
pancreatin
pancrelipase
ursodiol

COMBINATION PRODUCTS
BILRON: bile salts 150 mg and iron
300 mg.
DONNAZYME TABLETS: pancreatin
300 mg, pepsin 150 mg, bile salts
150 mg, hyoscyamine sulfate 0.0518
mg, atropine sulfate 0.0097 mg, scopolamine hydrobromide 0.0033 mg,
and phenobarbital 8.1 mg.
ENTOZYME TABLETS: pancreatin
300 mg, pepsin 250 mg, and bile salts
150 mg.
PANCREASE CAPSULES: lipase 4,000
units, protease 25,000 units, amylase
20,000 units, in enteric-coated microspheres.

---

chenodiol
(chenodeoxycholic acid)
Chenix

Pregnancy Risk Category: X

HOW SUPPLIED
Tablets: 250 mg

MECHANISM OF ACTION
Suppresses hepatic synthesis of both
cholesterol and cholic acid. These actions contribute to biliary cholesterol
desaturation and gradual dissolution
of gallstones.

INDICATIONS & DOSAGE
*Dissolution of radiolucent cholesterol
stones (gallstones) when systemic disease or age precludes surgery—*
Adults: 250 mg P.O. b.i.d. for the
first 2 weeks, followed, as tolerated,
by weekly increases of 250 mg/day,
up to 13 to 16 mg/kg/day for up to 24
months.

ADVERSE REACTIONS
GI: *diarrhea,* cramps, heartburn,
constipation, nausea, vomiting, anorexia, epigastric distress.
Hepatic: reversible elevated hepatic
enzymes, possible liver toxicity.

INTERACTIONS
*Cholestyramine, colestinol, estrogens,
oral contraceptives, clofibrate:* decreased chenodiol effect. Monitor patient carefully.

NURSING CONSIDERATIONS
• Contraindicated in known hepato-
cyte dysfunction; a gallbladder confirmed as nonvisualizing after two
consecutive single doses of dye; radi-
opaque or radiolucent bile pigment
stones; or gallstone complications or
compelling reasons for gallbladder
surgery, including unremitting acute
cholecystitis, cholangitis, biliary obstruction, gallstone pancreatitis, or
biliary GI fistula.
• Chenodiol treatment should be reserved for carefully selected patients.
• The drug is particularly effective in
the dissolution of small, floatable
gallstones.
• Monitor serum transaminase
monthly for the first 3 months and

Italicized adverse reactions are common or life-threatening.
*Liquid form contains alcohol.   **May contain tartrazine.

thereafter every 3 months for duration of therapy.

• The final dosage shouldn't be less than 10 mg/kg/day; lower dosages are usually ineffective.

• Diarrhea occurs in 30% to 40% of all patients. Doctor may reduce dosage until diarrhea subsides. Antidiarrheals may also be prescribed. In some patients, however, persistent diarrhea will require discontinuation of chenodiol therapy.

• Monitor oral cholecystogram or ultrasonogram every 6 to 9 months to observe for gallstone dissolution.

monooctanoin
Moctanin

Pregnancy Risk Category: C

HOW SUPPLIED
Infusion: 120-ml bottles

MECHANISM OF ACTION
Dissolves gallstones by rendering them more soluble.

INDICATIONS & DOSAGE
To solubilize cholesterol gallstones that are retained in the biliary tract after cholecystectomy—
Adults: Administered as a continuous infusion through a catheter inserted directly into the common bile duct via a T tube. Rate should not exceed 3 to 5 ml/hour at a pressure of 10 cm H_2O. Duration of infusion is 7 to 21 days.

ADVERSE REACTIONS
GI: *GI pain and discomfort, nausea, vomiting,* diarrhea, anorexia, indigestion.
Other: metabolic acidosis.

INTERACTIONS
None reported.

NURSING CONSIDERATIONS
• Contraindicated in clinical jaundice, significant biliary tract infec-

tion, or a history of recent duodenal ulcer or jejunitis.

• Because impaired liver function may lead to metabolic acidosis during administration of this drug, routine liver function tests should be done before perfusion therapy begins.

• Monooctanoin should only be started by individuals experienced in infusion therapy.

• Not to be administered parenterally. For biliary tract infusion only.

• Pressure *must* be kept below 15 cm H_2O. Keeping the pressure at 10 cm H_2O will help minimize GI and biliary tract irritation.

• Use a peristaltic infusion pump to regulate the infusion. Outpatients may use a battery-operated portable pump.

• Warm the solution to 60° to 80° F. (16° to 27° C.) before perfusion. Temperature of the solution should not fall below 65° F. (18° C.) during administration.

• GI symptoms may be reduced by slowing the infusion rate or discontinuing the infusion during meals.

pancreatin
Dizymes Tablets◇, Hi-Vegi-Lip Tablets◇, Pancreatin Enseals◇, Pancreatin Tablets◇

Pregnancy Risk Category: C

HOW SUPPLIED
Dizymes
Tablets (enteric-coated): 250 mg pancreatin, 6,750 units lipase, 41,250 units protease, 43,750 units amylase◇
Hi-Vegi-Lip
Tablets (enteric-coated): 2,400 mg pancreatin, 12,000 units lipase, 60,000 units protease, and 60,000 units amylase◇
Pancreatin Enseals
Tablets (enteric-coated): 1,000 mg pancreatin, 2,000 units lipase, 25,000 units protease, 25,000 units amylase◇
Pancreatin Tablets
Tablets (enteric-coated)◇: 325 mg

pancreatin, 650 units lipase, 8,125 units protease, 8,125 units amylase◦

MECHANISM OF ACTION
Replaces endogenous exocrine pancreatic enzymes and aids digestion of starches, fats, and proteins.

INDICATIONS & DOSAGE
Exocrine pancreatic secretion insufficiency, digestive aid in cystic fibrosis—
Adults and children: 1 to 3 tablets P.O. with meals.

ADVERSE REACTIONS
GI: nausea, *diarrhea* with high doses.
Other: hyperuricosuria (with high doses).

INTERACTIONS
Antacids: may negate pancreatin's beneficial effect. Don't use together.

NURSING CONSIDERATIONS
• Use cautiously in patients who are hypersensitive to pork. Bovine preparations are available for these patients, but are less effective.
• Minimal USP standards dictate that each milligram of bovine or porcine pancreatin contains lipase 2 units, protease 25 units, and amylase 25 units.
• Balance fat, protein, and starch intake properly to avoid indigestion. Dosage varies according to degree of maldigestion and malabsorption, amount of fat in diet, and enzyme activity of individual preparations.
• Adequate replacement decreases number of bowel movements and improves stool consistency.
• Use only after confirmed diagnosis of exocrine pancreatic insufficiency. Not effective in GI disorders unrelated to pancreatic enzyme deficiency.
• For infants, mix powder with applesauce and give with meals. Avoid inhalation of powder. Older children may swallow capsules with food.

• Enteric coating on some products may reduce availability of enzyme in upper portion of jejunum.
• Store in airtight containers at room temperature.

---

pancrelipase
Cotazym Capsules, Cotazym-S Capsules, Creon Capsules, Festal II Tablets◦, Ilozyme Tablets, Ku-Zyme HP Capsules, Pancrease Capsules, Pancrease MT4, Pancrease MT10, Pancrease MT16, Viokase Powder, Viokase Tablets

Pregnancy Risk Category: C

HOW SUPPLIED
Cotazym
Capsules: 8,000 units lipase, 30,000 units protease, 30,000 units amylase, 25 mg calcium carbonate
Cotazym-S
Capsules (enteric-coated spheres): 5,000 units lipase, 20,000 units protease, 20,000 units amylase
Creon
Capsules (enteric-coated microspheres): 8,000 units lipase, 13,000 units protease, 30,000 units amylase
Festal II
Tablets (enteric-coated): 6,000 units lipase, 20,000 units protease, 30,000 units amylase◦
Ilozyme
Tablets: 11,000 units lipase, 30,000 units protease, 30,000 units amylase
Ku-Zyme HP
Capsules: 8,000 units lipase, 30,000 units protease, 30,000 units amylase
Pancrease
Capsules (enteric-coated microspheres): 4,000 units lipase, 25,000 units protease, 20,000 units amylase
Pancrease MT4
Capsules (enteric-coated microtablets): 4,000 units lipase, 12,000 units protease, 30,000 units amylase
Pancrease MT10
Capsules (enteric-coated microtab-

---

lets): 10,000 units lipase, 30,000 units protease, 30,000 units amylase
Pancrease MT16
Capsules (enteric-coated microtablets): 16,000 units lipase, 48,000 units protease, 48,000 units amylase
Viokase
Tablets: 8,000 units lipase, 30,000 units protease, 30,000 units amylase
Powder: 16,800 units lipase, 70,000 units protease, 70,000 units amylase

MECHANISM OF ACTION
A combination of digestive enzymes that replaces endogenous exocrine pancreatic enzymes and aids digestion of starches, fats, and proteins.

INDICATIONS & DOSAGE
Dose must be titrated to patient's response. Exocrine pancreatic secretion insufficiency, cystic fibrosis in adults and children, steatorrhea and other disorders of fat metabolism secondary to insufficient pancreatic enzymes—
Adults and children: dosage ranges from 1 to 3 capsules or tablets P.O. before or with meals and 1 capsule or tablet with snack; or 1 to 2 powder packets before meals or snacks.

ADVERSE REACTIONS
GI: *nausea,* diarrhea with high doses.

INTERACTIONS
Antacids: may negate pancrelipase's beneficial effect. Don't use together.

NURSING CONSIDERATIONS
• Contraindicated in patients with severe pork hypersensitivity.
• Minimal USP standards dictate that each mg of pancrelipase contains 24 units lipase, 100 units protease, and 100 units amylase.
• Use only after confirmed diagnosis of exocrine pancreatic insufficiency. Not effective in GI disorders unrelated to enzyme deficiency.
• Lipase activity greater than with other pancreatic enzymes.

• For infants, mix powder with applesauce and give with meals. Avoid inhalation of powder. Older children may swallow capsules with food.
• Dosage varies with degree of maldigestion and malabsorption, amount of fat in diet, and enzyme activity of individual preparations.
• Adequate replacement decreases number of bowel movements and improves stool consistency.
• Enteric coating on some products may reduce availability of enzyme in upper portion of jejunum.
• Crushing or chewing of capsule interferes with the enteric coating.

ursodiol
Actigall
Pregnancy Risk Category: B

HOW SUPPLIED
Capsules: 300 mg

MECHANISM OF ACTION
A naturally occurring bile acid that suppresses hepatic synthesis and secretion of cholesterol as well as intestinal cholesterol absorption. After long-term administration, it can solubilize cholesterol from gallstones.

INDICATIONS & DOSAGE
Dissolution of gallstones less than 20 mm in diameter in patients who are poor surgical candidates or refuse surgery—
Adults: 8 to 10 mg/kg P.O. daily in two or three divided doses. Most patients receive 300 mg P.O. b.i.d. Therapy is usually long-term, with ultrasound images of the gall bladder at 6 month intervals. If partial stone dissolution is not seen within 12 months, eventual success is unlikely. Safety of use for longer than 24 months has not been established.

ADVERSE REACTIONS
CNS: headache, fatigue, anxiety, depression, sleep disorders.
EENT: cough, rhinitis.
GI: nausea, vomiting, dyspepsia, metallic taste, abdominal pain, biliary pain, cholecystitis, diarrhea, constipation, stomatitis, flatulence.
Skin: pruritus, rash, dry skin, urticaria, itching, hair thinning.
Other: arthralgia, myalgia, back pain.

INTERACTIONS
Aluminum-containing antacids, cholestyramine, colestipol: bind ursodiol and prevent its absorption.
Estrogens, oral contraceptives, clofibrate: increase hepatic cholesterol secretion and may counteract the effects of ursodiol.

NURSING CONSIDERATIONS
• Contraindicated in patients with hypersensitivity to ursodiol or other bile acids. Also contraindicated in chronic liver disease, acute cholecystitis, cholangitis, biliary obstruction, gallstone pancreatitis, or biliary-GI fistulae.
• Ursodiol will not dissolve calcified cholesterol stones, radiolucent bile pigment stones, or radio-opaque stones.
• Ursodiol therapy is long-term, requiring several months to produce an effect. The relapse rate after bile acid therapy may be as high as 50% after 5 years. Patients should be aware of alternative therapies, including 'watchful waiting' (no intervention) and cholecystectomy.
• Monitor liver function tests, including AST (SGOT) and ALT (SGPT) at the beginning of therapy, and after 1 month, 3 months and every 6 months while taking ursodiol. Abnormal tests may indicate a worsening of the disease. There is a theoretical risk of a hepatotoxic metabolite of ursodiol being formed in some patients.
• Ultrasound images of the gallbladder should be reviewed at least once every 6 months for the first year of therapy. Most patients who respond to ursodiol show significant improvement after 6 months of therapy.

Italicized adverse reactions are common or life-threatening.
*Liquid form contains alcohol.   **May contain tartrazine.

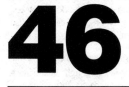

Antidiarrheals

bismuth subgallate
bismuth subsalicylate
calcium polycarbophil
(See Chapter 47, LAXATIVES.)
difenoxin hydrochloride
diphenoxylate hydrochloride
kaolin and pectin mixtures
loperamide
opium tincture
opium tincture, camphorated

COMBINATION PRODUCTS

DONNAGEL-PG*: powdered opium
24 mg, kaolin 6 g, pectin 142.8 mg,
hyoscyamine sulfate 0.1037 mg, atropine sulfate 0.0194 mg, scopolamine
hydrobromide 0.0065 mg, and alcohol 5% in 30-ml suspension.
DONNAGEL SUSPENSION*: kaolin 6 g,
pectin 142.8 mg, hyoscyamine sulfate
0.1037 mg, atropine sulfate 0.0194
mg, scopolamine hydrobromide
0.0065 mg, and alcohol 3.8% in 30-
ml suspension.
PAREPECTOLIN*: opium 15 mg
(equivalent to Paregoric 3.7 ml), kaolin 5.85 g, pectin 162 mg, and alcohol 0.69% in 30-ml suspension.

---

bismuth subgallate
Devrom◇

bismuth subsalicylate
Maximum Strength Pepto-Bismol
Liquid◇, Pepto-Bismol◇

*Pregnancy Risk Category: C (D in
third trimester)*

HOW SUPPLIED
subgallate
Tablets (chewable): 200 mg◇
subsalicylate
Tablets (chewable): 262 mg◇
Oral suspension: 262 mg/15 ml◇, 525
mg/15 ml◇

MECHANISM OF ACTION
Has a mild water-binding capacity;
also may adsorb toxins and provide
protective coating for mucosa.

INDICATIONS & DOSAGE
Mild, nonspecific diarrhea—
Adults: 1 to 2 tablets P.O. chewed or
swallowed whole t.i.d. (subgallate).
Adults: 30 ml or 2 tablets P.O. q ½ to 1
hour up to a maximum of 8 doses and
for no longer than 2 days (subsalicylate).
Children 9 to 12 years: 20 ml or 1
tablet P.O.
Children 6 to 9 years: 10 ml or ⅔
tablet P.O.
Children 3 to 6 years: 5 ml or ⅓ tablet
P.O.
*Prevention and treatment of traveler's
diarrhea (turista)—*
Adults: prophylactically, 60 ml (bismuth subsalicylate) P.O. q.i.d. during
the first 2 weeks of travel. During
acute illness, 30 to 60 ml P.O. q 30
minutes for a total of 8 doses. Alternatively, 2 tablets P.O. q.i.d. for up to
3 weeks.

ADVERSE REACTIONS
GI: temporary darkening of tongue
and stools.
Other: salicylism (high doses).

INTERACTIONS
Oral anticoagulants, oral hypoglycemic agents: theoretical risk of increased effects of these agents following high doses of bismuth subsalicylate. Monitor patient closely.
Probenecid: theoretical risk of decreased uricosuric effects following high doses of bismuth subsalicylate. Monitor patient closely.

NURSING CONSIDERATIONS
• Warn patient that bismuth subsalicylate contains a large amount of salicylate (each tablet provides 102 mg salicylate; the regular strength liquid provides 130 mg/15 ml, and the extra strength liquid yields 230 mg/15 ml). Should be used cautiously in patients already taking aspirin. Discontinue if tinnitus occurs.
• Consult with doctor before giving bismuth subsalicylate to children or teenagers during or after recovery from the flu or chicken pox.
• Instruct patient to chew tablets well.
• Both the liquid and tablet forms of Pepto-Bismol are effective against traveler's diarrhea. Tablets may be more convenient to carry.

---

difenoxin hydrochloride
Lyspafen‡, Motofen

Pregnancy Risk Category: C

HOW SUPPLIED
Tablets: 0.5 mg (with atropine sulphate, 0.025 mg)‡, 1 mg (with atropine sulfate, 0.025 mg)

MECHANISM OF ACTION
Exerts a direct effect on the intestinal wall to slow motility.

INDICATIONS AND DOSAGE
Adjunct in acute nonspecific diarrhea, and acute exacerbations of chronic functional diarrhea—
Adults: initially, 2 mg P.O., then 1 mg P.O. after each loose bowel movement. Total dosage should not exceed 8 mg daily. Not recommended for use longer than 2 days.

ADVERSE REACTIONS
CNS: dizziness and light-headedness, drowsiness, headache, fatigue, nervousness, insomnia, confusion.
EENT: burning eyes, blurred vision.
GI: nausea, vomiting, dry mouth, epigastric distress, constipation.

INTERACTIONS
Alcohol, CNS depressants, tranquilizers, narcotics, barbiturates: enhanced CNS depression. Closely monitor patients.
MAO inhibitors: potential hypertensive crisis. Avoid concomitant use.

NURSING CONSIDERATIONS
• Contraindicated in patients with hypersensitivity to difenoxin or atropine, in children under 2 years, and in patients with diarrhea from pseudomembranous colitis associated with antibiotics. Also contraindicated in patients with jaundice, or diarrhea from organisms that may penetrate the intestinal mucosa (including toxigenic *Escherichia coli, Salmonella,* or *Shigella*).
• Difenoxin is the principal metabolite of diphenoxylate (Lomotil) and is chemically related to meperidine. Use cautiously in patients with a history of drug abuse, or in those currently receiving drugs with a high abuse potential.
• Atropine has been added to difenoxin to prevent abuse. The small dosage of atropine is unlikely to cause any significant clinical problems, but patients may experience dry mouth, tachycardia, urine retention, and flushing. Monitor for these effects.
• Advise patients to avoid hazardous activities that may require mental alertness, such as driving or operating heavy machinery, until the CNS effects of the drug are known.

Italicized adverse reactions are common or life-threatening.
*Liquid form contains alcohol.   **May contain tartrazine.

• Monitor patients closely for fluid and electrolyte imbalance. Difenoxin-induced decreases in peristalsis may result in fluid retention in the colon, with subsequent dehydration and possibly delayed difenoxin intoxication.
• Advise patient to adhere to dosing schedule. Overdose with difenoxin may result in respiratory depression and coma. Encourage proper storage to keep drug out of children's reach.
• Patients who overdose with difenoxin should be observed for at least 48 hours. Respiratory depression may occur up to 30 hours after ingestion. Gastric lavage, establishment of a patent airway, and mechanically assisted ventilation are advised. Naloxone will reverse the respiratory depression. Because difenoxin has a longer duration of action than naloxone, repeated injections of naloxone will be necessary.

diphenoxylate hydrochloride
Diphenatol, Lofene, Logen, Lomanate, Lomotil*, Lonox, Lo-Trol, Low-Quel, Nor-Mil
Controlled Substance Schedule V

Pregnancy Risk Category: C

HOW SUPPLIED
Tablets: 2.5 mg (with atropine sulfate, 0.025 mg)
Liquid: 2.5 mg/5 ml (with atropine sulfate, 0.025 mg/5 ml)

MECHANISM OF ACTION
Increases smooth muscle tone in the GI tract, inhibits motility and propulsion, and diminishes secretions.

INDICATIONS & DOSAGE
Acute, nonspecific diarrhea—
Adults: initially, 5 mg P.O. q.i.d., then adjust dosage.
Children 2 to 12 years: 0.3 to 0.4 mg/kg P.O. daily in 4 divided doses, using liquid form only. For mainte-

nance, initial dose may be reduced by as much as 75%.
Don't use in children under 2 years.

ADVERSE REACTIONS
CNS: *sedation, dizziness,* headache, drowsiness, lethargy, restlessness, depression, euphoria.
CV: tachycardia.
EENT: mydriasis.
GI: *dry mouth,* nausea, vomiting, abdominal discomfort or distention, *paralytic ileus,* anorexia, fluid retention in bowel (may mask depletion of extracellular fluid and electrolytes, especially in young children treated for acute gastroenteritis).
GU: urine retention.
Skin: pruritus, giant urticaria, rash.
Other: possibly physical dependence in long-term use, angioedema, respiratory depression.

INTERACTIONS
None significant.

NURSING CONSIDERATIONS
• Contraindicated in acute diarrhea resulting from poison until toxic material is eliminated from GI tract; acute diarrhea caused by organisms that penetrate intestinal mucosa; diarrhea resulting from antibiotic-induced pseudomembranous enterocolitis; and in jaundiced patients. Use cautiously in children, in hepatic disease and narcotic dependence, and in pregnant women. Use cautiously in acute ulcerative colitis. Stop therapy immediately if abdominal distention or other signs of toxic megacolon develop.
• Risk of physical dependence increases with high dosage and long-term use. Atropine sulfate is included to discourage abuse.
• Not likely to be effective if there is no response within 48 hours.
• Patient should not use to treat acute diarrhea for longer than 2 days and should seek medical attention if diarrhea continues.

• Warn patient not to exceed recommended dosage.
• Dehydration, especially in young children, may increase risk of delayed toxicity. Correct fluid and electrolyte disturbances before starting drug.
• Dose of 2.5 mg is as effective as 5 ml camphorated tincture of opium.
• Not indicated in treatment of antibiotic-induced diarrhea.

kaolin and pectin mixtures
Donnagel-MB*†, Kao-Con†, Kaopectate◊, Kaopectate Concentrate◊, Kao-tin◊, Kapectolin◊, K-P◊, K-Pek◊

Pregnancy Risk Category: C

HOW SUPPLIED
Oral suspension: 5.2 mg kaolin and 260 mg pectin per 30 ml◊ (K-P◊); 5.85 g kaolin and 130 mg pectin per 30 ml◊ (Kaopectate◊, Kao-tin◊, Kapectolin◊, K-Pek◊); 5.91 g kaolin and 132 mg pectin per 30 ml◊ (Kaopectate◊), 6 g kaolin and 130 mg pectin per 30 ml◊ (Kaopectate†◊); 6 g kaolin and 143 mg pectin per 30 ml◊, with 3.8% alcohol (Donnagel-MB*†); 8.7 g kaolin and 195 mg pectin per 30 ml◊ (Kaopectate Concentrate◊); 8.8 g kaolin and 195 mg pectin per 30 ml◊ (Kaopectate Concentrate†◊, Kao-Con†)

MECHANISM OF ACTION
Decrease the stool's fluid content, although *total* water loss seems to remain the same.

INDICATIONS & DOSAGE
Mild, nonspecific diarrhea—
Adults: 60 to 120 ml P.O. after each bowel movement.
Children over 12 years: 60 ml P.O. after each bowel movement.
Children 6 to 12 years: 30 to 60 ml P.O. after each bowel movement.
Children 3 to 6 years: 15 to 30 ml P.O. after each bowel movement.

ADVERSE REACTIONS
GI: drug absorbs nutrients, drugs, and enzymes; fecal impaction or ulceration in infants and elderly or debilitated patients after chronic use; constipation.

INTERACTIONS
None significant.

NURSING CONSIDERATIONS
• Contraindicated in suspected obstructive bowel lesions.
• Don't use for more than 2 days.
• Don't use in place of specific therapy for underlying cause.
• May reduce absorption of other P.O. drugs, requiring dosage adjustments.
• It is a GI absorbent.

loperamide
Imodium, Imodium A-D◊

Pregnancy Risk Category: B

HOW SUPPLIED
Capsules: 2 mg
Oral liquid: 1 mg/5 ml◊

MECHANISM OF ACTION
Inhibits peristaltic activity, prolonging transit of intestinal contents.

INDICATIONS & DOSAGE
Acute, nonspecific diarrhea—
Adults: initially, 4 mg P.O., then 2 mg after each unformed stool. Maximum 16 mg daily.
Children 8 to 12 years: 10 ml t.i.d. P.O. on first day. (Subsequent doses of 5 ml per 10 kg of body weight may be administered after each unformed stool.)
Children 5 to 8 years: 10 ml P.O. b.i.d. on first day.
Children 2 to 5 years: 5 ml P.O. t.i.d. on first day.
Chronic diarrhea—
Adults: initially, 4 mg P.O., then 2 mg after each unformed stool until diarrhea subsides. Adjust dosage to individual response.

Italicized adverse reactions are common or life-threatening.
*Liquid form contains alcohol.   **May contain tartrazine.

ADVERSE REACTIONS
CNS: drowsiness, fatigue, dizziness.
GI: dry mouth; abdominal pain, distention, or discomfort; *constipation;* nausea; vomiting.
Skin: rash.

INTERACTIONS
None significant.

NURSING CONSIDERATIONS
• Contraindicated in acute diarrhea resulting from poison until toxic material is removed from GI tract, in acute diarrhea caused by organisms that penetrate intestinal mucosa, and when constipation must be avoided. Use cautiously in severe prostatic hypertrophy, hepatic disease, and history of narcotic dependence.
• Stop drug immediately if abdominal distention or other symptoms develop in acute colitis.
• In acute diarrhea, discontinue drug and seek medical attention if no improvement occurs within 48 hours; in chronic diarrhea, discontinue drug if no improvement occurs after giving 16 mg daily for at least 10 days.
• Warn patient not to exceed recommended dosage.
• Produces antidiarrheal action similar to diphenoxylate hydrochloride but without as many adverse CNS effects.

---

opium tincture*
Controlled Substance Schedule II

opium tincture, camphorated* (Paregoric)
Controlled Substance Schedule III

Pregnancy Risk Category: B (D for prolonged use or high doses at term)

HOW SUPPLIED
opium tincture
Oral solution: equivalent to morphine 10 mg/ml
opium tincture, camphorated
Oral solution: Each 5 ml contains morphine, 2 mg; anise oil, 0.2 ml; benzoic acid, 20 mg; camphor, 20 mg; glycerin, 0.2 ml; and ethanol to make 5 ml

MECHANISM OF ACTION
Increases smooth muscle tone in the GI tract, inhibits motility and propulsion, and diminishes secretions.

INDICATIONS & DOSAGE
Acute, nonspecific diarrhea—
Adults: 0.6 ml opium tincture (range 0.3 to 1 ml) P.O. q.i.d. Maximum dosage 6 ml daily; or 5 to 10 ml camphorated opium tincture daily b.i.d., t.i.d., or q.i.d. until diarrhea subsides.
Children: 0.25 to 0.5 ml/kg camphorated opium tincture P.O. daily, b.i.d., t.i.d., or q.i.d. until diarrhea subsides.

ADVERSE REACTIONS
GI: nausea, vomiting.
Other: physical dependence after long-term use.

INTERACTIONS
None significant.

NURSING CONSIDERATIONS
• Contraindicated in acute diarrhea resulting from poison until toxic material is removed from GI tract, and diarrhea caused by organisms that penetrate intestinal mucosa. Use cautiously in asthma, prostatic hypertrophy, hepatic disease, and narcotic dependence.
• Risk of physical dependence increases with long-term use.
• Don't use for more than 2 days.
• An effective and prompt-acting antidiarrheal; but unique because dos-

age can be adjusted precisely to patient's needs.

• Opium content of opium tincture 25 times greater than camphorated tincture of opium. Camphorated opium tincture is more dilute, and teaspoonful doses are easier to measure than dropper quantities of opium tincture.

• Milky fluid forms when camphorated opium tincture is added to water.

• Camphorated opium tincture 0.06 to 0.5 ml daily has been used to treat infants with mild narcotic physical dependence.

• Store in tightly capped, light-resistant container.

• Mix with sufficient water to ensure passage to stomach.

• Narcotic antagonist naloxone can reverse the respiratory depression resulting from overdose.

47

Laxatives

bisacodyl
calcium polycarbophil
cascara sagrada
cascara sagrada aromatic fluid extract
cascara sagrada fluid extract
castor oil
docusate calcium
docusate potassium
docusate sodium
glycerin
lactulose
magnesium citrate
magnesium hydroxide
magnesium sulfate
methylcellulose
mineral oil
phenolphthalein, white
phenolphthalein, yellow
polyethylene glycol-electrolyte solution
psyllium
senna
sodium phosphates

COMBINATION PRODUCTS
AGORAL◇: mineral oil 28% and white phenolphthalein 1.3% in emulsion, with tragacanth, agar, egg albumin, acacia, and glycerin.
DIALOSE-PLUS◇: docusate potassium 100 mg and casanthranol 30 mg.
DIOLAX◇: docusate sodium 100 mg and casanthranol 50 mg.
DOXIDAN◇: docusate calcium 60 mg and phenolphthalein 65 mg.
D-S-S PLUS◇: docusate sodium 100 mg and casanthranol 30 mg.
HALEY'S M-O◇: mineral oil (25%) and magnesium hydroxide.
KONDREMUL WITH CASCARA◇: heavy mineral oil 55%, cascara sagrada extract 660 mg/15 ml, and Irish moss as emulsifier.
KONDREMUL WITH PHENOLPHTHALEIN◇: heavy mineral oil 55%, white phenolphthalein 150 mg/15 ml, and Irish moss as emulsifier.
MODANE PLUS◇: docusate sodium 100 mg and phenolphthalein 60 mg.
PERI-COLACE◇(capsules): docusate sodium 100 mg and casanthranol 30 mg.
PERI-COLACE◇(syrup): docusate sodium 60 mg and casanthranol 30 mg/15 ml.
SENOKOT-S◇: docusate sodium 50 mg and standardized senna concentrate 187 mg.

bisacodyl

Bisacolax†◇, Bisalax‡, Bisco-Lax**◇, Dacodyl◇, Deficol◇, Dulcolax◇, Durolax‡, Fleet Bisacodyl◇, Laxit†◇, Theralax◇

Pregnancy Risk Category: C

HOW SUPPLIED
Tablets (enteric-coated): 5 mg◇
Enema: 0.33 mg/dl◇, 10 mg/5 ml (microenema)‡
Powder for rectal solution (bisacodyl tannex): 1.5 mg bisacodyl and 2.5 g tannic acid
Suppositories: 10 mg◇

MECHANISM OF ACTION
Increases peristalsis by direct effect on the smooth muscle of the intestine. Thought either to irritate the musculature or to stimulate the colonic in-

†Available in Canada only. ‡Available in Australia only. ◇Available OTC.

tramural plexus. Also promotes fluid accumulation in the colon and small intestine. A stimulant laxative.

INDICATIONS & DOSAGE
Chronic constipation; preparation for delivery, surgery, or rectal or bowel examination—
Adults: 10 to 15 mg P.O. in evening or before breakfast. Up to 30 mg may be used for thorough evacuation needed for examinations or surgery.
Children 6 years and older: 5 to 10 mg P.O.
Adults and children over 2 years: 10 mg rectally.
Children under 2 years: 5 mg rectally.

ADVERSE REACTIONS
CNS: muscle weakness in excessive use.
GI: *nausea, vomiting, abdominal cramps,* diarrhea with high doses, *burning sensation in rectum with suppositories.*
Metabolic: alkalosis, hypokalemia, tetany, protein-losing enteropathy in excessive use, fluid and electrolyte imbalance.
Other: laxative dependence in long-term or excessive use.

INTERACTIONS
None significant.

NURSING CONSIDERATIONS
• Contraindicated in patients with abdominal pain, nausea, vomiting, or other symptoms of appendicitis or acute surgical abdomen, or in rectal fissures or ulcerated hemorrhoids.
• Tell patient to swallow enteric-coated tablet whole to avoid GI irritation. Don't give within one hour of milk or antacid intake. Begins to act 6 to 12 hours after oral administration.
• Soft, formed stool usually produced 15 to 60 minutes after rectal administration. Time administration of drug

so as not to interfere with scheduled activities or sleep.
• Tablets and suppositories may be used together to cleanse colon before and after surgery and before barium enema.
• Insert suppository as high as possible into the rectum, and try to position the suppository against the rectal wall. Avoid embedding within fecal material because this may delay the onset of action.
• Use for short-term treatment. A stimulant laxative, this type of laxative is most abused. Discourage excessive use.
• Before giving for constipation, determine if patient has adequate fluid intake, exercise, and diet. Tell him that dietary sources of bulk include bran and other cereals, fresh fruit, and vegetables.
• Store tablets and suppositories at temperature below 86° F. (30° C.).
• Tell patient to report adverse effects to the doctor.

---

calcium polycarbophil
Equalactin◇, FiberCon◇, Mitrolan◇
Pregnancy Risk Category: C

HOW SUPPLIED
Tablets: 500 mg◇ (FiberCon◇)
Tablets (chewable): 500 mg◇ (Equalactin◇, Mitrolan◇)

MECHANISM OF ACTION
Absorbs water and expands to increase bulk and moisture content of the stool. The increased bulk encourages peristalsis and bowel movement. A bulk-forming laxative. As an antidiarrheal, absorbs free fecal water, thereby producing formed stools.

INDICATIONS & DOSAGE
Constipation (Equalactin and Mitrolan must be chewed before swallowing)—

Italicized adverse reactions are common or life-threatening.
*Liquid form contains alcohol.   **May contain tartrazine.

Adults: 1 g P.O. q.i.d. as required. Maximum 6 g in 24-hour period.
Children 6 to 12 years: 500 mg P.O. t.i.d. as required. Maximum 3 g in 24-hour period.
Children 2 to 6 years: 500 mg P.O. b.i.d. as required. Maximum 1.5 g in 24-hour period.
Diarrhea associated with irritable bowel syndrome, as well as acute nonspecific diarrhea (Mitrolan must be chewed before swallowing)—
Adults: 1 g P.O. q.i.d. as required. Maximum 6 g in 24-hour period.
Children 6 to 12 years 500 mg P.O. t.i.d. as required. Maximum 3 g in 24-hour period.
Children 2 to 6 years: 500 mg P.O. b.i.d. as required. Maximum 1.5 g in 24-hour period.

ADVERSE REACTIONS
GI: abdominal fullness and increased flatus, intestinal obstruction.
Other: laxative dependence in longterm or excessive use.

INTERACTIONS
None significant.

NURSING CONSIDERATIONS
• Contraindicated in signs of GI obstruction.
• Rectal bleeding or failure to respond to therapy may indicate need for surgery.
• Before giving for constipation, determine if patient has adequate fluid intake, exercise, and diet. Tell him that dietary sources of bulk include bran and other cereals, fresh fruit, and vegetables.
• Advise patient to chew the Equalactin or Mitrolan tablets thoroughly and drink a full glass of water with each dose. However, when used as an antidiarrheal, tell patient *not* to drink a glass of water.
• For episodes of severe diarrhea, the dose may be repeated every half hour,

but maximum daily dosage should not be exceeded.

---

cascara sagrada

cascara sagrada aromatic fluid extract*

cascara sagrada fluid extract*

Pregnancy Risk Category: C

HOW SUPPLIED
Tablets: 150 mg◊, 325 mg◊
Aromatic fluid extract: 1 g/ml◊
Fluidextract: 1 g/ml◊

MECHANISM OF ACTION
Increases peristalsis by direct effect on the smooth muscle of the intestine. Thought either to irritate the musculature or to stimulate the colonic intramural plexus. Also promotes fluid accumulation in the colon and small intestine. A stimulant laxative.

INDICATIONS & DOSAGE
Acute constipation; preparation for bowel or rectal examination—
Adults: 325 mg cascara sagrada tablets P.O. h.s.; or 1 ml fluid extract daily; or 5 ml aromatic fluid extract daily.
Children 2 to 12 years: ½ adult dose.
Children under 2 years: ¼ adult dose.

ADVERSE REACTIONS
GI: *nausea;* vomiting; diarrhea; loss of normal bowel function with excessive use; *abdominal cramps,* especially in severe constipation; malabsorption of nutrients; "cathartic colon" (syndrome resembling ulcerative colitis radiologically and pathologically) after chronic misuse; discoloration of rectal mucosa after long-term use.
Metabolic: hypokalemia, protein en-

---

teropathy, electrolyte imbalance in excessive use.
Other: laxative dependence in long-term or excessive use.

INTERACTIONS
None significant.

NURSING CONSIDERATIONS
• Contraindicated in abdominal pain, nausea, vomiting, or other symptoms of appendicitis or acute surgical abdomen; acute surgical delirium, fecal impaction, intestinal obstruction or perforation. Use cautiously when rectal bleeding is present.
• Aromatic cascara fluidextract is less active and less bitter than nonaromatic fluid extract.
• Liquid preparations more reliable than solid dosage forms.
• Before giving for constipation, determine if patient has adequate fluid intake, exercise, and diet. Tell him that dietary sources of bulk include bran and other cereals, fresh fruit, and vegetables.
• May turn alkaline urine red-pink and acidic urine yellow-brown.
• Monitor serum electrolytes during prolonged use.
• Onset of action is 6 to 12 hours.

castor oil
Alphamul◇, Emulsoil◇, Fleet Flavored Castor Oil◇, Kellogg's Castor Oil◇, Minims Castor Oil‡◇, Neoloid◇, Purge◇

Pregnancy Risk Category: X

HOW SUPPLIED
Capsules: 0.62 ml oil◇
Oral liquid◇: 36.4% (Neoloid◇), 60% (Alphamul◇), 67% (Fleet◇), 95% (Purge◇, Emulsoil◇), 100% (Kellogg's◇, Minims◇).

MECHANISM OF ACTION
Increases peristalsis by direct effect on the smooth muscle of the intestine.

Thought either to irritate the musculature or to stimulate the colonic intramural plexus. Also promotes fluid accumulation in the colon and small intestine. A stimulant laxative.

INDICATIONS & DOSAGE
Preparation for rectal or bowel examination, or surgery; acute constipation (rarely)—
Adults: 15 to 60 ml P.O.
Children over 2 years: 5 to 15 ml P.O.
Children under 2 years: 1.25 to 7.5 ml P.O.
Infants: up to 4 ml P.O. Increased dose produces no greater effect.

ADVERSE REACTIONS
GI: *nausea;* vomiting; diarrhea; loss of normal bowel function with excessive use; *abdominal cramps,* especially in severe constipation; malabsorption of nutrients; "cathartic colon" (syndrome resembling ulcerative colitis radiologically and pathologically) in chronic misuse. May cause constipation after catharsis.
GU: pelvic congestion in menstruating women.
Metabolic: hypokalemia, protein-losing enteropathy, other electrolyte imbalance in excessive use.
Other: laxative dependence in long-term or excessive use.

INTERACTIONS
None significant.

NURSING CONSIDERATIONS
• Contraindicated in ulcerative bowel lesions; during menstruation; in abdominal pain, nausea, vomiting, or other symptoms of appendicitis or acute surgical abdomen; in anal or rectal fissures, fecal impaction, intestinal obstruction or perforation; and in pregnancy. Use cautiously in rectal bleeding.
• Failure to respond may indicate acute condition requiring surgery.

Italicized adverse reactions are common or life-threatening.
*Liquid form contains alcohol.   **May contain tartrazine.

• Give with juice or carbonated beverage to mask oily taste. Patient should stir mixture and drink it promptly. Ice held in mouth before taking drug will help prevent tasting it.

• Shake emulsion well. Store below 40° F. (4.4° C.). Don't freeze.

• Give on empty stomach for best results.

• Produces complete evacuation after 3 hours. Tell patient that after castor oil has emptied bowel he will not have bowel movement for 1 to 2 days.

• Time drug administration so that it doesn't interfere with scheduled activities or sleep.

• Monitor serum electrolytes during prolonged use.

• Generally used before diagnostic testing or therapy requiring thorough evacuation of GI tract.

• Use for short-term treatment. Not recommended for routine use; useful for acute constipation not responsive to milder laxatives.

• Before giving for constipation, determine if patient has adequate fluid intake, exercise, and diet. Tell him that dietary sources of bulk include bran and other cereals, fresh fruit, and vegetables.

• Increased intestinal motility lessens absorption of concomitantly administered P.O. drugs. Reschedule dose.

• Castor oil affects the small intestine. Regular use may cause excessive loss of water and salt.

• Castor oil emulsion is better tolerated but is more expensive.

docusate calcium (dioctyl calcium sulfosuccinate)
Pro-Cal-Sof◊, Surfak◊

docusate potassium (dioctyl potassium sulfosuccinate)
Dialose◊, Diocto-K◊, Kasof◊

docusate sodium (dioctyl sodium sulfosuccinate)
Afko-Lube◊, Colace◊, Coloxyl‡, Coloxyl Enema Concentrate‡, Diocto◊, Dioeze◊, Diosuccin◊, Dio-Sul◊, Disonate◊, Di-Sosul◊, DOK-250◊, DOK Liquid◊, Doss 300◊, Doxinate◊, D-S-S◊, Duosol◊, Genasoft◊, Laxinate 100◊, Modane Soft◊, Pro-Sof◊, Pro-Sof 250◊, Pro-Sof Liquid Concentrate◊, Regulax SS◊, Regutol◊, Stulex◊

Pregnancy Risk Category: C

HOW SUPPLIED
calcium
Capsules: 50 mg◊, 240 mg◊
potassium
Capsules: 100 mg◊, 240 mg◊
sodium
Tablets: 50 mg◊, 100 mg◊
Capsules◊: 50 mg, 60 mg, 100 mg, 240 mg, 250 mg, 300 mg
Oral liquid: 50 mg/ml◊
Syrup: 50 mg/15 ml◊, 60 mg/15 ml◊
Enema concentrate: 18 g/100 ml (must be diluted)‡

MECHANISM OF ACTION
Reduces surface tension of interfacing liquid contents of the bowel. This detergent activity promotes incorporation of additional liquid into the stool, forming a softer mass. A stool softener.

INDICATIONS & DOSAGE
Stool softener—
Adults and older children: 50 to 300 mg (docusate sodium) P.O. daily or

---

50 to 300 mg (docusate calcium and docusate potassium) P.O. daily until bowel movements are normal. Alternatively, give enema (where available). Dilute 1:24 with sterile water before administration, and give 100 to 150 ml (retention enema), 300 to 500 ml (evacuation enema), or 0.5 to 1.5 liters (flushing enema).

Children 6 to 12 years: 40 to 120 mg (docusate sodium) P.O. daily.

Children 3 to 6 years: 20 to 60 mg (docusate sodium) P.O. daily.

Children under 3 years: 10 to 40 mg (docusate sodium) P.O. daily.

Higher dosages are for initial therapy. Adjust dosage to individual response. Usual dosage in children and adults with minimal needs: 50 to 150 mg (docusate calcium) P.O. daily.

ADVERSE REACTIONS
EENT: throat irritation.
GI: bitter taste, mild abdominal cramping, diarrhea.
Other: laxative dependence in long-term or excessive use.

INTERACTIONS
Mineral oil: may increase mineral oil absorption and cause lipoid pneumonia. Don't administer together.

NURSING CONSIDERATIONS
• Should only be used occasionally. Don't use for more than 1 week without doctor's knowledge.
• Give liquid in milk, fruit juice, or infant formula to mask bitter taste.
• Not for use in treating existing constipation, but prevents constipation from developing.
• Laxative of choice in patients who should not strain during defecation, such as those recovering from myocardial infarction or rectal surgery; in disease of rectum and anus that makes passage of firm stool difficult; or in postpartum constipation.
• Acts within 24 to 48 hours to produce firm, semisolid stool.

• Instruct patient that dietary sources of bulk include bran and other cereals, fresh fruit, and vegetables.
• Doesn't stimulate intestinal peristaltic movements.
• Discontinue if severe cramping occurs.
• Store at 59° to 86° F. (15° to 30° C.). Protect liquid from light.
• Many doctors feel that the minimum effective dosage is 300 mg daily. A lower dosage may not produce satisfactory results.

glycerin
Fleet Babylax◇, Sani-Supp◇
Pregnancy Risk Category: C

HOW SUPPLIED
Enema (pediatric): 4 ml/applicator◇
Suppositories: adult, children, and infant sizes◇

MECHANISM OF ACTION
Draws water from the tissues into the feces and thus stimulates evacuation. A hyperosmolar laxative.

INDICATIONS & DOSAGE
Constipation—
Adults and children over 6 years: 3 g as a rectal suppository; or 5 to 15 ml as an enema.
Children under 6 years: 1 to 1.5 g as a rectal suppository; or 2 to 5 ml as an enema.

ADVERSE REACTIONS
GI: *cramping pain,* rectal discomfort, hyperemia of rectal mucosa.

INTERACTIONS
None significant.

NURSING CONSIDERATIONS
• A hyperosmolar laxative used mainly to reestablish proper toilet habits in laxative-dependent patients.
• Must be retained for at least 15 minutes; usually acts within 1 hour.

Italicized adverse reactions are common or life-threatening.
*Liquid form contains alcohol.   **May contain tartrazine.

Entire suppository need not melt to be effective.

lactulose
Cephulac, Cholac, Chronulac, Constilac, Duphalac, Lactulax†

Pregnancy Risk Category: B

HOW SUPPLIED
Syrup: 10 g/15 ml

MECHANISM OF ACTION
Produces an osmotic effect in the colon. Resultant distention promotes peristalsis. Also decreases blood ammonia, probably as a result of bacterial degradation, which decreases the pH of colon contents.

INDICATIONS & DOSAGE
Treatment of constipation—
Adults: 15 to 30 ml P.O. daily.
To prevent and treat portal-systemic encephalopathy, including hepatic precoma and coma in patients with severe hepatic disease—
Adults: initially, 20 to 30 g P.O. (30 to 45 ml) t.i.d. or q.i.d., until two or three soft stools are produced daily. Usual dosage is 60 to 100 g daily in divided doses. Can also be given by retention enema in at least 100 ml of fluid.

ADVERSE REACTIONS
GI: abdominal cramps, belching, diarrhea, gaseous distention, flatulence.
Metabolic: hypernatremia.

INTERACTIONS
None significant.

NURSING CONSIDERATIONS
• Contraindicated in low-galactose diet. Use cautiously in diabetes mellitus.
• Reduce dosage if diarrhea occurs. Replace fluid loss.
• Monitor serum sodium for possible hypernatremia, especially when giving in higher doses to treat hepatic encephalopathy.
• Minimize drug's sweet taste by diluting with water or fruit juice or giving with food.
• Store at room temperature, preferably below 86° F. (30° C.). Don't freeze.

magnesium citrate (citrate of magnesia)
Citroma◊, Citro-Nesia◊

magnesium hydroxide (milk of magnesia)
M.O.M.◊

magnesium sulfate (epsom salts)◊

Pregnancy Risk Category: B

HOW SUPPLIED
citrate
Oral solution: approximately 168 mEq magnesium/240 ml◊
hydroxide
Oral suspension: 7% to 8.5% (approximately 80 mEq magnesium/30 ml)◊
sulfate
Granules: approximately 40 mEq magnesium/5 g◊

MECHANISM OF ACTION
Produces an osmotic effect in the small intestine by drawing water into the intestinal lumen. A saline laxative.

INDICATIONS & DOSAGE
Constipation, to evacuate bowel before surgery—
Adults and children over 6 years: 15 g magnesium sulfate P.O. in glass of water; or 10 to 20 ml concentrated milk of magnesia P.O.; or 15 to 60 ml milk of magnesia P.O.; or 5 to 10 oz magnesium citrate h.s.

---

†Available in Canada only. ‡Available in Australia only. ◊ Available OTC.

Children 2 to 6 years: 5 to 15 ml milk of magnesia P.O.
Antacid—
Adults: 5 to 15 ml milk of magnesia P.O. t.i.d. or q.i.d.

ADVERSE REACTIONS
GI: *abdominal cramping, nausea.*
Metabolic: fluid and electrolyte disturbances if used daily.
Other: laxative dependence in long-term or excessive use.

INTERACTIONS
None significant.

NURSING CONSIDERATIONS
• Contraindicated in abdominal pain, nausea, vomiting, or other symptoms of appendicitis or acute surgical abdomen; and in myocardial damage, heart block, imminent delivery, fecal impaction, rectal fissures, intestinal obstruction or perforation, or renal disease. Use cautiously in rectal bleeding.
• Shake suspension well; give with large amount of water when used as laxative. When administering through nasogastric tube, make sure tube is placed properly and is patent. After instilling, flush tube with water to ensure passage to stomach and maintain tube patency.
• For short-term therapy; don't use longer than 1 week.
• When used as laxative, don't give oral drugs 1 to 2 hours before or after administration.
• As a saline laxative, drug produces watery stool in 3 to 6 hours. Time drug administration so that it doesn't interfere with scheduled activities or sleep.
• Magnesium sulfate is more potent than other saline laxatives.
• Before giving for constipation, determine if patient has adequate fluid intake, exercise, and diet. Tell him that dietary sources of bulk include bran and other cereals, fresh fruit, and vegetables.
• Magnesium may accumulate in renal insufficiency.
• Chilling before use may make magnesium citrate more palatable.
• Monitor serum electrolytes during prolonged use.
• Frequent or prolonged use as a laxative may cause dependence.

methylcellulose
Citrucel◊, Cologel◊

Pregnancy Risk Category: C

HOW SUPPLIED
Oral liquid: 450 mg/5 ml◊
Powder: 2 g/heaping tablespoon◊

MECHANISM OF ACTION
Absorbs water and expands to increase bulk and moisture content of the stool. The increased bulk encourages peristalsis and bowel movement. A bulk-forming laxative.

INDICATIONS & DOSAGE
Chronic constipation—
Adults: 5 to 20 ml liquid P.O. t.i.d. with a glass of water; or 15 ml syrup P.O. morning and evening.
Children: 5 to 10 ml P.O. daily or b.i.d.

ADVERSE REACTIONS
GI: *nausea,* vomiting, diarrhea (all after excessive use); esophageal, gastric, small intestinal, or colonic strictures when drug is chewed or taken in dry form; *abdominal cramps,* especially in severe constipation.
Other: laxative dependence in long-term or excessive use.

INTERACTIONS
None significant.

NURSING CONSIDERATIONS
• Contraindicated in abdominal pain, nausea, vomiting, or other symptoms

---

Italicized adverse reactions are common or life-threatening.
*Liquid form contains alcohol.   **May contain tartrazine.

of appendicitis or acute surgical abdomen; and in intestinal obstruction or ulceration, disabling adhesion, or difficulty swallowing.

• Laxative effect usually takes 12 to 24 hours, but may be delayed 3 days.

• Tell patient to take drug with at least 8 oz (240 ml) of pleasant-tasting liquid to mask grittiness.

• Especially useful in postpartum constipation, debilitated patients, chronic laxative abuse, irritable bowel syndrome, diverticular disease, colostomies, and to empty colon before barium enema examinations.

• Before giving for constipation, determine if patient has adequate fluid intake, exercise, and diet. Tell him that dietary sources of bulk include bran and other cereals, fresh fruit, and vegetables.

• Not absorbed systemically; nontoxic.

mineral oil (liquid petrolatum)
Agoral Plain◊, Fleet Mineral Oil◊, Kondremul Plain◊, Milkinol◊, Neo-Cultol◊, Zymenol◊

Pregnancy Risk Category: C

HOW SUPPLIED
Emulsion: 50%◊
Jelly: 55%◊
Oral liquid: in pints, quarts, gallons◊

MECHANISM OF ACTION
Increases water retention in the stool by creating a barrier between colon wall and feces that prevents colonic reabsorption of fecal water. A lubricant laxative.

INDICATIONS & DOSAGE
Constipation; preparation for bowel studies or surgery—
Adults: 15 to 30 ml P.O. h.s.; or 120 ml enema.
Children: 5 to 15 ml P.O. h.s.; or 30 to 60 ml enema.

ADVERSE REACTIONS
GI: *nausea;* vomiting; diarrhea in excessive use; *abdominal cramps,* especially in severe constipation; decreased absorption of nutrients and fat-soluble vitamins, resulting in deficiency; and slowed healing after hemorrhoidectomy.
Other: laxative dependence in long-term or excessive use, pruritus.

INTERACTIONS
Docusate salts: may increase mineral oil absorption and cause lipid pneumonia. Don't administer together.
Fat soluble vitamins (A,D,E,K): absorption may be decreased after prolonged administration.

NURSING CONSIDERATIONS
• Contraindicated in abdominal pain, nausea, vomiting, or other symptoms of appendicitis or acute surgical abdomen; and in fecal impaction, or intestinal obstruction or perforation. Use cautiously in young children; in elderly or debilitated patients because of susceptibility to lipid pneumonitis through aspiration, absorption, and transport from intestinal mucosa; and in rectal bleeding. Enema contraindicated in children under 2 years.

• Don't give drug with meals or immediately after, as it delays passage of food from stomach. More active on an empty stomach.

• To be taken only at bedtime. Warn patient not to take for more than 1 week.

• Give with fruit juices or carbonated drinks to disguise taste.

• Use when patient needs to ease the strain of evacuation.

• Warn patient of possible rectal leakage from excessive dosages so he can avoid soiling clothing.

• Before giving for constipation, determine if patient has adequate fluid intake, exercise, and diet. Tell him that dietary sources of bulk include

---

†Available in Canada only.   ‡Available in Australia only.   ◊ Available OTC.

bran and other cereals, fresh fruit, and vegetables.
• Onset of action is 6 to 8 hours.

phenolphthalein, white
Alophen Pills◇, Medilax◇, Modane◇, Modane Mild◇, Phenolax Wafers**◇, Prulet◇

phenolphthalein, yellow
Feen-A-Mint Gum◇, Evac-U-Gen◇, Evac-U-Lax◇, Ex-Lax◇, Lax-Pills◇

Pregnancy Risk Category: C

HOW SUPPLIED
phenolphthalein, white
Tablets: 60 mg◇
Tablets (chewable): 60 mg◇, 64.8 mg◇
phenolphthalein, yellow
Tablets (chewable): 80 mg◇, 90 mg◇, 97.2 mg◇
Chewing gum: 97.2 mg◇

MECHANISM OF ACTION
Increases peristalsis by direct effect on the smooth muscle of the intestine. Thought either to irritate the musculature or to stimulate the colonic intramural plexus. Also promotes fluid accumulation in the colon and small intestine. A stimulant laxative.

INDICATIONS & DOSAGE
Constipation—
Adults and children over 12 years: 30 to 270 mg P.O., preferably h.s.
Children 6 to 11 years: 30 to 60 mg P.O. h.s.
Children 2 to 5 years: 15 to 30 mg P.O. h.s.

ADVERSE REACTIONS
GI: diarrhea; *colic in large doses;* factitious nausea; vomiting; loss of normal bowel function in excessive use; *abdominal cramps,* especially in severe constipation; malabsorption of nutrients; "cathartic colon" (syndrome resembling ulcerative colitis radiologically and pathologically) in chronic misuse; reddish discoloration in alkaline feces or urine.
Skin: dermatitis, pruritus, rash, pigmentation.
Other: laxative dependence in long-term or excessive use, *hypersensitivity.*

INTERACTIONS
None significant.

NURSING CONSIDERATIONS
• Contraindicated in abdominal pain, nausea, vomiting, or other symptoms of appendicitis or acute surgical abdomen; in fecal impaction, or intestinal obstruction or perforation. Use cautiously in rectal bleeding.
• Laxative effect may last up to 3 to 4 days.
• Produces semisolid stool within 6 to 8 hours. Time drug administration so that it doesn't interfere with scheduled activities or sleep.
• Warn patient with rash to avoid sun and discontinue use. Don't use any other product containing phenolphthalein.
• Before giving for constipation, determine if patient has adequate fluid intake, exercise, and diet. Tell him that dietary sources of bulk include bran and other cereals, fresh fruit, and vegetables.
• May discolor alkaline urine red-pink and acidic urine yellow-brown.
• Drug is available in many dosage forms. Most popular OTC laxative.
• Children may mistake for candy. Keep out of reach.
• Yellow phenolphthalein is two to three times as potent as white phenolphthalein.

Italicized adverse reactions are common or life-threatening.
*Liquid form contains alcohol. **May contain tartrazine.

polyethylene glycol-electrolyte solution
CoLyte, Glycoprep‡, GoLYTELY

Pregnancy Risk Category: C

HOW SUPPLIED
Powder for oral solution: polyethylene glycol (PEG) 3350 (120 g), sodium sulfate (3.36 g), sodium chloride (2.92 g), potassium chloride (1.49 g) per 2 liters (CoLyte); PEG 3350 (60 g), sodium chloride (1.46 g), potassium chloride (745 mg), sodium bicarbonate (1.68 g), sodium sulfate (5.68 g) per liter (Glycoprep‡); PEG 3350 (236 g), sodium sulfate (22.74 g), sodium bicarbonate (6.74g), sodium chloride (5.86 g), potassium chloride (2.97 g), per 4.8 liter (GoLYTELY)

MECHANISM OF ACTION
PEG 3350, a nonabsorbable solution, acts as an osmotic agent. Using sodium sulfate as the major sodium source, sodium absorption is greatly reduced. The electrolyte concentration results in virtually no net absorption or secretion of ions.

INDICATIONS & DOSAGE
Bowel preparation before GI examination—
Adults: 240 ml P.O. q 10 minutes until 4 liters are consumed. Usually administered 4 hours before examination, allowing 3 hours for drinking and 1 hour for bowel evacuation.

ADVERSE REACTIONS
GI: *nausea, bloating, cramps, vomiting.*

INTERACTIONS
None significant.

NURSING CONSIDERATIONS
• Contraindicated in GI obstruction or perforation, gastric retention, toxic colitis, or megacolon.

• If administered to semiconscious patients or to patients with impaired gag reflex, take care to prevent aspiration.
• No major shifts in fluid and electrolytes have been reported.
• Orally administered solution induces a diarrhea (onset 30 to 60 minutes) which rapidly cleanses the bowel, usually within 4 hours. The solution may be administered in the early morning, if the patient is scheduled for a mid-morning exam.
• May be less useful as a preparation for barium enema, because it may interfere with the barium coating of the colonic mucosa. To avoid such interference, administer solution the evening before the examination.
• Patient should fast for 3 to 4 hours before taking the solution, and thereafter ingest only clear fluids until the examination is complete.
• Tap water may be used to reconstitute powder. Shake vigorously to ensure that all powder is dissolved. Reconstituted solution may be refrigerated but should be used within 48 hours.
• Do not add flavoring or additional ingredients to the solution, and do not administer chilled solution. Hypothermia has been reported after ingestion of large amounts of chilled solution.

psyllium
Cillium◇, Konsyl◇, Metamucil◇, Metamucil Instant Mix◇, Metamucil Sugar Free◇, Naturacil◇, Perdiem Plain◇, Siblin◇, Syllact◇

Pregnancy Risk Category: C

HOW SUPPLIED
Chewable pieces: 1.7 g/piece◇
Effervescent powder: 3.4 g/packet◇, 3.7 g/packet◇
Granules: 2.5 g/tsp, 4.03 g/tsp◇
Powder: 3.3 g/tsp◇, 3.4 g/tsp◇, 3.5 g/tsp◇, 4.94 g/tsp◇
Wafers: 3.4 g/wafer◇

---

†Available in Canada only.   ‡Available in Australia only.   ◇Available OTC.

MECHANISM OF ACTION
Absorbs water and expands to increase bulk and moisture content of the stool. The increased bulk encourages peristalsis and bowel movement. A bulk-forming laxative.

INDICATIONS & DOSAGE
Constipation; bowel management—
Adults: 1 to 2 rounded teaspoonfuls P.O. in full glass of liquid daily, b.i.d. or t.i.d., followed by second glass of liquid; or 1 packet P.O. dissolved in water daily, b.i.d. or t.i.d.
Children over 6 years: 1 level teaspoonful P.O. in half a glass of liquid h.s.

ADVERSE REACTIONS
GI: *nausea, vomiting, diarrhea,* all after excessive use; esophageal, gastric, small intestinal, or colonic strictures when drug taken in dry form; abdominal cramps, especially in severe constipation.

INTERACTIONS
None significant.

NURSING CONSIDERATIONS
• Contraindicated in abdominal pain, nausea, vomiting, or other symptoms of appendicitis; and in intestinal obstruction or ulceration, disabling adhesion, or difficulty swallowing.
• In diabetic patients, use brand of psyllium that does not contain sugar. Check label.
• Mix with at least 8 oz (240 ml) of cold, pleasant-tasting liquid such as orange juice to mask grittiness, and stir only a few seconds. Patient should drink it immediately or mixture will congeal. Follow with additional glass of liquid.
• Before giving for constipation, determine if patient has adequate fluid intake, exercise, and diet. Tell him that dietary sources of bulk include bran and other cereals, fresh fruit, and vegetables.

• May reduce appetite if taken before meals.
• Laxative effect usually seen in 12 to 24 hours, but may be delayed 3 days.
• Not absorbed systemically; nontoxic. Especially useful in postpartum constipation, debilitated patients, chronic laxative abuse, irritable bowel syndrome, diverticular disease, and in combination with other laxatives to empty colon before barium enema examinations.

senna
Black-Draught◇, Senokot◇, X-Prep Liquid*◇
Pregnancy Risk Category: C

HOW SUPPLIED
Tablets: 187 mg◇, 217 mg◇, 600 mg◇
Granules: 326 mg/tsp◇, 1.65 g/½ tsp◇
Suppositories: 652 mg◇
Syrup: 218 mg/5 ml◇

MECHANISM OF ACTION
Increases peristalsis by direct effect on the smooth muscle of the intestine. Thought either to irritate the musculature or to stimulate the colonic intramural plexus. Also promotes fluid accumulation in the colon and small intestine. A stimulant laxative.

INDICATIONS & DOSAGE
Acute constipation, preparation for bowel or rectal examination—
Adults: Dosage range for Senokot: 1 to 8 tablets P.O.; ½ to 4 teaspoonfuls of granules added to liquid; 1 to 2 suppositories h.s.; 1 to 4 teaspoonfuls syrup h.s. Black-Draught: 2 tablets or ¼ to ½ level teaspoonfuls of granules mixed with water.
Children over 27 kg: half adult dose of tablets, granules, or syrup (except Black-Draught tablets and granules not recommended for children).
Children 1 month to 1 year: 1.25 to 2.5 ml Senokot syrup P.O. h.s.

Italicized adverse reactions are common or life-threatening.
*Liquid form contains alcohol.   **May contain tartrazine.

X-Prep Liquid used solely as single dose for preradiographic bowel evacuation. Give 20 g powder dissolved in juice or 75 ml liquid between 2 p.m. and 4 p.m. on day before X-ray procedure. May be given in divided doses for elderly or debilitated patients.

ADVERSE REACTIONS
GI: *nausea;* vomiting; diarrhea; loss of normal bowel function in excessive use; *abdominal cramps,* especially in severe constipation; malabsorption of nutrients; "cathartic colon" (syndrome resembling ulcerative colitis radiologically) in chronic misuse; may cause constipation after catharsis; yellow, yellow-green cast to feces; diarrhea in nursing infants of mothers receiving senna; darkened pigmentation of rectal mucosa in long-term use, which is usually reversible within 4 to 12 months after stopping drug.
GU: red-pink discoloration in alkaline urine; yellow-brown color to acidic urine.
Metabolic: hypokalemia, protein-losing enteropathy, electrolyte imbalance with excessive use.
Other: laxative dependence in long-term or excessive use.

INTERACTIONS
None significant.

NURSING CONSIDERATIONS
• Contraindicated in ulcerative bowel lesions; in nausea, vomiting, abdominal pain, or other symptoms of appendicitis or acute surgical abdomen; fecal impaction; or intestinal obstruction or perforation.
• Use for short-term treatment.
• More potent than cascara sagrada. Acts in 6 to 10 hours. X-Prep Liquid gives thorough, strong bowel action beginning in 6 hours.
• Avoid exposing to excessive heat or light.
• Before giving for constipation, determine if patient has adequate fluid

intake, exercise, and diet. Tell him that dietary sources of bulk include bran and other cereals, fresh fruit, and vegetables.
• After X-Prep Liquid is taken, diet should be confined to clear liquids.
• Senna is one of the most effective laxatives for counteracting constipation caused by narcotic analgesics.

---

sodium phosphates
Fleet Phospho-Soda◊

Pregnancy Risk Category: C

HOW SUPPLIED
Liquid: 2.4 g/5 ml sodium phosphate and 900 mg sodium biphosphate/5 ml◊
Enema: 160 mg/ml sodium phosphate and 60 mg/ml sodium biphosphate◊

MECHANISM OF ACTION
Produces an osmotic effect in the small intestine by drawing water into the intestinal lumen. A saline laxative.

INDICATIONS & DOSAGE
Constipation—
Adults: 5 to 20 ml liquid P.O. with water; or 4 g powder dissolved in warm water P.O.; or 20 to 30 ml solution mixed with 120 ml cold water P.O.; or 60 to 135 ml enema.

ADVERSE REACTIONS
GI: *abdominal cramping.*
Metabolic: fluid and electrolyte disturbances (hypernatremia, hyperphosphatemia) if used daily.
Other: laxative dependence in long-term or excessive use.

INTERACTIONS
None significant.

NURSING CONSIDERATIONS
• Contraindicated in abdominal pain, nausea, vomiting, or other symptoms of appendicitis or acute surgical abdo-

men; intestinal obstruction or perforation; edema; congestive heart failure; megacolon; impaired renal function; and in patients on salt-restricted diets.
• Use with caution in patients with large hemorrhoids or anal excoriations.
• Available in oral and rectal forms.
• Before giving for constipation, determine if patient has adequate fluid intake, exercise, and diet. Tell him that dietary sources of bulk include bran and other cereals, fresh fruit, and vegetables.
• Saline laxative; up to 10% of sodium content may be absorbed.
• Enema form elicits response in 5 to 10 minutes.
• Used in preparation for barium enema, sigmoidoscopy, and for treatment of fecal impaction.
• Also prescribed to treat hypercalcemia or as a phosphate replacement.

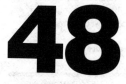

Antiemetics

benzquinamide hydrochloride
buclizine hydrochloride
chlorpromazine hydrochloride
(See Chapter 32, ANTIPSYCHOTICS.)
cyclizine hydrochloride
cyclizine lactate
dimenhydrinate
diphenidol hydrochloride
dronabinol
meclizine hydrochloride
metoclopramide hydrochloride
nabilone
prochlorperazine
prochlorperazine edisylate
prochlorperazine maleate
scopolamine
thiethylperazine maleate
trimethobenzamide
   hydrochloride

COMBINATION PRODUCTS
None.

---

benzquinamide hydrochloride
Emete-Con

Pregnancy Risk Category: C

HOW SUPPLIED
Injection: 50 mg/vial

MECHANISM OF ACTION
Acts on the chemoreceptor trigger
zone to inhibit nausea and vomiting.

INDICATIONS & DOSAGE
*Nausea and vomiting associated with
anesthesia and surgery—*
Adults: 50 mg I.M. (0.5 mg/kg to 1
mg/kg). May repeat in 1 hour, and
thereafter q 3 to 4 hours, p.r.n.; or 25
mg (0.2 mg/kg to 0.4 mg/kg) I.V. as
single dose, administered slowly.

ADVERSE REACTIONS
CNS: *drowsiness,* fatigue, insomnia,
restlessness, headache, excitation,
tremors, twitching, dizziness.
CV: sudden rise in blood pressure and
transient arrhythmias (premature
atrial and ventricular contractions,
atrial fibrillation) after I.V. administration; hypertension; hypotension.
EENT: dry mouth, salivation,
blurred vision.
GI: anorexia, nausea.
Skin: urticaria, rash.
Other: muscle weakness, flushing,
hiccups, sweating, chills, fever. May
mask symptoms of ototoxicity, brain
tumor, or intestinal obstruction.

INTERACTIONS
None significant.

NURSING CONSIDERATIONS
• I.V. use contraindicated in cardiovascular disease. Don't give I.V.
within 15 minutes of preanesthetic or
cardiovascular drugs.
• Give I.M. injections in large muscle mass. Use deltoid area only if well
developed. Be sure to aspirate syringe
for I.M. injection to avoid inadvertent
I.V. injection.
• Reconstituted solution is stable for
14 days at room temperature. Store
dry powder and reconstituted solution
in a light-resistant container.
• Precipitation occurs if reconstituted
with 0.9% sodium chloride injection.

---

†Available in Canada only.   ‡Available in Australia only.   ◊Available OTC.

- Monitor blood pressure frequently.
- Excellent alternative if prochlorperazine (Compazine) is contraindicated.

buclizine hydrochloride
Bucladin-S**

Pregnancy Risk Category: C

HOW SUPPLIED
Tablets: 50 mg

MECHANISM OF ACTION
May affect neural pathways originating in the labyrinth to inhibit nausea and vomiting, but the exact mechanism of action is unknown.

INDICATIONS & DOSAGE
Motion sickness (prevention)—
Adults: 50 mg P.O. at least one half hour before beginning travel. If needed, may repeat another 50 mg P.O. after 4 to 6 hours.
Vertigo—
Adults: 50 mg P.O., up to 150 mg P.O. daily in severe cases. Maintenance dose is 50 mg b.i.d.

ADVERSE REACTIONS
CNS: *drowsiness,* headache, dizziness, jitters.
EENT: blurred vision, dry mouth.
GU: urine retention.
Other: may mask symptoms of ototoxicity, intestinal obstruction, or brain tumor.

INTERACTIONS
None significant.

NURSING CONSIDERATIONS
- Use cautiously in patients with glaucoma, GU or GI obstruction, and in elderly males with possible prostatic hypertrophy.
- Warn patient against driving and other activities that require alertness until CNS effects of the drug are known.
- Tablets may be placed in mouth and

allowed to dissolve without water. May also be chewed or swallowed whole.
- Classified as an antihistamine.

cyclizine hydrochloride
Marezine◇

cyclizine lactate
Marezine, Marzine†

Pregnancy Risk Category: B

HOW SUPPLIED
hydrochloride
Tablets: 50 mg◇
lactate
Injection: 50 mg/ml

MECHANISM OF ACTION
May affect neural pathways originating in the labyrinth to inhibit nausea and vomiting, but the exact mechanism of action is unknown.

INDICATIONS & DOSAGE
Motion sickness (prevention and treatment)—
Adults: 50 mg P.O. (hydrochloride) one half hour before travel, then q 4 to 6 hours, p.r.n., to maximum of 200 mg daily; or 50 mg I.M. (lactate) q 4 to 6 hours, p.r.n.
Postoperative vomiting (prevention)—
Adults: 50 mg I.M. (lactate) preoperatively or 20 to 30 minutes before expected termination of surgery; then postoperatively 50 mg I.M. (lactate) q 4 to 6 hours, p.r.n.
Motion sickness and postoperative vomiting—
Children 6 to 12 years: 3 mg/kg (lactate) I.M. divided t.i.d., or 25 mg (hydrochloride) P.O. q 4 to 6 hours p.r.n. to a maximum of 75 mg daily.

ADVERSE REACTIONS
CNS: *drowsiness,* dizziness, auditory and visual hallucinations.
CV: hypotension.
EENT: blurred vision, dry mouth.

Italicized adverse reactions are common or life-threatening.
*Liquid form contains alcohol.   **May contain tartrazine.

GI: constipation.
GU: urine retention.
Other: may mask symptoms of ototoxicity, brain tumor, or intestinal obstruction.

INTERACTIONS
None significant.

NURSING CONSIDERATIONS
• Use cautiously in glaucoma, GU or GI obstruction, and in elderly males with possible prostatic hypertrophy.
• Warn patient against driving and other activities that require alertness until CNS effects of the drug are known.
• Classified as an antihistamine.
• Store in cool place. When stored at room temperature, injection may turn slightly yellow, but this color change does not indicate loss of potency.

---

dimenhydrinate
Andrumin‡, Apo-Dimenhydrinate†, Calm X◊, Dimentabs, Dinate, Dommanate, Dramamine◊*, Dramamine Chewable◊**, Dramamine Liquid◊*, Dramanate, Dramilin, Dramocen, Dramoject, Dymenate, Gravol†, Hydrate, Marmine◊, Motion-Aid, Nauseatol†, Novodimenate†, PMS-Dimenhydrinate†, Reidamine, Tega-Vert◊, Travamine†, Travs‡, Triptone Caplets◊, Wehamine
Pregnancy Risk Category: B

HOW SUPPLIED
Tablets: 50 mg◊
Tablets (chewable): 50 mg◊
Capsules: 50 mg◊
Oral liquid◊: 12.5 mg/4 ml◊, 15.62 mg/5 ml
Injection: 50 mg/ml

MECHANISM OF ACTION
May affect neural pathways originating in the labyrinth to inhibit nausea and vomiting, but the exact mechanism of action is unknown.

INDICATIONS & DOSAGE
Nausea, vomiting, dizziness of motion sickness (treatment and prevention)—
Adults: 50 mg P.O. q 4 hours, or 100 mg q 4 hours if drowsiness is not objectionable; or 50 mg I.M., p.r.n.; or 50 mg I.V. diluted in 10 ml sodium chloride solution, injected over 2 minutes.
Children: 5 mg/kg P.O. or I.M., divided q.i.d. Maximum dosage is 300 mg daily. Don't use in children under 2 years.

ADVERSE REACTIONS
CNS: *drowsiness,* headache, incoordination, dizziness.
CV: palpitations, hypotension.
EENT: blurred vision, tinnitus, dry mouth and respiratory passages.
Other: may mask symptoms of ototoxicity, brain tumor, or intestinal obstruction.

INTERACTIONS
None significant.

NURSING CONSIDERATIONS
• Use cautiously in seizures, narrow-angle glaucoma, and enlargement of prostate gland.
• Undiluted solution is irritating to veins; may cause sclerosis.
• Classified as an antihistamine.
• Warn patient against driving and other activities that require alertness until CNS effects of the drug are known.
• May mask ototoxicity of aminoglycoside antibiotics.
• Avoid mixing parenteral preparation with other drugs; incompatible with many solutions.

---

diphenidol hydrochloride
Vontrol**

Pregnancy Risk Category: C

HOW SUPPLIED
Tablets: 25 mg

MECHANISM OF ACTION
Influences the chemoreceptor trigger zone to inhibit nausea and vomiting.

INDICATIONS & DOSAGE
Peripheral (labyrinthine) dizziness—
Adults: 25 to 50 mg P.O. q 4 hours, p.r.n.
Nausea and vomiting—
Adults: 25 to 50 mg P.O. q 4 hours, p.r.n.
Children over 23 kg: 0.88 mg/kg P.O. q 4 hours, not to exceed 5.5 mg/kg/24 hours. Usual dosage is 25 mg.

ADVERSE REACTIONS
CNS: *drowsiness,* dizziness, sleep disturbances, *confusion;* auditory and visual hallucinations, disorientation occur within 3 days of starting drug; subside within 3 days after stopping drug.
CV: transient hypotension.
GI: dry mouth, nausea, indigestion, heartburn.
Skin: urticaria.
Other: antiemetic effect may mask symptoms of ototoxicity, brain tumor, intestinal obstruction, or other conditions.

INTERACTIONS
None significant.

NURSING CONSIDERATIONS
• Contraindicated in anuria. Use cautiously in glaucoma, pyloric stenosis, pylorospasm, obstructive lesions of GI or GU tract, prostatic hypertrophy, or organic cardioaspasm.
• Used in Ménière's disease, following middle and inner ear surgery, labyrinthine disturbances, and to control nausea and vomiting associated with infectious diseases, cancers, radiation sickness, general anesthetics, and antineoplastic agents.
• Drug should be stopped if auditory or visual hallucinations or disorientation or confusion occurs.
• Closely supervise patient. Patients are usually hospitalized when receiving this drug. Monitor intake/output; report any changes.
• Treatment of toxicity is symptomatic and supportive.

dronabinol (tetrahydrocannabinol)
Controlled Substance Schedule II
Marinol

Pregnancy Risk Category: B

HOW SUPPLIED
Capsules: 2.5 mg, 5 mg, 10 mg

MECHANISM OF ACTION
Unknown.

INDICATIONS & DOSAGE
Treatment of nausea and vomiting associated with cancer chemotherapy—
Adults: 5 mg/m^2 P.O. 1 to 3 hours before administration of chemotherapy. Then give same dose q 2 to 4 hours after chemotherapy is administered for a total of four to six doses per day. Dosage may be increased in increments of 2.5 mg/m^2 to a maximum of 15 mg/m^2 per dose.

ADVERSE REACTIONS
CNS: *dizziness, ataxia,* depersonalization, disorientation, hallucinations, headache, irritability, memory lapse, muddled thinking, paranoia, perceptual difficulties, weakness, paresthesias.
CV: tachycardia, orthostatic hypotension.
Other: *dry mouth,* visual distortions.

Italicized adverse reactions are common or life-threatening.
*Liquid form contains alcohol.   **May contain tartrazine.

INTERACTIONS
Alcohol, CNS depressants, sedatives, psychotomimetic substances: additive effects. Don't use together.

NURSING CONSIDERATIONS
• Contraindicated for nausea and vomiting from any cause other than cancer chemotherapy; contraindicated in patients hypersensitive to sesame oil.
• Use cautiously in elderly patients and those with hypertension, heart disease, and psychiatric illness.
• Warn patients against hazardous activities that require alertness until CNS effects of the drug are known.
• This drug is to be prescribed only for patients who have not responded satisfactorily to other antiemetics.
• Effects of this drug may persist for days after treatment ends. Duration of persistent effect varies greatly among patients. Therefore, patient should be supervised for untoward responses until it's certain that he's no longer experiencing the drug's effects.
• Dronabinol is the principal active substance present in *Cannabis sativa* (marijuana). Therefore, this can produce both physical and psychic dependence and has high potential for abuse.
• CNS effects are intensified at higher drug dosages.
• To prevent panic and anxiety, tell patients this drug may induce unusual changes in mood or other adverse behavioral effects.
• Impress upon family members that patient should be under supervision by a responsible person during and immediately after the treatment.

meclizine hydrochloride (meclozine hydrochloride)
Ancolan‡, Antivert, Antivert/25◊, Antivert/50, Bonamine†, Bonine◊, Dizmiss◊, Meni-D, Ru-Vert M
Pregnancy Risk Category: B

HOW SUPPLIED
Tablets: 12.5 mg, 25 mg◊, 50 mg
Tablets (chewable): 25 mg◊
Capsules: 15 mg, 25 mg, 30 mg

MECHANISM OF ACTION
May affect neural pathways originating in the labyrinth to inhibit nausea and vomiting, but the exact mechanism of action is unknown.

INDICATIONS & DOSAGE
Dizziness—
Adults: 25 to 100 mg P.O. daily in divided doses. Dosage varies with patient response.
Motion sickness—
Adults: 25 to 50 mg P.O. 1 hour before travel, repeated daily for duration of journey.

ADVERSE REACTIONS
CNS: *drowsiness,* fatigue.
EENT: dry mouth, blurred vision.
Other: may mask symptoms of ototoxicity, brain tumor, or intestinal obstruction.

INTERACTIONS
CNS depressants: increased drowsiness.

NURSING CONSIDERATIONS
• Use cautiously in glaucoma, GU or GI obstruction, and in elderly males with possible prostatic hypertrophy.
• Warn patient against driving and other activities that require alertness until CNS effects of the drug are known.
• This antihistamine has a slower onset and longer duration of action than other antihistamine antiemetics.

metoclopramide hydrochloride
Maxeran†, Maxolon‡, Maxolon High Dose‡, Reglan

Pregnancy Risk Category: B

HOW SUPPLIED
Tablets: 5 mg, 10 mg
Syrup: 5 mg/5 ml
Injection: 5 mg/ml

MECHANISM OF ACTION
Stimulates motility of the upper GI tract by increasing lower esophageal sphincter tone. Also blocks dopamine receptors at the chemoreceptor trigger zone.

INDICATIONS & DOSAGE
Preventing or reducing nausea and vomiting induced by cisplatin and other chemotherapy—
Adults: 2 mg/kg I.V. q 2 hours for 5 doses, beginning 30 minutes prior to cisplatin administration.
To facilitate small-bowel intubation and to aid in radiologic examinations—
Adults: 10 mg (2 ml) I.V. as a single dose over 1 to 2 minutes.
Children 6 to 14 years: 2.5 to 5 mg I.V. (0.5 to 1 ml).
Children under 6 years: 0.1 mg/kg I.V.
Delayed gastric emptying secondary to diabetic gastroparesis—
Adults: 10 mg P.O. 30 minutes before meals and h.s. for 2 to 8 weeks, depending on response.
Treatment of gastroesophageal reflux—
Adults: 10 to 15 mg P.O. q.i.d., p.r.n. Take 30 minutes before meals.

ADVERSE REACTIONS
CNS: *restlessness, anxiety, drowsiness,* fatigue, *lassitude,* insomnia, headache, dizziness, *extrapyramidal symptoms, tardive dyskinesia, dystonic reactions,* sedation.

CV: transient hypertension.
GI: nausea, bowel disturbances.
Skin: rash.
Other: fever, prolactin secretion, loss of libido.

INTERACTIONS
Anticholinergics, narcotic analgesics: antagonize effects of metoclopramide. Use together cautiously.

NURSING CONSIDERATIONS
● Contraindicated whenever stimulation of GI motility might be dangerous (hemorrhage, obstruction, or perforation), and in pheochromocytoma or epilepsy.
● Diphenhydramine 25 mg I.V. may be prescribed to counteract the extrapyramidal side effects associated with high metoclopramide doses.
● Elderly patients are more likely to experience extrapyramidal symptoms and tardive dyskinesia.
● Safety and effectiveness have not been established for therapy that continues longer than 12 weeks.
● Monitor blood pressure frequently in patients receiving I.V. dosage.
● I.V. infusions should be given slowly over at least 15 minutes. Protection from light is unnecessary if the infusion mixture is administered within 24 hours.
● Warn patient to avoid activities requiring alertness for 2 hours after taking each dose.
● Oral form is being used investigationally to treat nausea and vomiting.

nabilone
Controlled Substance Schedule II
Cesamet

Pregnancy Risk Category: B

HOW SUPPLIED
Capsules: 1 mg

MECHANISM OF ACTION
Unknown.

Italicized adverse reactions are common or life-threatening.
*Liquid form contains alcohol.　　　**May contain tartrazine.

INDICATIONS & DOSAGE

Treatment of nausea and vomiting associated with cancer chemotherapy—
Adults: 1 to 2 mg P.O. b.i.d. On the day of chemotherapy, the first dose should be given 1 to 3 hours before chemotherapy is administered. Maximum daily dosage is 6 mg divided t.i.d.

ADVERSE REACTIONS

CNS: *drowsiness, vertigo, euphoria, anxiety, decreased ability to concentrate, disorientation, depression,* ataxia, headache, visual disturbances, paresthesias, hallucinations.
CV: orthostatic hypotension, tachycardia.
GI: *dry mouth,* increased appetite.

INTERACTIONS

CNS depressants: may increase CNS adverse reactions. Avoid concomitant use.

NURSING CONSIDERATIONS

• Contraindicated for nausea and vomiting from any cause other than cancer chemotherapy.
• Use cautiously in elderly patients and those with hypertension, heart disease, or psychiatric illness.
• Warn patients to avoid driving and other hazardous activities that require mental alertness until CNS effects of the drug are known.
• This drug is to be prescribed only for patients who have not responded satisfactorily to other antiemetics.
• Effects of nabilone may persist for a variable and unpredictable period of time after its administration. Adverse psychological reactions can persist for 48 to 72 hours after treatment ends.
• Nabilone is a synthetic cannabinoid. It is chemically similar to dronabinol (tetrahydrocannabinol), the active substance in marijuana.
• CNS effects are intensified at higher dosages.
• To prevent panic and anxiety, tell

patients this drug may induce unusual changes in mood or other adverse behavioral effects.
• Impress upon family members that patient should be under supervision by a responsible person during and immediately after the treatment.

---

prochlorperazine
Compazine, Stemetil†‡

prochlorperazine edisylate
Compazine

prochlorperazine maleate
Anti-Naus‡, Chlorpazine, Compazine, Stemetil†‡

Pregnancy Risk Category: C

HOW SUPPLIED
prochlorperazine
Injection: 5 mg/ml
Suppositories: 2.5 mg, 5 mg, 25 mg
prochlorperazine edisylate
Syrup: 1 mg/ml
prochlorperazine maleate
Tablets: 5 mg, 10 mg, 25 mg
Capsules (sustained-release): 10 mg, 15 mg, 30 mg

MECHANISM OF ACTION
Acts on the chemoreceptor trigger zone to inhibit nausea and vomiting, and in larger doses, partially depresses the vomiting center as well.

INDICATIONS & DOSAGE
Preoperative nausea control—
Adults: 5 to 10 mg I.M. 1 to 2 hours before induction of anesthetic, repeat once in 30 minutes, if necessary; or 5 to 10 mg I.V. 15 to 30 minutes before induction of anesthetic (repeat once if necessary); or 20 mg/liter dextrose 5% in water and 0.9% sodium chloride solution by I.V. infusion, added to infusion 15 to 30 minutes before induction. Maximum parenteral dosage is 40 mg daily.
Severe nausea, vomiting—

Adults: 5 to 10 mg P.O. t.i.d. or q.i.d.; or 15 mg sustained-release form P.O. on arising; or 10 mg sustained-release form P.O. q 12 hours; or 25 mg rectally b.i.d.; or 5 to 10 mg I.M. injected deeply into upper outer quadrant of gluteal region. Repeat q 3 to 4 hours, p.r.n. Maximum I.M. dosage is 40 mg daily.

Children 18 to 39 kg: 2.5 mg P.O. or rectally t.i.d.; or 5 mg P.O. or rectally b.i.d. Maximum dosage is 15 mg daily; or 0.132 mg/kg deep I.M. injection. (Control usually obtained with 1 dose.)

Children 14 to 17 kg: 2.5 mg P.O. or rectally b.i.d. or t.i.d. Maximum dosage is 10 mg daily; or 0.132 mg/kg deep I.M. injection. (Control usually obtained with 1 dose.)

Children 9 to 13 kg: 2.5 mg P.O. or rectally daily or b.i.d. Maximum dosage is 7.5 mg daily; or 0.132 mg/kg deep I.M. injection. (Control usually obtained with 1 dose.)

Symptomatic management of psychotic disorders—
Adults: 5 to 10 mg, P.O. t.i.d. or q.i.d.

Children 2 to 12 years: 2.5 mg P.O. or P.R. b.i.d. or t.i.d. Do not exceed 10 mg on day 1. Increase dosage gradually to recommended maximum (if necessary).

Children 6 to 10 years: maximum 25 mg P.O. daily.

Children 2 to 5 years: maximum 20 mg P.O. daily.

Symptomatic management of severe psychoses—
Adults: 10 to 20 mg I.M. May be repeated in 1 to 4 hours. Rarely, patients may receive 10 to 20 mg q 4 to 6 hours. Oral therapy should be instituted after symptoms are controlled.

Children: 0.13 mg/kg I.M.

Management of excessive anxiety—
Adults: 5 to 10 mg by deep I.M. injection every 3 to 4 hours, not to exceed 40 mg daily; or 5 to 10 mg P.O. t.i.d. or q.i.d.; alternatively, give 15 mg (as the extended-release capsule) once daily, or 10 mg (extended-release capsule) q 12 hours.

ADVERSE REACTIONS
Blood: *transient leukopenia, agranulocytosis.*
CNS: *extrapyramidal reactions,* sedation, pseudoparkinsonism, EEG changes, dizziness.
CV: *orthostatic hypotension,* tachycardia, ECG changes.
EENT: *ocular changes, blurred vision.*
GI: *dry mouth, constipation.*
GU: *urine retention,* dark urine, menstrual irregularities, gynecomastia, inhibited ejaculation.
Hepatic: *cholestatic jaundice.*
Metabolic: hyperprolactinemia.
Skin: *mild photosensitivity,* dermal allergic reactions, *exfoliative dermatitis.*
Other: weight gain, increased appetite.

INTERACTIONS
Antacids: inhibited absorption of oral phenothiazines. Separate antacid and phenothiazine doses by at least 2 hours.
Anticholinergics, including antidepressants and antiparkinsonian agents: increased anticholinergic activity and aggravated parkinsonian symptoms. Use together cautiously.
Barbiturates: may decrease phenothiazine effect. Monitor patient for decreased antiemetic effect.

NURSING CONSIDERATIONS
• Contraindicated in phenothiazine hypersensitivity, CNS depression, bone marrow suppression, or subcortical damage; during pediatric surgery, use of spinal or epidural anesthetic or adrenergic blocking agents, alcohol usage, and those in a coma or depression. Use with caution in combination with other CNS depressants; in hepatic disease, arteriosclerosis or car-

---

Italicized adverse reactions are common or life-threatening.
*Liquid form contains alcohol.   **May contain tartrazine.

diovascular disease (may cause sudden drop in blood pressure), exposure to extreme heat or cold (including antipyretic therapy), respiratory disorders, hypocalcemia, convulsive disorders or severe reactions to insulin or electroshock therapy, suspected brain tumor or intestinal obstruction, glaucoma, or prostatic hypertrophy; in acutely ill, dehydrated, or vomiting children; and in elderly or debilitated patients.

• Elderly patients should usually receive dosages in the lower range.

• Store in light-resistant container. Slight yellowing does not affect potency; discard very discolored solutions.

• Use only when vomiting can't be controlled by other measures, or when only a few doses are required. If more than 4 doses needed in 24-hour period, notify doctor.

• Not effective in motion sickness.

• To prevent contact dermatitis, avoid getting concentrate or injection solution on hands or clothing.

• Dilute oral solution with tomato or fruit juice, milk, coffee, carbonated beverage, tea, water, soup, or pudding.

• Monitor CBC and liver function studies during prolonged therapy. Warn patients to wear protective clothing when exposed to sunlight.

• Watch for orthostatic hypotension, especially when giving I.V.

• Do not give subcutaneously or mix in syringe with another drug. Give deep I.M.

---

scopolamine (hyoscine)
Transderm-Scōp, Transderm-V†

Pregnancy Risk Category: C

HOW SUPPLIED
Transdermal patch: 1.5 mg

MECHANISM OF ACTION
May affect neural pathways originating in the labyrinth to inhibit nausea and vomiting, but the exact mechanism of action is unknown.

INDICATIONS & DOSAGE
Prevention of nausea and vomiting associated with motion sickness—
Adults: One Transderm-Scōp system (a circular flat unit) programmed to deliver 0.5 mg scopolamine over 3 days (72 hours), applied to the skin behind the ear several hours before the antiemetic is required.

Not recommended for children.

ADVERSE REACTIONS
CNS: *drowsiness,* restlessness, disorientation, confusion.
EENT: *dry mouth,* transient impairment of eye accommodation.

INTERACTIONS
None significant.

NURSING CONSIDERATIONS
• Use cautiously in patients with glaucoma, pyloric obstruction, or urinary bladder-neck obstruction.

• Wash and dry hands thoroughly before applying the system on dry skin behind the ear. After removing the system, discard it, then wash both the hands and application site thoroughly.

• If the system becomes displaced, remove and replace it with another system on a fresh skin site in the postauricular area.

• Caution patient to wash hands after applying transdermal patch, particularly before touching eye. May cause pupil to dilate.

• A patient brochure is available with this product; tell patient to request it from the pharmacist.

• Warn patient against driving and other activities that require alertness until CNS effects of the drug are known.

• Sugarless hard candy may be helpful in minimizing dry mouth.

• Transderm-Scōp is effective if ap-

plied 2 to 3 hours before experiencing motion, but more effective if used 12 hours before. Therefore, advise patient to apply system the night before a planned trip.
• Transdermal method of administration releases a controlled therapeutic amount of scopolamine.

---

thiethylperazine maleate
Norzine, Torecan**

Pregnancy Risk Category: C

HOW SUPPLIED
Tablets: 10 mg
Injection: 5 mg/ml
Suppositories: 10 mg

MECHANISM OF ACTION
Acts on the chemoreceptor trigger zone to inhibit nausea and vomiting.

INDICATIONS & DOSAGE
Nausea and vomiting—
Adults: 10 mg P.O., I.M., or rectally daily, b.i.d., or t.i.d.

ADVERSE REACTIONS
Blood: *transient leukopenia, agranulocytosis.*
CNS: *extrapyramidal reactions (high incidence),* sedation (low incidence), pseudoparkinsonism, EEG changes, dizziness.
CV: *orthostatic hypotension,* tachycardia, EKG changes.
EENT: *ocular changes, blurred vision.*
GI: *dry mouth, constipation.*
GU: *urinary retention,* dark urine, menstrual irregularities, gyneocmastia, inhibited ejaculation.
Hepatic: *cholestatic jaundice.*
Metabolic: hyperprolactinemia.
Skin: *mild photosensitivity,* dermal allergic reactions.
Other: weight gain, increased appetite.

INTERACTIONS
Antacids: inhibited absorption of oral phenothiazines. Separate antacid and phenothiazine dosage by at least 2 hours.
Anticholinergics, including antidepressants and antiparkinsonian agents: increased anticholinergic activity, aggravated parkinson-like symptoms. Use together cautiously.
Barbiturates: may decrease phenothiazine effect. Monitor for decreased antiemetic effect.

NURSING CONSIDERATIONS
• Contraindicated in severe CNS depression, hepatic disease, coma, phenothiazine hypersensitivity.
• Don't give I.V. May cause severe hypotension.
• For nausea and vomiting associated with anesthesia and surgery, give deep I.M. injection on or shortly before terminating anesthesia.
• Possibly effective in dizziness; not effective in motion sickness.
• Use only when vomiting can't be controlled by other measures, or when only a few doses are required.
• Warn patient about hypotension. Advise him to stay in bed for 1 hour after receiving the drug.
• Store suppositories tightly covered and at temperatures below 77° F (25° C).
• If drug gets on skin, wash off at once to prevent contact dermatitis.

---

trimethobenzamide hydrochloride
Tebamide, Tegamide, Ticon, Tigan, Tiject-20

Pregnancy Risk Category: C

HOW SUPPLIED
Capsules: 100 mg, 250 mg
Injection: 100 mg/ml
Suppositories: 100 mg, 200 mg

MECHANISM OF ACTION
Acts on the chemoreceptor trigger zone to inhibit nausea and vomiting.

INDICATIONS & DOSAGE
Nausea and vomiting (treatment)—
Adults: 250 mg P.O. t.i.d. or q.i.d.; or 200 mg I.M. or rectally t.i.d. or q.i.d.
Postoperative nausea and vomiting (prevention)—
Adults: 200 mg I.M. or rectally (single dose) before or during surgery; may repeat 3 hours after termination of anesthesia, p.r.n.
Children 13 to 40 kg: 100 to 200 mg P.O. or rectally t.i.d. or q.i.d.
Children under 13 kg: 100 mg rectally t.i.d. or q.i.d. Limited to prolonged vomiting of known etiology.

ADVERSE REACTIONS
CNS: *drowsiness,* dizziness (in large doses).
CV: hypotension.
GI: diarrhea, exaggeration of preexisting nausea (in large doses).
Hepatic: *liver toxicity.*
Skin: skin hypersensitivity reactions.
Local: pain, stinging, burning, redness, swelling at I.M. injection site.
Other: antiemetic effect may mask signs of overdosage of toxic agents, or intestinal obstruction, brain tumor, or other conditions.

INTERACTIONS
None significant.

NURSING CONSIDERATIONS
• Contraindicated in children with viral illness (a possible cause of vomiting in children); may contribute to the development of Reye's syndrome, a potentially fatal acute childhood encephalopathy, characterized by fatty degeneration of the liver.
• Suppositories contraindicated in hypersensitivity to benzocaine hydrochloride or similar local anesthetic.
• Stop drug if allergic skin reaction occurs.
• Give I.M. dose by deep injection into upper outer quadrant of gluteal region to reduce pain and local irritation.
• Warn patient of the possibility of drowsiness and dizziness, and caution him against driving or other activities requiring alertness until CNS effects of the drug are known.
• Store suppositories in refrigerator.
• Has little or no value in preventing motion sickness; limited value as antiemetic.

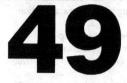

Gastrointestinal anticholinergics

Belladonna alkaloids
atropine sulfate
(See Chapter 20, ANTIARRHYTHMICS.)
belladonna leaf
hyoscyamine
hyoscyamine sulfate
leverotatory alkaloids of
   belladonna

Quaternary anticholinergics
anisotropine methylbromide
clidinium bromide
glycopyrrolate
(See Chapter 36, CHOLINERGIC BLOCKERS [PARASYMPATHOLYTICS].)
hexocyclium methylsulfate
isopropamide iodide
mepenzolate bromide
methantheline bromide
methscopolamine bromide
oxyphenonium bromide
propantheline bromide

Tertiary synthetics
   (antispasmodics)
dicyclomine hydrochloride
oxyphencyclimine hydrochloride

COMBINATION PRODUCTS

BARBIDONNA ELIXIR*: atropine sulfate 0.034 mg/5 ml, phenobarbital 21.6 mg/5 ml, hyoscyamine hydrobromide or sulfate 0.174 mg/5 ml, scopolamine hydrobromide 0.01 mg/5 ml, and alcohol 15%.

BARBIDONNA TABLETS: atropine sulfate 0.025 mg, scopolamine hydrobromide 0.0074 mg, hyoscyamine hydrobromide or sulfate 0.1286 mg, and phenobarbital 16 mg.

BARBIDONNA NO. 2 TABLETS: atropine sulfate 0.025 mg, scopolamine hydrobromide 0.0074 mg, hyoscyamine hydrobromide or sulfate 0.1286 mg, and phenobarbital 32 mg.

BELLADENAL TABLETS: L-alkaloids of belladonna 0.25 mg and phenobarbital 50 mg.

CHARDONNA-2: belladonna extract 15 mg and phenobarbital 15 mg.

DONNATAL ELIXIR*: atropine sulfate 0.0194 mg/5 ml, scopolamine hydrobromide 0.0065 mg/5 ml, alcohol 23%, hyoscyamine hydrobromide or sulfate 0.1037 mg/5 ml, and phenobarbital 16 mg/5 ml.

DONNATAL EXTENTABS: atropine sulfate 0.0582 mg, scopolamine hydrobromide 0.0195 mg, hyoscyamine sulfate 0.3111 mg, and phenobarbital 48.6 mg.

DONNATAL TABLETS AND CAPSULES: atropine sulfate 0.0194 mg, scopolamine hydrobromide 0.0065 mg, hyoscyamine hydrobromide or sulfate 0.1037 mg, and phenobarbital 16 mg.

DONNATAL NO. 2 TABLETS: atropine sulfate 0.0194 mg, scopolamine hydrobromide 0.0065 mg, hyoscyamine hydrobromide or sulfate 0.1037 mg, and phenobarbital 32.4 mg.

KINESED TABLETS: atropine sulfate 0.02 mg, scopolamine hydrobromide 0.007 mg, hyoscyamine hydrobromide or sulfate 0.1 mg, and phenobarbital 16 mg.

LIBRAX CAPSULES: clidinium bromide 2.5 mg and chlordiazepoxide hydrochloride 5 mg.

ROBINUL FORTE TABLETS: glycopyrrolate 2 mg and phenobarbital 16.2 mg.

Italicized adverse reactions are common or life-threatening.
*Liquid form contains alcohol.   **May contain tartrazine.

ROBINUL TABLETS: glycopyrrolate 1 mg and phenobarbital 16.2 mg.
VISTRAX 10 TABLETS: oxyphencyclimine hydrochloride 10 mg and hydroxyzine hydrochloride 25 mg.

---

anisotropine methylbromide
Valpin 50

Pregnancy Risk Category: C

HOW SUPPLIED
Tablets: 50 mg

MECHANISM OF ACTION
Competitively blocks acetylcholine, which decreases GI motility and inhibits gastric acid secretion.

INDICATIONS & DOSAGE
Adjunctive treatment of peptic ulcer—
Adults: 50 mg P.O. t.i.d. To be effective, should be titrated to individual patient's needs.

ADVERSE REACTIONS
CNS: headache, insomnia, drowsiness, dizziness, *confusion or excitement in elderly patients,* nervousness, weakness.
CV: *palpitations,* tachycardia.
EENT: *blurred vision,* mydriasis, increased ocular tension, cycloplegia, photophobia.
GI: *dry mouth,* dysphagia, heartburn, loss of taste, nausea, vomiting, *paralytic ileus, constipation.*
GU: *urinary hesitancy, urine retention,* impotence.
Skin: urticaria, decreased sweating and possible anhidrosis, other dermal manifestations.
Other: fever, allergic reactions.
Overdosage may cause curare-like symptoms.

INTERACTIONS
None significant.

NURSING CONSIDERATIONS
• Contraindicated in narrow-angle glaucoma, obstructive uropathy, obstructive disease of the GI tract, severe ulcerative colitis, myasthenia gravis, hypersensitivity to anticholinergics, paralytic ileus, intestinal atony, unstable cardiovascular status in acute hemorrhage, or toxic megacolon. Use cautiously in autonomic neuropathy, hyperthyroidism, coronary artery disease, cardiac arrhythmias, CHF, hypertension, hiatal hernia associated with reflux esophagitis, hepatic or renal disease, and ulcerative colitis, or in patients over 40 years because of increased incidence of glaucoma.
• Use with caution in hot or humid environments. Drug-induced heatstroke can develop.
• Give 30 minutes to 1 hour before meals.
• Administer smaller doses to elderly patients.
• Monitor patient's vital signs and urine output carefully.
• Instruct patient to avoid driving and other hazardous activities if he is drowsy, dizzy, or has blurred vision; to drink plenty of fluids to help prevent constipation; to report any skin rash or local eruption.
• Gum or sugarless hard candy may relieve dry mouth.

---

belladonna leaf
(used to prepare extract and tincture)
Belladonna Tincture USP*

Pregnancy Risk Category: C

HOW SUPPLIED
Tablets: 15 mg
Oral solution: 27 to 33 mg belladonna alkaloids/100 ml

MECHANISM OF ACTION
Competitively blocks acetylcholine,

---

which decreases GI motility and inhibits gastric acid secretion.

INDICATIONS & DOSAGE
Adjunctive therapy for peptic ulcer, irritable bowel syndrome, functional gastrointestinal disorders, and neurogenic bowel disturbances—
Adults: 15 mg P.O. t.i.d. or q.i.d. of the extract; 0.3 to 1 ml t.i.d. or q.i.d. of tincture.

ADVERSE REACTIONS
CNS: headache, insomnia, drowsiness, dizziness, *confusion or excitement in elderly patients,* nervousness, weakness.
CV: *palpitations,* tachycardia.
EENT: *blurred vision,* mydriasis, increased ocular tension, cycloplegia, photophobia.
GI: *dry mouth,* dysphagia, heartburn, loss of taste, *constipation,* nausea, vomiting.
GU: *urinary hesitancy, urine retention,* impotence.
Skin: urticaria, decreased sweating or possible anhidrosis, other dermal manifestations.
Other: fever, allergic reactions.
Overdosage may cause curare-like symptoms.

INTERACTIONS
None significant.

NURSING CONSIDERATIONS
• Contraindicated in narrow-angle glaucoma, obstructive uropathy, obstructive disease of GI tract, severe ulcerative colitis, myasthenia gravis, hypersensitivity to anticholinergics, paralytic ileus, intestinal atony, unstable cardiovascular status in acute hemorrhage, or toxic megacolon. Use cautiously in autonomic neuropathy, hyperthyroidism, coronary artery disease, cardiac arrhythmias, CHF, hypertension, hiatal hernia associated with reflux esophagitis, hepatic or renal disease, and ulcerative colitis,

or in patients over 40 years because of increased incidence of glaucoma.
• Give 30 minutes to 1 hour before meals and at bedtime. Bedtime dose can be larger and should be given at least 2 hours after last meal of day.
• Administer smaller doses to elderly patients.
• Use with caution in hot or humid environments. Drug-induced heatstroke can develop.
• Monitor patient's vital signs and urine output carefully.
• Instruct patient to avoid driving and other hazardous activities if he is drowsy, dizzy, or has blurred vision; to drink plenty of fluids to help prevent constipation; to report any skin rash or local eruption.
• Gum or sugarless hard candy may relieve dry mouth.

---

clidinium bromide
Quarzan

Pregnancy Risk Category: C

HOW SUPPLIED
Capsules: 2.5 mg, 5 mg

MECHANISM OF ACTION
Competitively blocks acetylcholine, which decreases GI motility and inhibits gastric acid secretion.

INDICATIONS & DOSAGE
Adjunctive therapy for peptic ulcers—
Dosage should be individualized according to severity of symptoms and occurrence of adverse reactions.
Elderly or debilitated patients: 2.5 to 5 mg P.O. t.i.d. or q.i.d. before meals and h.s.

ADVERSE REACTIONS
CNS: headache, insomnia, drowsiness, dizziness, *confusion or excitement in elderly patients,* nervousness, weakness.
CV: *palpitations,* tachycardia.
EENT: *blurred vision,* mydriasis, in-

Italicized adverse reactions are common or life-threatening.
*Liquid form contains alcohol.   **May contain tartrazine.

creased ocular tension, cycloplegia, photophobia.

GI: *dry mouth,* dysphagia, heartburn, loss of taste, nausea, vomiting, *paralytic ileus, constipation.*

GU: *urinary hesitancy, urine retention,* impotence.

Skin: urticaria, decreased sweating or possible anhidrosis, other dermal manifestations.

Other: fever, allergic reactions.

Overdosage may cause curare-like symptoms.

INTERACTIONS
None significant.

NURSING CONSIDERATIONS
• Contraindicated in narrow-angle glaucoma, obstructive uropathy, obstructive disease of GI tract, severe ulcerative colitis, myasthenia gravis, hypersensitivity to anticholinergics, paralytic ileus, intestinal atony, unstable cardiovascular status in acute hemorrhage, or toxic megacolon. Use cautiously in autonomic neuropathy, hyperthyroidism, coronary artery disease, cardiac arrhythmias, CHF, hypertension, hiatal hernia associated with reflux esophagitis, hepatic or renal disease, and ulcerative colitis, or in patients over 40 years, because of increased incidence of glaucoma.

• Give 30 minutes to 1 hour before meals and at bedtime. Bedtime dose can be larger and should be given at least 2 hours after last meal of day.

• Use with caution in hot or humid environments. Drug-induced heatstroke may develop.

• Monitor patient's vital signs and urine output carefully.

• Instruct patient to avoid driving and other hazardous activities if he is drowsy, dizzy, or has blurred vision; to drink plenty of fluids to help prevent constipation; and to report any rash or skin eruption.

• Gum or sugarless hard candy may relieve dry mouth.

• Dysphagia may cause aspiration.

• There is no conclusive evidence that clidinium aids in healing, decreases recurrence of, or prevents complications of peptic ulcers.

---

dicyclomine hydrochloride
Antispas, Bemote, Bentyl, Bentylol†, Byclomine, Dibent, Di-Cyclonex, Dilomine, Di-Spaz, Formulex†, Lomine†, Merbentyl‡, Neoquess Injection, Or-Tyl, Spasmoban†, Spasmoject, Viscerol†

Pregnancy Risk Category: B

HOW SUPPLIED
Tablets: 10 mg‡, 20 mg
Capsules: 10 mg, 20 mg
Syrup: 5 mg/5 ml‡, 10 mg/5 ml
Injection: 10 mg/ml

MECHANISM OF ACTION
Exerts a nonspecific, direct spasmolytic action on smooth muscle. Also possesses local anesthetic properties that may be partly responsible for spasmolysis.

INDICATIONS & DOSAGE
Adjunctive therapy for peptic ulcers and other functional GI disorders—
Adults: 10 to 20 mg P.O. t.i.d. or q.i.d.; 20 mg I.M. q 4 to 6 hours.

Always adjust dosage according to patient's needs and response.

ADVERSE REACTIONS
CNS: *headache,* insomnia, drowsiness, *dizziness.*
CV: *palpitations,* tachycardia.
GI: nausea, *constipation,* vomiting, *paralytic ileus.*
GU: *urinary hesitancy, urine retention, impotence.*
Skin: urticaria, decreased sweating or possible anhidrosis, other dermal manifestations.
Other: fever, allergic reactions.

Overdosage may cause curare-like symptoms.

INTERACTIONS
None significant.

NURSING CONSIDERATIONS
• Contraindicated in obstructive uropathy, obstructive disease of GI tract, severe ulcerative colitis, myasthenia gravis, hypersensitivity to anticholinergics, paralytic ileus, intestinal atony, unstable cardiovascular status in acute hemorrhage, or toxic megacolon. Use cautiously in autonomic neuropathy, narrow-angle glaucoma, hyperthyroidism, coronary artery disease, cardiac arrhythmias, CHF, hypertension, hiatal hernia associated with reflux esophagitis, hepatic or renal disease, and ulcerative colitis.
• Use with caution in hot or humid environments. Drug-induced heatstroke can develop.
• Give 30 minutes to 1 hour before meals and at bedtime. Bedtime dose can be larger and should be given at least 2 hours after last meal of day.
• Monitor patient's vital signs and urine output carefully.
• Instruct patient to avoid driving and other hazardous activities if he is drowsy, dizzy, or has blurred vision; to drink plenty of fluids to help prevent constipation; and to report any rash or skin eruption.
• Gum or sugarless hard candy may relieve dry mouth.
• A synthetic tertiary derivative that may have fewer atropine-like adverse reactions.
• Not for I.V. use.

---

hexocyclium methylsulfate
Tral Filmtabs**

Pregnancy Risk Category: C

HOW SUPPLIED
Tablets: 25 mg

MECHANISM OF ACTION
Competitively blocks acetylcholine, which decreases GI motility and inhibits gastric acid secretion.

INDICATIONS & DOSAGE
Adjunctive therapy in peptic ulcer and other GI disorders—
Adults: 25 mg P.O. q.i.d. before meals and h.s.

ADVERSE REACTIONS
CNS: headache, insomnia, drowsiness, dizziness, *confusion or excitement in elderly patients,* nervousness, weakness.
CV: *palpitations,* tachycardia.
EENT: *blurred vision,* mydriasis, increased ocular tension, cycloplegia, photophobia.
GI: *dry mouth,* dysphagia, heartburn, loss of taste, nausea, *constipation,* vomiting, *paralytic ileus.*
GU: *urinary hesitancy, urine retention,* impotence.
Skin: urticaria, decreased sweating or possible anhidrosis, other dermal manifestations.
Other: fever, allergic reactions.
   Overdosage may cause curare-like symptoms.

INTERACTIONS
None significant.

NURSING CONSIDERATIONS
• Contraindicated in narrow-angle glaucoma, obstructive uropathy, obstructive disease of GI tract, severe ulcerative colitis, myasthenia gravis, hypersensitivity to anticholinergics, paralytic ileus, intestinal atony, unstable cardiovascular status in acute hemorrhage, or toxic megacolon. Use cautiously in autonomic neuropathy, hyperthyroidism, coronary artery disease, cardiac arrhythmias, CHF, hypertension, hiatal hernia associated with reflux esophagitis, hepatic or renal disease, and ulcerative colitis,

---

or in patients over 40 years because of increased incidence of glaucoma.

• Use with caution in hot or humid environments. Drug-induced heat-stroke can develop.

• Give 30 minutes to 1 hour before meals and at bedtime. Bedtime dose can be larger and should be given at least 2 hours after last meal of day.

• Monitor patient's vital signs and urine output carefully.

• Instruct patient to avoid driving and other hazardous activities if he is drowsy, dizzy, or has blurred vision; to drink plenty of fluids to help prevent constipation; and to report any rash or skin eruption.

• Gum or sugarless hard candy may relieve dry mouth.

hyoscyamine
Cystospaz

hyoscyamine sulfate
Anaspaz, Cystospaz, Cystospaz-M, Levsin*, Levsinex Timecaps, Neoquess

Pregnancy Risk Category: C

HOW SUPPLIED
hyoscyamine
Tablets: 150 mcg
hyoscyamine sulfate
Tablets: 125 mcg, 130 mcg, 150 mcg
Capsules (timed-release): 375 mcg
Elixir: 125 mcg/5 ml
Injection: 500 mcg/ml

MECHANISM OF ACTION
Competitively blocks acetylcholine, which decreases GI motility and inhibits gastric acid secretion.

INDICATIONS & DOSAGE
Treatment of GI tract disorders caused by spasm; adjunctive therapy for peptic ulcers—
Adults: 0.125 to 0.25 mg P.O. or sublingually t.i.d. or q.i.d. before meals and h.s.; sustained-release form

0.375 mg P.O. q 12 hours; or 0.25 to 0.5 mg (1 or 2 ml) I.M., I.V., or S.C. q 6 hours. (Substitute oral medication when symptoms are controlled.)
Children 2 to 10 years: half of adult dose P.O.

ADVERSE REACTIONS
CNS: headache, insomnia, drowsiness, dizziness, *confusion or excitement in elderly patients,* nervousness, weakness.
CV: *palpitations,* tachycardia.
EENT: *blurred vision,* mydriasis, increased ocular tension, cycloplegia, photophobia.
GI: *dry mouth,* dysphagia, *constipation,* heartburn, loss of taste, nausea, vomiting, *paralytic ileus.*
GU: *urinary hesitancy, urine retention,* impotence.
Skin: urticaria, decreased sweating or possible anhidrosis, other dermal manifestations.
Other: fever, allergic reactions.
Overdosage may cause curare-like symptoms.

INTERACTIONS
None significant.

NURSING CONSIDERATIONS
• Contraindicated in narrow-angle glaucoma, obstructive uropathy, obstructive disease of GI tract, severe ulcerative colitis, myasthenia gravis, hypersensitivity to anticholinergics, paralytic ileus, intestinal atony, unstable cardiovascular status in acute hemorrhage, or toxic megacolon. Use cautiously in autonomic neuropathy, hyperthyroidism, coronary artery disease, cardiac arrhythmias, CHF, hypertension, hiatal hernia associated with reflux esophagitis, hepatic or renal disease, and ulcerative colitis, or in patients over 40 years, because of the increased incidence of glaucoma.

• Use with caution in hot or humid

environments. Drug-induced heat-stroke can develop.
- Give 30 minutes to 1 hour before meals and at bedtime. Bedtime dose can be larger and should be given at least 2 hours after the last meal of the day.
- Monitor patient's vital signs and urine output carefully.
- Instruct patient to avoid driving and other hazardous activities if he is drowsy, dizzy, or has blurred vision; to drink plenty of fluids to help prevent constipation; and to report any rash or skin eruption.
- Gum or sugarless hard candy may relieve dry mouth.

---

isopropamide iodide
Darbid, Tyrimide‡

Pregnancy Risk Category: C

HOW SUPPLIED
Tablets: 5 mg

MECHANISM OF ACTION
Competitively blocks acetylcholine, which decreases GI motility and inhibits gastric acid secretion.

INDICATIONS & DOSAGE
Adjunctive therapy for peptic ulcer, irritable bowel syndrome—
Adults and children over 12 years: 5 mg P.O. q 12 hours. Some patients may require 10 mg or more b.i.d.

   Dosage should be individualized to patient's need.

ADVERSE REACTIONS
CNS: headache, insomnia, drowsiness, dizziness, *confusion or excitement in elderly patients,* nervousness, weakness.
CV: *palpitations,* tachycardia.
EENT: *blurred vision,* mydriasis, increased ocular tension, cycloplegia, photophobia.
GI: *dry mouth,* dysphagia, heartburn,

loss of taste, nausea, vomiting, *constipation, paralytic ileus.*
GU: *urinary hesitancy, urine retention,* impotence.
Skin: urticaria, decreased sweating or possible anhidrosis, other dermal manifestations, iodine skin rash.
Other: fever, allergic reactions.

   Overdosage may cause curare-like symptoms.

INTERACTIONS
None significant.

NURSING CONSIDERATIONS
- Contraindicated in hypersensitivity to iodine, narrow-angle glaucoma, obstructive uropathy, obstructive disease of GI tract, severe ulcerative colitis, myasthenia gravis, hypersensitivity to anticholinergics, paralytic ileus, intestinal atony, unstable cardiovascular status in acute hemorrhage, or toxic megacolon. Use cautiously in autonomic neuropathy, hyperthyroidism, coronary artery disease, cardiac arrhythmias, CHF, hypertension, hiatal hernia associated with reflux esophagitis, hepatic or renal disease, and ulcerative colitis, or in patients over 40 years because of increased incidence of glaucoma.
- Use with caution in hot or humid environments. Drug-induced heat-stroke can develop.
- Give 30 minutes to 1 hour before meals and at bedtime. Bedtime dose can be larger and should be given at least 2 hours after the last meal of the day.
- Monitor patient's vital signs and urine output carefully.
- Instruct patient to avoid driving and other hazardous activities if he is drowsy, dizzy, or has blurred vision; to drink plenty of fluids to help prevent constipation; and to report any rash or skin eruption.
- Gum or sugarless hard candy may relieve dry mouth.
- Single dose produces 10- to 12-hour

Italicized adverse reactions are common or life-threatening.
*Liquid form contains alcohol.   **May contain tartrazine.

antisecretory effect and GI antispasmodic effect.
• Discontinue 1 week before thyroid function tests.

levorotatory alkaloids of belladonna
Bellafoline

Pregnancy Risk Category: C

HOW SUPPLIED
Tablets: 0.25 mg

MECHANISM OF ACTION
Competitively blocks acetylcholine, which decreases GI motility and inhibits gastric acid secretion.

INDICATIONS & DOSAGE
Adjunctive therapy for peptic ulcer, irritable bowel syndrome, and functional GI disorders—
Adults: 0.25 to 0.5 mg P.O. t.i.d.
Children over 6 years: 0.125 to 0.25 mg P.O. t.i.d.

ADVERSE REACTIONS
CNS: headache, insomnia, drowsiness, dizziness, *confusion or excitement in elderly patients,* nervousness, weakness.
CV: *palpitations,* tachycardia.
EENT: *blurred vision,* mydriasis, increased ocular tension, cycloplegia, photophobia.
GI: *dry mouth,* dysphagia, heartburn, loss of taste, *constipation, paralytic ileus.*
GU: *urinary hesitancy, urine retention,* impotence.
Skin: urticaria, decreased sweating or possible anhidrosis, other dermal manifestations.
Other: fever, allergic reactions.
Overdosage may cause curare-like symptoms.

INTERACTIONS
None significant.

NURSING CONSIDERATIONS
• Contraindicated in narrow-angle glaucoma, obstructive uropathy, obstructive disease of GI tract, severe ulcerative colitis, myasthenia gravis, hypersensitivity to anticholinergics, paralytic ileus, intestinal atony, unstable cardiovascular status in acute hemorrhage, or toxic megacolon. Use cautiously in autonomic neuropathy, hyperthyroidism, coronary artery disease, cardiac arrhythmias, CHF, hypertension, hiatal hernia associated with reflux esophagitis, hepatic or renal disease, and ulcerative colitis, or in patients over 40 years because of increased incidence of glaucoma.
• Use with caution in hot or humid environments. Drug-induced heatstroke can develop.
• Administer 30 minutes to 1 hour before meals.
• Monitor patient's vital signs and urine output carefully.
• Instruct patient to avoid driving and other hazardous activities if he is drowsy, dizzy, or has blurred vision; to drink plenty of fluids to help prevent constipation; to report any rash or skin eruption.
• Gum or sugarless hard candy may relieve dry mouth.

mepenzolate bromide
Cantil**

Pregnancy Risk Category: C

HOW SUPPLIED
Tablets: 25 mg

MECHANISM OF ACTION
Competitively blocks acetylcholine, which decreases GI motility and inhibits gastric acid secretion.

INDICATIONS & DOSAGE
Adjunctive therapy in treating peptic ulcer, irritable bowel syndrome, and neurologic bowel disturbances—
Adults: 25 to 50 mg P.O. q.i.d. with

meals and at bedtime. Adjust dosage to individual patient's needs.

ADVERSE REACTIONS
CNS: headache, insomnia, drowsiness, dizziness, *confusion or excitement in elderly patients,* nervousness, weakness.
CV: *palpitations,* tachycardia.
EENT: *blurred vision,* mydriasis, increased ocular tension, cycloplegia, photophobia.
GI: *dry mouth,* dysphagia, heartburn, loss of taste, nausea, *constipation,* vomiting, *paralytic ileus.*
GU: *urinary hesitancy, urine retention,* impotence.
Skin: urticaria, decreased sweating or possible anhidrosis, other dermal manifestations.
Other: fever, allergic reactions.
   Overdosage may cause curare-like symptoms.

INTERACTIONS
None significant.

NURSING CONSIDERATIONS
• Contraindicated in narrow-angle glaucoma, obstructive uropathy, obstructive disease of GI tract, severe ulcerative colitis, myasthenia gravis, hypersensitivity to anticholinergics, paralytic ileus, intestinal atony, unstable cardiovascular status in acute hemorrhage, or toxic megacolon. Use cautiously in autonomic neuropathy, hyperthyroidism, coronary artery disease, cardiac arrhythmias, CHF, hypertension, hiatal hernia associated with reflux esophagitis, hepatic or renal disease, and ulcerative colitis, or in patients over 40 years, because of increased incidence of glaucoma.
• Use with caution in hot or humid environments. Drug-induced heatstroke can develop.
• Give with meals and at bedtime.
• Monitor patient's vital signs and urine output carefully.
• Instruct patient to avoid driving and

other hazardous activities if he is drowsy, dizzy, or has blurred vision; to drink plenty of fluids to help prevent constipation; and to report any rash or skin eruption.
• Gum or sugarless hard candy may relieve dry mouth.

methantheline bromide
Banthine

Pregnancy Risk Category: C

HOW SUPPLIED
Tablets: 50 mg

MECHANISM OF ACTION
Competitively blocks acetylcholine, which decreases GI motility and inhibits gastric acid secretion.

INDICATIONS & DOSAGE
Adjunctive therapy in peptic ulcer, pylorospasm, spastic colon, biliary dyskinesia, pancreatitis, and certain forms of gastritis—
Adults: 50 to 100 mg P.O. q 6 hours.
Children over 1 year: 12.5 to 50 mg P.O. q.i.d.
Children under 1 year: 12.5 to 25 mg P.O. q.i.d.
Neonates: 12.5 mg P.O. b.i.d.

ADVERSE REACTIONS
CNS: headache, insomnia, drowsiness, dizziness, *confusion or excitement in elderly patients,* nervousness, weakness.
CV: *palpitations,* tachycardia.
EENT: *blurred vision,* mydriasis, increased ocular tension, cycloplegia, photophobia.
GI: *dry mouth,* dysphagia, *constipation,* heartburn, loss of taste, nausea, vomiting, *paralytic ileus.*
GU: *urinary hesitancy, urine retention,* impotence.
Skin: urticaria, decreased sweating or possible anhidrosis, other dermal manifestations.
Other: fever, allergic reactions.

Italicized adverse reactions are common or life-threatening.
*Liquid form contains alcohol.   **May contain tartrazine.

Overdosage may cause curare-like symptoms.

INTERACTIONS
None significant.

NURSING CONSIDERATIONS
• Contraindicated in narrow-angle glaucoma, obstructive uropathy, obstructive disease of GI tract, severe ulcerative colitis, myasthenia gravis, hypersensitivity to anticholinergics, paralytic ileus, intestinal atony, unstable cardiovascular status in acute hemorrhage, or toxic megacolon. Use cautiously in autonomic neuropathy, hyperthyroidism, coronary artery disease, cardiac arrhythmias, CHF, hypertension, hiatal hernia associated with reflux esophagitis, hepatic or renal disease, and ulcerative colitis, or in patients over 40 years because of the increased incidence of glaucoma.
• Use with caution in hot or humid environments. Drug-induced heatstroke can develop.
• Give 30 minutes to 1 hour before meals and at bedtime. Bedtime dose can be larger and should be given at least 2 hours after the last meal of the day.
• If patient is also taking antihistamines, he may experience increased dryness of mouth.
• Monitor patient's vital signs and urine output carefully.
• Instruct patient to avoid driving and other hazardous activities if he is drowsy, dizzy, or has blurred vision; to drink plenty of fluids to help prevent constipation; and to report any rash or skin eruption.
• Gum or sugarless hard candy may relieve dry mouth.
• Therapeutic effects appear in 30 to 45 minutes; persist for 4 to 6 hours after oral administration.

methscopolamine bromide
Pamine

Pregnancy Risk Category: C

HOW SUPPLIED
Tablets: 2.5 mg

MECHANISM OF ACTION
Competitively blocks acetylcholine, which decreases GI motility and inhibits gastric acid secretion.

INDICATIONS & DOSAGE
Adjunctive therapy in peptic ulcer—
Adults: 2.5 to 5 mg P.O. half hour before meals and h.s.

ADVERSE REACTIONS
CNS: headache, insomnia, dizziness, *confusion or excitement in elderly patients,* nervousness, weakness.
CV: *palpitations,* tachycardia.
EENT: *blurred vision,* mydriasis, increased ocular tension, cycloplegia, photophobia.
GI: *dry mouth,* dysphagia, *constipation,* heartburn, loss of taste, nausea, vomiting, *paralytic ileus.*
GU: *urinary hesitancy, urine retention,* impotence.
Skin: urticaria, decreased sweating or possible anhidrosis, other dermal manifestations.
Other: fever, allergic reactions.
    Overdosage may cause curare-like symptoms.

INTERACTIONS
None significant.

NURSING CONSIDERATIONS
• Contraindicated in narrow-angle glaucoma, obstructive uropathy, obstructive disease of GI tract, severe ulcerative colitis, myasthenia gravis, hypersensitivity to anticholinergics, paralytic ileus, intestinal atony, unstable cardiovascular status in acute hemorrhage, or toxic megacolon. Use cautiously in autonomic neuropathy,

hyperthyroidism, coronary artery disease, cardiac arrhythmias, CHF, hypertension, hiatal hernia associated with reflux esophagitis, hepatic or renal disease, and ulcerative colitis, or in patients over 40 years because of increased incidence of glaucoma.

• Use with caution in hot or humid environments. Drug-induced heatstroke can develop.

• Give 30 minutes to 1 hour before meals and at bedtime. Bedtime dose can be larger and should be given at least 2 hours after the last meal of the day.

• Monitor patient's vital signs and urine output carefully.

• Instruct patient to avoid driving and other hazardous activities if he is drowsy, dizzy, or has blurred vision; to drink plenty of fluids to help prevent constipation; and to report any rash or skin eruption.

• Gum or sugarless hard candy may relieve dry mouth.

---

oxyphencyclimine hydrochloride
Daricon

Pregnancy Risk Category: C

HOW SUPPLIED
Tablets: 10 mg

MECHANISM OF ACTION
Exerts a nonspecific, direct spasmolytic action on smooth muscle. Also possesses local anesthetic properties that may be partly responsible for spasmolysis.

INDICATIONS & DOSAGE
Adjunctive treatment of peptic ulcer—
Adults: 10 mg P.O. b.i.d. in the morning and at bedtime, or 5 mg b.i.d. or t.i.d.

ADVERSE REACTIONS
CNS: *headache,* insomnia, drowsiness, *dizziness.*

CV: *palpitations,* tachycardia.
EENT: *blurred vision,* mydriasis, increased ocular tension, cycloplegia, photophobia.
GI: *constipation,* nausea, vomiting, *paralytic ileus.*
GU: *urinary hesitancy, urine retention, impotence.*
Skin: urticaria, decreased sweating or possible anhidrosis, other dermal manifestations.
Other: fever, allergic reactions.
  Overdosage may cause curare-like symptoms.

INTERACTIONS
None significant.

NURSING CONSIDERATIONS
• Contraindicated in narrow-angle glaucoma, obstructive uropathy, obstructive disease of GI tract, severe ulcerative colitis, myasthenia gravis, hypersensitivity to anticholinergics, paralytic ileus, intestinal atony, unstable cardiovascular status in acute hemorrhage, or toxic megacolon.

• Use cautiously in autonomic neuropathy, hyperthyroidism, coronary artery disease, cardiac arrhythmias, CHF, hypertension, hiatal hernia associated with reflux esophagitis, hepatic or renal disease, and ulcerative colitis, or in patients over 40 years because of increased incidence of glaucoma.

• Use with caution in hot or humid environments. Drug-induced heatstroke can develop.

• Give 30 minutes to 1 hour before breakfast and at bedtime.

• Monitor patient's vital signs and urine output carefully.

• Instruct patient to avoid driving and other hazardous activities if he is drowsy, dizzy, or has blurred vision; to drink plenty of fluids to help prevent constipation; and to report any rash or skin eruption.

• Gum or sugarless hard candy may relieve dry mouth.

Italicized adverse reactions are common or life-threatening.
*Liquid form contains alcohol.   **May contain tartrazine.

• A synthetic tertiary derivative that may have fewer atropine-like adverse reactions.

---

oxyphenonium bromide
Antrenyl

Pregnancy Risk Category: C

HOW SUPPLIED
Tablets: 5 mg

MECHANISM OF ACTION
Competitively blocks acetylcholine, which decreases GI motility and inhibits gastric acid secretion.

INDICATIONS & DOSAGE
Adjunctive treatment of peptic ulcer—
Adults: 10 mg P.O. q.i.d. for several days, then reduced according to patient response.

ADVERSE REACTIONS
CNS: headache, insomnia, drowsiness, dizziness, *confusion or excitement in elderly patients,* nervousness, weakness.
CV: *palpitations,* tachycardia.
EENT: *blurred vision,* mydriasis, increased ocular tension, cycloplegia, photophobia.
GI: *dry mouth,* dysphagia, *constipation,* heartburn, loss of taste, nausea, vomiting, *paralytic ileus.*
GU: *urinary hesitancy, urine retention,* impotence.
Skin: urticaria, decreased sweating or possible anhidrosis, other dermal manifestations.
Other: fever, allergic reactions.
Overdosage may cause curare-like symptoms.

INTERACTIONS
None significant.

NURSING CONSIDERATIONS
• Contraindicated in narrow-angle glaucoma, obstructive uropathy, obstructive disease of GI tract, severe ulcerative colitis, myasthenia gravis, hypersensitivity to anticholinergics, paralytic ileus, intestinal atony, unstable cardiovascular status in acute hemorrhage, or toxic megacolon.
• Use cautiously in autonomic neuropathy, hyperthyroidism, coronary artery disease, cardiac arrhythmias, CHF, hypertension, hiatal hernia associated with reflux esophagitis, hepatic or renal disease, and ulcerative colitis, or in patients over 40 years because of increased incidence of glaucoma.
• Use with caution in hot or humid environments. Drug-induced heatstroke can develop.
• Give 30 minutes to 1 hour before meals and at bedtime. Bedtime dose can be larger and should be given at least 2 hours after the last meal of the day.
• Monitor patient's vital signs and urine output carefully.
• Instruct patient to avoid driving and other hazardous activities if he is drowsy, dizzy, or has blurred vision; to drink plenty of fluids to help prevent constipation; and to report any skin rash or local eruption.
• Gum or sugarless hard candy may relieve dry mouth.

---

propantheline bromide
Norpanth, Pantheline‡, Pro-Banthine, Propanthel†

Pregnancy Risk Category: C

HOW SUPPLIED
Tablets: 7.5 mg, 15 mg

MECHANISM OF ACTION
Competitively blocks acetylcholine, which decreases GI motility and inhibits gastric acid secretion.

INDICATIONS & DOSAGE
Adjunctive treatment of peptic ulcer, irritable bowel syndrome, and other gastrointestinal disorders; to reduce

duodenal motility during diagnostic radiologic procedures—
Adults: 15 mg P.O. t.i.d. before meals, and 30 mg h.s. up to 60 mg q.i.d. For elderly patients, 7.5 mg P.O. t.i.d. before meals.

ADVERSE REACTIONS
CNS: headache, insomnia, drowsiness, dizziness, *confusion or excitement in elderly patients,* nervousness, weakness.
CV: *palpitations,* tachycardia.
EENT: *blurred vision,* mydriasis, increased ocular tension, cycloplegia, photophobia.
GI: *dry mouth,* dysphagia, constipation, heartburn, loss of taste, nausea, vomiting, paralytic ileus.
GU: *urinary hesitancy, urine retention,* impotence.
Skin: urticaria, decreased sweating or possible anhidrosis, other dermal manifestations.
Other: fever, allergic reactions.
Overdosage may cause curare-like symptoms.

INTERACTIONS
None significant.

NURSING CONSIDERATIONS
• Contraindicated in narrow-angle glaucoma, obstructive uropathy, obstructive disease of GI tract, severe ulcerative colitis, myasthenia gravis, hypersensitivity to anticholinergics, paralytic ileus, intestinal atony, unstable cardiovascular status in acute hemorrhage, or toxic megacolon. Use cautiously in autonomic neuropathy, hyperthyroidism, coronary artery disease, cardiac arrhythmias, congestive heart failure, hypertension, hiatal hernia associated with reflux esophagitis, hepatic or renal disease, and ulcerative colitis, or in patients over 40 years because of the increased incidence of glaucoma.
• Use with caution in hot or humid

environments. Drug-induced heatstroke can develop.
• Give 30 minutes to 1 hour before meals and at bedtime. Bedtime dose can be larger and should be given at least 2 hours after the last meal of the day.
• Monitor patient's vital signs and urine output carefully.
• Instruct patient to avoid driving and other hazardous activities if he is drowsy, dizzy, or has blurred vision; to drink plenty of fluids to help prevent constipation; and to report any rash or skin eruption.
• Gum or sugarless hard candy may relieve dry mouth.

Italicized adverse reactions are common or life-threatening.
*Liquid form contains alcohol.   **May contain tartrazine.

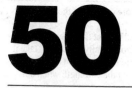

Antiulcer agents

cimetidine
famotidine
misoprostol
nizatidine
omeprazole
ranitidine hydrochloride
sucralfate

COMBINATION PRODUCTS
None.

cimetidine
Doractin‡, Tagamet

Pregnancy Risk Category: B

HOW SUPPLIED
Tablets: 200 mg, 300 mg, 400 mg, 800 mg
Oral liquid: 300 mg/5 ml
Injection: 150 mg/ml, 200 mg/2 ml‡

MECHANISM OF ACTION
Competitively inhibits the action of histamine (H_2) at receptor sites of the parietal cells, decreasing gastric acid secretion.

INDICATIONS & DOSAGE
Duodenal ulcer (short-term treatment)—
Adults and children over 16 years: 800 mg P.O. h.s. Alternatively, 400 mg P.O. b.i.d., or 300 mg P.O. q.i.d. (with meals and h.s.). Continue treatment for 4 to 6 weeks unless endoscopy shows healing. Maintenance therapy: 400 mg h.s. Parenteral: 300 mg diluted to 20 ml with 0.9% normal saline solution or other compatible I.V. solution by I.V. push over 1 to 2 minutes q 6 hours. Or 300 mg diluted in 50 ml dextrose 5% solution or other compatible I.V. solution by I.V. infusion over 15 to 20 minutes q 6 hours. Or 300 mg I.M. q 6 hours (no dilution necessary). To increase dose, give 300 mg doses more frequently to maximum daily dosage of 2,400 mg.
Duodenal ulcer prophylaxis—
Adults and children over 16 years: 400 mg P.O. h.s.
Active benign gastric ulcer—
Adults: 300 mg P.O. q.i.d. with meals and h.s. for up to 8 weeks.
Pathologic hypersecretory conditions (such as Zollinger-Ellison syndrome, systemic mastocytosis, and multiple endocrine adenomas)—
Adults and children over 16 years: 300 mg P.O. q.i.d. with meals and h.s.; adjust to individual needs. Maximum daily dosage is 2,400 mg. Parenteral: 300 mg diluted to 20 ml with 0.9% normal saline solution or other compatible I.V. solutions by I.V. push over 1 to 2 minutes q 6 hours. Or 300 mg diluted in 50 ml dextrose 5% solution or other compatible I.V. solution by I.V. infusion over 15 to 20 minutes q 6 hours. To increase dosage, give 300-mg doses more frequently to maximum daily dosage of 2,400 mg.

ADVERSE REACTIONS
Blood: *agranulocytosis, neutropenia, thrombocytopenia, aplastic anemia (rare).*
CNS: mental confusion, dizziness, headaches, peripheral neuropathy.
CV: bradycardia.

GI: *mild and transient diarrhea.*
GU: transient elevations in serum creatinine.
Hepatic: jaundice (rare).
Skin: acne-like rash, urticaria.
Other: hypersensitivity, muscle pain, mild gynecomastia after use longer than 1 month.

INTERACTIONS
Antacids: interfere with absorption of cimetidine. Separate cimetidine and antacids by at least 1 hour if possible.

Cimetidine may inhibit hepatic microsomal enzyme metabolism of some drugs, like warfarin, phenytoin, some benzodiazepines, lidocaine, theophylline, and propranolol. Monitor serum levels of these drugs closely during cimetidine therapy.

NURSING CONSIDERATIONS
• I.M. route of administration may be painful.
• I.V. solutions compatible for dilution with cimetidine: 0.9% sodium chloride solution, dextrose 5% and 10% (and combinations of these) in water solutions, lactated Ringer's solution, and 5% sodium bicarbonate injection. Do not dilute with sterile water for injection.
• Hemodialysis reduces blood levels of cimetidine. Schedule cimetidine dose at end of hemodialysis treatment.
• Up to 10 g overdosage has been reported without adverse reactions.
• Effectiveness in treatment of gastric ulcers not as great as in duodenal ulcer. Cimetidine may prove useful but is still unapproved in pancreatic insufficiency, short-bowel syndrome, psoriasis, prevention and treatment of GI bleeding, relief of symptoms and acid sensitivity in reflux esophagitis, and prevention of gastric inactivation of oral enzyme preparations by gastric acid and pepsin.
• Taking tablets with meals will en-

sure a more consistent therapeutic effect.
• Remind patient that if he's taking cimetidine once daily, he should take it at bedtime for best results.
• Identify tablet strength when obtaining a drug history.
• Elderly or debilitated patients may be more susceptible to cimetidine-induced mental confusion.
• I.V. cimetidine often used in critically ill patients prophylactically to prevent GI bleeding.
• Don't infuse I.V. too rapidly. May cause bradycardia.
• Urge patient to avoid cigarette smoking, as this may increase gastric acid secretion and worsen disease.
• When administering cimetidine I.V. in 100 ml of diluent solution, do not infuse so rapidly that circulatory overload is produced. Some authorities recommend that the drug be infused over at least 30 minutes, to minimize the risk of adverse cardiac effects. Sometimes administered as continuous I.V. infusion.
• Has many investigational uses. Used before anesthesia for prophylaxis of aspiration pneumonitis; also used to treat hyperparathyroidism, herpes zoster, chronic hives, and as an adjunct in the treatment of acetaminophen overdose.

famotidine
Pepcid, Pepcidine‡
Pregnancy Risk Category: B

HOW SUPPLIED
Tablets: 20 mg, 40 mg
Powder for oral suspension: 40 mg/5 ml after reconstituting
Injection: 10 mg/ml

MECHANISM OF ACTION
Competitively inhibits the action of histamine (H_2) at receptor sites of the parietal cells, decreasing gastric acid secretion.

Italicized adverse reactions are common or life-threatening.
*Liquid form contains alcohol.   **May contain tartrazine.

INDICATIONS & DOSAGE

Duodenal ulcer—

Adults: For acute therapy, 40 mg P.O. once daily h.s. For maintenance therapy, 20 mg P.O. once daily h.s.

Pathologic hypersecretory conditions (such as Zollinger-Ellison syndrome)—

Adults: 20 mg P.O. q 6 hours. As much as 160 mg q 6 hours may be administered.

Hospitalized patients with intractable ulcers or hypersecretory conditions, or patients who cannot take oral medication—

Adults: 20 mg I.V. q 12 hours.

ADVERSE REACTIONS

Blood: thrombocytopenia (rare).
CNS: *headache,* dizziness, hallucinations.
GI: diarrhea, constipation, nausea, flatulence.
GU: increased BUN and creatinine.
Skin: acne, pruritus, rash.
Local: transient irritation at I.V. site.

INTERACTIONS

None significant.

NURSING CONSIDERATIONS

• Gastric cancer must be ruled out before famotidine therapy.

• Advise patient not to take the drug for longer than 8 weeks unless doctor specifically orders it.

• Especially at the beginning of therapy when pain is severe and with doctor's knowledge, patient may take antacids concomitantly.

• Store reconstituted suspension below 86° F. (30° C.). Discard after 30 days.

• Store I.V. injection in refrigerator at 35.6° to 46.4° F. (2° to 8° C.)

• Urge patient to avoid cigarette smoking as this may increase gastric acid secretion and worsen disease.

• Patient may take famotidine with a snack if he desires. Remind patient that this drug is most effective if taken at bedtime.

• Some patients may have this drug prescribed to be taken 20 mg twice daily instead of 40 mg at bedtime. This alternate dosing schedule is also effective. However, at least one dose should be taken at bedtime.

• To prepare I.V. injection, dilute 2 ml (20 mg) famotidine with compatible I.V. solution to a total volume of either 5 or 10 ml, and inject slowly (over at least 2 minutes). Compatible solutions include sterile water for injection, 0.9% Sodium Chloride injection, 5% or 10% Dextrose injection, 5% Sodium Bicarbonate injection, or lactated Ringer's Injection.

• Alternatively, famotidine may be given by I.V. infusion. Dilute 20 mg (2 ml) famotidine in 100 ml of compatible solution, and infuse over 15 to 30 minutes. Solution is stable for 48 hours at room temperature after dilution.

misoprostol
Cytotec

Pregnancy Risk Category: X

HOW SUPPLIED

Tablets: 200 mcg

MECHANISM OF ACTION

A synthetic prostaglandin E$_1$ analog, misoprostol replaces gastric prostaglandins that are depleted by NSAID therapy. It also decreases basal and stimulated gastric acid secretion, and may increase gastric mucus and bicarbonate production.

INDICATIONS & DOSAGE

Prevention of NSAID-induced gastric ulcers in elderly or debilitated patients at high risk of complications from gastric ulcer, and patients with a history of NSAID-induced ulcers—

Adults: 200 mcg P.O. q.i.d. with food. If this dosage isn't tolerated, it may be decreased to 100 mcg P.O. q.i.d.

ADVERSE REACTIONS
CNS: headache.
GI: diarrhea, abdominal pain, nausea, flatulence, dyspepsia, vomiting, constipation.
GU: hypermenorrhea, dysmenorrhea, spotting, cramps, menstrual disorders.

INTERACTIONS
Antacids: reduced plasma levels when administered concomitantly. Not considered significant.

NURSING CONSIDERATIONS
• Misoprostol is an abortifacient and is contraindicated for use in pregnant women. Misoprostol is also contraindicated in patients who have a history of an allergic response to prostaglandins.
• Misoprostol should not be routinely administered to women of childbearing age unless they are at high risk of developing ulcers or complications from NSAID-induced ulcers.
• Special precautions must be taken to prevent the use of this drug during pregnancy. The patient must be fully aware of the dangers of misoprostol to a fetus, and must receive both oral and written warnings regarding these dangers. She must be capable of complying with effective contraceptive means, and must have a negative serum pregnancy test within 2 weeks of initiating therapy.
• Misoprostol therapy must not begin until the second or third day of the next normal menstrual period.
• Instruct *ALL* patients not to share misoprostol with anyone else. They should be aware that when taken by a pregnant patient this drug may cause miscarriage, often with potentially life threatening bleeding. Concomitant ingestion of food or antacids seems to reduce maximal plasma concentrations of misoprostol, but this doesn't appear to impair the drug's effectiveness.

• Misoprostol appears to reduce the bioavailability of concomitantly administered aspirin, but this effect is not considered clinically significant.

---

nizatidine
Axid

Pregnancy Risk Category: C

HOW SUPPLIED
Capsules: 150 mg, 300 mg

MECHANISM OF ACTION
Competitively inhibits the action of histamine at H_2 receptor sites of the parietal cells, decreasing gastric acid secretion.

INDICATIONS & DOSAGE
Active duodenal ulcer treatment—
Adults: 300 mg P.O. once daily at bedtime. Alternatively, patient may receive 150 mg b.i.d.
Maintenance therapy of duodenal ulcer—
Adults: 150 mg once daily h.s.

ADVERSE REACTIONS
Blood: *thrombocytopenia.*
CNS: *somnolence.*
CV: arrhythmias.
Skin: *sweating,* rash, urticaria, *exfoliative dermatitis.*
Other: hepatic damage, hyperuricemia, gynecomastia.

INTERACTIONS
Aspirin: nizatidine may elevate serum salicylate levels in patients taking high doses of aspirin.

NURSING CONSIDERATIONS
• Contraindicated in patients with hypersensitivity to H_2-receptor antagonists.
• Dosage should be reduced in patients with impaired renal function. Patients with a creatinine clearance of 20 to 50 ml/minute should receive 150 mg daily for treatment of active

---

duodenal ulcer, or 150 mg every other day for maintenance therapy. Patients with a creatinine clearance below 20 ml/minute should receive 150 mg every other day for treatment or 150 mg every third day for maintenance.

• False-positive test results for urobilinogen may occur.

• Nizatidine has not been associated with antiandrogenic activity and does not appear to affect hepatic drug-metabolizing enzyme systems.

• Urge patient to avoid cigarette smoking, which will increase gastric acid secretion and worsen disease.

omeprazole
Losec

Pregnancy Risk Category: C

HOW SUPPLIED
Capsules (delayed-release): 20 mg

MECHANISM OF ACTION
Inhibits the activity of the acid (proton) pump, $H+/K+$ ATPase, located at the secretory surface of the gastric parietal cell. This blocks the formation of gastric acid.

INDICATIONS & DOSAGE
Severe erosive esophagitis; symptomatic, poorly responsive gastroesophageal reflux disease (GERD)—
Adults: 20 mg P.O. daily for 4 to 8 weeks. Patients with GERD should have failed initial therapy with a histamine H_2 antagonist.
Pathologic hypersecretory conditions (such as Zollinger-Ellison syndrome)—
Adults: initially, 60 mg P.O. daily, with dosage titrated according to patient response. Daily dosage exceeding 80 mg should be administered in divided doses. Dosages up to 120 mg t.i.d. have been administered. Therapy should continue as long as clinically indicated.

ADVERSE REACTIONS
CNS: headache, dizziness.
GI: diarrhea, abdominal pain, nausea, vomiting, constipation, flatulence.
Respiratory: cough.
Skin: rash.
Other: back pain.

INTERACTIONS
Diazepam, warfarin, and phenytoin: Decreased hepatic clearance possibly leading to increased serum levels. Monitor closely.
Ketoconazole, iron derivatives, and ampicillin esters: may exhibit poor bioavailability in patients taking omeprazole because optimal absorption of these drugs requires a low gastric pH.

NURSING CONSIDERATIONS
• Contraindicated in patients hypersensitive to the drug or any component of the enteric formulation.

• Prolonged (2-year) studies in rats revealed a dose-related increase in gastric carcinoid tumors; studies in humans have not detected a risk from short-term exposure to the drug. Further study is needed to assess the impact of sustained hypergastrinemia and hypochlorhydria. The manufacturer recommends that therapy with omeprazole not exceed the indicated duration.

• Capsules should be swallowed whole and not opened or crushed.

• Omeprazole increases its own bioavailability with repeated administration. The drug is labile in gastric acid, and less drug is lost to hydrolysis as the drug increases gastric pH.

• Dosage adjustments are not required for renal or hepatic impairment.

ranitidine hydrochloride
Zantac*

Pregnancy Risk Category: B

HOW SUPPLIED
Tablets: 150 mg, 300 mg
Dispersible tablets: 150 mg‡
Syrup: 15 mg/ml
Injection: 25 mg/ml
Infusion: 0.5 mg/ml in 100-ml containers

MECHANISM OF ACTION
Competitively inhibits the action of histamine (H_2) at receptor sites of the parietal cells, decreasing gastric acid secretion.

INDICATIONS & DOSAGE
Duodenal and gastric ulcer (short-term treatment); pathological hypersecretory conditions, such as Zollinger-Ellison syndrome—
Adults: 150 mg P.O. b.i.d. or 300 mg once daily h.s. Dosages up to 6 g/day may be prescribed in patients with Zollinger-Ellison syndrome. May also be administered parenterally: 50 mg I.V. or I.M. q 6 to 8 hours. When administering I.V. push, dilute to a total volume of 20 ml and inject over a period of 5 minutes. No dilution necessary when administering I.M. May also be administered by intermittent I.V. infusion. Dilute 50 mg ranitidine in 100 ml of dextrose 5% in water and infuse over 15 to 20 minutes.
Maintenance therapy of duodenal ulcer—
Adults: 150 mg P.O. h.s.
Gastroesophageal reflux disease (GERD)—
Adults: 150 mg P.O. b.i.d.

ADVERSE REACTIONS
Blood: neutropenia, thrombocytopenia.
CNS: headache, malaise, dizziness, confusion.
CV: bradycardia.
GI: nausea, constipation.
Hepatic: elevated liver enzymes, jaundice.
Skin: rash.
Local: burning and itching at injection site.

INTERACTIONS
Antacids: may interfere with absorption of ranitidine (conflicting data). Stagger doses if possible.
Diazepam: decreased absorption when administered concomitantly with ranitidine.
Glipizide: possibly increased hypoglycemic effect. Dosage adjustment of glipizide may be necessary.
Procainamide: ranitodine may decrease renal clearance (conflicting data).
Warfarin: ranitidine may interfere with warfarin clearance (conflicting data).

NURSING CONSIDERATIONS
• Use cautiously in hepatic dysfunction. Dosage should be adjusted in patients with impaired renal function.
• Can be taken without regard to meals. Absorption not affected by food.
• Remind patient that if he's taking ranitidine once daily, he should take it at bedtime for best results.
• Urge patient to avoid smoking, as this may increase gastric acid secretion and worsen disease.
• When administering premixed I.V. infusion, give by slow I.V. drip (over 15 to 20 minutes). Do not add other drugs to the solution. If used with a primary I.V. fluid system, the primary solution should be discontinued during the infusion.
• To prepare I.V. injection, dilute 50 mg (2 ml) in 100 ml of compatible solution and infuse over 15 to 20 minutes. Compatible solutions include 0.9% Sodium Chloride injection, 5% or 10% Dextrose injection, 5% So-

---

Italicized adverse reactions are common or life-threatening.
*Liquid form contains alcohol.   **May contain tartrazine.

dium Bicarbonate injection, or lactated Ringer's Injection.

---

sucralfate
Carafate, Sulcrate†

Pregnancy Risk Category: B

HOW SUPPLIED
Tablets: 1 g

MECHANISM OF ACTION
Adheres to and protects the ulcer surface by forming a barrier.

INDICATIONS & DOSAGE
Short-term (up to 8 weeks) treatment of duodenal ulcer—
Adults: 1 g P.O. q.i.d. 1 hour before meals and h.s.

ADVERSE REACTIONS
CNS: dizziness, sleepiness.
GI: *constipation,* nausea, gastric discomfort, diarrhea, bezoar formation.

INTERACTIONS
Antacids: may decrease binding of drug to gastroduodenal mucosa, impairing effectiveness. Don't give within 30 minutes of each other.

NURSING CONSIDERATIONS
● No known contraindications.
● Drug is minimally absorbed. Incidence of adverse reactions is low.
● Tell patient for best results to take sucralfate on an empty stomach (1 hour before each meal and at bedtime).
● Pain and ulcer symptoms may subside within first few weeks of therapy. However, for complete healing, be sure patient continues on prescribed regimen.
● Monitor for severe, persistent constipation.
● Studies suggest that drug is as effective as cimetidine in healing duodenal ulcers.
● Drug has been used to treat gastric ulcers, but effectiveness of this use is still under investigation.
● Drug contains aluminum but isn't classified as an antacid.
● Urge patient to avoid smoking, as this may increase gastric acid secretion and worsen disease.

Corticosteroids

Glucocorticoids
beclomethasone dipropionate
betamethasone
**betamethasone acetate and
betamethasone sodium
phosphate**
**betamethasone sodium
phosphate**
cortisone acetate
dexamethasone
dexamethasone acetate
**dexamethasone sodium
phosphate**
flunisolide
hydrocortisone
hydrocortisone acetate
hydrocortisone cypionate
**hydrocortisone sodium
phosphate**
**hydrocortisone sodium
succinate**
methylprednisolone
methylprednisolone acetate
**methylprednisolone sodium
succinate**
paramethasone acetate
prednisolone
prednisolone acetate
prednisolone sodium phosphate
prednisolone steaglate
prednisolone tebutate
prednisone
triamcinolone
triamcinolone acetonide
triamcinolone diacetate
triamcinolone hexacetonide

Mineralocorticoid
fludrocortisone acetate

COMBINATION PRODUCT
DECADRON WITH XYLOCAINE: dexamethasone phosphate 4 mg and lidocaine hydrochloride 10 mg/ml.

beclomethasone dipropionate
Aldecin Aqueous Nasal Spray‡, Aldecin Inhaler‡, Becloforte Inhaler‡, Beclovent, Beclovent Rotacaps†, Vanceril

Pregnancy Risk Category: C

HOW SUPPLIED
Oral inhalation aerosol: 42 mcg/metered spray, 50 mcg/metered spray‡, 250 mcg/metered spray‡

MECHANISM OF ACTION
Decreases inflammation, mainly by stabilizing leukocyte lysosomal membranes. Also suppresses the immune response, stimulates bone marrow, and influences protein, fat, and carbohydrate metabolism.

INDICATIONS & DOSAGE
Steroid-dependent asthma—
Adults: 2 to 4 inhalations t.i.d. or q.i.d. Maximum dosage is 20 inhalations daily.
Children 6 to 12 years: 1 to 2 inhalations t.i.d. or q.i.d. Maximum dosage is 10 inhalations daily.

ADVERSE REACTIONS
EENT: hoarseness, fungal infections of mouth and throat, throat irritation.
GI: dry mouth.

Italicized adverse reactions are common or life-threatening.
*Liquid form contains alcohol.   **May contain tartrazine.

INTERACTIONS
None significant.

NURSING CONSIDERATIONS
• Contraindicated in status asthmaticus. Not for use in asthma controlled by bronchodilators or other noncorticosteroids alone, or for nonasthmatic bronchial diseases.
• Oral glucocorticoid therapy should be tapered slowly. Acute adrenal insufficiency and death have occurred in asthmatics who changed abruptly from oral corticosteroids to beclomethasone.
• During times of stress (trauma, surgery, or infection) systemic corticosteroids may be needed to prevent adrenal insufficiency in previously steroid-dependent patients.
• Instruct patient to carry a card indicating his need for supplemental systemic glucocorticoids during stress.
• Patient requiring bronchodilator should use it several minutes before beclomethasone.
• Tell patient to allow 1 minute to elapse before taking subsequent puffs of medication, and to hold breath for a few seconds to enhance action of drug.
• Inform patient that beclomethasone doesn't provide relief for emergency asthma attacks. Patients using nasal form should understand that full therapeutic effect may take from a few days to a couple of weeks.
• Instruct patient to contact doctor if he notices a decreased response or if symptoms don't improve within 3 weeks of initiating therapy. Dose may have to be adjusted. Patient shouldn't exceed recommended dose on his own.
• Check mucous membranes frequently for signs of fungal infection.
• Oral fungal infections can be prevented by following inhalations with glass of water.
• Tell patient to keep inhaler clean and unobstructed. Wash with warm water and dry thoroughly.
• Use of a spacer device with the Becloforte Inhaler is not recommended.

---

betamethasone
Betnelan†, Celestone*

betamethasone acetate and betamethasone sodium phosphate
Celestone Chronodose‡, Celestone Soluspan

betamethasone sodium phosphate
Betameth, Betnesol†, B.S.P., Celestone Phosphate, Cel-U-Jec, Prelestone, Selestoject

Pregnancy Risk Category: C

HOW SUPPLIED
betamethasone
Tablets: 600 mcg
Tablets (extended-release): 1 mg
Syrup: 600 mcg/5 ml
betamethasone acetate and betamethasone sodium phosphate
Injection: betamethasone acetate 3 mg and betamethasone sodium phosphate (equivalent to 3-mg base)/ml.
betamethasone sodium phosphate
Effervescent tablets: 500 mcg*
Injection: 4 mg (3-mg base)/ml in 5-ml vials

MECHANISM OF ACTION
Decreases inflammation, mainly by stabilizing leukocyte lysosomal membranes. Also suppresses the immune response, stimulates bone marrow, and influences protein, fat, and carbohydrate metabolism.

INDICATIONS & DOSAGE
Severe inflammation or immunosuppression—
Adults: 0.6 to 7.2 mg P.O. daily; or 0.5 to 9 mg (sodium phosphate) I.M., I.V., or into joint or soft tissue daily;

---

or 1.5 to 12 mg (sodium phosphate-acetate suspension) into joint or soft tissue q 1 to 2 weeks, p.r.n.
Prevention of neonatal respiratory distress syndrome—
Adults (pregnant women): 12 mg I.M. Celestone Soluspan 36 to 48 hours before premature delivery. Repeat in 24 hours.

ADVERSE REACTIONS
Most adverse reactions of corticosteroids are dose- or duration-dependent.
CNS: *euphoria, insomnia,* psychotic behavior, pseudotumor cerebri.
CV: *CHF,* hypertension, edema.
EENT: cataracts, glaucoma.
GI: *peptic ulcer,* GI irritation, increased appetite.
Metabolic: *possible hypokalemia, hyperglycemia and carbohydrate intolerance,* growth suppression in children.
Skin: delayed wound healing, acne, various skin eruptions.
Other: muscle weakness, pancreatitis, hirsutism, susceptibility to infections. Acute adrenal insufficiency may follow increased stress (infection, surgery, or trauma) or abrupt withdrawal after long-term therapy. *Withdrawal symptoms:* rebound inflammation, fatigue, weakness, arthralgia, fever, dizziness, lethargy, depression, fainting, orthostatic hypotension, dyspnea, anorexia, hypoglycemia. *Sudden withdrawal may be fatal.*

INTERACTIONS
Barbiturates, phenytoin, rifampin: decreased corticosteroid effect. Corticosteroid dose may need to be increased.
Indomethacin, aspirin: increased risk of GI distress and bleeding. Give together cautiously.

NURSING CONSIDERATIONS
• Contraindicated in systemic fungal infections. Use cautiously in patients with GI ulceration or renal disease, hypertension, osteoporosis, varicella, vaccinia, exanthema, diabetes mellitus, Cushing's syndrome, thromboembolic disorders, seizures, myasthenia gravis, CHF, tuberculosis, ocular herpes simplex, hypoalbuminemia, emotional instability, and psychotic tendencies.
• Don't use for alternate-day therapy.
• Adrenal suppression may last up to 1 year after drug is stopped. Gradually reduce drug dosage after long-term therapy. Tell patient not to stop drug abruptly or without doctor's consent.
• Always titrate to lowest effective dose.
• To prevent muscle atrophy, give I.M. injection deeply.
• Monitor blood sugar and serum potassium regularly. Diabetic patients may require adjustments in insulin dosage.
• Teach patients about the effects of the drug. Warn those on long-term therapy about cushingoid symptoms.
• Observe for signs of infection, especially after steroid withdrawal. Tell patients to report slow healing.
• Instruct patient to carry a card indicating his need for supplemental glucocorticoids during stress.
• Give a daily dosage in the morning for better results and less toxicity.
• Give with milk or food to reduce GI irritation.
• A glucocorticoid with little mineralocorticoid effect.
• Watch for additional potassium depletion from diuretics and amphotericin B.
• Immunizations may show decreased antibody response.
• Obtain baseline weight before starting therapy, and weigh patient daily; report any sudden weight gain to doctor.
• Betamethasone sometimes prescribed to treat respiratory distress syndrome in premature infants.

Italicized adverse reactions are common or life-threatening.
*Liquid form contains alcohol.   **May contain tartrazine.

cortisone acetate
Cortate‡, Cortone Acetate

Pregnancy Risk Category: D

HOW SUPPLIED
Tablets: 5 mg, 10 mg, 25 mg
Injection (suspension): 25 mg/ml, 50 mg/ml

MECHANISM OF ACTION
Decreases inflammation, mainly by stabilizing leukocyte lysosomal membranes. Also suppresses the immune response, stimulates bone marrow, and influences protein, fat, and carbohydrate metabolism.

INDICATIONS & DOSAGE
Adrenal insufficiency, allergy, inflammation—
Adults: 25 to 300 mg P.O. or I.M. daily or on alternate days. Dosages highly individualized, depending on severity of disease.

ADVERSE REACTIONS
Most adverse reactions of corticosteroids are dose- or duration-dependent.
CNS: *euphoria, insomnia,* psychotic behavior, pseudotumor cerebri.
CV: *CHF,* hypertension, edema.
EENT: cataracts, glaucoma.
GI: *peptic ulcer,* GI irritation, increased appetite.
Metabolic: *possible hypokalemia, hyperglycemia and carbohydrate intolerance,* growth suppression in children.
Skin: delayed wound healing, acne, various skin eruptions.
Local: atrophy at I.M. injection sites.
Other: muscle weakness, pancreatitis, hirsutism, susceptibility to infections. Acute adrenal insufficiency may follow increased stress (infection, surgery, or trauma) or abrupt withdrawal after long-term therapy.
Withdrawal symptoms: rebound inflammation, fatigue, weakness, arthralgia, fever, dizziness, lethargy, depression, fainting, orthostatic hypotension, dyspnea, anorexia, hypoglycemia. *Sudden withdrawal may be fatal.*

INTERACTIONS
Barbiturates, phenytoin, rifampin: decreased corticosteroid effect. Corticosteroid dose may need to be increased.
Indomethacin, aspirin: increased risk of GI distress and bleeding. Give together cautiously.

NURSING CONSIDERATIONS
• Contraindicated in systemic fungal infections. Use cautiously in patients with GI ulceration or renal disease, hypertension, osteoporosis, varicella, vaccinia, exanthema, diabetes mellitus, Cushing's syndrome, thromboembolic disorders, seizures, myasthenia gravis, congestive heart failure, tuberculosis, ocular herpes simplex, hypoalbuminemia, emotional instability, and psychotic tendencies.
• Gradually reduce drug dosage after long-term therapy. Tell patient not to discontinue drug abruptly or without doctor's consent.
• Always titrate to lowest effective dose.
• Patient may need low-sodium diet and potassium supplement.
• I.M. route causes slow onset of action. Don't use in acute conditions where rapid effect required. May use on a twice-daily schedule matching diurnal variation.
• A glucocorticoid with potent mineralocorticoid effect; report sudden weight gain or edema to doctor.
• Observe for signs of infection, especially after steroid withdrawal. Tell patient to report slow healing.
• Drug of choice for replacement therapy in adrenal insufficiency.
• Monitor serum electrolytes and blood sugar.
• Warn patients on long-term therapy about cushingoid symptoms.

---

†Available in Canada only.   ‡Available in Australia only.   ◊Available OTC.

- Give with milk or food to reduce GI irritation.
- Instruct patient to carry a card indicating his need for supplemental glucocorticoids during stress.
- Give a daily dosage in the morning for better results and less toxicity.
- Not for I.V. use.
- Watch for additional potassium depletion from diuretics and amphotericin B.
- Immunizations may show decreased antibody response.

---

dexamethasone
Decadron, Deronil, Dexasone†, Dexone, Hexadrol, Mymethasone

dexamethasone acetate
Dalalone D.P., Dalalone L.A., Decadron L.A., Decaject-L.A., Decameth L.A., Dexacen LA, Dexasone-LA, Dexone LA, Dexon LA, Solurex-LA

dexamethasone sodium phosphate
Ak-Dex, Dalalone, Decadrol, Decadron Phosphate, Decaject, Decameth, Dex, Dexacen, Dexasone, Dexon, Dexone, Hexadrol Phosphate, Solurex

Pregnancy Risk Category: C

HOW SUPPLIED
dexamethasone
Tablets: 0.25 mg, 0.5 mg, 0.75 mg, 1 mg, 1.5 mg, 2 mg, 4 mg, 6 mg
Oral solution: 0.5 mg/5 ml, 0.5 mg/0.5 ml
Elixir: 0.5 mg/5 ml
dexamethasone acetate
Injection: 8 mg/ml, 16 mg/ml suspension
dexamethasone sodium phosphate
Injection: 4 mg/ml, 10 mg/ml, 20 mg/ml, 24 mg/ml

MECHANISM OF ACTION
Decreases inflammation, mainly by stabilizing leukocyte lysosomal membranes. Also suppresses the immune response, stimulates bone marrow, and influences protein, fat, and carbohydrate metabolism.

INDICATIONS & DOSAGE
Cerebral edema—
Adults: initially, 10 mg (phosphate) I.V., then 4 to 6 mg I.M. q 6 hours for 2 to 4 days, then tapered over 5 to 7 days.
Children: initially, 0.5 to 1.5 mg/kg I.V. daily; then 0.2 to 0.5 mg/kg I.V. daily in divided doses q 6 hours.
Inflammatory conditions, allergic reactions, neoplasias—
Adults: 0.25 to 4 mg P.O. b.i.d., t.i.d., or q.i.d.; or 4 to 16 mg (acetate) I.M. into joint or soft tissue q 1 to 3 weeks; or 0.8 to 1.6 mg (acetate) into lesions q 1 to 3 weeks.
Shock—
Adults: 1 to 6 mg/kg (phosphate) I.V. single dosage; or 40 mg I.V. q 2 to 6 hours, p.r.n.
Dexamethasone suppression test—
Adults: 0.5 mg P.O. q 6 hours for 48 hours.

ADVERSE REACTIONS
Most adverse reactions of corticosteroids are dose- or duration-dependent.
CNS: *euphoria, insomnia,* psychotic behavior, pseudotumor cerebri.
CV: *CHF,* hypertension, edema.
EENT: cataracts, glaucoma.
GI: *peptic ulcer,* GI irritation, increased appetite.
Metabolic: *possible hypokalemia, hyperglycemia and carbohydrate intolerance,* growth suppression in children.
Skin: delayed wound healing, acne, various skin eruptions.
Local: atrophy at I.M. injection sites.
Other: muscle weakness, pancreatitis, hirsutism, susceptibility to infections. Acute adrenal insufficiency may follow increased stress (infec-

---

Italicized adverse reactions are common or life-threatening.
*Liquid form contains alcohol.   **May contain tartrazine.

tion, surgery, or trauma) or abrupt withdrawal after long-term therapy. *Withdrawal symptoms:* rebound inflammation, fatigue, weakness, arthralgia, fever, dizziness, lethargy, depression, fainting, orthostatic hypotension, dyspnea, anorexia, hypoglycemia. *Sudden withdrawal may be fatal.*

INTERACTIONS
Barbiturates, phenytoin, rifampin: decreased corticosteroid effect. Corticosteroid dose may need to be increased.
Indomethacin, aspirin: increased risk of GI distress and bleeding. Give together cautiously.

NURSING CONSIDERATIONS
• Contraindicated in systemic fungal infections and for alternate-day therapy. Use cautiously in GI ulceration or renal disease, hypertension, osteoporosis, varicella, vaccinia, exanthema, diabetes mellitus, Cushing's syndrome, thromboembolic disorders, seizures, myasthenia gravis, metastatic cancer, CHF, tuberculosis, ocular herpes simplex, hypoalbuminemia, emotional instability, and psychotic tendencies, and in children.
• Gradually reduce drug dosage after long-term therapy. Tell patient not to discontinue drug abruptly or without doctor's consent.
• Always titrate to lowest effective dose.
• Monitor patient's weight, blood pressure, serum electrolytes.
• Instruct patient to carry a card indicating his need for supplemental systemic glucocorticoids during stress, especially as dosage is decreased.
• Give a daily dosage in the morning for better results and less toxicity.
• Teach patient signs of early adrenal insufficiency: fatigue, muscular weakness, joint pain, fever, anorexia, nausea, dyspnea, dizziness, and fainting.

• May mask or exacerbate infections.
• Watch for depression or psychotic episodes, especially in high-dose therapy.
• Inspect patient's skin for petechiae. Warn patient about easy bruising.
• Patients with diabetes may need increased insulin; monitor blood glucose.
• Monitor growth in infants and children on long-term therapy.
• Give I.M. injection deep into gluteal muscle. Avoid S.C. injection, as atrophy and sterile abscesses may occur.
• Give P.O. dose with food when possible.
• Warn patients on long-term therapy about cushingoid symptoms.
• Watch for additional potassium depletion from diuretics and amphotericin B.
• Immunizations may show decreased antibody response.
• Not used for alternate-day therapy.
• Dexamethasone most recently used in the diagnosis of depression. It is also an effective antiemetic.

fludrocortisone acetate
Florinef

Pregnancy Risk Category: C

HOW SUPPLIED
Tablets: 0.1 mg

MECHANISM OF ACTION
Increases sodium reabsorption, and potassium and hydrogen secretion at the nephron's distal convoluted tubule.

INDICATIONS & DOSAGE
Adrenal insufficiency (partial replacement), adrenogenital syndrome—
Adults: 0.1 to 0.2 mg P.O. daily.

ADVERSE REACTIONS
CV: *sodium and water retention,* hy-

pertension, cardiac hypertrophy, edema.
Metabolic: hypokalemia.

INTERACTIONS
None significant.

NURSING CONSIDERATIONS
• Contraindicated in hypertension, CHF, or cardiac disease. Use cautiously in Addison's disease.
• Monitor patient's blood pressure and serum electrolytes. Weigh patient daily; report sudden weight gain to doctor.
• Warn patient that mild peripheral edema is common.
• Unless contraindicated, give low-sodium diet high in potassium and protein. Potassium supplement may be needed.
• Has potent mineralocorticoid effects. Little glucocorticoid effect with usual doses.
• Used with cortisone or hydrocortisone in adrenal insufficiency.
• Watch for additional potassium depletion from diuretics and amphotericin B.
• Fludrocortisone is also prescribed to treat severe orthostatic hypotension.

flunisolide
AeroBid Inhaler

Pregnancy Risk Category: C

HOW SUPPLIED
Oral inhalant: 250 mcg/metered spray, 50 doses/inhaler

MECHANISM OF ACTION
Decreases inflammation, mainly by stabilizing leukocyte lysosomal membranes. Also suppresses the immune response, stimulates bone marrow, and influences protein, fat, and carbohydrate metabolism.

INDICATIONS & DOSAGE
Steroid-dependent asthma—
Adults and children over 6 years:
AeroBid Inhaler 2 inhalations (500 mcg) b.i.d. Don't exceed 4 inhalations b.i.d.

ADVERSE REACTIONS
CNS: headache.
EENT: watery eyes, throat irritation, hoarseness.
GI: nausea, vomiting, dry mouth.
Other: development of nasopharyngeal fungal infections.

INTERACTIONS
None significant.

NURSING CONSIDERATIONS
• Contraindicated in status asthmaticus. Not recommended for use in asthma controlled by bronchodilators or other noncorticosteroids alone, or for nonasthmatic bronchial diseases.
• Oral glucocorticoid therapy should be tapered slowly.
• During times of stress (trauma, surgery, or infection), systemic corticosteroids may be needed to prevent adrenal insufficiency in previously steroid-dependent patients.
• Instruct patient to carry a card indicating his need for supplemental systemic glucocorticoids during stress.
• Check mucous membranes frequently for signs of fungal infection. Tell patient to follow inhalations with glass of water to help prevent fungal infections.
• Tell patient to keep inhaler clean and unobstructed. Wash with warm water and dry thoroughly after use.
• Patient requiring bronchodilator should use it several minutes before flunisolide.
• Tell patient to allow 1 minute to elapse before repeating inhalations, and to hold breath for a few seconds to enhance action of drug.
• Inform patient that flunisolide

---

doesn't relieve emergency asthma attacks.

---

hydrocortisone
Cortef, Cortenema, Hycortt,
Hydrocortone

hydrocortisone acetate
Biosone, Cortifoam, Cortamed,
Hydrocortone Acetate

hydrocortisone cypionate
Cortef

hydrocortisone sodium phosphate
Hydrocortone Phosphate

hydrocortisone sodium succinate
A-HydroCort, Solu-Cortef

Pregnancy Risk Category: C

HOW SUPPLIED
hydrocortisone
Tablets: 5 mg, 10 mg, 20 mg
Injection: 25 mg/ml, 50 mg/ml suspension
Enema: 100 mg/60 ml
hydrocortisone acetate
Injection: 25 mg/ml, 50 mg/ml suspension
Enema: 10% aerosol foam (provides 90 mg/application)
hydrocortisone cypionate
Oral suspension: 10 mg/5 ml
hydrocortisone sodium phosphate
Injection: 50 mg/ml solution
hydrocortisone sodium succinate
Injection: 100 mg, 250 mg, 500 mg, 1,000 mg/vial

MECHANISM OF ACTION
Decreases inflammation, mainly by stabilizing leukocyte lysosomal membranes. Also suppresses the immune response, stimulates bone marrow, and influences protein, fat, and carbohydrate metabolism.

INDICATIONS & DOSAGE
Severe inflammation, adrenal insufficiency—
Adults: 5 to 30 mg P.O. b.i.d., t.i.d., or q.i.d. (as much as 80 mg P.O. q.i.d. may be given in acute situations); or initially, 100 to 250 mg (succinate) I.M. or I.V., then 50 to 100 mg I.M., as indicated; or 15 to 240 mg (phosphate) I.M. or I.V. q 12 hours; or 5 to 75 mg (acetate) into joints and soft tissue. Dosage varies with size of joint. Often local anesthetics are injected with dose.
Shock—
Adults: 500 mg to 2 g (succinate) q 2 to 6 hours.
Children: 0.16 to 1 mg/kg (phosphate or succinate) I.M. or I.V., b.i.d. or t.i.d.
Adjunctive treatment of ulcerative colitis and proctitis—
Adults: 1 enema (100 mg) nightly for 21 days.

ADVERSE REACTIONS
Most adverse reactions of corticosteroids are dose- or duration-dependent.
CNS: *euphoria, insomnia,* psychotic behavior, pseudotumor cerebri.
CV: *CHF,* hypertension, edema.
EENT: cataracts, glaucoma.
GI: *peptic ulcer,* GI irritation, increased appetite.
Metabolic: *possible hypokalemia, hyperglycemia and carbohydrate intolerance,* growth suppression in children.
Skin: delayed wound healing, acne, various skin eruptions.
Other: muscle weakness, pancreatitis, hirsutism, susceptibility to infections. Acute adrenal insufficiency may occur with increased stress (infection, surgery, or trauma) or abrupt withdrawal after long-term therapy.
Withdrawal symptoms: rebound inflammation, fatigue, weakness, arthralgia, fever, dizziness, lethargy, depression, fainting, orthostatic hypotension, dyspnea, anorexia, hypo-

---

†Available in Canada only.   ‡Available in Australia only.   ◇ Available OTC.

glycemia. *Sudden withdrawal may be fatal.*

INTERACTIONS
Barbiturates, phenytoin, rifampin: decreased corticosteroid effect. Corticosteroid dose may need to be increased.

Indomethacin, aspirin: increased risk of GI distress and bleeding. Give together cautiously.

NURSING CONSIDERATIONS
• Contraindicated in systemic fungal infections. Use cautiously in patients with GI ulceration or renal disease, hypertension, osteoporosis, varicella, vaccinia, exanthema, diabetes mellitus, Cushing's syndrome, thromboembolic disorders, seizures, myasthenia gravis, metastatic cancer, CHF, tuberculosis, ocular herpes simplex, hypoalbuminemia, emotional instability, and psychotic tendencies, and in children.
• Gradually reduce drug dosage after long-term therapy. Tell patient not to discontinue drug abruptly or without doctor's consent.
• Always titrate to lowest effective dose.
• Has a glucocorticoid and mineralocorticoid effect.
• Monitor patient's weight, blood pressure, and serum electrolytes.
• May mask or exacerbate infections.
• Stress (fever, trauma, surgery, and emotional problems) may increase adrenal insufficiency. Dose may have to be increased.
• Instruct patient to carry a card identifying his need for supplemental systemic glucocorticoids during stress.
• Give a daily dosage in the morning for better results and less toxicity.
• Teach patient signs of early adrenal insufficiency: fatigue, muscular weakness, joint pain, fever, anorexia, nausea, dyspnea, dizziness, and fainting.
• Watch for depression or psychotic episodes, especially in high-dose therapy.
• Inspect patient's skin for petechiae. Warn patient about easy bruising.
• Patients with diabetes may need increased insulin; monitor blood glucose.
• Monitor growth in infants and children on long-term therapy.
• Give I.M. injection deep into gluteal muscle. Avoid S.C. injection as atrophy and sterile abscesses may occur.
• Unless contraindicated, give low-sodium diet high in potassium and protein. Potassium supplement may be needed. Watch for additional potassium depletion from diuretics and amphotericin B.
• Give P.O. dose with food when possible.
• Warn patients on long-term therapy about cushingoid symptoms, regardless of route of administration.
• Acetate form not for I.V. use.
• Enema may produce same systemic effects as other forms of hydrocortisone. If enema therapy must exceed 21 days, discontinue gradually by reducing administration to every other night for 2 or 3 weeks.
• Immunizations may show decreased antibody response.
• Do not confuse Solu-Cortef with Solu-Medrol.
• Injectable forms not used for alternate-day therapy.

Italicized adverse reactions are common or life-threatening.
*Liquid form contains alcohol.   **May contain tartrazine.

methylprednisolone
Medrol**, Meprolone

methylprednisolone acetate
depMedalone, Depoject, Depo-Medrol, Depopred, Depo-Predate, D-Med, Duralone, Durameth, Medralone, Medrol Enpak, Medrone, Methylone, M-Prednisol, Rep-Pred

methylprednisolone sodium succinate
A-Metha-pred, Medrol†, Solu-Medrol,

Pregnancy Risk Category: C

HOW SUPPLIED
methylprednisolone
Tablets: 2 mg, 4 mg, 8 mg, 16 mg, 24 mg, 32 mg
methylprednisolone acetate
Injection (suspension): 20 mg/ml, 40 mg/ml, 80 mg/ml
methylprednisolone sodium succinate
Injection: 40 mg, 125 mg, 500 mg, 1,000 mg, 2,000 mg/vial

MECHANISM OF ACTION
Decreases inflammation, mainly by stabilizing leukocyte lysosomal membranes. Also suppresses the immune response, stimulates bone marrow, and influences protein, fat, and carbohydrate metabolism.

INDICATIONS & DOSAGE
Severe inflammation or immunosuppression—
Adults: 2 to 60 mg P.O. in four divided doses; or 40 to 80 mg (acetate) daily, I.M. or 10 to 250 mg (succinate) I.M. or I.V. q 4 hours; or 4 to 30 mg (acetate) into joints and soft tissue, p.r.n.
Children: 117 mcg to 1.66 mg/kg (succinate) I.V. in three or four divided doses.
Shock—

Adults: 100 to 250 mg (succinate) I.V. at 2- to 6-hour intervals.
To decrease residual damage following spinal cord trauma—
Adults: 30 mg/kg I.V. as a bolus injection within 8 hours of the injury, followed by a continous infusion of 5.4 mg/hour for the next 23 hours.

ADVERSE REACTIONS
Most adverse reactions of corticosteroids are dose- or duration-dependent.
CNS: *euphoria, insomnia,* psychotic behavior, pseudotumor cerebri.
CV: *CHF,* hypertension, edema.
EENT: cataracts, glaucoma.
GI: *peptic ulcer,* GI irritation, increased appetite.
Metabolic: *possible hypokalemia, hyperglycemia and carbohydrate intolerance,* growth suppression in children.
Skin: delayed wound healing, acne, various skin eruptions.
Other: muscle weakness, pancreatitis, hirsutism, susceptibility to infections. Acute adrenal insufficiency may occur with increased stress (infection, surgery, or trauma) or abrupt withdrawal after long-term therapy. *Withdrawal symptoms:* rebound inflammation, fatigue, weakness, arthralgia, fever, dizziness, lethargy, depression, fainting, orthostatic hypotension, dyspnea, anorexia, hypoglycemia. *Sudden withdrawal may be fatal.*

INTERACTIONS
Barbiturates, phenytoin, rifampin: decreased corticosteroid effect. Corticosteroid dose may need to be increased.
Indomethacin, aspirin: increased risk of GI distress and bleeding. Give together cautiously.

NURSING CONSIDERATIONS
• Contraindicated in systemic fungal infections. Use cautiously in patients with GI ulceration or renal disease,

hypertension, osteoporosis, varicella, vaccinia, exanthema, diabetes mellitus, Cushing's syndrome, thromboembolic disorders, seizures, myasthenia gravis, metastatic cancer, CHF, tuberculosis, ocular herpes simplex, hypoalbuminemia, emotional instability, and psychotic tendencies.

• Gradually reduce drug dosage after long-term therapy. Tell patient not to discontinue drug abruptly or without doctor's consent.

• Always titrate to lowest effective dose.

• A glucocorticoid with little mineralocorticoid effect.

• Discard reconstituted solutions after 48 hours.

• Don't use acetate salt when immediate onset of action is needed.

• Dermal atrophy may occur with large doses of acetate salt. Use multiple small injections rather than a single large dose.

• Monitor weight, blood pressure, serum electrolytes, and sleep patterns. Euphoria may initially interfere with sleep, but patient generally adjusts to the medication after 1 to 3 weeks.

• May mask or exacerbate infections.

• Instruct patient to carry a card identifying his need for supplemental systemic glucocorticoids during stress.

• Give a daily dosage in the morning for better results and less toxicity.

• Teach patient signs of early adrenal insufficiency: fatigue, muscular weakness, joint pain, fever, anorexia, nausea, dyspnea, dizziness, and fainting.

• Watch for depression or psychotic episodes, especially in high-dose therapy.

• Patients with diabetes may need increased insulin; monitor blood glucose.

• Give I.M. injection deep into gluteal muscle. Avoid S.C. injection, as atrophy and sterile abscesses may occur.

• Unless contraindicated, give low-sodium diet high in potassium and protein. Potassium supplement may be needed. Watch for additional potassium depletion from diuretics and amphotericin B.

• Give P.O. dose with food when possible. Critically ill patients may require concomitant antacid therapy.

• Give I.V. dose slowly over 1 minute; in shock, give massive I.V. doses over at least 10 minutes to prevent cardiac arrhythmias and circulatory collapse.

• Warn patients on long-term therapy about cushingoid symptoms.

• Acetate form not for I.V. use.

• Do not confuse Solu-Medrol with Solu-Cortef.

• Immunizations may show decreased antibody response.

• May be used for alternate-day therapy.

paramethasone acetate
Haldrone
Pregnancy Risk Category: C

HOW SUPPLIED
Tablets: 1 mg, 2 mg

MECHANISM OF ACTION
Decreases inflammation, mainly by stabilizing leukocyte lysosomal membranes. Also suppresses the immune response, stimulates bone marrow, and influences protein, fat, and carbohydrate metabolism.

INDICATIONS & DOSAGE
Inflammatory conditions—
Adults: 0.5 to 6 mg P.O. t.i.d. or q.i.d.
Children: 58 to 800 mcg/kg P.O. daily divided t.i.d. or q.i.d.

ADVERSE REACTIONS
Most adverse reactions of corticosteroids are dose- or duration-dependent.

Italicized adverse reactions are common or life-threatening.
*Liquid form contains alcohol.   **May contain tartrazine.

CNS: *euphoria, insomnia,* psychotic behavior, pseudotumor cerebri.
CV: *CHF,* hypertension, edema.
EENT: cataracts, glaucoma.
GI: *peptic ulcer,* GI irritation, increased appetite.
Metabolic: *possible hypokalemia, hyperglycemia and carbohydrate intolerance,* growth suppression in children.
Skin: delayed wound healing, acne, various skin eruptions.
Other: muscle weakness, pancreatitis, hirsutism, susceptibility to infections. Acute adrenal insufficiency may occur with increased stress (infection, surgery, or trauma) or abrupt withdrawal after long-term therapy. *Withdrawal symptoms:* rebound inflammation, fatigue, weakness, arthralgia, fever, dizziness, lethargy, depression, fainting, orthostatic hypotension, dyspnea, anorexia, hypoglycemia. *Sudden withdrawal may be fatal.*

INTERACTIONS
Barbiturates, phenytoin, rifampin: decreased corticosteroid effect. Corticosteroid dose may need to be increased.
Indomethacin, aspirin: increased risk of GI distress and bleeding. Give together cautiously.

NURSING CONSIDERATIONS
• Contraindicated in systemic fungal infections and alternate-day therapy. Use cautiously in GI ulceration or renal disease, hypertension, osteoporosis, varicella, vaccinia, exanthema, diabetes mellitus, Cushing's syndrome, thromboembolic disorders, seizures, myasthenia gravis, metastatic cancer, CHF, tuberculosis, ocular herpes simplex, hypoalbuminemia, emotional instability, and psychotic tendencies.
• Gradually reduce drug dosage after long-term therapy. Tell patient not to discontinue drug abruptly or without doctor's consent.

• Titrate to lowest effective dose.
• Has little mineralocorticoid effect.
• Monitor patient's weight, blood pressure, and serum electrolytes.
• May mask or exacerbate infections.
• Instruct patient to carry a card identifying his need for supplemental systemic glucocorticoids during stress.
• Give a daily dosage in the morning for better results and less toxicity.
• Teach patient signs of early adrenal insufficiency: fatigue, muscular weakness, joint pain, fever, anorexia, nausea, dyspnea, dizziness, and fainting.
• Watch for depression or psychotic episodes with high-dose therapy.
• Patients with diabetes may need increased insulin; monitor blood glucose.
• Monitor growth in infants and children on long-term therapy.
• Unless contraindicated, give low-sodium diet high in potassium and protein. Potassium supplement may be needed.
• Watch for additional hypokalemia from diuretics and amphotericin B.
• Give P.O. dose with food when possible, especially if GI irritation occurs.
• Warn patients on long-term therapy about cushingoid symptoms.
• Immunizations may show decreased antibody response.

---

†Available in Canada only.　　　‡Available in Australia only.　　　◊ Available OTC.

prednisolone
Cortalone, Delta-Cortef,
Deltasolone‡, Novo-prednisolone†,
Panafcortelone‡, Prelone, Solone‡

prednisolone acetate
Articulose, Key-Pred, Niscort,
Predaject, Predalone, Predate,
Predcor, Predicort

prednisolone sodium phosphate
Codesol, Hydeltrasol, Key-Pred-SP,
Pediapred, Predate-S, Predicort
RP, Predsol Retention Enema‡,
Predsol Suppositories‡

prednisolone steaglate
Sintisone‡

prednisolone tebutate
Hydeltra-TBA, Metalone-TBA, Nor-
Pred TBA, Predalone TBA, Predate
TBA, Predcor TBA, Prednisol TBA

Pregnancy Risk Category: B

HOW SUPPLIED
prednisolone
Tablets: 1 mg‡, 5 mg, 25 mg‡
Syrup: 15 mg/5 ml
prednisolone acetate
Injection (suspension): 25 mg/ml, 50
mg/ml, 100 mg/ml
**prednisolone acetate and predniso-
lone sodium phosphate**
Injection (suspension): 80 mg acetate
and 20 mg sodium phosphate/ml
prednisolone sodium phosphate
Oral liquid: 6.7 mg (5-mg base)/5 ml
Injection: 20 mg/ml
Retention enema: 20 mg/100 ml‡
Suppositories: 5 mg‡
prednisolone steaglate
Tablets: 6.65 mg (equal to 3.5 mg
prednisolone)‡
prednisolone tebutate
Injection (suspension): 20 mg/ml

MECHANISM OF ACTION
Decreases inflammation, mainly by
stabilizing leukocyte lysosomal membranes. Also suppresses the immune
response, stimulates bone marrow,
and influences protein, fat, and carbohydrate metabolism.

INDICATIONS & DOSAGE
*Severe inflammation or immunosup-
pression—*
Adults: 2.5 to 15 mg P.O. b.i.d.,
t.i.d., or q.i.d.; 2 to 30 mg I.M. (acetate, phosphate), or I.V. (phosphate) q
12 hours; or 2 to 30 mg (phosphate)
into joints, lesions, and soft tissue; or
4 to 40 mg (tebutate) into joints and
lesions; or 0.25 to 1 ml (acetate-phos-
phate suspension) into joints weekly,
p.r.n.
Treatment of proctitis‡—
Adults: 1 suppository b.i.d., preferably in the morning and h.s.
Treatment of ulcerative colitis‡—
Adults: 1 retention enema h.s. nightly
for 2 to 4 weeks. The contents of the
enema should be retained overnight.

ADVERSE REACTIONS
Most adverse reactions of corticosteroids are dose- or duration-dependent.
CNS: *euphoria, insomnia,* psychotic
behavior, pseudotumor cerebri.
CV: *CHF,* hypertension, edema.
EENT: cataracts, glaucoma.
GI: *peptic ulcer,* GI irritation, increased appetite.
Metabolic: *possible hypokalemia, hyperglycemia and carbohydrate intolerance,* growth suppression in children.
Skin: delayed wound healing, acne,
various skin eruptions.
Other: muscle weakness, pancreatitis, hirsutism, susceptibility to infections. Acute adrenal insufficiency
may occur with increased stress (infection, surgery, or trauma) or abrupt
withdrawal after long-term therapy.
Withdrawal symptoms: rebound inflammation, fatigue, weakness, arthralgia, fever, dizziness, lethargy,
depression, fainting, orthostatic hy-

Italicized adverse reactions are common or life-threatening.
*Liquid form contains alcohol.   **May contain tartrazine.

potension, dyspnea, anorexia, hypoglycemia. *Sudden withdrawal may be
fatal.*

INTERACTIONS
Barbiturates, phenytoin, rifampin: decreased corticosteroid effect. Corticosteroid dose may need to be increased.
Indomethacin, aspirin: increased risk
of GI distress and bleeding. Give together cautiously.

NURSING CONSIDERATIONS
• Contraindicated in systemic fungal
infections. Use cautiously in GI ulceration or renal disease, hypertension,
osteoporosis, varicella, vaccinia, exanthema, diabetes mellitus, Cushing's
syndrome, thromboembolic disorders,
seizures, myasthenia gravis, metastatic cancer, CHF, tuberculosis, ocular herpes simplex, hypoalbuminemia, emotional instability, and psychotic tendencies.
• Don't confuse with prednisone.
• Gradually reduce drug dosage after
long-term therapy. Tell patient not to
discontinue drug abruptly or without
doctor's consent.
• Always titrate to lowest effective
dose.
• A glucocorticoid with slight mineralocorticoid action.
• Prednisolone salts (acetate, sodium
phosphate, and tebutate) are used parenterally less often than other corticosteroids that have more potent anti-inflammatory action.
• May be used for alternate-day therapy.
• Monitor patient's weight, blood
pressure, and serum electrolytes.
• May mask or exacerbate infections.
Tell patient to report slow healing.
• Instruct patient to carry a card identifying his need for supplemental systemic glucocorticoids during stress.
• Teach patient signs of early adrenal
insufficiency: fatigue, muscular
weakness, joint pain, fever, anorexia,

nausea, dyspnea, dizziness, and fainting.
• Watch for depression or psychotic
episodes, especially in high-dose therapy.
• Patients with diabetes may need increased insulin; monitor blood glucose.
• Give I.M. injection deep into gluteal muscle. Avoid S.C. injection, as
atrophy and sterile abscesses may occur.
• Unless contraindicated, give low-
sodium diet high in potassium and
protein. Potassium supplement may
be needed.
• Give P.O. dose with food when possible to reduce GI irritation.
• Warn patients on long-term therapy
about cushingoid symptoms.
• Acetate form not for I.V. use.
• Watch for additional potassium depletion from diuretics and amphotericin B.
• Immunizations may show decreased antibody response.

prednisone
Apo-Prednisone†, Deltasone,
Liquid Pred*, Meticorten, Novo-
prednisone†, Orasone, Panafcort‡,
Panasol, Prednicen-M, Prednisone
Intensol*, Sone‡, Sterapred,
Winpred†

Pregnancy Risk Category: B

HOW SUPPLIED
Tablets: 1 mg, 2.5 mg, 5 mg, 10 mg,
20 mg, 25 mg, 50 mg
Oral solution: 5 mg/5 ml*, 5 mg/ml
(concentrate)*
Syrup: 5 mg/5 ml*

MECHANISM OF ACTION
Decreases inflammation, mainly by
stabilizing leukocyte lysosomal membranes. Also suppresses the immune
response, stimulates bone marrow,
and influences protein, fat, and carbohydrate metabolism.

INDICATIONS & DOSAGE

Severe inflammation or immunosuppression—
Adults: 2.5 to 15 mg P.O. b.i.d., t.i.d., or q.i.d. Maintenance dosage given once daily or every other day. Dosage must be individualized.
Children: 0.14 to 2 mg/kg P.O. daily divided q.i.d.
Acute exacerbations of multiple sclerosis—
Adults: 200 mg P.O. daily for 1 week, then 80 mg every other day for 1 month.

ADVERSE REACTIONS

Most adverse reactions of corticosteroids are dose- or duration-dependent.
CNS: *euphoria, insomnia,* psychotic behavior, pseudotumor cerebri.
CV: *CHF,* hypertension, edema.
EENT: cataracts, glaucoma.
GI: *peptic ulcer,* GI irritation, increased appetite.
Metabolic: *possible hypokalemia, hyperglycemia and carbohydrate intolerance,* growth suppression in children.
Skin: delayed wound healing, acne, various skin eruptions.
Other: muscle weakness, pancreatitis, hirsutism, susceptibility to infections. Acute adrenal insufficiency may occur with increased stress (infection, surgery, or trauma) or abrupt withdrawal after long-term therapy. *Withdrawal symptoms:* rebound inflammation, fatigue, weakness, arthralgia, fever, dizziness, lethargy, depression, fainting, orthostatic hypotension, dyspnea, anorexia, hypoglycemia. *Sudden withdrawal may be fatal.*

INTERACTIONS

Barbiturates, phenytoin, rifampin: decreased corticosteroid effect. Corticosteroid dose may need to be increased.
Indomethacin, aspirin: increased risk of GI distress and bleeding. Give together cautiously.

NURSING CONSIDERATIONS

• Contraindicated in systemic fungal infections. Use cautiously in GI ulceration or renal disease, hypertension, osteoporosis, varicella, vaccinia, exanthema, diabetes mellitus, Cushing's syndrome, thromboembolic disorders, seizures, myasthenia gravis, metastatic cancer, CHF, tuberculosis, ocular herpes simplex, hypoalbuminemia, emotional instability, and psychotic tendencies.
• Don't confuse with prednisolone.
• Gradually reduce drug dosage after long-term therapy. Tell patient not to discontinue drug abruptly or without doctor's consent.
• Always titrate to lowest effective dose.
• Monitor patient's blood pressure, sleep patterns, and serum potassium.
• Weigh patient daily; report sudden weight gain to doctor.
• May mask or exacerbate infections. Tell patient to report slow healing.
• Instruct patient to carry a card identifying his need for supplemental systemic glucocorticoids during stress.
• Give a daily dosage in the morning for better results and less toxicity.
• Teach patient signs of early adrenal insufficiency: fatigue, muscular weakness, joint pain, fever, anorexia, nausea, dyspnea, dizziness, and fainting.
• Watch for depression or psychotic episodes, especially in high-dose therapy.
• Patients with diabetes may need increased insulin; monitor blood glucose.
• Monitor growth in infants and children on long-term therapy.
• Unless contraindicated, give low-sodium diet high in potassium and protein. Potassium supplement may be needed.
• Unless contraindicated, give P.O.

Italicized adverse reactions are common or life-threatening.
*Liquid form contains alcohol.   **May contain tartrazine.

dose with food when possible to reduce GI irritation.
- May be used for alternate-day therapy.
- Watch for additional potassium depletion from diuretics and amphotericin B.
- Warn patients on long-term therapy about cushingoid symptoms.
- Immunizations may show decreased antibody response.

---

triamcinolone
Aristocort, Atolone, Kenacort**, Tricilone

triamcinolone acetonide
Cenocort A, Cinonide, Kenaject, Kenalog, Kenalone, Tramacort, Triam-A, Triamonide, Tri-Kort, Trilog

triamcinolone diacetate
Amcort, Aristocort Forte, Aristocort Intralesional, Articulose-L.A., Cenocort Forte, Cinalone, Kenacort, Triam-Forte, Trilone, Tristoject

triamcinolone hexacetonide
Aristospan Intra-articular, Aristospan Intralesional

Pregnancy Risk Category: C

HOW SUPPLIED
triamcinolone
Tablets: 1 mg, 2 mg, 4 mg, 8 mg
Syrup: 2 mg/ml, 4 mg/ml
triamcinolone acetonide
Injection (suspension): 10 mg/ml, 40 mg/ml
triamcinolone diacetate
Injection (suspension): 25 mg/ml, 40 mg/ml
triamcinolone hexacetonide
Injection (suspension): 5 mg/ml, 20 mg/ml
Oral inhalation aerosol: 100 mcg/metered spray, 240 doses/inhaler

MECHANISM OF ACTION
Decreases inflammation, mainly by stabilizing leukocyte lysosomal membranes. Also suppresses the immune response, stimulates bone marrow, and influences protein, fat, and carbohydrate metabolism.

INDICATIONS & DOSAGE
Severe inflammation or immunosuppression—
Adults: 4 to 48 mg P.O. daily divided b.i.d., t.i.d., or q.i.d., or 40 mg I.M. (diacetate or acetonide) weekly; or 5 to 48 mg (diacetate or acetonide) into lesions; or 2 to 40 mg (diacetate or acetonide) into joints and soft tissue; or up to 0.5 mg (hexacetonide) per square inch of affected skin intralesional; or 2 to 20 mg (hexacetonide) intra-articular or intrasynovial into soft tissue or into joint or lesion. Often, a local anesthetic is injected into the joint with triamcinolone.
Steroid-dependent asthma—
Adults: 2 inhalations t.i.d. to q.i.d. Maximum 16 inhalations daily.
Children 6 to 12 years: 1 to 2 inhalations t.i.d. to q.i.d. Maximum 12 inhalations daily.

ADVERSE REACTIONS
Most adverse reactions of corticosteroids are dose- or duration-dependent.
CNS: *euphoria, insomnia,* psychotic behavior, pseudotumor cerebri.
CV: *CHF,* hypertension, edema.
EENT: cataracts, glaucoma.
GI: *peptic ulcer,* GI irritation, increased appetite.
Metabolic: *possible hypokalemia, hyperglycemia and carbohydrate intolerance,* growth suppression in children.
Skin: delayed wound healing, acne, various skin eruptions.
Other: muscle weakness, pancreatitis, hirsutism, susceptibility to infections. Acute adrenal insufficiency may occur with increased stress (in-

---

†Available in Canada only.   ‡Available in Australia only.   ◊ Available OTC.

fection, surgery, or trauma) or abrupt withdrawal after long-term therapy. *Withdrawal symptoms:* rebound inflammation, fatigue, weakness, arthralgia, fever, dizziness, lethargy, depression, fainting, orthostatic hypotension, dyspnea, anorexia, hypoglycemia. *Sudden withdrawal may be fatal.*
Inhalation:
EENT: hoarseness, fungal infections of mouth and throat.
GI: dry mouth.

INTERACTIONS
Systemic:
Barbiturates, phenytoin, rifampin: decreased corticosteroid effect. Corticosteroid dose may need to be increased.
Indomethacin, aspirin: increased risk of GI distress and bleeding. Give together cautiously.

NURSING CONSIDERATIONS
Systemic:
• Contraindicated in systemic fungal infections. Use cautiously in GI ulceration or renal disease, hypertension, osteoporosis, varicella, vaccinia, exanthema, diabetes mellitus, Cushing's syndrome, thromboembolic disorders, seizures, myasthenia gravis, metastatic cancer, CHF, tuberculosis, ocular herpes simplex, hypoalbuminemia, emotional instability, and psychotic tendencies.
• Gradually reduce drug dosage after long-term therapy. Tell patient not to discontinue drug abruptly or without doctor's consent.
• Always titrate to lowest effective dose.
• Monitor patient's weight, blood pressure, and serum electrolytes.
• May mask or exacerbate infections. Tell patient to report slow healing.
• Instruct patient to carry a card identifying his need for supplemental systemic glucocorticoids during stress.

• Give a daily dosage in the morning for better results and less toxicity.
• Teach patient signs of early adrenal insufficiency: fatigue, muscular weakness, joint pain, fever, anorexia, nausea, dyspnea, dizziness, and fainting.
• Watch for depression or psychotic episodes, especially in high-dose therapy.
• Patients with diabetes may need increased insulin; monitor blood glucose.
• Give I.M. injection deep into gluteal muscle.
• Unless contraindicated, give low-sodium diet high in potassium and protein. Potassium supplement may be needed. Watch for additional potassium depletion from diuretics and amphotericin B.
• Give P.O. dose with food when possible to reduce GI irritation.
• Don't use diluents that contain preservatives. Flocculation may occur.
• Warn patients on long-term therapy about cushingoid symptoms.
• Immunizations may show decreased antibody response.
• Not used for alternate-day therapy.
• Parenteral form is *not* for I.V. use.
Inhalation:
• Contraindicated in status asthmaticus. Not for use in asthma controlled by bronchodilators or other noncorticosteroids alone, or for nonasthmatic bronchial diseases.
• Oral therapy should be tapered slowly.
• Instruct patient to carry a card indicating his need for supplemental systemic glucocorticoids during stress.
• Patient requiring bronchodilator should use it several minutes before triamcinolone.
• Tell patient to allow 1 minute to elapse before repeat inhalations, and hold breath for a few seconds to enhance action of drug.
• Inform patient that triamcinolone

Italicized adverse reactions are common or life-threatening.
*Liquid form contains alcohol.   **May contain tartrazine.

doesn't provide relief for emergency asthma attacks.
• Instruct patient to contact doctor if he notices a decreased response. Dose may have to be adjusted. Patient shouldn't exceed recommended dose on his own.
• Check mucous membranes frequently for signs of fungal infection. Tell patient to follow inhalations with glass of water to help prevent fungal infections.
• Tell patient to keep inhaler clean and unobstructed. Wash with warm water and dry thoroughly after use.

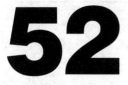

52

Androgens and anabolic steroids

danazol
ethylestrenol
fluoxymesterone
methyltestosterone
nandrolone decanoate
nandrolone phenpropionate
oxandrolone
oxymetholone
stanozolol
testosterone
testosterone cypionate
testosterone enanthate
testosterone propionate

COMBINATION PRODUCTS
DELADUMONE : testosterone enanthate 90 mg/ml, estradiol valerate 4
mg/ml, and chlorobutanol 0.5% in sesame oil.
DEPO-TESTADIOL (oil): testosterone
cypionate 50 mg, estradiol cypionate
2 mg, and chlorobutanol 0.5%.
DITATE-DS: estradiol valerate 8 mg,
and testosterone enanthate 180 mg.
ESTRATEST: esterified estrogens 1.25
mg, and methyltestosterone 2.5 mg.
ESTRATEST H.S.: esterified estrogens
0.625 mg, and methyltestosterone
1.25 mg.
HALODRIN: fluoxymesterone 1 mg
with ethinyl estradiol 0.02 mg
PREMARIN WITH METHYLTESTOSTER-
ONE: conjugated estrogens 0.625 mg
and methyltestosterone 5 mg.

---

danazol
Cycloment†, Danocrine
Pregnancy Risk Category: C

HOW SUPPLIED
Capsules: 50 mg, 100 mg, 200 mg

MECHANISM OF ACTION
Gonadotropin inhibitor that suppresses the pituitary-ovarian axis.
Also acts on estrogen receptors to inhibit estrogenic effects.

INDICATIONS & DOSAGE
Mild endometriosis—
Women: initially, 100 to 200 mg P.O.
b.i.d. Subsequent dosage based upon
patient response.
Moderate to severe endometriosis—
Women: 400 mg P.O. b.i.d. uninterrupted for 3 to 6 months; may continue for 9 months.
Fibrocystic breast disease—
Women: 100 to 400 mg P.O. daily in
2 divided doses uninterrupted for 2 to
6 months.
*Prevention of hereditary angio-
edema—*
Adults: 200 mg P.O. 2 to 3 times a
day, continued until favorable response is achieved. Then dosage
should be decreased by half at 1- to 3-
month intervals.

ADVERSE REACTIONS
Androgenic: in women—acne,
edema, *weight gain, hirsutism,*
hoarseness, clitoral enlargement, *decrease in breast size,* changes in li-

---

bido, male pattern baldness, *oiliness of skin or hair*.
Blood: thrombocytopenia.
CNS: dizziness, headache, sleep disorders, fatigue, tremor, irritability, excitation, lethargy, mental depression, chills, paresthesias.
CV: elevated blood pressure.
EENT: visual disturbances.
GI: gastric irritation, nausea, vomiting, diarrhea, constipation, change in appetite.
GU: hematuria.
Hepatic: reversible jaundice.
Hypoestrogenic: flushing; sweating; vaginitis, including itching, dryness, burning, and vaginal bleeding; nervousness, emotional lability, menstrual irregularities.
Other: muscle cramps or spasms.

INTERACTIONS
None significant.

NURSING CONSIDERATIONS
• Contraindicated in undiagnosed abnormal genital bleeding; impaired renal, cardiac, or hepatic function. Use cautiously in epilepsy or migraine headache.
• Use with diet high in calories and protein unless contraindicated.
• Monitor closely for signs of virilization. Some androgenic effects, such as deepening of voice, may not be reversible upon discontinuation of drug.
• Advise patient who is taking danazol for fibrocystic disease to examine breasts regularly. If breast nodule enlarges during treatment, tell patient to call doctor immediately.
• Instruct patient to wear cotton underwear only.
• Washing after intercourse is recommended to decrease the risk of vaginitis.
• Has been used investigationally with impressive results in treating hemophilia and Christmas disease; has also been used to decrease symptoms of systemic lupus erythematosus in

women and to treat gynecomastia in men.

---

ethylestrenol
(ethyloestrenol)
Maxibolin*, Orabolin‡

Pregnancy Risk Category: X

HOW SUPPLIED
Tablets: 2 mg
Elixir: 2 mg/5 ml

MECHANISM OF ACTION
Anabolic steroid that promotes tissue-building processes and reverses catabolism. Also stimulates erythropoiesis.

INDICATIONS & DOSAGE
Promote weight gain and combat tissue depletion, refractory anemias, catabolic effects of corticosteroid therapy, osteoporosis, prolonged immobilization, and debilitated states—
Adults: 4 to 8 mg P.O. daily, reduced to minimum levels at first evidence of clinical response.
Children: 1 to 3 mg P.O. daily; dosage is highly individualized.
    A single course of therapy in both adults and children should not exceed 6 weeks; may be reinstituted after 4-week interval.

ADVERSE REACTIONS
Androgenic: in women—*acne, edema, oily skin, weight gain, hirsutism, hoarseness,* clitoral enlargement, changes in libido. In men—prepubertal: premature epiphyseal closure, acne, priapism, growth of body and facial hair, phallic enlargement; postpubertal: testicular atrophy, oligospermia, decreased ejaculatory volume, impotence, gynecomastia, epididymitis.
CV: edema.
GI: gastroenteritis, nausea, vomiting, diarrhea, constipation, change in appetite.
GU: bladder irritability.

Hepatic: reversible jaundice, hepato-toxicity.
Hypoestrogenic: in women—flushing; sweating; vaginitis with itching, drying, burning, or bleeding; menstrual irregularities.
Other: hypercalcemia.

INTERACTIONS
None significant.

NURSING CONSIDERATIONS
• Contraindicated in prostatic hypertrophy with obstruction; carcinoma of male breast; hypercalcemia; prostatic cancer; cardiac, hepatic, or renal decompensation; nephrosis; and in premature infants. Use cautiously in prepubertal males; patients with diabetes or coronary disease; patients taking ACTH, corticosteroids, or anticoagulants.
• Hypercalcemia symptoms may be difficult to distinguish from symptoms of condition being treated unless anticipated and thought of as a symptom cluster. Hypercalcemia is particularly likely to occur in patients with metastatic breast cancer and may indicate bone metastases.
• Tell women to report menstrual irregularities; therapy should be discontinued pending etiologic determination.
• Watch for signs of virilization; may be irreversible despite prompt discontinuation of therapy. Doctor must decide if benefits outweigh effects.
• Closely monitor boys under 7 years for precocious development of male sexual characteristics.
• In children: therapy should be preceded by X-ray of wrist bones to establish level of bone maturation. During treatment, bone maturation may proceed more rapidly than linear growth; dosage should be intermittent and X-rays taken periodically.
• Edema is generally controllable with salt restriction or diuretics. Monitor weight routinely.

• Watch for symptoms of jaundice. Dosage adjustment may reverse condition. If liver function tests are abnormal, discontinue therapy.
• Observe patient on concomitant anticoagulant therapy for ecchymotic areas, petechiae, or abnormal bleeding. Monitor prothrombin time.
• Watch for symptoms of hypoglycemia in patients with diabetes. Dosage of antidiabetic drug may need adjustment.
• Use with diet high in calories and protein unless contraindicated. Give small, frequent feedings.
• Take with food or meals if GI upset occurs.
• Anabolic steroids may alter many laboratory studies during therapy and for 2 to 3 weeks after therapy is stopped.
• Involve the patient, family members, and a dietitian in developing a dietary regimen suitable to the anorexic or debilitated patient.

---

fluoxymesterone
Android F, Halotestin**, Ora-Testryl
Pregnancy Risk Category: X

HOW SUPPLIED
Tablets: 2 mg, 5 mg, 10 mg

MECHANISM OF ACTION
Stimulates target tissues to develop normally in androgen-deficient men.

INDICATIONS & DOSAGE
Hypogonadism and impotence caused by testicular deficiency—
Adults: 2 to 10 mg P.O. daily.
Palliation of breast cancer in women—
Adults: 15 to 30 mg P.O. daily in divided doses. All dosages should be individualized and reduced to minimum when effect is noted.
Postpartum breast engorgement—
Adults: 2.5 mg P.O. followed by 5 to 10 mg daily for 5 days.

Italicized adverse reactions are common or life-threatening.
*Liquid form contains alcohol.   **May contain tartrazine.

ADVERSE REACTIONS

Androgenic: in women—*acne, edema, oily skin, weight gain, hirsutism, hoarseness,* clitoral enlargement, change in libido. In men—prepubertal: premature epiphyseal closure, acne, priapism, growth of body and facial hair, phallic enlargement; postpubertal: testicular atrophy, oligospermia, decreased ejaculatory volume, impotence, gynecomastia, epididymitis.

CV: edema.

GI: gastroenteritis, nausea, vomiting, constipation, change in appetite, diarrhea.

GU: bladder irritability.

Hepatic: reversible jaundice.

Hypoestrogenic: in women—flushing; sweating; vaginitis with itching, drying, burning, or bleeding; menstrual irregularities; emotional lability.

Other: hypercalcemia.

INTERACTIONS

None significant.

NURSING CONSIDERATIONS

• Contraindicated in prostatic hypertrophy with obstruction; carcinoma of male breast; prostatic cancer; cardiac, hepatic, or renal decompensation; nephrosis; hypercalcemia; and in premature infants. Use cautiously in prepubertal males; patients with diabetes or coronary disease; and patients taking ACTH, corticosteroids, or anticoagulants.

• Hypercalcemia symptoms may be difficult to distinguish from symptoms associated with condition being treated unless anticipated and thought of as a symptom cluster. Hypercalcemia is particularly likely to occur in patients with metastatic breast cancer and may indicate bone metastases.

• Explain to patient on drug for palliation of breast cancer that virilization usually occurs at dosage used. Give emotional support. Tell patient to report androgenic effects immediately. Stopping drug will prevent further androgenic changes but will probably not reverse those already existing.

• When used in breast cancer, subjective effects may not be seen for about 1 month; objective symptoms not for 3 months.

• Tell women to report menstrual irregularities; therapy should be discontinued pending etiologic determination.

• Edema is generally controllable with salt restriction or diuretics. Monitor weight routinely.

• Watch for symptoms of jaundice. Dosage adjustment may reverse condition. If liver function tests are abnormal, therapy should be stopped.

• Observe patient on concomitant anticoagulant therapy for ecchymotic areas, petechiae, or abnormal bleeding. Monitor prothrombin time.

• Watch for symptoms of hypoglycemia in patients with diabetes. Dosage of antidiabetic drug may need adjustment.

• Use with diet high in calories and protein unless contraindicated. Give small, frequent feedings.

• Take with food or meals if GI upset occurs.

---

methyltestosterone

Android, Metandren**, Metandren Linguets, Oreton Methyl, Testomet‡, Testred, Virilon

Pregnancy Risk Category: X

HOW SUPPLIED

Tablets: 5 mg‡, 10 mg, 25 mg, 50 mg‡
Tablets (buccal): 5 mg, 10 mg
Capsules: 10 mg

MECHANISM OF ACTION

Stimulates target tissues to develop normally in androgen-deficient males.

INDICATIONS & DOSAGE

Breast engorgement of nonnursing mothers—
Adults: 80 mg P.O. daily, or 40 mg buccal daily for 3 to 5 days.
Breast cancer in women 1 to 5 years postmenopausal—
Adults: 200 mg P.O. daily; or 100 mg buccal daily.
Eunuchoidism and eunuchism, male climacteric symptoms—
Adults: 10 to 40 mg P.O. daily; or 5 to 20 mg buccal daily.
Postpubertal cryptorchidism—
Adults: 30 mg P.O. daily; or 15 mg buccal daily.

ADVERSE REACTIONS

Androgenic: in women—*acne, edema, oily skin, weight gain, hirsutism, hoarseness,* clitoral enlargement, changes in libido. In men—prepubertal: premature epiphyseal closure, acne, priapism, growth of body and facial hair, phallic enlargement; postpubertal: testicular atrophy, oligospermia, decreased ejaculatory volume, impotence, gynecomastia, epididymitis.
CV: edema.
GI: gastroenteritis, constipation, nausea, vomiting, diarrhea, change in appetite.
GU: bladder irritability.
Hepatic: reversible jaundice.
Hypoestrogenic: in women—flushing; sweating; vaginitis with itching, drying, burning, or bleeding; menstrual irregularities.
Local: irritation of oral mucosa with buccal administration.
Other: hypercalcemia.

INTERACTIONS

None significant.

NURSING CONSIDERATIONS

• Contraindicated in women of childbearing potential (possible masculinization of female infant); in elderly, asthenic men who may react adversely to androgen overstimulation; in hypercalcemia; cardiac, hepatic, or renal decompensation; prostatic or breast cancer in men; benign prostatic hypertrophy with obstruction; conditions aggravated by fluid retention; hypertension; and in premature infants. Use cautiously in myocardial infarction or coronary artery disease.
• Treatment of breast cancer usually restricted to patients 1 to 5 years postmenopausal.
• Edema is generally controllable with salt restriction or diuretics.
• Periodic serum cholesterol and calcium determinations, and cardiac and liver function tests recommended. Usually only used for intermittent therapy. Because of the potential for hepatotoxicity, watch closely for jaundice.
• In metastatic breast cancer, hypercalcemia may indicate progression of bone metastases. Report signs of hypercalcemia.
• Therapeutic response in breast cancer is usually apparent within 3 months. Therapy should be stopped if signs of disease progression appear.
• Enhances hypoglycemia; teach patient signs of hypoglycemia, and instruct him to report immediately if they occur.
• Watch for ecchymoses, petechiae, and abnormal bleeding in patients receiving concomitant anticoagulants.
• Promptly report signs of virilization in women.
• Use with diet high in calories and protein unless contraindicated. Give small, frequent feedings.
• Buccal tablets twice as potent as oral tablets. Tell patient to avoid eating, drinking, chewing, or smoking while buccal tablet is in place, and that tablet is not to be swallowed. Place in upper or lower buccal pouch between cheek and gum. Tablet requires 30 to 60 minutes to dissolve. Instruct patient to change tablet ab-

---

Italicized adverse reactions are common or life-threatening.
*Liquid form contains alcohol.   **May contain tartrazine.

sorption site with each dose to minimize risk of buccal irritation.
• Erroneously thought to enhance athletic ability.

nandrolone decanoate
Anabolin LA, Androlone-D, Deca-Durabolin, Decolone, Hybolin Decanoate, Kabolin, Nandrobolic L.A., Neo-Durabolic

nandrolone phenpropionate
Anabolin IM, Androlone, Durabolin, Hybolin Improved, Nandrobolic

Pregnancy Risk Category: X

HOW SUPPLIED
decanoate
Injection (in oil): 50 mg/ml, 100 mg/ml, 200 mg/ml
phenpropionate
Injection (in oil): 25 mg/ml, 50 mg/ml

MECHANISM OF ACTION
Anabolic steroid that promotes tissue-building processes and reverses catabolism. Also stimulates erythropoiesis.

INDICATIONS & DOSAGE
Severe debility or disease states, refractory anemias (decanoate)—
Adults: 100 to 200 mg I.M. weekly. Therapy should be intermittent.
Tissue-building (decanoate)—
Adults: 50 to 100 mg I.M. q 3 to 4 weeks.
Children 2 to 13 years: 25 to 50 mg I.M. q 3 to 4 weeks.
Control of metastatic breast cancer (phenpropionate)—
Adults: 25 to 50 mg I.M. weekly.
Children 2 to 13 years: 12.5 to 25 mg I.M. every 2 to 4 weeks.

ADVERSE REACTIONS
Androgenic: in women—*acne, edema, oily skin, weight gain, hirsutism, hoarseness,* clitoral enlargement, decreased or increased libido. In men—prepubertal: premature epiphyseal closure, acne, priapism, growth of body and facial hair, phallic enlargement; postpubertal: testicular atrophy, oligospermia, decreased ejaculatory volume, impotence, gynecomastia, epididymitis.
CV: edema.
GI: gastroenteritis, nausea, vomiting, diarrhea, change in appetite.
GU: bladder irritability.
Hepatic: reversible jaundice, hepatotoxicity.
Hypoestrogenic: in women—flushing; sweating; vaginitis with itching, drying, burning, or bleeding; menstrual irregularities with large doses.
Local: pain at injection site, induration.
Other: hypercalcemia, hypercalciuria.

INTERACTIONS
None significant.

NURSING CONSIDERATIONS
• Contraindicated in prostatic hypertrophy with obstruction; male breast and prostatic cancer; cardiac, hepatic, or renal decompensation; nephrosis; and in premature infants. Use cautiously in prepubertal males; patients with diabetes or coronary disease; patients taking ACTH, corticosteroids, or anticoagulants.
• Inject drug deep I.M., preferably into upper outer quadrant of gluteal muscle in adults.
• Hypercalcemia is most likely to occur in patients with mammary carcinoma; these patients should have quantitative urine and serum calcium level determinations.
• Tell women to report menstrual irregularities; therapy should be discontinued pending etiologic determination.
• Watch for signs of virilization; they may be irreversible despite prompt discontinuation of therapy.
• Closely observe boys under 7 years

for precocious development of male sexual characteristics.
- In children, therapy should be preceded by X-ray of wrist bones to establish level of bone maturation. During treatment, bone maturation may proceed more rapidly than linear growth; dosage should be intermittent and X-rays taken periodically.
- Edema is generally controllable with salt restrictions or diuretics.
- Watch for symptoms of jaundice. Dosage adjustment may reverse condition. If liver function tests are abnormal, therapy should be stopped.
- Observe patients receiving concomitant anticoagulant therapy for ecchymotic areas, petechiae, or abnormal bleeding. Monitor prothrombin time.
- Watch for symptoms of hypoglycemia in patients with diabetes. Dosage of antidiabetic drug may need adjustment.
- Use with diet high in calories and protein unless contraindicated. Give small, frequent feedings.
- Erroneously thought to enhance athletic ability.
- Considered an adjunctive therapy.
- Anabolic steroids may alter many laboratory studies during therapy and for 2 to 3 weeks after therapy is stopped.

---

oxandrolone
Anavar, Lonavar‡

Pregnancy Risk Category: X

HOW SUPPLIED
Tablets: 2.5 mg

MECHANISM OF ACTION
Anabolic steroid that promotes tissue-building processes and reverses catabolism. Also stimulates erythropoiesis.

INDICATIONS & DOSAGE
To combat catabolic effects of corticosteroid therapy, osteoporosis, pro-longed immobilization and debilitated states—
Adults: 2.5 mg P.O. b.i.d., t.i.d., or q.i.d.; up to 20 mg daily for 2 to 4 weeks.
Children: 0.25 mg/kg daily P.O. for 2 to 4 weeks.
Continuous therapy should not exceed 3 months.

ADVERSE REACTIONS
Androgenic: in women—*acne, edema, oily skin, weight gain, hirsutism, hoarseness,* clitoral enlargement, decreased or increased libido. In men—prepubertal: premature epiphyseal closure, acne, priapism, growth of body and facial hair, phallic enlargement; postpubertal: testicular atrophy, oligospermia, decreased ejaculatory volume, impotence, gynecomastia, epididymitis.
CV: edema.
GI: gastroenteritis, nausea, vomiting, constipation or diarrhea, change in appetite.
GU: bladder irritability.
Hepatic: reversible jaundice, hepatotoxicity.
Hypoestrogenic: in women—flushing; sweating; vaginitis with itching, drying, burning, or bleeding; menstrual irregularities.
Other: hypercalcemia.

INTERACTIONS
None significant.

NURSING CONSIDERATIONS
- Contraindicated in prostatic hypertrophy with obstruction; prostatic and male breast cancer; cardiac, hepatic, or renal decompensation; nephrosis; and in premature infants. Use cautiously in prepubertal males; patients with diabetes or coronary disease; patients taking ACTH, corticosteroids, or anticoagulants.
- Hypercalcemia symptoms may be difficult to distinguish from symptoms of condition being treated unless

---

Italicized adverse reactions are common or life-threatening.
*Liquid form contains alcohol.   **May contain tartrazine.

anticipated and thought of as a cluster. Hypercalcemia most likely to occur with metastatic breast cancer and may indicate bone metastases.

• Tell women to report menstrual irregularities; therapy should be discontinued pending etiologic determination.

• Watch for signs of virilization; may be irreversible despite prompt discontinuation of therapy. Doctor must decide if benefits outweigh effects.

• Boys under 7 years should be closely observed for precocious development of male sexual characteristics.

• In children, therapy should be preceded by X-ray of wrist bones to establish level of bone maturation. During treatment, bone maturation may proceed more rapidly than linear growth; dosage should be intermittent and X-rays taken periodically.

• Edema is generally controllable with salt restriction or diuretics. Monitor weight routinely.

• Watch for symptoms of jaundice. Dosage adjustment may reverse condition. Periodic liver function tests are recommended.

• Observe patient on concomitant anticoagulant therapy for ecchymotic areas, petechiae, or abnormal bleeding. Monitor prothrombin time.

• Watch for symptoms of hypoglycemia in patients with diabetes. Dosage of antidiabetic drug may need adjustment.

• Use with diet high in calories and protein unless contraindicated. Give small, frequent feedings.

• Take with food or meals if GI upset occurs.

• Erroneously thought to enhance athletic ability.

• Anabolic steroids may alter many laboratory studies during therapy and for 2 to 3 weeks after therapy is stopped.

oxymetholone
Anadrol-50, Anapolon†, Anapolon 50†‡

Pregnancy Risk Category: X

HOW SUPPLIED
Tablets: 50 mg

MECHANISM OF ACTION
Anabolic steroid that promotes tissue-building processes and reverses catabolism. Also stimulates erythropoiesis.

INDICATIONS & DOSAGE
Aplastic anemia—
Adults and children: 1 to 5 mg/kg P.O. daily. Dosage highly individualized; response not immediate. Trial of 3 to 6 months required.
Osteoporosis, catabolic conditions—
Adults: 5 to 15 mg P.O. daily, or up to 30 mg P.O. daily.
Children over 6 years: up to 10 mg P.O. daily.
Children under 6 years: 1.25 mg P.O. daily or up to q.i.d. Continuous therapy should not exceed 30 days in children; 90 days in any patient.

ADVERSE REACTIONS
Androgenic: in women—*acne, edema, oily skin, weight gain, hirsutism, hoarseness,* clitoral enlargement, decreased or increased libido, male pattern baldness. In men—prepubertal: premature epiphyseal closure, acne, priapism, growth of body and facial hair, phallic enlargement; postpubertal: testicular atrophy, oligospermia, decreased ejaculatory volume, impotence, gynecomastia, epididymitis.
CV: edema.
GI: gastroenteritis, nausea, vomiting, constipation, diarrhea, change in appetite.
GU: bladder irritability.
Hepatic: reversible jaundice, hepatotoxicity.
Hypoestrogenic: in women—flush-

ing; sweating; vaginitis with itching, drying, burning, or bleeding; menstrual irregularities.
Other: hypercalcemia.

INTERACTIONS
None significant.

NURSING CONSIDERATIONS
• Contraindicated in prostatic hypertrophy with obstruction; prostatic and male breast cancer; cardiac, hepatic, or renal decompensation; nephrosis; and in premature infants. Use cautiously in prepubertal males; patients with diabetes or coronary diseases; patients taking ACTH, corticosteroids, or anticoagulants.
• Hypercalcemia symptoms may be difficult to distinguish from symptoms of condition being treated unless anticipated and thought of as a cluster. Hypercalcemia most likely to occur in metastatic breast cancer and may indicate bone metastases.
• Supportive treatment of anemias (transfusions, correction of iron, folic acid, vitamin B_{12}, or pyridoxine deficiency). Give 3 to 6 months for response.
• Effects in osteoporosis usually seen in 4 to 6 weeks.
• Tell women to report menstrual irregularities; therapy should be discontinued pending etiologic determination.
• Watch for signs of virilization; may be irreversible despite prompt discontinuation of therapy. Doctor must decide if benefits outweigh effects.
• Boys under 7 years should be closely observed for precocious development of male sexual characteristics.
• In children, therapy should be preceded by X-ray of wrist bones to establish level of bone maturation. During treatment, bone maturation may proceed more rapidly than linear growth; dosage should be intermittent and X-rays taken periodically. Epiph-

yseal development may continue 6 months after stopping therapy.
• Edema is generally controllable with salt restriction or diuretics. Monitor weight routinely.
• Watch for symptoms of jaundice. Dosage adjustment may reverse condition; if liver function tests are abnormal, therapy should be stopped.
• Observe patient on concomitant anticoagulant therapy for ecchymotic areas, petechiae, or abnormal bleeding. Monitor prothrombin time.
• Watch for symptoms of hypoglycemia in patients with diabetes. Dosage of antidiabetic drug may need adjustment.
• Use with diet high in calories and protein unless contraindicated. Give small, frequent feedings.
• Take with food or meals if GI upset occurs.
• Erroneously thought to enhance athletic ability.
• Anabolic steroids may alter many laboratory studies during therapy and for 2 to 3 weeks after therapy is stopped.
• Has also been used to prevent hereditary angioedema.

---

stanozolol
Winstrol

Pregnancy Risk Category: X

HOW SUPPLIED
Tablets: 2 mg

MECHANISM OF ACTION
Anabolic steroid that promotes tissue-building processes and reverses catabolism. Also stimulates erythropoiesis.

INDICATIONS & DOSAGE
Prevention of hereditary angioedema—
Adults: 2 mg P.O. t.i.d. to 4 mg P.O. q.i.d for 5 days initially. Dosage is gradually reduced at intervals of 1 to 3 months to a dosage of 2 mg daily.

Children age 6 to 12: Administer up to 2 mg P.O. daily.
Children under age 6: 1 mg P.O. daily
Note: Stanozolol should be used in children only during an acute attack.

ADVERSE REACTIONS
Androgenic: in women—*acne, edema, oily skin, weight gain, hirsutism, hoarseness,* clitoral enlargement, decreased or increased libido. In men— prepubertal: premature epiphyseal closure, acne, priapism, growth of body and facial hair, phallic enlargement; postpubertal: testicular atrophy, oligospermia, decreased ejaculatory volume, impotence, gynecomastia, epididymitis.
CV: edema.
GI: gastroenteritis, nausea, vomiting, constipation, diarrhea, change in appetite.
GU: bladder irritability.
Hepatic: reversible jaundice, hepatotoxicity.
Hypoestrogenic: in women—flushing; sweating; vaginitis with itching, drying, burning or bleeding; menstrual irregularities.
Other: hypercalcemia.

INTERACTIONS
None significant.

NURSING CONSIDERATIONS
• Contraindicated in prostatic hypertrophy with obstruction; prostatic and male breast cancer; cardiac, hepatic, or renal decompensation; nephrosis; and in premature infants. Use cautiously in prepubertal males; patients with diabetes or coronary disease; patients taking ACTH, corticosteroids, or anticoagulants.
• A lower dosage in young women (2 mg b.i.d.) is recommended to avoid virilization. Watch for these adverse reactions; may be irreversible despite prompt discontinuation of therapy.

Doctor must decide if benefits outweigh adverse effects.
• Tell women to report menstrual irregularities; therapy should be discontinued pending etiologic determination.
• Boys under 7 years should be closely observed for precocious development of male sexual characteristics.
• In children, therapy should be preceded by X-ray of wrist bones to establish level of bone maturation. During treatment, bone maturation may proceed more rapidly than linear growth; dosage should be intermittent and X-rays taken periodically.
• Edema is generally controllable with salt restriction or diuretics. Monitor weight routinely.
• Watch for symptoms of jaundice. Dosage adjustment may reverse condition; check liver function tests regularly. If abnormal, therapy should be discontinued.
• Observe patient on concomitant anticoagulant therapy for ecchymotic areas, petechiae, or abnormal bleeding. Monitor prothrombin time.
• Watch for symptoms of hypoglycemia in patients with diabetes. Dosage of antidiabetic drug may need adjustment.
• Use with diet high in calories and protein unless contraindicated. Give small, frequent feedings.
• Administer before or with meals to minimize GI distress.
• Monitor serum cholesterol in cardiac patients.
• Erroneously thought to enhance athletic ability.
• Anabolic steroids may alter many laboratory studies during therapy and for 2 to 3 weeks after therapy is stopped.

---

†Available in Canada only.　　‡Available in Australia only.　　◊ Available OTC.

testosterone
Andro, Andronaq, Histerone, Malogen, Testaqua, Testoject

Pregnancy Risk Category: X

HOW SUPPLIED
Injection (aqueous suspension): 25 mg/ml, 50 mg/ml, 100 mg/ml
Pellets (sterile) for subcutaneous implantation: 75 mg

MECHANISM OF ACTION
Stimulates target tissues to develop normally in androgen-deficient men.

INDICATIONS & DOSAGE
Eunuchoidism, eunuchism, male climacteric symptoms—
Adults: 10 to 25 mg I.M. 2 to 5 times weekly.
Breast engorgement of nonnursing mothers—
25 to 50 mg I.M. daily for 3 to 4 days, starting at delivery.
Breast cancer in women 1 to 5 years postmenopausal—
100 mg I.M. 3 times weekly as long as improvement maintained.

ADVERSE REACTIONS
Androgenic: in women—*acne, edema, oily skin, weight gain, hirsutism, hoarseness,* clitoral enlargement, decreased or increased libido. In men—prepubertal: premature epiphyseal closure, acne, priapism, growth of body and facial hair, phallic enlargement; postpubertal: testicular atrophy, oligospermia, decreased ejaculatory volume, impotence, gynecomastia, epididymitis.
CV: edema.
GI: gastroenteritis, nausea, vomiting, constipation, diarrhea, change in appetite.
GU: bladder irritability.
Hepatic: reversible jaundice.
Hypoestrogenic: in women—flushing; sweating; vaginitis with itching, drying, burning, or bleeding; menstrual irregularities.
Local: pain at injection site, induration, irritation and sloughing with pellet implantation, edema.
Other: hypercalcemia.

INTERACTIONS
None significant.

NURSING CONSIDERATIONS
• Contraindicated in women of childbearing potential (possible masculinization of female infant); in elderly, asthenic men who may react adversely to androgen overstimulation; in hypercalcemia; cardiac, hepatic, or renal decompensation; prostatic or breast cancer in males; benign prostatic hypertrophy with obstruction; conditions aggravated by fluid retention; hypertension; and in premature infants. Use cautiously in myocardial infarction or coronary artery disease, and in prepubertal males.
• Periodic liver function tests should be performed.
• In metastatic breast cancer, hypercalcemia usually indicates progression of bone metastases. Report signs of hypercalcemia.
• Therapeutic response in breast cancer is usually apparent within 3 months. Stop therapy if signs of disease progression appear.
• Enhances hypoglycemia; tell patient to report signs of hyperinsulinism.
• Instruct men to report priapism, reduced ejaculatory volume, and gynecomastia. Withdraw drug if these occur.
• Report signs of virilization in females; reevaluate treatment.
• Monitor prepubertal men by X-ray for rate of bone maturation.
• Edema is generally controllable with salt restriction or diuretics. Monitor weight routinely.
• Use with diet high in calories and protein unless contraindicated. Give small, frequent feedings.

Italicized adverse reactions are common or life-threatening.
*Liquid form contains alcohol.   **May contain tartrazine.

• Store I.M. preparations at room temperature. If crystals appear, warming and shaking the bottle will usually disperse them.
• Inject deep into upper outer quadrant of gluteal muscle.
• Watch for ecchymotic areas, petechiae, or abnormal bleeding in patients on concomitant anticoagulant therapy. Monitor prothrombin time.
• Many laboratory studies may be altered during therapy and for 2 to 3 weeks after therapy is stopped.

testosterone cypionate
Andro-Cyp, Andronaq-LA, Andronate, dep Andro, Depotest, Depo-Testosterone, Duratest, T-Cypionate, Tesionate, Testa-C, Testoject-LA, Testred Cypionate, Virilon IM

testosterone enanthate
Android-T, Andro-LA, Andryl, Delatestryl, Durathate, Everone, Malogex†, Testone LA, Testrin PA

testosterone propionate
Malogen†, Testex

Pregnancy Risk Category: X

HOW SUPPLIED
cypionate
Injection (in oil): 50 mg/ml, 100 mg/ml, 200 mg/ml
enanthate
Injection (in oil): 100 mg/ml, 200 mg/ml
propionate
Injection (in oil): 25 mg/ml, 50 mg/ml, 100 mg/ml

MECHANISM OF ACTION
Stimulates target tissues to develop normally in androgen-deficient men.

INDICATIONS & DOSAGE
Eunuchism, eunuchoidism, deficiency after castration and male climacteric—

Adults: 200 to 400 mg (cypionate or enanthate) I.M. q 4 weeks.
Oligospermia—
Adults: 100 to 200 mg (cypionate or enanthate) I.M. q 4 to 6 weeks for development and maintenance of testicular function.
Eunuchism and eunuchoidism, male climacteric, impotence—
Adults: 10 to 25 mg (propionate) I.M. 2 to 4 times weekly.
Metastatic breast cancer in women—
50 to 100 mg (propionate) I.M. 3 times weekly. 200 to 400 mg (cypionate or enanthate) I.M. q 2 to 4 weeks.
Postmenopausal or primary osteoporosis—
Adults: 200 to 400 mg (enanthate) I.M. q 4 weeks.

ADVERSE REACTIONS
Androgenic: in women—*acne, edema, oily skin, weight gain, hirsutism, hoarseness,* clitoral enlargement, changes in libido. In men—prepubertal: premature epiphyseal closure, acne, priapism, growth of body and facial hair, phallic enlargement; postpubertal: testicular atrophy, oligospermia, decreased ejaculatory volume, impotence, gynecomastia, epididymitis.
CV: edema.
GI: gastroenteritis, nausea, vomiting, constipation, diarrhea, change in appetite.
GU: bladder irritability.
Hepatic: reversible jaundice.
Local: pain at injection site, induration, postinjection furunculosis.
Other: hypercalcemia.

INTERACTIONS
None significant.

NURSING CONSIDERATIONS
• Contraindicated in women of childbearing potential (possible masculinization of female infant); in patients with hypercalcemia; cardiac, hepatic,

or renal decompensation; prostatic or breast cancer in men; benign prostatic hypertrophy with obstruction; conditions aggravated by fluid retention; hypertension; elderly, asthenic men who may react adversely to androgen overstimulation; and in premature infants. Use cautiously in myocardial infarction or coronary artery disease, and in prepubertal males.

• Periodic liver function tests should be performed.

• In metastatic breast cancer, hypercalcemia usually indicates progression of bone metastases. Report signs of hypercalcemia.

• Response in breast cancer is usually apparent within 3 months. Stop therapy if signs of disease progression appear.

• Enhances hypoglycemia; teach signs of hypoglycemia, and instruct the patient to report immediately if they occur.

• Instruct men to report priapism, reduced ejaculatory volume, and gynecomastia. Withdraw drug.

• Watch for signs of ecchymoses, petechiae with concomitant anticoagulant therapy. Monitor prothrombin time.

• Inject deep into upper outer quadrant of gluteal muscle. Report soreness at site; possibility of postinjection furunculosis.

• Report signs of virilization in women; reevaluate treatment.

• Monitor prepubertal males by X-ray for rate of bone maturation.

• Edema is generally controllable with salt restriction or diuretics. Monitor weight routinely.

• Use with diet high in calories and protein unless contraindicated. Give small, frequent feedings.

• Daily requirements best administered in divided doses.

• May alter many laboratory studies during therapy and for 2 to 3 weeks after therapy is stopped.

Italicized adverse reactions are common or life-threatening.
*Liquid form contains alcohol.   **May contain tartrazine.

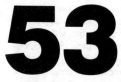

Estrogens and progestins

Estrogens
chlorotrianisene
dienestrol
diethylstilbestrol
diethylstilbestrol diphosphate
esterified estrogens
estradiol
estradiol cypionate
estradiol valerate
estrogens, conjugated
estrone
estropipate
ethinyl estradiol
quinestrol

Estrogen and progestin
ethinyl estradiol and
    ethynodiol diacetate
ethinyl estradiol and
    levonorgestrel
ethinyl estradiol and
    norethindrone
ethinyl estradiol and
    norethindrone acetate
ethinyl estradiol and
    norgestrel
ethinyl estradiol, norethindrone
    acetate, and ferrous fumarate
mestranol and norethindrone

Progestins
hydroxyprogesterone caproate
medroxyprogesterone acetate
norethindrone
norethindrone acetate
norgestrel
progesterone

COMBINATION PRODUCTS
MENRIUM 5-2: chlordiazepoxide 5 mg
and esterified estrogens 0.2 mg.
MENRIUM 5-4: chlordiazepoxide 5 mg
and esterified estrogens 0.4 mg.
MENRIUM 10-4: chlordiazepoxide
10 mg and esterified estrogens 0.4
mg.
MILPREM-200: conjugated estrogens
0.45 mg and meprobamate 200 mg.
MILPREM-400: conjugated estrogens
0.45 mg and meprobamate 400 mg.
PMB 200: conjugated estrogens 0.45
mg and meprobamate 200 mg.
PMB 400: conjugated estrogens 0.45
mg and meprobamate 400 mg.

chlorotrianisene
TACE**

Pregnancy Risk Category: X

HOW SUPPLIED
Capsules: 12 mg, 25 mg

MECHANISM OF ACTION
Increases the synthesis of DNA,
RNA, and protein in responsive tissues. Also reduces FSH and LH release from the pituitary.

INDICATIONS & DOSAGE
Prostatic cancer—
Men: 12 to 25 mg P.O. daily.
Atrophic vaginitis—
Women: 12 to 25 mg P.O. daily for 30
to 60 days.
Female hypogonadism—
Women: 12 to 25 mg P.O. for 21
days, followed by 1 dose of progester-
one 100 mg I.M. or 5 days of oral
progestogen given concurrently with
last 5 days of chlorotrianisene (for ex-

---

†Available in Canada only.   ‡Available in Australia only.   ◊ Available OTC.

ample, medroxyprogesterone 5 to 10 mg).

Menopausal symptoms—
Women: 12 to 25 mg P.O. daily for 30 days or cyclic (3 weeks on, 1 week off).

ADVERSE REACTIONS
CNS: headache, dizziness, chorea, migraine, depression, libido changes.
CV: thrombophlebitis; *thromboembolism;* hypertension; edema; *increased risk of stroke, pulmonary embolism, and myocardial infarction.*
EENT: worsening of myopia or astigmatism, intolerance to contact lenses.
GI: *nausea,* vomiting, abdominal cramps, bloating, diarrhea, constipation, anorexia, increased appetite, excessive thirst, weight changes, pancreatitis.
GU: in women—breakthrough bleeding, altered menstrual flow, dysmenorrhea, amenorrhea, cervical erosion or abnormal secretions, enlargement of uterine fibromas, vaginal candidiasis. In men—*gynecomastia, testicular atrophy, impotence.*
Hepatic: cholestatic jaundice.
Metabolic: hyperglycemia, hypercalcemia, folic acid deficiency.
Skin: melasma, urticaria, acne, seborrhea, oily skin, hirsutism or loss of hair.
Other: leg cramps, purpura, breast changes (tenderness, enlargement, secretion).

INTERACTIONS
None significant.

NURSING CONSIDERATIONS
• Contraindicated in thrombophlebitis or thromboembolic disorders; cancer of breast, reproductive organs, or genitals; undiagnosed abnormal genital bleeding; and pregnancy. Use cautiously in hypertension, asthma, mental depression, bone diseases, blood dyscrasias, gallbladder disease, migraine, seizures, diabetes mellitus, amenorrhea, heart failure, hepatic or renal dysfunction, and family history (mother, grandmother, sister) of breast or genital tract cancer. Development or worsening of these conditions may require discontinuation of the drug.

• Patient package insert that describes estrogen's adverse reactions is available. However, provide verbal explanation also.

• Warn patient to report immediately: abdominal pain; pain, numbness, or stiffness in legs or buttocks; pressure or pain in chest; shortness of breath; severe headaches; visual disturbances, such as blind spots, flashing lights, blurriness; vaginal bleeding or discharge; breast lumps; swelling of hands or feet; yellow skin and sclera; dark urine; and light-colored stools.

• Not used for menstrual disorders because duration of action is very long.

• Pathologist should be advised of estrogen therapy when specimen is sent.

• Patients with diabetes should report elevated blood glucose test results so antidiabetic medication dose can be adjusted.

• Teach women how to perform routine breast self-examination.

• Explain to patient on cyclic therapy for postmenopausal symptoms that, although withdrawal bleeding may occur during week off drug, fertility has not been restored. Pregnancy is not possible since she has not ovulated.

---

dienestrol (dienoestrol)
DV, Ortho Dienestrol
Pregnancy Risk Category: X

HOW SUPPLIED
Vaginal cream: 0.01%

MECHANISM OF ACTION
Increases the synthesis of DNA, RNA, and protein in responsive tis-

---

Italicized adverse reactions are common or life-threatening.
*Liquid form contains alcohol.   **May contain tartrazine.

sues. Also reduces FSH and LH release from the pituitary.

INDICATIONS & DOSAGE
Atrophic vaginitis and kraurosis vulvae—
Postmenopausal women: 1 to 2 intravaginal applications of vaginal cream daily for 1 to 2 weeks (as directed), then half that dose for the same period. A maintenance dosage of 1 applicatorful one to three times a week may be ordered.

ADVERSE REACTIONS
GU: vaginal discharge; with excessive use, uterine bleeding.
Local: increased discomfort, burning sensation. Systemic effects possible.
Other: breast tenderness.

INTERACTIONS
None significant.

NURSING CONSIDERATIONS
• Contraindicated in thrombophlebitis or thromboembolic disorders; cancer of breast, reproductive organs, or genitals; undiagnosed abnormal genital bleeding; and pregnancy. Use cautiously in menstrual irregularities or endometriosis.
• Instruct patient to apply drug at bedtime to increase effectiveness.
• Prolonged therapy with estrogen-containing products is contraindicated.
• Patient package insert that describes estrogen's adverse reactions is available. However, provide verbal explanation also.
• Systemic reactions possible with normal intravaginal use. Monitor closely.
• Warn patient not to exceed the prescribed dose.
• Withdrawal bleeding may occur if estrogen is suddenly stopped.
• Patient shouldn't wear tampon while receiving vaginal therapy. She may need to wear sanitary pad to protect clothing.
• Teach patient how to insert suppositories or cream. Wash vaginal area with soap and water before application.
• Instruct patient to remain recumbent for 30 minutes after administration to prevent loss of drug.
• Teach patient how to perform breast self-examination.

diethylstilbestrol (stilboestrol)
DES

diethylstilbestrol diphosphate
Honvol†

Pregnancy Risk Category: X

HOW SUPPLIED
diethylstilbestrol
Tablets: 1 mg, 2.5 mg, 5 mg
Tablets (enteric-coated): 1 mg, 5 mg
diethylstilbestrol diphosphate
Tablets: 83 mg†
Injection: 50 mg/ml

MECHANISM OF ACTION
Increases the synthesis of DNA, RNA, and protein in responsive tissues. Also reduces FSH and LH release from the pituitary.

INDICATIONS & DOSAGE
Hypogonadism, castration, primary ovarian failure—
Women: 0.2 to 0.5 mg P.O. daily.
Menopausal symptoms—
Women: 0.1 to 2 mg P.O. daily in cycles of 3 weeks on and 1 week off.
Postcoital contraception ("morning-after pill")—
Women: 25 mg P.O. b.i.d. for 5 days, starting within 72 hours after coitus.
Postpartum breast engorgement—
Women: 5 mg P.O. daily or t.i.d. up to total dose of 30 mg.
Prostatic cancer—

Men: initially, 1 to 3 mg P.O. daily; may be reduced to 1 mg P.O. daily, or 5 mg I.M. twice weekly initially, followed by up to 4 mg I.M. twice weekly. Or 50 to 200 mg (diphosphate) P.O. t.i.d.; or 0.25 to 1 g I.V. daily for 5 days, then once or twice weekly.

Breast cancer—

Men and postmenopausal women: 15 mg P.O. daily.

ADVERSE REACTIONS

CNS: headache, dizziness, chorea, depression, lethargy.

CV: *thrombophlebitis; thromboembolism;* hypertension; edema; *increased risk of stroke, pulmonary embolism, and myocardial infarction.*

EENT: worsening of myopia or astigmatism, intolerance to contact lenses.

GI: *nausea,* vomiting, abdominal cramps, bloating, diarrhea, constipation, anorexia, increased appetite, excessive thirst, weight changes, pancreatitis.

GU: in women—breakthrough bleeding, altered menstrual flow, dysmenorrhea, amenorrhea, cervical erosion, altered cervical secretions, enlargement of uterine fibromas, vaginal candidiasis, loss of libido. In men—gynecomastia, testicular atrophy, impotence.

Hepatic: cholestatic jaundice.

Metabolic: hyperglycemia, hypercalcemia, folic acid deficiency.

Skin: melasma, urticaria, acne, seborrhea, oily skin, hirsutism or loss of hair.

Other: leg cramps, breast tenderness or enlargement.

INTERACTIONS

None significant.

NURSING CONSIDERATIONS

• Contraindicated in thrombophlebitis or thromboembolic disorders; undiagnosed abnormal genital bleeding; and pregnancy. Use cautiously in hypertension, asthma, mental depression, bone disease, migraine, seizures, blood dyscrasias, diabetes mellitus, gallbladder disease, amenorrhea, heart failure, hepatic or renal dysfunction, and family history (mother, grandmother, sister) of breast or genital tract cancer. Development or worsening of these conditions may require discontinuation of the drug.

• Patient package insert that describes estrogen's adverse reactions is available. However, provide verbal explanation also.

• Only the 25-mg tablet is approved by FDA as the "morning-after pill." To be effective, it must be taken within 72 hours after coitus. Nausea and vomiting are common with this large dose.

• Warn patient to stop taking drug immediately if she becomes pregnant, since it can affect the fetus adversely.

• Warn patient to report immediately: abdominal pain; pain, numbness, or stiffness in legs or buttocks; pressure or pain in chest; shortness of breath; severe headache; visual disturbances, such as blind spots, flashing lights, or blurriness; vaginal bleeding or discharge; breast lumps; sudden weight gain; swelling of hands or feet; yellow sclera or skin; dark urine or light-colored stools.

• Pathologist should be advised of estrogen therapy when specimen is sent.

• Patients with diabetes should report elevated blood glucose test results so antidiabetic medication dose can be adjusted.

• High incidence of gross nonmalignant genital changes in offspring of women taking drug during pregnancy. Female offspring have higher than normal risk of developing cervical and vaginal adenocarcinoma. Male offspring may have higher than normal risk of developing testicular tumors, epididymal cysts, and impaired fertility.

Italicized adverse reactions are common or life-threatening.
*Liquid form contains alcohol.   **May contain tartrazine.

- Increased number of cardiovascular deaths reported in men taking diethylstilbestrol tablet (5 mg daily) for prostatic cancer over long period of time. This effect not associated with 1-mg daily dose.
- Teach women how to perform routine breast self-examination.
- Explain to patient on cyclic therapy for postmenopausal symptoms that, although withdrawal bleeding may occur during week off drug, fertility has not been restored. Pregnancy is not possible since she has not ovulated.
- Use of estrogens associated with increased risk of endometrial cancer. Possible increased risk of breast cancer.

esterified estrogens
Estratab, Estromed†, Menest, Neo-Estrone†

Pregnancy Risk Category: X

HOW SUPPLIED
Tablets: 0.3 mg, 0.625 mg, 1.25 mg, 2.5 mg

MECHANISM OF ACTION
Increases the synthesis of DNA, RNA, and protein in responsive tissues. Also reduces FSH and LH release from the pituitary.

INDICATIONS & DOSAGE
Inoperable prostatic cancer—
Men: 1.25 to 2.5 mg P.O. t.i.d.
Breast cancer—
Men and postmenopausal women: 10 mg P.O. t.i.d. for 3 or more months.
Hypogonadism, castration, primary ovarian failure—
Women: 2.5 mg P.O. daily to t.i.d. in cycles of 3 weeks on, 1 week off.
Menopausal symptoms—
Women: average 0.3 to 3.75 mg P.O. daily in cycles of 3 weeks on, 1 week off.

ADVERSE REACTIONS
CNS: headache, dizziness, chorea, depression, libido changes, lethargy.
CV: thrombophlebitis; *thromboembolism;* hypertension; edema; *increased risk of stroke, pulmonary embolism, and myocardial infarction.*
EENT: worsening of myopia or astigmatism, intolerance to contact lenses.
GI: *nausea,* vomiting, abdominal cramps, bloating, diarrhea, constipation, anorexia, increased appetite, weight changes, pancreatitis.
GU: in women—breakthrough bleeding, altered menstrual flow, dysmenorrhea, amenorrhea, cervical erosion, altered cervical secretions, enlargement of uterine fibromas, vaginal candidiasis. In men—gynecomastia, testicular atrophy, impotence.
Hepatic: cholestatic jaundice.
Metabolic: hyperglycemia, hypercalcemia, folic acid deficiency.
Skin: melasma, rash, acne, hirsutism or hair loss, seborrhea, oily skin.
Other: breast changes (tenderness, enlargement, secretion).

INTERACTIONS
None significant.

NURSING CONSIDERATIONS
- Contraindicated in thrombophlebitis or thromboembolic disorders; undiagnosed abnormal genital bleeding; and pregnancy. Use cautiously in patients with history of hypertension, mental depression, gallbladder disease, migraine, seizures, diabetes mellitus, amenorrhea, or family history (mother, grandmother, sister) of breast or genital tract cancer. Development or worsening of these conditions may require discontinuation of the drug.
- Patient package insert that describes estrogen's adverse reactions is available. However, provide verbal explanation also.
- Warn patient to report immediately: abdominal pain; pain, numbness, or

stiffness in legs or buttocks; pressure or pain in chest; shortness of breath; severe headaches; visual disturbances, such as blind spots, flashing lights, or blurriness; vaginal bleeding or discharge; breast lumps; swelling of hands or feet; yellow skin or sclera; dark urine or light-colored stools.

• Pathologist should be advised of estrogen therapy when specimen is sent.

• Patients with diabetes should report elevated blood glucose test results so antidiabetic medication dosage can be adjusted.

• Explain to patient on cyclic therapy for postmenopausal symptoms that, although she may experience withdrawal bleeding during week off drug, fertility has not been restored. Pregnancy cannot occur since she has not ovulated.

• Teach women how to perform routine breast self-examination.

estradiol (oestradiol)
Estrace**, Estrace Vaginal Cream, Estraderm

estradiol cypionate
depGynogen, Depo-Estradiol, Dura-Estrin, E-Cypionate, Estro-Cyp, Estrofem, Estroject-L.A., Estronol-LA

estradiol valerate (oestradiol valerate)
Delestrogen, Dioval, Duragen 10, Duragen 20, Duragen 40, Estradiol L.A., Estraval, Estraval P.A., Estra-L 20, Estra-L 40, Feminate, Femogex, Gynogen L.A., L.A.E., Menaval, Primogyn Depot‡, Ru-Est-Span 20, Ru-Est-Span 40, Valergen 10, Valergen 20, Valergen 40

Pregnancy Risk Category: X

HOW SUPPLIED
estradiol
Tablets (micronized): 1 mg, 2 mg
Transdermal: 4 mg/10 cm² (delivers 0.05 mg/24 hours); 8 mg/20 cm² (delivers 0.1 mg/24 hours)
Vaginal cream: (in nonliquefying base): 0.1 mg/g
estradiol cypionate
Injection (in oil): 1 mg/ml, 5 mg/ml
estradiol valerate
Injection (in oil): 10 mg/ml, 20 mg/ml, 40 mg/ml

MECHANISM OF ACTION
Increases the synthesis of DNA, RNA, and protein in responsive tissues. Also reduces FSH and LH release from the pituitary.

INDICATIONS & DOSAGE
Menopausal symptoms, hypogonadism, castration, primary ovarian failure—
Women: 1 to 2 mg P.O. daily, in cycles of 21 days on and 7 days off, or cycles of 5 days on and 2 days off; or 0.2 to 1 mg I.M. weekly.
Kraurosis vulvae—
Women: 1 to 1.5 mg I.M. once or more per week.
Atrophic vaginitis—
Women: 2 to 4 g intravaginal applications of cream daily for 1 to 2 weeks. When vaginal mucosa is restored, begin maintenance dosage of 1 g one to three times weekly.
Menopausal symptoms—
Women: 1 to 5 mg (cypionate) I.M. q 3 to 4 weeks. Or 5 to 20 mg (valerate) I.M., repeated once after 2 to 3 weeks.
Postpartum breast engorgement—
Women: 10 to 25 mg (valerate) I.M. at end of first stage of labor.
Inoperable breast cancer—
Women: 10 mg P.O. (oral estradiol) t.i.d. for 3 months.
Treatment of moderate to severe symptoms of menopause, female hypogonadism, female castration, primary ovarian failure, and atrophic conditions caused by deficient endogenous estrogen production—
Women: place one Estraderm trans-

---

dermal patch on trunk of the body twice weekly. Administer on an intermittent cyclic schedule (3 weeks of therapy followed by discontinuation for 1 week).

Inoperable prostatic cancer—
Men: 30 mg (valerate) I.M. q 1 to 2 weeks. Or, 1 to 2 mg (oral estradiol) t.i.d.

ADVERSE REACTIONS
CNS: headache, dizziness, chorea, depression, libido changes, lethargy.
CV: thrombophlebitis, *thromboembolism,* hypertension, edema.
EENT: worsening of myopia or astigmatism, intolerance to contact lenses.
GI: *nausea,* vomiting, abdominal cramps, bloating, diarrhea, constipation, anorexia, increased appetite, weight changes, pancreatitis.
GU: in women—breakthrough bleeding, altered menstrual flow, dysmenorrhea, amenorrhea, cervical erosion, altered cervical secretions, enlargement of uterine fibromas, vaginal candidiasis. In men—gynecomastia, testicular atrophy, impotence.
Hepatic: cholestatic jaundice.
Metabolic: hyperglycemia, hypercalcemia, folic acid deficiency.
Skin: melasma, urticaria, acne, seborrhea, oily skin, hirsutism or hair loss.
Other: breast changes (tenderness, enlargement, secretion), leg cramps.

INTERACTIONS
None significant.

NURSING CONSIDERATIONS
• Contraindicated in thrombophlebitis or thromboembolic disorders; cancer of breast, reproductive organs; undiagnosed abnormal genital bleeding; and pregnancy. Use cautiously in hypertension, mental depression, bone diseases, blood dyscrasias, migraine, seizures, diabetes mellitus, amenorrhea, heart failure, hepatic or renal dysfunction, or family history (mother, grandmother, sister) of breast or genital tract cancer. Development or worsening of these conditions may require discontinuation of the drug.
• Patient package insert that describes estrogen's adverse reactions is available. However, provide verbal explanation also.
• Warn patient to report immediately: abdominal pain; pain, numbness, or stiffness in legs or buttocks; pressure or pain in chest; shortness of breath; severe headaches; visual disturbances, such as blind spots, flashing lights, or blurriness; vaginal bleeding or discharge; breast lumps; swelling of hands or feet; yellow skin or sclera; dark urine or light-colored stools.
• Risk of endometrial cancer is increased in postmenopausal women who take estrogens for more than 1 year.
• Patients with diabetes should report elevated blood glucose test results so antidiabetic medication dosage can be adjusted.
• Pathologist should be advised of estrogen therapy when specimen is sent.
• Ask patient about allergies, especially to foods or plants. Estradiol is available as an aqueous solution or as a solution in peanut oil. Estradiol cypionate is available as a solution in cottonseed oil or vegetable oil. Estradiol valerate is available as a solution in castor oil, sesame oil, or vegetable oil.
• Before injection, make sure drug is well dispersed in solution by rolling vial between palms. Inject deep I.M. into large muscle. Drug should never be given I.V.
• In women who are currently taking oral estrogen, treatment with the Estraderm transdermal patch can begin 1 week after withdrawal of oral therapy or sooner if symptoms appear before the end of the week.
• Teach women how to perform routine breast self-examination.

• Explain to patient on cyclic therapy for postmenopausal symptoms that, although withdrawal bleeding may occur during week off drug, fertility has not been restored. Pregnancy cannot occur since she has not ovulated.

---

estrogens, conjugated (estrogenic substances, conjugated; oestrogens, conjugated)

C.E.S.†, Conjugated Estrogens C.S.D.†, Premarin, Premarin Intravenous, Progens

Pregnancy Risk Category: X

HOW SUPPLIED

Tablets: 0.3 mg, 0.625 mg, 0.9 mg, 1.25 mg, 2.5 mg
Injection: 25 mg/5 ml
Vaginal cream: 0.625 mg/g

MECHANISM OF ACTION

Increases the synthesis of DNA, RNA, and protein in responsive tissues. Also reduces FSH and LH release from the pituitary.

INDICATIONS & DOSAGE

Abnormal uterine bleeding (hormonal imbalance)—
Women: 25 mg I.V. or I.M. Repeat in 6 to 12 hours.
Breast cancer (at least 5 years after menopause)—
Women: 10 mg P.O. t.i.d. for 3 months or more.
Castration, primary ovarian failure, and osteoporosis—
Women: 1.25 mg P.O. daily in cycles of 3 weeks on, 1 week off.
Hypogonadism—
Women: 2.5 mg P.O. b.i.d. or t.i.d. for 20 consecutive days each month.
Menopausal symptoms—
Women: 0.3 to 1.25 mg P.O. daily in cycles of 3 weeks on, 1 week off.
Postpartum breast engorgement—
Women: 3.75 mg P.O. q 4 hours for

five doses or 1.25 mg q 4 hours for 5 days.
Treatment of atrophic vaginitis, kraurosis vulvae associated with menopause—
Women: 2 to 4 g intravaginally on a cyclical basis (3 weeks on, 1 week off).
Inoperable prostatic cancer—
Men: 1.25 to 2.5 mg P.O. t.i.d.

ADVERSE REACTIONS

CNS: headache, dizziness, chorea, depression, libido changes, lethargy.
CV: thrombophlebitis; *thromboembolism;* hypertension; edema; *increased risk of stroke, pulmonary embolism, and myocardial infarction.*
EENT: worsening of myopia or astigmatism, intolerance to contact lenses.
GI: *nausea,* vomiting, abdominal cramps, bloating, diarrhea, constipation, anorexia, increased appetite, weight changes, pancreatitis.
GU: in women—breakthrough bleeding, altered menstrual flow, dysmenorrhea, amenorrhea, cervical erosion, altered cervical secretions, enlargement of uterine fibromas, vaginal candidiasis. In men—gynecomastia, testicular atrophy, impotence.
Hepatic: cholestatic jaundice.
Metabolic: hyperglycemia, hypercalcemia, folic acid deficiency.
Skin: melasma, urticaria, acne, seborrhea, oily skin, flushing (when given rapidly I.V.), hirsutism or loss of hair.
Other: breast changes (tenderness, enlargement, secretion), leg cramps.

INTERACTIONS

None significant.

NURSING CONSIDERATIONS

• Contraindicated in thrombophlebitis or thromboembolic disorders; undiagnosed abnormal genital bleeding; and pregnancy. Use cautiously in hypertension, gallbladder disease, bone diseases, blood dyscrasias, migraine,

---

Italicized adverse reactions are common or life-threatening.
*Liquid form contains alcohol.   **May contain tartrazine.

seizures, diabetes mellitus, amenorrhea, heart failure, hepatic or renal dysfunction, or family history (mother, grandmother, sister) of breast or genital tract cancer. Development or worsening of these conditions may require discontinuation of the drug.

• Patient package insert that describes estrogen's adverse reactions is available. However, provide verbal explanation also.

• Warn patient to report immediately: abdominal pain; pain, numbness, or stiffness in legs or buttocks; pressure or pain in chest; shortness of breath; severe headaches; visual disturbances, such as blind spots, flashing lights, or blurriness; vaginal bleeding or discharge; breast lumps; swelling of hands or feet; yellow skin or sclera; dark urine or light-colored stools.

• I.M. or I.V. use preferred for rapid treatment of dysfunctional uterine bleeding or reduction of surgical bleeding.

• Refrigerate before reconstituting. Agitate gently after adding diluent.

• Pathologist should be advised of estrogen therapy when specimen is sent.

• Patients with diabetes should report elevated blood glucose test results so antidiabetic medication dosage can be adjusted.

• Use associated with increased risk of endometrial cancer. Possible increased risk of breast cancer.

• Teach women how to perform routine breast self-examination.

• Explain to patient on cyclic therapy for postmenopausal symptoms that, although withdrawal bleeding may occur during week off drug, fertility has not been restored. Pregnancy cannot occur since she has not ovulated.

estrone (oestrone)
Estrone "5", Estrone Aqueous, Estronol, Kestrone, Theelin Aqueous

Pregnancy Risk Category: X

HOW SUPPLIED
Injection (aqueous suspension): 2 mg/ml, 5 mg/ml

MECHANISM OF ACTION
Increases the synthesis of DNA, RNA, and protein in responsive tissues. Also reduces FSH and LH release from the pituitary.

INDICATIONS & DOSAGE
Atrophic vaginitis and menopausal symptoms—
Women: 0.1 to 0.5 mg I.M. two or three times weekly.
Female hypogonadism and primary ovarian failure—
Women: 0.1 to 1 mg I.M. weekly in single or divided doses.
Inoperable prostatic cancer—
Men: 2 to 4 mg I.M. 2 to 3 times weekly.

ADVERSE REACTIONS
CNS: headache, dizziness, chorea, depression, libido changes, lethargy.
CV: thrombophlebitis, *thromboembolism,* hypertension, edema.
EENT: worsening of myopia or astigmatism, intolerance to contact lenses.
GI: *nausea,* vomiting, abdominal cramps, bloating, diarrhea, constipation, anorexia, increased appetite, weight changes, pancreatitis.
GU: in women—breakthrough bleeding, altered menstrual flow, dysmenorrhea, amenorrhea, cervical erosion, altered cervical secretions, enlargement of uterine fibromas, vaginal candidiasis. In men—gynecomastia, testicular atrophy, impotence.
Hepatic: cholestatic jaundice.
Metabolic: hyperglycemia, hypercalcemia, folic acid deficiency.

Skin: melasma, urticaria, acne, seborrhea, oily skin, hirsutism or hair loss.
Other: breast changes (tenderness, enlargement, secretion), leg cramps.

INTERACTIONS
None significant.

NURSING CONSIDERATIONS
• Contraindicated in thrombophlebitis or thromboembolic disorders; cancer of breast or reproductive organs; undiagnosed abnormal genital bleeding; and pregnancy. Use cautiously in hypertension, mental depression, migraine, seizures, diabetes mellitus, amenorrhea, hepatic or renal dysfunction, or family history (mother, grandmother, sister) of breast or genital tract cancer. Development or worsening of these conditions may require discontinuation of the drug.
• Estrone must be administered I.M.
• Patient package insert that describes estrogen's adverse reactions is available. However, provide verbal explanation also.
• Warn patient to report immediately: abdominal pain; pain, numbness, or stiffness in legs or buttocks; pressure or pain in chest; shortness of breath; severe headaches; visual disturbances, such as blind spots, flashing lights, or blurriness; vaginal bleeding or discharge; breast lumps; swelling of hands and feet.
• Pathologist should be advised of estrogen therapy when specimen is sent.
• Patients with diabetes should report elevated blood glucose test results so antidiabetic medication dosage can be adjusted.
• Teach women how to perform routine breast self-examination.
• Use of estrogens associated with increased risk of endometrial cancer. Possible increased risk of breast cancer.
• Explain to patient on cyclic therapy for postmenopausal symptoms that, although withdrawal bleeding may occur during week off drug, fertility has not been restored. Pregnancy cannot occur since she has not ovulated.

estropipate (piperazine estrone sulfate)
Ogen
Pregnancy Risk Category: X

HOW SUPPLIED
Tablets: 0.625 mg, 1.25 mg, 2.5 mg, 5 mg
Vaginal cream: 1.5 mg estropipate/g

MECHANISM OF ACTION
Increases the synthesis of DNA, RNA, and proteins in responsive tissues.

INDICATIONS & DOSAGE
Atrophic vaginitis, kraurosis vulvae, or moderate to severe vasomotor symptoms associated with menopause—
Women: 0.625 to 5 mg P.O. daily. Dosage is usually given on a cyclical, short-term basis.
Primary ovarian failure, female castration, or female hypogonadism—
Women: administer on a cyclical basis—1.25 to 7.5 mg P.O. daily for the first 3 weeks, followed by a rest period of 8 to 10 days. If bleeding does not occur by the end of the rest period, repeat cycle.
Atrophic vaginitis or kraurosis vulvae—
Women: 2 to 4 g of vaginal cream daily. Administration should be cyclic and short term (3 weeks on and 1 week off)

ADVERSE REACTIONS
CNS: depression, headache, dizziness, migraine, changes in libido.
CV: edema.
GI: nausea, vomiting, abdominal cramps, bloating, cholestatic jaundice.

Italicized adverse reactions are common or life-threatening.
*Liquid form contains alcohol.   **May contain tartrazine.

GU: increased size of uterine fibro-myomata, vaginal candidiasis, cysti-tis-like syndrome, dysmenorrhea, amenorrhea, breakthrough bleeding, premenstrual-like syndrome.
Skin: hemorrhagic eruption, ery-thema nodosum, erythema multi-forme, hirsutism, chloasma, hair loss.
Other: breast engorgement or en-largement, weight changes, aggrava-tion of porphyria.

INTERACTIONS
None significant.

NURSING CONSIDERATIONS
• Contraindicated in thrombophlebi-tis or thromboembolic disorders; can-cer of the breast, reproductive organs, or genitals; undiagnosed genital bleeding; and pregnancy. Use cau-tiously in hypertension, asthma, men-tal depression, bone diseases, blood dyscrasias, gallbladder disease, mi-graine, seizures, diabetes mellitus, amenorrhea, heart failure, hepatic or renal dysfunction, and a family his-tory of breast or genital cancer. De-velopment or worsening of any of these conditions may require discon-tinuation of the drug.
• A patient package insert is available to describe the adverse reactions of estrogens, including the increased risk of endometrial carcinoma. However, provide a verbal explanation as well.
• Warn patient to report any of the following conditions immediately: ab-dominal pain, pain, stiffness or numb-ness in the legs or buttocks, pressure or pain in the chest, shortness of breath, severe headaches, visual dis-turbances (blind spots, flashing lights), vaginal bleeding or discharge, breast lumps, swelling of the hands or feet, yellow skin or sclera, dark urine, or light-colored stools.
• Teach patient how to perform breast self-examination.
• When used to treat hypogonadism, the duration of therapy necessary to

produce withdrawal bleeding depends upon the individual's endometrial re-sponse to the drug. If satisfactory withdrawal bleeding does not occur, an oral progestin may have to be added to the regimen. Explain to the patient that, despite the return of withdrawal bleeding, pregnancy is not possible since she is not ovulating.

---

ethinyl estradiol (ethinyloestradiol)
Estinyl**, Feminone

Pregnancy Risk Category: X

HOW SUPPLIED
Tablets: 0.02 mg, 0.05 mg, and 0.5 mg

MECHANISM OF ACTION
Increases the synthesis of DNA, RNA, and protein in responsive tis-sues. Also reduces FSH and LH re-lease from the pituitary.

INDICATIONS & DOSAGE
Breast cancer (at least 5 years after menopause)—
Women: 1 mg P.O. t.i.d.
Hypogonadism—
Women: 0.05 mg P.O. daily to t.i.d. for 2 weeks a month, followed by 2 weeks progesterone therapy; continue for 3 to 6 monthly dosing cycles, fol-lowed by 2 months off.
Menopausal symptoms—
Women: 0.02 to 0.05 mg P.O. daily for cycles of 3 weeks on, 1 week off.
Postpartum breast engorgement—
Women: 0.5 to 1 mg P.O. daily for 3 days, then taper over 7 days to 0.1 mg and discontinue.
Inoperable prostatic cancer—
Men: 0.15 to 2 mg P.O. daily.

ADVERSE REACTIONS
CNS: headache, dizziness, chorea, depression, libido changes, lethargy.
CV: thrombophlebitis, *thromboembo-lism,* hypertension, edema.

EENT: worsening of myopia or astigmatism, intolerance to contact lenses.
GI: *nausea,* vomiting, abdominal cramps, bloating, diarrhea, constipation, anorexia, increased appetite, weight changes.
GU: in women—breakthrough bleeding, altered menstrual flow, dysmenorrhea, amenorrhea, cervical erosion, altered cervical secretions, enlargement of uterine fibromas, vaginal candidiasis. In men—gynecomastia, testicular atrophy, impotence.
Hepatic: cholestatic jaundice.
Metabolic: hyperglycemia, hypercalcemia, folic acid deficiency.
Skin: melasma, urticaria, acne, seborrhea, oily skin, hirsutism or hair loss.
Other: breast changes (tenderness, enlargement, secretion), leg cramps.

INTERACTIONS
None significant.

NURSING CONSIDERATIONS
• Contraindicated in thrombophlebitis or thromboembolic disorders; undiagnosed abnormal genital bleeding; and pregnancy. Use cautiously in hypertension, mental depression, bone diseases, migraine, seizures, blood dyscrasias, diabetes mellitus, amenorrhea, heart failure, hepatic or renal dysfunction, or family history (mother, grandmother, sister) of breast or genital tract cancer. Development or worsening of these conditions may require discontinuation of the drug.
• Patient package insert that describes estrogen's adverse reactions is available. However, provide verbal explanation also.
• Warn patient to report immediately: abdominal pain; pain, numbness, or stiffness in legs or buttocks; pressure or pain in chest; shortness of breath; severe headaches; visual disturbances, such as blind spots, flashing lights, or blurriness; vaginal bleeding or discharge; breast lumps; swelling of hands or feet; yellow skin or sclera; dark urine or light-colored stools.
• Pathologist should be advised of estrogen therapy when specimen is sent.
• Patients with diabetes should report elevated blood glucose test results so antidiabetic medication dosage can be adjusted.
• Teach women how to perform routine breast self-examination.
• Use of estrogens associated with increased risk of endometrial cancer. Possible increased risk of breast cancer.
• Explain to patient on cyclic therapy for postmenopausal symptoms that, although withdrawal bleeding may occur during week off drug, fertility has not been restored. Pregnancy cannot occur because she has not ovulated.

ethinyl estradiol and ethynodiol diacetate
monophasic: Demulen 1/35, Demulen 1/50

ethinyl estradiol and levonorgestrel
monophasic: Levlen, Nordette
triphasic: Tri-Levlen, Triphasil

ethinyl estradiol and norethindrone
monophasic: Brevicon, Genora 0.5/35, Genora 1/35, Modicon, N.E.E. 1/35, Nelova 0.5/35 E, Nelova 1/35 E, Norcept-E 1/35, Norethin 1/35 E, Norinyl 1 + 35, Ortho-Novum 1/35, Ovcon-35, Ovcon-50
biphasic: Nelova 10/11, Ortho Novum 10/11
triphasic: Ortho Novum 7/7/7, Tri-Norinyl

---

ethinyl estradiol and norethindrone acetate
monophasic: Loestrin 21 1/20, Loestrin 21 1.5/30, Norlestrin 21 1/50, Norlestrin 21 2.5/50

ethinyl estradiol and norgestrel
monophasic: Lo/Ovral, Ovral

ethinyl estradiol, norethindrone acetate, and ferrous fumarate
monophasic: Loestrin Fe 1/20, Loestrin Fe 1.5/30, Norlestrin Fe 1/50, Norlestrin Fe 2.5/50

mestranol and norethindrone
monophasic: Genora 1/50, Nelova 1/50 M, Norethin 1/50 M, Norinyl 1 + 50, Ortho-Novum 1/50

Pregnancy Risk Category: X

HOW SUPPLIED
Monophasic oral contraceptives
ethinyl estradiol and ethynodiol diacetate
Tablets: ethinyl estradiol 35 mcg and ethynodiol diacetate 1 mg (Demulen 1/35); ethinyl estradiol 50 mcg and ethynodiol diacetate 1 mg (Demulen 1/50)
ethinyl estradiol and levonorgestrel
Tablets: ethinyl estradiol 30 mcg and levonorgestrel 0.15 mg (Levlen, Nordette)
ethinyl estradiol and norethindrone
Tablets: ethinyl estradiol 35 mcg and norethindrone 0.4 mg (Ovcon-35); ethinyl estradiol 35 mcg and norethindrone 0.5 mg (Brevicon, Genora 0.5/35, Modicon, Nelova 0.5/35E); ethinyl estradiol 35 mcg and norethindrone 1 mg (Genora 1/35, N.E.E 1/35, Nelova 1/35 E, Norcept-E 1/35, Norethin 1/35 E, Norinyl 1 + 35, Ortho-Novum 1/35), ethinyl estradiol 50 mcg and norethindrone 1 mg (Ovcon-50)

ethinyl estradiol and norethindrone acetate
Tablets: ethinyl estradiol 20 mcg and norethindrone acetate 1 mg (Loestrin 21 1/20); ethinyl estradiol 30 mcg and norethindrone acetate 1.5 mg (Loestrin 21 1.5/30); ethinyl estradiol 50 mcg and norethindrone acetate 1 mg (Norlestrin 21 1/50); ethinyl estradiol 50 mcg and norethindrone acetate 2.5 mg (Norlestrin 21 2.5/50)
ethinyl estradiol and norgestrel
Tablets: ethinyl estradiol 30 mcg and norgestrel 0.3 mg (Lo/Ovral); ethinyl estradiol 50 mcg and norgestrel 0.5 mg (Ovral)
ethinyl estradiol, norethindrone acetate, and ferrous fumarate
Tablets: ethinyl estradiol 20 mcg, norethindrone acetate 1 mg, and ferrous fumarate 75 mg (Loestrin Fe 1/20); ethinyl estradiol 30 mcg, norethindrone acetate 1.5 mg, and ferrous fumarate 75 mg (Loestrin Fe 1.5/30); ethinyl estradiol 50 mcg, norethindrone acetate 1 mg, and ferrous fumarate 75 mg (Norlestrin Fe 1/50); ethinyl estradiol 50 mcg, norethindrone acetate 2.5 mg, and ferrous fumarate 75 mg (Norlestrin Fe 2.5/50)
mestranol and norethindrone
Tablets: mestranol 50 mcg and norethindrone 1 mg Genora 1/50, Nelova 1/50 M, Norethin 1/50 M, Norinyl 1 + 50, Ortho-Novum 1/50)
Biphasic oral contraceptives
ethinyl estradiol and norethindrone
Tablets: ethinyl estradiol 35 mcg and norethindrone 0.5 mg during phase 1 [10 days]; ethinyl estradiol 35 mcg and norethindrone 1 mg during phase 2 [11 days] (Nelova 10/11, Ortho Novum 10/11)
Triphasic oral contraceptives
ethinyl estradiol and levonorgestrel
Tablets: (Tri-Levlen, Triphasil) ethinyl estradiol 35 mcg and levonorgestrel 0.05 mg during phase 1 [6 days]; ethinyl estradiol 35 mcg and levonorgestrel 0.075 mg during phase 2 [5 days]; ethinyl estradiol 35 mcg and le-

vonorgestrel 0.125 mg during phase 3 [10 days]

ethinyl estradiol and norethindrone
Tablets: (Tri-Norinyl) ethinyl estradiol 35 mcg and norethindrone 0.5 mg during phase 1 [7 days]; ethinyl estradiol 35 mcg and norethindrone 1 mg during phase 2 [9 days]; ethinyl estradiol 35 mcg and norethindrone 0.5 mg during phase 3 [5 days]; (Ortho Novum 7/7/7) ethinyl estradiol 35 mcg and norethindrone 0.5 mg during phase 1 [7 days]; ethinyl estradiol 35 mcg and norethindrone 0.75 mg during phase 2 [7 days] ; ethinyl estradiol 35 mcg and norethindrone 1 mg during phase 3 [7 days]

MECHANISM OF ACTION
Oral contraceptives inhibit ovulation through a negative feedback mechanism directed at the hypothalamus. They may also prevent transport of the ovum through the fallopian tubes.

Estrogen suppresses secretion of follicle-stimulating hormone, blocking follicular development and ovulation.

Progestin suppresses luteinizing hormone secretion so ovulation can't occur even if the follicle develops. Progestin thickens cervical mucus, which interferes with sperm migration, and also causes endometrial changes that prevent implantation of the fertilized ovum.

INDICATIONS & DOSAGE
Contraception—
Women: 1 tablet P.O. daily, beginning on day 5 of menstrual cycle (first day of menstrual flow is day 1). With 20- and 21-tablet packages, new dosing cycle begins 7 days after last tablet taken. With 28-tablet packages, dosage is 1 tablet daily without interruption; extra tablets are placebos or contain iron. If only 1 or 2 doses are missed, dosage may continue on schedule. If 3 or more doses are missed, remaining tablets in monthly package must be discarded and another contraceptive method substituted. If next menstrual period doesn't begin on schedule, rule out pregnancy before starting new dosing cycle. If menstrual period begins, start new dosing cycle 7 days after last tablet was taken. If all doses have been taken on schedule and 1 menstrual period is missed, continue dosing cycle. If 2 consecutive menstrual periods are missed, pregnancy test is required before new dosing cycle is started.
Biphasic oral contraceptives—
1 color tablet P.O. daily for 10 days, then next color tablet for 11 days.
Triphasic oral contraceptives—
1 tablet P.O. daily in the sequence specified by the brand.
Endometriosis—
Women: Enovid 5 mg or 10 mg—1 tablet P.O. daily for 2 weeks starting on day 5 of menstrual cycle. Continue without interruption for 6 to 9 months, increasing dose by 5 to 10 mg q 2 weeks, up to 20 mg daily. Up to 40 mg daily may be needed if breakthrough bleeding occurs.

ADVERSE REACTIONS
CNS: *headache, dizziness,* depression, libido changes, lethargy, migraine.
CV: *thromboembolism,* hypertension, edema.
EENT: worsening of myopia or astigmatism, intolerance to contact lenses.
GI: *nausea,* vomiting, abdominal cramps, bloating, diarrhea, constipation, anorexia, changes in appetite, weight gain, *bowel ischemia,* pancreatitis.
GU: *breakthrough bleeding, granulomatous colitis,* dysmenorrhea, amenorrhea, cervical erosion or abnormal secretions, enlargement of uterine fibromas, vaginal candidiasis.
Hepatic: gallbladder disease, cholestatic jaundice, liver tumors.

Italicized adverse reactions are common or life-threatening.
*Liquid form contains alcohol.   **May contain tartrazine.

Metabolic: hyperglycemia, hypercalcemia, folic acid deficiency.
Skin: rash, acne, seborrhea, oily skin, erythema multiforme, hyperpigmentation.
Other: *breast tenderness,* enlargement, secretion.

Adverse reactions may be more serious, frequent, and rapid in onset with high-dose than with low-dose combinations.

INTERACTIONS
Barbiturates, anticonvulsants, rifampin: may diminish contraceptive effectiveness. Use supplemental form of contraception.

NURSING CONSIDERATIONS
• Contraindicated in thromboembolic disorders, cerebrovascular or coronary artery disease, myocardial infarction, known or suspected cancer of breasts or reproductive organs, benign or malignant liver tumors, undiagnosed abnormal vaginal bleeding, known or suspected pregnancy, lactation; and in adolescents with incomplete epiphyseal closure. Also contraindicated in women 35 years or older who smoke more than 15 cigarettes a day, and in all women over 40 years. Use cautiously in patients with systemic lupus erythematosus, hypertension, mental depression, migraine, epilepsy, asthma, diabetes mellitus, amenorrhea, scanty or irregular periods, fibrocystic breast disease, family history (mother, grandmother, sister) of breast or genital tract cancer, renal or gallbladder disease. Report development or worsening of these conditions to doctor. Prolonged therapy inadvisable in women who plan to become pregnant.
• Discontinue if patient develops granulomatous colitis while on oral contraceptives.
• Discontinue at least 1 week before surgery to decrease risk of thromboembolism. Use an alternate method of birth control.
• If one menstrual period is missed and tablets have been taken on schedule, tell patient to continue taking them. If two consecutive menstrual periods are missed, tell patient to stop drug and to have pregnancy test. Progestogens may cause birth defects if taken early in pregnancy.
• Missed doses in midcycle greatly increase likelihood of pregnancy.
• If one tablet is missed, tell patient to take it as soon as remembered, or take two tablets the next day and continue regular schedule. If patient misses 2 consecutive days, she should take two tablets daily for 2 days, and resume normal schedule. Patient should use an additional method of birth control for 7 days after two missed doses.
• Warn patient that headache, nausea, dizziness, breast tenderness, spotting, and breakthrough bleeding are common at first. These should diminish after 3 to 6 dosing cycles (months). However, breakthrough bleeding in patients taking high-dose estrogen-progestogen combinations for menstrual disorders may necessitate dosage adjustment.
• Warn patient to immediately report abdominal pain; numbness, stiffness, or pain in legs or buttocks; pressure or pain in chest; shortness of breath; severe headache; visual disturbances, such as blind spots, blurriness, or flashing lights; undiagnosed vaginal bleeding or discharge; two consecutive missed menstrual periods; lumps in the breast; swelling of hands or feet; severe pain in the abdomen (tumor rupture in the liver).
• Advise patient to use an additional method of birth control for the first week of administration in the initial cycle. Some doctors instruct patients to also use condoms or a diaphragm with spermicide.
• Tell patient to take tablets at same

time each day; nighttime dosing may reduce nausea and headaches.
• Advise patient not to take same drug for longer than 18 months without consulting doctor. Stress importance of Pap smears and annual gynecologic examinations.
• Warn the patient of possible delay in achieving pregnancy when drug is discontinued.
• Many doctors recommend that women not become pregnant within 2 months after stopping drug. Advise patient to check with her doctor about how soon pregnancy may be attempted after hormonal therapy is stopped.
• Teach the patient how to perform a breast self-examination.
• Advise the patient of increased risks associated with simultaneous use of cigarettes and oral contraceptives.
• Many laboratory tests are affected by oral contraceptives; some include: increase in serum bilirubin, alkaline phosphatase, AST (SGOT), ALT (SGPT), and protein-bound iodine; decrease in glucose tolerance and urinary excretion of 17-hydroxycorticosteroids (17-OHCS).
• Estrogens and progestins may alter glucose tolerance, thus changing requirements for antidiabetic drugs. Monitor blood glucose levels.
• Instruct patient to weigh herself at least twice a week and to report any sudden weight gain or edema to doctor.
• Warn patient to avoid exposure to ultraviolet light or prolonged exposure to sunlight.
• Many doctors advise women on prolonged therapy with oral contraceptives (5 years or longer) to stop drug and use other birth control methods in order to periodically reassess patient while off hormone therapy.
• The Centers for Disease Control (CDC) reports that the use of oral contraceptives *may decrease* the incidence of ovarian and endometrial cancers. Also, oral contraceptives do not appear to increase a woman's risk of breast cancer. However, FDA reports that they may be linked to an increased risk of cervical cancer.
• Ovral has been prescribed as a postcoital contraceptive ("morning-after" pill). Patients are given 2 tablets at the initial visit and 2 tablets 12 hours later.
• Triphasic oral contraceptives may cause fewer adverse reactions such as breakthrough bleeding and spotting.

hydroxyprogesterone caproate
Delalutin†, Duralutin, Gesterol L.A., Hy-Gesterone, Hylutin, Hyprogest, Hyproval P.A., Hyroxon, Pro-Depo, Prodrox

Pregnancy Risk Category: X

HOW SUPPLIED
Injection: 125 mg/ml, 250 mg/ml

MECHANISM OF ACTION
Suppresses ovulation, possibly by inhibiting pituitary gonadotropin secretion. Also forms a thick cervical mucus.

INDICATIONS & DOSAGE
Menstrual disorders—
Women: 125 to 375 mg I.M. q 4 weeks. Stop after 4 cycles.
Uterine cancer—
Women: 1 to 5 g I.M. weekly.

ADVERSE REACTIONS
CNS: dizziness, migraine headache, lethargy, depression.
CV: hypertension, thrombophlebitis, *pulmonary embolism, edema.*
GI: nausea, vomiting, abdominal cramps.
GU: breakthrough bleeding, dysmenorrhea, amenorrhea, cervical erosion, or abnormal secretions, uterine fibromas, vaginal candidiasis.

Italicized adverse reactions are common or life-threatening.
*Liquid form contains alcohol.   **May contain tartrazine.

Hepatic: cholestatic jaundice.
Metabolic: hyperglycemia.
Skin: melasma, rash.
Local: irritation and pain at injection site.
Other: breast tenderness, enlargement, or secretion; decreased libido.

INTERACTIONS
Rifampin: decreased progestogen effects. Monitor for diminished therapeutic response.

NURSING CONSIDERATIONS
• Contraindicated in thromboembolic disorders, breast cancer, undiagnosed abnormal vaginal bleeding, severe hepatic disease, missed abortion, or in pregnant women. Use cautiously in diabetes mellitus, seizure disorder, migraine, cardiac or renal disease, asthma, and mental illness.
• FDA regulations require that, before receiving first dose, patients read package insert explaining possible progestin adverse reactions. Provide verbal explanation also. Patient should report any unusual symptoms immediately and should stop drug and call doctor if visual disturbances or migraine occurs.
• Hydroxyprogesterone should not be used to induce withdrawal bleeding or as a test for pregnancy; drug may cause birth defects and masculinization of female fetus.
• Warn patient that edema and weight gain are likely.
• Give oil solutions (sesame oil and castor oil) deep I.M. in gluteal muscle.
• Effect lasts 7 to 14 days.
• Teach patient how to perform a monthly breast self-examination.
• Instruct patient that normal menstrual cycles may not resume for 2 to 3 months after drug is stopped.

medroxyprogesterone acetate
Amen, Curretab, Cycrin, Depo-Provera, Provera

Pregnancy Risk Category: X

HOW SUPPLIED
Tablets: 2.5 mg, 5 mg, 10 mg
Injection (suspension): 100 mg/ml, 400 mg/ml

MECHANISM OF ACTION
Suppresses ovulation, possibly by inhibiting pituitary gonadotropin secretion. Also forms a thick cervical mucus.

INDICATIONS & DOSAGE
Abnormal uterine bleeding due to hormonal imbalance—
Women: 5 to 10 mg P.O. daily for 5 to 10 days beginning on the 16th day of menstrual cycle. If patient has received estrogen—10 mg P.O. daily for 10 days beginning on 16th day of cycle.
Secondary amenorrhea—
Women: 5 to 10 mg P.O. daily for 5 to 10 days.
Endometrial or renal carcinoma—
Adults: 400 to 1,000 mg/week I.M.

ADVERSE REACTIONS
CNS: dizziness, migraine headache, lethargy, depression.
CV: hypertension, thrombophlebitis, *pulmonary embolism, edema.*
GI: nausea, vomiting, abdominal cramps.
GU: breakthrough bleeding, dysmenorrhea, amenorrhea, cervical erosion, or abnormal secretions, uterine fibromas, vaginal candidiasis.
Hepatic: cholestatic jaundice.
Metabolic: hyperglycemia.
Skin: melasma, rash.
Local: pain, induration, sterile abscesses.
Other: breast tenderness, enlargement, or secretion; decreased libido.

INTERACTIONS
Rifampin: decreased progestogen effects. Monitor for diminished therapeutic response.

NURSING CONSIDERATIONS
• Contraindicated in thromboembolic disorders, breast cancer, undiagnosed abnormal vaginal bleeding, missed abortion, hepatic dysfunction, or in pregnant women. Use cautiously in diabetes mellitus, seizure disorder, migraine, cardiac or renal disease, asthma, and mental illness.
• I.M. injection may be painful. Monitor sites for evidence of sterile abscess.
• FDA regulations require that, before receiving first dose, patients read package insert explaining possible progestin adverse reactions. Provide verbal explanation also. Patient should report any unusual symptoms immediately and should stop drug and call doctor if visual disturbances or migraine occurs.
• Don't use as test for pregnancy; drug may cause birth defects and masculinization of female fetus.
• Teach patient how to perform a monthly breast self-examination.
• Has been used effectively to treat obstructive sleep apnea.

---

norethindrone
Micronor, Norlutin, Nor-Q.D.

Pregnancy Risk Category: X

HOW SUPPLIED
Tablets: 0.35 mg, 5 mg

MECHANISM OF ACTION
Suppresses ovulation, possibly by inhibiting pituitary gonadotropin secretion. Also forms a thick cervical mucus.

INDICATIONS & DOSAGE
Amenorrhea, abnormal uterine bleeding—

Adults: 5 to 20 mg P.O. daily on days 5 to 25 of menstrual cycle.
Endometriosis—
Adults: 10 mg P.O. daily for 14 days, then increase by 5 mg P.O. daily q 2 weeks up to 30 mg daily.
Contraception (norethindrone)—
Adults: initiate therapy with 0.35 mg P.O. on the first day of menstruation. Then, 0.35 mg P.O. daily.

ADVERSE REACTIONS
CNS: dizziness, migraine headache, lethargy, depression.
CV: hypertension, thrombophlebitis, *pulmonary embolism, edema.*
GI: nausea, vomiting, abdominal cramps.
GU: breakthrough bleeding, dysmenorrhea, amenorrhea, cervical erosion, or abnormal secretions, uterine fibromas, vaginal candidiasis.
Hepatic: cholestatic jaundice.
Metabolic: hyperglycemia.
Skin: melasma, rash.
Other: breast tenderness, enlargement, or secretion; decreased libido.

INTERACTIONS
Rifampin: decreased progestogen effects. Monitor for diminished therapeutic response.

NURSING CONSIDERATIONS
• Contraindicated in thromboembolic disorders, breast cancer, undiagnosed abnormal vaginal bleeding, severe hepatic disease, missed abortion, or in pregnant women. Use cautiously in diabetes mellitus, seizure disorder, migraine, cardiac or renal disease, asthma, and mental illness.
• Don't use as test for pregnancy; drug may cause birth defects and masculinization of female fetus.
• FDA regulations require that, before receiving first dose, patients read package insert explaining possible progestin adverse reactions. Provide verbal explanation also. Patient should report any unusual symptoms

---

Italicized adverse reactions are common or life-threatening.
*Liquid form contains alcohol.   **May contain tartrazine.

immediately and should stop drug and call doctor if visual disturbances or migraine occurs.

• Watch patient carefully for signs of edema.

• Preliminary estrogen treatment is usually needed in menstrual disorders.

• Teach the patient how to perform a monthly breast self-examination.

norethindrone acetate
Aygestin, Aygestin Cycle Pack, Norlutate

Pregnancy Risk Category: X

HOW SUPPLIED
Tablets: 5 mg

MECHANISM OF ACTION
Suppresses ovulation, possibly by inhibiting pituitary gonadotropin secretion. Also forms a thick cervical mucus.

INDICATIONS & DOSAGE
Amenorrhea, abnormal uterine bleeding—
Women: 2.5 to 10 mg P.O. daily on days 5 to 25 of menstrual cycle.
Endometriosis—
Women: 5 mg P.O. daily for 14 days, then increase by 2.5 mg daily q 2 weeks up to 15 mg daily.

ADVERSE REACTIONS
CNS: dizziness, migraine headache, lethargy, depression.
CV: hypertension, thrombophlebitis, *pulmonary embolism, edema.*
GI: nausea, vomiting, abdominal cramps.
GU: breakthrough bleeding, dysmenorrhea, amenorrhea, cervical erosion, or abnormal secretions, uterine fibromas, vaginal candidiasis.
Hepatic: cholestatic jaundice.
Metabolic: hyperglycemia.
Skin: melasma, rash.

Other: breast tenderness, enlargement, or secretion; decreased libido.

INTERACTIONS
Rifampin: decreased progestogen effects. Monitor for diminished therapeutic response.

NURSING CONSIDERATIONS
• Contraindicated in thromboembolic disorders, breast cancer, undiagnosed abnormal vaginal bleeding, severe hepatic disease, missed abortion, or in pregnant women. Use cautiously in diabetes mellitus, seizure disorder, migraine, cardiac or renal disease, asthma, and mental illness.

• FDA regulations require that, before receiving first dose, patients read package insert explaining possible progestin adverse reactions. Provide verbal explanation also. Patient should report any unusual symptoms immediately and should stop drug and call doctor if visual disturbances or migraine occurs.

• Don't use as test for pregnancy; drug may cause birth defects and masculinization of female fetus.

• Preliminary estrogen treatment is usually needed in menstrual disorders.

• Twice as potent as norethindrone.

• Teach patient how to perform a monthly breast self-examination.

norgestrel
Ovrette**

Pregnancy Risk Category: X

HOW SUPPLIED
Tablets: 0.075 mg

MECHANISM OF ACTION
Suppresses ovulation, possibly by inhibiting pituitary gonadotropin secretion. Also forms a thick cervical mucus.

INDICATIONS & DOSAGE
Contraception—
Women: 0.075 mg P.O. daily.

ADVERSE REACTIONS
CNS: cerebral thrombosis or hemorrhage, migraine headache, lethargy, depression.
CV: hypertension, thrombophlebitis, *pulmonary embolism, edema.*
GI: nausea, vomiting, abdominal cramps, gallbladder disease.
GU: *breakthrough bleeding, change in menstrual flow,* dysmenorrhea, spotting, amenorrhea, cervical erosion, vaginal candidiasis.
Hepatic: cholestatic jaundice.
Skin: melasma, rash.
Other: breast tenderness, enlargement, or secretion.

INTERACTIONS
Rifampin: decreased progestogen effects. Monitor for diminished therapeutic response.

NURSING CONSIDERATIONS
• Contraindicated in thromboembolic disorders, breast cancer, undiagnosed abnormal vaginal bleeding, severe hepatic disease, missed abortion, or in pregnant women. Use cautiously in diabetes mellitus, seizure disorder, migraine, cardiac or renal disease, asthma, and mental illness.
• FDA regulations require that, before receiving first dose, patients read package insert explaining possible progestin adverse reactions. Provide verbal explanation also. Patient should report any unusual symptoms immediately and should stop drug and call doctor if visual disturbances, migraine, or numbness or tingling in limbs occurs.
• Tell patient to take pill every day, even if menstruating. Pill should be taken at the same time every day.
• A progestogen-only oral contraceptive known as "minipill."

• Teach the patient how to perform a monthly breast self-examination.
• Women using oral contraceptives should be advised of the increased risk of serious cardiovascular adverse reactions associated with heavy cigarette smoking (15 or more cigarettes per day). These risks are quite marked in women over 35 years.
• Risk of pregnancy increases with each tablet missed. A patient who misses one tablet should take it as soon as she remembers; she should then take the next tablet at the regular time. A patient who misses two tablets should take one as soon as she remembers and then take the next regular dose at the usual time; she should use a nonhormonal method of contraception in addition to norgestrel until 14 tablets have been taken. A patient who misses three or more tablets should discontinue the drug and use a nonhormonal method of contraception until after her menses. If her menstrual period does not occur within 45 days, pregnancy testing is necessary.
• Instruct the patient to immediately report excessive bleeding or bleeding between menstrual cycles.

---

progesterone
Gesterol 50, Progestaject, Progestilin†

Pregnancy Risk Category: X

HOW SUPPLIED
Injection (in oil): 50 mg/ml

MECHANISM OF ACTION
Suppresses ovulation, possibly by inhibiting pituitary gonadotropin secretion. Also forms a thick cervical mucus.

INDICATIONS & DOSAGE
Amenorrhea—
Women: 5 to 10 mg I.M. daily for 6 to 8 days.

Italicized adverse reactions are common or life-threatening.
*Liquid form contains alcohol.   **May contain tartrazine.

Dysfunctional uterine bleeding—
Women: 5 to 10 mg I.M. daily for 6 doses.
Management of premenstrual syndrome (PMS)—
Women: 200 to 400 mg as a suppository administered either rectally or vaginally.

ADVERSE REACTIONS
CNS: dizziness, migraine headache, lethargy, depression.
CV: hypertension, thrombophlebitis, *pulmonary embolism, edema.*
GI: nausea, vomiting, abdominal cramps.
GU: breakthrough bleeding, dysmenorrhea, amenorrhea, cervical erosion, or abnormal secretions, uterine fibromas, vaginal candidiasis.
Hepatic: cholestatic jaundice.
Local: pain at injection site.
Metabolic: hyperglycemia.
Skin: melasma, rash.
Other: breast tenderness, enlargement, or secretion; decreased libido.

INTERACTIONS
Rifampin: decreased progestogen effects. Monitor for diminished therapeutic response.

NURSING CONSIDERATIONS
• Contraindicated in thromboembolic disorders, breast cancer, undiagnosed abnormal vaginal bleeding, severe hepatic disease, or missed abortion. Use cautiously in diabetes mellitus, seizure disorder, migraine, cardiac or renal disease, asthma, and mental illness.
• FDA regulations require that, before receiving first dose, patients read package insert explaining possible progestin adverse reactions. Provide verbal explanation also. Patient should report any unusual symptoms immediately and should stop drug and call doctor if visual disturbances or migraine occurs.
• Give oil solutions (peanut oil or se-

same oil) deep I.M. Check sites frequently for irritation. Rotate injection sites.
• Preliminary estrogen treatment is usually needed in menstrual disorders.
• Teach the patient how to perform a monthly breast self-examination.

---

quinestrol
Estrovis

Pregnancy Risk Category: X

HOW SUPPLIED
Tablets: 100 mcg

MECHANISM OF ACTION
Increases the synthesis of DNA, RNA, and protein in responsive tissues. Also reduces FSH and LH release from the pituitary.

INDICATIONS & DOSAGE
Moderate to severe vasomotor symptoms associated with menopause, and for atrophic vaginitis, kraurosis vulvae, female hypogonadism, female castration, and primary ovarian failure—
Women: 100 mcg P.O. once daily for 7 days, followed by 100 mcg weekly as maintenance dosage beginning 2 weeks after start of treatment. Dosage may be increased to 200 mcg weekly.

ADVERSE REACTIONS
CNS: headache, dizziness, chorea, migraine, depression, libido changes.
CV: thrombophlebitis; *thromboembolism;* hypertension; edema; *increased risk of stroke, pulmonary embolism, and myocardial infarction.*
EENT: worsening of myopia or astigmatism, intolerance to contact lenses.
GI: *nausea,* vomiting, abdominal cramps, bloating, diarrhea, constipation, anorexia, increased appetite, excessive thirst, weight changes.
GU: breakthrough bleeding, altered menstrual flow, dysmenorrhea, amen-

orrhea, cervical erosion or abnormal secretions, enlargement of uterine fibromas, vaginal candidiasis.

Hepatic: cholestatic jaundice.

Metabolic: hyperglycemia, hypercalcemia, folic acid deficiency.

Skin: melasma, urticaria, acne, seborrhea, oily skin, hirsutism or loss of hair.

Other: leg cramps, purpura, breast changes (tenderness, enlargement, secretion).

INTERACTIONS
None significant.

NURSING CONSIDERATIONS
• Contraindicated in thrombophlebitis or thromboembolic disorders; cancer of breast or reproductive organs; undiagnosed abnormal genital bleeding; and pregnancy. Use cautiously in hypertension, mental depression, migraine, seizures, diabetes mellitus, amenorrhea, hepatic or renal dysfunction, or family history (mother, grandmother, sister) of breast or genital tract cancer. Development or worsening of these may require discontinuation of the drug.

• Patient package insert that describes estrogen's adverse reactions is available. However, provide verbal explanation also.

• Warn patient to report immediately: abdominal pain; pain, numbness, or stiffness in legs or buttocks; pressure or pain in chest; shortness of breath; severe headaches; visual disturbances, such as blind spots, flashing lights, or blurriness; vaginal bleeding or discharge; breast lumps; swelling of hands or feet; yellow skin or sclera; dark urine or light-colored stools.

• Pathologist should be advised of estrogen therapy when specimen is sent.

• Patients with diabetes should report elevated blood glucose test results so antidiabetic medication dosage can be adjusted.

• Attempts to discontinue medication should be made at 3- to 6-month intervals.

• Similar in effectiveness to conjugated estrogens in treating postmenopausal symptoms. Biggest advantage is that quinestrol can be taken once a week.

• Use of estrogens associated with increased risk of endometrial cancer.

• Explain to patients on replacement therapy for postmenopausal symptoms that, although menstrual-like bleeding or spotting may occur, fertility has not been restored.

• Teach women how to perform breast self-examination.

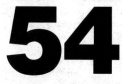

Gonadotropins

gonadorelin acetate
gonadorelin hydrochloride
gonadotropin, chorionic
menotropins
nafarelin acetate

COMBINATION PRODUCTS
None.

---

gonadorelin acetate
Lutrepulse

Pregnancy Risk Category: B

HOW SUPPLIED
Injection: 0.8-mg/10-ml, 3.2-mg/
10-ml vials; supplied as a kit with I.V.
supplies and ambulatory infusion
pump

MECHANISM OF ACTION
Mimics the action of gonadotropin releasing hormone, which results in the
synthesis and release of luteinizing
hormone (LH) from the anterior pituitary. LH subsequently acts upon the
reproductive organs to regulate hormone synthesis.

INDICATIONS & DOSAGE
*Induction of ovulation in women with
primary hypothalamic amenorrhea—*
Women: 5 mcg I.V. q 90 minutes for
21 days. If no response follows three
treatment intervals, dosage may be increased.

ADVERSE REACTIONS
GU: ovarian hyperstimulation.
Local: hematoma, infection, inflam-
mation, mild phlebitis.

Other: multiple pregnancy.

INTERACTIONS
None reported.

NURSING CONSIDERATIONS
• Contraindicated in patients hypersensitive to the drug, in any women
with conditions that could be complicated by pregnancy (such as pituitary
prolactinoma), in patients who are anovulatory from any cause other than a
hypothalamic disorder, and in patients with ovarian cysts.
• Anaphylaxis has been reported with
similar drugs. Teach the patient how
to recognize the signs and symptoms
of hypersensitivity reactions (hives,
wheezing, difficulty breathing) and
encourage her to report these as soon
as possible.
• Patients should understand that a
multiple pregnancy is possible (incidence about 12%). Close monitoring
of dosage as well as ultrasonograpy of
the ovaries to monitor drug response
is necessary.
• Patients usually require pelvic ultrasound on days 7 and 14 after establishment of a baseline scan. Some clinicians prefer shorter intervals between scans.
• Encourage patients to adhere to the
close monitoring schedule required by
the therapy. Regular pelvic examinations, midluteal phase serum progesterone determinations, and multiple
ovarian ultrasound scans are necessary. Inspect the I.V. site at each visit.
• To mimic the naturally occurring
hormone, gonadorelin acetate must be

---

administered in a pulsatile fashion with the available ambulatory infusion pump. The pulse period is set at 1 minute (drug is infused over 1 minute) and pulse interval is set at 90 minutes.
• To administer 2.5 mcg/pulse, reconstitute the 0.8-mg vial with 8 ml of supplied diluent, and set the pump to deliver 25 microliters/pulse. To administer 5 mcg/pulse, use the same dosage strength and dilution but set the pump to deliver 50 microliters/pulse.
• Some patients may require higher doses. To administer 10 mcg/pulse, reconstitute the 3.2-mg vial with 8 ml of supplied diluent, and set the pump to deliver 25 microliters/pulse. To administer 20 mcg/pulse, use the same dosage strength and dilution but set the pump to deliver 50 microliters/pulse.
• Instruct the patient about proper aseptic technique and care of the I.V. site. Cannula and I.V. site should be changed every 48 hours. Written instructions are available for the patient.

---

gonadorelin hydrochloride (luteinizing hormone-releasing hormone, LHRH; gonadotropin releasing hormone, GnRH)
Factrel

Pregnancy Risk Category: B

HOW SUPPLIED
Injection: 100 mcg, 500 mcg

MECHANISM OF ACTION
A synthetic luteinizing hormone that releases LHRH.

INDICATIONS & DOSAGE
Evaluation of the functional capacity and response of gonadotropic hormones—
Adults: 100 mcg S.C. or I.V. In women for whom the phase of the menstrual cycle can be established, perform the test between day 1 and day 7.

ADVERSE REACTIONS
CNS: headache, flushing, light-headedness.
GI: nausea, abdominal discomfort.
Local: swelling, occasionally with pain and pruritus when administered S.C.; skin rash after chronic S.C. administration.

INTERACTIONS
Digoxin, oral contraceptives: may depress gonadotropin levels. Monitor results carefully.
Levodopa, spironolactone: may elevate gonadotropin levels. Monitor results carefully.

NURSING CONSIDERATIONS
• Although no hypersensitivity reactions have been reported to date, use cautiously in patients who are allergic to other drugs. Keep epinephrine readily available.
• The gonadorelin test can be performed concomitantly with other post-treatment evaluations.
• For specific test methodology and interpretation of test results, refer to the manufacturer's full product information. Ask pharmacist for a copy.
• Reconstitute vial with 1 ml of accompanying sterile diluent. Prepare solution immediately before use. After reconstitution, store at room temperature and use within 1 day. Discard unused reconstituted solution and diluent.
• As a single injection, gonadorelin can evaluate the functional capacity and response of the gonadotropins of the anterior pituitary. Prolonged or repeated administration may be necessary to measure pituitary gonadotropic reserve.

Italicized adverse reactions are common or life-threatening.
*Liquid form contains alcohol.   **May contain tartrazine.

gonadotropin, chorionic (HCG)
Antuitrin, A.P.L., Chorex, Follutein, Pregnyl, Profasi HP

Pregnancy Risk Category: C

HOW SUPPLIED
Injection: 200 units/ml, 500 units/ml, 1,000 units/ml, 2,000 units/ml (after reconstitution)

MECHANISM OF ACTION
Serves as a substitute for luteinizing hormone to stimulate ovulation of an human menopausal gonadotropin–prepared follicle. Also promotes secretion of gonadal steroid hormones by stimulating production of androgen by the interstitial cells of the testes (Leydig's cells).

INDICATIONS & DOSAGE
Anovulation and infertility—
Women: 10,000 units I.M. 1 day after last dose of menotropins.
Hypogonadism—
Men: 500 to 1,000 units I.M. three times weekly for 3 weeks, then twice weekly for 3 weeks; or 4,000 units I.M. three times weekly for 6 to 9 months, then 2,000 units three times weekly for 3 more months.
Nonobstructive cryptorchidism—
Boys 4 to 9 years: 5,000 units I.M. every other day for four doses.

ADVERSE REACTIONS
CNS: headache, fatigue, irritability, restlessness, depression.
GU: early puberty (growth of testes, penis, pubic and axillary hair; voice change; down on upper lip; growth of body hair).
Local: *pain at injection site*.
Other: gynecomastia, edema.

INTERACTIONS
None significant.

NURSING CONSIDERATIONS
• Contraindicated in pituitary hypertrophy or tumor, prostatic cancer, and early puberty (usual onset between 10 and 13 years of age). Use cautiously in epilepsy, migraine, asthma, and cardiac or renal disease.
• When used with menotropins to induce ovulation, multiple births are possible.
• Usually used only after failure of clomiphene in anovulatory patients.
• In infertility, encourage daily intercourse from day before chorionic gonadotropin is given until ovulation occurs.
• Inspect genitalia of boys for signs of early puberty.
• Be alert to symptoms of ectopic pregnancy. Usually evident between week 8 to 12 of gestation.

menotropins
Pergonal

Pregnancy Risk Category: C

HOW SUPPLIED
Injection: 75 IU of luteinizing hormone (LH) and 75 IU of follicle-stimulating hormone (FSH) activity/ ampule; 150 IU of LH and 150 IU of FSH activity/ampule

MECHANISM OF ACTION
Menotropins, when administered to women who have not had primary ovarian failure, mimics follicle-stimulating hormone (FSH) in inducing follicular growth and luteinizing hormone (LH) in aiding follicular maturation.

INDICATIONS & DOSAGE
Anovulation—
Women: 75 IU each FSH and LH I.M. daily for 9 to 12 days, followed by 10,000 units chorionic gonadotropin I.M. 1 day after last dose of menotropins. Repeat for one to three menstrual cycles until ovulation occurs.

Infertility with ovulation—
Women: 75 IU each of FSH and LH
I.M. daily for 9 to 12 days, followed
by 10,000 units chorionic gonadotropin I.M. 1 day after last dose of menotropins. Repeat for two menstrual
cycles and then increase to 150 IU
each FSH and LH I.M. daily for 9 to
12 days, followed by 10,000 units
chorionic gonadotropin I.M. 1 day after last dose of menotropins. Repeat
for two menstrual cycles.
Infertility—
Men: 1 ampule I.M. three times
weekly (given concomitantly with
HCG 2,000 units twice weekly) for at
least 4 months.

Menotropins are available in ampules containing 75 IU each FSH and
LH.

ADVERSE REACTIONS
Blood: hemoconcentration with fluid
loss into abdomen.
GI: nausea, vomiting, diarrhea.
GU: in women—*ovarian enlargement
with pain and abdominal distention,*
multiple births, ovarian hyperstimulation syndrome (sudden ovarian enlargement, ascites with or without
pain, or pleural effusion); in men—
gynecomastia.
Other: fever.

INTERACTIONS
None significant.

NURSING CONSIDERATIONS
• Contraindicated in ovarian failure,
high urinary gonadotropin levels, thyroid or adrenal dysfunction, pituitary
tumor, abnormal uterine bleeding,
ovarian cysts or enlargement, and
pregnancy.
• Close monitoring of patient response is critical to ensure adequate
ovarian stimulation without hyperstimulation.
• Tell patient that there is a possibility of multiple births.
• In infertility, encourage daily inter-

course from day before chorionic gonadotropin is given until ovulation occurs.
• Pregnancy usually occurs 4 to 6
weeks after therapy.
• Reconstitute with 1 to 2 ml sterile
saline injection. Use immediately.

nafarelin acetate
Synarel
Pregnancy Risk Category: X

HOW SUPPLIED
Nasal solution: 200 mcg/spray in metered-dose spray bottle (2 mg/ml)

MECHANISM OF ACTION
A gonadotropin-releasing hormone
(GnRH) analog that acts on the pituitary to decrease the release of follicle-stimulating hormone (FSH) and
luteinizing hormone (LH). The result
is decreased ovarian stimulation, lowered circulating estrogens, and improvement of the symptoms associated with endometriosis.

INDICATIONS & DOSAGE
Management of endometriosis—
Women 18 years and older: 1 spray
in one nostril b.i.d. Maximum duration of therapy is 6 months.

ADVERSE REACTIONS
CNS: *headaches, emotional lability,
insomnia,* depression.
CV: edema.
EENT: *nasal irritation.*
GU: *vaginal dryness.*
Skin: *acne,* seborrhea, hirsutism.
Other: *hot flashes, decreased libido,
myalgia,* reduced breast size, weight
gain or loss, increased libido, de-
creased bone density.

INTERACTIONS
None reported.

NURSING CONSIDERATIONS
• Contraindicated in patients hyper-

Italicized adverse reactions are common or life-threatening.
*Liquid form contains alcohol.   **May contain tartrazine.

sensitive to GnRH analogs or any components of the formulation (benzalkonium chloride, sorbitol, purified water, glacial acetic acid, hydrochloric acid, or sodium hydroxide). Also contraindicated in the presence of undiagnosed vaginal bleeding, in breastfeeding women, and during pregnancy. Nafarelin may cause fetal harm if administered to a pregnant woman.

• Studies have confirmed a small loss in bone density after 6 months of therapy, probably caused by the hypoestrogenic state induced by the drug. Patients with major risk factors for osteoporosis (chronic alcohol or tobacco users, strong family history of osteoporosis, or patients who are using drugs that may reduce bone mass such as anticonvulsants or corticosteroids) should not receive additional courses of therapy and should strongly weigh risk/benefit before an initial trial of the drug.

• Advise the patient that she should contact her doctor if she develops a cold or rhinitis during therapy. If she requires a topical nasal decongestant, the manufacturer suggests that it be used at least 30 minutes after nafarelin treatment to reduce the possibility of interference with nafarelin absorption.

• Advise the patient to use a mechanical form of contraception (such as barrier contraception). Although the drug will usually inhibit ovulation and stop menstruation, it is not a reliable contraceptive, particularly if the patient misses a few doses. She should stop the drug immediately and contact her doctor if she believes that she is pregnant.

• Teach the patient that menstruation will stop with regular use of the drug. She should contact her doctor if menstruation persists or breakthrough bleeding occurs.

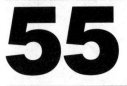

Antidiabetic agents and glucagon

acetohexamide
chlorpropamide
glipizide
glucagon
glyburide
insulins
tolazamide
tolbutamide

COMBINATION PRODUCT
MIXTARD INJECTION◇: 100 mg/ml isophane purified pork insulin suspension and purified pork insulin injection.

---

acetohexamide
Dimelor†, Dymelor

Pregnancy Risk Category: D

HOW SUPPLIED
Tablets: 250 mg, 500 mg

MECHANISM OF ACTION
Stimulates insulin release from the pancreatic beta cells and reduces glucose output by the liver. An extrapancreatic effect increases peripheral sensitivity to insulin. A sulfonylurea.

INDICATIONS & DOSAGE
Adjunct to diet to lower the blood glucose in patients with non-insulin-dependent diabetes mellitus (type II)—
Adults: initially, 250 mg P.O. daily before breakfast; may increase dosage q 5 to 7 days (by 250 to 500 mg) as needed to maximum of 1.5 g daily, divided b.i.d. to t.i.d. before meals.
To replace insulin therapy—
Adults: if insulin dosage is less than 20 units daily, insulin may be stopped and oral therapy started with 250 mg P.O. daily, before breakfast, increased as above if needed. If insulin dosage is 20 to 40 units daily, start oral therapy with 250 mg P.O. daily, before breakfast, while reducing insulin dosage 25% to 30% daily or every other day, depending on response to oral therapy.

ADVERSE REACTIONS
GI: nausea, heartburn, vomiting.
Metabolic: sodium loss, *hypoglycemia.*
Skin: rash, pruritus, facial flushing.
Other: hypersensitivity reactions.

INTERACTIONS
Anabolic steroids, chloramphenicol, clofibrate, guanethidine, MAO inhibitors, oral anticoagulants, phenylbutazone, salicylates, sulfonamides: increased hypoglycemic activity. Monitor blood glucose level.
Beta blockers, clonidine: prolonged hypoglycemic effect and masked symptoms of hypoglycemia. Use together cautiously.
Corticosteroids, glucagon, rifampin, thiazide diuretics: decreased hypoglycemic response. Monitor blood glucose level.

NURSING CONSIDERATIONS
• Contraindicated in treating type I (insulin-dependent) diabetes mellitus (IDDM); in diabetes adequately controlled by diet; and in type II diabetes complicated by ketosis, acidosis, diabetic coma, Raynaud's disease, gan-

---

Italicized adverse reactions are common or life-threatening.
*Liquid form contains alcohol.   **May contain tartrazine.

grene, renal or hepatic impairment, or thyroid or other endocrine dysfunction. Use cautiously in patients with sulfonamide hypersensitivity.

• Instruct patient about nature of disease; importance of following therapeutic regimen, adhering to specific diet, weight reduction, exercise, and personal hygiene programs, and avoiding infection; how and when to perform self-monitoring of blood glucose level; and recognition of hypoglycemia and hyperglycemia.

• Make sure patient understands that therapy relieves symptoms but doesn't cure the disease.

• Patient transferring from another oral sulfonylurea antidiabetic drug usually needs no transition period.

• Patient transferring from insulin therapy to an oral antidiabetic requires blood glucose monitoring at least t.i.d. before meals. Patient may require hospitalization during transition.

• During periods of increased stress, such as infection, fever, surgery, or trauma, patient may require insulin therapy. Monitor patient closely for hyperglycemia in these situations.

• Advise patient to avoid moderate to large intake of alcohol; disulfiram-like reaction possible.

• The possibility of increased cardiovascular mortality is associated with the use of sulfonylureas.

chlorpropamide

Apo-Chlorpropamide†, Diabinese, Glucamide, Novo-propamide†

Pregnancy Risk Category: D

HOW SUPPLIED
Tablets: 100 mg, 250 mg

MECHANISM OF ACTION
Stimulates insulin release from the pancreatic beta cells and reduces glucose output by the liver. An extrapancreatic effect increases peripheral

sensitivity to insulin. Also exerts an antidiuretic effect in patients with pituitary-deficient diabetes insipidus. A sulfonylurea.

INDICATIONS & DOSAGE
Adjunct to diet to lower blood glucose in patients with non-insulin-dependent diabetes mellitus (type II)—
Adults: 250 mg P.O. daily with breakfast or in divided doses if GI disturbances occur. First dosage increase may be made after 5 to 7 days because of extended duration of action, then dosage may be increased q 3 to 5 days by 50 to 125 mg, if needed, to maximum of 750 mg daily.
Adults over 65 years: initial dose should be in the range of 100 to 125 mg P.O. daily.
To change from insulin to oral therapy—
Adults: if insulin dosage is less than 40 units daily, insulin may be stopped and oral therapy started as above. If insulin dosage is 40 units or more daily, start oral therapy as above with insulin reduced 50%. Further insulin reductions should be made according to patient response.

ADVERSE REACTIONS
GI: nausea, heartburn, vomiting.
GU: tea-colored urine.
Metabolic: prolonged hypoglycemia, *dilutional hyponatremia.*
Skin: rash, pruritus, facial flushing.
Other: *hypersensitivity reactions.*

INTERACTIONS
Anabolic steroids, chloramphenicol, clofibrate, guanethidine, MAO inhibitors, oral anticoagulants, phenylbutazone, salicylates, sulfonamides: increased hypoglycemic activity. Monitor blood glucose level.
Beta blockers, clonidine: prolonged hypoglycemic effect and masked symptoms of hypoglycemia. Use together cautiously.
Corticosteroids, glucagon, rifampin,

thiazide diuretics: decreased hypoglycemic response. Monitor blood glucose level.

NURSING CONSIDERATIONS
• Contraindicated in treating type I (insulin-dependent) diabetes mellitus (IDDM); in diabetes adequately controlled by diet; and in type II diabetes complicated by fever, ketosis, acidosis, diabetic coma, major surgery, severe trauma, Raynaud's disease, gangrene, renal or hepatic impairment, or thyroid or other endocrine dysfunction. Use cautiously in patients with sulfonamide hypersensitivity.
• Elderly patients may be more sensitive to this drug's adverse reactions.
• Instruct patient about nature of the disease; importance of following therapeutic regimen, adhering to specific diet, weight reduction, exercise, and personal hygiene programs, and avoiding infection; how and when to perform self-monitoring of blood glucose level; and recognition of and intervention for hypoglycemia and hyperglycemia.
• Make sure patient understands that therapy relieves symptoms but doesn't cure the disease.
• Adverse effects, especially hypoglycemia, may be more frequent or severe than with some other sulfonylurea drugs (acetohexamide, tolazamide, and tolbutamide) because of its long duration of effect (36 hours).
• If hypoglycemia occurs, patient should be monitored closely for a minimum of 3 to 5 days.
• Patient transferring from another oral sulfonylurea antidiabetic drug usually needs no transition period.
• Patient may require hospitalization during transition from insulin therapy to an oral antidiabetic. Monitor patient for blood glucose levels at least t.i.d., before meals; emphasize the need for a double-voided specimen.

• Drug may accumulate in patients with renal insufficiency.
• Advise patient to avoid intake of alcohol. Chlorpropamide-alcohol flush (CPAF) is characterized by facial flushing, light-headedness, headache, and occasional breathlessness. Even very small amounts of alcohol can produce this reaction.
• Watch for signs of impending renal insufficiency, such as dysuria, anuria, and hematuria, and report them to the doctor immediately.
• May potentiate antidiuretic hormone. Sometimes used to treat diabetes insipidus.
• The possibility of increased cardiovascular mortality is associated with the use of sulfonylureas.

glipizide
Glucotrol, Minidiab‡

Pregnancy Risk Category: C

HOW SUPPLIED
Tablets: 5 mg, 10 mg

MECHANISM OF ACTION
Stimulates insulin release from the pancreatic beta cells and reduces glucose output by the liver. An extrapancreatic effect increases peripheral sensitivity to insulin. A sulfonylurea.

INDICATIONS & DOSAGE
Adjunct to diet to lower the blood glucose in patients with non-insulin-dependent diabetes mellitus (type II)—
Adults: initially, 5 mg P.O. daily given before breakfast. Elderly patients or those with liver disease may be started on 2.5 mg. Usual maintenance dosage is 10 to 15 mg. Maximum recommended daily dosage is 40 mg.
To replace insulin therapy—
Adults: if insulin dosage is more than 20 units daily, patient may be started at usual dosage in addition to 50% of the insulin. If insulin dosage is less

---

than 20 units, insulin may be discontinued.

ADVERSE REACTIONS
CNS: dizziness.
GI: nausea, vomiting, constipation.
Hepatic: *cholestatic jaundice*.
Metabolic: *hypoglycemia*.
Skin: rash, pruritus, facial flushing.

INTERACTIONS
Anabolic steroids, chloramphenicol, clofibrate, guanethidine, MAO inhibitors, oral anticoagulants, phenylbutazone, salicylates, sulfonamides: increased hypoglycemic activity. Monitor blood glucose level.
Beta blockers, clonidine: prolonged hypoglycemic effect and masked symptoms of hypoglycemia. Use together cautiously.
Corticosteroids, glucagon, rifampin, thiazide diuretics: decreased hypoglycemic response. Monitor blood glucose level.

NURSING CONSIDERATIONS
• Contraindicated in diabetic ketoacidosis, with or without coma. Use cautiously in renal and hepatic disease and sulfonamide hypersensitivity.
• Elderly patients may be more sensitive to this drug's adverse reactions.
• Patient transferring from insulin therapy to an oral antidiabetic requires blood glucose monitoring at least t.i.d. before meals. Patient may require hospitalization during transition.
• During periods of increased stress, such as infection, fever, surgery, or trauma, patient may require insulin therapy. Monitor patient closely for hyperglycemia in these situations.
• Instruct patient about nature of disease; importance of following therapeutic regimen, adhering to specific diet, weight reduction, exercise, and personal hygiene programs, and avoiding infection; how and when to perform self-monitoring of blood glucose level; recognition of hypoglycemia and hyperglycemia.
• Some patients taking glipizide may be effectively controlled on a once-daily regimen, while others show better response with divided dosing.
• Give approximately 30 minutes before meals.
• Glipizide is a second-generation sulfonylurea oral hypoglycemic. The frequency of adverse reactions appears to be lower than with first-generation drugs such as chlorpropamide and tolbutamide.
• Glipizide has a mild diuretic effect. May be useful in patients who have CHF or cirrhosis.
• The possibility of increased cardiovascular mortality is associated with the use of sulfonylureas.

glucagon
Pregnancy Risk Category: B

HOW SUPPLIED
Powder for injection: 1 mg (1 unit)/vial, 10 mg (10 units)/vial

MECHANISM OF ACTION
Raises blood glucose level by promoting catalytic depolymerization of hepatic glycogen to glucose.

INDICATIONS & DOSAGE
Coma of insulin-shock therapy—
Adults: 0.5 to 1 mg S.C., I.M., or I.V. 1 hour after coma develops; may repeat within 25 minutes, if necessary. In very deep coma, also give glucose 10% to 50% I.V. for faster response. When patient responds, give additional carbohydrate immediately.
Severe insulin-induced hypoglycemia during diabetic therapy—
Adults and children: 0.5 to 1 mg S.C., I.M., or I.V.; may repeat q 20 minutes for 2 doses, if necessary. If coma persists, give glucose 10% to 50% I.V.

---

†Available in Canada only.   ‡Available in Australia only.   ◊Available OTC.

Diagnostic aid for radiologic examination—
Adults: 0.25 to 2 mg I.V. or I.M. before initiation of radiologic procedure.

ADVERSE REACTIONS
GI: nausea, vomiting.
Other: hypersensitivity.

INTERACTIONS
Phenytoin: inhibited glucagon-induced insulin release. Use cautiously.

NURSING CONSIDERATIONS
• Unstable hypoglycemic diabetics may not respond to glucagon. Give dextrose I.V. instead.
• It is vital to arouse the patient from coma as quickly as possible and to give additional carbohydrates orally to prevent secondary hypoglycemic reactions.
• For I.V. drip infusion, glucagon is compatible with dextrose solution, but forms a precipitate in chloride solutions.
• Instruct the patient and family in proper glucagon administration, recognition of hypoglycemia, and urgency of calling a doctor immediately in emergencies.
• May be used as diagnostic aid in radiologic examination of the stomach, duodenum, small bowel, and colon when a hypotonic state is advantageous.
• Has a positive inotropic and chronotropic action on the heart. May be used to treat overdosage of beta-adrenergic blockers.

glyburide
DiaBeta**, Euglucon†, Micronase
Pregnancy Risk Category: B

HOW SUPPLIED
Tablets: 1.25 mg, 2.5 mg, 5 mg

MECHANISM OF ACTION
Stimulates insulin release from the pancreatic beta cells and reduces glucose output by the liver. An extrapancreatic effect increases peripheral sensitivity to insulin. A sulfonylurea.

INDICATIONS & DOSAGE
Adjunct to diet to lower the blood glucose in patients with non-insulin-dependent diabetes mellitus (type II)—
Adults: initially, 2.5 to 5 mg P.O. daily administered with breakfast. Patients who are more sensitive to hypoglycemic drugs should be started at 1.25 mg daily. Usual maintenance dosage is 1.25 to 20 mg daily, given either as a single dose or in divided doses.
To replace insulin therapy—
Adults: if insulin dosage is more than 40 units daily, patient may be started on 5 mg glyburide daily in addition to 50% of the insulin dosage.

ADVERSE REACTIONS
GI: nausea, epigastric fullness, heartburn.
Hepatic: *cholestatic jaundice.*
Metabolic: *hypoglycemia.*
Skin: rash, pruritus, facial flushing.

INTERACTIONS
Anabolic steroids, chloramphenicol, clofibrate, guanethidine, MAO inhibitors, oral anticoagulants, phenylbutazone, salicylates, sulfonamides: increased hypoglycemic activity. Monitor blood glucose level.
Beta blockers, clonidine: prolonged hypoglycemic effect and masked symptoms of hypoglycemia. Use together cautiously.
Corticosteroids, glucagon, rifampin, thiazide diuretics: decreased hypoglycemic response. Monitor blood glucose level.

NURSING CONSIDERATIONS
• Contraindicated in diabetic ketoacidosis, with or without coma. Use cau-

---

Italicized adverse reactions are common or life-threatening.
*Liquid form contains alcohol.   **May contain tartrazine.

tiously in sulfonamide hypersensitivity and severe renal impairment.

• Elderly patients may be more sensitive to this drug's adverse reactions.

• Patient transferring from insulin therapy to an oral antidiabetic requires blood glucose monitoring at least t.i.d. before meals. Patient may require hospitalization during transition.

• During periods of increased stress, such as infection, fever, surgery, or trauma, patient may require insulin therapy. Monitor patient closely for hyperglycemia in these situations.

• Instruct patient about nature of disease; importance of following therapeutic regimen, adhering to specific diet, weight reduction, exercise, and personal hygiene programs, and avoiding infection; how and when to perform self-monitoring of blood glucose level; recognition of hypoglycemia and hyperglycemia.

• A maintenance dosage of 5 mg glyburide provides approximately the same degree of blood glucose control as 250 to 375 mg chlorpropamide, 250 to 375 mg tolazamide, 500 to 750 mg acetohexamide, or 1,000 to 1,500 mg tolbutamide.

• Although most patients may take glyburide once daily, patients taking more than 10 mg daily may achieve better results with twice-daily dosage.

• Glyburide is a second-generation sulfonylurea oral hypoglycemic. The frequency of adverse effects appears to be lower than with first-generation drugs such as chlorpropamide and tolbutamide.

• Glyburide exerts a mild diuretic effect. May be useful in patients who have CHF or cirrhosis.

• The possibility of increased cardiovascular mortality is associated with the use of sulfonylureas.

insulins

insulin injection (regular insulin, crystalline zinc insulin)

Actrapid HM‡, Actrapid HM Penfill‡, Actrapid MC‡, Actrapid MC Penfill‡, Beef Regular Iletin II◇, Humulin R◇, Hypurin Neutral‡, Insulin 2‡, Novolin R◇, Novolin R Penfill◇, Pork Regular Iletin II◇, Regular (Concentrated) Iletin II, Regular Iletin I◇, Regular Purified Pork Insulin◇, Velosulin◇, Velosulin Human‡, Velosulin Insuject◇

insulin zinc suspension, prompt (semilente)

Semilente Iletin I◇, Semilente Insulin◇, Semilente MC Pork‡, Semilente Purified Pork◇

isophane insulin suspension (neutral protamine Hagedorn insulin, NPH)

Beef NPH Iletin II◇, Humulin N◇, Humulin NPH‡, Hypurin Isophane‡, Insulatard‡, Insulatard Human‡, Insulatard NPH◇, Isotard MC‡, Novolin N◇, NPH Iletin I◇, NPH Insulin◇, NPH Purified Pork◇, Pork NPH Iletin II◇, Protaphane HM‡, Protaphane HM Penfill‡, Protaphane MC‡

isophane insulin suspension with insulin injection

Actraphane HM‡, Actraphane HM Penfill‡, Actraphane MC‡, Mixtard◇, Mixtard Human‡, Novolin 70/30

insulin zinc suspension (lente)

Humulin L◇, Lente Iletin I◇, Lente Iletine II◇, Lente Insulin◇, Lente MC‡, Lente Purified Pork Insulin◇,

---

Monotard HM‡, Monotard MC‡, Novolin L◇

protamine zinc suspension (PZI)

Protamine, Zinc & Iletin I◇;
Protamine, Zinc & Iletin II (Beef)◇;
Protamine, Zinc & Iletin II (Pork)◇;
Protamine Zinc Insulin MC‡

insulin zinc suspension, extended (ultralente)

Ultralente Iletin I◇, Ultralente Insulin◇, Ultralente Purified Beef◇, Ultratard HM‡, Ultratard MC‡

Pregnancy Risk Category: B

HOW SUPPLIED
insulin injection
Injection (from beef and pork): 40 units/ml◇, 100 units/ml◇ (Regular Iletin I◇)
Injection (human): 100 units/ml (Actrapid HM‡, Humulin R◇, Novolin R◇, Velosulin◇, Velosulin Human‡); 100 units/ml in 1.5-ml cartridge system◇ (Actrapid HM Penfill‡, Novolin R Penfill◇)
Injection (from pork): 100 units/ml◇
Injection (purified beef): 100 units/ml (Beef Regular Iletin II◇, Hypurin Neutral‡, Insulin 2‡)
Injection (purified pork): 100 units/ml (Actrapid MC‡, Pork Regular Iletin II◇, Regular Purified Pork Insulin◇, Velosulin◇); 100 units/ml in 1.5-ml cartridge system‡ (Actrapid MC Penfill‡); 100 units/ml in 2-ml cartridge system‡ (Velosulin Insuject‡); 500 units/ml (Regular [Concentrated] Iletin II)
insulin zinc suspension, prompt
Injection (from beef): 100 units/ml◇ (Semilente Insulin◇)
Injection (from beef and pork): 40 units/ml◇, 100 units/ml◇ (Semilente Iletin◇)
Injection (purified pork): 100 units/ml◇ (Semilente MC‡, Semilente Purified Pork◇)
isophane insulin suspension

Injection (from beef): 100 units/ml◇ (NPH Insulin◇)
Injection (from beef and pork): 40 units/ml◇, 100 units/ml◇ (NPH Iletin I◇)
Injection (human, recombinant): 100 units/ml (Humulin N◇, Humulin NPH‡, Insulatard Human†, Insulatard NPH◇, Novolin N◇, Protaphane HM‡); 100 units/ml in 1.5-ml cartridge system‡ (Protaphane HM Penfill‡)
Injection (purified beef): 100 units/ml (Beef NPH Iletin II◇, Hypurin Isophane†, Isotard MC†)
Injection (purified pork): 100 units/ml (Insulatard‡, Insulatard NPH◇, NPH Purified Pork◇, Pork NPH Iletin II, Protaphane MC‡)
isophane insulin suspension with insulin injection
Injection (human): 100 units/ml (Actraphane HM‡, Mixtard Human‡, Novolin 70/30◇); 100 units/ml in 1.5-ml cartridge system‡ (Actraphane HM Penfill‡)
Injection (purified pork): 100 units/ml (Actraphane MC‡, Mixtard◇, Lente MC‡)
insulin zinc suspension
Injection (beef): 100 units/ml (Lente Insulin◇, Lente MC‡)
Injection (from beef and pork): 40 units/ml◇, 100 units/ml◇ (Lente Iletin I◇)
Injection: (purified beef): 100 units/ml (Lente Iletin II◇, Lente MC‡)
Injection (purified pork): 100 units/ml (Monotard MC‡, Lente Purified Pork Insulin◇)
Injection (human): 100 units/ml◇ (Humulin L◇, Monotard HM◇, Novolin I◇)
protamine zinc suspension
Injection (from beef and pork): 40 units/ml◇, 100 units/ml◇ (Protamine, Zinc & Iletin I◇)
Injection (purified beef): 100 units/ml◇ (Protamine, Zinc & Iletin II [Beef]◇)
Injection (purified pork): 100 units/ml

Italicized adverse reactions are common or life-threatening.
*Liquid form contains alcohol.   **May contain tartrazine.

(Protamine, Zinc & Iletin II [Pork]◊,
Protamine Zinc Insulin MC‡)
insulin zinc suspension, extended
Injection (from beef): 100 units/ml◊
(Ultralente Purified Beef◊)
Injection (from beef and pork): 40
units/ml◊, 100 units/ml◊ (Ultralente
Iletin I◊)
Injection (human): 100 units/ml‡ (Ul-
tratard HM‡)
Injection (purified pork): 100 units/
ml‡ (Ultralente MC‡)

MECHANISM OF ACTION

Increases glucose transport across
muscle and fat cell membranes to reduce blood glucose level. Promotes
conversion of glucose to its storage
form, glycogen; triggers amino acid
uptake and conversion to protein in
muscle cells and inhibits protein degradation; stimulates triglyceride formation and inhibits release of free
fatty acids from adipose tissue; and
stimulates lipoprotein lipase activity,
which converts circulating lipoproteins to fatty acids.

INDICATIONS & DOSAGE

*Diabetic ketoacidosis (use regular in-
sulin only)—*
Adults: 25 to 150 units I.V. immediately, then additional doses may be
given q 1 hour based on blood sugar
level until patient is out of acidosis;
then give S.C. q 6 hours thereafter.
Alternative dosage schedule: 50 to
100 units I.V. and 50 to 100 units S.C.
stat; additional doses may be given q 2
to 6 hours based on blood sugar levels; or 0.33 units/kg I.V. bolus, followed by 7 to 10 units/hour I.V. by
continuous infusion. Continue infusion until blood sugar drops to 250
mg/dl, then start S.C. insulin q 6
hours.
Children: 0.5 to 1 unit/kg in two divided doses, 1 given I.V. and the other
S.C., followed by 0.5 to 1 unit/kg I.V.
q 1 to 2 hours; or 0.1 unit/kg I.V.
bolus, then 0.1 unit/kg hourly contin-

uous I.V. infusion until blood sugar
drops to 250 mg/dl, then start S.C. insulin. Preparation of infusion: add
100 units regular insulin and 1 g albumin to 100 ml 0.9% saline solution.
Insulin concentration will be 1 unit/
ml. (The albumin will adsorb to plastic, preventing loss of the insulin to
plastic.)
*Type I (insulin-dependent) diabetes
mellitus, ketosis-prone diabetics, diabetes mellitus inadequately controlled
by diet and oral hypoglycemics—*
Adults and children: therapeutic regimen prescribed by doctor and adjusted according to patient's blood
and urine glucose concentrations.

ADVERSE REACTIONS

Metabolic: *hypoglycemia, hyperglycemia (rebound, or Somogyi, effect).*
Skin: *urticaria.*
Local: *lipoatrophy, lipohypertrophy,
itching, swelling, redness, stinging,
warmth at site of injection.*
Other: *anaphylaxis.*

INTERACTIONS

*Alcohol, beta blockers, clofibrate, fen-
fluramine, MAO inhibitors, salicylates, tetracycline:* prolonged hypoglycemic effect. Monitor blood glucose level carefully.
Corticosteroids, thiazide diuretics: diminished insulin response. Monitor
for hyperglycemia.

NURSING CONSIDERATIONS

• Use only regular insulin in patients
with circulatory collapse, diabetic ketoacidosis, or hyperkalemia. Do not
use regular insulin concentrated I.V.
Do not use intermediate or long-
acting insulins for coma or other
emergency requiring rapid drug action.
• Accuracy of measurement is very
important, especially with regular insulin concentrated. Aids, such as
magnifying sleeve, dose magnifier, or

---

†Available in Canada only.   ‡Available in Australia only.   ◊ Available OTC.

cornwall syringe, may help improve accuracy.

• Dosage is always expressed in USP units.

• Don't interchange single-source beef or pork insulins; a dosage adjustment may be required.

• Lente, semilente, and ultralente insulins may be mixed in any proportion.

• Regular insulin may be mixed with NPH or lente insulins in any proportion.

• Regular insulin *should not* be mixed with globin insulin.

• Advise patient not to alter the order of mixing insulins or change the model or brand of syringe or needle.

• Note that switching from separate injections to a prepared mixture may alter patient's response. Whenever NPH or lente is mixed with regular insulin in the same syringe, be sure to administer immediately to avoid binding.

• Store insulin in cool area. Refrigeration desirable but not essential, except with regular insulin concentrated.

• Don't use insulin that has changed color or becomes clumped or granular in appearance.

• Check expiration date on vial before using contents.

• Administration route is S.C. because absorption rate and pain are less than with I.M. injections.

• Ketosis-prone type I diabetics, severely ill, and newly diagnosed diabetics with very high blood sugar level may require hospitalization and I.V. treatment with regular fast-acting insulin.

• Ketosis-resistant diabetics may be treated as outpatients with intermediate-acting insulin and instructions on how to alter dosage according to self-performed blood glucose determinations.

• Instruct patients on proper use of equipment for performing self-monitoring of blood glucose.

• Press but do not rub site after injection. Rotate injection sites and chart to avoid overuse of one area. However, unstable diabetics may achieve better control if injection site is rotated within same anatomic region.

• To mix insulin suspension, swirl vial gently or rotate between palms or between palm and thigh. Don't shake vigorously: this causes bubbling and air in syringe.

• Insulin requirements increase, sometimes drastically, in pregnant diabetics, then decline immediately postpartum.

• Be sure the patient knows that therapy relieves symptoms but doesn't cure the disease.

• Instruct patient about nature of disease; the importance of following the therapeutic regimen, adhering to specific diet, weight reduction, exercise, and personal hygiene programs, and avoiding infection; and timing of injection and eating. Emphasize that meals must not be omitted. Teach that self-monitoring of blood glucose tests and urine ketone tests are essential guides to dosage and success of therapy; important to recognize hypoglycemic symptoms because insulin-induced hypoglycemia is hazardous and may cause brain damage if prolonged; most adverse effects are self-limiting and temporary.

• Advise patient to wear medical identification alert at all times; to carry ample insulin supply and syringes on trips; to have carbohydrates (lump of sugar or candy) on hand for emergency; to take note of time zone changes for dose schedule when traveling.

• Marijuana use may increase insulin requirements.

• Cigarette smoking decreases the amount of absorption of insulin administered subcutaneously. Advise

---

Italicized adverse reactions are common or life-threatening.
*Liquid form contains alcohol.   **May contain tartrazine.

patient not to smoke within 30 minutes after insulin injection.
• Some patients may develop insulin resistance and require large insulin doses to control symptoms of diabetes. U-500 insulin is available as Regular (Concentrated) Iletin I for such patients. Although every pharmacy may not normally stock it, it is readily available. Patient should notify pharmacist several days before refill of prescription is needed. Nurse should give hospital pharmacy sufficient notice before needing to refill in-house prescription. Never store U-500 insulin in same area with other insulin preparations because of danger of severe overdose if given accidentally to other patients. U-500 insulin must be administered with a U-100 syringe since no syringes are made for this drug.
• Humulin is synthesized by a strain of *Escherichia coli* that has been genetically altered. Novolin is derived from enzymatic alteration of pork insulin.

---

tolazamide
Ronase, Tolamide, Tolinase
Pregnancy Risk Category: C

HOW SUPPLIED
Tablets: 100 mg, 250 mg, 500 mg

MECHANISM OF ACTION
Stimulates insulin release from the pancreatic beta cells and reduces glucose output by the liver. An extrapancreatic effect increases peripheral sensitivity to insulin. A sulfonylurea.

INDICATIONS & DOSAGE
Adjunct to diet to lower the blood glucose in patients with non-insulin-dependent diabetes mellitus (type II)—
Adults: initially, 100 mg P.O. daily with breakfast if fasting blood sugar (FBS) under 200 mg/dl; or 250 mg if FBS is over 200 mg/dl. May adjust

dosage at weekly intervals by 100 to 250 mg. Maximum dosage is 500 mg b.i.d. before meals.
Adults over 65: 100 mg P.O. once daily.
To change from insulin to oral therapy—
Adults: if insulin dosage is under 20 units daily, insulin may be stopped and oral therapy started at 100 mg P.O. daily with breakfast. If insulin dosage is 20 to 40 units daily, insulin may be stopped and oral therapy started at 250 mg P.O. daily with breakfast. If insulin dosage is over 40 units daily, decrease insulin 50% and start oral therapy at 250 mg P.O. daily with breakfast. Increase dosages as above.

ADVERSE REACTIONS
GI: nausea, vomiting.
Metabolic: hypoglycemia.
Skin: rash, urticaria, facial flushing.
Other: hypersensitivity reactions.

INTERACTIONS
Anabolic steroids, chloramphenicol, clofibrate, guanethidine, MAO inhibitors, oral anticoagulants, phenylbutazone, salicylates, sulfonamides: increased hypoglycemic activity. Monitor blood glucose level.
Beta blockers, clonidine: prolonged hypoglycemic effect and masked symptoms of hypoglycemia. Use together cautiously.
Corticosteroids, glucagon, rifampin, thiazide diuretics: decreased hypoglycemic response. Monitor blood glucose level.

NURSING CONSIDERATIONS
• Contraindicated in treating type I (insulin-dependent) diabetes mellitus (IDDM); in diabetes adequately controlled by diet; and in type II diabetes complicated by fever, ketosis, acidosis, or coma, major surgery, severe trauma, Raynaud's disease, renal or hepatic impairment, or thyroid or

---

†Available in Canada only.　　‡Available in Australia only.　　◊ Available OTC.

other endocrine dysfunction. Use cautiously in sulfonamide hypersensitivity and in elderly, debilitated, or malnourished patients.
• Elderly patients may be more sensitive to this drug's adverse reactions.
• Instruct patient about nature of disease; importance of following therapeutic regimen, adhering to specific diet, weight reduction, exercise, and personal hygiene programs, and avoiding infection; how and when to perform self-monitoring of blood glucose level; and recognition of hypoglycemia and hyperglycemia.
• Be sure patient knows that therapy relieves symptoms but doesn't cure disease.
• Patient transferring from another oral sulfonylurea antidiabetic drug usually needs no transition period.
• Patient transferring from insulin therapy to an oral hypoglycemic should test for blood glucose at least t.i.d. before meals. Hospitalization may be required during the transition.
• Advise patient to avoid moderate to large intake of alcohol; disulfiram-like reaction possible.
• The possibility of increased cardiovascular mortality is associated with the use of sulfonylureas.

tolbutamide
Apo-Tolbutamide, Mobenol†, Novobutamide†, Oramide, Orinase
Pregnancy Risk Category: C

HOW SUPPLIED
Tablets: 250 mg, 500 mg

MECHANISM OF ACTION
Stimulates insulin release from the pancreatic beta cells and reduces glucose output by the liver. An extrapancreatic effect increases peripheral sensitivity to insulin. A sulfonylurea.

INDICATIONS & DOSAGE
Stable, maturity-onset (Type II) nonke-totic diabetes mellitus uncontrolled by diet alone and previously untreated—
Adults: initially, 1 to 2 g P.O. daily as single dose or divided b.i.d. to t.i.d. May adjust dosage to maximum of 3 g daily.
To change from insulin to oral therapy—
Adults: if insulin dosage is under 20 units daily, insulin may be stopped and oral therapy started at 1 to 2 g P.O. daily. If insulin dosage is 20 to 40 units daily, insulin is reduced 30% to 50% and oral therapy started as above. If insulin dosage is over 40 units daily, insulin is decreased 20% and oral therapy started as above. Further reductions in insulin are based on patient's response to oral therapy.

ADVERSE REACTIONS
GI: nausea, heartburn.
Metabolic: hypoglycemia, dilutional hyponatremia.
Skin: rash, pruritus, facial flushing.
Other: hypersensitivity reactions.

INTERACTIONS
Anabolic steroids, chloramphenicol, clofibrate, guanethidine, MAO inhibitors, oral anticoagulants, phenylbutazone, salicylates, sulfonamides: increased hypoglycemic activity. Monitor blood glucose level.
Beta blockers, clonidine: prolonged hypoglycemic effect and masked symptoms of hypoglycemia. Use together cautiously.
Corticosteroids, glucagon, rifampin, thiazide diuretics: decreased hypoglycemic response. Monitor blood glucose level.

NURSING CONSIDERATIONS
• Contraindicated in treating type I (insulin-dependent) diabetes mellitus (IDDM); in diabetes mellitus adequately controlled by diet; and in type II diabetes complicated by fever, ketosis, acidosis, or coma, major surgery,

---

Italicized adverse reactions are common or life-threatening.
*Liquid form contains alcohol.   **May contain tartrazine.

severe trauma, Raynaud's disease, renal or hepatic impairment, thyroid or other endocrine dysfunction, or pregnancy. Use cautiously in patients with sulfonamide hypersensitivity.

• Elderly patients may be more sensitive to this drug's adverse reactions.

• Instruct patient about nature of disease; importance of following therapeutic regimen, adhering to specific diet, weight reduction, exercise, and personal hygiene program, and avoiding infection; how and when to perform self-monitoring of blood glucose level; and recognition of hypoglycemia and hyperglycemia.

• Be sure patient knows that therapy relieves symptoms but doesn't cure disease.

• Patient transferring from another oral sulfonylurea antidiabetic drug usually needs no transition period.

• Patient transferring from insulin therapy to an oral hypoglycemic should test for blood glucose at least t.i.d. before meals. Hospitalization may be required during the transition.

• Advise patient to avoid moderate to large intake of alcohol: disulfiram-like reaction possible.

• The possibility of increased cardiovascular mortality is associated with the use of sulfonylureas.

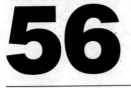

Thyroid hormones

levothyroxine sodium
liothyronine sodium
liotrix
thyroglobulin
thyroid desiccated
thyrotropin

COMBINATION PRODUCTS

EUTHROID-½: levothyroxine sodium 30 mcg and liothyronine sodium 7.5 mcg.
EUTHROID-1: levothyroxine sodium 60 mcg and liothyronine sodium 15 mcg.
EUTHROID-2: levothyroxine sodium 120 mcg and liothyronine sodium 30 mcg.
EUTHROID-3: levothyroxine sodium 180 mcg and liothyronine sodium 45 mcg.
THYROLAR-¼: levothyroxine sodium 12.5 mcg and liothyronine sodium 3.1 mcg.
THYROLAR-½: levothyroxine sodium 25 mcg and liothyronine sodium 6.25 mcg.
THYROLAR-1: levothyroxine sodium 50 mcg and liothyronine sodium 12.5 mcg.
THYROLAR-2: levothyroxine sodium 100 mcg and liothyronine sodium 25 mcg.
THYROLAR-3: levothyroxine sodium 150 mcg and liothyronine sodium 37.5 mcg.

levothyroxine sodium (T_4 or L-thyroxine sodium)

Eltroxin†, Levoid, Levothroid, Levoxine, Oroxine‡, Synthroid**, Synthrox

Pregnancy Risk Category: A

HOW SUPPLIED

Tablets: 25 mcg, 50 mcg, 75 mcg, 100 mcg, 125 mcg, 150 mcg, 175 mcg, 200 mcg, 300 mcg
Injection: 200 mcg/vial, 500 mcg/vial

MECHANISM OF ACTION

Stimulates the metabolism of all body tissues by accelerating the rate of cellular oxidation.

INDICATIONS & DOSAGE

Cretinism—
Children under 1 year: initially, 0.025 to 0.05 mg P.O. daily, increased by 0.05 mg P.O. q 2 to 3 weeks to total daily dosage of 0.1 to 0.4 mg P.O.
Myxedema coma—
Adults: 0.2 to 0.5 mg I.V. If no response in 24 hours, additional 0.1 to 0.3 mg I.V. After condition stabilized, oral maintenance.
Thyroid hormone replacement—
Adults: initially, 0.025 to 0.1 mg P.O. daily, increased by 0.05 to 0.1 mg P.O. q 1 to 4 weeks until desired response. Maintenance dosage is 0.1 to 0.4 mg daily. May be administered I.V. or I.M. when P.O. ingestion is precluded for long periods.
Adults over 65 years: 0.025 mg P.O. daily. May be increased by 0.025 mg

---

Italicized adverse reactions are common or life-threatening.
*Liquid form contains alcohol.   **May contain tartrazine.

at 3- to 4-week intervals depending on response.

Children: initially, maximum 0.05 mg P.O. daily, gradually increased by 0.025 to 0.05 mg P.O. q 1 to 4 weeks until desired response.

ADVERSE REACTIONS

Adverse reactions of thyroid hormones are extensions of their pharmacologic properties and reflect patient sensitivity to them.

Signs of overdosage:
CNS: *nervousness, insomnia, tremor.*
CV: *tachycardia, palpitations, arrhythmias, angina pectoris,* hypertension.
GI: change in appetite, nausea, diarrhea.
Other: headache, leg cramps, weight loss, sweating, heat intolerance, fever, menstrual irregularities.

INTERACTIONS

Cholestyramine and colestipol: levothyroxine absorption impaired. Separate doses by 4 to 5 hours.
I.V. phenytoin: free thyroid released. Monitor for tachycardia.

NURSING CONSIDERATIONS

• Contraindicated in myocardial infarction, thyrotoxicosis (except with antithyroid drugs), or uncorrected adrenal insufficiency (thyroid hormones increase tissue demand for adrenocortical hormone and may cause acute adrenal crisis). Use with extreme caution in angina pectoris, hypertension, or other cardiovascular disorders; renal insufficiency; and ischemic states.
• Thyroid hormone replacement requirements are about 25% lower in patients over 60 years than in young adults.
• Use carefully in myxedema; patients are unusually sensitive to thyroid hormone. Dose varies widely among patients; start at lowest and titrate in higher doses according to pa-

tient's symptoms and laboratory data until euthyroid state is reached.
• Rapid replacement in patients with arteriosclerosis may precipitate angina, coronary occlusion, or stroke. Use cautiously in these patients.
• In patients with coronary artery disease who must receive thyroid, observe carefully for possible coronary insufficiency if catecholamines must be given.
• Potentially dangerous; not indicated to relieve such vague symptoms as physical and mental sluggishness, irritability, depression, nervousness, and ill-defined pains; to treat obesity in euthyroid persons; to treat metabolic insufficiency not associated with thyroid insufficiency; or to treat menstrual disorders or male infertility, unless associated with hypothyroidism.
• When changing from levothyroxine to liothyronine, stop levothyroxine and begin liothyronine. Increase in small increments after residual effects of levothyroxine have disappeared. When changing from liothyronine to levothyroxine, start levothyroxine several days before withdrawing liothyronine to avoid relapse.
• Warn patient (especially elderly patients) to tell doctor at once if chest pain, palpitations, sweating, nervousness, shortness of breath, or other signs of overdosage or aggravated cardiovascular disease occur.
• Tell patient to take thyroid hormones at the same time each day to maintain constant hormone levels.
• Suggest morning dosage to prevent insomnia.
• Monitor pulse rate and blood pressure.
• Prepare I.V. dosage immediately before injection.
• Thyroid hormones alter thyroid function test results. Monitor prothrombin time; patients taking these hormones usually require less antico-

---

agulant. Alert patients to report unusual bleeding and bruising.
• Patients taking levothyroxine who need to have radioactive iodine uptake studies must discontinue drug 4 weeks before test.

---

liothyronine sodium (T₃)
Cyronine, Cytomel, Tertroxin‡

Pregnancy Risk Category: A

HOW SUPPLIED
Tablets: 5 mcg, 25 mcg, 50 mcg

MECHANISM OF ACTION
Stimulates the metabolism of all body tissues by accelerating the rate of cellular oxidation.

INDICATIONS & DOSAGE
Cretinism—
Children 3 years and older: 50 to 100 mcg P.O. daily.
Children under 3 years: 5 mcg P.O. daily, increased by 5 mcg q 3 to 4 days until desired response occurs.
Myxedema—
Adults: initially, 5 mcg P.O. daily, increased by 5 to 10 mcg q 1 or 2 weeks. Maintenance dosage is 50 to 100 mcg daily.
Nontoxic goiter—
Adults: initially, 5 mcg P.O. daily; may be increased by 12.5 to 25 mcg daily q 1 to 2 weeks. Usual maintenance dosage is 75 mcg daily.
Adults over 65 years: initially, 5 mcg P.O. daily, increased by 5-mcg increments at weekly intervals until desired response.
Children: initially, 5 mcg P.O. daily, increased by 5-mcg increments at weekly intervals until desired response.
Thyroid hormone replacement—
Adults: initially, 25 mcg P.O. daily, increased by 12.5 to 25 mcg q 1 to 2 weeks until satisfactory response.

Usual maintenance dosage is 25 to 75 mcg daily.
T₃ suppression test to differentiate hyperthyroidism from euthyroidism—
Adults: 75 to 100 mcg P.O. daily for 7 days.

ADVERSE REACTIONS
Adverse reactions of thyroid hormones are extensions of their pharmacologic properties and reflect patient sensitivity to them.
CNS: hyperirritability, *nervousness, insomnia,* twitching, *tremors,* headache.
CV: increased cardiac output, *tachycardia,* cardiac arrhythmias, *angina pectoris,* increased blood pressure, *cardiac decompensation and collapse.*
GI: diarrhea, abdominal cramps, vomiting.
Other: weight loss, heat intolerance, hyperhidrosis, menstrual irregularities; in infants and children—accelerated rate of bone maturation.

INTERACTIONS
Cholestyramine and colestipol: liothyronine absorption impaired. Separate doses by 4 to 5 hours.
I.V. phenytoin: free thyroid released. Monitor for tachycardia.

NURSING CONSIDERATIONS
• Contraindicated in myocardial infarction, thyrotoxicosis (except with antithyroid drugs), or uncorrected adrenal insufficiency (thyroid hormones increase tissue demand for adrenocortical hormone and may cause acute adrenal crisis). Use with extreme caution in angina pectoris, hypertension, or other cardiovascular disorders; renal insufficiency; and ischemic states.
• Thyroid hormone replacement requirements are about 25% lower in patients over 60 years than in young adults.
• Rapid replacement in patients with arteriosclerosis may precipitate an-

---

Italicized adverse reactions are common or life-threatening.
*Liquid form contains alcohol.   **May contain tartrazine.

gina, coronary occlusion, or stroke. Use cautiously in these patients.
• In patients with coronary artery disease who must receive thyroid hormones, observe carefully for possible coronary insufficiency if catecholamines must be given.
• Use carefully in myxedema; these patients are unusually sensitive to thyroid hormone.
• Potentially dangerous; not indicated to relieve vague symptoms, such as physical and mental sluggishness, irritability, depression, nervousness, and ill-defined aches and pains; to treat obesity in euthyroid persons; to treat metabolic insufficiency; or to treat menstrual disorders or male infertility, unless asssociated with hypothyroidism.
• When changing from levothyroxine to liothyronine, stop levothyroxine and begin liothyronine. Increase in small increments after residual effects of levothyroxine have disappeared. When changing from liothyronine to levothyroxine, start levothyroxine several days before withdrawing liothyronine to avoid relapse.
• Warn patient (especially elderly patients) to tell doctor at once if chest pain, palpitations, sweating, nervousness, or other signs of overdosage occur. Also notify doctor immediately if any signs of aggravated cardiovascular disease develop (chest pain, dyspnea, and tachycardia).
• Tell patient to take thyroid hormones at the same time each day, to maintain constant hormone levels.
• Suggest morning dosage to prevent insomnia.
• Monitor pulse rate and blood pressure.
• Thyroid hormones alter thyroid function tests. Monitor prothrombin time; patients taking these hormones usually require less anticoagulant. Alert patients to report unusual bleeding and bruising.
• Patients taking liothyronine who need to have radioactive iodine uptake studies must discontinue drug 7 to 10 days before test.

liotrix
Euthroid**, Thyrolar
Pregnancy Risk Category: A

HOW SUPPLIED
Tablets: levothyroxine sodium 30 mcg and liothyronine sodium 7.5 mcg (Euthroid-½); levothyroxine sodium 60 mcg and liothyronine sodium 15 mcg (Euthroid-1); levothyroxine sodium 120 mcg and liothyronine sodium 30 mcg (Euthroid-2); levothyroxine sodium 180 mcg and liothyronine sodium 45 mcg (Euthroid-3); levothyroxine sodium 12.5 mcg and liothyronine sodium 3.1 mcg (Thyrolar-¼); levothyroxine sodium 25 mcg and liothyronine sodium 6.25 mcg (Thyrolar-½); levothyroxine sodium 50 mcg and liothyronine sodium 12.5 mcg (Thyrolar-1); levothyroxine sodium 100 mcg and liothyronine sodium 25 mcg (Thyrolar-2); levothyroxine sodium 150 mcg and liothyronine sodium 37.5 mcg (Thyrolar-3)

MECHANISM OF ACTION
Stimulates the metabolism of all body tissues by accelerating the rate of cellular oxidation.

INDICATIONS & DOSAGE
Dosages are expressed in thyroid equivalents and must be individualized to approximate the deficit in the patient's thyroid secretion.
Hypothroidism—
Adults and children: initially, 15 to 30 mg P.O. daily, increasing by 15 to 30 mg q 1 to 2 weeks to desired response; increments in children's dosage q 2 weeks.
Adults over 65 years: initially, 15 to 30 mg P.O. Usual adult dosage doubled q 6 to 8 weeks to desired response.

---

†Available in Canada only.   ‡Available in Australia only.   ◊Available OTC.

ADVERSE REACTIONS

Adverse reactions of thyroid hormones are extensions of their pharmacologic properties and reflect patient sensitivity to them.

CNS: hyperirritability, *nervousness, insomnia,* twitching, *tremors.*

CV: increased cardiac output, *tachycardia,* cardiac arrhythmias, *angina pectoris,* increased blood pressure, *cardiac decompensation and collapse.*

GI: diarrhea, abdominal cramps, vomiting.

Other: weight loss, menstrual irregularities, heat intolerance, hyperhidrosis; infants and children—accelerated rate of bone maturation.

INTERACTIONS

Cholestyramine and colestipol: liotrix absorption impaired. Separate doses by 4 to 5 hours.

I.V. phenytoin: free thyroid released. Monitor for tachycardia.

NURSING CONSIDERATIONS

• Contraindicated in myocardial infarction, thyrotoxicosis (except with antithyroid drugs), or uncorrected adrenal insufficiency (thyroid hormones increase tissue demand for adrenocortical hormone and may cause acute adrenal crisis). Use with extreme caution in angina pectoris, hypertension, or other cardiovascular disorders; renal insufficiency; and ischemic states.

• Thyroid hormone replacement requirements are about 25% lower in patients over 60 years than in young adults.

• Rapid replacement in arteriosclerosis may precipitate angina, coronary occlusion, or stroke. Use cautiously in these patients.

• Use carefully in myxedema; these patients are unusually sensitive to thyroid hormone.

• In patients with coronary artery disease who must receive thyroid hormones, observe carefully for possible coronary insufficiency if catecholamines must be given. Also observe carefully during surgery, since cardiac arrhythmias can be precipitated.

• Potentially dangerous; not indicated to relieve vague symptoms, such as physical and mental sluggishness, irritability, depression, nervousness, and ill-defined pains; to treat obesity in euthyroid persons; to treat metabolic insufficiency not associated with thyroid insufficiency; or to treat menstrual disorders for male infertility, unless associated with hypothyroidism.

• Tell patient to take thyroid hormones at the same time each day, preferably before breakfast, to maintain constant hormone levels.

• Warn patient (especially elderly patients) to tell doctor at once if chest pain, palpitations, sweating, nervousness, or other signs of overdosage occur. Also notify doctor immediately if any signs of aggravated cardiovascular disease develop (chest pain, dyspnea, and tachycardia).

• The two commercially prepared liotrix drugs contain different amounts of each ingredient; do not change from one brand to the other without considering the differences in potency: Thyrolar-½ contains 25 mcg T_4 and 6.25 mcg T_3; Euthroid-½ contains 30 mcg T_4 and 7.5 mcg T_3.

• Monitor pulse rate and blood pressure.

• Thyroid hormones alter thyroid function test results. Monitor prothrombin time; patients taking these hormones usually require less anticoagulant. Alert patients to report unusual bleeding and bruising.

Italicized adverse reactions are common or life-threatening.
*Liquid form contains alcohol.   **May contain tartrazine.

thyroglobulin
Proloid

Pregnancy Risk Category: A

HOW SUPPLIED
Tablets: 32 mg, 65 mg, 100 mg, 130 mg, 200 mg

MECHANISM OF ACTION
Stimulates the metabolism of all body tissues by accelerating the rate of cellular oxidation.

INDICATIONS & DOSAGE
Cretinism and juvenile hypothyroidism—

Children 1 year and older: dosage may approach adult dosage (60 to 180 mg P.O. daily), depending on response.
Children 4 to 12 months: 60 to 80 mg P.O. daily.
Children 1 to 4 months: initially, 15 to 30 mg P.O. daily, increased at 2-week intervals. Usual maintenance dosage is 30 to 45 mg P.O. daily.
Hypothyroidism or myxedema—
Adults: initially, 15 to 30 mg P.O. daily, increased by 15 to 30 mg at 2-week intervals until desired response. Usual maintenance dosage is 60 to 180 mg P.O. daily, as a single dose.
Adults over 65 years: initially, 7.5 to 15 mg P.O. daily; dosage is doubled at 6- to 8-week intervals until desired response is obtained.

ADVERSE REACTIONS
Adverse reactions of thyroid hormones are extensions of their pharmacologic properties and reflect patient sensitivity to them.
CNS: hyperirritability, *nervousness, insomnia,* twitching, *tremors,* headache.
CV: increased cardiac output, *tachycardia,* cardiac arrhythmias, *angina pectoris,* increased blood pressure, *cardiac decompensation and collapse.*

GI: diarrhea, abdominal cramps, vomiting.
Other: weight loss, heat intolerance, hyperhidrosis, menstrual irregularities; in infants and children—accelerated rate of bone maturation.

INTERACTIONS
Cholestyramine and colestipol: thyroglobulin absorption impaired. Separate doses by 4 to 5 hours.
I.V. phenytoin: free thyroid released. Monitor for tachycardia.

NURSING CONSIDERATIONS
• Contraindicated in myocardial infarction, thyrotoxicosis (except with antithyroid drugs), or uncorrected adrenal insufficiency (thyroid hormones increase tissue demand for adrenocortical hormone and may cause acute adrenal crisis). Use with extreme caution in angina pectoris, hypertension, or other cardiovascular disorders; renal insufficiency; and ischemic states.
• Thyroid hormone replacement requirements are about 25% lower in patients over 60 years than in young adults.
• In patients with coronary artery disease who must receive thyroid hormones, observe carefully for possible coronary insufficiency if catecholamines must be given.
• Use carefully in myxedema; these patients are unusually sensitive to thyroid hormone.
• Potentially dangerous; not indicated to relieve vague symptoms, such as physical and mental sluggishness, irritability, depression, nervousness, and ill-defined pains; to treat obesity in euthyroid persons; to treat metabolic insufficiency not associated with thyroid insufficiency; or to treat menstrual disorders or male infertility, unless associated with hypothyroidism.
• Tell patient to take thyroid hor-

---

mones at the same time each day, to maintain constant hormone levels.
• Warn patient (especially elderly patients) to tell doctor at once if chest pain, palpitations, sweating, nervousness, or other signs of overdosage occur. Also notify doctor immediately if any signs of aggravated cardiovascular disease develop (chest pain, dyspnea, and tachycardia).
• Suggest morning dosage to prevent insomnia.
• Monitor pulse rate and blood pressure.
• Thyroid hormones alter thyroid function test results. Monitor prothrombin time; patients taking these hormones usually require less anticoagulant. Alert patients to report unusual bleeding and bruising.

thyroid dessicated
Armour Thyroid, S-P-T, Thyrar, Thyroid Strong, Thyroid USP Enseals, Thyro-Teric

Pregnancy Risk Category: A

HOW SUPPLIED
Tablets: 16 mg, 32 mg, 65 mg, 98 mg, 130 mg, 195 mg, 260 mg, 325 mg
Tablets (bovine origin): 32 mg, 65 mg, 130 mg
Tablets (enteric-coated): 32 mg, 65 mg, 130 mg
Strong tablets (50% stronger than thyroid USP, and containing 0.3% iodine): 32 mg, 65 mg, 130 mg, 195 mg
Capsules (porcine origin): 65 mg, 130 mg, 195 mg, 325 mg

MECHANISM OF ACTION
Stimulates the metabolism of all body tissues by accelerating the rate of cellular oxidation.

INDICATIONS & DOSAGE
Adult hypothyroidism—
Adults: initially, 60 mg P.O. daily, increased by 60 mg q 30 days until desired response. Usual maintenance

dosage is 60 to 180 mg P.O. daily, as a single dose.
Adults over 65 years: 7.5 to 15 mg P.O. daily; dosage is doubled at 6- to 8-week intervals.
Adult myxedema—
Adults: 16 mg P.O. daily. May double dosage q 2 weeks to maximum 120 mg.
Cretinism and juvenile hypothyroidism—
Children 1 year and older: dosage may approach adult dosage (60 to 180 mg P.O.) daily, depending on response.
Children 4 to 12 months: 30 to 60 mg P.O. daily.
Children 1 to 4 months: initially, 15 to 30 mg P.O. daily, increased at 2-week intervals. Usual maintenance dosage is 30 to 45 mg P.O. daily.

ADVERSE REACTIONS
Adverse reactions of thyroid hormones are extensions of their pharmacologic properties and reflect patient sensitivity to them.
CNS: *hyperirritability, nervousness, insomnia,* twitching, tremors, headache.
CV: increased cardiac output, *tachycardia,* cardiac arrhythmias, *angina pectoris,* increased blood pressure, *cardiac decompensation and collapse.*
GI: diarrhea, abdominal cramps, vomiting.
Other: weight loss, heat intolerance, hyperhidrosis, menstrual irregularities; in infants and children—accelerated rate of bone maturation.

INTERACTIONS
Cholestyramine: thyroid absorption impaired. Separate doses by 4 to 5 hours.
I.V. phenytoin: free thyroid released. Monitor for tachycardia.

NURSING CONSIDERATIONS
• Contraindicated in myocardial infarction, thyrotoxicosis (except with

---

Italicized adverse reactions are common or life-threatening.
*Liquid form contains alcohol.   **May contain tartrazine.

antithyroid drugs), or uncorrected adrenal insufficiency (thyroid hormones increase tissue demand for adrenocortical hormone and may cause acute adrenal crisis). Use with extreme caution in angina pectoris, hypertension, or other cardiovascular disorders; renal insufficiency; and ischemic states.

• Thyroid hormone replacement requirements are about 25% lower in patients over 60 years than in young adults.

• Use carefully in myxedema; these patients are unusually sensitive to thyroid hormone.

• In patients with coronary artery disease who must receive thyroid hormones, observe carefully for possible coronary insufficiency if catecholamines must be given.

• Potentially dangerous; not indicated to relieve vague symptoms, such as physical and mental sluggishness, irritability, depression, nervousness, and ill-defined pains; to treat obesity in euthyroid persons; to treat metabolic insufficiency not associated with thyroid insufficiency; or to treat menstrual disorders or male infertility, unless associated with hypothyroidism.

• Tell patient to take thyroid hormones at the same time each day to maintain constant hormone levels.

• Warn patient (especially elderly patients) to tell doctor at once if chest pain, palpitations, sweating, nervousness, or other signs of overdosage occur. Also notify doctor immediately if any signs of aggravated cardiovascular disease develop (chest pain, dyspnea, and tachycardia).

• Suggest morning dosage to prevent insomnia.

• Monitor pulse rate and blood pressure.

• In children, sleeping pulse rate and basal morning temperature are guides to treatment.

• Thyroid hormones alter thyroid function test results. Monitor prothrombin time; patients taking these hormones usually require less anticoagulant. Alert patients to report unusual bleeding and bruising.

thyrotropin (thyroid-stimulating hormone, or TSH)
Thytropar

Pregnancy Risk Category: C

HOW SUPPLIED
Powder for injection: 10 IU/vial

MECHANISM OF ACTION
Stimulates the uptake of radioactive iodine in patients with thyroid carcinoma. Also promotes thyroid hormone production by the anterior pituitary.

INDICATIONS & DOSAGE
Diagnosis of thyroid cancer remnant with ^{131}I after surgery—
Adults: 10 IU I.M. or S.C. for 3 to 7 days.
Differential diagnosis of primary and secondary hypothyroidism—
Adults: 10 IU I.M. or S.C. for 1 to 3 days.
In PBI or ^{131}I uptake determinations for differential diagnosis of subclinical hypothyroidism or low thyroid reserve—
Adults: 10 IU I.M. or S.C.
Therapy for thyroid carcinoma (local or metastatic) with ^{131}I—
Adults: 10 IU I.M. or S.C. for 3 to 8 days.
To determine thyroid status of patient receiving thyroid—
Adults: 10 units I.M. or S.C. for 1 to 3 days.

ADVERSE REACTIONS
CNS: headache.
CV: *tachycardia,* atrial fibrillation, *angina pectoris, CHF,* hypotension.
GI: nausea, vomiting.

Other: thyroid hyperplasia (large doses), fever, menstrual irregularities, allergic reactions (postinjection flare, urticaria, *anaphylaxis*).

INTERACTIONS
None significant.

NURSING CONSIDERATIONS
• Contraindicated in coronary thrombosis and untreated Addison's disease. Use cautiously in angina pectoris, CHF, hypopituitarism, and adrenocortical suppression.
• May cause thyroid hyperplasia.
• Diagnostic use: to identify subclinical hypothyroidism or low thyroid reserve, to evaluate need for thyroid therapy, to distinguish between primary and secondary hypothyroidism, and to detect thyroid remnants and metastases of thyroid carcinoma.
• Three-day dosage schedule may be used in long-standing pituitary myxedema or with prolonged use of thyroid medication.

Italicized adverse reactions are common or life-threatening.
*Liquid form contains alcohol.   **May contain tartrazine.

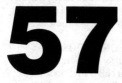

Thyroid hormone antagonists

methimazole
potassium iodide
propylthiouracil
radioactive iodine (sodium
iodide) ¹³¹I

COMBINATION PRODUCTS
None.

methimazole
Tapazole

Pregnancy Risk Category: D

HOW SUPPLIED
Tablets: 5 mg, 10 mg

MECHANISM OF ACTION
Inhibits oxidation of iodine in the thyroid gland, blocking iodine's ability to combine with tyrosine to form thyroxine. May also prevent the coupling of monoiodotyrosine and diiodotyrosine to form thyroxine and triiodothyronine.

INDICATIONS & DOSAGE
Hyperthyroidism—
Adults: 5 mg P.O. t.i.d. if mild; 10 to 15 mg P.O. t.i.d. if moderately severe; and 20 mg P.O. t.i.d. if severe. Continue until patient is euthyroid, then start maintenance dosage of 5 mg daily to t.i.d. Maximum dosage 150 mg daily.
Children: 0.4 mg/kg P.O. daily divided q 8 hours. Continue until patient is euthyroid, then start maintenance dosage of 0.2 mg/kg daily divided q 8 hours.
Preparation for thyroidectomy—

Adults and children: same doses as for hyperthyroidism until patient is euthyroid; then iodine may be added for 10 days before surgery.
Thyrotoxic crisis—
Adults and children: same doses as for hyperthyroidism, with concomitant iodine therapy and propranolol.

ADVERSE REACTIONS
Blood: *agranulocytosis,* leukopenia, granulopenia, thrombocytopenia (appear to be dose-related).
CNS: headache, drowsiness, vertigo.
GI: diarrhea, nausea, vomiting (may be dose-related).
Hepatic: jaundice.
Skin: rash, urticaria, skin discoloration.
Other: arthralgia, myalgia, salivary gland enlargement, loss of taste, drug fever, lymphadenopathy.

INTERACTIONS
None significant.

NURSING CONSIDERATIONS
• Use cautiously in pregnancy. Pregnant women may require less drug as pregnancy progresses. Monitor thyroid function studies closely. Thyroid may be added to regimen. Drugs may be stopped during last few weeks of pregnancy.
• Watch for signs of hypothyroidism (mental depression; cold intolerance; hard, nonpitting edema). Dosage may need to be adjusted.
• Monitor CBC periodically to detect impending leukopenia, thrombocytopenia, and agranulocytosis.

---

†Available in Canada only.   ‡Available in Australia only.   ◊ Available OTC.

• Doses of over 30 mg/day increase the risk of agranulocytosis.
• Warn patient to report immediately: fever, sore throat, or mouth sores (possible signs of developing agranulocytosis). Agranulocytosis can develop too rapidly to be detected by periodic blood cell counts. Tell patient also to immediately report skin eruptions (sign of hypersensitivity).
• Drug should be stopped if severe rash or enlarged cervical lymph nodes develop.
• Tell patient to ask doctor about using iodized salt and eating shellfish during treatment.
• Warn patient against over-the-counter cough medicines; many contain iodine.
• Give with meals to reduce GI adverse reactions.
• Store in light-resistant container.

---

potassium iodide
Pima

potassium iodide, saturated solution (SSKI)

strong iodine solution (Lugol's solution)

Pregnancy Risk Category: D

HOW SUPPLIED
potassium iodide
Tablets (enteric-coated): 300 mg
Oral solution: 500 mg/15 ml
Syrup: 325 mg/5 ml
potassium iodide, saturated solution
Oral solution: 1 g/ml
strong iodine solution
Oral solution: iodine 50 mg/ml and potassium iodide 100 mg/ml

MECHANISM OF ACTION
Inhibits thyroid hormone formation by blocking iodotyrosine and iodothyronine synthesis. It also limits iodide transport into the thyroid gland and blocks thyroid hormone release.

INDICATIONS & DOSAGE
Preparation for thyroidectomy—
Adults and children: Strong Iodine Solution, USP, 0.1 to 0.3 ml P.O. t.i.d., or Potassium Iodide Solution, USP, 5 drops in water P.O. t.i.d. after meals for 2 to 3 weeks before surgery.
Thyrotoxic crisis—
Adults and children: Strong Iodine Solution, USP, 1 ml in water P.O. t.i.d. after meals.
Radiation protectant for thyroid gland—
Adults: 100 to 150 mg P.O. 24 hours before and for 3 to 10 days after radiation exposure
Expectorant—
Adults: 0.3 to 0.6 ml SSKI diluted in water three or four times a day.

ADVERSE REACTIONS
EENT: acute rhinitis, inflammation of salivary glands, periorbital edema, conjunctivitis, hyperemia.
GI: burning, irritation, *nausea,* vomiting, *metallic taste.*
Skin: acneiform rash, mucous membrane ulceration.
Other: fever, frontal headache, tooth discoloration, *hypersensitivity, including symptoms resembling serum sickness.*

INTERACTIONS
Lithium carbonate: hypothyroidism may occur. Use with caution.

NURSING CONSIDERATIONS
• Contraindicated in tuberculosis, iodide hypersensitivity, hyperkalemia; after meals that contain excessive starch; in laryngeal edema, swelling of salivary glands.
• Earliest signs of delayed hypersensitivity caused by iodides are irritation and swelling of the eyelids.
• Dilute oral doses in water, milk, or fruit juice, and give after meals to

---

Italicized adverse reactions are common or life-threatening.
*Liquid form contains alcohol.   **May contain tartrazine.

prevent gastric irritation, to hydrate the patient, and to mask the very salty taste.
• Tell patient to ask the doctor about using iodized salt and eating shellfish during treatment. Iodine-rich foods may not be permitted.
• Warn the patient that sudden withdrawal may precipitate thyroid storm.
• Avoid using enteric-coated tablets, which have been associated with small bowel lesions and can lead to serious complications, including perforation, hemorrhage, or obstruction.
• Store in light-resistant container.
• Give iodides through straw to avoid tooth discoloration.
• Usually given with other antithyroid drugs.

propylthiouracil (PTU)
Propyl-Thyracil†

Pregnancy Risk Category: D

HOW SUPPLIED
Tablets: 50 mg, 100 mg†

MECHANISM OF ACTION
Inhibits oxidation of iodine in the thyroid gland, blocking iodine's ability to combine with tyrosine to form thyroxine. May also prevent the coupling of monoiodotyrosine and diiodotyrosine to form thyroxine and triiodothyronine.

INDICATIONS & DOSAGE
Hyperthyroidism—
Adults: 100 mg P.O. t.i.d.; up to 300 mg q 8 hours have been used in severe cases. Continue until patient is euthyroid, then start maintenance dosage of 100 mg daily to t.i.d.
Children over 10 years: 100 mg P.O. t.i.d. Continue until patient is euthyroid, then start maintenance dosage of 25 mg t.i.d. to 100 mg b.i.d.
Children 6 to 10 years: 50 to 150 mg P.O. divided doses q 8 hours.
Preparation for thyroidectomy—

Adults and children: same doses as for hyperthyroidism, then iodine may be added 10 days before surgery.
Thyrotoxic crisis—
Adults and children: same doses as for hyperthyroidism, with concomitant iodine therapy and propranolol.

ADVERSE REACTIONS
Blood: *agranulocytosis,* leukopenia, thrombocytopenia (appear to be dose-related).
CNS: headache, drowsiness, vertigo.
EENT: visual disturbances.
GI: diarrhea, *nausea, vomiting* (may be dose-related).
Hepatic: jaundice, *hepatotoxicity.*
Skin: rash, urticaria, skin discoloration, pruritus.
Other: arthralgia, myalgia, salivary gland enlargement, loss of taste, drug fever, lymphadenopathy, vasculitis.

INTERACTIONS
None significant.

NURSING CONSIDERATIONS
• Use cautiously in pregnancy. Pregnant women may require less drug as pregnancy progresses. Monitor thyroid function studies closely. Thyroid may be added to regimen. Drugs may be stopped during last few weeks of pregnancy.
• Watch for signs of hypothyroidism (mental depression; cold intolerance; hard, nonpitting edema). Dosage may need to be adjusted.
• Monitor CBC periodically to detect impending leukopenia, thrombocytopenia, and agranulocytosis.
• Warn patient to report immediately: fever, sore throat, or mouth sores (possible signs of developing agranulocytosis). Agranulocytosis can develop too rapidly to be detected by periodic blood cell counts. Tell patient to also report skin eruptions (sign of hypersensitivity) immediately.
• Drug should be stopped if severe

rash or enlarged cervical lymph nodes develop.

• Tell patient to ask doctor about using iodized salt and eating shellfish during treatment.

• Warn patient against over-the-counter cough medicines; many contain iodine.

• Give with meals to reduce GI adverse reactions.

• Store in light-resistant container.

radioactive iodine (sodium iodide) 131I
Iodotope Therapeutic, Sodium Iodide 131I Therapeutic

Pregnancy Risk Category: X

HOW SUPPLIED
All radioactivity concentrations are determined at the time of calibration; 131I has a physical half-life of about 8 days.

Iodotope Therapeutic
Capsules: radioactivity range is 1 to 50 millicuries (mCi)/capsule at time of calibration.
Oral solution: radioactivity concentration is 7.05 mCi/ml at time of calibration; in vials containing approximately 7, 14, 28, 70, or 106 mCi at time of calibration
Sodium Iodide 131I Therapeutic
Capsules: radioactivity range is 0.8 to 100 mCi/capsule
Oral solution: radioactivity range is 3.5 to 150 mCi/vial

MECHANISM OF ACTION
Limits thyroid hormone secretion by destroying thyroid tissue. The affinity of thyroid tissue for radioactive iodine facilitates uptake of the drug by cancerous thyroid tissue that has metastasized to other sites in the body.

INDICATIONS & DOSAGE
Hyperthyroidism—
Adults: usual dosage is 4 to 10 mCi P.O. Dosage based on estimated weight of thyroid gland and thyroid uptake. Treatment may be repeated after 6 weeks, according to serum thyroxine.
Thyroid cancer—
Adults: 50 to 150 mCi P.O. Dosage based on estimated malignant thyroid tissue and metastatic tissue as determined by total body scan. Treatment may be repeated according to clinical status.

ADVERSE REACTIONS
EENT: *feeling of fullness in neck,* metallic taste, "radiation mumps."
Endocrine: hypothyroidism, radiation thyroiditis.
Other: possible increased risk of developing leukemia later in life after sufficient 131I dose for thyroid ablation following cancer surgery; possible increased risk of birth defects in offspring after sufficient 131I dose for thyroid ablation following cancer surgery.

INTERACTIONS
Lithium carbonate: hypothyroidism may occur. Use with caution.

NURSING CONSIDERATIONS
• Contraindicated in pregnancy and lactation unless used to treat thyroid cancer.
• Stop all antithyroid medications, thyroid preparations, and iodine-containing preparations 1 week before 131I dose. If medications are not stopped, patient may receive thyroid-stimulating hormone for 3 days before 131I dose. When treating women of childbearing age, give dose during menstruation or within 7 days after menstruation.
• Food may delay absorption. Patient should fast overnight before administration.
• After therapy for hyperthyroidism, patient should not resume antithyroid drugs, but should continue propranolol or other drugs used to treat symp-

---

Italicized adverse reactions are common or life-threatening.
*Liquid form contains alcohol.   **May contain tartrazine.

toms of hyperthyroidism until onset of full ^{131}I effect (usually 6 weeks).
• Monitor thyroid function with serum thyroxine.
• After dose for hyperthyroidism, patient's urine and saliva are slightly radioactive for 24 hours; vomitus is highly radioactive for 6 to 8 hours. Institute full radiation precautions during this time. Instruct patient to use appropriate disposal methods when coughing and expectorating.
• After dose for thyroid cancer, patient's urine, saliva, and perspiration remain radioactive for 3 days. Isolate patient and observe the following precautions: pregnant personnel should not take care of patient; disposable eating utensils and linens should be used; instruct patient to save all urine in lead containers for 24 to 48 hours so amount of radioactive material excreted can be determined. Patient should drink as much fluid as possible for 48 hours after drug administration to facilitate excretion. Limit contact with patient to 30 minutes per shift per person the first day. May increase time to 1 hour second day and longer on third day.
• If patient is discharged less than 7 days after ^{131}I dose for thyroid cancer, warn him to avoid close, prolonged contact with small children (for example, holding children on lap), and instruct him not to sleep in same room with spouse for 7 days after treatment because of increased risk of thyroid cancer in persons exposed to ^{131}I. Tell patient he may use same bathroom facilities as rest of family.

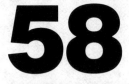

Pituitary hormones

corticotropin
cosyntropin
desmopressin acetate
lypressin
somatrem
vasopressin
vasopressin tannate

COMBINATION PRODUCTS
None.

corticotropin (adrenocorticotropic hormone, ACTH)

ACTH, Acthar, Acthar Gel (H.P.)†, ACTH Gel, Cortigel-40, Cortigel-80, Cortrophin Gel, Cortropic-Gel-40, Cortropic-Gel-80, H.P. Acthar Gel

Pregnancy Risk Category: C

HOW SUPPLIED
Aqueous injection: 25 units/vial, 40 units/vial
Repository injection: 40 units/ml, 80 units/ml

MECHANISM OF ACTION
By replacing the body's own tropic hormone, stimulates the adrenal cortex to secrete its entire spectrum of hormones.

INDICATIONS & DOSAGE
Diagnostic test of adrenocortical function—
Adults: up to 80 units I.M. or S.C. in divided doses; or a single dose of repository form; or 10 to 25 units (aqueous form) in 500 ml dextrose 5% in water I.V. over 8 hours, between blood samplings.

Individual dosages generally vary with adrenal glands' sensitivity to stimulation as well as with specific disease. Infants and younger children require larger doses per kilogram than do older children and adults.
For therapeutic use—
Adults: 40 units S.C. or I.M. in 4 divided doses (aqueous); 40 units q 12 to 24 hours (gel or repository form).

ADVERSE REACTIONS
CNS: *seizures, dizziness,* papilledema, headache, *euphoria, insomnia,* mood swings, personality changes, depression, psychosis.
EENT: cataracts, glaucoma.
GI: peptic ulcer with perforation and hemorrhage, pancreatitis, abdominal distention, ulcerative esophagitis, nausea, vomiting.
GU: menstrual irregularities.
Metabolic: *sodium and fluid retention,* calcium and potassium loss, hypokalemic alkalosis, negative nitrogen balance.
Skin: *impaired wound healing,* thin fragile skin, petechiae, ecchymoses, facial erythema, increased sweating, acne, hyperpigmentation, allergic skin reactions, hirsutism.
Other: muscle weakness, steroid myopathy, loss of muscle mass, osteoporosis, vertebral compression fractures, cushingoid state, suppression of growth in children, *activation of latent diabetes mellitus,* progressive increase in antibodies, loss of ACTH

Italicized adverse reactions are common or life-threatening.
*Liquid form contains alcohol.   **May contain tartrazine.

stimulatory effect, and *hypersensitivity*.

INTERACTIONS
None significant.

NURSING CONSIDERATIONS
• Contraindicated in scleroderma, osteoporosis, systemic fungal infections, ocular herpes simplex, recent surgery, peptic ulcer, congestive heart failure, hypertension, sensitivity to pork and pork products, concomitant smallpox vaccination, adrenocortical hyperfunction or primary insufficiency, or Cushing's syndrome. Use with caution in pregnant women or breast-feeding mothers and in women of childbearing age; patients being immunized; latent tuberculosis or tuberculin reactivity; hypothyroidism; cirrhosis; infection (use anti-infective therapy during and after ACTH treatment); acute gouty arthritis (limit ACTH treatment to a few days, and use conventional therapy during and for several days after ACTH treatment); emotional instability or psychotic tendencies; diabetes; abscess; pyogenic infections; renal insufficiency; myasthenia gravis.
• ACTH treatment should be preceded by verification of adrenal responsiveness and test for hypersensitivity and allergic reactions.
• ACTH should be adjunctive; not sole therapy. Oral agents are preferred for long-term therapy.
• Unusual stress may require additional use of rapidly acting corticosteroids. When possible, gradually reduce ACTH dosage to smallest effective dose to minimize induced adrenocortical insufficiency. Reinstitute therapy if stressful situation (trauma, surgery, severe illness) occurs shortly after stopping drug.
• Watch neonates of ACTH-treated mothers for signs of hypoadrenalism.
• Counteract edema by low-sodium, high-potassium intake; nitrogen loss by high-protein diet; and psychotic changes by reducing ACTH dosage or administering sedatives.
• ACTH may mask signs of chronic disease and decrease host resistance and ability to localize infection.
• Note and record weight changes, fluid exchange, and resting blood pressures until minimal effective dose is achieved.
• Refrigerate reconstituted solution and use within 24 hours.
• If administering gel, warm it to room temperature, draw into large needle, and give slowly deep I.M. with 21G or 22G needle. Warn patient that injection is painful.

cosyntropin
Cortrosyn
Pregnancy Risk Category: C

HOW SUPPLIED
Injection: 0.25 mg/vial

MECHANISM OF ACTION
By replacing the body's own tropic hormone, stimulates the adrenal cortex to secrete its entire spectrum of hormones.

INDICATIONS & DOSAGE
Diagnostic test of adrenocortical function—
Adults and children: 0.25 to 1 mg I.M. or I.V. (unless label prohibits I.V. administration) between blood samplings.
Children under 2 years: 0.125 mg I.M. or I.V.

ADVERSE REACTIONS
Skin: pruritus.
Other: flushing, hypersensitivity.

INTERACTIONS
None significant.

NURSING CONSIDERATIONS
• Use cautiously in patients with hy-

persensitivity to natural corticotropin.

• Drug is synthetic duplication of the biologically active part of the ACTH molecule. It is less likely to produce sensitivity than natural ACTH from animal sources.

---

desmopressin acetate
DDAVP, Minirin‡, Stimate

Pregnancy Risk Category: B

HOW SUPPLIED
Nasal solution: 0.1 mg/ml
Injection: 4 mcg/ml

MECHANISM OF ACTION
Increases the permeability of the renal tubular epithelium to adenosine monophosphate and water; the epithelium promotes reabsorption of water and produces a concentrated urine (antidiuretic hormone effect). Desmopressin also increases Factor VIII activity by releasing endogenous Factor VIII from plasma storage sites.

INDICATIONS & DOSAGE
Nonnephrogenic diabetes insipidus, temporary polyuria and polydipsia associated with pituitary trauma—
Adults: 0.1 to 0.4 ml intranasally daily in 1 to 3 doses. Adjust morning and evening doses separately for adequate diurnal rhythm of water turnover. Alternatively, may administer injectable form in dosage of 0.5 to 1 ml I.V. or S.C. daily, usually in two divided doses.
Children 3 months to 12 years: 0.05 to 0.3 ml intranasally daily in 1 or 2 doses.
Treatment of hemophilia A and von Willebrand's disease—
Adults and children: 0.3 mcg/kg diluted in normal saline and infused I.V. slowly over 15 to 30 minutes. May repeat dose if necessary as indicated by laboratory response and the patient's clinical condition.

Primary nocturnal enuresis—
Children 5 years and over: initially, 20 mcg intranasally h.s. Adjust dose according to response. Maximum recommended dose is 40 mcg daily.

ADVERSE REACTIONS
CNS: headache.
CV: slight rise in blood pressure at high dosage.
EENT: nasal congestion, rhinitis.
GI: nausea.
GU: vulval pain.
Other: flushing.

INTERACTIONS
None significant.

NURSING CONSIDERATIONS
• Use with caution in coronary artery insufficiency or hypertensive cardiovascular disease.
• Adjust fluid intake to reduce risk of water intoxication and sodium depletion, especially in children or elderly patients.
• Overdose may cause oxytocic or vasopressor activity. Withhold drug until effects subside. Furosemide may be used if fluid retention is excessive.
• Some patients may have difficulty measuring and inhaling drug into nostrils. Teach patient correct method of administration.
• For treating nocturnal enuresis, the recommended method of administration is one-half of the calculated dose in each nostril.
• Intranasal use can cause changes in the nasal mucosa resulting in erratic, unreliable absorption. Report any patient's worsening condition to doctor, who may prescribe injectable DDAVP.
• Desmopressin injection should not be used to treat hemophilia A with Factor VIII levels of 0% to 5%, or severe cases of von Willebrand's disease.
• In patients treated for hemophilia A and von Willebrand's disease, use of

---

Italicized adverse reactions are common or life-threatening.
*Liquid form contains alcohol.   **May contain tartrazine.

desmopressin may avoid the hazards of using blood products.
• Has been used successfully to reduce blood loss during cardiac surgery.

lypressin
Diapid

Pregnancy Risk Category: B

HOW SUPPLIED
Nasal spray: 0.185 mg/ml

MECHANISM OF ACTION
Increases the permeability of the renal tubular epithelium to adenosine monophosphate and water; the epithelium promotes reabsorption of water and produces a concentrated urine (antidiuretic hormone effect).

INDICATIONS & DOSAGE
Nonnephrogenic diabetes insipidus—
Adults and children: 1 or 2 sprays (approximately 2 USP posterior pituitary pressor units/spray) in either or both nostrils q.i.d. and an additional dose at bedtime, if needed, to prevent nocturia. If usual dosage is inadequate, increase frequency rather than number of sprays.

ADVERSE REACTIONS
CNS: headache, dizziness.
EENT: nasal congestion or ulceration, irritation, pruritus of nasal passages, rhinorrhea, conjunctivitis.
GI: heartburn due to drip of excess spray into pharynx, abdominal cramps, frequent bowel movements.
GU: possible transient fluid retention from overdose.
Skin: hypersensitivity reaction.

INTERACTIONS
None significant.

NURSING CONSIDERATIONS
• Use with caution in coronary artery disease.

• Particularly useful if diabetes insipidus is unresponsive to other therapy, or if antidiuretic hormones of animal origin cause adverse effects.
• Nasal congestion, allergic rhinitis, or upper respiratory infections may diminish drug absorption and require larger dose or adjunctive therapy.
• Instruct patient to clear nasal passage before inhaling drug.
• Inadvertent inhalation of spray may cause tightness in chest, coughing, and transient dyspnea.
• Test patients sensitive to antidiuretic hormone for sensitivity to lypressin.
• To administer a uniform, well-diffused spray, hold bottle upright with patient in vertical position holding head upright.
• Instruct the patient to carry the medication with him at all times because of its fairly short duration.

somatrem
Protropin

Pregnancy Risk Category: C

HOW SUPPLIED
Injectable lyophilized powder: 5 mg (10 IU)/vial

MECHANISM OF ACTION
Purified growth hormone of recombinant DNA origin that stimulates linear, skeletal muscle, and organ growth.

INDICATIONS & DOSAGE
Long-term treatment of children who have growth failure because of lack of adequate endogenous growth hormone secretion—
Children (pre-puberty): 0.1 mg/kg I.M. or S.C. given three times weekly.

ADVERSE REACTIONS
Endocrine: *hypothyroidism, hyperglycemia.*

Other: *antibodies to growth hormone*.

INTERACTIONS
Glucocorticoids: may inhibit growth-promoting action of somatrem. Glucocorticoid dose may need to be adjusted.

NURSING CONSIDERATIONS
• Contraindicated in patients with closed epiphyses (drug is of no value for enhancing athletic performance), an active underlying intracranial lesion, or known sensitivity to benzyl alcohol.
• Use cautiously in patients whose growth hormone deficiency results from an intracranial lesion. Patient should be examined frequently for progression or recurrence of the underlying disease.
• Drug is of no value for enhancing athletic performance.
• Observe patient for signs of glucose intolerance and hyperglycemia.
• Monitor periodic thyroid function tests for hypothyroidism, which may require treatment with a thyroid hormone.
• This drug replaces pituitary-derived human growth hormone, which was removed from the market in 1985 because of an association with a rare but fatal virus infection (Jakob-Creutzfeldt disease). Reassure your patient and his family that somatrem is *pure* and that it is *safe*.
• To prepare the solution, inject the bacteriostatic water for injection (which is supplied) into the vial containing the drug. Then swirl the vial with a gentle rotary motion until the contents are completely dissolved. *Don't shake* the vial.
• After reconstitution, vial solution should be clear. Don't inject into the patient if the solution is cloudy or contains any particles.
• Store reconstituted vial in refrigerator. Must use within 7 days.

• Be sure to check this product's expiration date.

---

vasopressin (antidiuretic hormone)
Pitressin

vasopressin tannate
Pitressin Tannate

Pregnancy Risk Category: B

HOW SUPPLIED
vasopressin
Injection: 0.5-ml and 1-ml ampules, 20 units/ml
vasopressin tannate
Injection: 1-ml ampules, 5 units/ml

MECHANISM OF ACTION
Increases the permeability of the renal tubular epithelium to adenosine monophosphate and water; the epithelium promotes reabsorption of water and produces a concentrated urine (antidiuretic hormone effect).

INDICATIONS & DOSAGE
Nonnephrogenic, nonpsychogenic diabetes insipidus—
Adults: 5 to 10 units I.M. or S.C. b.i.d. to q.i.d., p.r.n.; or intranasally (aqueous solution used as spray or applied to cotton balls) in individualized doses, based on response. For chronic therapy, inject 2.5 to 5 units Pitressin Tannate in oil suspension I.M. or S.C. q 2 to 3 days.
Children: 2.5 to 10 units I.M. or S.C. b.i.d. to q.i.d., p.r.n.; or intranasally (aqueous solution used as spray or applied to cotton balls) in individualized doses. For chronic therapy, inject 1.25 to 2.5 units Pitressin Tannate in oil suspension I.M. or S.C. q 2 to 3 days.
Postoperative abdominal distention—
Adults: 5 units (aqueous) I.M. initially, then q 3 to 4 hours, increasing dose to 10 units, if needed. Reduce dose proportionately for children.

Italicized adverse reactions are common or life-threatening.
*Liquid form contains alcohol.   **May contain tartrazine.

To expel gas before abdominal X-ray—
Adults: inject 10 units S.C. at 2 hours, then again at 30 minutes before X-ray. Enema before first dose may also help to eliminate gas.
Upper GI tract hemorrhage—
Adults: 0.2 to 0.4 units/minute by intraarterial injection. Do not use tannate in oil suspension.

ADVERSE REACTIONS
CNS: tremor, dizziness, headache.
CV: *angina in patients with vascular disease,* vasoconstriction. Large doses may cause hypertension, electrocardiographic changes. (With intraarterial infusion: *bradycardia, cardiac arrhythmias, pulmonary edema.*)
GI: abdominal cramps, nausea, vomiting, diarrhea, intestinal hyperactivity.
GU: uterine cramps, anuria.
Skin: circumoral pallor.
Other: water intoxication (drowsiness, listlessness, headache, confusion, weight gain), hypersensitivity reactions (urticaria, angioneurotic edema, bronchoconstriction, fever, rash, wheezing, dyspnea, *anaphylaxis),* sweating.

INTERACTIONS
Chlorpropamide: increased antidiuretic response. Use together cautiously.
Lithium, demeclocycline: reduced antidiuretic activity. Use together cautiously.

NURSING CONSIDERATIONS
• Contraindicated in chronic nephritis with nitrogen retention. Use cautiously in children, elderly persons, pregnant women, and patients with epilepsy, migraine, asthma, cardiovascular disease, or fluid overload.
• Never inject vasopressin tannate in oil I.V.
• Never inject during first stage of labor; may cause ruptured uterus.

• Monitor specific gravity of urine and intake and output to aid evaluation of drug effectiveness.
• Place tannate in oil in warm water for 10 to 15 minutes. Then shake thoroughly to make suspension uniform before withdrawing I.M. injection dose. Small brown particles must be seen in suspension. Use absolutely dry syringe to avoid dilution.
• Give with 1 to 2 glasses of water to reduce adverse reactions and to improve therapeutic response.
• To prevent possible seizures, coma, and death, observe patient closely for early signs of water intoxication.
• Overhydration more likely with long-acting tannate oil suspension than with aqueous vasopressin solution.
• Use minimum effective dosage to reduce adverse reactions.
• May be used for transient polyuria resulting from antidiuretic hormone deficiency related to neurosurgery or head injury.
• Synthetic desmopressin is sometimes preferred because of longer duration and less frequent adverse reactions. Desmopressin is also commercially available as a nasal solution.
• Monitor blood pressure of patient on vasopressin twice daily. Watch for excessively elevated blood pressure or lack of response to drug, which may be indicated by hypotension. Also monitor fluid intake and output and daily weights.
• A rectal tube will facilitate gas expulsion following vasopressin injection.

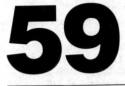

Parathyroid-like agents

calcifediol
calcitonin (human)
calcitonin (salmon)
calcitriol
dihydrotachysterol
etidronate disodium

COMBINATION PRODUCTS
None.

---

calcifediol
Calderol

Pregnancy Risk Category: A

HOW SUPPLIED
Capsules: 20 mcg, 50 mcg

MECHANISM OF ACTION
Stimulates calcium absorption from the GI tract and promotes secretion of calcium from bone to blood.

INDICATIONS & DOSAGE
Treatment and management of metabolic bone disease associated with chronic renal failure—
Adults: initially, 300 to 350 mcg P.O. weekly, given on a daily or alternate-day schedule. Dosage may be increased at 4-week intervals. Optimal dosage must be carefully determined for each patient.

ADVERSE REACTIONS
Vitamin D intoxication associated with hypercalcemia:
CNS: headache, somnolence.
EENT: conjunctivitis, photosensitivity, rhinorrhea.
GI: nausea, vomiting, constipation, metallic taste, dry mouth, anorexia, diarrhea.
GU: polyuria.
Other: weakness, bone and muscle pain.

INTERACTIONS
Cholestyramine: may impair absorption of calcifediol.

NURSING CONSIDERATIONS
• Contraindicated in hypercalcemia or vitamin D toxicity. Withhold all preparations containing vitamin D in patients taking calcifediol. Use cautiously in patients on digitalis because hypercalcemia may precipitate cardiac arrhythmias.
• Monitor serum calcium; serum calcium times serum phosphate should not exceed 70. During titration, serum calcium should be determined at least weekly. If hypercalcemia occurs, calcifediol should be discontinued but resumed after serum calcium returns to normal.
• Patient should receive adequate daily intake of calcium.
• Advise patient to adhere to diet and calcium supplementation and to avoid nonprescription drugs.
• Teach patient to report signs and symptoms of hypercalcemia.

Italicized adverse reactions are common or life-threatening.
*Liquid form contains alcohol.   **May contain tartrazine.

calcitonin (human)
Cibacalcin

calcitonin (salmon)
Calcimar, Miacalcin

Pregnancy Risk Category: B

HOW SUPPLIED
Injection: salmon—100 IU/ml, 1-ml ampules; 200 IU/ml, 2-ml ampules; human—0.5 mg/vial

MECHANISM OF ACTION
Decreases osteoclastic activity by inhibiting osteocytic osteolysis. Also decreases mineral release and matrix or collagen breakdown in bone.

INDICATIONS & DOSAGE
Paget's disease of bone (osteitis deformans)—
Adults: initially, 100 IU of calcitonin (salmon) daily S.C. or I.M. Maintenance dosage is 50 to 100 IU daily or every other day. Alternatively, give calcitonin (human) 0.5 mg S.C. daily. If patient obtains sufficient improvement, dosage may be reduced to 0.25 mg. daily 2 or 3 times per week. Some patients may need as much as 1 mg daily.
Hypercalcemia—
Adults: 4 IU/kg of calcitonin (salmon) q 12 hours I.M.
Postmenopausal osteoporosis—
Adults: 100 of calcitonin (salmon) daily I.M. or S.C.

ADVERSE REACTIONS
CNS: headaches.
GI: transient nausea with or without vomiting, diarrhea, anorexia.
GU: transient diuresis.
Metabolic: hyperglycemia.
Local: inflammation at injection site, skin rashes.
Other: *facial flushing;* hypocalcemia; swelling, tingling, and tenderness of hands; unusual taste sensation; *anaphylaxis.*

INTERACTIONS
None significant.

NURSING CONSIDERATIONS
• Contraindicated in allergy to gelatin diluent used to prepare drug. Not recommended for breast-feeding mothers, or women who are or may become pregnant. Safe use in children not established.
• Periodic serum alkaline phosphatase and 24-hour urine hydroxyproline levels should be determined to evaluate drug effect.
• Skin test is usually done before beginning therapy.
• Systemic allergic reactions possible since hormone is protein. Keep epinephrine handy when administering.
• Patients with good initial clinical response to calcitonin who suffer relapse should be evaluated for antibody formation response to the hormone protein.
• Tell patient in whom calcitonin loses its hypocalcemic activity that further medication or increased dosages will be of no value.
• Facial flushing and warmth occur in 20% to 30% of all patients within minutes of injection; usually last about 1 hour. Reassure patient that this is a transient effect.
• Observe patient for signs of hypocalcemic tetany during therapy (muscle twitching, tetanic spasms, and seizures if hypocalcemia is severe).
• Monitor calcium closely. Watch for signs of hypercalcemic relapse: bone pain, renal calculi, polyria, anorexia, nausea, vomiting, thirst, constipation, lethargy, bradycardia, muscle hypotonicity, pathologic fracture, psychosis, and coma.
• Periodic examinations of urine sediment are advisable.
• Calcitonin (human) is indicated especially in patients who have developed resistance to calcitonin (salmon). Calcitonin (human) is associated with risk of diminishing effi-

---

cacy caused by antibody formation or hypersensitivity reactions.

• Administer the drug at bedtime when possible to minimize nausea and vomiting.

• Treatment should continue for at least 6 months. Then, if symptoms have been relieved, it may be discontinued until symptoms or radiologic signs recur.

• Be sure to use the freshly reconstituted solution within 2 hours.

• When administered for postmenopausal osteoporosis, remind patient to take adequate calcium and vitamin D supplementation.

calcitriol (1,25-dihydroxycholecalciferol)
Rocaltrol

Pregnancy Risk Category: A (D if used in doses > RDA)

HOW SUPPLIED
Capsules: 0.25 mcg, 0.5 mcg

MECHANISM OF ACTION
Stimulates calcium absorption from the GI tract and promotes secretion of calcium from bone to blood.

INDICATIONS & DOSAGE
Management of hypocalcemia in patients undergoing chronic dialysis—
Adults: initially, 0.25 mcg P.O. daily. Dosage may be increased by 0.25 mcg daily at 2- to 4-week intervals. Maintenance dosage is 0.25 mcg every other day up to 0.5 to 1.25 mcg daily.
Management of hypoparathyroidism and pseudohypoparathyroidism—
Adults and children over 1 year: initially, 0.25 mcg P.O. daily. Dosage may be increased at 2- to 4-week intervals. Maintenance dosage is 0.25 to 2 mcg daily.

ADVERSE REACTIONS
Vitamin D intoxication associated with hypercalcemia:

CNS: headache, somnolence.
EENT: conjunctivitis, photophobia, rhinorrhea.
GI: nausea, vomiting, constipation, metallic taste, dry mouth, anorexia.
GU: polyuria.
Other: weakness, bone and muscle pain.

INTERACTIONS
None significant.

NURSING CONSIDERATIONS
• Contraindicated in hypercalcemia or vitamin D toxicity. Withhold all preparations containing vitamin D in patients taking calcitriol. Not recommended in breast-feeding mothers. Use cautiously in patients on digitalis; hypercalcemia may precipitate cardiac arrhythmias.

• Monitor serum calcium; serum calcium times serum phosphate should not exceed 70. During titration, determine serum calcium twice weekly. If hypercalcemia occurs, discontinue, but resume after serum calcium returns to normal. Patient should receive adequate daily intake of calcium—1,000 mg.

• Protect from heat and light.

• Instruct patient to adhere to diet and calcium supplementation and to avoid unapproved nonprescription drugs.

• Patients should not use magnesium-containing antacids while taking this drug.

• Patients should report to doctor immediately any of the following symptoms: weakness, nausea, vomiting, dry mouth, constipation, muscle or bone pain, or metallic taste—early symptoms of vitamin D intoxication.

• Tell patient that although this drug is a vitamin, it must not be taken by anyone for whom it was not prescribed because of its potentially serious toxicities.

• Most potent form of vitamin D available.

Italicized adverse reactions are common or life-threatening.
*Liquid form contains alcohol.   **May contain tartrazine.

dihydrotachysterol
AT-10‡, DHT*, Hytakerol

Pregnancy Risk Category: A (D if used in doses > RDA)

HOW SUPPLIED
Tablets: 0.125 mg, 0.2 mg, 0.4 mg
Capsules: 0.125 mg
Oral solution: 0.2 mg/5 ml, 0.2 mg/ml (Intensol), 0.25 mg/ml (in sesame oil)

MECHANISM OF ACTION
Stimulates calcium absorption from the GI tract and promotes secretion of calcium from bone to blood.

INDICATIONS & DOSAGE
Familial hypophosphatemia—
Adults and children: 0.5 to 2 mg P.O. daily. Maintenance dosage is 0.3 to 1.5 mg daily.
Hypocalcemia associated with hypoparathyroidism and pseudohypoparathyroidism—
Adults: initially, 0.8 to 2.4 mg P.O. daily for several days. Maintenance dosage is 0.2 to 2 mg daily, as required for normal serum calcium. Average dose is 0.6 mg daily.
Children: initially, 1 to 5 mg P.O. for several days. Maintenance dosage is 0.2 to 1 mg daily, as required for normal serum calcium.
Renal osteodystrophy in chronic uremia—
Adults: 0.1 to 0.6 mg P.O. daily.
Prophylaxis of hypocalcemic tetany following thyroid surgery—
Adults: 0.25 mg P.O. daily (with calcium supplements).

ADVERSE REACTIONS
Vitamin D intoxication associated with hypercalcemia:
CNS: headache, somnolence.
EENT: conjunctivitis, photophobia, rhinorrhea.
GI: nausea, vomiting, constipation, metallic taste, dry mouth, anorexia, diarrhea.
GU: polyuria.
Other: weakness, bone and muscle pain.

INTERACTIONS
Thiazide diuretics: possible hypercalcemia in hypoparathyroid patients. Avoid concomitant use.

NURSING CONSIDERATIONS
• Contraindicated in hypercalcemia, hypocalcemia associated with renal insufficiency and hyperphosphatemia, renal stones, hypersensitivity to vitamin D, and in breast-feeding mothers.
• Monitor serum and urine calcium. Watch for signs of hypercalcemia.
• Adequate dietary calcium intake is necessary; usually supplemented with 10 to 15 g oral calcium lactate or gluconate daily.
• Report hypercalcemia reactions to doctor. Early signs of hypercalcemia include thirst, headache, vertigo, tinnitus, anorexia.
• 1 mg equal to 120,000 units ergocalciferol (vitamin D_2).
• Store in tightly closed, light-resistant container. Don't refrigerate.

etidronate disodium
Didronel

Pregnancy Risk Category: B

HOW SUPPLIED
Tablets: 200 mg, 400 mg

MECHANISM OF ACTION
Decreases osteoclastic activity by inhibiting osteocytic osteolysis. Also decreases mineral release and matrix or collagen breakdown in bone.

INDICATIONS & DOSAGE
Symptomatic Paget's disease—
Adults: 5 mg/kg P.O. daily as a single dose 2 hours before a meal with water or juice. Patient should not eat for 2

hours after dose. May give up to 10 mg/kg daily in severe cases. Maximum dosage is 20 mg/kg daily.
Heterotopic ossification in spinal cord injuries—
Adults: 20 mg/kg P.O. daily for 2 weeks, then 10 mg/kg daily for 10 weeks. Total treatment period is 12 weeks.
Heterotopic ossification after total hip replacement—
Adults: 20 mg/kg daily P.O. for 1 month before total hip replacement and for 3 months afterward.

ADVERSE REACTIONS
GI: (seen most frequently at 20 mg/kg daily) diarrhea, increased frequency of bowel movements, nausea.
Other: increased or recurrent bone pain at pagetic sites, pain at previously asymptomatic sites, increased risk of fracture, *elevated serum phosphate.*

INTERACTIONS
None significant.

NURSING CONSIDERATIONS
• Use cautiously in enterocolitis, impaired renal function.
• Therapy should not last more than 6 months. After 3 months, resume if needed. Don't give longer than 3 months at doses above 10 mg/kg daily.
• Don't give drug with food, milk, or antacids; may reduce absorption.
• Monitor renal function before and during therapy.
• Elevated serum phosphate may occur, especially in patients receiving higher doses. However, serum phosphate usually returns to normal 2 to 4 weeks after drug's discontinued.
• Monitor drug effect by serum alkaline phosphatase and urinary hydroxyproline excretion (both lowered if therapy effective).
• Tell patient that improvement may not occur for up to 3 months but may continue for months after drug is stopped. Stress importance of good nutrition, especially diet high in calcium and vitamin D.

Italicized adverse reactions are common or life-threatening.
*Liquid form contains alcohol.   **May contain tartrazine.

60

Diuretics

Carbonic anhydrase inhibitors
acetazolamide
acetazolamide sodium
dichlorphenamide
methazolamide

Loop diuretics
bumetanide
ethacrynate sodium
ethacrynic acid
furosemide

Osmotic diuretics
mannitol
urea

Potassium-sparing diuretics
amiloride hydrochloride
spironolactone
triamterene

Thiazide diuretics
bendroflumethiazide
benzthiazide
chlorothiazide
chlorothiazide sodium
cyclothiazide
hydrochlorothiazide
hydroflumethiazide
methyclothiazide
polythiazide
trichlormethiazide

Thiazide-like diuretics
chlorthalidone
indapamide
metolazone
quinethazone

COMBINATION PRODUCTS
ALAZIDE: spironolactone 25 mg and hydrochlorothiazide 25 mg.
ALDACTAZIDE: spironolactone 25 mg and hydrochlorothiazide 25 mg.
ALDACTAZIDE 50/50: spironolactone 50 mg and hydrochlorothiazide 50 mg.
ALTEXIDE: spironolactone 25 mg and hydrochlorothiazide 25 mg.
DYAZIDE: triamterene 50 mg and hydrochlorothiazide 25 mg.
MAXZIDE: triamterene 75 mg and hydrochlorothiazide 50 mg.
MODURETIC: amiloride hydrochloride 5 mg and hydrochlorothiazide 50 mg.
SPIRONAZIDE: spironolactone 25 mg and hydrochlorothiazide 25 mg.
SPIROZIDE: spironolactone 25 mg and hydrochlorothiazide 25 mg.

---

acetazolamide
Acetazolam†, Ak-Zol, Apo-Acetazolamide†, Dazamide, Diamox, Diamox Sequels

acetazolamide sodium
Diamox Parenteral, Diamox Sodium†

Pregnancy Risk Category: C

HOW SUPPLIED
Tablets: 125 mg, 250 mg
Capsules (extended-release): 500 mg
Injection: 500 mg/vial

MECHANISM OF ACTION
Blocks the action of carbonic anhydrase, thereby promoting the renal excretion of sodium, potassium, bicar-

---

bonate, and water. Bicarbonate ion excretion makes the urine alkaline. Also decreases secretion of aqueous humor in the eye, thereby lowering intraocular pressure. As an anticonvulsant, may inhibit carbonic anhydrase in the CNS and decrease abnormal paroxysmal or excessive neuronal discharge.

INDICATIONS & DOSAGE

Narrow-angle glaucoma—
Adults: 250 mg q 4 hours; or 250 mg P.O., I.M., or I.V. b.i.d. for short-term therapy.
Edema in congestive heart failure—
Adults: 250 to 375 mg P.O., I.M., or I.V. daily in a.m.
Children: 5 mg/kg daily in a.m.
Open-angle glaucoma—
Adults: 250 mg daily to 1 g P.O., I.M., or I.V. divided q.i.d.
Prevention or amelioration of acute mountain sickness—
Adults: 250 mg P.O. q 8 to 12 hours.
Myoclonic, refractory generalized tonic-clonic (grand mal) or absence (petit mal), or mixed seizures—
Adults: 375 mg P.O., I.M., or I.V. daily up to 250 mg q.i.d. Alternatively, use sustained-release form 250 to 500 mg P.O. daily or b.i.d. Initial dosage when used with other anticonvulsants usually is 250 mg daily.
Children: 8 to 30 mg/kg P.O. daily, divided t.i.d. or q.i.d. Maximum dosage is 1.5 g daily, or 300 to 900 mg/m² daily.

ADVERSE REACTIONS

Blood: *aplastic anemia,* hemolytic anemia, leukopenia.
CNS: drowsiness, paresthesias, confusion.
EENT: transient myopia.
GI: nausea, vomiting, anorexia.
GU: crystalluria, renal calculi, hematuria.
Metabolic: *hyperchloremic acidosis,* hypokalemia, asymptomatic hyperuricemia.

Skin: rash.
Local: *pain at injection site,* sterile abscesses.

INTERACTIONS

None significant.

NURSING CONSIDERATIONS

• Contraindicated in long-term therapy for chronic noncongestive narrow-angle glaucoma; also in hyponatremia or hypokalemia, renal or hepatic disease or dysfunction, adrenal gland failure, or hyperchloremic acidosis. Use cautiously in respiratory acidosis, emphysema, chronic pulmonary disease, and in those patients receiving other diuretics.
• Monitor intake/output and electrolytes, especially serum potassium. When used in diuretic therapy, consult with doctor and dietitian to provide high-potassium diet.
• Weigh patient daily. Rapid or excessive fluid loss cuases weight loss and hypotension.
• Diuretic effect is decreased when acidosis occurs but can be reestablished by withdrawing drug for several days and then restarting, or by using intermittent administration schedules.
• Reconstitute 500-mg vial with at least 5 ml sterile water for injection. Use within 24 hours of reconstitution.
• I.M. injection is painful because of alkalinity of solution. Direct I.V. administration is preferred (100 to 500 mg/minute).
• Elderly patients are especially susceptible to excessive diuresis.
• May cause false-positive urine protein tests by alkalinizing the urine.
• To make an oral liquid: soften 1 tablet in 2 teaspoonfuls of very warm water and add to 2 teaspoonfuls honey or syrup (chocolate or cherry). Don't use fruit juice.

Italicized adverse reactions are common or life-threatening.
*Liquid form contains alcohol.   **May contain tartrazine.

amiloride hydrochloride
Kaluril‡, Midamor

Pregnancy Risk Category: B

HOW SUPPLIED
Tablets: 5 mg

MECHANISM OF ACTION
A potassium-sparing diuretic that inhibits sodium reabsorption and potassium excretion by direct action on the distal tubule.

INDICATIONS & DOSAGE
Hypertension; edema associated with congestive heart failure, usually in patients who are also taking thiazide or other potassium-wasting diuretics—
Adults: usual dosage is 5 mg P.O. daily. Dosage may be increased to 10 mg daily, if necessary. As much as 20 mg daily can be given.

ADVERSE REACTIONS
CNS: *headache,* weakness, dizziness.
CV: orthostatic hypotension.
GI: *nausea, anorexia, diarrhea, vomiting,* abdominal pain, constipation.
GU: impotence.
Metabolic: hyperkalemia.

INTERACTIONS
None significant.

NURSING CONSIDERATIONS
• Contraindicated in patients with elevated serum potassium level (greater than 5.5 mEq/liter). Don't administer to patients receiving other potassium-sparing diuretics, such as spironolactone and triamterene. Also contraindicated in anuria.
• Use cautiously in patients with renal impairment, because potassium retention is increased.
• Risk of hyperkalemia is greater when a potassium-wasting drug is not taken concurrently. When amiloride is taken this way, be sure to monitor daily potassium.
• Discontinue immediately if potassium level exceeds 6.5 mEq/liter.
• Advise patient to avoid sudden posture changes and rise slowly to avoid orthostatic hypotension.
• Warn patient to avoid excessive ingestion of potassium-rich foods or potassium-containing salt substitutes. Concomitant potassium supplement can lead to serious hyperkalemia.
• Administer amiloride with meals to prevent nausea.

bendroflumethiazide (bendrofluazide)
Aprinox‡, Aprinox-M‡, Benzide‡, Naturetin

Pregnancy Risk Category: B

HOW SUPPLIED
Tablets: 2.5 mg, 5 mg, 10 mg

MECHANISM OF ACTION
A thiazide diuretic that increases urine excretion of sodium and water by inhibiting sodium reabsorption in the cortical diluting site of the ascending loop of Henle.

INDICATIONS & DOSAGE
Edema, hypertension—
Adults: 5 to 20 mg P.O. daily or divided b.i.d.
Children: initially, 0.1 to 0.4 mg/kg (3 to 12 mg/m^2) P.O. daily or divided b.i.d.
Maintenance: 0.05 to 0.1 mg/kg (1.5 to 3 mg/m^2) P.O. daily or divided b.i.d.

ADVERSE REACTIONS
Blood: *aplastic anemia, agranulocytosis,* leukopenia, thrombocytopenia.
CV: *volume depletion and dehydration,* orthostatic hypotension.
GI: anorexia, nausea, pancreatitis.
Hepatic: hepatic encephalopathy.
Metabolic: *hypokalemia, asymptomatic hyperuricemia, hyperglycemia and impairment of glucose tolerance,*

---

fluid and electrolyte imbalances including dilutional hyponatremia and hypochloremia, metabolic alkalosis, hypercalcemia, gout.
Skin: dermatitis, photosensitivity, rash.
Other: hypersensitivity reactions, such as pneumonitis and vasculitis.

INTERACTIONS
Cholestyramine, colestipol: intestinal absorption of thiazides decreased. Keep doses as separate as possible.
Diazoxide: increased antihypertensive, hyperglycemic, and hyperuricemic effects. Use together cautiously.

NURSING CONSIDERATIONS
• Contraindicated in anuria or hypersensitivity to other thiazides or other sulfonamide-derived drugs. Use cautiously in severe renal disease and impaired hepatic function.
• Monitor intake/output, weight, and serum electrolytes regularly. Monitor serum creatinine and BUN regularly. Not as effective if these are more than twice normal.
• Consult with doctor and dietitian to provide high-potassium diet. Watch for signs of hypokalemia (for example, muscle weakness and cramps). Patients on digitalis have an increased risk of digitalis toxicity from potassium-depleting adverse effect of this diuretic. May be used with potassium-sparing diuretic to prevent potassium loss.
• Foods rich in potassium include citrus fruits, bananas, tomatoes, dates, and apricots.
• Monitor blood sugar. Check insulin requirements in patients with diabetes. May treat severe hyperglycemia with oral antidiabetic agents.
• Monitor blood uric acid, especially in patients with a history of gout.
• Elderly patients are especially susceptible to excessive diuresis.
• Give in a.m. to prevent nocturia.

• In hypertension, therapeutic response may be delayed several days.
• Thiazides and thiazide-like diuretics should be discontinued before tests for parathyroid function are performed.
• Advise patient to avoid sudden posture changes and rise slowly to avoid orthostatic hypotension.
• Advise patient to wear a sunscreen.

---

benzthiazide
Aquatag**, Exna**, Hydrex, Proaqua**
Pregnancy Risk Category: D

HOW SUPPLIED
Tablets: 50 mg

MECHANISM OF ACTION
A thiazide diuretic that increases urine excretion of sodium and water by inhibiting sodium reabsorption in the cortical diluting site of the nephron.

INDICATIONS & DOSAGE
Edema—
Adults: 50 to 200 mg P.O. daily or in divided doses.
Children: 1 to 4 mg/kg P.O. daily in three divided doses.
Hypertension—
Adults: 50 mg P.O. daily b.i.d., t.i.d., or q.i.d., adjusted to patient response.

ADVERSE REACTIONS
Blood: *aplastic anemia, agranulocytosis,* leukopenia, thrombocytopenia.
CV: *volume depletion and dehydration,* orthostatic hypotension.
GI: anorexia, nausea, pancreatitis.
Hepatic: hepatic encephalopathy.
Metabolic: *hypokalemia, asymptomatic hyperuricemia, hyperglycemia and impairment of glucose tolerance,* fluid and electrolyte imbalances including dilutional hyponatremia and

---

hypochloremia, metabolic alkalosis, hypercalcemia, gout.
Skin: dermatitis, photosensitivity, rash.
Other: hypersensitivity reactions, such as pneumonitis and vasculitis.

INTERACTIONS
Cholestyramine, colestipol: intestinal absorption of thiazides decreased. Keep doses as separate as possible.
Diazoxide: increased antihypertensive, hyperglycemic, and hyperuricemic effects. Use together cautiously.

NURSING CONSIDERATIONS
• Contraindicated in anuria or hypersensitivity to other thiazides or other sulfonamide-derived drugs. Use cautiously in severe renal disease and impaired hepatic function.
• Monitor intake/output, weight, and serum electrolytes regularly. Consult with doctor and dietitian to provide high-potassium diet. Watch for signs of hypokalemia (for example, muscle weakness and cramps). Patients on digitalis have an increased risk of digitalis toxicity from the potassium-depleting adverse effect of this diuretic. May use with potassium-sparing diuretic to prevent potassium loss.
• Foods rich in potassium include citrus fruits, bananas, tomatoes, dates, and apricots.
• Monitor blood pressure routinely. If possible, teach patient or family how to check blood pressure.
• Monitor serum creatinine and BUN regularly. Not as effective if these levels are more than twice normal.
• Monitor blood sugar. Check insulin requirements in patients with diabetes. May treat severe hyperglycemia with oral antidiabetic agents.
• Monitor blood uric acid level, especially in patients with a history of gout.
• Give in a.m. to prevent nocturia.

• Elderly patients are especially susceptible to excessive diuresis.
• In hypertension, therapeutic response may be delayed several days.
• Thiazides and thiazide-like diuretics should be discontinued before tests for parathyroid function are performed.
• Advise patient to avoid sudden posture changes and rise slowly to avoid orthostatic hypotension.
• Advise patient to wear a sunscreen.

---

bumetanide
Bumex, Burinex‡
Pregnancy Risk Category: C

HOW SUPPLIED
Tablets: 0.5 mg, 1 mg, 2 mg
Injection: 0.25 mg/ml

MECHANISM OF ACTION
A loop diuretic that inhibits reabsorption of sodium and chloride at the proximal portion of the ascending loop of Henle.

INDICATIONS & DOSAGE
Edema (congestive heart failure, hepatic and renal disease)—
Adults: 0.5 to 2 mg P.O. once daily. If diuretic response not adequate, a second or third dose may be given at 4- to 5-hour intervals. Maximum dosage is 10 mg/day. May be administered parenterally when P.O. not feasible. Usual initial dose is 0.5 to 1 mg I.V. or I.M. If response is not adequate, a second or third dose may be given at 2- to 3-hour intervals. Maximum dosage is 10 mg/day.

ADVERSE REACTIONS
CNS: dizziness, headache.
CV: *volume depletion and dehydration, orthostatic hypotension,* ECG changes.
EENT: transient deafness.
GI: nausea.
Metabolic: *hypokalemia; hypochlore-*

mic alkalosis; asymptomatic hyperuricemia; fluid and electrolyte imbalances, including dilutional hyponatremia, hypocalcemia, hypomagnesemia; hyperglycemia and impairment of glucose tolerance.
Skin: rash.
Other: muscle pain and tenderness.

INTERACTIONS

Aminoglycoside antibiotics: potentiated ototoxicity. Use together cautiously.
Probenecid, indomethacin: inhibited diuretic response. Use cautiously.

NURSING CONSIDERATIONS

• Contraindicated in anuria, hepatic coma, or in states of severe electrolyte depletion.
• Use cautiously in patients with hepatic cirrhosis and ascites. Supplemental potassium or potassium-sparing diuretics may be used to prevent hypokalemia and metabolic alkalosis in these patients. Use cautiously in patients with depressed renal function.
• Use cautiously in patients allergic to sulfonamides. These patients may show hypersensitivity to bumetanide.
• Potent loop diuretic; can lead to profound water and electrolyte depletion. Monitor blood pressure and pulse rate during rapid diuresis.
• If oliguria or azotemia develops or increases, may require stopping drug.
• Monitor serum electrolytes, BUN, and CO_2 frequently.
• Watch for signs of hypokalemia (for example, muscle weakness and cramps). Patients also receiving digitalis have an increased risk of digitalis toxicity from the potassium-depleting effect of this diuretic.
• Consult with doctor and dietitian to provide high-potassium diet.
• Foods rich in potassium include citrus fruits, tomatoes, bananas, dates, and apricots.
• Monitor blood sugar in patients

with diabetes. May treat severe hyperglycemia with oral antidiabetic agents.
• Monitor blood uric acid, especially in patients with a history of gout.
• Give I.V. doses over 1 to 2 minutes.
• Advise patients taking bumetanide to stand up slowly to prevent dizziness and to limit alcohol intake and strenuous exercise in hot weather since these exacerbate orthostatic hypotension.
• Bumetanide can be safely prescribed in patients allergic to furosemide.
• 1 mg of bumetanide is equal to 40 mg of furosemide.
• May be less ototoxic than furosemide, but the clinical relevance of this has not been determined.
• Give in a.m. to prevent nocturia. If second dose is necessary, give in the early afternoon.
• Intermittent dosage given on alternate days, or for 3 to 4 days with 1 or 2 days intervening, is recommended as the safest and most effective dosage schedule for control of edema.

chlorothiazide
Azide‡, Chlotride‡, Diachlor, Diuret‡, Diurigen, Diuril

chlorothiazide sodium
Diuril Sodium

Pregnancy Risk Category: D

HOW SUPPLIED
Tablets: 250 mg, 500 mg
Oral suspension: 250 mg/5 ml
Injection: 500-mg vial

MECHANISM OF ACTION
A thiazide diuretic that increases urine excretion of sodium and water by inhibiting sodium reabsorption in the cortical diluting site of the nephron.

INDICATIONS & DOSAGE

Edema, hypertension—
Adults: 500 mg to 2 g P.O. or I.V. daily or in two divided doses.
Diuresis—
Children over 6 months: 20 mg/kg P.O. or I.V. daily in divided doses.
Children under 6 months: may require 30 mg/kg P.O. or I.V. daily in two divided doses.

ADVERSE REACTIONS

Blood: *aplastic anemia, agranulocytosis,* leukopenia, thrombocytopenia.
CV: *volume depletion and dehydration,* orthostatic hypotension.
GI: anorexia, nausea, pancreatitis.
Hepatic: hepatic encephalopathy.
Metabolic: *hypokalemia, asymptomatic hyperuricemia, hyperglycemia and impairment of glucose tolerance,* fluid and electrolyte imbalances including dilutional hyponatremia and hypochloremia, metabolic alkalosis, hypercalcemia, gout.
Skin: dermatitis, photosensitivity, rash.
Other: hypersensitivity reactions such as pneumonitis and vasculitis.

INTERACTIONS

Cholestyramine, colestipol: intestinal absorption of thiazides decreased. Keep doses as separate as possible.
Diazoxide: increased antihypertensive, hyperglycemic, and hyperuricemic effects. Use together cautiously.

NURSING CONSIDERATIONS

• Contraindicated in anuria; hypersensitivity to other thiazides or other sulfonamide-derived drugs; impaired hepatic function; or progressive hepatic disease. Use cautiously in severe renal disease.
• Monitor intake/output, weight, blood pressure, and serum electrolytes regularly.
• Consult with doctor and dietitian to provide high-potassium diet. Watch for signs of hypokalemia (for example, muscle weakness, and cramps). Patients on digitalis have an increased risk of digitalis toxicity from the potassium-depleting effect of the diuretic. May use with potassium-sparing diuretic to prevent potassium loss.
• Foods rich in potassium include citrus fruits, tomatoes, bananas, dates, and apricots.
• Monitor blood sugar. Check insulin requirements in patients with diabetes. May treat severe hyperglycemia with oral antidiabetic agents.
• Monitor serum creatinine and BUN regularly. Not as effective if these levels are more than twice normal.
• Monitor blood uric acid, especially in patients with a history of gout.
• Monitor serum calcium and watch for progressive renal impairment.
• Only injectable thiazide. For I.V. use only—not I.M. or S.C. Reconstitute 500 mg with 18 ml of sterile water for injection. May store reconstituted solutions at room temperature up to 24 hours. Compatible with I.V. dextrose or sodium chloride solutions.
• Avoid I.V. infiltration; can be very painful.
• Give in a.m. to prevent nocturia.
• In hypertension, therapeutic response may be delayed several days.
• Elderly patients are especially susceptible to excessive diuresis.
• Thiazides and thiazide-like diuretics should be stopped before tests for parathyroid function are performed.
• Advise patient to avoid sudden posture changes and rise slowly to avoid orthostatic hypotension.
• Advise patient to wear a sunscreen.

---

chlorthalidone
Apo-Chlorthalidone†, Hygroton, Novothalidone†, Thalitone, Uridon†
Pregnancy Risk Category: D

HOW SUPPLIED
Tablets: 25 mg, 50 mg, 100 mg

MECHANISM OF ACTION
Although not a thiazide, chlorthalidone acts in a similar fashion. It increases urine excretion of sodium and water by inhibiting sodium reabsorption in the cortical diluting site of the nephron.

INDICATIONS & DOSAGE
Edema, hypertension—
Adults: 25 to 100 mg P.O. daily, or 100 mg 3 times weekly or on alternate days.
Children: 2 mg/kg P.O. 3 times weekly.

ADVERSE REACTIONS
Blood: *aplastic anemia, agranulocytosis,* leukopenia, thrombocytopenia.
CV: *volume depletion and dehydration,* orthostatic hypotension.
GI: anorexia, nausea, pancreatitis.
GU: impotence.
Hepatic: hepatic encephalopathy.
Metabolic: *hypokalemia, asymptomatic hyperuricemia, hyperglycemia and impairment of glucose tolerance,* fluid and electrolyte imbalances including dilutional hyponatremia and hypochloremia, metabolic alkalosis, hypercalcemia, gout.
Skin: dermatitis, photosensitivity, rash.
Other: hypersensitivity reactions, such as pneumonitis and vasculitis.

INTERACTIONS
Cholestyramine, colestipol: intestinal absorption of thiazides decreased. Keep doses as separate as possible.
Diazoxide: increased antihypertensive, hyperglycemic, and hyperuricemic effects. Use together cautiously.

NURSING CONSIDERATIONS
• Contraindicated in anuria or in hypersensitivity to thiazides or other sulfonamide-derived drugs. Use cautiously in severe renal disease, progressive hepatic disease, and impaired hepatic function.
• Monitor intake/output, weight, blood pressure, and serum electrolytes regularly.
• Consult with doctor and dietitian to provide high-potassium diet. Watch for signs of hypokalemia (for example, muscle weakness, and cramps). Patients on digitalis have an increased risk of digitalis toxicity from the potassium-depleting effect of this diuretic. May use with potassium-sparing diuretic to prevent potassium loss.
• Foods rich in potassium include citrus fruits, tomatoes, bananas, dates, and apricots.
• Monitor serum creatinine and BUN regularly. Not as effective if these levels are more than twice normal.
• Monitor blood uric acid, especially in patients with a history of gout.
• Monitor blood sugar. Check insulin requirements in patients with diabetes. May treat severe hyperglycemia with oral antidiabetic agents.
• In hypertension, therapeutic response may be delayed several days.
• Give in a.m. to prevent nocturia.
• Elderly patients are especially susceptible to excessive diuresis.
• Thiazides and thiazide-like diuretics should be stopped before tests for parathyroid function are performed.
• Advise patient to avoid sudden posture changes and rise slowly to avoid orthostatic hypotension.
• Advise patient to wear a sunscreen.
• Notice that Uridon tablets (available in Canada only) should not be confused with the urinary anti-infective Uridon Modified (available in the United States).

---

cyclothiazide
Anhydron, Fluidil
Pregnancy Risk Category: D

HOW SUPPLIED
Tablets: 2 mg

MECHANISM OF ACTION

A thiazide diuretic that increases urine excretion of sodium and water by inhibiting sodium reabsorption in the cortical diluting site of the nephron.

INDICATIONS & DOSAGE

Edema—
Adults: 1 to 2 mg P.O. daily. May be used on alternate days as maintenance dosage.
Children: 0.02 to 0.04 mg/kg P.O. daily.
Hypertension—
Adults: 2 mg P.O. daily; up to 2 mg b.i.d. or t.i.d.

ADVERSE REACTIONS

Blood: *aplastic anemia, agranulocytosis,* leukopenia, thrombocytopenia.
CV: *volume depletion and dehydration,* orthostatic hypotension.
GI: anorexia, nausea, pancreatitis.
Hepatic: hepatic encephalopathy.
Metabolic: *hypokalemia, asymptomatic hyperuricemia, hyperglycemia and impairment of glucose tolerance,* fluid and electrolyte imbalances including dilutional hyponatremia and hypochloremia, metabolic alkalosis, hypercalcemia, gout.
Skin: dermatitis, photosensitivity, rash.
Other: hypersensitivity reactions, such as pneumonitis and vasculitis.

INTERACTIONS

Cholestyramine, colestipol: intestinal absorption of thiazides decreased. Keep doses as separate as possible.
Diazoxide: increased antihypertensive, hyperglycemic, and hyperuricemic effects. Use together cautiously.

NURSING CONSIDERATIONS

• Contraindicated in anuria or in hypersensitivity to other thiazides or other sulfonamide-derived drugs. Use cautiously in severe renal disease, impaired hepatic function, and progressive hepatic disease.
• Monitor intake/output, weight, blood pressure, and serum electrolytes regularly.
• Consult with doctor and dietitian to provide high-potassium diet. Watch for signs of hypokalemia (for example, muscle weakness and cramps). Patients on digitalis have an increased risk of digitalis toxicity from the potassium-depleting effect of this diuretic. May use with potassium-sparing diuretic to prevent potassium loss.
• Foods rich in potassium include citrus fruits, tomatoes, bananas, dates, and apricots.
• Monitor blood sugar. Check insulin requirements in patients with diabetes. May treat severe hyperglycemia with oral antidiabetic agents.
• Monitor serum creatinine and BUN regularly. Not as effective if these levels are more than twice normal.
• Monitor blood uric acid, especially in patients with a history of gout.
• In hypertension, therapeutic response may be delayed several days.
• Give in a.m. to prevent nocturia.
• Elderly patients are especially susceptible to excessive diuresis.
• Thiazides and thiazide-like diuretics should be stopped before tests for parathyroid function are performed.
• Advise patient to avoid sudden posture changes and rise slowly to avoid orthostatic hypotension.
• Advise patient to wear a sunscreen.

dichlorphenamide
Daranide

Pregnancy Risk Category: C

HOW SUPPLIED

Tablets: 50 mg

MECHANISM OF ACTION

A carbonic anhydrase inhibitor that decreases secretion of aqueous humor

---

in the eye, thereby lowering intraocular pressure.

INDICATIONS & DOSAGE
Adjunct in glaucoma—
Adults: initially, 100 to 200 mg P.O., followed by 100 mg q 12 hours until desired response obtained. Maintenance dosage is 25 to 50 mg P.O. daily b.i.d. or t.i.d. Give miotics concomitantly.

ADVERSE REACTIONS
Blood: *aplastic anemia,* hemolytic anemia, leukopenia.
CNS: drowsiness, paresthesias.
EENT: transient myopia.
GI: nausea, vomiting, anorexia.
GU: crystalluria, renal calculi.
Metabolic: *hyperchloremic acidosis,* hypokalemia, asymptomatic hyperuricemia.
Skin: rash.

INTERACTIONS
None significant.

NURSING CONSIDERATIONS
• Contraindicated in hepatic insufficiency, renal failure, adrenocortical insufficiency, hyperchloremic acidosis, depressed sodium or potassium levels, severe pulmonary obstruction with inability to increase alveolar ventilation, or Addison's disease. Long-term use contraindicated in severe, absolute, or chronic noncongestive narrow-angle glaucoma. Use cautiously in respiratory acidosis, monitoring blood pH and blood gases.
• Monitor electrolytes, especially serum potassium in initial treatment. Usually no problem in long-term glaucoma therapy unless risk of hypokalemia from other causes; potassium supplements may be necessary.
• May cause false-positive results in urine protein tests.
• Anticipate that drug will be given every day for glaucoma but intermittently for edema.

• Evaluate patient with glaucoma for eye pain to make sure drug is effective in decreasing intraocular pressure.

---

ethacrynate sodium
Edecrin Sodium

ethacrynic acid
Edecril‡, Edecrin
Pregnancy Risk Category: D

HOW SUPPLIED
Tablets: 25 mg, 50 mg
Injection: 50 mg (with 62.5 mg of mannitol and 0.1 mg of thimerosal)

MECHANISM OF ACTION
A loop diuretic that inhibits reabsorption of sodium and chloride at the proximal portion of the ascending loop of Henle.

INDICATIONS & DOSAGE
Acute pulmonary edema—
Adults: 50 to 100 mg of ethacrynate sodium I.V. slowly over several minutes.
Edema—
Adults: 50 to 200 mg P.O. daily. Refractory cases may require up to 200 mg b.i.d.
Children: initial dose is 25 mg P.O., cautiously, increased in 25-mg increments daily until desired effect is achieved.

ADVERSE REACTIONS
Blood: *agranulocytosis,* neutropenia, thrombocytopenia.
CV: *volume depletion and dehydration,* orthostatic hypotension.
EENT: transient deafness with too-rapid I.V. injection.
GI: abdominal discomfort and pain, diarrhea.
Metabolic: *hypokalemia; hypochloremic alkalosis; asymptomatic hyperuricemia; fluid and electrolyte imbalances including dilutional hyponatremia, hypocalcemia, hypomagnesemia;*

---

hyperglycemia and impairment of glucose tolerance.
Skin: dermatitis.

INTERACTIONS
Aminoglycoside antibiotics: potentiated ototoxic adverse reactions of both ethacrynic acid and aminoglycosides. Use together cautiously.
Warfarin: potentiated anticoagulant effect. Use together cautiously.

NURSING CONSIDERATIONS
• Contraindicated in anuria and in infants. Use cautiously in electrolyte abnormalities. If electrolyte imbalance, azotemia, or oliguria develops, may require stopping drug.
• This drug is a very potent diuretic.
• Monitor intake/output, weight, blood pressure, and serum electrolytes regularly.
• Consult with doctor and dietitian to provide high-potassium diet. Watch for signs of hypokalemia (for example, muscle weakness and cramps).
• Foods rich in potassium include citrus fruits, tomatoes, bananas, dates, and apricots.
• Patients also on digitalis have an increased risk of digitalis toxicity from the potassium-depleting effect.
• I.V. injection painful; may cause thrombophlebitis. Don't give subcutaneously or I.M. Give slowly through tubing of running infusion over several minutes.
• Sodium and potassium chloride supplement may be needed during therapy.
• Reconstitute vacuum vial with 50 ml of dextrose 5% injection or sodium chloride injection. Discard unused solution after 24 hours. Don't use cloudy or opalescent solutions.
• Elderly patients are especially susceptible to excessive diuresis.
• Give P.O. doses in a.m. to prevent nocturia.
• Severe diarrhea may necessitate discontinuing drug.

• Monitor blood uric acid, especially in patients with a history of gout.
• Advise patient to avoid sudden posture changes and rise slowly to avoid orthostatic hypotension.

---

furosemide (frusemide)
Apo-Furosemide†, Furoside†, Lasix*, Lasix Special†, Myrosemide*, Novosemide†, Urex‡, Urex-M‡, Uritol†
Pregnancy Risk Category: C

HOW SUPPLIED
Tablets: 20 mg, 40 mg, 80 mg, 500 mg†
Oral solution: 8 mg/ml, 10 mg/ml, 50 mg/ml
Injection: 10 mg/ml

MECHANISM OF ACTION
A loop diuretic that inhibits reabsorption of sodium and chloride at the proximal portion of the ascending loop of Henle.

INDICATIONS & DOSAGE
Acute pulmonary edema—
Adults: 40 mg I.V. injected slowly; then 40 mg I.V. in 1 to 1½ hours if needed.
Edema—
Adults: 20 to 80 mg P.O. daily in a.m., second dose can be given in 6 to 8 hours; carefully titrated up to 600 mg daily if needed; or 20 to 40 mg I.M. or I.V. Increase by 20 mg q 2 hours until desired response is achieved. I.V. dose should be given slowly over 1 to 2 minutes.
Hypertension—
Adults: 40 mg P.O. b.i.d. Adjust dose according to response.
Infants and children: 2 mg/kg P.O. daily; dose increased by 1 to 2 mg/kg in 6 to 8 hours if needed; carefully titrated up to 6 mg/kg daily if needed.
Hypertensive crisis, acute renal failure—

Adults: 100 to 200 mg I.V. over 1 to 2 minutes.
Chronic renal failure—
Adults: initially, 80 mg P.O. daily. Increase by 80 to 120 mg daily until desired response is achieved.

ADVERSE REACTIONS
Blood: *agranulocytosis,* leukopenia, thrombocytopenia.
CV: *volume depletion and dehydration,* orthostatic hypotension.
EENT: transient deafness with too rapid I.V. injection.
GI: abdominal discomfort and pain, diarrhea (with oral solution).
Metabolic: *hypokalemia; hypochloremic alkalosis; asymptomatic hyperuricemia, fluid and electrolyte imbalances including dilutional hyponatremia, hypocalcemia, hypomagnesemia;* hyperglycemia and impairment of glucose tolerance.
Skin: dermatitis.

INTERACTIONS
Aminoglycoside antibiotics: potentiated ototoxicity. Use together cautiously.
Chloral hydrate: sweating, flushing with I.V. furosemide.
Clofibrate: enhanced furosemide effects. Use cautiously.
Indomethacin: inhibited diuretic response. Use cautiously.

NURSING CONSIDERATIONS
• Use cautiously in cardiogenic shock complicated by pulmonary edema, anuria, hepatic coma, or electrolyte imbalances. Drug is not routinely administered to women of childbearing age because its safety in pregnancy hasn't been established.
• Potent loop diuretic; can lead to profound water and electrolyte depletion. Monitor blood pressure and pulse rate during rapid diuresis and routinely with chronic use.
• Sulfonamide-sensitive patients may have allergic reactions to furosemide.

• If oliguria or azotemia develops or increases, may require stopping drug.
• Monitor serum electrolyte, BUN, and CO_2 frequently.
• Monitor serum potassium level. Watch for signs of hypokalemia (for example, muscle weakness and cramps). Patients also on digitalis have an increased risk of digitalis toxicity from the potassium-depleting effect.
• Consult with doctor and dietitian to provide high-potassium diet.
• Foods rich in potassium include citrus fruits, tomatoes, bananas, dates, and apricots.
• Monitor blood sugar in patients with diabetes. May treat severe hyperglycemia with oral antidiabetic agents.
• Monitor blood uric acid, especially in patients with a history of gout.
• Give I.V. doses over 1 to 2 minutes.
• Don't use parenteral route in infants and children unless oral dosage form is not practical.
• Give P.O. and I.M. preparations in a.m. to prevent nocturia. Give second doses in early afternoon.
• Elderly patients are especially susceptible to excessive diuresis, with potential for circulatory collapse and thromboembolic complications.
• Store tablets in light-resistant container to prevent discoloration (doesn't affect potency). Don't use discolored (yellow) injectable preparation. Oral furosemide solution should be stored in the refrigerator to ensure stability of the drug.
• Promotes calcium excretion. I.V. furosemide often used to treat hypercalcemia.
• Advise patients taking furosemide to stand slowly to prevent dizziness, and to limit alcohol intake and strenuous exercise in hot weather because these exacerbate orthostatic hypotension.
• Advise patients to report immediately ringing in ears, severe abdomi-

---

Italicized adverse reactions are common or life-threatening.
*Liquid form contains alcohol.   **May contain tartrazine.

nal pain, or sore throat and fever; may indicate furosemide toxicity.

• Discourage patients receiving furosemide therapy at home from storing different types of medication in the same container. This increases the risk of drug errors, especially for patients taking both furosemide and digoxin, since the most popular strengths of these drugs' pills are white tablets approximately equal in size.

• To prepare parenteral furosemide for I.V. infusion, mix drug with dextrose 5% in water, 0.9% sodium chloride solution, or lactated Ringer's solution. Use prepared infusion solution within 24 hours.

hydrochlorothiazide
Apo-Hydro†, Dichlotride‡, Diuchlor H†, Esidrix, HydroDIURIL, Mictrin, Natrimax†, Novohydrazide†, Oretic, Thiuretic, Urozide†

Pregnancy Risk Category: D

HOW SUPPLIED
Tablets: 25 mg, 50 mg, 100 mg
Oral solution: 10 mg/ml, 100 mg/ml

MECHANISM OF ACTION
A thiazide diuretic that increases urine excretion of sodium and water by inhibiting sodium reabsorption in the cortical diluting site of the nephron.

INDICATIONS & DOSAGE
Edema—
Adults: initially, 25 to 100 mg P.O. daily or intermittently for maintenance dosage.
Children over 6 months: 2.2 mg/kg P.O. daily divided b.i.d.
Children under 6 months: up to 3.3 mg/kg P.O. daily divided b.i.d.
Hypertension—
Adults: 25 to 100 mg P.O. daily or divided dosage. Daily dosage increased

or decreased according to blood pressure.

ADVERSE REACTIONS
Blood: *aplastic anemia, agranulocytosis,* leukopenia, thrombocytopenia.
CV: *volume depletion and dehydration,* orthostatic hypotension.
GI: anorexia, nausea, pancreatitis.
Hepatic: hepatic encephalopathy.
Metabolic: *hypokalemia, asymptomatic hyperuricemia, hyperglycemia and impairment of glucose tolerance,* fluid and electrolyte imbalances including dilutional hyponatremia and hypochloremia, metabolic alkalosis, hypercalcemia, gout.
Skin: dermatitis, photosensitivity, rash.
Other: hypersensitivity reactions, such as pneumonitis and vasculitis.

INTERACTIONS
Cholestyramine, colestipol: intestinal absorption of thiazides decreased. Keep doses as separate as possible.
Diazoxide: increased antihypertensive, hyperglycemic, and hyperuricemic effects. Use together cautiously.

NURSING CONSIDERATIONS
• Contraindicated in anuria or hypersensitivity to other thiazides or other sulfonamide derivatives. Use cautiously in severe renal disease, impaired hepatic function, and progressive hepatic disease.
• Monitor intake/output, weight, blood pressure, and serum electrolytes regularly.
• Consult with doctor and dietitian to provide high-potassium diet. Watch for hypokalemia (for example, muscle weakness and cramps). Patients also on digitalis have an increased risk of digitalis toxicity from the potassium-depleting effect of this diuretic. May use with potassium-sparing diuretic to prevent potassium loss.
• Foods rich in potassium include cit-

rus fruits, tomatoes, bananas, dates, and apricots.
• Monitor serum creatinine and BUN regularly. Not as effective if these levels are more than twice normal.
• Monitor blood uric acid, especially in patients with a history of gout.
• Check insulin requirements in patients with diabetes. May treat severe hyperglycemia with oral antidiabetic agents.
• In hypertension, therapeutic response may be delayed several days.
• Give in a.m. to prevent nocturia. Studies have shown that the drug is as effective when administered once daily as it is when given more frequently.
• Elderly patients are especially susceptible to excessive diuresis.
• Thiazides and thiazide-like diuretics should be stopped before tests for parathyroid function are performed.
• Advise patient to avoid sudden posture changes and rise slowly to avoid orthostatic hypotension.
• Advise patient to wear a sunscreen.

---

hydroflumethiazide
Diucardin, Saluron

Pregnancy Risk Category: B

HOW SUPPLIED
Tablets: 50 mg

MECHANISM OF ACTION
A thiazide diuretic that increases urine excretion of sodium and water by inhibiting sodium reabsorption in the cortical diluting site of the ascending loop of Henle.

INDICATIONS & DOSAGE
Edema—
Adults: 25 to 200 mg P.O. daily in divided doses. Maintenance dosages may be on intermittent or alternate-day schedule.
Children: 1 mg/kg P.O. daily.
Hypertension—

Adults: 50 to 100 mg P.O. daily or b.i.d.

ADVERSE REACTIONS
Blood: *aplastic anemia, agranulocytosis,* leukopenia, thrombocytopenia.
CV: *volume depletion and dehydration,* orthostatic hypotension.
GI: anorexia, nausea, pancreatitis.
Hepatic: hepatic encephalopathy.
Metabolic: *hypokalemia, asymptomatic hyperuricemia, hyperglycemia and impairment of glucose tolerance,* fluid and electrolyte imbalances including dilutional hyponatremia and hypochloremia, metabolic alkalosis, hypercalcemia, gout.
Skin: dermatitis, photosensitivity, rash.
Other: hypersensitivity reactions, such as pneumonitis and vasculitis.

INTERACTIONS
Cholestyramine, colestipol: intestinal absorption of thiazides decreased. Keep doses as separate as possible.
Diazoxide: increased antihypertensive, hyperglycemic, and hyperuricemic effects. Use together cautiously.

NURSING CONSIDERATIONS
• Contraindicated in anuria or hypersensitivity to other thiazides or other sulfonamide-derived drugs. Use cautiously in severe renal disease, impaired hepatic function, and progressive hepatic disease.
• Monitor intake/output, weight, blood pressure, and serum electrolytes regularly.
• Consult with doctor and dietitian to provide high-potassium diet. Foods rich in potassium include citrus fruits, tomatoes, bananas, dates, and apricots. Watch for hypokalemia (for example, muscle weakness and cramps). May use with potassium-sparing diuretic to prevent potassium loss. Patients also on digitalis have an increased risk of digitalis toxicity from

---

Italicized adverse reactions are common or life-threatening.
*Liquid form contains alcohol.   **May contain tartrazine.

the potassium-depleting effects of this diuretic.
• Monitor serum creatinine and BUN regularly. Not as effective if these levels are more than twice normal.
• Monitor blood uric acid, especially in patients with a history of gout.
• Check insulin requirements in patients with diabetes. May treat severe hyperglycemia with oral antidiabetic agents.
• Give in a.m. to prevent nocturia.
• In hypertension, therapeutic response may be delayed several days.
• Elderly patients are especially susceptible to excessive diuresis.
• Thiazides and thiazide-like diuretics should be stopped before tests for parathyroid function are performed.
• Advise patient to avoid sudden posture changes and rise slowly to avoid orthostatic hypotension.
• Advise patient to wear a sunscreen.

indapamide
Lozide†, Lozol, Natrilix‡
Pregnancy Risk Category: B

HOW SUPPLIED
Tablets: 2.5 mg

MECHANISM OF ACTION
A thiazide-like diuretic that inhibits sodium reabsorption in the cortical diluting site of the nephron. Also has a direct vasodilating effect that may be a result of calcium channel-blocking action.

INDICATIONS & DOSAGE
Edema, hypertension—
Adults: 2.5 mg P.O. as a single daily dose taken in the morning. Dosage may be increased to 5 mg daily.

ADVERSE REACTIONS
CNS: headache, irritability, nervousness.
CV: *volume depletion and dehydration,* orthostatic hypotension.

GI: anorexia, nausea, pancreatitis.
Metabolic: *hypokalemia; asymptomatic hyperuricemia;* fluid and electrolyte imbalances, including dilutional hyponatremia and hypochloremia; metabolic alkalosis; gout.
Skin: dermatitis, photosensitivity, rash.
Other: muscle cramps and spasms.

INTERACTIONS
Diazoxide: increased antihypertensive, hyperglycemic, and hyperuricemic effects. Use together cautiously.

NURSING CONSIDERATIONS
• Contraindicated in anuria or hypersensitivity to other sulfonamide-derived drugs.
• Use cautiously in severe renal disease, impaired hepatic function, and progressive hepatic disease.
• Monitor intake/output, weight, blood pressure, and serum electrolytes regularly.
• Consult with doctor and dietitian to provide high-potassium diet. Foods rich in potassium include citrus fruits, tomatoes, bananas, dates, and apricots. Watch for symptoms of hypokalemia (for example, muscle weakness and cramps). May use with potassium-sparing diuretic to prevent potassium loss. Patients also receiving digitalis have an increased risk of digitalis toxicity from the potassium-depleting effects of this diuretic.
• Monitor serum creatinine and BUN regularly. Not as effective if these levels are more than twice normal.
• Monitor blood uric acid level, especially in patients with a history of gout.
• Check insulin requirements in patients with diabetes. May treat severe hyperglycemia with oral antidiabetic agents.
• Give in a.m. to prevent nocturia.
• In hypertension, therapeutic response may be delayed several days.

- Elderly patients are especially susceptible to excessive diuresis.
- Thiazides and thiazide-like diuretics should be stopped before tests for parathyroid function are performed.
- Advise patient to avoid sudden posture changes and rise slowly to avoid orthostatic hypotension.
- Advise patient to wear a sunscreen.

---

mannitol
Osmitrol†

Pregnancy Risk Category: C

HOW SUPPLIED
Injection: 5%, 10%, 15%, 20%, 25%

MECHANISM OF ACTION
An osmotic diuretic that increases the osmotic pressure of glomerular filtrate, inhibiting tubular reabsorption of water and electrolytes. Also elevates blood plasma osmolality, resulting in enhanced flow of water into extracellular fluid.

INDICATIONS & DOSAGE
Test dose for marked oliguria or suspected inadequate renal function—
Adults and children over 12 years: 200 mg/kg or 12.5 g as a 15% or 20% solution I.V. over 3 to 5 minutes. Response adequate if 30 to 50 ml urine/hour is excreted over 2 to 3 hours.
Treatment of oliguria—
Adults and children over 12 years: 50 to 100 g I.V. as a 15% to 20% solution over 90 minutes to several hours.
Prevention of oliguria or acute renal failure—
Adults and children over 12 years: 50 to 100 g I.V. of a concentrated (5% to 25%) solution. Exact concentration is determined by fluid requirements.
Edema—
Adults and children over 12 years: 100 g I.V. as a 10% to 20% solution over 2- to 6-hour period.
To reduce intraocular pressure or intracranial pressure—

Adults and children over 12 years: 1.5 to 2 g/kg as a 15% to 25% solution I.V. over 30 to 60 minutes.
To promote diuresis in drug intoxication—
Adults and children over 12 years: 5% to 10% solution continuously up to 200 g I.V., while maintaining 100 to 500 ml urine output/hour and a positive fluid balance.

ADVERSE REACTIONS
CNS: rebound increase in intracranial pressure 8 to 12 hours after diuresis, headache, confusion.
CV: *transient expansion of plasma volume during infusion causing circulatory overload and pulmonary edema,* tachycardia, angina-like chest pain.
EENT: blurred vision, rhinitis.
GI: thirst, nausea, vomiting.
GU: urine retention.
Metabolic: *fluid and electrolyte imbalance, water intoxication, cellular dehydration.*

INTERACTIONS
None significant.

NURSING CONSIDERATIONS
- Contraindicated in anuria, severe pulmonary congestion, frank pulmonary edema, severe congestive heart disease, severe dehydration, metabolic edema, progressive renal disease or dysfunction, progressive heart failure during administration, or active intracranial bleeding except during craniotomy.
- Monitor vital signs (including central venous pressure) at least hourly; intake/output hourly (report increasing oliguria). Monitor: weight, renal function, fluid balance, serum and urine sodium and potassium levels daily.
- Solution often crystallizes, especially at low temperatures. To redissolve, warm bottle in hot water bath, shake vigorously. Cool to body tem-

---

Italicized adverse reactions are common or life-threatening.
*Liquid form contains alcohol. **May contain tartrazine.

perature before giving. Concentrations greater than 15% have greater tendency to crystallize. Do not use solution with undissolved crystals.
• Infusions should always be given I.V. via an in-line filter.
• Avoid infiltration; if it occurs, observe for inflammation, edema, and necrosis.
• For maximum intraocular pressure reduction before surgery, give 1 to 1½ hours preoperatively.
• Can be used to measure glomerular filtration rate.
• Give frequent mouth care or fluids as permitted to relieve thirst.
• Urethral catheter is inserted in comatose or incontinent patients because therapy is based on strict evaluation of intake and output. In patients with urethral catheters, use an hourly urometer collection bag to facilitate accurate evaluation of output.

methazolamide
Neptazane

Pregnancy Risk Category: C

HOW SUPPLIED
Tablets: 25 mg, 50 mg

MECHANISM OF ACTION
A carbonic anhydrase inhibitor that decreases secretion of aqueous humor in the eye, thereby lowering intraocular pressure.

INDICATIONS & DOSAGE
Glaucoma (open-angle, or preoperatively in obstructive or narrow-angle)—
Adults: 50 to 100 mg b.i.d. or t.i.d.

ADVERSE REACTIONS
Blood: *aplastic anemia,* hemolytic anemia, leukopenia.
CNS: drowsiness, paresthesias.
EENT: transient myopia.
GI: nausea, vomiting, anorexia.
GU: crystalluria, renal calculi.

Metabolic: *hyperchloremic acidosis,* hypokalemia, asymptomatic hyperuricemia.
Skin: rash.

INTERACTIONS
None significant.

NURSING CONSIDERATIONS
• Contraindicated in severe or absolute glaucoma; for long-term use in chronic noncongestive narrow-angle glaucoma; in patients with depressed sodium or potassium serum, renal or hepatic disease or dysfunction, adrenal gland dysfunction, or hyperchloremic acidosis. Use cautiously in respiratory acidosis, emphysema, chronic pulmonary disease.
• Monitor intake/output, weight, and serum electrolytes frequently.
• May cause false-positive urine protein tests by alkalinizing urine.
• Elderly patients are especially susceptible to excessive diuresis.
• Diuretic effect decreases in acidosis.
• Anticipate that drug will be given every day for glaucoma but intermittently for edema. Caution patient to comply with prescribed dosage and schedule to lessen risk of metabolic acidosis.
• Carefully evaluate the patient with glaucoma for eye pain to make sure drug is effective in decreasing intraocular pressure.

methyclothiazide
Aquatensen, Duretic†, Enduron, Enduron M‡

Pregnancy Risk Category: D

HOW SUPPLIED
Tablets: 2.5 mg, 5 mg

MECHANISM OF ACTION
A thiazide diuretic that increases urine excretion of sodium and water by inhibiting sodium reabsorption in

the cortical diluting site of the nephron.

INDICATIONS & DOSAGE
Edema, hypertension—
Adults: 2.5 to 10 mg P.O daily.

ADVERSE REACTIONS
Blood: *aplastic anemia, agranulocytosis,* leukopenia, thrombocytopenia.
CV: *volume depletion and dehydration,* orthostatic hypotension.
GI: anorexia, nausea, pancreatitis.
Hepatic: hepatic encephalopathy.
Metabolic: *hypokalemia, asymptomatic hyperuricemia, hyperglycemia and impairment of glucose tolerance,* fluid and electrolyte imbalances including dilutional hyponatremia and hypochloremia, metabolic alkalosis, hypercalcemia, gout.
Skin: dermatitis, photosensitivity, rash.
Other: hypersensitivity reactions, such as pneumonitis and vasculitis.

INTERACTIONS
Cholestyramine, colestipol: intestinal absorption of thiazides decreased. Keep doses as separate as possible.
Diazoxide: increased antihypertensive, hyperglycemic, and hyperuricemic effects. Use together cautiously.

NURSING CONSIDERATIONS
• Contraindicated in renal decompensation; anuria; or hypersensitivity to other thiazides or other sulfonamide-derived drugs. Use cautiously in potassium depletion, renal disease or dysfunction, impaired hepatic function, and progressive hepatic disease.
• Monitor intake/output, weight, blood pressure, and serum electrolytes regularly.
• Consult with doctor and dietitian to provide high-potassium diet. Foods rich in potassium include citrus fruits, tomatoes, bananas, dates, and apricots. Watch for hypokalemia (for ex-

ample, muscle weakness and cramps). Patients also on digitalis have an increased risk of digitalis toxicity from the potassium-depleting effect of this diuretic. May use with potassium-sparing diuretic to prevent potassium loss.
• Check insulin requirements in patients with diabetes. May treat severe hyperglycemia with oral antidiabetic agents.
• Monitor serum creatinine and BUN regularly. Not as effective if these level are more than twice normal.
• Monitor blood uric acid, especially in patients with a history of gout.
• In hypertension, therapeutic response may be delayed several days.
• Give in a.m. to prevent nocturia.
• Elderly patients are especially susceptible to excessive diuresis.
• Thiazides and thiazide-like diuretics should be stopped before tests for parathyroid function are performed.
• Advise patient to avoid sudden posture changes and rise slowly to avoid orthostatic hypotension.
• Advise patient to wear a sunscreen.

metolazone
Diulo, Mykrox, Zaroxolyn**
Pregnancy Risk Category: D

HOW SUPPLIED
Tablets: 2.5 mg, 5 mg, 10 mg

MECHANISM OF ACTION
Although not a thiazide diuretic, metolazone acts in a similar fashion. It increases urine excretion of sodium and water by inhibiting sodium reabsorption in the cortical diluting site of the ascending loop of Henle.

INDICATIONS & DOSAGE
Edema (heart failure)—
Adults: 5 to 10 mg P.O. daily.
Edema (renal disease)—
Adults: 5 to 20 mg P.O. daily.
Hypertension—

Italicized adverse reactions are common or life-threatening.
*Liquid form contains alcohol.   **May contain tartrazine.

Adults: 2.5 to 5 mg P.O. daily. Maintenance dosage determined by patient's blood pressure.

ADVERSE REACTIONS
Blood: *aplastic anemia, agranulocytosis,* leukopenia, thrombocytopenia.
CV: *volume depletion and dehydration,* orthostatic hypotension.
GI: anorexia, nausea, pancreatitis.
Hepatic: hepatic encephalopathy.
Metabolic: *hypokalemia, asymptomatic hyperuricemia, hyperglycemia and impairment of glucose tolerance,* fluid and electrolyte imbalances including dilutional hyponatremia and hypochloremia, metabolic alkalosis, hypercalcemia, gout.
Skin: dermatitis, photosensitivity, rash.
Other: hypersensitivity reactions, such as pneumonitis and vasculitis.

INTERACTIONS
Cholestyramine, colestipol: intestinal absorption of thiazides decreased. Keep doses as separate as possible.
Diazoxide: increased antihypertensive, hyperglycemic, and hyperuricemic effects. Use together cautiously.

NURSING CONSIDERATIONS
• Contraindicated in anuria; hepatic coma or precoma; or hypersensitivity to thiazides or other sulfonamide-derived drugs. Use cautiously in hyperuricemia or gout and severely impaired renal function.
• Monitor intake/output, weight, blood pressure, and serum electrolytes regularly.
• Consult with doctor and dietitian to provide high-potassium diet. Foods rich in potassium include citrus fruits, tomatoes, bananas, dates, and apricots. Watch for hypokalemia (for example, muscle weakness and cramps). Patients also on digitalis may have an increased risk of digitalis toxicity from the potassium-depleting effect of this diuretic. May use with potassium-sparing diuretic to prevent potassium loss.
• Check insulin requirements in patients with diabetes. May treat severe hyperglycemia with oral antidiabetic agents.
• Monitor blood uric acid, especially in patients with a history of gout.
• In hypertension, therapeutic response may be delayed several days.
• Give in a.m. to prevent nocturia.
• Elderly patients are especially susceptible to excessive diuresis.
• A thiazide-related diuretic. However, unlike thiazide diuretics, metolazone is effective in patients with decreased renal function.
• Used as an adjunct in furosemide-resistant edema.
• Thiazides and thiazide-like diuretics should be stopped before tests for parathyroid function are performed.
• Mykrox tablets are more rapidly and completely absorbed than other brands, and their absorption characteristics mimic those of an oral solution.
• Advise patient to avoid sudden posture changes and rise slowly to avoid orthostatic hypotension.
• Advise patient to wear a sunscreen.

polythiazide
Renese

Pregnancy Risk Category: D

HOW SUPPLIED
Tablets: 1 mg, 2 mg, 4 mg

MECHANISM OF ACTION
A thiazide diuretic that increases urine excretion of sodium and water by inhibiting sodium reabsorption in the cortical diluting site of the nephron.

INDICATIONS & DOSAGE
Hypertension—
Adults: 2 to 4 mg P.O. daily.

Edema (heart failure, renal failure)—
Adults: 1 to 4 mg P.O. daily.
Children: 0.02 to 0.08 mg/kg P.O. daily.

ADVERSE REACTIONS
Blood: *aplastic anemia, agranulocytosis,* leukopenia, thrombocytopenia.
CV: *volume depletion and dehydration,* orthostatic hypotension.
GI: anorexia, nausea, pancreatitis.
Hepatic: hepatic encephalopathy.
Metabolic: *hypokalemia, asymptomatic hyperuricemia, hyperglycemia and impairment of glucose tolerance,* fluid and electrolyte imbalances including dilutional hyponatremia and hypochloremia, metabolic alkalosis, hypercalcemia, gout.
Skin: dermatitis, photosensitivity, rash.
Other: hypersensitivity reactions, such as pneumonitis and vasculitis.

INTERACTIONS
Cholestyramine, colestipol: intestinal absorption of thiazides decreased. Keep doses as separate as possible.
Diazoxide: increased antihypertensive, hyperglycemic, and hyperuricemic effects. Use together cautiously.

NURSING CONSIDERATIONS
• Contraindicated in anuria or hypersensitivity to other thiazides or other sulfonamide-derived drugs. Use cautiously in severe renal disease, impaired hepatic function, and allergies.
• Monitor intake/output, weight, blood pressure, and serum electrolytes regularly.
• Consult with doctor and dietitian to provide high-potassium diet. Foods rich in potassium include citrus fruits, tomatoes, bananas, dates, and apricots. Watch for hypokalemia (for example, muscle weakness and cramps). Patients also on digitalis may have an increased risk of digitalis toxicity from the potassium-depleting effect of

this diuretic. May use with potassium-sparing diuretic to prevent potassium loss.
• Monitor blood uric acid, especially in patients with a history of gout.
• Check insulin requirements in patients with diabetes. May treat severe hyperglycemia with oral antidiabetic agents.
• In hypertension, therapeutic response may be delayed several days.
• Give in a.m. to prevent nocturia.
• Elderly patients are especially susceptible to excessive diuresis.
• Thiazides and thiazide-like diuretics should be stopped before tests for parathyroid function are performed.
• Advise patient to avoid sudden posture changes and rise slowly to avoid orthostatic hypotension.
• Advise patient to wear a sunscreen.

quinethazone
Aquamox‡, Hydromox
Pregnancy Risk Category: D

HOW SUPPLIED
Tablets: 50 mg

MECHANISM OF ACTION
Although not a thiazide diuretic, quinethazone acts in a similar fashion. It increases urine excretion of sodium and water by inhibiting sodium reabsorption in the cortical diluting site of the nephron.

INDICATIONS & DOSAGE
Management of edema or hypertension—
Adults: 50 to 100 mg P.O. daily or 50 mg P.O. b.i.d. Occasionally, up to 150 to 200 mg P.O. daily may be needed.

ADVERSE REACTIONS
Blood: *aplastic anemia, agranulocytosis,* leukopenia, thrombocytopenia.
CV: *volume depletion and dehydration,* orthostatic hypotension.

Italicized adverse reactions are common or life-threatening.
*Liquid form contains alcohol.   **May contain tartrazine.

GI: anorexia, nausea, pancreatitis.
Hepatic: hepatic encephalopathy.
Metabolic: *hypokalemia, asymptomatic hyperuricemia, hyperglycemia and impairment of glucose tolerance,* fluid and electrolyte imbalances including dilutional hyponatremia and hypochloremia, metabolic alkalosis, hypercalcemia, gout.
Skin: dermatitis, photosensitivity, rash.
Other: hypersensitivity reactions, such as pneumonitis and vasculitis.

INTERACTIONS
Cholestyramine, colestipol: intestinal absorption of thiazides decreased. Keep doses as separate as possible.
Diazoxide: increased antihypertensive, hyperglycemic, and hyperuricemic effects. Use together cautiously.

NURSING CONSIDERATIONS
• Contraindicated in anuria or hypersensitivity to quinethazones, thiazides, or other sulfonamide-derived drugs. Use cautiously in severe renal disease, impaired hepatic function, and allergies.
• Monitor intake/output, weight, blood pressure, and serum electrolytes regularly.
• Consult with doctor and dietitian to provide high-potassium diet. Foods rich in potassium include citrus fruits, tomatoes, bananas, dates, and apricots. Watch for hypokalemia (for example, muscle weakness and cramps). Patients also on digitalis have an increased risk of digitalis toxicity from the potassium-depleting effect of this diuretic. May use with potassium-sparing diuretic to prevent potassium loss.
• Monitor serum creatinine and BUN regularly.
• Check insulin requirements in patients with diabetes. May treat severe hyperglycemia with oral hypoglycemics.

• Monitor blood uric acid, especially in patients with a history of gout.
• In hypertension, therapeutic response may be delayed several days.
• Give in a.m. to prevent nocturia.
• Elderly patients are especially susceptible to excessive diuresis.
• Thiazides and thiazide-like diuretics should be stopped before tests for parathyroid function are performed.
• Advise patient to avoid sudden posture changes and rise slowly to avoid orthostatic hypotension.
• Advise patient to wear a sunscreen.

spironolactone
Aldactone, Novospiroton†, Sincomen†, Spirotone‡

Pregnancy Risk Category: D

HOW SUPPLIED
Tablets: 25 mg, 50 mg, 100 mg

MECHANISM OF ACTION
A potassium-sparing diuretic that antagonizes aldosterone in the distal tubule, increasing excretion of sodium and water but sparing potassium.

INDICATIONS & DOSAGE
Edema—
Adults: 25 to 200 mg P.O. daily in divided doses.
Children: initially, 3.3 mg/kg P.O. daily in divided doses.
Hypertension—
Adults: 50 to 100 mg P.O. daily in divided doses.
Treatment of diuretic-induced hypokalemia—
Adults: 25 to 100 mg P.O. daily when oral potassium supplements are considered inappropriate.
Detection of primary hyperaldosteronism—
Adults: 400 mg P.O. daily for 4 days (short test) or 3 to 4 weeks (long test). If hypokalemia and hypertension are corrected, a presumptive diagnosis of primary hyperaldosteronism is made.

ADVERSE REACTIONS
CNS: headache.
GI: anorexia, nausea, diarrhea.
Metabolic: *hyperkalemia,* dehydration, hyponatremia, transient elevation in BUN, acidosis.
Skin: urticaria.
Other: gynecomastia in men, breast soreness and menstrual disturbances in women.

INTERACTIONS
Aspirin: possible blocked spironolactone effect. Watch for diminished spironolactone response.

NURSING CONSIDERATIONS
• Contraindicated in anuria, acute or progressive renal insufficiency, or hyperkalemia. Use cautiously in fluid or electrolyte imbalances, impaired renal function, and hepatic disease.
• A mild acidosis may occur during therapy. This may be dangerous in patients with hepatic cirrhosis.
• Monitor serum electrolytes, intake/output, weight, and blood pressure regularly.
• Potassium-sparing diuretic; useful as an adjunct to other diuretic therapy. Less potent diuretic than thiazide and loop types. Diuretic effect delayed 2 to 3 days when used alone.
• Maximum antihypertensive response may be delayed up to 2 weeks.
• Warn patient to avoid excessive ingestion of potassium-rich foods or potassium-containing salt substitutes. Concomitant potassium supplement can lead to serious hyperkalemia.
• Elderly patients are more susceptible to excessive diuresis.
• Protect drug from light.
• Breast cancer reported in some patients taking spironolactone, but cause-and-effect relationship not confirmed. Warn against taking drug indiscriminately.
• Give with meals to enhance absorption.
• Because of its antiandrogenic properties, spironolactone has been prescribed to treat hirsutism. The dose for this indication is 200 mg daily.

triamterene
Dyrenium, Dytac‡

Pregnancy Risk Category: D

HOW SUPPLIED
Tablets: 50 mg, 100 mg

MECHANISM OF ACTION
A potassium-sparing diuretic that inhibits sodium reabsorption and potassium excretion by direct action on the distal tubule.

INDICATIONS & DOSAGE
Diuresis—
Adults: initially, 100 mg P.O. b.i.d. after meals. Total daily dosage should not exceed 300 mg.

ADVERSE REACTIONS
Blood: megaloblastic anemia related to low folic acid levels.
CNS: dizziness.
CV: hypotension.
EENT: sore throat.
GI: dry mouth, nausea, vomiting.
Metabolic: *hyperkalemia,* dehydration, hyponatremia, transient elevation in BUN, acidosis.
Skin: photosensitivity, rash.
Other: *anaphylaxis,* muscle cramps.

INTERACTIONS
None significant.

NURSING CONSIDERATIONS
• Contraindicated in anuria, severe or progressive renal disease or dysfunction, severe hepatic disease, or hyperkalemia. Use cautiously in impaired hepatic function, diabetes mellitus, pregnancy, or lactation.
• Watch for blood dyscrasias.
• Monitor blood pressure, BUN, and serum electrolytes.
• A potassium-sparing diuretic, use-

Italicized adverse reactions are common or life-threatening.
*Liquid form contains alcohol.   **May contain tartrazine.

ful as an adjunct to other diuretic therapy. Less potent than thiazides and loop diuretics. Full diuretic effect delayed 2 to 3 days when used alone.
• Warn patients to avoid excessive ingestion of potassium-rich foods or potassium-containing salt substitutes. Concomitant potassium supplement can lead to serious hyperkalemia.
• Give medication after meals to prevent nausea.
• Withdraw gradually to prevent excessive rebound potassium excretion.

---

trichlormethiazide
Aquazide, Diurese, Metahydrin**, Naqua

Pregnancy Risk Category: D

HOW SUPPLIED
Tablets: 2 mg, 4 mg

MECHANISM OF ACTION
A thiazide diuretic that increases urine excretion of sodium and water by inhibiting sodium reabsorption in the cortical diluting site of the nephron.

INDICATIONS & DOSAGE
Edema—
Adults: 1 to 4 mg P.O. daily or in two divided doses.
Hypertension—
Adults: 2 to 4 mg P.O. daily.

ADVERSE REACTIONS
Blood: *aplastic anemia, agranulocytosis,* leukopenia, thrombocytopenia.
CV: *volume depletion and dehydration,* orthostatic hypotension.
GI: anorexia, nausea, pancreatitis.
Hepatic: hepatic encephalopathy.
Metabolic: *hypokalemia, asymptomatic hyperuricemia, hyperglycemia and impairment of glucose tolerance,* fluid and electrolyte imbalances including dilutional hyponatremia and hypochloremia, metabolic alkalosis, hypercalcemia, gout.

Skin: dermatitis, photosensitivity, rash.
Other: hypersensitivity reactions, such as pneumonitis and vasculitis.

INTERACTIONS
Cholestyramine, colestipol: intestinal absorption of thiazides decreased. Keep doses as separate as possible.
Diazoxide: increased antihypertensive, hyperglycemic, and hyperuricemic effects. Use together cautiously.

NURSING CONSIDERATIONS
• Contraindicated in anuria or hypersensitivity to other thiazides or other sulfonamide-derived drugs. Use cautiously in severe renal disease, and impaired hepatic function.
• Monitor intake/output, weight, blood pressure, and serum electrolytes regularly.
• Consult with doctor and dietitian to provide high-potassium diet. Foods rich in potassium include citrus fruits, tomatoes, bananas, dates, and apricots. Watch for hypokalemia (for example, muscle weakness and cramps). Patients also on digitalis have an increased risk of digitalis toxicity from the potassium-depleting effect of this diuretic. May use with potassium-sparing diuretic to prevent hypokalemia.
• Monitor serum creatinine and BUN regularly. Not as effective if these levels are more than twice normal.
• Check insulin requirements in patients with diabetes. May treat severe hyperglycemia with oral antidiabetic agents. Monitor blood sugar.
• Monitor blood uric acid, especially in patients with a history of gout.
• In hypertension, therapeutic response may be delayed several days.
• Give in a.m. to prevent nocturia.
• Elderly patients are especially susceptible to excessive diuresis.
• Thiazides and thiazide-like diuret-

---

ics should be stopped before tests for parathyroid function are performed.
• Advise patient to avoid sudden posture changes and rise slowly to avoid orthostatic hypotension.
• Advise patient to wear a sunscreen.

urea (carbamide)
Ureaphil

Pregnancy Risk Category: C

HOW SUPPLIED
Injection: 40 g/150 ml

MECHANISM OF ACTION
An osmotic diuretic that increases the osmotic pressure of glomerular filtrate, inhibiting tubular reabsorption of water and electrolytes. Also elevates blood plasma osmolality, resulting in enhanced flow of water into extracellular fluid.

INDICATIONS & DOSAGE
Intracranial or intraocular pressure—
Adults: 1 to 1.5 g/kg as a 30% solution by slow I.V. infusion over 1 to 2.5 hours.
Children over 2 years: 0.5 to 1.5 g/kg slow I.V. infusion.
Children under 2 years: as little as 0.1 g/kg slow I.V. infusion. Maximum rate is 4 ml/minute.
   Maximum adult daily dosage is 120 g. To prepare 135 ml 30% solution, mix contents of 40-g vial of urea with 105 ml dextrose 5% or 10% in water or 10% invert sugar in water. Each ml of 30% solution provides 300 mg urea.

ADVERSE REACTIONS
CNS: *headache.*
CV: tachycardia, CHF, *pulmonary edema.*
GI: *nausea, vomiting.*
Metabolic: sodium and potassium depletion.
Local: irritation or necrotic sloughing may occur with extravasation.

INTERACTIONS
None significant.

NURSING CONSIDERATIONS
• Contraindicated in severely impaired renal function, marked dehydration, frank hepatic failure, or active intracranial bleeding. Use cautiously in pregnancy, lactation, cardiac disease, hepatic impairment, and sickle cell disease with CNS involvement.
• Avoid rapid I.V. infusion; may cause hemolysis or increased capillary bleeding. Avoid extravasation; may cause reactions ranging from mild irritation to necrosis.
• Don't infuse into leg veins; may cause phlebitis or thrombosis, especially in elderly patients.
• Watch for hyponatremia or hypokalemia (muscle weakness, lethargy); may indicate electrolyte depletion before serum levels are reduced.
• Maintain adequate hydration; monitor blood pressure, intake/output, and serum electrolytes.
• In renal disease, monitor BUN frequently.
• Indwelling urethral catheter should be used in comatose patients to ensure bladder emptying. Use an hourly urometer collection bag to facilitate accurate evaluation of diuresis.
• If satisfactory diuresis does not occur in 6 to 12 hours, urea should be discontinued and renal function reevaluated.
• Use freshly reconstituted urea only for I.V. infusion; solution becomes ammonia upon standing.
• Use within minutes of reconstitution.
• Assess breath sounds for crackles, indicating pulmonary edema.

Italicized adverse reactions are common or life-threatening.
*Liquid form contains alcohol.   **May contain tartrazine.

61

Electrolytes and replacement solutions

calcium carbonate
calcium chloride
calcium citrate
calcium glubionate
calcium gluceptate
calcium gluconate
calcium lactate
calcium phosphate, dibasic
calcium phosphate, tribasic
dextran (low molecular weight)
dextran (high molecular weight)
hetastarch
magnesium sulfate
potassium acetate
potassium bicarbonate
potassium chloride
potassium gluconate
Ringer's injection
Ringer's injection, lactated
sodium chloride

COMBINATION PRODUCTS

KAOCHLOR-EFF: 20 mEq potassium, 20 mEq chloride (from potassium chloride, potassium citrate, potassium bicarbonate, and betaine hydrochloride).

KLORVESS*: 20 mEq each potassium and chloride (from potassium chloride, potassium bicarbonate, and l-lysine monohydrochloride).

KOLYUM: 20 mEq potassium, 3.4 mEq chloride (from potassium gluconate and potassium chloride).

NEUTRA-PHOS: phosphorus 250 mg, sodium 164 mg, potassium 278 mg (from dibasic and monobasic sodium and potassium phosphate).

TWIN-K-CL: 15 ml supplies 15 mEq of potassium ions as a combination of potassium gluconate, potassium citrate, and ammonium chloride.

---

calcium carbonate
Alka-Mints◊, Amitone◊, Chooz◊, Dicarbosil◊, Equilet◊, Mallamint◊, Rolaids Calcium Rich◊, Tums◊, Tums Extra Strength◊, Tums E-X Extra Strength◊

calcium chloride◊

calcium citrate◊

calcium glubionate◊

calcium gluceptate◊

calcium gluconate
Kalcinate◊

calcium lactate◊

calcium phosphate, dibasic◊

calcium phosphate, tribasic
Posture◊

Pregnancy Risk Category: C

HOW SUPPLIED
calcium carbonate
Tablets◊: 650 mg, 667 mg, 750 mg, 1.25 g, 1.5 g (contains 400 mg calcium/g)
Tablets (chewable)◊: 350 mg, 420 mg, 500 mg, 625 mg, 750 mg, 850 mg, 1.25 g
Capsules: 1.512 g◊
Oral suspension: 1.25 g/5 ml (con-

tains 400 mg of elemental calcium/
g)◊
Chewy squares: 1.5 g
calcium chloride
Injection: 10% solution in 10-ml ampules, vials, and syringes
calcium citrate
Tablets: 950 mg (contains 211 mg of
elemental calcium/g)◊
calcium glubionate
Syrup: 1.8 g/5 ml (contains 64 mg of
elemental calcium/g)
calcium gluceptate
Injection: 1.1 g/5 ml in 5-ml ampules
or 50-ml vials
calcium gluconate
Tablets: 500 mg◊, 650 mg◊, 975
mg◊, 1 g◊ (contains 90 mg of elemental calcium/g)
Injection: 10% solution in 10-ml ampules and vials, 10-ml or 20-ml vials
calcium lactate
Tablets: 325 mg, 650 mg (contains
130 mg of elemental calcium/g)
calcium phosphate, dibasic
Tablets: 468 mg (contains 230 mg of
elemental calcium/g)◊
calcium phosphate, tribasic
Tablets: 300 mg◊, 600 mg◊ (contains
400 mg of elemental calcium/g)

MECHANISM OF ACTION
Replaces and maintains calcium.

INDICATIONS & DOSAGE
*Hypocalcemia, hypocalcemic tetany,
hypocalcemia during exchange transfusions, cardiac resuscitation for inotropic effect when epinephrine has
failed; magnesium intoxication; hypoparathyroidism—*
Adults and children: initially, 500
mg to 1 g calcium salt I.V., with further dosage based on serum calcium
determinations and specific calcium
salt. See below for dosages with specific calcium salts.
    Dosage with calcium chloride (1 g
[10 ml] yields 13.5 mEq Ca^{++}):
Magnesium intoxication—
Adults and children: initially, 500

mg I.V., with further doses based on
calcium and magnesium determinations.
Cardiac arrest—
0.5 to 1 g I.V., not to exceed 1 ml/
minute; or 200 to 800 mg into the
ventricular cavity.
Hypocalcemia—
500 mg to 1 g I.V. at intervals of 1 to 3
days, determined by serum calcium
levels.
    Dosage with calcium gluconate (1 g
[10 ml] yields 4.5 mEq Ca^{++}):
Hypocalcemia—
Adults: 500 mg to 1 g I.V., repeated q
1 to 3 days p.r.n. as determined by
serum calcium levels. Further doses
depend on serum calcium determinations.
Children: 100 to 150 mg/kg I.V.
three to four times daily. Rate of infusion should not exceed 0.5 ml/minute.
    Dosage with calcium gluceptate
(1.1 g [5 ml] yields 4.5 mEq Ca^{++})
and calcium salts (18 mg [1 ml] yields
0.898 mEq Ca^{++}):
Hypocalcemia—
Adults: initially, 5 to 20 ml I.V., with
further doses based on serum calcium
determinations. If I.V. injection is impossible, 2 to 5 ml I.M. Average adult
oral dose is 1 to 2 g elemental calcium
P.O. daily, divided t.i.d. or q.i.d. Average oral dose for children is 45 to 65
mg/kg P.O. daily, divided t.i.d. or
q.i.d.
During exchange transfusions—
Adults and children: 0.5 ml I.V. after each 100 ml blood exchanged.

ADVERSE REACTIONS
CNS: from I.V. use, tingling sensations, sense of oppression or heat
waves; with rapid I.V. injection, syncope.
CV: mild fall in blood pressure; with
rapid I.V. injection, vasodilation, *bradycardia, cardiac arrhythmias, cardiac arrest.*
GI: with oral ingestion, irritation,
hemorrhage, *constipation;* with I.V.

Italicized adverse reactions are common or life-threatening.
*Liquid form contains alcohol.   **May contain tartrazine.

administration, chalky taste; with oral calcium chloride, GI hemorrhage, nausea, vomiting, thirst, abdominal pain.
GU: hypercalcemia, polyuria, renal calculi.
Skin: local reaction if calcium salts given I.M., burning, necrosis, tissue sloughing, cellulitis, soft tissue calcification.
Local: with S.C. injection, pain and irritation; *with I.V., vein irritation*.

INTERACTIONS
Cardiac glycosides: increased digitalis toxicity; administer calcium very cautiously (if at all) to digitalized patients.

NURSING CONSIDERATIONS
• Contraindicated in ventricular fibrillation, hypercalcemia, or renal calculi. Use cautiously in patients with sarcoidosis and renal or cardiac disease, and in digitalized patients. Use calcium chloride cautiously in cor pulmonale, respiratory acidosis, and respiratory failure.
• Monitor ECG when giving calcium I.V. Such injections should not exceed 0.7 to 1.5 mEq/minute. Stop if patient complains of discomfort. Following I.V. injection, patient should remain recumbent for a short while.
• I.M. injection should be given in the gluteal region in adults; lateral thigh in infants. I.M. route used only in emergencies when no I.V. route available.
• Monitor blood calcium frequently. Report abnormalities.
• Hypercalcemia may result after large doses in chronic renal failure.
• If possible, administer I.V. into a large vein.
• I.V. route usually recommended in children, but not by scalp vein (can cause tissue necrosis).
• Solutions should be warmed to

body temperature before administration.
• Calcium chloride should be given I.V. only. When adding to parenteral solutions that contain other additives, observe closely for precipitate.
• Severe necrosis and tissue sloughing follow extravasation. Calcium gluconate is less irritating to veins and tissues than calcium chloride.
• Following injection, patient should be recumbent for 15 minutes.
• If GI upset occurs, give oral calcium products 1 to 1½ hours after meals.
• Oxalic acid (found in rhubarb and spinach), phytic acid (in bran and whole cereals), and phosphorus (in milk and dairy products) may interfere with absorption of calcium.
• Crash carts usually contain both gluconate and chloride. Make sure doctor specifies form he wants administered.

---

dextran
(low molecular weight)
Dextran 40, Gentran 40, Rheomacrodex

Pregnancy Risk Category: C

HOW SUPPLIED
Injection: 10% Dextran 40 in dextrose 5% or 0.9% sodium chloride

MECHANISM OF ACTION
Expands plasma volume and provides fluid replacement.

INDICATIONS & DOSAGE
Plasma volume expansion—
Dosage of 10% solution by I.V. infusion depends on amount of fluid loss.
First 500 ml of Dextran 40 may be infused rapidly with central venous pressure monitoring. Infuse remaining dose slowly. Total daily dosage not to exceed 2 g/kg body weight. If therapy continued past 24 hours, do not ex-

ceed 1 g/kg daily. Continue for no longer than 5 days.
Reduction of blood sludging—
500 ml of 10% solution by I.V. infusion.
Prophylaxis of venous thrombosis—
Adults: 10 ml/kg (500 to 1,000 ml) of a 10% solution I.V. on the day of the procedure; 500 ml on days 2 and 3.

ADVERSE REACTIONS
Blood: *decreased level of hemoglobin and hematocrit;* with higher doses, increased bleeding time.
GI: nausea, vomiting.
GU: tubular stasis and blocking, increased viscosity of urine.
Hepatic: increased AST (SGOT) and ALT (SGPT) levels.
Skin: hypersensitivity reaction, urticaria.
Other: *anaphylaxis.*

INTERACTIONS
None significant.

NURSING CONSIDERATIONS
• Contraindicated in marked hemostatic defects; marked cardiac decompensation or pulmonary edema; renal disease with severe oliguria or anuria; or extreme dehydration. Use cautiously in active hemorrhage; may cause additional blood loss. Evaluate patient's hydration status before administration.
• Doctor may order dextran 1 (Promit) to protect against dextran-induced anaphylaxis. Administer Promit, 20 ml I.V. over 60 seconds, 1 to 2 minutes before the I.V. infusion of Dextran 40.
• Hazardous when given to patients with heart failure, especially if in saline solution. Use dextrose in water solution instead.
• Works as plasma expander via colloidal osmotic effect, thereby drawing fluid from interstitial to intravascular space. Provides plasma expansion slightly greater than volume infused.

Watch for circulatory overload and a rise in central venous pressure readings.
• Monitor urine flow rate during administration. If oliguria or anuria occurs or is not relieved by infusion, stop dextran and give loop diuretic.
• Hydration should be assessed before starting therapy; otherwise, use urine or serum osmolarity because urine specific gravity is affected by urine dextran concentration.
• Check hemoglobin and hematocrit; don't allow to fall below 30% by volume.
• Observe patient closely during early phase of infusion; most anaphylactoid reactions occur during this time.
• May interfere with analyses of blood grouping, cross matching, bilirubin, blood glucose, and protein.
• Store at constant 77° F. (25° C.). May precipitate in storage, but can be heated to dissolve if necessary.

dextran
(high molecular weight)
Dextran 70, Dextran 75, Gentran 75, Macrodex
Pregnancy Risk Category: C

HOW SUPPLIED
Injection: 6% Dextran 70 in 0.9% sodium chloride or dextrose 5%; 6% Dextran 75 in 0.9% sodium chloride or dextrose 5%

MECHANISM OF ACTION
Expands plasma volume and provides fluid replacement.

INDICATIONS & DOSAGE
Plasma expander—
Adults: usual dose 30 g (500 ml of 6% solution) I.V. In emergency situations, may be administered at rate of 1.2 to 2.4 g (20 to 40 ml) per minute. In normovolemic or nearly normovolemic patients, rate of infusion should not exceed 240 mg (4 ml)/minute.

Italicized adverse reactions are common or life-threatening.
*Liquid form contains alcohol.   **May contain tartrazine.

Total dosage during first 24 hours not to exceed 1.2 g/kg; actual dosage depends on amount of fluid loss and resultant hemoconcentration, and must be determined for each patient.

ADVERSE REACTIONS
Blood: *decreased level of hemoglobin and hematocrit;* with doses of 15 ml/kg body weight, prolonged bleeding time and significant suppression of platelet function.
GI: nausea, vomiting.
GU: increased specific gravity and viscosity of urine, tubular stasis and blocking.
Hepatic: increased AST (SGOT) and ALT (SGPT) levels.
Skin: hypersensitivity reaction, urticaria.
Other: fever, arthralgia, nasal congestion, *anaphylaxis.*

INTERACTIONS
None significant.

NURSING CONSIDERATIONS
• Contraindicated in marked hemostatic defects; marked cardiac decompensation or pulmonary edema; renal disease with severe oliguria or anuria; or extreme dehydration. Use cautiously in active hemorrhage; may cause additional blood loss.
• Doctor may order dextran 1 (Promit) to protect against dextran-induced anaphylaxis. Administer Promit, 20 ml I.V. over 60 seconds, 1 to 2 minutes before the I.V. infusion of Dextran 70.
• Hazardous when given to patients with heart failure, especially if in saline solution. Use dextrose in water solution instead.
• Works as plasma expander via colloidal osmotic effect, thereby drawing fluid from interstitial to intravascular space. Provides plasma expansion slightly greater than volume infused. Watch for circulatory overload.
• Monitor urine flow rate during administration. If oliguria or anuria occurs or is not relieved by infusion, stop dextran and give loop diuretic.
• Hydration should be assessed before starting therapy; otherwise, use urine or serum osmolarity because urine specific gravity is affected by the urine dextran concentration.
• Check hemoglobin and hematocrit; don't allow to fall below 30% by volume.
• Draw blood samples *before* starting infusion.
• Observe patient closely during early phase of infusion; most anaphylactoid reactions occur during this time.
• May interfere with analyses of blood grouping, cross matching, bilirubin, blood glucose, and protein.
• May precipitate in storage, but can be heated to dissolve if necessary.

hetastarch
Hespan

Pregnancy Risk Category: C

HOW SUPPLIED
Injection: 500 ml (6 g/100 ml in 0.9% sodium chloride solution)

MECHANISM OF ACTION
Expands plasma volume and provides fluid replacement.

INDICATIONS & DOSAGE
Plasma expander—
Adults: 500 to 1,000 ml I.V. depending on amount of blood lost and resultant hemoconcentration. Total dosage usually not to exceed 1,500 ml/day. Up to 20 ml/kg hourly may be used in hemorrhagic shock.

ADVERSE REACTIONS
CNS: headaches.
CV: peripheral edema of lower extremities.
EENT: periorbital edema.
GI: nausea, vomiting.
Skin: urticaria.

Other: wheezing, mild fever.

INTERACTIONS
None significant.

NURSING CONSIDERATIONS
• Contraindicated in severe bleeding disorders, with severe congestive heart failure, or renal failure with oliguria and anuria.
• To avoid circulatory overload, monitor patients with impaired renal function carefully.
• Discontinue if allergic or sensitivity reactions occur. If necessary, administer an antihistamine.
• When used in continuous-flow centrifugation, leukapheresis ratio is usually 1 part hetastarch to 8 parts venous whole blood.
• Hetastarch is *not* a substitute for blood or plasma.
• Available in 500-ml I.V. infusion bottles.
• Discard partially used bottles.

---

magnesium sulfate
Pregnancy Risk Category: B

HOW SUPPLIED
Injectable solutions: 10%, 12.5%, 25%, 50% in 2-ml, 5-ml, 10-ml, 20-ml, and 30-ml ampules, vials, and prefilled syringes

MECHANISM OF ACTION
Replaces and maintains magnesium levels. As an anticonvulsant, reduces muscle contractions by interfering with the release of acetylcholine at the myoneural junction.

INDICATIONS & DOSAGE
Hypomagnesemia—
Adults: 1 g, or 8.12 mEq, of 50% solution (2 ml) I.M. q 6 hours for 4 doses, depending on serum magnesium level.
Severe hypomagnesemia (serum magnesium 0.8 mEq/liter or less, with symptoms)—
6 g, or 50 mEq, of 50% solution I.V. in 1 liter of solution over 4 hours.
  Subsequent doses depend on serum magnesium levels.
Magnesium supplementation in hyperalimentation—
Adults: 8 to 24 mEq I.V. daily added to hyperalimentation solution.
Children over 6 years: 2 to 10 mEq I.V. daily added to hyperalimentation solution.
  Each 2 ml of 50% solution contains 1 g, or 8.12 mEq, magnesium sulfate.
Acute treatment of preeclampsia and eclampsia—
Adults: loading dose: 2 to 4 g (4 to 8 ml of 50% solution) given by slow I.V. bolus (over 5 minutes).
Maintenance dosage: 1 to 2 g hourly as a constant infusion. Prepare by adding 8 ml of 50% solution to 250 ml dextrose 5% in water.
Hypomagnesemic seizures—
Adults: 1 to 2 g (as 10% solution) I.V. over 15 minutes, then 1 g I.M. q 4 to 6 hours, based on patient response and magnesium blood level.
Seizures secondary to hypomagnesemia in acute nephritis—
Adults: 0.2 ml/kg of 50% solution I.M. q 4 to 6 hours, p.r.n. or 100 mg/kg of 10% solution I.V. very slowly. Titrate dosage according to magnesium blood level and seizure response.
Paroxysmal atrial tachycardia—
Adults: 3 to 4 g I.V. (as a 10% solution) over 30 seconds, with close monitoring of ECG.

ADVERSE REACTIONS
CNS: toxicity: *weak or absent deep tendon reflexes,* flaccid paralysis, hypothermia, drowsiness, hypocalcemia (perioral paresthesias, twitching carpopedal spasm, tetany, and seizures).
CV: slow, weak pulse; cardiac arrhythmias (hypocalcemia); *hypotension.*
Skin: flushing, sweating.

Italicized adverse reactions are common or life-threatening.
*Liquid form contains alcohol.   **May contain tartrazine.

Other: *respiratory paralysis,* hypocalcemia.

INTERACTIONS
Neuromuscular blocking agents: may cause increased neuromuscular blockage. Use cautiously.

NURSING CONSIDERATIONS
• Contraindicated in impaired renal function, myocardial damage, or heart block, and in actively progressing labor. Use parenteral magnesium with extreme caution in patients receiving digitalis preparations. Treating magnesium toxicity with calcium in such patients could cause serious alterations in cardiac conduction; heart block may result.
• I.V. bolus dose *must* be injected slowly in order to avoid respiratory or cardiac arrest.
• If available, use a continual infusion pump when administering infusion.
• Maximum infusion rate is 150 mg/ minute. Rapid drip causes feeling of heat.
• Keep I.V. calcium available to reverse magnesium intoxication.
• Monitor vital signs every 15 minutes when giving I.V. for severe hypomagnesemia. Watch for respiratory depression and signs of heart block. Respirations should be more than 16/ minute before dose is given.
• Monitor intake/output. Output should be 100 ml or more during 4-hour period before dose.
• Test knee-jerk and patellar reflexes before each additional dose. If absent, give no more magnesium until reflexes return; otherwise, patient may develop temporary respiratory failure and need cardiopulmonary resuscitation or I.V. administration of calcium.
• Check magnesium level after repeated doses.
• After giving to toxemic mothers within 24 hours before delivery, watch neonate for signs of magnesium toxicity, including neuromuscular and respiratory depression.

potassium acetate
Pregnancy Risk Category: C

HOW SUPPLIED
Injection: 2 mEq/ml in 20-ml, 30-ml vials.

MECHANISM OF ACTION
Replaces and maintains potassium level.

INDICATIONS & DOSAGE
Potassium replacement—
I.V. should be used for life-threatening hypokalemia or when oral replacement not feasible. Give no more than 20 mEq hourly in concentration of 40 mEq/liter or less. Total 24-hour dosage should not exceed 150 mEq (3 mEq/kg in children). Potassium replacement should be done with ECG monitoring and frequent serum potassium determinations.
Prevention of hypokalemia—
Adults: dosage is individualized according to patient's needs. In most cases, dosage should not exceed 150 mEq/day. Administer as an additive to I.V. infusions. Usual dose is 40 mEq/ liter, and solutions are usually infused at a rate not to exceed 20 mEq/hour.
Children: individualize dose. Usual dose should not exceed 3 mEq/kg/day. Administer as an additive to I.V. infusions.

ADVERSE REACTIONS
Signs of hyperkalemia:
CNS: paresthesias of the extremities, listlessness, mental confusion, weakness or heaviness of legs, flaccid paralysis.
CV: *peripheral vascular collapse with fall in blood pressure, cardiac arrhythmias,* heart block, possible cardiac arrest, ECG changes (prolonged P-R intervals; wide QRS complex; ST

segment depression; tall, tented T waves).
GI: nausea, vomiting, abdominal pain, diarrhea, bowel ulceration.
GU: oliguria.
Skin: cold skin, gray pallor.

INTERACTIONS
None significant.

NURSING CONSIDERATIONS
• Contraindicated in severe renal impairment with oliguria, anuria, azotemia; untreated Addison's disease; or in acute dehydration, hyperkalemia, hyperkalemic form of familial periodic paralysis, and conditions associated with extensive tissue breakdown. Use cautiously in patients with cardiac disease, patients receiving potassium-sparing diuretics, and those with renal impairment.
• During therapy, monitor ECG, renal function, intake/output, serum potassium, serum creatinine, and BUN. Never give potassium postoperatively until urine flow is established.
• Give slowly as diluted solution; potentially fatal hyperkalemia may result from too-rapid infusion.
• Parenteral potassium given by infusion only; never I.V. push or I.M.
• Observe for pain and redness at infusion site. Large-bore needle reduces local irritation.
• Watch for signs of GI ulceration: obstruction, hemorrhage, pain, distention, severe vomiting, and bleeding.
• Reconstitute potassium acetate powder with liquids; give after meals with a full glass of water or fruit juice to minimize GI irritation.
• To prevent serious hyperkalemia, potassium deficits must be replaced gradually.

potassium bicarbonate
K + Care ET, Klor-Con/EF

Pregnancy Risk Category: A

HOW SUPPLIED
Effervescent tablets: 25 mEq

MECHANISM OF ACTION
Replaces and maintains potassium.

INDICATIONS & DOSAGE
Hypokalemia—
25 to 50 mEq dissolved in ½ to a full glass of water (120 to 240 ml) once daily to q.i.d.

ADVERSE REACTIONS
CNS: paresthesias of the extremities, listlessness, mental confusion, weakness or heaviness of legs, flaccid paralysis.
CV: *cardiac arrhythmias,* ECG changes (prolonged P-R interval; wide QRS complex; ST segment depression; tall, tented T waves).
GI: *nausea, vomiting, abdominal pain,* diarrhea, ulcerations, hemorrhage, obstruction, perforation.

INTERACTIONS
None significant.

NURSING CONSIDERATIONS
• Contraindicated in severe renal impairment with oliguria, anuria, azotemia, and untreated Addison's disease; also in acute dehydration, hyperkalemia, hyperkalemic form of familial periodic paralysis, and conditions associated with extensive tissue breakdown. Use with caution in cardiac disease and patients receiving potassium-sparing diuretics.
• Monitor serum potassium, BUN, serum creatinine, and intake/output.
• Never switch potassium products without a doctor's order.
• Dissolve potassium bicarbonate tablets in 6 to 8 ounces of cold water.

Italicized adverse reactions are common or life-threatening.
*Liquid form contains alcohol.   **May contain tartrazine.

Dissolve completely to minimize GI irritation.

• Have patient take with meals and sip slowly over a 5- to 10-minute period.

• Potassium bicarbonate cannot be given instead of potassium chloride.

• Potassium bicarbonate does not correct hypochloremic alkalosis.

• Available in lime and orange flavors. Check for patient's flavor preference.

---

potassium chloride

K-Lor, K-Lyte/Cl, Kaochlor 10%*, Kaochlor S-F 10%*, Kaon-Cl, Kaon-Cl 20%*, Kato Powder, Kay Ciel*, Klor-10%*, Klor-Con, Kloride***, Klorvess, Klotrix, K-Tab, Micro-K Extencaps, SK-Potassium Chloride, Slow-K, Ten-K

Pregnancy Risk Category: A

HOW SUPPLIED
Tablets: 1.22 mEq (99 mg), 8 mEq (600 mg), 10 mEq (750 mg), 20 mEq (1,500 mg), 25 mEq (1,875 mg)
Tablets (controlled-release): 6.7 mEq (500 mg), 8 mEq (600 mg), 10 mEq (750 mg), 20 mEq (1,500 mg)
Tablets (enteric-coated): 4 mEq (300 mg), 13.4 mEq (1,000 mg)
Capsules (controlled-release): 8 mEq (600 mg), 10 mEq (750 mg)
Oral liquid: 5% (10 mEq/15 ml), 7.5% (15 mEq/15 ml), 10% (20 mEq/15 ml), 15% (30 mEq/15 ml), 20% (40 mEq/15 ml)
Powder for oral use: 15 mEq/packet, 20 mEq/packet, 25 mEq/packet, 25 mEq/dose
Injection: 20 mEq, 40 mEq ampules; additive syringes containing 30 mEq or 40 mEq; 10 mEq, 20 mEq, 30 mEq, 40 mEq, 45 mEq, 60 mEq, 100 mEq, 200 mEq, 400 mEq, or 1,000 mEq vials.

MECHANISM OF ACTION
Replaces and maintains potassium level.

INDICATIONS & DOSAGE
Hypokalemia—
40 to 100 mEq P.O. daily in three or four divided doses for treatment; 20 mEq for prevention. Further dosage based on serum potassium.

I.V. route when oral replacement not feasible or when hypokalemia life-threatening. Usual dose 20 mEq hourly in concentration of 40 mEq/liter or less. Total daily dosage not to exceed 150 mEq (3 mEq/kg in children). Potassium replacement should be done only with ECG monitoring and frequent serum potassium determinations.

ADVERSE REACTIONS
Signs of hyperkalemia:
CNS: paresthesias of the extremities, listlessness, mental confusion, weakness or heaviness of limbs, flaccid paralysis.
CV: *peripheral vascular collapse with fall in blood pressure, cardiac arrhythmias, heart block, possible cardiac arrest, ECG changes (prolonged P-R interval; wide QRS; ST segment depression; tall, tented T waves).*
GI: *nausea, vomiting, abdominal pain,* diarrhea, GI ulcerations (possible stenosis, hemorrhage, obstruction, perforation).
GU: oliguria.
Skin: cold skin, gray pallor.
Local: *postinfusion phlebitis.*

INTERACTIONS
None significant.

NURSING CONSIDERATIONS
• Contraindicated in severe renal impairment with oliguria, anuria, azotemia, and untreated Addison's disease; also in acute dehydration, hyperkalemia, hyperkalemic form of fa-

---

milial periodic paralysis, and conditions associated with extensive tissue breakdown. Use with caution in cardiac disease, and those patients receiving potassium-sparing diuretics.
• Potassium should not be given during immediate postoperative period until urine flow is established.
• Parenteral potassium given by infusion only; never I.V. push or I.M.
• Small amounts of lidocaine injection (1 to 3 ml of the 1% strength) may be added directly to the potassium chloride solution. This will help reverse postinfusion phlebitis.
• Give slowly as dilute solution; potentially fatal hyperkalemia may result from too rapid infusion.
• Give oral potassium supplements with extreme caution because its many forms deliver varying amounts of potassium. Never switch products without a doctor's order.
• Sugar-free liquid available (Kaochlor S-F 10%).
• Use a liquid preparation for potassium supplement if tablet or capsule passage is likely to be delayed, such as in GI obstruction.
• Have patient sip liquid potassium slowly to minimize GI irritation.
• Give with or after meals with full glass of water or fruit juice to lessen GI distress.
• Patient should make sure powders are completely dissolved before ingesting.
• Enteric-coated tablets not recommended due to potential for GI bleeding and small-bowel ulcerations.
• Tablets in wax matrix sometimes lodge in esophagus and cause ulceration in cardiac patients who have esophageal compression from enlarged left atrium. In such patients and in those with esophageal stasis or obstruction, use liquid form.
• Microencapsulated form (Micro-K) has been shown in one study to cause less GI bleeding than the wax matrix

tablets. However, this hasn't been completely confirmed.
• Often used orally with diuretics that cause potassium excretion. Potassium chloride most useful since diuretics waste chloride ion. Hypokalemic alkalosis treated best with potassium chloride.
• Monitor ECG and serum electrolytes during therapy.
• Don't crush sustained-release potassium products.

potassium gluconate
Kaon Liquid*, Kaon Tablets, Kayliker*, K-G Elixir*, Potassium Rougier†

Pregnancy Risk Category: A

HOW SUPPLIED
Tablets: 500 mg (2mEq K$^+$), 1,170 mg (5 mEq K$^+$)†
Elixir: 4.68 g (20 mEq K$^+$)/15 ml

MECHANISM OF ACTION
Replaces and maintains potassium.

INDICATIONS & DOSAGE
Hypokalemia—
40 to 100 mEq P.O. daily in three or four divided doses for treatment; 20 mEq daily for prevention. Further dosage based on serum potassium determinations.

ADVERSE REACTIONS
CNS: paresthesias of the extremities, listlessness, mental confusion, weakness or heaviness of legs, flaccid paralysis.
CV: cardiac arrhythmias, ECG changes (prolonged P-R interval; wide QRS complex; ST segment depression; tall, tented T waves).
GI: *nausea, vomiting, abdominal pain,* diarrhea, GI ulcerations with oral products (especially enteric-coated tablets); ulcerations may be accompanied by stenosis, hemorrhage, obstruction, perforation.

Italicized adverse reactions are common or life-threatening.
*Liquid form contains alcohol.   **May contain tartrazine.

INTERACTIONS
None significant.

NURSING CONSIDERATIONS
• Contraindicated in severe renal impairment with oliguria, anuria, azotemia, and untreated Addison's disease; also in acute dehydration, hyperkalemia, hyperkalemic form of familial periodic paralysis, and conditions associated with extensive tissue breakdown. Use with caution in patients with cardiac disease and in those receiving potassium-sparing diuretics.
• Monitor serum potassium, BUN, serum creatinine, and intake/output.
• Give oral potassium supplements with extreme caution because their many forms deliver varying amounts of potassium. Never switch products without a doctor's order.
• Have patient sip liquid potassium slowly to minimize GI irritation.
• Give with or after meals with full glass of water or fruit juice to lessen GI distress.
• Potassium gluconate does not correct hypokalemic hypochloremic alkalosis.
• Enteric-coated tablets not recommended because of potential for GI bleeding and small-bowel ulcerations.
• Monitor ECG and serum electrolytes during therapy.

Ringer's injection
Pregnancy Risk Category: C

HOW SUPPLIED
Injection: 250 ml, 500 ml, 1,000 ml

MECHANISM OF ACTION
Replaces fluids and electrolytes.

INDICATIONS & DOSAGE
Fluid and electrolyte replacement—
Adults and children: dose highly individualized, but usually 1.5 to 3 liters (2% to 6% body weight) infused I.V. over 18 to 24 hours.

ADVERSE REACTIONS
CV: fluid overload.

INTERACTIONS
None significant.

NURSING CONSIDERATIONS
• Contraindicated in renal failure, except as emergency volume expander. Use cautiously in congestive heart failure, circulatory insufficiency, renal dysfunction, hypoproteinemia, and pulmonary edema.
• Ringer's injection contains sodium, 147 mEq/liter; potassium, 4 mEq/liter; calcium, 4.5 mEq/liter; and chloride, 155.5 mEq/liter. This electrolyte content is insufficient for treating severe electrolyte deficiencies, although it does provide electrolytes in levels approximately equal to those of the blood.

Ringer's injection, lactated
(Hartmann's solution, Ringer's lactate solution)
Pregnancy Risk Category: C

HOW SUPPLIED
Injection: 250 ml, 500 ml, 1,000 ml

MECHANISM OF ACTION
Replaces fluids and electrolytes.

INDICATIONS & DOSAGE
Fluid and electrolyte replacement—
Adults and children: dosage highly individualized, but usually 1.5 to 3 liters (2% to 6% body weight) infused I.V. over 18 to 24 hours.

ADVERSE REACTIONS
CV: fluid overload.

INTERACTIONS
None significant.

NURSING CONSIDERATIONS

• Contraindicated in renal failure, except as emergency volume expander. Use cautiously in congestive heart failure, circulatory insufficiency, renal dysfunction, hypoproteinemia, and pulmonary edema.
• Ringer's injection, lactated, contains sodium, 130 mEq/liter; potassium, 4 mEq/liter; calcium, 3 mEq/liter; chloride, 109.7 mEq/liter; and lactate, 28 mEq/liter.
• Approximates more closely the electrolyte concentration in blood plasma than Ringer's injection.

sodium chloride
Pregnancy Risk Category: C

HOW SUPPLIED
Tablets (enteric-coated): 1 g
Tablets (slow-release): 600 mg
Injection: 0.45% sodium chloride 500 ml, 1,000 ml; 0.9% sodium chloride 50 ml, 100 ml, 150 ml, 250 ml, 500 ml, 1,000 ml; 3% sodium chloride 500 ml; 5% sodium chloride 500 ml

MECHANISM OF ACTION
Replaces and maintains sodium and chloride levels.

INDICATIONS & DOSAGE
Highly individualized fluid and electrolyte replacement in hyponatremia caused by electrolyte loss or in severe salt depletion—
Adults: 400 ml of 3% or 5% solution only with frequent electrolyte determination and only if given slow I.V.; *with 0.45% solution:* 3% to 8% of body weight, according to deficiencies, over 18 to 24 hours; *with 0.9% solution:* 2% to 6% of body weight, according to deficiencies, over 18 to 24 hours.
Management of "heat cramp" caused by excessive perspiration—
Adults: 1 g P.O. with every glass of water.

ADVERSE REACTIONS
CV: aggravation of congestive heart failure; edema and pulmonary edema if too much given or given too rapidly.
Metabolic: hypernatremia and aggravation of existing acidosis with excessive infusion; serious electrolyte disturbance, loss of potassium.

INTERACTIONS
None significant.

NURSING CONSIDERATIONS
• Use with caution in congestive heart failure, circulatory insufficiency, renal dysfunction, and hypoproteinemia.
• Infuse 3% and 5% solutions very slowly and with caution to avoid pulmonary edema. Use only for critical situations. Observe patient continually.
• Concentrates available for addition to parenteral nutrient solutions. Don't confuse these small volumes of parenterals with normal saline injection. *Read label carefully.*
• Monitor serum electrolytes.

Italicized adverse reactions are common or life-threatening.
*Liquid form contains alcohol.   **May contain tartrazine.

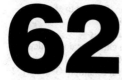

Acidifier and alkalinizers

Acidifier
ammonium chloride

Alkalinizers
sodium bicarbonate
sodium lactate
tromethamine

COMBINATION PRODUCTS
None.

ammonium chloride◊

Pregnancy Risk Category: B

HOW SUPPLIED
Tablets: 500 mg◊
Tablets (enteric-coated): 500 mg◊,
1,000 mg◊
Injection: 2.14% (0.4 mEq/ml),
26.75% (5 mEq/ml)

MECHANISM OF ACTION
Increases free hydrogen ion (H^+) concentration. Also acts as an expectorant by causing reflex stimulation of bronchial mucous glands.

INDICATIONS & DOSAGE
Metabolic alkalosis—
Adults and children: I.V. dose (in mEq) is equal to the serum chloride deficit (in mEq/ml) multiplied by the extracellular fluid volume (estimated as 20% of the body weight in kilograms). One-half the calculated volume should be given, then patient should be reassessed.
As an acidifying agent—
Adults: 4 to 12 g P.O. daily in divided doses.

Children: 75 mg/kg P.O. daily in four divided doses.
As expectorant—
Adults: 250 to 500 mg P.O. q 2 to 4 hours.

ADVERSE REACTIONS
Adverse reactions usually result from ammonia toxicity or too-rapid I.V. administration.
CNS: headache, confusion, progressive drowsiness, excitement alternating with coma, hyperventilation, *calcium-deficient tetany, twitching, hyperreflexia, EEG abnormalities.*
CV: bradycardia.
GI: (with oral dose) *gastric irritation, nausea, vomiting,* thirst, anorexia, retching.
GU: glycosuria.
Metabolic: *acidosis, hyperchloremia, hypokalemia,* hyperglycemia.
Skin: rash, pallor.
Local: pain at injection site.
Other: irregular respirations with periods of apnea.

INTERACTIONS
Spironolactone: systemic acidosis. Use together cautiously.

NURSING CONSIDERATIONS
• Contraindicated in severe hepatic or renal dysfunction. Use cautiously in pulmonary insufficiency or cardiac edema and in infants.
• Dilute concentrated form (26.75%) before administration. Add 100 to 200 mEq (20 to 40 ml of the 26.75% solution) to 500 or 1,000 ml of normal saline injection. Administer via infusion

pump not exceeding 5 ml/min in adults.

• Give oral form after meals to decrease GI adverse reactions. Enteric-coated tablets may also minimize GI symptoms but are absorbed erratically.

• Do not administer drug with milk or other alkaline solutions because they are not compatible.

• Pain of I.V. injection may be lessened by decreasing infusion rate.

• Determine CO_2 combining power and serum electrolytes before and during therapy to prevent acidosis.

• Monitor urine pH and output. Diuresis is normal for first 2 days.

• Monitor rate and depth of respirations frequently.

• When using as an expectorant, give with full glass of water.

---

sodium bicarbonate ◇

Pregnancy Risk Category: C

HOW SUPPLIED
Tablets: 300 mg◇, 325 mg◇, 600 mg◇, 650 mg◇
Injection: 4% (2.4 mEq/5 ml), 4.2% (5 mEq/10 ml), 5% (297.5 mEq/500 ml), 7.5% (8.92 mEq/10 ml and 44.6 mEq/50 ml), 8.4% (10 mEq/10 ml and 50 mEq/50 ml)

MECHANISM OF ACTION
Restores buffering capacity of the body. Also neutralizes excess acid.

INDICATIONS & DOSAGE
Cardiac arrest—
Adults and children: as a 7.5% or 8.4% solution, 1 mEq/kg I.V. followed by 0.5 mEq/kg I.V. every 10 minutes depending on blood gases. Further dosages based on blood gases. If blood gases unavailable, use 0.5 mEq/kg I.V. q 10 minutes until spontaneous circulation returns.
Infants up to 2 years: 4.2% solution,

I.V. infusion. Rate not to exceed 8 mEq/kg daily.
Metabolic acidosis—
Adults and children: dosage depends on blood CO_2 content, pH, and patient's clinical condition. Generally, 2 to 5 mEq/kg I.V. infused over 4- to 8-hour period.
Systemic or urinary alkalinization—
Adults: 325 mg to 2 g P.O. q.i.d.
Children: 12 to 120 mg/kg P.O. daily.
Antacid—
Adults: 300 mg to 2 g P.O. chewed and taken with glass of water.

ADVERSE REACTIONS
GI: gastric distention, belching, flatulence.
GU: renal calculi or crystals.
Metabolic: (with overdose) *alkalosis, hypernatremia, hyperkalemia, hyperosmolarity.*

INTERACTIONS
None significant.

NURSING CONSIDERATIONS
• No contraindications for use in life-threatening emergencies. Contraindicated in hypertension, in patients with tendency toward edema, in patients who are losing chlorides by vomiting or from continuous GI suction, in patients receiving diuretics known to produce hypochloremic alkalosis, and in patients on sodium-restricted diets or with renal disease.

• May be added to other I.V. fluids.

• Because sodium bicarbonate inactivates such catecholamines as norepinephrine and dopamine, do not mix with I.V. solutions of these agents.

• To avoid risk of alkalosis, determine blood pH, PaO_2, $PaCO_2$, and serum electrolytes. Keep doctor informed of serum laboratory results.

• Tell patient not to take with milk. May cause hypercalcemia, alkalosis, and possibly renal calculi.

• Discourage use as an antacid. Offer

Italicized adverse reactions are common or life-threatening.
*Liquid form contains alcohol.   **May contain tartrazine.

a nonabsorbable alternative antacid if it is to be used repeatedly.
• May cause enteric-coated drugs to be prematurely released in the stomach.
• Sodium bicarbonate is not routinely recommended for use in cardiac arrest because it may produce a paradoxical acidosis from CO_2 production. It should not be routinely administered during the early stages of resuscitation unless preexisting acidosis is clearly present. May be used at team leader's discretion after such interventions as defibrillation, cardiac compression, and administration of first-line drugs.
• If sodium bicarbonate is being used to produce an alkaline urine, monitor urine pH q 4 to 6 hours (should be >7.0).

sodium lactate
Pregnancy Risk Category: C

HOW SUPPLIED
Injection: ⅙ molar solution
Injection (for preparations of I.V. admixtures): 2.5 mEq/ml

MECHANISM OF ACTION
Metabolized to sodium bicarbonate. Then produces buffering effect.

INDICATIONS & DOSAGE
Alkalinize urine—
Adults: 30 ml of ⅙ molar solution/kg of body weight I.V. given in divided doses over 24 hours.
Metabolic acidosis—
Adults: usually given as ¹/₆ molar injection (167 mEq lactate/liter I.V.). Dosage depends on degree of bicarbonate deficit.

ADVERSE REACTIONS
Metabolic: (with overdose) alkalosis, hypernatremia, hyperosmolarity.

INTERACTIONS
None significant.

NURSING CONSIDERATIONS
• Contraindicated in severe hepatic and renal disease, respiratory alkalosis, or acidosis associated with congenital heart disease with persistent cyanosis.
• Monitor serum electrolytes to avoid alkalosis.

tromethamine
Tham
Pregnancy Risk Category: C

HOW SUPPLIED
Injection: 18 g/500 ml

MECHANISM OF ACTION
Combines with hydrogen ions and associated acid anions; the resulting salts are excreted.

INDICATIONS & DOSAGE
Metabolic acidosis (associated with cardiac bypass surgery or with cardiac arrest)—
Adults: dosage depends on bicarbonate deficit. Calculate as follows: ml of 0.3 M tromethamine solution required = wt in kg × bicarbonate deficit (mEq/liter). Additional therapy based on serial determinations of existing bicarbonate deficit.
Children: calculate dosage as above. Give slowly over 3 to 6 hours. Additional therapy based on degree of acidosis. Total 24-hour dosage should not exceed 33 to 40 ml/kg.

ADVERSE REACTIONS
CNS: respiratory depression.
Metabolic: hypoglycemia, hyperkalemia (with decreased urine output).
Local: venospasm; I.V. thrombosis; inflammation, necrosis, and sloughing if extravasation occurs.

INTERACTIONS
None significant.

NURSING CONSIDERATIONS
• Contraindicated in anuria, uremia, chronic respiratory acidosis, or pregnancy (except in acute, life-threatening situations). Use cautiously in renal disease and poor urine output. Monitor ECG and serum potassium in these patients.
• To prevent blood pH from rising above normal, adjust dosage carefully.
• Give slowly through large needle (18G to 20G) into largest antecubital vein or by indwelling I.V. catheter.
• Before, during, and after therapy make the following determinations: blood pH; carbon dioxide tension; bicarbonate, glucose, and electrolyte levels.
• When giving drug to patient with associated respiratory acidosis, mechanical ventilation should be readily available.
• Except in life-threatening situations, do not use longer than 1 day.
• If extravasation occurs, infiltrate area with 1% procaine and hyaluronidase 150 units; may reduce vasospasm and dilute remaining drug in local area.

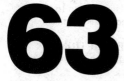

Hematinics

ferrous fumarate
ferrous gluconate
ferrous sulfate
iron dextran

COMBINATION PRODUCTS
FERMALOX◊: ferrous sulfate 200 mg, and magnesium hydroxide and dried aluminum hydroxide gel 200 mg.
FEROCYL◊: iron (as fumarate) 50 mg and docusate sodium 100 mg.
FERRO-SEQUELS◊: iron (as fumarate) 50 mg and docusate sodium 100 mg.
SIMRON◊: iron (as gluconate) 10 mg and polysorbate 20, 400 mg.

---

ferrous fumarate
Eldofe◊, Feostat◊, Ferranol◊, Fersamal†, Fumasorb◊, Fumerin◊, Hemocyte◊, Ircon◊, Maniron◊, Novofumar†, Palafer†, Span-FF◊

Pregnancy Risk Category: A

HOW SUPPLIED
Tablets◊*:* 63 mg, 195 mg, 200 mg, 324 mg, 325 mg
Tablets (chewable): 100 mg◊
Capsules (controlled-release): 325 mg◊
Oral suspension: 100 mg/5 ml◊
Drops: 45 mg/0.6 ml◊

MECHANISM OF ACTION
Provides elemental iron, an essential component in the formation of hemoglobin. Each 100 mg of ferrous fumarate provides 33 mg of elemental iron.

INDICATIONS & DOSAGE
Iron deficiency—
Adults: 200 mg P.O. t.i.d. or q.i.d.
Children: 3 mg/kg P.O. t.i.d., increased to 6 mg/kg P.O. t.i.d. as needed and tolerated.

ADVERSE REACTIONS
GI: *nausea,* vomiting, *constipation, black stools.*
Other: elixir may stain teeth.

INTERACTIONS
Antacids, cholestyramine resin, pancreatic extracts, vitamin E: decreased iron absorption. Separate doses if possible.
Chloramphenicol: watch for delayed response to iron therapy.
Vitamin C: concurrent administration may increase iron absorption. Beneficial drug interaction.

NURSING CONSIDERATIONS
• Contraindicated in hemosiderosis and hemochromatosis. Use cautiously in peptic ulcer, regional enteritis, and ulcerative colitis. Also use cautiously on long-term basis.
• GI upset related to dose. Between-meal dosing preferable, but can be given with some foods although absorption may be decreased. Enteric-coated products reduce GI upset but also reduce amount of iron absorbed.
• Iron is toxic; parents should be aware of iron poisoning in children.
• Tablets may be given with juice or water, but not in milk or antacids. Give with orange juice to promote iron absorption.

• To avoid staining teeth, give elixir iron preparations with straw; patient may take with water or fruit juice.
• Check for constipation; record color and amount of stool. Teach dietary measures for preventing constipation.
• Oral iron may turn stools black. This unabsorbed iron is harmless; however, it could mask the presence of melena.
• Monitor hemoglobin and reticulocyte counts during therapy.
• Combination products—Simron, Ferro-Sequels, Ferocyl, Fer-Regules—contain stool softeners to help prevent constipation. Fermalox contains antacids to help relieve GI upset, if present; don't use this product unless absolutely necessary because of decreased iron absorption. Usually, combination iron products should be avoided.

ferrous gluconate
Fergon*◊, Ferralet◊, Fertinic†, Novoferrogluc†

Pregnancy Risk Category: A

HOW SUPPLIED
Tablets: 300 mg◊, 320 mg◊, 325 mg◊ (320-mg tablet contains 37 mg Fe⁺)
Capsules: 86 mg◊, 325 mg◊, 435 mg◊
Elixir: 300 mg/5 ml (contains 35 mg Fe⁺)◊

MECHANISM OF ACTION
Provides elemental iron, an essential component in the formation of hemoglobin. Each 100 mg of ferrous gluconate provides 11.6 mg of elemental iron.

INDICATIONS & DOSAGE
Iron deficiency—
Adults: 300 to 325 mg P.O. q.i.d., increased to 650 mg q.i.d. as needed and tolerated.
Children 2 years or older: 8 mg/kg

P.O. t.i.d., increased to 16 mg P.O. t.i.d. as needed and tolerated.

ADVERSE REACTIONS
GI: *nausea,* vomiting, *constipation, black stools.*
Other: elixir may stain teeth.

INTERACTIONS
Antacids, cholestyramine resin, pancreatic extracts, vitamin E: decreased iron absorption. Separate doses if possible.
Chloramphenicol: watch for delayed response to iron therapy.
Vitamin C: may increase iron absorption. Beneficial drug interaction.

NURSING CONSIDERATIONS
• Contraindicated in peptic ulcer, regional enteritis, ulcerative colitis, hemosiderosis, and hemochromatosis. Use cautiously on long-term basis.
• GI upset related to dose. Between-meal dosing preferable, but can be given with some foods although absorption may be decreased. Enteric-coated products reduce GI upset but also reduce amount of iron absorbed.
• Tell patient to continue regular dosing schedule if he misses a dose. Patient shouldn't double the dose.
• Iron is toxic; parents should be aware of iron poisoning in children.
• Dilute liquid preparations in juice (preferably orange juice) or water, but not in milk or antacids. Give tablets with orange juice to promote absorption.
• To avoid staining teeth, give elixir iron preparations with straw; patient may take with water or fruit juice.
• Check for constipation; record color and amount of stool. Teach dietary measures for preventing constipation.
• Oral iron may turn stools black. This unabsorbed iron is harmless; however, it could mask melena.
• Monitor hemoglobin and reticulocyte counts during therapy.

ferrous sulfate

Feosol*◊, Fer-In-Sol*◊, Feritard‡,
Fero-Grad†, Fero-Gradumet◊,
Ferolix*◊, Ferospace◊, Ferralyn◊,
Fespan‡, Irospan◊, Mol-Iron*◊,
Novoferrosulfa†, Slow-Fe, Telefon◊

Pregnancy Risk Category: A

HOW SUPPLIED

Ferrous sulfate is 20% elemental iron;
dried and powdered (exsiccated), it is
about 32% elemental iron.
Tablets: 195 mg◊, 300 mg◊, 325
mg◊; 200 mg (exsiccated)◊
Tablets (extended-release): 160 mg
(exsiccated)◊
Capsules: 150 mg◊, 225 mg◊, 250
mg◊, 390 mg◊, 190 mg (exsiccated)◊
Capsules (extended-release): 525
mg◊, 150 mg◊, 167 mg (exsiccated)◊
Elixir: 220 mg/5 ml◊
Liquid: 75 mg/0.6 ml◊
Syrup: 90 mg/5 ml◊

MECHANISM OF ACTION

Provides elemental iron, an essential
component in the formation of hemoglobin.

INDICATIONS & DOSAGE

Iron deficiency—
Adults: 325 mg P.O. t.i.d. or q.i.d.
Alternatively, give 1 delayed release
capsule (160 or 525 mg) P.O. twice
daily.
Children: 5 mg/kg P.O. t.i.d., increased to 10 mg/kg P.O. t.i.d. as
needed and tolerated.
*Prophylaxis for iron deficiency ane-
mia—*
Pregnant women: 150 to 300 mg
P.O. daily in divided doses.
**Premature or undernourished in-
fants:** 1 to 2 mg/kg P.O. daily (as elemental iron) in divided doses.

ADVERSE REACTIONS

GI: *nausea,* vomiting, *constipation,
black stools.*
Other: elixir may stain teeth.

INTERACTIONS

*Antacids, cholestyramine resin, pan-
creatic extracts, vitamin E:* decreased
iron absorption. Separate doses if possible.
Chloramphenicol: watch for delayed
response to iron therapy.
Vitamin C: may increase iron absorption. Beneficial drug interaction.

NURSING CONSIDERATIONS

• Contraindicated in hemosiderosis
and hemochromatosis. Use cautiously
in peptic ulcer, ulcerative colitis, and
regional enteritis. Also use cautiously
on long-term basis.
• GI upset related to dose. Between-
meal dosing preferable, but can be
given with some foods although absorption may be decreased. Enteric-
coated products reduce GI upset but
also reduce amount of iron absorbed.
• Tell patient to continue regular dosing schedule if he misses a dose. Patient shouldn't double the dose.
• Iron is toxic; parents should be
aware of potential for iron poisoning
in children.
• Dilute liquid preparations in juice
or water, but not in milk or antacids.
Dilute liquids in orange juice; give
tablets with orange juice to promote
iron absorption.
• To avoid staining teeth, give elixir
iron preparations with straw.
• Check for constipation; record
color and amount of stool. Teach dietary measures for preventing constipation.
• Oral iron may turn stools black.
This unabsorbed iron is harmless;
however, it could mask melena.
• Monitor hemoglobin and reticulocyte counts during therapy.

iron dextran

Hydextran, Imferon, K-FeRON

Pregnancy Risk Category: C

HOW SUPPLIED
Injection: 50 mg elemental iron/ml

MECHANISM OF ACTION
Provides elemental iron, an essential component in the formation of hemoglobin; 1 ml iron dextran provides 50 mg elemental iron.

INDICATIONS & DOSAGE
Iron deficiency anemia—
Adults: I.M. or I.V. injections of iron are advisable only for patients for whom oral administration is impossible or ineffective. Test dose (0.5 ml) required before administration.
I.M. (by Z-track): inject 0.5 ml test dose. If no reactions next daily dose should ordinarily not exceed 0.5 ml (25 mg) for infants under 5 kg; 1 ml (50 mg) for children under 9 kg; 2 ml (100 mg) for patients under 50 kg; 5 ml (250 mg) for patients over 50 kg.
I.V. push: inject 0.5 ml test dose. If no reaction, within 2 to 3 days the dosage may be raised to 2 ml daily I.V., 1 ml/minute undiluted and infused slowly until total dose is achieved. No single dose should exceed 100 mg.
I.V. infusion: dosages are expressed in terms of elemental iron. Dilute in 250 to 1,000 ml of normal saline solution; dextrose increases local vein irritation. Infuse test dose of 25 mg slowly over 5 minutes. If no reaction occurs in 5 minutes, infusion may be started. Infuse total dose slowly over approximately 6 to 12 hours.

ADVERSE REACTIONS
CNS: headache, transitory paresthesias, arthralgia, myalgia, dizziness, malaise, syncope.
CV: *hypotensive reaction, peripheral vascular flushing with overly rapid I.V. administration, tachycardia.*
GI: nausea, vomiting, metallic taste, transient loss of taste perception.
Local: *soreness and inflammation at injection site (I.M.); brown skin discoloration at injection site (I.M.); local phlebitis at injection site (I.V.).*
Skin: rash, urticaria.
Other: *anaphylaxis.*

INTERACTIONS
None significant.

NURSING CONSIDERATIONS
• Contraindicated in all anemias other than iron deficiency anemia. Use with extreme caution in patients with impaired hepatic function and rheumatoid arthritis.
• Monitor vital signs for drug reaction. Reactions are varied, ranging from pain, inflammation, and myalgia to hypotension, shock, and death.
• Inject deeply into upper outer quadrant of buttock—never into arm or other exposed area—with a 2- to 3-inch, 19G or 20G needle. Use Z-track technique to avoid leakage into subcutaneous tissue and staining of skin.
• Skin staining may be minimized by using a separate needle to withdraw the drug from its container.
• Monitor hemoglobin concentration, hematocrit, and reticulocyte count.
• Use I.V. in these situations: insufficient muscle mass for deep intramuscular injection; impaired absorption from muscle due to stasis or edema; possibility of uncontrolled intramuscular bleeding from trauma (as may occur in hemophilia); and with massive and prolonged parenteral therapy (as may be necessary in cases of chronic substantial blood loss).
• Upon completion of I.V. iron dextran infusion, flush the vein with 10 ml of 0.9% sodium chloride solution.
• Patient should rest 15 to 30 minutes after I.V. administration.
• Check hospital policy before administering I.V. Some do not permit infusion method because its safety is controversial.
• Not removed by hemodialysis.

Italicized adverse reactions are common or life-threatening.
*Liquid form contains alcohol.   **May contain tartrazine.

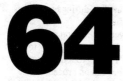

64

Anticoagulants

dicumarol
heparin calcium
heparin sodium
intravascular perfluorochemical
    emulsion
warfarin sodium

COMBINATION PRODUCTS
None.

---

dicumarol
(bishydroxycoumarin)

Pregnancy Risk Category: D

HOW SUPPLIED
Tablets: 25 mg, 50 mg

MECHANISM OF ACTION
Inhibits vitamin K-dependent activation of clotting factors II, VII, IX, and X, which are formed in the liver.

INDICATIONS & DOSAGE
Treatment of pulmonary emboli; prevention and treatment of deep vein thrombosis, myocardial infarction, rheumatic heart disease with heart valve damage, atrial arrhythmias—
Adults: 200 to 300 mg P.O. on first day, 25 to 200 mg P.O. daily thereafter, based on prothrombin times.

ADVERSE REACTIONS
Blood: *hemorrhage with excessive dosage,* leukopenia, *agranulocytosis.*
GI: anorexia, nausea, vomiting, cramps, *diarrhea,* mouth ulcers.
GU: hematuria.
Skin: dermatitis, urticaria, alopecia, *rash.*

Other: *fever.*

INTERACTIONS
Acetaminophen: increased bleeding possible with chronic (greater than 2 weeks) therapy with acetaminophen. Monitor very carefully.
Allopurinol, amiodarone, chloramphenicol, clofibrate, diflunisal, thyroid drugs, heparin, anabolic steroids, cimetidine, disulfiram, glucagon, inhalation anesthetics, metronidazole, quinidine, influenza vaccine, sulindac, sulfinpyrazone, sulfonamides, tricyclic antidepressants: increased prothrombin time. Monitor patient carefully for bleeding. Consider anticoagulant dosage reduction.
Barbiturates: inhibition of hypoprothrombinemic effect of anticoagulants. If barbiturates are withdrawn, reduce anticoagulant dosage; inhibition may last weeks after barbiturate is withdrawn, but fatal hemorrhage can occur when inhibiting effect disappears.
Cholestyramine: decreased response when administered too close together. Administer 6 hours after oral anticoagulants.
Ethacrynic acid, indomethacin, mefenamic acid, oxyphenbutazone, phenylbutazone, salicylates: increased prothrombin time; ulcerogenic effects. Don't use together.
Glutethimide, chloral hydrate, sulfinpyrazone, triclofos sodium: increased or decreased prothrombin time. Avoid use if possible, or monitor patient carefully.
Griseofulvin, haloperidol, ethchlorvy-

---

nol, carbamazepine, rifampin: decreased prothrombin time with reduced anticoagulant effect. Monitor patient carefully.

NURSING CONSIDERATIONS
• Contraindicated in hemophilia, thrombocytopenic purpura, leukemia with pronounced bleeding tendency, open wounds or ulcers, impaired hepatic or renal function, severe hypertension, acute nephritis, subacute bacterial endocarditis. Use cautiously during menses, during use of any drainage tube, and in any patient in whom slight bleeding is dangerous. Use with extreme caution (if at all) in psychiatric patients, debilitated patients, or cachectic patients.
• Use caution when adding or stopping any drug for patient receiving anticoagulants. May change the clotting status and result in hemorrhage.
• Fever and skin rash signal severe adverse reactions. Withhold drug and call doctor.
• Give drug at same time daily. Stress importance of complying with recommended dosage and keeping follow-up appointments. Patient should carry a card that identifies him as a potential bleeder.
• Regularly inspect patient for bleeding gums, bruises on arms or legs, petechiae, nosebleeds, melena, tarry stools, hematuria, hematemesis. Tell patient and family to watch for these signs and notify doctor immediately.
• Warn patient to avoid OTC products containing aspirin, other salicylates, or drugs that may interact with dicumarol.
• Because onset of action is delayed, heparin sodium is often given during first few days of treatment. When heparin is being given simultaneously, don't draw blood for prothrombin time within 5 hours of intermittent I.V. heparin administration. However, prothrombin time may be drawn at any time during continuous heparin infusion.
• Dose given depends on prothrombin time (PT). Doctors usually try to maintain PT at 1.5 to 2 times normal. PT values depend on procedure and reagents used in individual laboratory.
• Tell patient to notify doctor if menses is heavier than usual.
• Tell patient to use electric razor when shaving to avoid scratching skin and to brush teeth with a soft toothbrush.
• May turn alkaline urine red-orange.
• Duration of action 2 to 6 days.
• Light to moderate alcohol intake does not significantly affect prothrombin times.
• Tell patient to eat a consistent amount of leafy green vegetables every day. These contain vitamin K, and eating different amounts daily may alter anticoagulant effect.

heparin calcium
Calcilean†, Calciparine, Caprin‡, Uniparin-Ca‡

heparin sodium
Hepalean†, Heparin Lock Flush Solution (Tubex), Hep Lock, Liquaemin Sodium, Uniparin‡

Pregnancy Risk Category: C

HOW SUPPLIED
Products are derived from beef lung or porcine intestinal mucosa.
calcium
Ampule: 12,500 units/0.5 ml; 20,000 units/0.8 ml
Syringe: 5,000 units/0.2 ml
sodium
Carpuject: 5,000 units/ml
Disposable syringes: 1,000 units/ml, 2,500 units/ml, 5,000 units/ml, 7,500 units/ml, 10,000 units/ml, 20,000 units/ml, 40,000 units/ml
Premixed I.V. solutions: 1,000 units in 500 ml normal saline solution;

Italicized adverse reactions are common or life-threatening.
*Liquid form contains alcohol.   **May contain tartrazine.

2,000 units in 1,000 ml normal saline solution; 12,500 units in 250 ml 0.45% saline solution; 25,000 units in 250 ml 0.45% saline solution; 25,000 units in 500 ml 0.45% saline solution; 10,000 units in 100 ml 5% dextrose in water (D_5W); 12,500 units in 250 ml D_5W; 25,000 units in 250 ml D_5W; 25,000 units in 500 ml D_5W
Unit-dose ampules: 1,000 units/ml, 5,000 units/ml, 10,000 units/ml
Vials: 1,000 units/ml, 2,500 units/ml, 5,000 units/ml, 7,500 units/ml, 10,000 units/ml, 15,000 units/ml, 20,000 units/ml, 40,000 units/ml
heparin sodium flush
Disposable syringes: 10 units/ml, 100 units/ml
Vials: 10 units/ml, 100 units/ml

MECHANISM OF ACTION
Accelerates formation of an antithrombin III–thrombin complex. It inactivates thrombin and prevents conversion of fibrinogen to fibrin.

INDICATIONS & DOSAGE
Treatment of deep vein thrombosis, myocardial infarction—
Adults: initially, 5,000 to 7,500 units I.V. push, then adjust dose according to PTT results and give dose I.V. q 4 hours (usually 4,000 to 5,000 units); or 5,000 to 7,500 units I.V. bolus, then 1,000 units/hour by I.V. infusion pump. Wait 8 hours following bolus dose, and adjust hourly rate according to PTT.
Treatment of pulmonary embolism—
Adults: initially, 7,500 to 10,000 units I.V. push, then adjust dose according to PTT results and give dose I.V. q 4 hours (usually 4,000 to 5,000 units); or 7,500 to 10,000 units I.V. bolus, then 1,000 units hourly by I.V. infusion pump. Wait 8 hours following bolus dose, and adjust hourly rate according to PTT.
Prophylaxis of embolism—
Adults: 5,000 units S.C. q 12 hours.
Open heart surgery—
Adults: (total body perfusion) 150 to 300 units/kg continuous I.V infusion.
Treatment of pulmonary emboli; prevention and treatment of deep vein thrombosis—
Children: initially, 50 units/kg I.V. drip. Maintenance dose is 100 units/kg I.V. drip q 4 hours. Constant infusion: 20,000 units/m² daily. Dosages adjusted according to PTT.
As an I.V. flush to maintain patency of I.V. indwelling catheters—
10 to 100 units as an I.V. flush. Not intended for therapeutic use.
Heparin dosing is highly individualized, depending upon disease state, age, renal and hepatic status.

ADVERSE REACTIONS
Blood: *hemorrhage with excessive dosage, overly prolonged clotting time, thrombocytopenia.*
Local: irritation, mild pain.
Other: *"white clot" syndrome,* hypersensitivity reactions including chills, fever, pruritus, rhinitis, burning of feet, conjunctivitis, lacrimation, arthralgia, urticaria.

INTERACTIONS
Anticoagulants, oral: additive anticoagulation. Monitor prothrombin time and partial thromboplastin time.
Salicylates: increased anticoagulant effect. Don't use together.

NURSING CONSIDERATIONS
● Conditionally contraindicated in active bleeding; blood dyscrasias; or bleeding tendencies such as hemophilia, thrombocytopenia, or hepatic disease with hypoprothrombinemia; suspected intracranial hemorrhage; suppurative thrombophlebitis; inaccessible ulcerative lesions (especially of GI tract); open ulcerative wounds; extensive denudation of skin; ascorbic acid deficiency and other conditions causing increased capillary permeability; during or after brain, eye, or spinal cord surgery; during continu-

ous tube drainage of stomach or small intestine; in subacute bacterial endocarditis; shock; advanced renal disease; threatened abortion; severe hypertension. Although the use of heparin is clearly hazardous in these conditions, a decision to use it depends on the comparative risk in failure to treat the coexisting thromboembolic disorder.

• Use cautiously during menses; in mild hepatic or renal disease; alcoholism; in patients in occupations with the risk of physical injury; immediately postpartum; and in patients with history of allergies, asthma, or GI ulcers.

• Monitor platelet counts regularly. Thrombocytopenia caused by heparin may be associated with a type of arterial thrombosis known as "white clot" syndrome.

• Measure partial thromboplastin time (PTT) carefully and regularly. Anticoagulation present when PTT values are 1.5 to 2 times control values.

• Drug requirements are higher in early phases of thrombogenic diseases and febrile states; lower when patient becomes stabilized.

• Regularly inspect patient for bleeding gums, bruises on arms or legs, petechiae, nosebleeds, melena, tarry stools, hematuria, hematemesis. Tell patient and family to watch for these signs and notify doctor immediately.

• Tell patient to avoid OTC medications containing aspirin, other salicylates, or drugs that may interact with heparin.

• Heparin comes in various concentrations. Check order and vial carefully.

• Low-dose injections given sequentially between iliac crests in lower abdomen deep into subcutaneous fat. Inject drug slowly subcutaneously into fat pad. Leave needle in place for 10 seconds after injection; then withdraw needle. Alternate site every 12 hours—right for a.m., left for p.m.

• Don't massage after subcutaneous injection. Watch for signs of bleeding at injection site. Rotate sites and keep accurate record.

• Check constant I.V. infusions regularly, even when pumps are in good working order, to prevent overdosage or underdosage.

• I.M. administration not recommended.

• I.V. administration preferred because of long-term effect and irregular absorption when given subcutaneously. Whenever possible, administer I.V. heparin using infusion pump to provide maximum safety.

• Concentrated heparin solutions (greater than 100 units/ml) can irritate blood vessels.

• Place notice above patient's bed to inform I.V. team or lab personnel to apply pressure dressings after taking blood.

• Avoid excessive I.M. injections of other drugs to prevent or minimize hematomas. If possible, don't give I.M. injections at all.

• Elderly patients should usually start at lower doses.

• When intermittent I.V. therapy is utilized, always draw blood ½ hour before next scheduled dose to avoid falsely elevated PTT.

• Blood for PTT can be drawn any time after 8 hours of initiation of continuous I.V. heparin therapy. Never draw blood for PTT from the I.V. tubing of the heparin infusion, or from vein of infusion. Falsely elevated PTT will result. Always draw blood from opposite arm.

• Give on time; try not to skip a dose or "catch up" with an I.V. containing heparin. If I.V. is out, get it restarted as soon as possible, and reschedule bolus dose immediately.

• Never piggyback other drugs into an infusion line while heparin infusion is running. Many antibiotics and

---

Italicized adverse reactions are common or life-threatening.
*Liquid form contains alcohol.   **May contain tartrazine.

other drugs inactivate heparin. Never mix any drug with heparin in syringe when bolus therapy is used.
• Abrupt withdrawal may cause increased coagulability. Usually, heparin therapy is followed by oral anticoagulants for prophylaxis.

intravascular perfluorochemical emulsion
Fluosol

Pregnancy Risk Category: B

HOW SUPPLIED
Emulsion for injection: 20%; supplied in kit form with additive solutions (1 and 2) and materials to provide continuous oxygenation.

MECHANISM OF ACTION
An emulsion of synthetic perfluorochemicals that acts as a carrier of oxygen.

INDICATIONS & DOSAGE
To prevent or decrease myocardial ischemia during percutaneous transluminal coronary angioplasty (PTCA) in patients at high risk for ischemic complications of angioplasty (including patients with a low baseline ejection fraction; patients with large areas of the myocardium at risk; patients with recent myocardial infarction; patients with unstable angina or refractory angina requiring hospitalization)—
Adults: first, a test dose of 0.5 ml should be withdrawn from the prepared solution and injected into a peripheral vein. If no adverse reactions occur within 10 minutes, warmed, oxygenated emulsion may be administered by intracoronary injection at a rate of 60 to 90 ml/minute. Administer through the central lumen of an angioplasty balloon catheter without removing the guide wire. Use an an-

giographic power injector with a warming jacket.

ADVERSE REACTIONS
CV: *ventricular tachycardia or fibrillation,* bradycardia, chest discomfort, hypotension.
Respiratory: dyspnea, increased respiratory rate, coughing.
Skin: mild pruritus.

INTERACTIONS
Anesthetics: may prolong the action of lipid soluble anesthetics.
Hepatotoxic agents: animal studies revealed that perfluorochemicals enhanced the hepatotoxic effects of carbon tetrachloride.

NURSING CONSIDERATIONS
• Contraindicated in patients who are hypersensitive to any components of the compound and in patients with functionally critical secondary stenosis in areas distal to the site of the lesion being treated.
• Reportedly, this drug will accumulate in the body after repeated dosage. Intravascular perfluorochemical emulsion should not be given more than once every 6 months.
• Drug should be administered only by physicians familiar with PTCA. Follow institutional policy regarding emergency surgical procedures for coronary artery bypass graft surgery.
• When used with an angiographic power injector reservoir of 260 ml and a flow rate of 60 ml/minute, more than 4 minutes of perfusion time will be allowed. Perfusion time should be limited by patient tolerance and physician judgment.
• In the unlikely event that the patient reacts adversely to the test dose (1.2% of the patients in clinical trials reacted), the drug should not be given. Severe reactions can be managed with methylprednisolone or diphenhydramine.
• The emulsion must be oxygenated

and warmed to approximately 98.6° F. (37° C.) before administration. Infusion of solutions at room temperature has been associated with ventricular fibrillation.

• The container of intravascular perfluorochemical emulsion must be stored in the freezer (between 23° and −22° F. [−5° and −30° C.). Emulsions that appear to have thawed partially during storage should not be used. Use a warming cabinet or water bath set at 98.6° F. to thaw the solution (do not use a microwave oven because this may cause uneven heating of the solution). Do not refreeze thawed solutions. Allow at least 30 minutes for thawing of the solution.

• The additive solutions (solutions 1 and 2) should not be frozen; they may be stored at room temperature not exceeding 86° F. (30° C.).

• Do not add anything other than solutions 1 and 2 or carbogen gas (95% oxygen, 5% carbon dioxide) to the emulsion. Do not oxygenate with 100% oxygen, because this will adversely affect the solution's final pH. When administering, do not use a filter. Never administer any solution that has evidence of emulsion separation.

• Studies have shown that perfluorochemicals are excreted in breast milk. Breast-feeding after administration of intravascular perfluorochemical emulsion is not recommended.

warfarin sodium
Coumadin, Panwarfin**, Warfilone Sodium†

Pregnancy Risk Category: D

HOW SUPPLIED
Tablets: 2 mg, 2.5 mg, 5 mg, 7.5 mg, 10 mg
Injection: 50 mg/vial

MECHANISM OF ACTION
Inhibits vitamin K–dependent activa-

tion of clotting factors II, VII, IX, and X, which are formed in the liver.

INDICATIONS & DOSAGE
Treatment of pulmonary emboli; prevention and treatment of deep vein thrombosis, myocardial infarction, rheumatic heart disease with heart valve damage, atrial arrhythmias—
Adults: 10 to 15 mg P.O. for 3 days, then dosage based on daily prothrombin (PT) times. Usual maintenance dosage is 2 to 10 mg P.O. daily. Alternate regimen: initially, 40 to 60 mg P.O. daily; then 2 to 10 mg daily based on PT determinations.

Warfarin sodium also available for I.V. use (50 mg/vial). Reconstitute with sterile water for injection. I.V. form rarely used and may be in periodic short supply.

ADVERSE REACTIONS
Blood: *hemorrhage with excessive dosage,* leukopenia.
GI: paralytic ileus, intestinal obstruction (both resulting from hemorrhage), diarrhea, vomiting, cramps, nausea.
GU: excessive uterine bleeding.
Skin: dermatitis, urticaria, *rash,* necrosis, alopecia.
Other: *fever.*

INTERACTIONS
Acetaminophen: increased bleeding possible with chronic (greater than 2 weeks) therapy with acetaminophen. Monitor very carefully.
Amiodarone, chloramphenicol, clofibrate, diflunisal, thyroid drugs, heparin, anabolic steroids, cimetidine, disulfiram, glucagon, inhalation anesthetics, metronidazole, quinidine, influenza vaccine, sulindac, sulfinpyrazone, sulfonamides: increased prothrombin time. Monitor patient carefully for bleeding. Consider anticoagulant dosage reduction.
Barbiturates: inhibition of hypoprothrombinemic effect of anticoagu-

---

Italicized adverse reactions are common or life-threatening.
*Liquid form contains alcohol.   **May contain tartrazine.

lants. If barbiturates are withdrawn, reduce anticoagulant dose; inhibition may last weeks after barbiturate is withdrawn, but fatal hemorrhage can occur when inhibiting effect disappears.

Cholestyramine: decreased response when administered too close together. Administer 6 hours after oral anticoagulants.

Ethacrynic acid, indomethacin, mefenamic acid, oxyphenbutazone, phenylbutazone, salicylates: increased prothrombin time; ulcerogenic effects. Don't use together.

Glutethimide, chloral hydrate, triclofos sodium: increased or decreased prothrombin time. Avoid use if possible, or monitor patient carefully.

Griseofulvin, haloperidol, ethchlorvynol, carbamazepine, paraldehyde, rifampin: decreased prothrombin time with reduced anticoagulant effect. Monitor patient carefully.

NURSING CONSIDERATIONS

• Contraindicated in bleeding or hemorrhagic tendencies resulting from open wounds, visceral cancer, GI ulcers, severe hepatic or renal disease, severe uncontrolled hypertension, subacute bacterial endocarditis, vitamin K deficiency; after recent operations in eye, brain, or spinal cord. Use cautiously in diverticulitis, colitis, mild or moderate hypertension, mild or moderate hepatic or renal disease, lactation; with drainage tubes in any orifice; with regional or lumbar block anesthesia; or in any condition increasing risk of hemorrhage.

• Observe nursing infants of mothers on drug for unexpected bleeding.

• PT determinations essential for proper control. High incidence of bleeding when PT exceeds 2.5 times control values. Doctors usually try to maintain PT at 1.5 to 2 times normal.

• Give at same time daily. Stress importance of complying with recommended dosage and keeping follow-up appointments. Patient should carry a card that identifies him as a potential bleeder.

• Elderly patients and patients with renal or hepatic failure are especially sensitive to warfarin effect.

• Half-life of warfarin's anticoagulant effect is 36 to 44 hours.

• Warfarin effect can be neutralized by vitamin K injections.

• Regularly inspect patient for bleeding gums, bruises on arms or legs, petechiae, nosebleeds, melena, tarry stools, hematuria, hematemesis. Tell patient and family to watch for these signs and notify doctor immediately.

• Warn patient to avoid OTC products containing aspirin, other salicylates, or drugs that may interact with warfarin sodium.

• Food and enteral feedings that contain vitamin K may cause inadequate anticoagulation. Warn patient to read labels.

• Because onset of action is delayed, heparin sodium is often given during first few days of treatment. When heparin is being given simultaneously, don't draw blood for prothrombin time within 5 hours of intermittent I.V. heparin administration. However, blood for prothrombin time may be drawn at any time during continuous heparin infusion.

• Fever and skin rash signal severe adverse reactions. Withhold drug and call doctor immediately.

• Tell patient to notify doctor if menses is heavier than usual. May require dosage adjustment.

• Tell patient to use electric razor when shaving to avoid scratching skin and to brush teeth with a soft toothbrush.

• Best oral anticoagulant when patient must receive antacids or phenytoin.

• Light to moderate alcohol intake does not significantly affect prothrombin time.

● Possibly effective in treatment of transient cerebral ischemic attacks.
● Tell patient to eat a consistent amount of leafy green vegetables every day. These contain vitamin K, and eating different amounts daily may alter anticoagulant effects.

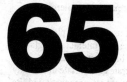

Hemostatics

absorbable gelatin sponge
antihemophilic factor
Factor IX complex
microfibrillar collagen hemostat
oxidized cellulose
thrombin

COMBINATION PRODUCTS
None.

absorbable gelatin sponge
Gelfoam

HOW SUPPLIED
Sponges: 20 mm × 60 mm × 3 mm,
20 mm × 60 mm × 7 mm, 80 mm ×
62.5 mm × 10 mm, 80 mm × 125
mm × 10 mm, 80 mm × 250 mm ×
10 mm, 80 mm × 125 mm (compressed)
Packs: 40 cm × 2 cm, 40 cm × 6 cm
Dental packs: 10 mm × 20 mm × 7
mm, 20 mm × 20 mm × 7 mm
Prostatectomy cones: 13 cm (5″) diameter, 18 cm (7″) diameter

MECHANISM OF ACTION
Absorbs and holds many times its
weight in blood. Also provides a
framework for growth of granulation
tissue.

INDICATIONS & DOSAGE
Decubitus ulcers—
Adults: place aseptically deep into ulcer. Don't disturb or remove; may add
extra p.r.n.
To provide hemostasis in surgery (adjunct)—
Adults: apply saturated with isotonic
sodium chloride injection or thrombin
solution. Hold in place for 10 to 15
seconds. When oozing is controlled,
allow material to remain in place.

ADVERSE REACTIONS
None reported.

INTERACTIONS
None significant.

NURSING CONSIDERATIONS
• Contraindicated in frank infection,
or postpartum bleeding or hemorrhage; also for use as a sole hemostatic agent in abnormal bleeding.
• Avoid overpacking when placed
into body cavities or closed tissue
spaces.
• Systemically absorbed within 4 to 6
weeks; no need to remove.

antihemophilic factor (AHF)
Hemofil M, Koate-HS, Koate-HT,
Monoclate

Pregnancy Risk Category: C

HOW SUPPLIED
Injection: vials, with diluent. Number
of units on label.
A new porcine product is now
available for patients with congenital
hemophilia A who have antibodies to
human Factor VIII:C.

MECHANISM OF ACTION
Directly replaces deficient clotting
factor.

INDICATIONS & DOSAGE

Prophylaxis of spontaneous hemorrhage in patients with hemophilia A (Factor VIII deficiency)—
Adults and children: dosage must be calculated using the formula:

$$\text{AHF required (IU)} = \text{body weight (kg)} \times \text{desired Factor VIII increase (\% of normal)} \times 0.5$$

To prevent spontaneous hemorrhage, the desired level of Factor VIII is 5% of normal. Following trauma and surgery, the desired level is 30%.
Treatment of bleeding in patients with hemophilia A (Factor VIII deficiency)—
Adults and children: 15 to 25 units/kg by slow I.V. injection or I.V. infusion, followed by 8 to 15 units/kg q 8 to 12 hours for 3 to 4 days as necessary.

ADVERSE REACTIONS

CNS: headache, paresthesias, clouding or loss of consciousness.
CV: tachycardia, hypotension, possible intravascular hemolysis in patients with blood type A, B, or AB.
EENT: visual disturbances.
GI: nausea, vomiting.
Skin: erythema, *urticaria*.
Other: *chills, fever, backache, flushing,* chest constriction; hypersensitivity.

INTERACTIONS

None significant.

NURSING CONSIDERATIONS

• Use cautiously in neonates, infants, and patients with hepatic disease because of susceptibility to hepatitis, which may be transmitted in antihemophilic factor.
• Monitor vital signs regularly. Take baseline pulse rate before I.V. administration. If pulse rate increases significantly, flow rate should be reduced or administration stopped.

• Monitor patient for allergic reactions.
• For I.V. use only. Use plastic syringe; drug may interact with glass syringe and bind to its surface.
• Refrigerate concentrate until ready to use, but not after reconstituted. Refrigeration after reconstitution may cause the active ingredient to precipitate. Before reconstituting, concentrate and diluent bottles should be warmed to room temperature. To mix drug, gently roll vial between hands. Reconstituted solution unstable; use within 3 hours. Store away from heat. Don't shake or mix with other I.V. solutions.
• As ordered, administer hepatitis B vaccine before administering antihemophilic factor.
• Monitor coagulation studies before and during therapy.

Factor IX complex
Konyne-HT, Profilnine Heat-Treated, Proplex T

Pregnancy Risk Category: C

HOW SUPPLIED

Injection: vials, with diluents. Units specified on label.

MECHANISM OF ACTION

Directly replaces deficient clotting factor.

INDICATIONS & DOSAGE

Factor IX deficiency (hemophilia B or Christmas disease), anticoagulant overdosage—
Adults and children: units required equal 0.8 to 1 × body weight in kg × percentage of desired increase of Factor IX level, by slow I.V. infusion or I.V. push. Dosage is highly individualized, depending on degree of deficiency, level of Factor IX desired, weight of patient, and severity of bleeding.

Italicized adverse reactions are common or life-threatening.
*Liquid form contains alcohol.   **May contain tartrazine.

ADVERSE REACTIONS
CNS: headache.
CV: *thromboembolic reactions,* possible intravascular hemolysis in patients with blood type A, B, or AB.
Other: *transient fever, chills, flushing, tingling,* hypersensitivity.

INTERACTIONS
None significant.

NURSING CONSIDERATIONS
• Contraindicated in hepatic disease, intravascular coagulation, or fibrinolysis. Use cautiously in neonates and infants because of susceptibility to hepatitis, which may be transmitted with Factor IX complex.
• Observe patient for allergic reactions, and monitor vital signs regularly.
• As ordered, administer hepatitis B vaccine before administering Factor IX complex.
• Avoid rapid infusion. If tingling sensation, fever, chills, or headache develops during I.V. infusion, decrease flow rate and notify the doctor.
• Reconstitute with 20 ml sterile water for injection for each vial of lyophilized drug. Keep refrigerated until ready to use; warm to room temperature before reconstituting. Use within 3 hours of reconstitution. Unstable in solution. Don't shake, refrigerate, or mix reconstituted solution with other I.V. solutions. Store away from heat.

---

microfibrillar collagen hemostat
Avitene

Pregnancy Risk Category: C

HOW SUPPLIED
Nonwoven web: 70 mm × 70 mm × 1 mm, 70 mm × 35 mm × 1 mm

MECHANISM OF ACTION
Attracts and aggregates platelets.

INDICATIONS & DOSAGE
To provide hemostasis in surgery (adjunct)—
Adults and children: amount depends on severity of bleeding. Compress area with dry sponges. Apply drug directly to bleeding site for 1 to 5 minutes. Gently remove excess. Reapply if needed.

ADVERSE REACTIONS
Blood: hematoma.
Local: exacerbation of wound dehiscence, abscess formation, foreign body reaction, adhesion formation.
Other: enhanced infection in contaminated wounds, mediastinitis, hypersensitivity.

INTERACTIONS
None significant.

NURSING CONSIDERATIONS
• Contraindicated in closure of skin incisions; it may interfere with healing.
• Not for injection.
• Don't spill on nonbleeding surfaces.
• Don't dilute. Always apply dry.
• Adheres to wet gloves, instruments, or tissue surfaces. Handle and apply with smooth, dry forceps. Apply directly to source of bleeding.

---

oxidized cellulose
Oxycel, Surgicel

HOW SUPPLIED
Pads: 3″ × 3″, 8 ply
Pledgets: 2″ × 1″ × 1″
Strips: ½ × 2″, ½ × 5″, ½ × 36″;
2″ × 3″, 2″ × 14″, 2″ × 18″; 4″ × 8″

MECHANISM OF ACTION
Absorbs and holds many times its weight in blood.

INDICATIONS & DOSAGE
To provide hemostasis in surgery (ad-

---

junct); external bleeding at tumor sites—

Adults and children: apply with sterile technique, p.r.n. Remove after hemostasis, if possible, with dry sterile forceps. Leave in place if necessary.

ADVERSE REACTIONS
CNS: headache when used as packing for epistaxis, or after rhinologic procedures or application to surface wounds.
EENT: sneezing, epistaxis, stinging, or burning when used as packing for rhinologic procedures; nasal membrane necrosis or septal perforation.
Local: encapsulation of fluid, foreign body reaction, burning or stinging after application to surface wounds.
Other: possible prolongation of drainage in cholecystectomies.

INTERACTIONS
Thrombin: may decrease blood clotting effectiveness.

NURSING CONSIDERATIONS
• Contraindicated in controlling hemorrhage from large arteries; for use on nonhemorrhagic, serous, oozing surfaces; in implantation in bone defects.
• Don't pack or wad unless it will be removed after hemostasis. Don't apply too tightly when used as wrap sheet in vascular surgery. Apply loosely against bleeding surface.
• Always remove after hemostasis when used in laminectomies or near optic nerve chain.
• Don't autoclave this product.
• Use only amount needed to produce hemostasis. Remove excess before surgical closure.
• Use minimal amounts in urologic procedures.
• In large wounds, don't overlap skin edges.
• Use sterile technique to remove from open wounds after hemostasis. Don't remove without irrigating mate-

rial first; otherwise, fresh bleeding may occur.
• Don't moisten. Hemostatic effect is greater when applied dry.
• Should not be used for permanent packing in fractures because it may result in cyst formation.

---

thrombin
Thrombinar, Thrombostat‡
Pregnancy Risk Category: C

HOW SUPPLIED
Powder: 1,000-, 5,000-, 10,000-, and 20,000-unit vials
Kit: 20,000-unit with sprayer assembly

MECHANISM OF ACTION
Clots to form fibrin in the presence of fibrinogen.

INDICATIONS & DOSAGE
Bleeding from parenchymatous tissue, cancellous bone, dental sockets, nasal and laryngeal surgery, and in plastic surgery and skin-grafting procedures—
Adults: apply 100 units per ml of sterile isotonic sodium chloride solution or sterile distilled water to area where clotting needed (or may apply dry powder in bone surgery); in major bleeding, apply 1,000 to 2,000 units/ml sterile isotonic sodium chloride solution. Sponge blood from area before application, but avoid sponging area after application.
GI hemorrhage—
Adults: give 60 ml (2 oz) of milk, followed by 60 ml of milk containing 10,000 to 20,000 units thrombin. Repeat t.i.d. for 4 to 5 days or until bleeding is controlled.

ADVERSE REACTIONS
Systemic: hypersensitivity and fever.

INTERACTIONS
None significant.

NURSING CONSIDERATIONS

• Contraindicated in patients with hypersensitivity to thrombin or bovine products.

• Obtain patient history of reactions to thrombin or bovine products.

• Observe patient for allergic reactions, and monitor vital signs regularly.

• Have blood typed and cross matched to treat possible hemorrhage.

• Don't inject topical thrombin or allow it to enter large blood vessels. I.V. injection may cause death because of severe intravascular clotting.

• May be used with absorbable gelatin sponge but not with oxidized cellulose. Check sponge labeling before use.

• Neutralize stomach acids before oral use in GI hemorrhage.

• Keep refrigerated, preferably frozen, until ready to use. Unstable in solution. Use within 24 hours of reconstitution; discard after 48 hours. Store away from heat.

• Broken down by diluted acid, alkali, and salts of heavy metals.

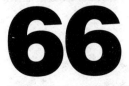

Blood derivatives

normal serum albumin 5%
normal serum albumin 25%
plasma protein fraction

COMBINATION PRODUCTS
None.

normal serum albumin 5%
Albuminar 5%, Albutein 5%,
Buminate 5%, Plasbumin 5%

normal serum albumin 25%
Albuminar 25%, Albumisol 25%,
Buminate 25%, Plasbumin 25%

Pregnancy Risk Category: C

HOW SUPPLIED
albumin 5%
Injection: 5%, in 50-ml, 250-ml, 500-ml, 1,000-ml bottles
albumin 25%
Injection: 25%, in 10-ml, 20-ml, 50-ml, 100-ml vials.

MECHANISM OF ACTION
Normal serum albumin 25% provides intravascular oncotic pressure in a 5:1 ratio, which causes a shift of fluid from interstitial spaces to the circulation and slightly increases plasma protein concentration. Normal serum albumin 5% supplies colloid to the blood and expands plasma volume.

INDICATIONS & DOSAGE
Shock—
Adults: initially, 500 ml (5% solution) by I.V. infusion, repeat q 30 minutes, p.r.n. Dosage varies with patient's condition and response.

Children: 25% to 50% adult dose in nonemergency.
Hypoproteinemia—
Adults: 1,000 to 1,500 ml 5% solution by I.V. infusion daily, maximum rate 5 to 10 ml/minute; or 25 to 100 g 25% solution by I.V. infusion daily, maximum rate 3 ml/minute. Dosage varies with patient's condition and response.
*Burns—*dosage varies according to extent of burn and patient's condition. Usually maintain plasma albumin at 2 to 3 g/100 ml.
Hyperbilirubinemia—
Infants: 1 g albumin (4 ml 25%)/kg before transfusion.

ADVERSE REACTIONS
CV: *vascular overload after rapid infusion,* hypotension, altered pulse rate.
GI: increased salivation, nausea, vomiting.
Skin: urticaria.
Other: chills, fever, altered respiration.

INTERACTIONS
None significant.

NURSING CONSIDERATIONS
• Contraindicated in severe anemia or heart failure. Use cautiously in low cardiac reserve, absence of albumin deficiency, and restricted sodium intake.
• Do not give more than 250 g in 48 hours.
• Watch for hemorrhage or shock if used after surgery or injury.

Italicized adverse reactions are common or life-threatening.
*Liquid form contains alcohol.   **May contain tartrazine.

• Monitor vital signs carefully.
• Watch for signs of vascular overload (heart failure or pulmonary edema).
• Patient should be properly hydrated before infusion of solution.
• Avoid rapid I.V. infusion. Specific rate is individualized according to patient's age, condition, and diagnosis.
• Dilute with sterile water for injection, 0.9% sodium chloride solution, or dextrose 5% in water injection. Use solution promptly; contains no preservatives. Discard unused solution.
• Don't use cloudy solutions or those containing sediment. Solution should be clear amber color.
• Freezing may cause bottle to break. Follow storage instructions on bottle.
• One volume of 25% albumin is equivalent to five volumes of 5% albumin in producing hemodilution and relative anemia.
• This product is very expensive, and random supply shortages occur often.
• Monitor intake/output, hemoglobin, hematocrit, and serum protein and electrolytes during therapy.

plasma protein fraction
Plasmanate, Plasma-Plex, Plasmatein, Protenate

Pregnancy Risk Category: C

HOW SUPPLIED
Injection: 5% solution in 50-ml, 250-ml, 500-ml vials

MECHANISM OF ACTION
Supplies colloid to the blood and expands plasma volume.

INDICATIONS & DOSAGE
Shock—
Adults: varies with patient's condition and response, but usual dose is 250 to 500 ml I.V. (12.5 to 25 g protein), usually no faster than 10 ml/minute.
Children: 22 to 33 ml/kg I.V. infused at rate of 5 to 10 ml/minute.

Hypoproteinemia—
Adults: 1,000 to 1,500 ml I.V. daily. Maximum infusion rate 8 ml/minute.

ADVERSE REACTIONS
CNS: headache.
CV: variable effects on blood pressure after rapid infusion or intraarterial administration; *vascular overload after rapid infusion.*
GI: nausea, vomiting, hypersalivation.
Skin: erythema, urticaria.
Other: flushing, chills, fever, back pain, dyspnea.

INTERACTIONS
None significant.

NURSING CONSIDERATIONS
• Contraindicated in patients with severe anemia or heart failure, and those patients undergoing cardiac bypass. Use cautiously in hepatic or renal failure, low cardiac reserve, and restricted sodium intake.
• Monitor blood pressure. Infusion should be slowed or stopped if hypotension suddenly occurs.
• Vital signs should return to normal gradually; monitor hourly.
• Watch for signs of vascular overload (heart failure or pulmonary edema).
• Monitor intake/output. Watch for decreased urine output. Notify doctor if this occurs.
• Check expiration date on container before using. Discard solutions in containers that have been opened for more than 4 hours. Solution contains no preservatives.
• Don't use solutions that are cloudy, contain sediment, or have been frozen.
• If patient is dehydrated, give additional fluids either P.O. or I.V.
• Do not give more than 250 g (5,000 ml 5%) in 48 hours.
• Contains 130 to 160 mEq sodium/liter.

67

Thrombolytic enzymes

alteplase
anistreplase
streptokinase
urokinase

COMBINATION PRODUCTS
None.

---

alteplase (tissue plasminogen activator, recombinant; t-PA)
Actilyse‡, Activase

Pregnancy Risk Category: C

HOW SUPPLIED
Injection: 20-mg (11.6 million–IU), 50-mg (29 million–IU) vials

MECHANISM OF ACTION
Binds to fibrin in a thrombus, and locally converts plasminogen to plasmin, which initiates local fibrinolysis.

INDICATIONS & DOSAGE
Lysis of thrombi obstructing coronary arteries in acute myocardial infarction—
Adults: 100 mg I.V. infusion over 3 hours as follows: 60 mg in the first hour, of which 6 to 10 mg is given as a bolus over the first 1 to 2 minutes. Then 20 mg/hr infusion for 2 hours. Smaller adults (<65 kg) should receive a dose of 1.25 mg/kg in a similar fashion (60% in the first hour, with 10% as a bolus; then 20% of the total dose per hour for 2 hours).

ADVERSE REACTIONS
Blood: *severe, spontaneous bleeding (cerebral, retroperitoneal, GU, GI).*
CNS: *cerebral hemorrhage,* fever.
CV: hypotension, arrhythmias.
GI: nausea, vomiting.
Local: bleeding at puncture sites.
Other: hypersensitivity, urticaria.

INTERACTIONS
Aspirin, dipyridamole, heparin, coumarin anticoagulants: increased risk of bleeding. Monitor patient carefully.

NURSING CONSIDERATIONS
• Contraindicated in active internal bleeding, intracranial neoplasm, arteriovenous malformation, aneurysm, and severe uncontrolled hypertension. Also contraindicated in a history of cardiovascular accident, recent (within 2 months) intraspinal or intracranial trauma or surgery, or known bleeding diathesis.
• Do not exceed dose of 100 mg. Higher doses are associated with an increased incidence of intracranial bleeding.
• Coronary thrombolysis is associated with arrhythmias induced by reperfusion of ischemic myocardium. Such arrhythmias are not different from those commonly associated with myocardial infarction. Have antiarrhythmic agents readily available and carefully monitor the ECG.
• Successful recanalization of occluded coronary arteries and improvement of heart function are time-dependent phenomena and require initiation of treatment with alteplase as

---

Italicized adverse reactions are common or life-threatening.
*Liquid form contains alcohol.   **May contain tartrazine.

soon as possible after the onset of symptoms.

• Bleeding is the most common adverse effect and may occur internally and at external puncture sites. Carefully monitor patient.

• Heparin therapy is frequently initiated after treatment with alteplase to decrease the risk of rethrombosis.

• Reconstitute drug with sterile water for injection (without preservatives) only. Do not use vial if the vacuum is not present. Reconstitute with a large bore (18G) needle, directing the stream of sterile water at the lyophilized cake. Slight foaming is common, and the resulting solution should be clear to pale yellow. Avoid excess agitation of solution.

• Drug may be administered as reconstituted (1 mg/ml) or diluted with an equal volume of normal saline or dextrose 5% in water to make a 0.5 mg/ml solution. Adding other to the infusion is not recommended.

• Reconstitute alteplase solution immediately before use, and administer it within 8 hours. The drug may be temporarily stored at 35° to 86° F. (2° to 30° C.), but it is stable for 8 hours at room temperature. Discard any solution unused after that time because it contains no preservatives.

---

anistreplase (anisoylated plasminogen-streptokinase activator complex; APSAC)
Eminase

Pregnancy Risk Category: C

HOW SUPPLIED
Injection: 30 units/vial

MECHANISM OF ACTION
Anistreplase is derived from Lys-plasminogen and streptokinase. It is formulated into a fibrinolytic enzyme plus activator complex with the activator temporarily blocked by an anisoyl group. The drug is activated in vivo by a nonenzymatic process that removes the anisoyl group. The active Lys-plasminogen-streptokinase activator complex is progressively formed in the bloodstream or within the thrombus.

INDICATIONS & DOSAGE
Lysis of conary artery thrombi following acute myocardial infarction—
Adults: 30 units I.V. over 2 to 5 minutes. Administer by direct injection.

ADVERSE REACTIONS
Blood: bleeding.
CNS: intracranial hemorrhage.
CV: arrhythmias, conduction disorders, hypotension.
EENT: hemoptysis, gum/mouth hemorrhage.
GI: *bleeding.*
GU: hematuria.
Skin: hematomas, urticaria, itching, flushing, delayed (2 weeks after therapy) purpuric rash.
Local: bleeding at puncture sites.
Other: *anaphylactoid reactions (rare).*

INTERACTIONS
Heparin, oral anticoagulants, and drugs that alter platelet function (including aspirin and dipyridamole): may increase the risk of bleeding.

NURSING CONSIDERATIONS
• Contraindicated in patients with active internal bleeding, history of cerebrovascular accident, recent (within the past 2 months) intraspinal and intracranial surgery or trauma, aneurysm, arteriovenous malformation, intracranial neoplasm, or known bleeding diathesis.

• Consider risk/benefit in patients with recent (within 10 days) major surgery, trauma (including cardiopulmonary resuscitation), GI or GU bleeding; patients with cerebrovascular disease or hypertension (systolic ≥180 mm Hg and/or diastolic ≥110 mm Hg; in patients with a mitral stenosis or atrial fibrillation or other condition that may lead to left heart thrombus; patients with acute pericarditis or subacute bacterial endocarditis; patients with septic thrombophlebitis; patients 75 years and older; diabetic hemorrhagic retinopathy; and in patients receiving anticoagulants.

• Unlike other thrombolytics that must be infused, anistreplase is given by direct injection over 2 to 5 minutes.

• Thrombolytic therapy is associated with the occurrence of reperfusion arrhythmias that may signify successful thrombolysis. These arrhythmias are similar to those seen in the course of an acute MI and may include sinus bradycardia, accelerated idioventricular rhythm, ventricular tachycardia, or premature ventricular depolarizations. Be prepared to treat bradycardia or ventricular irritability during anistreplase therapy. Carefully monitor ECG during treatment with anistreplase.

• Anistreplase is derived from human plasma. No cases of hepatitis or human immunodeficiency virus (HIV) infection have been reported to date. The manufacturing process is designed to purify the plasma used in the preparation of the drug.

• Reconstitute the drug by slowly adding 5 ml of sterile water for injection. Direct the stream against the side of the vial, not at the drug itself. Gently roll the vial to mix the dry powder and water. To avoid excessive foaming, don't shake the vial. The reconstituted solution should be colorless to pale yellow. Inspect for particulate matter.

• Do not mix the drug with other medications; do not dilute the solution after reconstitution.

• If the drug is not administered within 30 minutes of reconstituting, discard the vial.

• In vitro coagulation tests will be affected by the presence of anistreplase. This can be attenuated if blood samples are collected in the presence of aprotinin (150 to 200 units/ml).

• Bleeding is the most common adverse reaction and may occur internally and at external puncture sites. Carefully monitor patient.

• Heparin therapy is frequently initiated after treatment with thrombolytics to decrease the risk of rethrombosis.

• Teach the patient signs of internal bleeding. Tell him to report these immediately. Advise the patient about proper dental care to avoid excessive gum trauma.

---

streptokinase
Kabikinase, Streptase

Pregnancy Risk Category: C

HOW SUPPLIED
Injection: 100,000 IU, 250,000 IU, 600,000 IU, 750,000 IU, 1,500,000 IU in vials for reconstitution

MECHANISM OF ACTION
Activates plasminogen in two steps. Plasminogen and streptokinase form a complex that exposes the plasminogen-activating site. Plasminogen is converted to plasmin by cleavage of the peptide bond.

INDICATIONS & DOSAGE
Arteriovenous cannula occlusion—
Adults: 250,000 IU in 2 ml I.V. solution by I.V. pump infusion into each occluded limb of the cannula over 25 to 35 minutes. Clamp off cannula for 2 hours. Then aspirate contents of cannula; flush with saline solution and reconnect.
Venous thrombosis, pulmonary embolism, and arterial thrombosis and embolism—
Adults: loading dose is 250,000 IU I.V. infusion over 30 minutes. Sustaining dose is 100,000 IU/hour I.V.

Italicized adverse reactions are common or life-threatening.
*Liquid form contains alcohol.   **May contain tartrazine.

infusion for 72 hours for deep vein thrombosis and 100,000 IU/hour over 24 to 72 hours by I.V. infusion pump for pulmonary embolism.

Lysis of coronary artery thrombi following acute myocardial infarction—
Adults: loading dose is 20,000 IU via coronary catheter, followed by a maintenance dose. Maintenance dose is 2,000 IU/minute for 60 minutes as an infusion. Alternatively, may be administered as an I.V. infusion. Usual adult dose is 1.5 million units infused over 60 minutes.

ADVERSE REACTIONS
Blood: bleeding, low hematocrit.
CV: transient lowering or elevation of blood pressure.
EENT: periorbital edema.
Skin: urticaria.
Local: phlebitis at injection site.
Other: *hypersensitivity to drug, fever, anaphylaxis,* musculoskeletal pain, minor breathing difficulty, bronchospasms, angioneurotic edema.

INTERACTIONS
Anticoagulants: concurrent use with streptokinase is not recommended. Reversing the effects of oral anticoagulants must be considered before beginning therapy; heparin must be stopped and its effect allowed to diminish.
Aspirin, dipyridamole, indomethacin, phenylbutazone, drugs affecting platelet activity: increased risk of bleeding. Combined therapy with low-dose aspirin (162.5 mg) or dipyridamole has improved acute and long-term results.

NURSING CONSIDERATIONS
• Contraindicated in ulcerative wounds, active internal bleeding, and recent cerebrovascular accident; recent trauma with possible internal injuries; visceral or intracranial malignancy; ulcerative colitis; diverticulitis; severe hypertension; acute or chronic hepatic or renal insufficiency;

uncontrolled hypocoagulation; chronic pulmonary disease with cavitation; subacute bacterial endocarditis or rheumatic valvular disease; recent cerebral embolism, thrombosis, or hemorrhage. Also contraindicated within 10 days after intraarterial diagnostic procedure or any surgery, including liver or kidney biopsy, lumbar puncture, thoracentesis, paracentesis, or extensive or multiple cutdowns.
• Use cautiously when treating arterial emboli that originate from left side of heart because of danger of cerebral infarction.
• I.M. injections are contraindicated during streptokinase therapy.
• Before initiating therapy, draw blood to determine PTT and PT. Rate of I.V. infusion depends on thrombin time and streptokinase resistance.
• If the patient has had either a recent streptococcal infection or recent treatment with streptokinase, a higher loading dose may be necessary.
• Preparation of I.V. solution: reconstitute each vial with 5 ml normal saline solution for injection. Further dilute to 45 ml. Don't shake; roll gently to mix. Use within 24 hours. Store at room temperature in powder form; refrigerate after reconstitution.
• Monitor patient for excessive bleeding every 15 minutes for the first hour, every 30 minutes for the second through eighth hours, then once every shift. If bleeding is evident, stop therapy. Pretreatment with heparin or drugs affecting platelets causes high risk of bleeding, but may improve long-term results. Monitor closely.
• Monitor pulses, color, and sensation of extremities every hour.
• Have typed and crossmatched packed red cells and whole blood ready to treat possible hemorrhage.
• Keep aminocaproic acid available to treat bleeding. Corticosteroids are used to treat allergic reactions.
• Before using streptokinase to clear

---

an occluded arteriovenous cannula, try flushing with heparinized saline.
• Bruising more likely during therapy; avoid unnecessary handling of patient. Side rails should be padded.
• Maintain the involved extremity in straight alignment to prevent bleeding from the infusion site.
• Keep venipuncture sites to a minimum; use pressure dressing on puncture sites for at least 15 minutes.
• Keep a laboratory flow sheet on patient's chart to monitor partial thromboplastin time, prothrombin time, hemoglobin, and hematocrit.
• Monitor vital signs frequently.
• Watch for signs of hypersensitivity. Notify doctor immediately.
• Heparin by continuous infusion is usually started within an hour after stopping streptokinase. Use infusion pump to administer heparin.
• Should be used only by doctors with wide experience in thrombotic disease management where clinical and laboratory monitoring can be performed.
• Thrombolytic therapy in patients with acute myocardial infarction is associated with decreased infarct size, improved ventricular function, and decreased incidence of congestive heart failure. Streptokinase must be administered within 6 hours of the onset of symptoms for optimal effect.

---

urokinase
Abbokinase, Ukidan‡, Win-Kinase
Pregnancy Risk Category: B

HOW SUPPLIED
Injection: 5,000 IU/ml unit-dose vial; 250,000-IU vial

MECHANISM OF ACTION
Activates plasminogen by directly cleaving peptide bonds at two different sites.

INDICATIONS & DOSAGE
Lysis of acute massive pulmonary emboli and lysis of pulmonary emboli accompanied by unstable hemodynamics—
Adults: for I.V. infusion only by constant infusion pump that will deliver a total volume of 195 ml.
Priming dose: 4,400 IU/kg of urokinase–normal saline solution admixture given over 10 minutes. Follow with 4,400 IU/kg hourly for 12 to 24 hours. Total volume should not exceed 200 ml. Follow therapy with continuous I.V. infusion of heparin, then oral anticoagulants.
Coronary artery thrombosis—
Adults: following a bolus dose of heparin ranging from 2,500 to 10,000 units, infuse 6,000 IU/minute of urokinase into the occluded artery for up to 2 hours. Average total dosage is 500,000 IU.
Venous catheter occlusion—
Instill 5,000 IU into occluded line, wait 5 minutes, then aspirate. Repeat aspiration attempts q 5 minutes for 30 minutes. If not patent after 30 minutes, cap line and let urokinase work for 30 to 60 minutes before aspirating. May require second instillation.

ADVERSE REACTIONS
Blood: bleeding, low hematocrit.
Local: phlebitis at injection site.
Other: hypersensitivity (not as frequent as streptokinase), musculoskeletal pain, bronchospasm, *anaphylaxis.*

INTERACTIONS
Anticoagulants: concurrent use with urokinase is not recommended. Consider reversing the effects of oral anticoagulants before beginning therapy; heparin must be stopped and its effect allowed to diminish.
Aspirin, dipyridamole, indomethacin, phenylbutazone, other drugs affecting platelet activity: increased risk of bleeding.

Italicized adverse reactions are common or life-threatening.
*Liquid form contains alcohol.   **May contain tartrazine.

NURSING CONSIDERATIONS

• Contraindicated in ulcerative wounds, active internal bleeding, and cerebrovascular accident; recent trauma with possible internal injuries; visceral or intracranial malignancy; pregnancy and first 10 days postpartum; ulcerative colitis; diverticulitis; severe hypertension; acute or chronic hepatic or renal insufficiency; uncontrolled hypocoagulation; chronic pulmonary disease with cavitation; subacute bacterial endocarditis or rheumatic valvular disease; and recent cerebral embolism, thrombosis, or hemorrhage. Also contraindicated within 10 days after intraarterial diagnostic procedure or any surgery, including liver or kidney biopsy, lumbar puncture, thoracentesis, paracentesis, or extensive or multiple cutdowns.

• I.M. injections are contraindicated during urokinase therapy.

• Maintain the involved extremity in straight alignment to prevent bleeding from the infusion site.

• To prepare I.V. solution: add 5 ml sterile water for injection to vial. Dilute further with 0.9% sodium chloride or 5% dextrose in water solution before infusion. The total volume of fluid administered should not exceed 200 ml. Don't use bacteriostatic water for injection to reconstitute; it contains preservatives.

• Monitor patient for bleeding every 15 minutes for the first hour; every 30 minutes for the second through eighth hours; then once every shift. Pretreatment with drugs affecting platelets places patient at high risk of bleeding.

• Monitor pulses, color, and sensation of extremities every hour.

• Have typed and crossmatched red cells, whole blood, and aminocaproic acid available to treat bleeding. Corticosteroids are used to treat allergic reactions.

• Keep a laboratory flow sheet on patient's chart to monitor partial thromboplastin time, prothrombin time, hemoglobin, and hematocrit.

• Watch for signs of hypersensitivity.

• Monitor vital signs.

• Keep venipuncture sites to a minimum; use pressure dressing on puncture sites for at least 15 minutes.

• Heparin by continuous infusion is usually started within an hour after urokinase has been stopped.

• Bruising is more likely during therapy; avoid unnecessary handling of patient. Side rails should be padded.

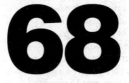

Alkylating agents

busulfan
carboplatin
carmustine
chlorambucil
cisplatin
cyclophosphamide
dacarbazine
ifosfamide
lomustine
mechlorethamine hydrochloride
melphalan
streptozocin
thiotepa
uracil mustard

COMBINATION PRODUCTS
None.

busulfan
Myleran
Pregnancy Risk Category: D

HOW SUPPLIED
Tablets: 2 mg

MECHANISM OF ACTION
Cross-links strands of cellular DNA
and interferes with RNA transcription, causing an imbalance of growth
that leads to cell death. Cell cycle-
nonspecific.

INDICATIONS & DOSAGE
*Chronic myelocytic (granulocytic)
leukemia—*
Adults: 4 to 8 mg P.O. daily up to 12
mg P.O. daily until WBC falls to
15,000/mm³; stop drug until WBC
rises to 50,000/mm³, then resume
treatment as before; or 4 to 8 mg P.O.

daily until WBC falls to 10,000 to
20,000/mm³, then reduce daily dosage as needed to maintain WBC at
this level (usually 2 mg daily).
Children: 0.06 to 0.12 mg/kg or 2.3
to 4.6 mg/m²/day P.O.; adjust dosage
to maintain WBC at 20,000/mm³, but
never less than 10,000/mm³.

ADVERSE REACTIONS
Blood: WBC falling after about 10
days and continuing to fall for 2
weeks after stopping drug; *thrombocytopenia,* leukopenia, anemia.
GI: nausea, vomiting, diarrhea, cheilosis, glossitis.
GU: amenorrhea, testicular atrophy,
impotence.
Metabolic: Addison-like wasting syndrome, profound hyperuricemia due
to increased cell lysis.
Skin: transient hyperpigmentation,
anhidrosis.
Other: gynecomastia; alopecia; *irreversible pulmonary fibrosis, commonly
termed "busulfan lung."*

INTERACTIONS
None significant.

NURSING CONSIDERATIONS
• Use cautiously in patients recently
given other myelosuppressive drugs or
radiation treatment, and in those with
depressed neutrophil or platelet
count.
• Warn patient to watch for signs of
infection (fever, sore throat, fatigue)
and bleeding (easy bruising, nosebleeds, bleeding gums, melena). Take
temperature daily.

Italicized adverse reactions are common or life-threatening.
*Liquid form contains alcohol.   **May contain tartrazine.

• Pulmonary fibrosis may occur as late as 4 to 6 months after treatment with busulfan.

• Persistent cough and progressive dyspnea with alveolar exudate may result from drug toxicity, not pneumonia. Instruct patient to report symptoms so dosage adjustments can be made.

• To prevent hyperuricemia with resulting uric acid nephropathy, allopurinol may be used with adequate hydration. Monitor serum uric acid.

• Patient response usually begins within 1 to 2 weeks (increased appetite, sense of well-being, decreased total leukocyte count, reduction in size of spleen).

• Anticoagulants and aspirin products should be used cautiously. Watch closely for signs of bleeding. Instruct patient to avoid any OTC product containing aspirin.

• Avoid all I.M. injections when platelets are below 100,000/mm³.

• Therapeutic effects are often accompanied by toxicity.

---

carboplatin
Paraplatin

Pregnancy Risk Category: D

HOW SUPPLIED
Injection: 50-mg, 150-mg, 450-mg vials

MECHANISM OF ACTION
A non-cell–cycle specific alkylating agent that produces cross-linking of strands of DNA.

INDICATIONS & DOSAGE
Palliative treatment of ovarian carcinoma—

Adults: 360 mg/m² I.V. on day 1 q 4 weeks; doses should not be repeated until platelet count exceeds 100,000/mm³ and neutrophil count exceeds 2,000/mm³. Subsequent doses are based on blood counts. Clinical trials have suggested the following dosage adjustments: if platelet count is above 100,000/mm³ and neutrophil count is above 2,000/mm³, dose administered should be 125% of the recommended starting dose. Dose should be reduced to 75% if platelet count falls below 50,000/mm³ or neutrophil count is below 500/mm³.

ADVERSE REACTIONS
Blood: *thrombocytopenia, leukopenia, neutropenia, anemia.*
CNS: dizziness, confusion, peripheral neuropathy, ototoxicity, central neurotoxicity.
GI: constipation, diarrhea, *nausea, vomiting.*
Other: alopecia, hypersensitivity, hepatotoxicity, *increased BUN, AST, or alkaline phosphatase.*

INTERACTIONS
Bone marrow depressants (including radiotherapy): increased hematologic toxicity.
Nephrotoxic agents: added nephrotoxicity of carboplatin.

NURSING CONSIDERATIONS
• Contraindicated in patients with a history of hypersensitivity to cisplatin, platinum-containing compounds, or mannitol.

• Carboplatin should be avoided in patients with severe bone marrow depression or bleeding.

• Administer this drug under the supervision of a doctor who is experienced in the use of chemotherapeutic agents.

• Determine serum electrolytes, creatinine, BUN, CBC, and creatinine clearance levels before the first infusion and before each course.

• Hydration or diuresis before or after treatment is not necessary.

• Transfusions may be necessary during treatment because of cumulative anemia.

• Bone marrow depression may be

---

more severe in patients with creatinine clearance below 60 ml/minute, and dosage adjustments are recommended for such patients. Patients with a creatinine clearance of 41 to 59 ml/minute should receive a starting dose of 250 mg/m^2; patients with a creatinine clearance of 16 to 40 ml/minute should receive a starting dose of 200 mg/m^2. Recommended dosage adjustments are not available for patients with a creatinine clearance of 15 ml/minute or less.

• Patients over 65 years are at greater risk for neurotoxicity.

• Dosage adjustments may be necessary in patients with decreased renal function.

• Exercise extreme caution when preparing or administering carboplatin to avoid mutagenic, teratogenic, and carcinogenic risks. Use a biological containment cabinet, wear gloves and mask, and use syringes with Luer-Lok fittings to prevent leakage of drug solution. Also correctly dispose of needles, vials, and unused drug, and avoid contaminating work surfaces. Avoid inhalation of dust or vapors and contact with skin or mucous membranes.

• Reconstitute with 5% dextrose in water (D$_5$W), 0.9% sodium chloride, or sterile water for injection to make a concentration of 10 mg/ml. Add 5 ml diluent to the 50-mg vial, 15 ml diluent to the 150-mg vial, or 45 ml diluent to the 450-mg vial. It can then be further diluted for infusion with 0.9% sodium chloride or D$_5$W. Concentration as low as 0.5 mg/ml can be prepared.

• Monitor CBC and platelet count frequently during therapy and, when indicated, until recovery. Leukocyte and platelet nadirs usually occur by day 21. Levels usually return to baseline by day 28. Don't repeat dose unless platelet count exceeds 100,000/mm^3.

• Unopened vials should be stored at room temperature. Once reconstituted and diluted as directed, drug is stable at room temperature for 8 hours. Because the drug does not contain antibacterial preservatives, unused drug should be discarded after 8 hours.

• Do not use needles or I.V. administration sets containing aluminum because carboplatin may precipitate and lose potency.

• Carboplatin can produce severe vomiting. Administer antiemetic therapy as ordered.

• Monitor vital signs during infusion.

• Check ordered dose against laboratory test results carefully. Only one increase in dosage is recommended. Subsequent doses should not exceed 125% of starting dose.

• Because of the possibility of infant toxicity, nursing mothers taking carboplatin should discontinue breast-feeding.

• Have epinephrine, corticosteroids, and antihistamines available when administering carboplatin because anaphylaxis-like reactions may occur within minutes of administration.

• Advise women of childbearing age to avoid becoming pregnant during therapy. Also recommend consulting with doctor before becoming pregnant.

carmustine (BCNU)
BiCNU

Pregnancy Risk Category: D

HOW SUPPLIED
Injection: 100-mg vial (lyophilized), with a 3-ml vial of absolute alcohol supplied as a diluent

MECHANISM OF ACTION
Cross-links strands of cellular DNA and interferes with RNA transcription, causing an imbalance of growth that leads to cell death. Cell cycle-nonspecific.

Italicized adverse reactions are common or life-threatening.
*Liquid form contains alcohol.   **May contain tartrazine.

INDICATIONS & DOSAGE

Brain, colon, and stomach cancer; Hodgkin's disease; non-Hodgkin's lymphomas; melanomas; multiple myeloma; and hepatoma—
Adults: 75 to 100 mg/m² I.V. by slow infusion daily for 2 days; repeat q 6 weeks if platelets are above 100,000/mm³ and WBC is above 4,000/mm³. Dosage is reduced 50% when WBC is less than 2,000/mm³ and platelets are less than 25,000/mm³.

Alternate therapy: 200 mg/m² I.V. slow infusion as a single dose, repeated q 6 to 8 weeks; or 40 mg/m² I.V. slow infusion for 5 consecutive days, repeated q 6 weeks.

ADVERSE REACTIONS

Blood: *cumulative bone marrow depression, delayed 4 to 6 weeks, lasting 1 to 2 weeks; leukopenia; thrombocytopenia.*
CNS: ataxia, drowsiness.
GI: *nausea, which begins in 2 to 6 hours (can be severe); vomiting.*
GU: nephrotoxicity.
Hepatic: hepatotoxicity.
Metabolic: possible hyperuricemia in lymphoma patients when rapid cell lysis occurs.
Skin: facial flushing.
Local: *intense pain at infusion site from venous spasm.*
Other: pulmonary fibrosis.

INTERACTIONS

Cimetidine: may increase carmustine's bone marrow toxicity. Avoid combination if possible.

NURSING CONSIDERATIONS

• To reduce pain on infusion, dilute further or slow infusion rate.
• Warn patient to watch for signs of infection (fever, sore throat, fatigue) and bleeding (easy bruising, nosebleeds, bleeding gums, melena). Take temperature daily.
• Monitor CBC.

• To reduce nausea, give antiemetic before administering.
• Don't mix with other drugs during administration.
• To reconstitute, dissolve 100 mg carmustine in 3 ml absolute alcohol provided by manufacturer. Dilute solution with 27 ml sterile water for injection. Resultant solution contains 3.3 mg carmustine/ml in 10% alcohol. Dilute in normal saline solution or dextrose 5% in water for I.V. infusion. Give at least 250 ml over 1 to 2 hours.
• May store reconstituted solution in refrigerator for 24 hours.
• May decompose at temperatures above 80° F. (26.6° C.).
• Solution is unstable in plastic I.V. bags. Administer only in glass containers.
• If powder liquefies or appears oily, it is a sign of decomposition. Discard.
• To prevent hyperuricemia with resulting uric acid nephropathy, allopurinol may be used with adequate hydration. Monitor serum uric acid.
• Avoid contact with skin, as carmustine will cause a brown stain. If drug comes into contact with skin, wash off thoroughly.
• Anticoagulants and aspirin products should be used cautiously. Watch closely for signs of bleeding. Instruct patient to avoid any OTC product containing aspirin.
• Avoid all I.M. injections when platelets are below 100,000/mm³.
• Since carmustine crosses the blood/brain barrier, it may be used to treat primary brain tumors.
• Preparation of parenteral form is associated with carcinogenic, mutagenic, and teratogenic risks for personnel. Follow institutional policy to reduce risks.
• Therapeutic effects are often accompanied by toxicity.

---

†Available in Canada only.   ‡Available in Australia only.   ◊ Available OTC.

chlorambucil
Leukeran

Pregnancy Risk Category: D

HOW SUPPLIED
Tablets: 2 mg

MECHANISM OF ACTION
Cross-links strands of cellular DNA and interferes with RNA transcription, causing an imbalance of growth that leads to cell death. Cell cycle-nonspecific.

INDICATIONS & DOSAGE
Chronic lymphocytic leukemia, diffuse lymphocytic lymphoma, nodular lymphocytic lymphoma, Hodgkin's disease, ovarian carcinoma, mycosis fungoides—
Adults: 0.1 to 0.2 mg/kg P.O. daily for 3 to 6 weeks, then adjust for maintenance (usually 2 mg daily).
Children: 0.1 to 0.2 mg/kg/day or 4.5 mg/m² P.O. daily as a single dose or in divided doses.

ADVERSE REACTIONS
Blood: leukopenia, delayed up to 3 weeks, lasting up to 10 days after last dose; thrombocytopenia; anemia; myelosuppression (usually moderate, gradual, and rapidly reversible).
CNS: seizures (with overdose).
GI: *nausea, vomiting.*
GU: *azoospermia, infertility.*
Metabolic: hyperuricemia, hepatotoxicity (rare).
Respiratory: interstitial pneumonitis or pulmonary fibrosis (rare).
Skin: *exfoliative dermatitis,* rash.
Other: allergic febrile reaction.

INTERACTIONS
None significant.

NURSING CONSIDERATIONS
• Place patient on neutropenia precautions if WBC falls below 2,000/

mm³ or granulocytes fall below 1,000/ mm³.
• Severe neutropenia reversible up to cumulative dosage of 6.5 mg/kg in a single course.
• Warn patient to watch for signs of infection (fever, sore throat, fatigue) and bleeding (easy bruising, nose-bleeds, bleeding gums, melena). Take temperature daily.
• Monitor CBC.
• To prevent hyperuricemia with resulting uric acid nephropathy, allopurinol may be used with adequate hydration. Monitor serum uric acid.
• Avoid all I.M. injections when platelets are below 100,000/mm³.
• Anticoagulants and aspirin products should be used cautiously. Watch closely for signs of bleeding. Instruct patient to avoid OTC products containing aspirin.
• Therapeutic effects are often accompanied by toxicity.

cisplatin (cis-platinum)
Platamine‡, Platinol

Pregnancy Risk Category: D

HOW SUPPLIED
Injection: 10-mg, 50-mg vials

MECHANISM OF ACTION
Cross-links strands of cellular DNA and interferes with RNA transcription, causing an imbalance of growth that leads to cell death. Cell cycle-nonspecific.

INDICATIONS & DOSAGE
Adjunctive therapy in metastatic testicular cancer—
Adults: 20 mg/m² I.V. daily for 5 days. Repeat every 3 weeks for 3 cycles or longer.
Adjunctive therapy in metastatic ovarian cancer—
100 mg/m² I.V. Repeat every 4 weeks; or 50 mg/m² I.V. every 3 weeks with concurrent doxorubicin HCl therapy.

Italicized adverse reactions are common or life-threatening.
*Liquid form contains alcohol.   **May contain tartrazine.

Give as I.V. infusion in 2 liters normal saline solution with 37.5 g mannitol over 6 to 8 hours.
Treatment of advanced bladder cancer—

Adults: 50 to 70 mg/m² I.V. once every 3 to 4 weeks. Patients who have received other antineoplastics or radiation therapy should receive 50 mg/m² every 4 weeks.

Note: Prehydration and mannitol diuresis may reduce renal toxicity and ototoxicity significantly.

ADVERSE REACTIONS
Blood: *mild myelosuppression in 25% to 30% of patients, leukopenia, thrombocytopenia,* anemia; nadirs in circulating platelets and leukocytes on days 18 to 23, with recovery by day 39.
CNS: peripheral neuritis, loss of taste, seizures.
EENT: *tinnitus, hearing loss.*
GI: *nausea, vomiting, beginning 1 to 4 hours after dose and lasting 24 hours; diarrhea;* metallic taste.
GU: *more prolonged and severe renal toxicity with repeated courses of therapy.*
Other: *anaphylactoid reaction.*

INTERACTIONS
Aminoglycoside antibiotics: additive nephrotoxicity. Monitor renal function studies very carefully.

NURSING CONSIDERATIONS
• Dosage modification may be required in preexisting renal impairment, myelosuppression, or hearing impairment.
• Hydrate patient with normal saline solution before giving drug. Maintain urine output of 100 ml/hour for 4 consecutive hours before therapy and for 24 hours after therapy.
• Mannitol may be given as 12.5 g I.V. bolus before starting cisplatin infusion. Follow, if ordered, by infusion of mannitol at rate of up to 10 g/hour

p.r.n. to maintain urine output during and 6 to 24 hours after cisplatin infusion.
• Some clinicians use I.V. sodium thiosulfate to minimize toxicity. Check current protocol.
• Do not repeat dosage unless platelets are over 100,000/mm³, WBC is over 4,000/mm³, creatinine is under 1.5 mg/dl, or BUN is under 25 mg/dl.
• Warn patient to watch for signs of infection (fever, sore throat, fatigue) and bleeding (easy bruising, nosebleeds, bleeding gums, melena). Take temperature daily.
• Monitor CBC, electrolytes (especially potassium and magnesium), platelets, and renal function studies before initial and subsequent dosages.
• To prevent deficiencies (10 to 20 mEq/L), potassium chloride is frequently added to I.V. fluids before and after cisplatin therapy.
• Tell patient to report tinnitus immediately to prevent permanent hearing loss. Do audiometry prior to initial dosage and subsequent courses.
• Nausea and vomiting may be severe and protracted (up to 24 hours). Antiemetics can be started 24 hours before therapy. Monitor intake/output. Continue I.V. hydration until patient can tolerate adequate oral intake.
• Delayed-onset vomiting (3 to 5 days after treatment) has been reported. Patients may need prolonged antiemetic treatment.
• Reconstitute with sterile water for injection. Stable for 24 hours in normal saline solution at room temperature. Don't refrigerate.
• Infusions are most stable in chloride-containing solutions (such as normal saline, 0.45% normal saline, and 0.22% normal saline).
• Given with bleomycin and vinblastine for testicular cancer and with doxorubicin for ovarian cancer.
• Renal toxicity is cumulative. Renal function must return to normal before next dose can be given.

• Avoid all I.M. injections when platelets are below 100,000/mm³.

• Metoclopramide has been used very effectively to treat and prevent nausea and vomiting.

• Anaphylactoid reaction usually responds to immediate treatment with epinephrine, corticosteroids, or antihistamines.

• Preparation of parenteral form is associated with carcinogenic, mutagenic, and teratogenic risks for personnel. Follow institutional policy to reduce risks.

• Therapeutic effects are often accompanied by toxicity.

cyclophosphamide
Cycoblastin‡, Cytoxan**, Cytoxan Lyophilized, Endoxan-Asta‡, Neosar, Procytox†

Pregnancy Risk Category: D

HOW SUPPLIED
Tablets: 25 mg, 50 mg
Injection: 100-mg, 200-mg, 500-mg, 1-g, 2-g vials

MECHANISM OF ACTION
Cross-links strands of cellular DNA and interferes with RNA transcription, causing an imbalance of growth that leads to cell death. Cell cycle-nonspecific.

INDICATIONS & DOSAGE
Breast, head, neck, lung, and ovarian cancer; Hodgkin's disease; chronic lymphocytic leukemia; chronic myelocytic leukemia; acute lymphoblastic leukemia; neuroblastoma; retinoblastoma; non-Hodgkin's lymphomas; multiple myeloma; mycosis fungoides; sarcomas—
Adults: initially, 40 to 50 mg/kg I.V. in divided doses over 2 to 5 days; then adjust for maintenance. Or 1 to 5 mg/kg P.O. daily, depending upon patient tolerance. Maintenance dosage is 1 to 5 mg/kg P.O. daily; or 10 to 15 mg/kg q 7 to 10 days I.V.; or 3 to 5 mg/kg I.V. twice weekly.
Children: 2 to 8 mg/kg daily or 60 to 250 mg/m² daily P.O. or I.V. for 6 days (dosage depends on susceptibility of neoplasm). Maintenance dosage 2 to 5 mg/kg or 50 to 150 mg/m² P.O. twice weekly.

ADVERSE REACTIONS
Blood: *leukopenia,* nadir between days 8 to 15, recovery in 17 to 28 days; thrombocytopenia; anemia.
CV: *cardiotoxicity* (with very high doses and in combination with doxorubicin).
GI: anorexia; *nausea and vomiting beginning within 6 hours, lasting 4 hours;* stomatitis; mucositis.
GU: gonadal suppression (may be irreversible), *hemorrhagic cystitis,* bladder fibrosis, nephrotoxicity.
Metabolic: hyperuricemia; syndrome of inappropriate antidiuretic hormone secretion (with high doses).
Other: *reversible alopecia in 50% of patients, especially with high doses;* secondary malignancies, *pulmonary fibrosis (high doses).*

INTERACTIONS
Barbiturates: increased pharmacologic effect and enhanced cyclophosphamide toxicity due to induction of hepatic enzymes.
Cardiotoxic drugs: additive adverse cardiac effects.
Corticosteroids, chloramphenicol: reduced activity of cyclophosphamide. Use cautiously.
Succinylcholine: may cause apnea. Don't use together.

NURSING CONSIDERATIONS
• Dosage modification may be required in severe leukopenia, thrombocytopenia, malignant cell infiltration of bone marrow, recent radiation therapy or chemotherapy, or hepatic or renal disease.
• Advise both male and female pa-

Italicized adverse reactions are common or life-threatening.
*Liquid form contains alcohol.   **May contain tartrazine.

tients to practice contraception while taking this drug and for 4 months after; drug is potentially teratogenic.
• Monitor CBC and renal and hepatic functions.
• Encourage fluid intake (3 liters daily) to prevent hemorrhagic cystitis. Don't give drug at bedtime, because voiding is too infrequent to avoid cystitis. If hemorrhagic cystitis occurs, discontinue drug. Cystitis can occur months after therapy has been stopped.
• Encourage patients to void every 1 to 2 hours while awake to minimize risk of hemorrhagic cystitis.
• Lyophilized preparation is much easier to reconstitute. Request this form from the pharmacy when preparing I.V.
• Reconstituted solution is stable 6 days refrigerated or 24 hours at room temperature.
• Check reconstituted solution for small particles. Filter solution if necessary.
• Avoid all I.M. injections when platelets are below 100,000/mm³.
• Can be given by direct I.V. push into a running I.V. line or by infusion in normal saline solution or dextrose 5% in water.
• To prevent hyperuricemia with resulting uric acid nephropathy, allopurinol may be used with adequate hydration. Monitor serum uric acid.
• Warn patient that alopecia is likely to occur, but that it is reversible.
• Monitor for cyclophosphamide toxicity if patient's corticosteroid therapy is discontinued.
• Preparation of parenteral form is associated with carcinogenic, mutagenic, and teratogenic risks for personnel. Follow institutional policy to reduce risks.
• Therapeutic effects are often accompanied by toxicity.

dacarbazine (DTIC)
DTIC-Dome
Pregnancy Risk Category: C

HOW SUPPLIED
Injection: 100-mg, 200-mg vials

MECHANISM OF ACTION
Cross-links strands of cellular DNA and interferes with RNA transcription, causing an imbalance of growth that leads to cell death. Cell cycle-nonspecific.

INDICATIONS & DOSAGE
Metastatic malignant melanoma—
Adults: 2 to 4.5 mg/kg or 70 to 160 mg/m² I.V. daily for 10 days, then repeat q 4 weeks as tolerated; or 250 mg/m² I.V. daily for 5 days, repeated at 3-week intervals.
Hodgkin's disease—
Adults: 150 mg/m² I.V. daily (in combination with other agents) for 5 days, repeated q 4 weeks; or 375 mg/m² on the first day of a combination regimen, repeated q 15 days.

ADVERSE REACTIONS
Blood: *leukopenia and thrombocytopenia,* nadir between 3 and 4 weeks.
GI: *severe nausea and vomiting begin within 1 to 3 hours in 90% of patients, last 1 to 12 hours; anorexia.*
Metabolic: increased liver enzymes, hepatotoxicity (rare).
Skin: phototoxicity.
Local: severe pain if I.V. infiltrates or if solution is too concentrated; tissue damage.
Other: *flu-like syndrome* (fever, malaise, myalgia beginning 7 days after treatment stopped and possibly lasting 7 to 21 days), alopecia, *anaphylaxis.*

INTERACTIONS
None significant.

NURSING CONSIDERATIONS
- Contraindicated in patients with hypersensitivity to the drug.
- Use lower dosage if renal or bone marrow function is impaired. Stop drug if WBC falls to 3,000/mm³ or platelets drop to 100,000/mm³. Monitor CBC.
- Warn patient to watch for signs of infection (fever, sore throat, fatigue) and bleeding (easy bruising, nosebleeds, bleeding gums, melena). Take temperature daily.
- Discard refrigerated solution after 72 hours and room temperature solution after 8 hours.
- Avoid all I.M. injections when platelets are below 100,000/mm³.
- Give I.V. infusion in 50 to 100 ml dextrose 5% in water over 30 minutes. May dilute further or slow infusion to decrease pain at infusion site. Make sure drug does not infiltrate.
- If I.V. infiltrates, discontinue immediately and apply ice to area for 24 to 48 hours.
- During infusion, protect bag from direct sunlight to avoid possible drug breakdown.
- For Hodgkin's disease, usually given with bleomycin, vinblastine, and doxorubicin.
- Advise patient to avoid sunlight and sunlamps for first 2 days after treatment.
- Anticoagulants and aspirin products should be used cautiously. Watch closely for signs of bleeding. Instruct patient to avoid OTC products containing aspirin.
- Administering antiemetics before giving dacarbazine may help decrease nausea. Nausea and vomiting may sometimes subside after several doses.
- Reassure patient that flulike syndrome may be treated with mild antipyretics, such as acetaminophen.
- Preparation of parenteral form is associated with carcinogenic, mutagenic, and teratogenic risks for personnel. Follow institutional policy to reduce risks.
- Therapeutic effects are often accompanied by toxicity.

ifosfamide
Ifex

Pregnancy Risk Category: D

HOW SUPPLIED
Injection: 1 g (supplied with 200-mg ampule of mesna), 2 g†, 3 g†

MECHANISM OF ACTION
Cross-links strands of cellular DNA, and interferes with RNA transcription causing an imbalance of growth that leads to cell death. Cell cycle-nonspecific.

INDICATIONS & DOSAGE
Testicular cancer—
Adults: 1.2 g/m²/day I.V. for 5 consecutive days. Treatment is repeated every 3 weeks or after the patient recovers from hematologic toxicity.

ADVERSE REACTIONS
Blood: leukopenia, thrombocytopenia, *myelosuppression.*
CNS: *lethargy, somnolence, confusion, depressive psychosis,* coma.
GI: *nausea, vomiting.*
GU: hemorrhagic cystitis *(dose-limiting adverse reaction occurring in up to 50% of patients), hematuria,* nephrotoxicity.
Hepatic: elevated liver enzymes.
Other: *alopecia.*

INTERACTIONS
Allopurinol: may produce excessive ifosfamide effect by prolonging half-life. Monitor for enhanced toxicity.
Barbiturates: induce hepatic enzymes, hastening the formation of toxic metabolites. Ifosfamide toxicity may be increased.
Corticosteroids: may inhibit hepatic enzymes, reducing ifosfamide's ef-

---

Italicized adverse reactions are common or life-threatening.
*Liquid form contains alcohol.   **May contain tartrazine.

fect. Monitor for enhanced ifosfamide toxicity if concurrent steroid dosage is suddenly reduced or discontinued. *Myelosuppressants:* enhanced hematologic toxicity. Dosage adjustment may be necessary.

NURSING CONSIDERATIONS
• Use cautiously in renal or hepatic impairment.
• Ifosfamide should be administered with a protecting agent (mesna) to prevent hemorrhagic cystitis. Adequate fluid intake (2 liters/day, either P.O. or I.V.) is essential.
• Obtain a urinalysis prior to each dose. If microscopic hematuria is present, drug should be witheld until it resolves.
• Bladder irrigation with normal saline solution may decrease the possibility of cystitis.
• Avoid giving the drug at bedtime, because infrequent voiding during the night may increase the possibility of cystitis. Stop the drug if patient develops cystitis.
• Warn patient to watch for signs of infection (fever, sore throat, fatigue) and bleeding (easy bruising, nosebleeds, bleeding gums, melena). Take temperature daily.
• Avoid all I.M. injections when platelets are below 100,000/mm³.
• Anticoagulants and aspirin products should be used cautiously. Watch closely for signs of bleeding. Instruct patient to avoid OTC products containing aspirin.
• Administering antiemetics before giving ifosfamide may help decrease nausea.
• Assess patient for changes in mental status and cerebellar dysfunction. Dosage may have to be decreased.
• Prepare I.V. solution by reconstituting 1 gram vial with 20 ml sterile water for injection or bacteriostatic water for injection to yield a solution of 50 mg/ml. It may then be further diluted with sterile water, dextrose

2.5% or 5% in water, 0.45% or 0.9% sodium chloride injection, 5% dextrose and 9% sodium chloride injection, or Ringer's lactated injection.
• Reconstituted solution is stable 1 week at room temperature or 3 weeks refrigerated. However, use solution within 6 hours if drug was reconstituted with sterile water without a preservative (such as benzyl alcohol or parabens).
• Infusing each dose slowly (over at least 30 minutes)will decrease possibility of cystitis.
• Monitor CBC and renal and liver function tests.
• Monitor patient for CNS changes.
• Preparation of parenteral form is associated with carcinogenic, mutagenic, and teratogenic risks for personnel. Follow institutional policy to reduce risks.

lomustine (CCNU)
CeeNU

Pregnancy Risk Category: D

HOW SUPPLIED
Capsules: 10 mg, 40 mg, 100 mg, dose pack (2 100-mg, 2 40-mg, 2 10-mg capsules)

MECHANISM OF ACTION
Cross-links strands of cellular DNA and interferes with RNA transcription, causing an imbalance of growth that leads to cell death. Cell cycle-nonspecific.

INDICATIONS & DOSAGE
Brain tumors, Hodgkin's disease—
Adults and children: 130 mg/m² P.O. as a single dose q 6 weeks. Reduce dosage according to degree of bone marrow suppression. Repeat doses should not be given until WBC is more than 4,000/mm³ and platelet count is more than 100,000/mm³.

ADVERSE REACTIONS

Blood: *leukopenia, delayed up to 6 weeks, lasting 1 to 2 weeks; thrombocytopenia, delayed up to 4 weeks, lasting 1 to 2 weeks.*
GI: *nausea and vomiting beginning within 4 to 5 hours, lasting 24 hours;* stomatitis.
GU: nephrotoxicity, progressive azotemia.

INTERACTIONS

None significant.

NURSING CONSIDERATIONS

• Dosage modification may be required in patients with decreased platelets, leukocytes, or erythrocytes, and in patients receiving other myelosuppressive drugs.
• Give 2 to 4 hours after meals. Lomustine will be more completely absorbed if taken when the stomach is empty. To avoid nausea, give antiemetic before administering.
• May be useful in cancer involving CNS, since cerebrospinal fluid level equals 30% to 50% of plasma level 1 hour after administration.
• Monitor CBC weekly. Usually not administered more often than every 6 weeks; bone marrow toxicity is cumulative and delayed.
• Warn patient to watch for signs of infection (fever, sore throat, fatigue) and bleeding (easy bruising, nosebleeds, bleeding gums, melena). Take temperature daily.
• Monitor serum uric acid.
• Periodically monitor liver function.
• Avoid all I.M. injections when platelets are below 100,000/mm³.
• Anticoagulants and aspirin products should be used cautiously. Watch closely for signs of bleeding. Instruct patient to avoid OTC products containing aspirin.
• Since lomustine crosses the blood/brain barrier, it may be used to treat primary brain tumors.

• Therapeutic effects are often accompanied by toxicity.

mechlorethamine hydrochloride (nitrogen mustard)

Mustargen

Pregnancy Risk Category: D

HOW SUPPLIED

Injection: 10-mg vials

MECHANISM OF ACTION

Cross-links strands of cellular DNA and interferes with RNA transcription, causing an imbalance of growth that leads to cell death. Cell cycle-nonspecific.

INDICATIONS & DOSAGE

Breast, lung, and ovarian cancer; Hodgkin's disease; non-Hodgkin's lymphomas; diffuse lymphocytic lymphoma—
Adults: 0.4 mg/kg or 10 mg/m² I.V. as a single dose or in divided doses q 3 to 6 weeks. Give through running I.V. infusion. Dosage reduced in prior radiation or chemotherapy to 0.2 to 0.4 mg/kg. Dosage based on ideal or actual body weight, whichever is less.
Neoplastic effusions—
Adults: 0.4 mg/kg intracavitarily.
Mycosis fungoides—
Adults: topical solution or ointment applied to lesion. Topical preparations must be compounded by pharmacist; drug concentration, frequency of application, and duration of therapy will vary according to patient tolerance and response. Mechlorethamine ointments of 0.01% to 0.02% and topical solutions containing 10 mg/50 to 60 ml have been used.

ADVERSE REACTIONS

Blood: *nadir of myelosuppression occurring by days 4 to 10, lasting 10 to 21 days;* mild anemia begins in 2 to 3 weeks, possibly lasting 7 weeks.

Italicized adverse reactions are common or life-threatening.
*Liquid form contains alcohol.   **May contain tartrazine.

CNS: headache.
EENT: tinnitus; *metallic taste* (immediately after dose); deafness with high doses.
GI: *nausea, vomiting, and anorexia* begin within minutes, last 8 to 24 hours.
Metabolic: hyperuricemia.
Skin: rash.
Local: *thrombophlebitis, sloughing, severe irritation if drug extravasates or touches skin.*
Other: *alopecia,* may precipitate herpes zoster, *anaphylaxis.*

INTERACTIONS
Procarbazine, cyclophosphamide: possible increased risk of hepatotoxicity.

NURSING CONSIDERATIONS
• Dosage modification may be required in severe anemia, depressed neutrophil or platelet count, or in patients recently treated with radiation or chemotherapy. Monitor CBC.
• Avoid contact with skin or mucous membranes. Wear gloves when preparing solution to prevent accidental skin contact. If contact occurs, wash with copious amounts of water.
• Mechlorethamine is a potent vesicant. Be sure I.V. doesn't infiltrate. If drug extravasates, apply cold compresses and infiltrate the area with isotonic sodium thiosulfate.
• When given intracavitarily for sclerosing effect, turn patient from side to side every 15 minutes to 1 hour to distribute drug.
• Very unstable solution. Prepare immediately before infusion. Use within 15 minutes. Discard unused solution.
• To prevent hyperuricemia with resulting uric acid nephropathy, mechlorethamine may be used with adequate hydration. Monitor serum uric acid.
• Avoid all I.M. injections when platelets are below 100,000/mm³.
• Warn patient to watch for signs of

infection (fever, sore throat, fatigue) and bleeding (easy bruising, nosebleeds, bleeding gums, melena). Take temperature daily.
• Anticoagulants and aspirin products should be used cautiously. Watch closely for signs of bleeding. Instruct patient to avoid OTC products containing aspirin.
• Any equipment used in the preparation and administration of mechlorethamine should be disposed of properly and according to institutional policy. Unused solution should be neutralized with an equal volume of 5% sodium bicarbonate and 5% sodium thiosulfate.
• Preparation of parenteral form is associated with carcinogenic, mutagenic, and teratogenic risks for personnel. Follow institutional policy to reduce risks.
• Therapeutic effects are often accompanied by toxicity.

melphalan (L-phenylalanine mustard)
Alkeran

Pregnancy Risk Category: D

HOW SUPPLIED
Tablets (scored): 2 mg

MECHANISM OF ACTION
Cross-links strands of cellular DNA and interferes with RNA transcription, causing an imbalance of growth that leads to cell death. Cell cycle-nonspecific.

INDICATIONS & DOSAGE
Multiple myeloma—
Adults: initially, 6 mg P.O. daily for 2 to 3 weeks, then stop drug for up to 4 weeks or until WBC and platelets stop dropping and begin to rise again; resume with maintenance dosage of 2 mg daily. Stop drug if WBC is below 3,000/mm³ or platelets are below 100,000/mm³. Alternate therapy:

0.15 mg/kg P.O. daily for 7 days, or 0.25 mg/kg for 4 days; repeat q 4 to 6 weeks.

Nonresectable advanced ovarian cancer—

Adults: 0.2 mg/kg P.O. daily for 5 days. Repeat q 4 to 5 weeks, depending on bone marrow recovery.

ADVERSE REACTIONS

Blood: *thrombocytopenia, leukopenia, agranulocytosis.*
Skin: rash, alopecia.
Other: *pneumonitis and pulmonary fibrosis, anaphylaxis.*

INTERACTIONS

None significant.

NURSING CONSIDERATIONS

• Not recommended in severe leukopenia, thrombocytopenia, or anemia; or in chronic lymphocytic leukemia.
• Monitor serum uric acid and CBC.
• Avoid all I.M. injections when platelets are below 100,000/mm³.
• May need dosage reduction in renal impairment.
• Therapeutic effects are often accompanied by toxicity.
• Drug of choice in multiple myeloma in combination with prednisone.
• Anticoagulants and aspirin products should be used cautiously. Watch closely for signs of bleeding. Instruct patient to avoid OTC products containing aspirin.
• Administer on empty stomach, because absorption is decreased by food.
• Warn patient to watch for signs of infection (fever, sore throat, fatigue) and bleeding (easy bruising, nosebleeds, bleeding gums, melena). Take temperature daily.

streptozocin
Zanosar
Pregnancy Risk Category: C

HOW SUPPLIED
Injection: 1-g vials

MECHANISM OF ACTION
Cross-links strands of cellular DNA and interferes with RNA transcription, causing an imbalance of growth that leads to cell death. Cell cycle-nonspecific.

INDICATIONS & DOSAGE
Treatment of metastatic islet cell carcinoma of the pancreas; colon cancer; exocrine pancreatic tumors; and carcinoid tumors—
Adults and children: 500 mg/m² I.V. for 5 consecutive days q 6 weeks until maximum benefit or until toxicity is observed. Alternatively, 1,000 mg/m² at weekly intervals for the first 2 weeks. Don't exceed a single dose of 1,500 mg/m².

ADVERSE REACTIONS
Blood: *leukopenia, thrombocytopenia.*
GI: *nausea, vomiting,* diarrhea.
Hepatic: elevated liver enzymes.
Metabolic: hyperglycemia and hypoglycemia.
Renal: *renal toxicity (evidenced by azotemia, glycosuria, and renal tubular acidosis),* mild proteinuria.
Local: *sloughing, severe irritation if extravasation occurs.*

INTERACTIONS
Doxorubicin: prolonged elimination half-life of doxorubicin if administered with streptozocin. Dose of doxorubicin should be reduced.
Other potentially nephrotoxic drugs such as aminoglycosides: increased risk of renal toxicity. Use cautiously.
Phenytoin: may decrease the effects of streptozocin. Monitor carefully.

Italicized adverse reactions are common or life-threatening.
*Liquid form contains alcohol.   **May contain tartrazine.

NURSING CONSIDERATIONS

• Dosage modification may be required in patients with preexisting renal or hepatic disease.

• Renal toxicity resulting from streptozocin therapy is dose-related and cumulative. Monitor renal function before and after each course of therapy. Urinalysis, BUN, creatinine, serum electrolytes, and creatinine clearance should be obtained before, and at least weekly during, drug administration. Weekly monitoring should continue for 4 weeks after each course.

• Mild proteinuria is one of the first signs of renal toxicity. Make sure doctor is aware if and when this occurs. The dosage of the drug may have to be reduced.

• Test urine for protein and glucose each nursing shift.

• Monitor CBC and liver function studies at least weekly.

• Warn patient to watch for signs of infection (fever, sore throat, fatigue) and bleeding (easy bruising, nosebleeds, bleeding gums, melena). Take temperature daily.

• Nausea and vomiting occurs in almost *all* patients. Make sure patient is being treated with an antiemetic.

• Reconstitute the streptozocin powder with 0.9% sodium chloride injection. This will produce a pale gold solution.

• Best to use within 12 hours of reconstitution. However, drug will remain stable for at least 48 hours, especially if kept refrigerated.

• The product contains no preservatives and is not intended as a multiple-dose vial.

• When preparing the solution, wear gloves to protect the skin from contact. If contact occurs, wash with copious amounts of water.

• Unopened and unreconstituted vials of streptozocin should be stored in the refrigerator.

• Preparation of parenteral form is associated with carcinogenic, mutagenic, and teratogenic risks for personnel. Follow institutional policy to reduce risks.

• Therapeutic effects are often accompanied by toxicity.

thiotepa
Thiotepa

Pregnancy Risk Category: D

HOW SUPPLIED
Injection: 15-mg vials

MECHANISM OF ACTION
Cross-links strands of cellular DNA and interferes with RNA transcription, causing an imbalance of growth that leads to cell death. Cell cycle-nonspecific.

INDICATIONS & DOSAGE
Breast and ovarian cancer; lymphomas and bronchogenic carcinomas—
Adults and children over 12 years:
0.2 mg/kg I.V. daily for 4 to 5 days at intervals of 2 to 4 weeks.
Bladder tumor—
Adults and children over 12 years:
60 mg in 60 ml water instilled in bladder for 2 hours once weekly for 4 weeks.
Neoplastic effusions—
Adults and children over 12 years:
0.6 to 0.8 mg/kg intracavitarily, p.r.n. Stop drug or decrease dosage if WBC is below 4,000/mm³ or if platelets are below 150,000/mm³.
Malignant meningeal neoplasms—
Adults: 1 to 10 mg/m² intrathecally once or twice weekly.

ADVERSE REACTIONS
Blood: *leukopenia begins within 5 to 30 days; thrombocytopenia; neutropenia.*
GI: *nausea, vomiting.*
GU: amenorrhea, decreased spermatogenesis.
Metabolic: hyperuricemia.

Skin: hives, rash.
Local: intense pain at administration site.
Other: headache, fever, tightness of throat, dizziness.

INTERACTIONS
Succinylcholine: prolonged neuromuscular blockade.

NURSING CONSIDERATIONS
• Use cautiously in bone marrow suppression and renal or hepatic dysfunction.
• Monitor CBC weekly for at least 3 weeks after last dosage. Warn patient to report even mild infections.
• GU adverse reactions reversible in 6 to 8 months.
• May require use of local anesthetic at injection site if intense pain occurs.
• For bladder instillation: Dehydrate patient 8 to 10 hours before therapy. Instill drug into bladder by catheter; ask patient to retain solution for 2 hours. Volume may be reduced to 30 ml if discomfort is too great with 60 ml. Reposition patient every 15 minutes for maximum area contact.
• Toxicity delayed and prolonged because drug binds to tissues and stays in body several hours.
• Refrigerate dry powder; protect from light.
• Use only sterile water for injection to reconstitute. Refrigerated solution is stable for 5 days.
• To prevent hyperuricemia with resulting uric acid nephropathy, allopurinol may be used with adequate hydration. Monitor serum uric acid.
• Avoid all I.M. injections when platelets are below 100,000/mm³.
• Warn patient to watch for signs of infection (fever, sore throat, fatigue) and bleeding (easy bruising, nosebleeds, bleeding gums, melena). Take temperature daily.
• Can be given by all parenteral routes, including direct injection into the tumor.

• Anticoagulants and aspirin products should be used cautiously. Watch closely for signs of bleeding. Instruct patient to avoid OTC products containing aspirin.
• Preparation of parenteral form is associated with carcinogenic, mutagenic, and teratogenic risks for personnel. Follow institutional policy to reduce risks.
• Therapeutic effects are often accompanied by toxicity.

uracil mustard
Uracil Mustard Capsules**
Pregnancy Risk Category: X

HOW SUPPLIED
Capsules: 1 mg

MECHANISM OF ACTION
Cross-links strands of cellular DNA and interferes with RNA transcription, causing an imbalance of growth that leads to cell death. Cell cycle-nonspecific.

INDICATIONS & DOSAGE
Chronic lymphocytic and myelocytic leukemia; Hodgkin's disease; non-Hodgkin's lymphomas of the histiocytic and lymphocytic types; reticulum cell sarcoma; lymphomas; mycosis fungoides; polycythemia vera; cancer of ovaries, cervix, and lungs—
Adults: 1 to 2 mg P.O. daily for 3 months or until desired response or toxicity; maintenance dosage is 1 mg daily for 3 out of 4 weeks until optimum response or relapse; or 3 to 5 mg P.O. for 7 days not to exceed total dosage of 0.5 mg/kg, then 1 mg daily until response, then 1 mg daily 3 out of 4 weeks.

ADVERSE REACTIONS
Blood: bone marrow suppression, delayed 2 to 4 weeks; *thrombocytopenia; leukopenia;* anemia.

Italicized adverse reactions are common or life-threatening.
*Liquid form contains alcohol.   **May contain tartrazine.

CNS: irritability, nervousness, mental cloudiness, and depression.
GI: *nausea, vomiting, diarrhea, epigastric distress,* abdominal pain, anorexia.
Metabolic: hyperuricemia.
Skin: pruritus, dermatitis, hyperpigmentation, alopecia.

INTERACTIONS
None significant.

NURSING CONSIDERATIONS
• Dosage modification may be required in severe thrombocytopenia, aplastic anemia, leukopenia, or acute leukemia.
• Give at bedtime to reduce nausea.
• Warn patient to watch for signs of infection (fever, sore throat, fatigue) and bleeding (easy bruising, nosebleeds, bleeding gums, melena). Take temperature daily.
• Monitor platelet count. Check CBC once or twice weekly for 4 weeks; then 4 weeks after stopping drug.
• To prevent hyperuricemia and resulting uric acid nephropathy, allopurinol may be used with adequate hydration. Monitor serum uric acid.
• Avoid all I.M. injections when platelets are below 100,000/mm³.
• Warn patient to watch for signs of infection (fever, sore throat, fatigue) and bleeding (easy bruising, nosebleeds, bleeding gums, melena). Take temperature daily.
• Anticoagulants and aspirin products should be used cautiously. Watch closely for signs of bleeding. Instruct patient to avoid OTC products containing aspirin.
• Therapeutic effects are often accompanied by toxicity.

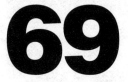

69

Antimetabolites

cytarabine
floxuridine
fluorouracil
hydroxyurea
mercaptopurine
methotrexate
methotrexate sodium
thioguanine
trimetrexate gluconate

COMBINATION PRODUCTS
None.

cytarabine (ara-C, cytosine arabinoside)
Alexan‡, Cytosar-U

Pregnancy Risk Category: D

HOW SUPPLIED
Injection: 40-mg‡, 100-mg, 500-mg vials

MECHANISM OF ACTION
Inhibits DNA synthesis.

INDICATIONS & DOSAGE
Acute myelocytic and other acute leukemias—
Adults and children: 200 mg/m² daily by continuous I.V. infusion for 5 days.
Meningeal leukemias and meningeal neoplasms—
Adults and children: 10 to 30 mg/m² intrathecally once every 4 days.

ADVERSE REACTIONS
Blood: WBC nadir 5 to 7 days after drug stopped; *leukopenia,* anemia, *thrombocytopenia,* reticulocytopenia; platelet nadir occurring on day 10; *megaloblastosis.*
CNS: neurotoxicity with high doses.
EENT: *keratitis.*
GI: *nausea, vomiting,* diarrhea, dysphagia; reddened area at juncture of lips, followed by sore mouth, oral ulcers in 5 to 10 days; high dose given via rapid I.V. may cause projectile vomiting.
Hepatic: hepatotoxicity (usually mild and reversible).
Metabolic: hyperuricemia.
Skin: rash.
Other: flulike syndrome.

INTERACTIONS
None significant.

NURSING CONSIDERATIONS
• Dosage modification may be required in thrombocytopenia, leukopenia, renal or hepatic disease, and after other chemotherapy or radiation therapy.
• Watch for signs of infection (cough, fever, sore throat) and bleeding (easy bruising, nosebleeds, bleeding gums). Monitor CBC.
• Excellent mouth care can help prevent stomatitis.
• Nausea and vomiting more frequent when large doses are administered rapidly by I.V. push. These reactions are less frequent with infusion. To reduce nausea, give antiemetic before administering.
• Steroid eye drops are prescribed to prevent drug-induced keratitis.
• Monitor intake/output carefully. Maintain high fluid intake and give

Italicized adverse reactions are common or life-threatening.
*Liquid form contains alcohol.   **May contain tartrazine.

allopurinol, if ordered, to avoid urate nephropathy in leukemia induction therapy. Monitor serum uric acid.
• Monitor hepatic function.
• Use preservative-free normal saline or Elliot's B solution for intrathecal use.
• Reconstituted solution is stable for 48 hours. Discard cloudy reconstituted solution.
• Avoid I.M. injections of any drugs in patients with thrombocytopenia to prevent bleeding.
• Warn patient to watch for signs of infection (fever, sore throat, fatigue) and bleeding (easy bruising, nosebleeds, bleeding gums, melena). Take temperature daily.
• Modify or discontinue therapy if polymorphonuclear granulocyte count is below 1,000/mm³ or if platelet count is below 50,000/mm³.
• Assess patients receiving high doses for neurotoxicity. May first appear as nystagmus, but can progress to ataxia and cerebellar dysfunction.
• Preparation of parenteral form is associated with carcinogenic, mutagenic, and teratogenic risks for personnel. Follow institutional policy to reduce risks.

floxuridine
FUDR

Pregnancy Risk Category: D

HOW SUPPLIED
Injection: 500-mg vials (50 mg/ml in 10-ml vials or 100 mg/ml in 5-ml vials)

MECHANISM OF ACTION
Inhibits DNA synthesis.

INDICATIONS & DOSAGE
Brain, breast, head, neck, liver, gallbladder, and bile duct cancer—
Adults: 0.1 to 0.6 mg/kg daily by intraarterial infusion (use pump for continuous, uniform rate); or 0.4 to 0.6 mg/kg daily into hepatic artery.

ADVERSE REACTIONS
Blood: *leukopenia, anemia,* thrombocytopenia.
CNS: cerebellar ataxia, vertigo, nystagmus, seizures, depression, hemiplegia, hiccups, lethargy.
EENT: blurred vision.
GI: *stomatitis, cramps, nausea, vomiting, diarrhea, bleeding, enteritis.*
Hepatic: cholangitis, jaundice, elevated liver enzymes.
Skin: *erythema,* dermatitis, pruritus, rash.

INTERACTIONS
None significant.

NURSING CONSIDERATIONS
• Dosage modification may be required in poor nutritional state, bone marrow suppression, or serious infection. Use cautiously following high-dose pelvic irradiation or use of alkylating agent, and in impaired hepatic or renal function.
• Severe skin and GI adverse reactions require stopping drug. Use of antacid eases but probably won't prevent GI distress.
• Excellent mouth care can help prevent stomatitis.
• Monitor intake/output, CBC, and renal and hepatic function.
• Discontinue if WBC falls below 3,500/mm³ or if platelet count below 100,000/mm³.
• Therapeutic effect may be delayed 1 to 6 weeks. Make sure patient is aware of time it may take for improvement to be noted.
• Reconstitute with sterile water for injection. Dilute further in dextrose 5% in water or normal saline solution for actual infusion.
• Avoid I.M. injections of any drugs in patients with thrombocytopenia to prevent bleeding.

• Refrigerated solution is stable for no more than 2 weeks.
• Check line for bleeding, blockage, displacement, or leakage.
• Preparation of parenteral form is associated with carcinogenic, mutagenic, and teratogenic risks for personnel. Follow institutional policy to reduce risks.

fluorouracil (5-fluorouracil, 5-FU)
Adrucil

Pregnancy Risk Category: D

HOW SUPPLIED
Injection: 50 mg/ml

MECHANISM OF ACTION
Inhibits DNA synthesis.

INDICATIONS & DOSAGE
Colon, rectal, breast, ovarian, cervical, bladder, liver, and pancreatic cancer—
Adults: 12.5 mg/kg I.V. daily for 3 to 5 days q 4 weeks; or 15 mg/kg weekly for 6 weeks. (Dosages recommended based on lean body weight.) Maximum single recommended dose is 800 mg, although higher single doses (up to 1.5 g) have been used. The injectable form has been given orally but is not recommended.

ADVERSE REACTIONS
Blood: *leukopenia,* thrombocytopenia, anemia; WBC nadir 9 to 14 days after first dose; platelet nadir in 7 to 14 days.
CNS: acute cerebellar syndrome.
GI: *stomatitis, GI ulcer may precede leukopenia, nausea, vomiting in 30% to 50% of patients; diarrhea.*
Skin: *dermatitis,* hyperpigmentation (especially in blacks), nail changes, pigmented palmar creases.
Other: *reversible alopecia in 5% to 20% of patients, weakness, malaise.*

INTERACTIONS
None significant.

NURSING CONSIDERATIONS
• Use cautiously following major surgery; when patient is in poor nutritional state; and with serious infections and bone marrow suppression. Use cautiously following high-dose pelvic irradiation or use of alkylating agents, in impaired hepatic or renal function, and in widespread neoplastic infiltration of bone marrow.
• Watch for stomatitis or diarrhea (signs of toxicity). May use topical oral anesthetic to soothe lesions. Discontinue if diarrhea occurs.
• Encourage good and frequent oral hygiene to prevent superinfection of denuded mucosa.
• Give antiemetic before administering drug to reduce nausea.
• Do WBC and platelet counts daily. Drug should be stopped when WBC is less than 3,500/mm³. Watch for ecchymoses, petechiae, easy bruising, and anemia. Drug should be stopped if platelet count is less than 100,000/mm³.
• Dermatologic side effects reversible when drug is stopped. Patient should use highly protective sun blockers to avoid inflammatory erythematous dermatitis.
• Therapeutic concentrations are not reached in cerebrospinal fluid.
• Slowing infusion rate so it takes from 2 to 8 hours lessens toxicity.
• Monitor intake/output, CBC, and renal and hepatic functions.
• Don't refrigerate fluorouracil.
• Don't use cloudy solution. If crystals form, redissolve by warming.
• Solution is more stable in plastic I.V. bags than in glass bottles. Use plastic I.V. containers for administering continuous infusions.
• Sometimes ordered as 5-fluorouracil or 5-FU. The numeral 5 is part of the drug name and should not be confused with dosage units.

Italicized adverse reactions are common or life-threatening.
*Liquid form contains alcohol.   **May contain tartrazine.

- Sometimes administered via hepatic arterial infusion in treatment of hepatic metastases.
- Warn patient that alopecia may occur but is reversible.
- To prevent bleeding, avoid I.M. injections of any drugs in patients with thrombocytopenia.
- Fluorouracil toxicity may be delayed for 1 to 3 weeks.
- Preparation of parenteral form is associated with carcinogenic, mutagenic, and teratogenic risks for personnel. Follow institutional policy to reduce risks.

hydroxyurea
Hydrea**

Pregnancy Risk Category: D

HOW SUPPLIED
Capsules: 500 mg

MECHANISM OF ACTION
Inhibits DNA synthesis.

INDICATIONS & DOSAGE
Melanoma; resistant chronic myelocytic leukemia; recurrent, metastatic, or inoperable ovarian cancer—
Adults: 80 mg/kg P.O. as single dose q 3 days; or 20 to 30 mg/kg P.O. daily.

ADVERSE REACTIONS
Blood: *leukopenia,* thrombocytopenia, anemia, *megaloblastosis; dose-limiting and dose-related bone marrow suppression, with rapid recovery.*
CNS: drowsiness, hallucinations.
GI: *anorexia, nausea, vomiting, diarrhea,* stomatitis.
GU: increased BUN and serum creatinine levels.
Metabolic: hyperuricemia.
Skin: rash, pruritus.

INTERACTIONS
None significant.

NURSING CONSIDERATIONS
- Dosage modification may be required following other chemotherapy or radiation therapy.
- Use with caution in renal dysfunction. Discontinue if WBC is less than 3,500/mm³ or if platelet count is less than 100,000/mm³.
- Warn patient to watch for signs of infection (fever, sore throat, fatigue) and bleeding (easy bruising, nosebleeds, bleeding gums, melena). Take temperature daily.
- If patient can't swallow capsule, he may empty contents into water and take immediately.
- Monitor intake/output; keep patient hydrated.
- Routinely measure BUN, uric acid, and serum creatinine.
- Drug crosses blood/brain barrier.
- Auditory and visual hallucinations and blood toxicity increase when decreased renal function exists.
- May exacerbate postirradiation erythema.
- Avoid all I.M. injections when platelets are below 100,000/mm³.

mercaptopurine (6-MP, 6-mercaptopurine)
Purinethol

Pregnancy Risk Category: D

HOW SUPPLIED
Tablets (scored): 50 mg

MECHANISM OF ACTION
Inhibits RNA and DNA synthesis.

INDICATIONS & DOSAGE
Acute lymphoblastic leukemia (in children), acute myeloblastic leukemia, chronic myelocytic leukemia—
Adults: 80 to 100 mg/m² P.O. daily as a single dose up to 5 mg/kg daily.
Children: 70 mg/m² P.O. daily.
  Usual maintenance for adults and children: 1.5 to 2.5 mg/kg daily.

ADVERSE REACTIONS
Blood: *decreased RBC; leukopenia, thrombocytopenia, and anemia; all may persist several days after drug is stopped.*
GI: *nausea, vomiting, and anorexia in 25% of patients;* painful oral ulcers.
Hepatic: *jaundice, hepatic necrosis.*
Metabolic: hyperuricemia.
Skin: rash, hyperpigmentation.

INTERACTIONS
Allopurinol: slowed inactivation of mercaptopurine. Decrease mercaptopurine to ¼ or ⅓ normal dose.
Hepatotoxic drugs: may enhance liver toxicity of mercaptopurine.
Warfarin: enhanced anticoagulant effect.

NURSING CONSIDERATIONS
● Dosage modifications may be required following chemotherapy or radiation therapy, in depressed neutrophil or platelet count, and in impaired hepatic or renal function.
● Observe for signs of bleeding and infection.
● Hepatic dysfunction is reversible when drug is stopped. Watch for jaundice, clay-colored stools, and frothy dark urine. Drug should be stopped if hepatic tenderness occurs.
● Do weekly blood counts; watch for precipitous fall.
● Warn patient to watch for signs of infection (fever, sore throat, fatigue) and bleeding (easy bruising, nosebleeds, bleeding gums, melena). Take temperature daily.
● Monitor intake/output. Encourage fluid intake (3 liters daily).
● Sometimes ordered as 6-mercaptopurine or 6-MP. The numeral 6 is part of drug name and does not signify number of dosage units.
● Warn patient that improvement may take 2 to 4 weeks or longer.
● GI adverse reactions less common in children than in adults.

● Avoid all I.M. injections when platelets are below 100,000/mm³.
● Monitor serum uric acid. If allopurinol is necessary, use cautiously.

methotrexate

methotrexate sodium
Folex, Mexate, Rheumatrex
Pregnancy Risk Category: D

HOW SUPPLIED
Tablets (scored): 2.5 mg
Injection: 20-mg, 25-mg, 50-mg, 100-mg, 250-mg vials, lyophilized powder, preservative-free; 25-mg/ml vials, preservative-free solution; 2.5-mg/ml, 25-mg/ml vials, lyophilized powder, preserved

MECHANISM OF ACTION
Prevents reduction of folic acid to tetrahydrofolate by binding to dihydrofolate reductase.

INDICATIONS & DOSAGE
Trophoblastic tumors (choriocarcinoma, hydatidiform mole)—
Adults: 15 to 30 mg P.O. or I.M. daily for 5 days. Repeat after 1 or more weeks, according to response or toxicity.
Acute lymphoblastic and lymphatic leukemia—
Adults and children: 3.3 mg/m² P.O., I.M., or I.V. daily for 4 to 6 weeks or until remission occurs; then 20 to 30 mg/m² P.O. or I.M. twice weekly.
Meningeal leukemia—
Adults and children: 10 to 15 mg/m² intrathecally q 2 to 5 days until cerebrospinal fluid is normal. Use only 20-, 50-, or 100-mg vials of powder with no preservatives; dilute using 0.9% sodium chloride injection *without* preservatives or Elliot's B solution. Use only new vials of drug and diluent. Use immediately.

Italicized adverse reactions are common or life-threatening.
*Liquid form contains alcohol.   **May contain tartrazine.

Burkitt's lymphoma (Stage I or Stage II)—
Adults: 10 to 25 mg P.O. daily for 4 to 8 days with 1-week rest intervals.
Lymphosarcoma (Stage III)—
Adults: 0.625 to 2.5 mg/kg daily P.O., I.M., or I.V.
Mycosis fungoides—
Adults: 2.5 to 10 mg P.O. daily or 50 mg I.M. weekly; or 25 mg I.M. twice weekly.
Psoriasis—
Adults: 10 to 25 mg P.O., I.M., or I.V. as single weekly dose.
Rheumatoid arthritis—
Adults: Initially 7.5 mg P.O. weekly, either in a single dose or divided as 2.5 mg P.O. q 12 hours for three doses once a week. Dosage may be gradually increased to a maximum of 20 mg weekly.

ADVERSE REACTIONS
Blood: WBC and platelet nadir occurring on day 7; anemia, *leukopenia, thrombocytopenia* (all dose-related).
CNS: *arachnoiditis within hours of intrathecal use;* subacute neurotoxicity which may begin a few weeks later; necrotizing demyelinating leukoencephalopathy a few years later.
GI: *stomatitis; diarrhea leading to hemorrhagic enteritis and intestinal perforation; nausea; vomiting.*
GU: nephropathy, *tubular necrosis.*
Hepatic: acute toxicity (elevated transaminases), *chronic toxicity* (cirrhosis, *hepatic fibrosis*).
Metabolic: hyperuricemia.
Skin: exposure to sun may aggravate psoriatic lesions, rash, photosensitivity.
Other: alopecia; *pulmonary interstitial infiltrates;* long-term use in children may cause osteoporosis.

INTERACTIONS
Folic acid derivatives: antagonized methotrexate effect.
Probenecid, phenylbutazone, NSAIDs, salicylates, sulfonamides: increased methotrexate toxicity; don't use together if possible.
Vaccines: immunizations may be ineffective; risk of disseminated infection with live virus vaccines.

NURSING CONSIDERATIONS
• Dosage modification may be required in impaired hepatic or renal function, bone marrow suppression, aplasia, leukopenia, thrombocytopenia, or anemia. Use cautiously in infection, peptic ulcer, ulcerative colitis, and in very young, elderly, or debilitated patients.
• Warn patient to avoid conception during and immediately after therapy because of possible abortion or congenital anomalies.
• GI adverse reactions may require stopping drug.
• Rash, redness, or ulcerations in mouth or pulmonary adverse reactions may signal serious complications.
• Monitor serum uric acid.
• Monitor intake/output daily. Encourage fluid intake (2 to 3 liters daily).
• Alkalinize urine by giving sodium bicarbonate tablets to prevent precipitation of drug, especially with high doses. Maintain urine pH at more than 6.5. Reduce dosage if BUN 20 to 30 mg% or creatinine 1.2 to 2 mg%. Stop drug if BUN more than 30 mg% or creatinine more than 2 mg%.
• Watch for increases in AST (SGOT), ALT (SGPT), alkaline phosphatase; may signal hepatic dysfunction.
• Watch for bleeding (especially GI) and infection.
• Warn patient to use highly protective sun screening agent when exposed to sunlight.
• Take temperature daily, and watch for cough, dyspnea, and cyanosis.
• Leucovorin rescue is necessary with high dose protocols (greater than 100-mg doses). Don't confuse with

folic acid. This rescue technique is effective against systemic toxicity but does not interfere with the tumor cells' absorption of the methotrexate.
• Avoid all I.M. injections in patients with thrombocytopenia.
• Advise patient not to discontinue leucovorin rescue if he experiences severe nausea and vomiting. Parenteral therapy may be necessary.
• Teach patient good oral care to prevent superinfection of oral cavity.
• Preparation of parenteral form is associated with carcinogenic, mutagenic, and teratogenic risks for personnel. Follow institutional policy to reduce risks.

NURSING CONSIDERATIONS
• Dosage modification may be required in renal or hepatic dysfunction.
• Stop drug if hepatotoxicity or hepatic tenderness occurs. Watch for jaundice; may be reversible if drug is stopped promptly.
• Do CBC daily during induction, then weekly during maintenance therapy.
• Monitor serum uric acid.
• Sometimes ordered as 6-thioguanine. The numeral 6 is part of drug name and does not signify dosage units.
• Avoid all I.M. injections when platelets are below 100,000/mm³.

---

thioguanine (6-thioguanine, 6-TG)
Lanvis†

Pregnancy Risk Category: D

HOW SUPPLIED
Tablets (scored): 40 mg

MECHANISM OF ACTION
Inhibits purine synthesis.

INDICATIONS & DOSAGE
Acute leukemia, chronic granulocytic leukemia—
Adults and children: initially, 2 mg/kg daily P.O. (usually calculated to nearest 20 mg); then increased gradually to 3 mg/kg daily if no toxic effects occur.

ADVERSE REACTIONS
Blood: *leukopenia,* anemia, *thrombocytopenia* (occurs slowly over 2 to 4 weeks).
GI: nausea, vomiting, stomatitis, diarrhea, anorexia.
Hepatic: hepatotoxicity, jaundice.
Metabolic: hyperuricemia.

INTERACTIONS
None significant.

---

trimetrexate gluconate
Pregnancy Risk Category: C

HOW SUPPLIED
Information about use of trimetrexate under the treatment IND available from the National Information Center for Orphan Drugs and Rare Diseases (NICODARD) at (800) 336-4797, or (202) 565-4167 in the Washington, D.C., metropolitan area.
Injection: 25-mg vials

MECHANISM OF ACTION
Prevents reduction of folic acid to tetrahydrofolate by binding to dihydrofolate reductase.

INDICATIONS & DOSAGE
Neoplastic disorders—
Adults: dosage and indication will vary with protocol.
Treatment of Pneumocystis carinii *pneumonia in patients with AIDS (approved as a treatment—IND)—*
Adults: dosage may vary with protocol. 30 mg/m² I.V. bolus daily for 21 days, administered with leucovorin (20 mg/m² I.V. or P.O. daily).

Italicized adverse reactions are common or life-threatening.
*Liquid form contains alcohol.   **May contain tartrazine.

ADVERSE REACTIONS
Blood: *neutropenia, thrombocytopenia.*
Skin: rash.
Other: *hepatotoxicity, peripheral neuropathy.*

INTERACTIONS
Leucovorin: precipitate will form if mixed with trimetrexate. Administer separately.

NURSING CONSIDERATIONS
• Avoid I.M. injections in patients with thrombocytopenia.
• Warn patient to watch for signs of infection (fever, sore throat, fatigue) and bleeding (easy bruising, nose-bleeds, bleeding gums, melena). Take temperature daily.
• Store intact vials in refrigerator.
• Reconstitute 25-mg vial with 2 ml sterile water for injection to yield a solution of 12.5 mg/ml.
• Incompatible with chloride-containing solutions (including normal saline solution). Only dextrose 5% in water is recommended for I.V. infusion.
• Preparation of parenteral form is associated with carcinogenic, mutagenic, and teratogenic risks for personnel. Follow institutional policy to reduce risks.

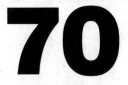

Antibiotic antineoplastic agents

bleomycin sulfate
dactinomycin
daunorubicin hydrochloride
doxorubicin hydrochloride
mitomycin
plicamycin
procarbazine hydrochloride

COMBINATION PRODUCTS
None.

---

bleomycin sulfate
Blenoxane

Pregnancy Risk Category: D

HOW SUPPLIED
Injection: 15-unit vials (1 unit = 1 mg)

MECHANISM OF ACTION
Inhibits DNA synthesis and causes scission of single- and double-stranded DNA.

INDICATIONS & DOSAGE
Dosage and indications may vary. Check patient's protocol with doctor.
Cervical, esophageal, head, neck, and testicular cancer—
Adults: 10 to 20 units/m² I.V., I.M., or S.C. 1 or 2 times weekly to total 300 to 400 units.
Hodgkin's disease—
Adults: 10 to 20 units/m² I.V., I.M., or S.C. 1 or 2 times weekly. After 50% response, maintenance 1 unit I.M. or I.V. daily or 5 units I.M. or I.V. weekly.
Lymphomas—
Adults: first two doses should be 2 units or less, and patient should be monitored for any allergic reaction. If no reaction occurs, then follow above dosing schedule.

ADVERSE REACTIONS
CNS: hyperesthesia of scalp and fingers, headache.
GI: *stomatitis, prolonged anorexia in 13% of patients, nausea, vomiting,* diarrhea.
Skin: *erythema, vesiculation, and hardening and discoloration of palmar and plantar skin in 8% of patients;* desquamation of hands, feet, and pressure areas; *hyperpigmentation;* acne.
Other: *reversible alopecia,* swelling of interphalangeal joints, *pulmonary fibrosis in 10% of patients, pulmonary adverse reactions (fine crackles, fever, dyspnea), leukocytosis and nonproductive cough, allergic reaction (fever up to 106° F. [41.1° C.] with chills up to 5 hours after injection; anaphylaxis in 1% to 6% of patients).*

INTERACTIONS
Digitalis glycosides: combination therapy that includes bleomycin may result in decreased serum digoxin levels.

NURSING CONSIDERATIONS
• Use cautiously in renal or pulmonary impairment.
• Pulmonary adverse reactions common in patients over 70 years. Fatal pulmonary fibrosis occurs in 1% of patients, especially when cumulative dose exceeds 400 units.

Italicized adverse reactions are common or life-threatening.
*Liquid form contains alcohol.   **May contain tartrazine.

• Pulmonary function tests should be performed to establish pre-treatment baseline. Drug should be stopped if pulmonary function test shows a marked decline.

• Monitor chest X-ray and listen to lungs.

• Monitor injection site for signs of irritation.

• Drug concentrates in keratin of squamous epithelium. To prevent linear streaking, don't use adhesive dressings on skin.

• Allergic reactions may be delayed for several hours, especially in lymphoma.

• Advise patient that alopecia may occur, but is usually reversible.

• Refrigerated, reconstituted solution is stable for 4 weeks; at room temperature, it's stable for 2 weeks. Bleomycin may adsorb to plastic (PVC) I.V. bags. For prolonged stability, use glass containers.

• Bleomycin-induced fever is common and may be treated with antipyretics. This reaction usually occurs within 3 to 6 hours of administration.

• Refrigerate unopened vials containing dry powder.

• Preparation of parenteral form is associated with carcinogenic, mutagenic, and teratogenic risks for personnel. Follow institutional policy to reduce risks.

---

dactinomycin (actinomycin D)
Cosmegen

Pregnancy Risk Category: C

HOW SUPPLIED
Injectable: 500 mcg/vial

MECHANISM OF ACTION
Interferes with DNA-dependent RNA synthesis by intercalation.

INDICATIONS & DOSAGE
Dosage and indications may vary. Check patient's protocol with doctor.
Melanomas, sarcomas, trophoblastic tumors in women, testicular cancer—
Adults: 500 mcg I.V. daily for 5 days not to exceed 15 mg/kg or 400 to 600 mg/m² daily; wait 2 to 4 weeks and repeat. Or 2 mg I.V. single weekly dose for 3 weeks; wait for bone marrow recovery, then repeat in 3 to 4 weeks.
Wilms' tumor, rhabdomyosarcoma, Ewing's sarcoma—
Children: 15 mcg/kg I.V. daily for 5 days. Maximum dosage 500 mcg daily. Wait for bone marrow recovery.

ADVERSE REACTIONS
Blood: anemia, *leukopenia, thrombocytopenia, pancytopenia.*
GI: *anorexia, nausea, vomiting,* abdominal pain, diarrhea, *stomatitis.*
Skin: *erythema;* desquamation; *hyperpigmentation of skin, especially in previously irradiated areas; acne-like eruptions (reversible).*
Local: phlebitis, severe damage to soft tissue.
Other: reversible alopecia, hepatotoxicity.

INTERACTIONS
None significant.

NURSING CONSIDERATIONS
• Contraindicated in renal, hepatic, or bone marrow impairment.

• Stomatitis, diarrhea, leukopenia, thrombocytopenia may require modifying dosage and schedule.

• Give antiemetic before administering to reduce nausea.

• Monitor renal and hepatic functions.

• Monitor CBC daily and platelet counts frequently.

• Warn patient to watch for signs of infection (fever, sore throat, fatigue) and bleeding (easy bruising, nosebleeds, bleeding gums, melena). Take temperature daily.

- Warn patient that alopecia may occur but is usually reversible.
- Use only sterile water (without preservatives) as diluent for injection. Discard unused solutions since they do not contain a preservative.
- Dactinomycin is a vesicant. Administer through a running I.V. with good blood return. If infiltration occurs, apply cold compresses to area.
- Preparation of parenteral form is associated with carcinogenic, mutagenic, and teratogenic risks for personnel. Follow institutional policy to reduce risks.

daunorubicin hydrochloride (DNR)
Cerubidin‡, Cerubidine

Pregnancy Risk Category: D

HOW SUPPLIED
Injection: 20 mg/vial

MECHANISM OF ACTION
Interferes with DNA-dependent RNA synthesis by intercalation.

INDICATIONS & DOSAGE
Dosage and indications may vary. Check patient's protocol with doctor.
Remission induction in acute nonlymphocytic leukemia (myelogenous, monocytic, erythroid)—
Adults: as a single agent, 60 mg/m² daily I.V. on days 1, 2, and 3 q 3 to 4 weeks; in combination, 45 mg/m² daily I.V. on days 1, 2, and 3 of the first course and on days 1 and 2 of subsequent courses with cytosine arabinoside infusions.
Note: Dose should be reduced if hepatic or renal function is impaired.

ADVERSE REACTIONS
Blood: *bone marrow suppression* (lowest blood counts 10 to 14 days after administration).
CV: *irreversible cardiomyopathy*
(dose-related), ECG changes, *arrhythmias,* pericarditis, myocarditis.
GI: *nausea, vomiting, stomatitis, esophagitis,* anorexia, diarrhea.
GU: nephrotoxicity, transient red urine.
Hepatic: hepatotoxicity.
Skin: rash, pigmentation of fingernails and toenails.
Local: *severe cellulitis or tissue sloughing if drug extravasates.*
Other: *generalized alopecia,* fever, chills.

INTERACTIONS
Heparin: don't mix. May form a precipitate.

NURSING CONSIDERATIONS
- Use cautiously in myelosuppression and impaired cardiac, renal, and liver function.
- Stop drug immediately in signs of CHF or cardiomyopathy. Prevent by limiting cumulative dose to 550 mg/m²; 450 mg/m² when patient has been receiving radiation therapy that encompasses the heart or any other cardiotoxic agent, such as cyclophosphamide.
- Monitor ECG before treatment, monthly during therapy.
- Note if resting pulse rate is high (a sign of cardiac adverse reactions).
- *Avoid extravasation;* inject into tubing of freely flowing I.V. *Never give* I.M. or S.C. If extravasation occurs, discontinue I.V. immediately and apply ice to area for 24 to 48 hours. Local infiltration with hydrocortisone sodium succinate injection (50 to 100 mg) and/or sodium bicarbonate (5 ml of 8.4% injection) may be ordered.
- Monitor CBC and hepatic function.
- Warn patient that urine may be red for 1 to 2 days and that it's a normal side effect, not hematuria.
- Advise patient that alopecia may occur but is usually reversible.
- Nausea and vomiting may be very severe and last 24 to 48 hours.

Italicized adverse reactions are common or life-threatening.
*Liquid form contains alcohol.   **May contain tartrazine.

• Reconstituted solution is stable for 24 hours at room temperature or 48 hours refrigerated. Optimally, use within 8 hours of preparation.
• Reddish color looks very similar to doxorubicin (Adriamycin). *Do not confuse the two drugs.*
• Preparation of parenteral form is associated with carcinogenic, mutagenic, and teratogenic risks for personnel. Follow institutional policy to reduce risks.

---

doxorubicin hydrochloride
Adriamycin‡, Adriamycin PFS, Adriamycin RDF

Pregnancy Risk Category: D

HOW SUPPLIED
Injection (preservative-free): 2 mg/ml
Powder for injection: 10-mg, 20-mg, 50-mg vials.

MECHANISM OF ACTION
Interferes with DNA-dependent RNA synthesis by intercalation.

INDICATIONS & DOSAGE
Dosage and indications may vary. Check patient's protocol with doctor.
Bladder, breast, cervical, head, neck, liver, lung, ovarian, prostatic, stomach, testicular, and thyroid cancer; Hodgkin's disease; acute lymphoblastic and myeloblastic leukemia; Wilms' tumor; neuroblastomas; lymphomas; sarcomas—
Adults: 60 to 75 mg/m² I.V. as single dose q 3 weeks; or 30 mg/m² I.V. in single daily dose, days 1 to 3 of 4-week cycle. Alternatively, 20 mg/m² I.V. once weekly or 30 mg/m² I.V. on 3 successive days, repeated every 4 weeks. Maximum cumulative dose 550 mg/m².

ADVERSE REACTIONS
Blood: *leukopenia, especially agranulocytosis, during days 10 to 15, with* recovery by day 21; thrombocytopenia.
CV: *cardiac depression, seen in such ECG changes as sinus tachycardia, T wave flattening, ST segment depression, voltage reduction; arrhythmias in 11% of patients; irreversible cardiomyopathy (sometimes with pulmonary edema) with mortality of 30% to 75%.*
GI: *nausea, vomiting,* diarrhea, *stomatitis,* esophagitis.
GU: enhancement of cyclophosphamide-induced bladder injury, transient red urine.
Skin: *hyperpigmentation of skin, especially in previously irradiated areas.*
Local: *severe cellulitis or tissue sloughing if drug extravasates.*
Other: hyperpigmentation of nails and dermal creases, *complete alopecia within 3 to 4 weeks;* hair may regrow 2 to 5 months after drug is stopped.

INTERACTIONS
Streptozocin: increased and prolonged blood levels. Dosage may have to be adjusted.
Heparin: don't mix together. May form a precipitate.

NURSING CONSIDERATIONS
• Dosage modification may be required in myelosuppression and in impaired cardiac or hepatic function.
• Stop drug or slow rate of infusion if tachycardia develops.
• Stop drug immediately in signs of CHF. Prevent by limiting cumulative dose to 550 mg/m²; 450 mg/m² when patient is also receiving cyclophosphamide or irradiation to cardiac area.
• Monitor ECG before treatment, monthly during therapy.
• *Avoid extravasation;* inject slowly by I.V. push into tubing of freely flowing I.V. *Never* give I.M. or S.C. If extravasation occurs, discontinue I.V.

---

immediately and apply ice to area for 24 to 48 hours.
• If vein streaking occurs, slow administration rate. However, if welts occur, stop administration and report to doctor.
• Monitor CBC and hepatic function.
• Warn patient to watch for signs of infection (fever, sore throat, fatigue) and bleeding (easy bruising, nosebleeds, bleeding gums, melena). Take temperature daily.
• Warn patient urine will be red for 1 to 2 days.
• Dosage should be reduced in hepatic dysfunction.
• Warn patient that alopecia will occur but is usually reversible.
• Refrigerated, reconstituted solution is stable for 48 hours; at room temperature, it's stable for 24 hours.
• If cumulative dose exceeds 550 mg/m² body surface area, 30% of patients develop cardiac adverse reactions, which begin 2 weeks to 6 months after stopping drug.
• The alternative dosage schedule (once-weekly dosing) has been found to cause a lower incidence of cardiomyopathy.
• Decrease dosage if serum bilirubin is increased: 50% dosage when bilirubin is 1.2 to 3 mg/100 ml; 25% dosage when bilirubin is greater than 3 mg/100 ml.
• Esophagitis is very common in patients who have also received radiation therapy.
• Premedicate with antiemetic to reduce nausea.
• Reddish color looks very similar to daunorubicin (Cerubidine). *Do not confuse the two drugs.*
• Preparation of parenteral form is associated with carcinogenic, mutagenic, and teratogenic risks for personnel. Follow institutional policy to reduce risks.

mitomycin (mitomycin-C)
Mutamycin

Pregnancy Risk Category: D

HOW SUPPLIED
Injection: 5-mg, 20-mg vials

MECHANISM OF ACTION
Acts like an alkylating agent, cross-linking strands of DNA. This causes an imbalance of cell growth, leading to cell death.

INDICATIONS & DOSAGE
Dosage and indications may vary. Check patient's protocol with doctor.
Breast, colon, head, neck, lung, pancreatic, and stomach cancer; malignant melanoma—
Adults: 2 mg/m² I.V. daily for 5 days. Stop drug for 2 days, then repeat dosage for 5 more days; or 20 mg/m² as a single dose. Repeat cycle 6 to 8 weeks. Stop drug if WBC less than 4,000/mm³ or platelets less than 75,000/mm³.

ADVERSE REACTIONS
Blood: *thrombocytopenia, leukopenia (may be delayed up to 8 weeks and may be cumulative with successive doses).*
CNS: paresthesias.
GI: *nausea, vomiting,* anorexia, stomatitis.
Local: desquamation, induration, pruritus, *pain at injection site.* Extravasation causes cellulitis, ulceration, sloughing.
Other: *reversible alopecia; purple coloration of nail beds;* fever; *microangiopathic hemolytic anemia, syndrome characterized by thrombocytopenia, renal failure, and hypertension; interstitial pneumonitis.*

INTERACTIONS
None significant.

Italicized adverse reactions are common or life-threatening.
*Liquid form contains alcohol.   **May contain tartrazine.

NURSING CONSIDERATIONS

• Dosage modification is required when platelet count is below 75,000/mm³, WBC is less than 4,000/mm³; in coagulation or bleeding disorders, serious infections, and impaired renal function.

• Continue CBC and blood studies at least 7 weeks after therapy is stopped.

• Warn patient to watch for signs of infection (fever, sore throat, fatigue) and bleeding (easy bruising, nosebleeds, bleeding gums, melena). Take temperature daily.

• Advise patient that alopecia may occur, but that it's usually reversible.

• Reconstituted solution stable 1 week at room temperature, 2 weeks refrigerated.

• Has been administered topically by bladder instillation and has been given intraarterially through the hepatic artery.

• Monitor renal function.

• Avoid all I.M. injections in patients with thrombocytopenia.

• Preparation of parenteral form is associated with carcinogenic, mutagenic, and teratogenic risks for personnel. Follow institutional policy to reduce risks.

---

plicamycin (mithramycin)
Mithracin

Pregnancy Risk Category: X

HOW SUPPLIED
Injection: 2.5-mg vials

MECHANISM OF ACTION
Forms a complex with DNA, thus inhibiting RNA synthesis. Also inhibits osteocytic activity, blocking calcium and phosphorus resorption from bone.

INDICATIONS & DOSAGE
Dosage and indications may vary. Check patient's protocol with doctor.
Hypercalcemia associated with advanced malignancy—

Adults: 25 mcg/kg I.V. daily for 1 to 4 days.
Testicular cancer—
Adults: 25 to 30 mcg/kg I.V. daily for up to 10 days (based on ideal body weight or actual weight, whichever is less).

ADVERSE REACTIONS
Blood: *thrombocytopenia; bleeding syndrome, from epistaxis to generalized hemorrhage; facial flushing.*
GI: *nausea, vomiting,* anorexia, diarrhea, stomatitis, metallic taste.
GU: proteinuria; increased BUN, serum creatinine.
Metabolic: *decreased serum calcium,* potassium, and phosphorus; elevated liver enzymes.
Skin: periorbital pallor, usually the day before toxic symptoms occur.
Local: extravasation causes irritation, cellulitis.

INTERACTIONS
None significant.

NURSING CONSIDERATIONS
• Contraindicated in thrombocytopenia and in coagulation and bleeding disorders. Dosage modification may be required in renal, hepatic, or bone marrow impairment.

• Slow infusion reduces nausea that develops with I.V. push.

• Monitor LDH, AST (SGOT), ALT (SGPT), alkaline phosphatase, BUN, creatinine, potassium, calcium, and phosphorus levels.

• Monitor platelet count and prothrombin time before and during therapy.

• Warn patient to watch for signs of infection (fever, sore throat, fatigue) and bleeding (easy bruising, nosebleeds, bleeding gums, melena). Take temperature daily.

• Facial flushing is an early indicator of bleeding.

• Give antiemetic before administering to reduce nausea.

• Avoid extravasation. Plicamycin is a vesicant. If I.V. infiltrates, stop immediately; use ice packs. Restart I.V.
• Avoid contact with skin or mucous membranes.
• Therapeutic effect in hypercalcemia may not be seen for 24 to 48 hours; may last 3 to 15 days.
• Precipitous drop in calcium possible. Monitor patient for tetany, carpopedal spasm, Chvostek's sign, muscle cramps; check serum calcium.
• Store lyophilized powder in refrigerator. Remains stable after reconstitution for 24 hours; 48 hours in refrigerator.
• Preparation of parenteral form is associated with carcinogenic, mutagenic, and teratogenic risks for personnel. Follow institutional policy to reduce risks.

procarbazine hydrochloride
Matulane, Natulan†‡

Pregnancy Risk Category: D

HOW SUPPLIED
Capsules: 50 mg

MECHANISM OF ACTION
Inhibits DNA, RNA, and protein synthesis.

INDICATIONS & DOSAGE
Dosage and indications may vary. Check patient's protocol with doctor.
Hodgkin's disease, lymphomas, brain and lung cancer—
Adults: 2 to 4 mg/kg P.O. daily in a single dose or divided doses for the first week. Then, 4 to 6 mg/kg daily until WBC falls below 4,000/mm³ or platelets fall below 100,000/mm³. After bone marrow recovers, resume maintenance dosage of 1 to 2 mg/kg/day.
Children: 50 mg/m² P.O. daily for first week, then 100 mg/m² until response or toxicity occurs. Mainte-

nance dosage is 50 mg/m² P.O. daily after bone marrow recovery.

ADVERSE REACTIONS
Blood: bleeding tendency, *thrombocytopenia, leukopenia,* anemia.
CNS: nervousness, depression, insomnia, nightmares, *hallucinations,* confusion.
EENT: retinal hemorrhage, nystagmus, photophobia.
GI: *nausea, vomiting, anorexia,* stomatitis, dry mouth, dysphagia, diarrhea, constipation.
Skin: dermatitis.
Other: reversible alopecia, pleural effusion.

INTERACTIONS
Alcohol: mild disulfiram-like reaction. Warn patient not to drink alcohol.
CNS depressants: additive depressant effects.
Meperidine: may cause severe hypotension and possible death. Don't give together.
Sympathomimetics, local anesthetics, antidepressants, foods high in tyramine content (chianti wine, cheese): possible tremors, palpitations, increased blood pressure.

NURSING CONSIDERATIONS
• Use cautiously in inadequate bone marrow reserve, leukopenia, thrombocytopenia, anemia, and impaired hepatic or renal function.
• Warn patient to watch for signs of infection (fever, sore throat, fatigue) and bleeding (easy bruising, nosebleeds, bleeding gums, melena). Take temperature daily.
• Nausea and vomiting may be decreased if taken at bedtime and in divided doses.
• Warn patient not to drink alcoholic beverages while taking this drug.
• Procarbazine inhibits MAO and can cause disulfiram-like reaction if taken with other MAO inhibitors, tricyclic

---

Italicized adverse reactions are common or life-threatening.
*Liquid form contains alcohol.   **May contain tartrazine.

antidepressants, or foods with a high tyramine content.

• Instruct patient to stop medication and check with doctor immediately if disulfiram-like reaction occurs (chest pains, rapid or irregular heartbeat, severe headache, stiff neck).

• Monitor CBC and platelet counts.

• Avoid all I.M. injections in patients with thrombocytopenia.

• Warn patient to avoid hazardous tasks such as driving or operating heavy machinery until the adverse CNS reactions of the drug are known.

Antineoplastics altering hormone balance

aminoglutethimide
estramustine phosphate sodium
flutamide
goserelin acetate
leuprolide acetate
megestrol acetate
mitotane
tamoxifen citrate
testolactone
trilostane

COMBINATION PRODUCTS
None.

aminoglutethimide
Cytadren

Pregnancy Risk Category: D

HOW SUPPLIED
Tablets: 250 mg

MECHANISM OF ACTION
Blocks conversion of cholesterol to
delta-5-pregnenolone in the adrenal
cortex, inhibiting the synthesis of glucocorticoids, mineralocorticoids, and
other steroids.

INDICATIONS & DOSAGE
*Suppression of adrenal function in
Cushing's syndrome and adrenal cancer; metastatic breast cancer—*
Adults: 250 mg P.O. q.i.d. at 6-hour
intervals. Dosage may be increased in
increments of 250 mg daily every 1 to
2 weeks to a maximum daily dosage
of 2 g.

ADVERSE REACTIONS
Blood: transient leukopenia, *severe
pancytopenia.*
CNS: *drowsiness,* headache, dizzi-
ness.
CV: hypotension, tachycardia.
Endocrine: adrenal insufficiency,
masculinization, hirsutism.
GI: nausea, anorexia.
Skin: *morbilliform skin rash,* pruri-
tus, urticaria.
Other: fever, myalgia.

INTERACTIONS
Alcohol: may potentiate the effects of
aminoglutethimide.
*Dexamethasone, medroxyprogester-
one, digitoxin, theophylline:* aminoglutethimide increases hepatic metabolism of these agents.
Oral anticoagulants: decreased anticoagulant effect.

NURSING CONSIDERATIONS
• May cause adrenal hypofunction,
especially under stressful conditions,
such as surgery, trauma, or acute illness. Patients may need hydrocortisone and mineralocorticoid supplements in these situations. Monitor
such patients carefully.
• Monitor blood pressure frequently.
Advise patient to stand up slowly in
order to minimize orthostatic hypotension.
• May cause a decrease in thyroid
hormone production. Monitor thyroid
function studies.
• Perform baseline hematologic studies and monitor CBC periodically.
• Warn patient to watch for signs of

Italicized adverse reactions are common or life-threatening.
*Liquid form contains alcohol.   **May contain tartrazine.

infection (fever, sore throat, fatigue) and bleeding (easy bruising, nosebleeds, bleeding gums, melena). Take temperature daily.

• Warn patient that drug can cause drowsiness and dizziness. Advise him to avoid activities that require alertness and good psychomotor coordination until CNS effects of the drug are known.

• Tell patient to report if skin rash persists for more than 8 days. Reassure patient that drowsiness, nausea, and loss of appetite will diminish within 2 weeks after start of aminoglutethimide therapy. However, if these symptoms persist, tell patient to notify doctor.

---

estramustine phosphate sodium
Emcyt, Estracyst‡

Pregnancy Risk Category: D

HOW SUPPLIED
Capsules: 140 mg

MECHANISM OF ACTION
A combination of estrogen and an alkylating agent; acts by its ability to bind selectively to a protein present in the human prostate.

INDICATIONS & DOSAGE
Palliative treatment of metastatic or progressive cancer of the prostate—
Adults: 10 to 16 mg/kg P.O. in three to four divided doses. Usual dosage is 14 mg/kg daily. Therapy should continue for up to 3 months and, if successful, be maintained as long as the patient responds.

ADVERSE REACTIONS
Blood: leukopenia, thrombocytopenia.
CV: *myocardial infarction, CVA, edema, pulmonary emboli,* thrombophlebitis, CHF, hypertension.
GI: *nausea, vomiting,* diarrhea.

Skin: rash, pruritus.
Other: *painful gynecomastia and breast tenderness,* thinning of hair, hyperglycemia, fluid retention.

INTERACTIONS
Calcium-rich foods (milk and dairy products): impaired absorption of estramustine.

NURSING CONSIDERATIONS
• Contraindicated in patients hypersensitive to estradiol and nitrogen mustard. Also contraindicated in active thrombophlebitis or thromboembolic disorders, except in those cases where the actual tumor mass is the cause of the thromboembolic phenomenon.

• Use cautiously in patients with history of thrombophlebitis or thromboembolic disorders and cerebrovascular or coronary artery disease.

• Estramustine may exaggerate preexisting peripheral edema or CHF. Weight gain should be monitored regularly in these patients.

• Monitor blood pressure and glucose tolerance periodically throughout therapy.

• Each 140-mg capsule contains 12.5 mg sodium.

• Because of the possibility of mutagenic effects, advise patient and spouse to use contraceptive measures if woman is of childbearing age.

• Estramustine is a combination of the estrogen estradiol and a nitrogen mustard. Shown to be effective in patients refractory to estrogen therapy alone.

• Patient may continue estramustine as long as he's responding favorably. Some patients have taken the drug for more than 3 years.

• Store capsules in refrigerator.

flutamide
Eulexin

Pregnancy Risk Category: D

HOW SUPPLIED
Capsules: 125 mg

MECHANISM OF ACTION
Inhibits androgen uptake or prevents binding of androgens in nucleus of cells within target tissues.

INDICATIONS & DOSAGE
Treatment of metastatic prostatic carcinoma (stage D_2) in combination with luteinizing hormone-releasing hormone analogs such as leuprolide acetate—
Adults: 250 mg P.O. q. 8 hours.

ADVERSE REACTIONS
CNS: *loss of libido.*
CV: edema, hypertension.
GI: *diarrhea, nausea, vomiting.*
GU: *impotence.*
Metabolic: gynecomastia, elevated of hepatic enzymes, hepatitis.
Skin: rash, photosensitivity.
Other: *hot flashes.*

INTERACTIONS
None reported.

NURSING CONSIDERATIONS
• Contraindicated in patients with hypersensitivity to flutamide.
• Periodic liver tests should be performed in patients receiving chronic therapy with flutamide.
• Patients should understand that flutamide must be taken continuously with the agent used for medical castration (such as leuprolide acetate) to allow the full benefit of therapy. Leuprolide suppresses testosterone production, while flutamide inhibits testosterone action at the cellular level. Together they can impair the growth of androgen-responsive tumors. Patients should not discontinue either drug without consulting the doctor.

goserelin acetate
Zoladex

Pregnancy Risk Category: X

HOW SUPPLIED
Implants: 3.6 mg

MECHANISM OF ACTION
A luteinizing hormone-releasing hormone (LHRH) analog that acts on the pituitary to decrease the release of follicle-stimulating hormone (FSH) and luteinizing hormone (LH). In males, the result is dramatically lowered serum levels of testosterone.

INDICATIONS & DOSAGE
Palliative treatment of advanced carcinoma of the prostate—
Adults: 1 implant S.C. q 28 days into the upper abdominal wall.

ADVERSE REACTIONS
Blood: anemia.
CNS: lethargy, pain (worsened in the first 30 days), dizziness, insomnia, anxiety, depression, headache, chills, fever.
CV: edema, CHF, arrhythmias, CVA, hypertension, myocardial infarction, peripheral vascular disorder, chest pain.
EENT: upper respiratory infection.
GI: nausea, vomiting, diarrhea, constipation, ulcer.
GU: *decreased erections, lower urinary tract symptoms,* renal insufficiency, urinary obstruction, urinary tract infection.
Skin: rash, sweating.
Other: *hot flashes, sexual dysfunction,* gout, hyperglycemia, weight increase, breast swelling and tenderness.

INTERACTIONS
None reported.

Italicized adverse reactions are common or life-threatening.
*Liquid form contains alcohol.   **May contain tartrazine.

NURSING CONSIDERATIONS
• Goserelin is contraindicated during pregnancy.
• At the beginning of therapy, LHRH analogs such as goserelin may cause a worsening of the symptoms of prostatic cancer because the drug initially causes an increase in testosterone serum levels. A few patients may experience increased bone pain. Rarely, disease exacerbation (either spinal cord compression or ureteral obstruction) has occurred.
• Advise the patient that he should report every 28 days for a new implant. A delay of a couple of days is permissible, however.
• The implant comes in a preloaded syringe. If the package is damaged, do not use the syringe. Make sure that the drug is visible in the translucent chamber of the syringe.
• The drug is administered into the upper abdominal wall using aseptic technique. After cleaning the area with an alcohol swab (and injecting a local anesthetic), stretch the patient's skin with one hand while grasping the barrel of the syringe with the other. Insert the needle into the S.C. fat, then change direction of the needle so that it parallels the abdominal wall. The needle should then be pushed in until the hub touches the patient's skin, then withdrawn about 1 cm (this creates a gap for the drug to be injected) before depressing the plunger completely.
• To avoid the need for a new syringe and injection site, do not aspirate after inserting the needle.

---

leuprolide acetate
Lucrin‡, Lupron, Lupron Depot
Pregnancy Risk Category: B

HOW SUPPLIED
Injection: 1 mg/0.2 ml (5 mg/ml) in 2.8-ml multiple-dose vials
Depot injection: 7.5 mg/ml

MECHANISM OF ACTION
Initially stimulates but then inhibits the release of follicle-stimulating and luteinizing hormone. This results in testosterone suppression.

INDICATIONS & DOSAGE
Management of advanced prostate cancer—
Adults: 1 mg S.C. daily. Alternatively, give 7.5 mg I.M. (depot injection) monthly.

ADVERSE REACTIONS
Endocrine: *hot flashes.*
GI: nausea, vomiting.
Local: skin reactions at injection site.
Other: pulmonary embolus, peripheral edema, decreased libido, transient bone pain during first week of treatment.

INTERACTIONS
None significant.

NURSING CONSIDERATIONS
• Never administer by I.V. injection.
• Leuprolide is a nonsurgical alternative to orchiectomy for prostate cancer.
• Studies show leuprolide is therapeutically equivalent to diethylstilbestrol in "medical castration" palliation treatment but has significantly milder and fewer adverse reactions.
• Reassure your patient who has had undesirable effects from other endocrine therapies that leuprolide is much easier to tolerate.
• Reassure patient that bone pain is transient and will disappear after about 1 week.
• Patients may be maintained on this drug for long-term treatment.
• If patient is going to self-administer S.C. injection, he should be carefully instructed about proper administration techniques, and he should be advised to use only the syringes provided by the manufacturer.
• If another syringe must be substi-

tuted, a low dose insulin syringe (U-100, 0.5 ml) may be an appropriate choice.

• Advise patients to store the drug at room temperature, protected from light and sources of heat.

• One monthly depot injection should be administered under medical supervision. Use supplied diluent to reconstitute drug. Draw 1 ml into a syringe with a 22G needle (extra diluent is provided and should be discarded). Inject into vial, then shake well. Suspension will appear milky.

---

megestrol acetate
Megace, Megostat‡

Pregnancy Risk Category: X

HOW SUPPLIED
Tablets: 20 mg, 40 mg

MECHANISM OF ACTION
Changes the tumor's hormonal environment and alters the neoplastic process.

INDICATIONS & DOSAGE
Breast cancer—
Women: 40 mg P.O. q.i.d.
Endometrial cancer—
Women: 40 to 320 mg P.O. daily in divided doses.

ADVERSE REACTIONS
GU: dysfunctional uterine bleeding when drug is discontinued.
Other: carpal tunnel syndrome, thrombophlebitis, alopecia, hirsutism, breast tenderness.

INTERACTIONS
None significant.

NURSING CONSIDERATIONS
• Use cautiously in patients with history of thrombophlebitis.
• Adequate trial is 2 months. Reassure patient that therapeutic response isn't immediate.

mitotane
Lysodren

Pregnancy Risk Category: C

HOW SUPPLIED
Tablets (scored): 500 mg

MECHANISM OF ACTION
Selectively destroys adrenocortical tissue and hinders extraadrenal metabolism of cortisol.

INDICATIONS & DOSAGE
Inoperable adrenocortical cancer—
Adults: initially, 1 to 6 g P.O. daily divided t.i.d. or q.i.d.; increased to 9 to 10 g P.O. daily, divided t.i.d. or q.i.d. Dosage is adjusted until maximum tolerated dosage is achieved (varies from 2 to 16 g daily but is usually 8 to 10 g daily).
Children: initially, 0.5 to 1 g P.O. daily in divided doses. Increase dosage based upon patient tolerance and response.

ADVERSE REACTIONS
CNS: *depression, somnolence, vertigo;* brain damage and dysfunction in long-term, high-dose therapy.
GI: *severe nausea, vomiting,* diarrhea, anorexia.
Metabolic: adrenal insufficiency.
Skin: dermatitis.

INTERACTIONS
None significant.

NURSING CONSIDERATIONS
• Dosage modification may be required in hepatic disease.
• Drug should not be used in a patient with shock or trauma. Use of corticosteroids may avoid acute adrenocorticoid insufficiency.
• Assess and record behavioral and neurologic signs for baseline data daily throughout therapy.
• Give antiemetic before administering to reduce nausea.

Italicized adverse reactions are common or life-threatening.
*Liquid form contains alcohol.   **May contain tartrazine.

- Dosage may be reduced if GI or skin adverse reactions are severe.
- Obese patients may need higher dosage and may have longer-lasting adverse reactions, since drug distributes mostly to body fat.
- Warn ambulatory patient of CNS adverse reactions; advise him to avoid hazardous tasks requiring mental alertness or physical coordination.
- Monitor effectiveness by reduction in pain, weakness, anorexia.
- Adequate trial is at least 3 months, but therapy can continue if clinical benefits are observed.

tamoxifen citrate
Nolvadex, Nolvadex D†‡, Tamofen†

Pregnancy Risk Category: C

HOW SUPPLIED
Tablets: 10 mg, 15.2 mg†
Tablets (film-coated): 30.4 mg†

MECHANISM OF ACTION
Acts as an estrogen antagonist.

INDICATIONS & DOSAGE
Advanced premenopausal and postmenopausal breast cancer—
Women: 10 mg P.O. b.i.d.

ADVERSE REACTIONS
Blood: transient fall in WBC or platelets.
GI: nausea in 10% of patients, vomiting, anorexia.
GU: vaginal discharge and bleeding.
Metabolic: hypercalcemia.
Skin: rash.
Other: temporary bone or tumor pain, hot flashes in 7% of patients. Brief exacerbation of pain from osseous metastases.

INTERACTIONS
None significant.

NURSING CONSIDERATIONS
- Monitor CBC closely in patients with preexisting leukopenia or thrombocytopenia.
- Acts as an "antiestrogen." Best results have been reported in patients with positive estrogen receptors.
- Adverse reactions are usually minor and well tolerated.
- Reassure patient that acute exacerbation of bone pain during tamoxifen therapy usually indicates drug will produce good response. Use analgesic to relieve pain.
- Short-term therapy induces ovulation in premenopausal women. *Mechanical* contraceptive recommended.
- Monitor serum calcium. Drug may compound hypercalcemia related to bone metastases.
- Also used to treat breast cancer in men and advanced ovarian cancer in women. Has been used to stimulate ovulation in women with oligomenorrhea or amenorrhea who previously used oral contraceptives.

testolactone
Teslac

Pregnancy Risk Category: C

HOW SUPPLIED
Tablets: 50 mg

MECHANISM OF ACTION
Changes the tumor's hormonal environment and alters the neoplastic process.

INDICATIONS & DOSAGE
Advanced postmenopausal breast cancer—
Women: 250 mg P.O. q.i.d.

ADVERSE REACTIONS
CNS: paresthesias.
CV: increased blood pressure, edema.
GI: nausea, vomiting, diarrhea.
Metabolic: hypercalcemia.
Other: alopecia.

INTERACTIONS
Oral anticoagulants: increased pharmacologic effects. Monitor carefully.

NURSING CONSIDERATIONS
• Contraindicated in male breast cancer and not recommended for premenopausal women.
• Adequate trial is 3 months. Reassure patient that therapeutic response isn't immediate.
• Monitor fluids and electrolytes, especially calcium.
• Immobilized patients are prone to hypercalcemia. Exercise may prevent it. Force fluids to aid calcium excretion.
• Drug causes less virilization than testosterone.
• Higher-than-recommended doses do not increase incidence of remission.
• Testolactone is an androgen.

---

trilostane
Modrastane

Pregnancy Risk Category: X

HOW SUPPLIED
Capsules: 30 mg, 60 mg

MECHANISM OF ACTION
Reversibly lowers elevated circulating levels of glucocorticoids by inhibiting the enzyme system essential for their production in the adrenal gland.

INDICATIONS & DOSAGE
Adrenal cortical hyperfunction in Cushing's syndrome—
Adults: 30 mg P.O. q.i.d. initially. May be increased at intervals of 3 to 4 days to maximum of 480 mg daily.

ADVERSE REACTIONS
CNS: headache.
CV: *orthostatic hypotension.*
EENT: burning of oral and nasal membranes.

GI: *diarrhea, upset stomach,* nausea, flatulence, bloating.
Metabolic: hyperkalemia.
Skin: flushing, rash.
Other: fever, fatigue.

INTERACTIONS
Aminoglutethimide, mitotane: may cause severe adrenocortical hypofunction.
Thiazides, loop diuretics: decreased potassium loss because trilostane inhibits aldosterone production.

NURSING CONSIDERATIONS
• Contraindicated in patients with severe renal or hepatic disease.
• Use cautiously in patients who are receiving other drugs that suppress adrenal function.
• Trilostane may prevent normal response to physiologic stressful situation. Therefore, patients who develop a severe illness or need surgery may need to have this drug temporarily discontinued.
• Because the drug may cause orthostatic hypotension by suppressing aldosterone production, monitor blood pressure regularly in all patients.
• Patient should show therapeutic response within 2 weeks. If no response has occurred, the doctor may discontinue the drug.
• Most patients show a therapeutic response at doses below 360 mg/day.
• Trilostane is prescribed when surgery or pituitary radiation is inappropriate or must be delayed. Explain to patient that the drug does not cure the underlying disease.

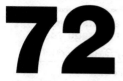

Miscellaneous antineoplastic agents

asparaginase
Erwinia asparaginase
etoposide
mitoxantrone hydrochloride
vinblastine sulfate
vincristine sulfate

COMBINATION PRODUCTS
None.

asparaginase
(L-asparaginase)
Elspar, Kidrolase†

Pregnancy Risk Category: C

HOW SUPPLIED
Injection: 10,000-IU vials

MECHANISM OF ACTION
Destroys the amino acid asparagine, which is needed for protein synthesis in acute lymphocytic leukemia. This leads to death of the leukemic cell.

INDICATIONS & DOSAGE
Acute lymphocytic leukemia (when used along with other drugs)—
Adults and children: 1,000 IU/kg I.V. daily for 10 days, injected over 30 minutes or by slow I.V. push; or 6,000 IU/m² I.M. at intervals specified in protocol.
Sole induction agent for acute lymphocytic leukemia—
200 IU/kg I.V. daily for 28 days.

ADVERSE REACTIONS
Blood: *hypofibrinogenemia* and depression of other clotting factors, thrombocytopenia, *leukopenia,* depression of serum albumin.
CNS: lethargy, somnolence.
GI: *vomiting (may last up to 24 hours), anorexia, nausea,* cramps, weight loss.
GU: *azotemia,* renal failure, uric acid nephropathy, glycosuria, polyuria.
Hepatic: elevated AST (SGOT), ALT (SGPT), *hepatotoxicity.*
Metabolic: elevated alkaline phosphatase and bilirubin (direct and indirect); increase or decrease in total lipids; *hyperglycemia; increased blood ammonia.*
Skin: *rash, urticaria.*
Other: *hemorrhagic pancreatitis and anaphylaxis (relatively common),* chills, fever.

INTERACTIONS
Methotrexate: decreased methotrexate effectiveness.
Vincristine, prednisone: concurrent use is associated with increased toxicity.

NURSING CONSIDERATIONS
• Contraindicated in pancreatitis and previous hypersensitivity unless desensitized. Use cautiously in preexisting hepatic dysfunction.
• Should be administered in hospital setting with close supervision.
• Keep epinephrine, diphenhydramine, and I.V. corticosteroids available for treatment of anaphylaxis.
• Don't use as sole agent to induce remission unless combination therapy is inappropriate. Not recommended for maintenance therapy.

---

†Available in Canada only. ‡Available in Australia only. ◇Available OTC.

• Risk of hypersensitivity increases with repeated dosages. Patient may be desensitized, but this doesn't rule out risk of allergic reactions. Routine administration of 2 IU I.V. test dose may identify high-risk patients.

• Give I.V. injection over 30-minute period through a running infusion of sodium chloride injection or dextrose 5% injection.

• For I.M. injection, limit dose at single injection site to 2 ml.

• Because of vomiting, patient may need parenteral fluids for 24 hours or until oral fluids are tolerated.

• Monitor CBC and bone marrow function. Bone marrow regeneration may take 5 to 6 weeks.

• Obtain frequent serum amylase determinations to check pancreatic status. If elevated, asparaginase should be discontinued.

• Tumor lysis can result in uric acid nephropathy. Prevent occurrence by increasing fluid intake. Allopurinol should be started before therapy begins.

• Warn patient to watch for signs of infection (fever, sore throat, fatigue) and bleeding (easy bruising, nosebleeds, bleeding gums, melena). Take temperature daily.

• Monitor blood and urine glucose before and during therapy. Watch for signs of hyperglycemia, such as glycosuria and polyuria.

• Reconstitute with either 2 to 5 ml sterile water for injection or sodium chloride injection.

• Don't shake vial; may cause loss of potency. Don't use cloudy solutions.

• Refrigerate unopened dry powder. Reconstituted solution is stable for 6 hours at room temperature, 24 hours refrigerated.

• Preparation of parenteral form is associated with carcinogenic, mutagenic, and teratogenic risks for personnel. Follow institutional policy to reduce risks.

Erwinia asparaginase (porton asparaginase)

Pregnancy Risk Category: C

HOW SUPPLIED
Available through National Cancer Institute
Injection: 10,000 IU/vial

MECHANISM OF ACTION
Destroys the amino acid asparagine, which is needed for protein synthesis.

INDICATIONS & DOSAGE
Acute lymphocytic leukemia (in combination with other drugs)—
Adults: 5,000 to 10,000 IU/m²/day for 7 days every 3 weeks or 10,000 to 40,000 IU/m² every 2 to 3 weeks.

Doses may be given I.V. over 15 to 30 minutes or by I.M. injection.
Children: 6,000 to 10,000 IU/m² I.V. or I.M. daily for 14 days; or 60,000 IU/m² every other day for a total of 12 doses; or 1,000 IU/kg for 10 days.

ADVERSE REACTIONS
Blood: *hypofibrinogenemia and depression of other clotting factors,* leukopenia (rare), and thrombocytopenia.
CNS: *lethargy,* somnolence.
GI: mild nausea and vomiting, anorexia, weight loss.
GU: (rare) azotemia and renal failure.
Hepatic: hepatotoxicity, elevated liver function tests, hypoalbuminemia.
Metabolic: *hyperglycemia.*
Skin: rash, urticaria.
Other: *acute pancreatitis, anaphylaxis, fever.*

INTERACTIONS
None significant.

NURSING CONSIDERATIONS
• Contraindicated in pancreatitis.
• *Erwinia strain* of asparaginase is usually reserved for those patients

---

Italicized adverse reactions are common or life-threatening.
*Liquid form contains alcohol.   **May contain tartrazine.

with previous reactions to *Escherichia coli* asparaginase. The two forms of the drug are not cross-reactive.
• Use cautiously in preexisting hepatic dysfunction.
• Monitor vital signs closely.
• Should be administered in a hospital setting with close supervision.
• Risk of hypersensitivity increases with repeated dosages.
• Keep epinephrine, diphenhydramine, and I.V. corticosteroids available for treatment of anaphylaxis.
• Don't use as sole agent to induce remission unless combination therapy is inappropriate. Not recommended for maintenance therapy.
• Give I.V. infusion or I.V. push over 30 minutes through a running infusion of normal saline solution or dextrose 5% in water.
• For I.M. injection, limit dose at single injection site to 2 ml.
• Reconstitute with 2 to 5 ml sterile water for injection or sodium chloride injection. For I.M. use, each 10,000 I.V. vial may be dissolved in 1 ml of diluent.
• Don't shake vial; may cause loss of potency. Don't use cloudy solutions.
• Reconstituted solutions are stable for 3 weeks at either room temperature or refrigerated. Solutions further diluted for infusion are stable at room temperature or refrigerated for at least 4 days.
• The reconstituted solution should be withdrawn from the vial within 15 minutes to minimize protein denaturation resulting from contact with the stopper.
• Monitor CBC and renal and liver function tests.
• Watch for signs of bleeding, such as petechiae and ecchymoses.
• Monitor blood sugar, and test urine for glycosuria before and during therapy.
• Obtain frequent serum amylase and lipase determinations to check pancreatic status. If serum levels are ele-

vated, asparaginase should be discontinued.
• Preparation of parenteral form is associated with carcinogenic, mutagenic, and teratogenic risks for personnel. Follow institutional policy to reduce risks.

etoposide (VP-16)
VePesid

Pregnancy Risk Category: D

HOW SUPPLIED
Capsules: 50 mg
Injection: 100-mg/5-ml multiple-dose vials

MECHANISM OF ACTION
A semi-synthetic derivative of podophyllotoxin that arrests cell mitosis.

INDICATIONS & DOSAGE
Small-cell carcinoma of the lung, acute nonlymphocytic leukemia, lymphosarcoma, Hodgkin's disease, testicular carcinoma—
Adults: 45 to 75 mg/m² daily I.V. or P.O. for 3 to 5 days repeated q 3 to 5 weeks; or 200 to 250 mg/m² I.V. or P.O. weekly; or 125 to 140 mg/m² daily I.V. or P.O. three times a week q 5 weeks.

ADVERSE REACTIONS
Blood: *myelosuppression (dose-limiting), leukopenia,* thrombocytopenia.
CV: hypotension from rapid infusion.
GI: nausea and vomiting.
Local: infrequent phlebitis.
Other: occasional headache and fever, *reversible alopecia, anaphylaxis* (rare).

INTERACTIONS
Warfarin: etoposide may further increase prothrombin time.

NURSING CONSIDERATIONS
• Intrapleural and intrathecal admin-

---

istration of this drug is contraindicated.

• Give drug by slow I.V. infusion (over at least 30 minutes) to prevent severe hypotension.

• Blood pressure should be monitored before infusion and at 30-minute intervals during infusion. If systolic blood pressure falls below 90 mm Hg, infusion should be stopped and doctor notified.

• Have diphenhydramine, hydrocortisone, epinephrine, and airway available in case of an anaphylactic reaction.

• Monitor CBC. Observe patient for signs of bone marrow suppression.

• The drug may be diluted in either dextrose 5% in water or normal saline solution to a concentration of 0.2 or 0.4 mg/ml. Higher concentrations may crystallize.

• Solutions diluted to 0.2 mg/ml are stable for 96 hours at room temperature in plastic or glass unprotected from light; solutions diluted to 0.4 mg/ml are stable for 48 hours under the same conditions.

• Do not administer through membrane-type in-line filters because the diluent may dissolve the filter.

• Etoposide has produced complete remissions in small-cell lung cancer and testicular cancer.

• Preparation of parenteral form is associated with carcinogenic, mutagenic, and teratogenic risks for personnel. Follow institutional policy to reduce risks.

---

mitoxantrone hydrochloride
Novantrone

Pregnancy Risk Category: D

HOW SUPPLIED
Injection: 2 mg/ml in 10-ml, 12.5-ml, 15-ml vials

MECHANISM OF ACTION
Not fully understood; probably non-

cell–cycle specific. Reacts with DNA, producing cytotoxic effect.

INDICATIONS & DOSAGE
Combination initial therapy for acute nonlymphocytic leukemia (ANL)—
Adults: 12 mg/m² I.V. daily on days 1 through 3, in combination with cytosine arabinoside 100 mg/m² daily on days 1 through 7. If a repeat course is necessary, mitoxantrone should be given on days 1 and 2 with cytosine arabinoside administered on days 1 through 5.

ADVERSE REACTIONS
Blood: *myelosuppression.*
CNS: seizures, headache.
CV: CHF, arrhythmias, tachycardia.
GI: *bleeding, abdominal pain, diarrhea, nausea, mucositis, stomatitis, vomiting.*
Respiratory: dyspnea, cough.
Other: alopecia, jaundice, fever, hyperuricemia.

INTERACTIONS
Heparin: incompatible when mixed together.

NURSING CONSIDERATIONS
• Contraindicated in patients with hypersensitivity to mitoxantrone.

• Uric acid nephropathy can be avoided by adequately hydrating the patient before and during therapy. Be prepared to administer allopurinol as ordered.

• Patients with significant myelosuppression should not receive mitoxantrone unless the benefits outweigh the risks. Mitoxantrone should be prescribed only by doctors experienced with chemotherapy.

• Hematologic and chemistry laboratory parameters should be monitored closely.

• Should be used cautiously in patients with prior exposure to anthracyclines or other cardiotoxic drugs.

• Available as an aqueous solution of

Italicized adverse reactions are common or life-threatening.
*Liquid form contains alcohol.   **May contain tartrazine.

2 mg/ml in volumes of 10, 12.5, and 15 ml. The dose should be diluted in at least 50 ml of 0.9% sodium chloride injection or 5% dextrose in water (D₅W) injection. The drug should be administered by direct injection into a free-flowing I.V. of 0.9% sodium chloride or D₅W injection over at least 3 minutes. Mixing with other drugs is not recommended.

• The undiluted solution should be stored at room temperature. Once diluted, the mixture is stable for 48 hours at room temperature.

• Exercise extreme caution when preparing or administering mitoxantrone to avoid mutagenic, teratogenic, and carcinogenic risks. Use a biological containment cabinet, wear gloves and mask, and use syringes with Luer-Lok fittings to prevent leakage of drug solution. Also correctly dispose of needles, vials, and unused drug, and avoid contaminating work surfaces. Avoid inhalation of dust or vapors and contact with skin or mucous membranes. If contact with the eye occurs, irrigate with water or saline and consult an ophthalmologist. If the drug comes in contact with the skin, irrigate the area with water. Mitoxantrone is not a vesicant.

• Infections should be treated with antibiotics, as ordered. If severe nonhematologic toxicity occurs during the first course of therapy, the second course should be delayed until patient recovers.

• Patients should be informed that the urine may appear blue-green within 24 hours after administration and some bluish discoloration of the sclera may occur, but that these effects are not harmful.

• Monitor left ventricular ejection fraction during administration.

vinblastine sulfate (VLB)
Alkaban-AQ, Velban, Velbe†‡, Velsar

Pregnancy Risk Category: D

HOW SUPPLIED
Injection: 10-mg vials (lyophilized powder), 10-mg/10-ml vials

MECHANISM OF ACTION
Arrests mitosis in metaphase, blocking cell division.

INDICATIONS & DOSAGE
Breast or testicular cancer, Hodgkin's and non-Hodgkin's lymphomas, choriocarcinoma, lymphosarcoma, neuroblastoma, mycosis fungoides, histiocytosis—
Adults and children: 0.1 mg/kg or 3.7 mg/m² I.V. weekly or q 2 weeks. May be increased to maximum dosage (adults) of 0.5 mg/kg or 18.5 mg/m² I.V. weekly according to response. Dosage should not be repeated if WBC less than 4,000/mm³.

ADVERSE REACTIONS
Blood: *leukopenia* (nadir days 4 to 10 and lasts another 7 to 14 days), *thrombocytopenia.*
CNS: depression, *paresthesias, peripheral neuropathy and neuritis, numbness, loss of deep tendon reflexes, muscle pain and weakness.*
CV: hypertension.
EENT: pharyngitis.
GI: *nausea, vomiting, stomatitis,* ulcer and bleeding, *constipation, ileus, anorexia, weight loss,* abdominal pain.
GU: oligospermia, aspermia, urine retention.
Skin: dermatitis, vesication.
Local: *irritation, phlebitis,* cellulitis, necrosis if I.V. extravasates.
Other: *acute bronchospasm,* reversible alopecia in 5% to 10% of patients, *pain in tumor site,* low fever.

INTERACTIONS
Mitomycin: increased risk of bronchospasm and shortness of breath.
Phenytoin: decreased plasma phenytoin levels.

NURSING CONSIDERATIONS
• Contraindicated in severe leukopenia or bacterial infection. Use cautiously in jaundice or hepatic dysfunction.
• After administering, monitor for life-threatening acute bronchospasm reaction. If this occurs, notify doctor immediately. Reaction most likely to occur in patient who is also receiving mitomycin.
• Give antiemetic before administering to reduce nausea.
• Drug should be stopped if stomatitis occurs.
• Assess bowel activity. Give laxatives as needed. May use stool softeners prophylactically.
• Don't repeat dosage more frequently than every 7 days or severe leukopenia will develop.
• Less neurotoxic than vincristine.
• Assess for numbness and tingling in hands and feet. Assess gait for early evidence of footdrop.
• Should be injected directly into vein or tubing of running I.V. over 1 minute. May also be given in a 50-ml dextrose 5% in water or normal saline solution and infused over 15 minutes. If extravasation occurs, stop infusion. The manufacturer recommends that moderate heat be applied to the area of leakage. Local injection of hyaluronidase may help disperse the drug. Some clinicians prefer to apply ice packs on and off every 2 hours for 24 hours, with local injection of hydrocortisone or 0.9% sodium chloride.
• Warn patient that alopecia may occur but is usually reversible.
• Adequate trial 12 weeks; reassure patient that therapeutic response isn't immediate.
• Reconstitute 10-mg vial with 10 ml of sodium chloride injection or sterile water. This yields 1 mg/ml.
• Refrigerate reconstituted solution. Discard after 30 days.
• Don't confuse vinblastine with vincristine or the investigational agent vindesine.
• Preparation of parenteral form is associated with carcinogenic, mutagenic, and teratogenic risks for personnel. Follow institutional policy to reduce risks.

vincristine sulfate
Oncovin, Vincasar PFS

Pregnancy Risk Category: D

HOW SUPPLIED
Injection: 1-mg/ml, 2-mg/2-ml, 5-mg/5-ml multiple-dose vials; 1-mg/1-ml, 2-mg/2-ml preservative-free vials

MECHANISM OF ACTION
Arrests mitosis in metaphase, blocking cell division.

INDICATIONS & DOSAGE
Acute lymphoblastic and other leukemias, Hodgkin's disease, lymphosarcoma, reticulum cell sarcoma, neuroblastoma, rhabdomyosarcoma, Wilms' tumor, osteogenic and other sarcomas, lung and breast cancer—
Adults: 1 to 2 mg/m² I.V. weekly.
Children: 1.5 to 2 mg/m² I.V. weekly. Maximum single dosage (adults and children) is 2 mg.

ADVERSE REACTIONS
Blood: rapidly reversible mild anemia and leukopenia.
CNS: *peripheral neuropathy,* sensory loss, *loss of deep tendon reflexes, paresthesias, wristdrop and footdrop,* ataxia, cranial nerve palsies (headache, *jaw pain,* hoarseness, vocal cord paralysis, visual disturbances), *muscle weakness and cramps,* depression, agitation, insomnia; some neurotoxicities may be permanent.

Italicized adverse reactions are common or life-threatening.
*Liquid form contains alcohol.   **May contain tartrazine.

EENT: diplopia, optic and extraocular neuropathy, ptosis.

GI: *constipation, cramps,* ileus that mimics surgical abdomen, *nausea, vomiting,* anorexia, *stomatitis,* weight loss, dysphagia.

GU: urine retention, syndrome of inappropriate antidiuretic hormone (SIADH).

Local: severe local reaction when extravasated, *phlebitis,* cellulitis.

Other: *acute bronchospasm, reversible alopecia (up to 71% of patients).*

INTERACTIONS

Asparaginase: decreased hepatic clearance of vincristine.

Calcium channel blockers: enhanced vincristine accumulation in cells.

Digoxin: decreased digoxin effects. Monitor serum digoxin.

Mitomycin: possibly increased frequency of bronchospasm and acute pulmonary reactions.

NURSING CONSIDERATIONS

• Use cautiously in jaundice or hepatic dysfunction, neuromuscular disease, infection, and with other neurotoxic drugs.

• After administering, monitor for life-threatening acute bronchospasm reaction. If this occurs, notify doctor immediately. Reaction most likely to occur in patient who is also receiving mitomycin.

• Because of neurotoxicity, don't give drug more than once a week. Children more resistant to neurotoxicity than adults. Neurotoxicity is dose-related and usually reversible.

• Should be given directly into vein or tubing of running I.V. slowly over 1 minute. May also be given in a 50-ml dextrose 5% in water or normal saline solution and infused over 15 minutes. If drug infiltrates, apply ice packs on and off every 2 hours for 24 hours.

• Check for depression of Achilles tendon reflex, numbness, tingling, footdrop or wristdrop, difficulty in walking, ataxia, and slapping gait. Also check ability to walk on heels. Support patient when walking.

• Monitor bowel function. Give stool softener, laxative, or water before dosing. Constipation may be an early sign of neurotoxicity.

• Warn patient that alopecia may occur but is usually reversible.

• Be extremely careful about doses. Don't confuse vincristine with vinblastine or the investigational agent vindesine.

• 5-mg vials are for multiple-dose use only. Don't administer entire vial to one patient as a single dose.

• All vials (1-mg, 2-mg, 5-mg) contain 1 mg/ml solution and should be refrigerated.

• Preparation of parenteral form is associated with carcinogenic, mutagenic, and teratogenic risks for personnel. Follow institutional policy to reduce risks.

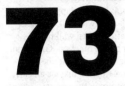

Immunosuppressants

**azathioprine
cyclosporine
lymphocyte immune globulin
muromonab-CD3**

COMBINATION PRODUCTS
None.

---

azathioprine
Imuran, Thioprine‡

Pregnancy Risk Category: D

HOW SUPPLIED
Tablets: 50 mg
Injection: 100 mg

MECHANISM OF ACTION
Inhibits purine synthesis.

INDICATIONS & DOSAGE
Immunosuppression in renal transplants—
Adults and children: initially, 3 to 5 mg/kg P.O. or I.V. daily usually beginning on the day of transplantation. Maintain at 1 to 3 mg/kg daily (dosage varies considerably according to patient response).
Treatment of severe, refractory rheumatoid arthritis—
Adults: initially, 1 mg/kg P.O. taken as a single dose or as two doses. If patient response is not satisfactory after 6 to 8 weeks, dosage may be increased by 0.5 mg/kg daily (up to a maximum of 2.5 mg/kg daily) at 4-week intervals.

ADVERSE REACTIONS
Blood: *leukopenia, bone marrow suppression,* anemia, pancytopenia, thrombocytopenia.
GI: nausea, vomiting, anorexia, *pancreatitis,* steatorrhea, mouth ulceration, esophagitis.
Hepatic: hepatotoxicity, jaundice.
Skin: rash.
Other: *immunosuppression (possibly profound),* arthralgia, muscle wasting, alopecia.

INTERACTIONS
Allopurinol: impaired inactivation of azathioprine. Decrease azathioprine dose to ¼ or ⅓ normal dose.
Nondepolarizing neuromuscular blocking agents: azathioprine may reverse the neuromuscular blockade.

NURSING CONSIDERATIONS
• Use cautiously in hepatic or renal dysfunction.
• Watch for clay-colored stools, dark urine, pruritus, and yellow skin and sclera; and for increased alkaline phosphatase, bilirubin, AST (SGOT), and ALT (SGPT).
• In renal homotransplants, start drug 1 to 5 days before surgery.
• Hemoglobin, WBC, and platelet count should be done at least once monthly; more often at beginning of treatment. Drug should be stopped immediately when WBC is less than 3,000/mm³ to prevent irreversible bone marrow suppression.
• This is a potent immunosuppressive. Warn patient to report even mild infections (colds, fever, sore throat, and malaise).
• Patient should avoid conception

Italicized adverse reactions are common or life-threatening.
*Liquid form contains alcohol.   **May contain tartrazine.

during therapy and 4 months after stopping therapy.
- Warn patient that some thinning of hair is possible.
- Avoid I.M. injections of any drugs in patients with severely depressed platelet counts (thrombocytopenia) to prevent bleeding.
- When used for refractory rheumatoid arthritis, inform patient that it may take up to 12 weeks to be effective.

---

cyclosporine (cyclosporin)
Sandimmun‡, Sandimmune

Pregnancy Risk Category: C

HOW SUPPLIED
Oral solution: 100 mg/ml
Injection: 50 mg/ml

MECHANISM OF ACTION
Inhibits the action of T lymphocytes.

INDICATIONS & DOSAGE
Prophylaxis of organ rejection in kidney, liver, bone marrow, and heart transplants—
Adults and children: 15 mg/kg P.O. (oral solution) 4 to 12 hours before transplantation. Continue this daily dosage postoperatively for 1 to 2 weeks. Then, gradually reduce dosage by 5%/week to maintenance level of 5 to 10 mg/kg/day. Alternatively, administer I.V. concentrate 4 to 5 mg/kg 4 to 12 hours before transplantation. Postoperatively, repeat this dosage daily until patient can tolerate oral solution.

ADVERSE REACTIONS
CNS: *tremor*, headache.
CV: hypertension.
GI: *gum hyperplasia*, nausea, vomiting, diarrhea, oral thrush.
GU: *nephrotoxicity*.
Hepatic: hepatotoxicity.
Skin: *hirsutism*, acne.
Other: sinusitis, flushing.

INTERACTIONS
Aminoglycosides, amphotericin B, cotrimoxazole, NSAIDs: increased risk of nephrotoxicity.
Azathioprine, corticosteroids, cyclophosphamide, verapamil: increased immunosuppression.
Carbamazepine, isoniazid, phenobarbital, phenytoin, rifampin: possible decreased immunosuppressant effect. May need to increase cyclosporine dosage.
Ketoconazole, amphotericin B, cimetidine, diltiazem, erythromycin, imipenem-cilastatin, metoclopramide, prednisolone: may increase blood levels of cyclosporine. Monitor for increased toxicity.

NURSING CONSIDERATIONS
- Cyclosporine may cause nephrotoxicity. Monitor BUN and serum creatinine levels. Nephrotoxicity may develop 2 to 3 months after transplant surgery. Report these findings to doctor. He may reduce the dosage.
- Differentiation between transplanted kidney rejection and cyclosporine-induced nephrotoxicity must be made.
- Monitor liver function tests for hepatotoxicity, which usually occurs during first month post–organ transplant.
- Cyclosporine should always be given concomitantly with adrenal corticosteroids.
- Absorption of cyclosporine oral solution can be erratic. Monitor cyclosporine blood levels at regular intervals.
- Measure oral doses carefully in an oral syringe. To increase palatability, mix with whole milk, chocolate milk, or fruit juice. Use a glass container to minimize adherence to container walls.
- Dosage should be given once daily in the morning. Encourage patient to take drug at the same time each day.
- Patient may take with meals if drug causes nausea.

- Stress to patient that therapy should not be stopped without doctor's approval.
- To prevent thrush, patient should swish and swallow nystatin four times daily.
- If hirsutism occurs, tell patient she may use a depilatory.

lymphocyte immune globulin (antithymocyte globulin [equine], ATG)
Atgam

Pregnancy Risk Category: C

HOW SUPPLIED
Injection: 50 mg of equine IgG/ml, 5-ml ampules

MECHANISM OF ACTION
Inhibits cell-mediated immune responses by either altering T cell function or eliminating antigen-reactive T cells.

INDICATIONS & DOSAGE
Prevention of acute renal allograft rejection—
Adults and children: 15 mg/kg I.V. daily for 14 days followed by alternate-day dosing for 14 days; the first dose should be given within 24 hours of transplantation.
Treatment of acute renal allograft rejection—
Adults and children: 10 to 15 mg/kg I.V. daily for 14 days followed by alternate-day dosing for 14 days. Therapy should be initiated when rejection is diagnosed.

ADVERSE REACTIONS
Blood: leukopenia, thrombocytopenia, *hemolysis,* hyperglycemia, elevated serum hepatic enzymes.
CNS: malaise, seizures, headache.
CV: *hypotension, chest pain,* thrombophlebitis, tachycardia, edema, *pulmonary edema,* iliac vein obstruction, renal artery stenosis.

EENT: *dyspnea, laryngospasm.*
GI: *nausea, vomiting,* diarrhea, stomatitis, hiccups, epigastric pain, abdominal distension.
Other: febrile reactions, serum sickness, *anaphylaxis,* rash, infections, arthralgia, night sweats, lymphadenopathy.

INTERACTIONS
None reported.

NURSING CONSIDERATIONS
- Use cautiously in patients receiving additional immunosuppressive therapy (e.g., corticosteroids, azathioprine) because of the increased potential for infection. ATG concentrate should not be diluted with dextrose solutions or solutions with a low salt concentration since a precipitate may form. The proteins in ATG can be denatured by air. ATG is unstable in acidic solutions.
- An intradermal skin test is recommended at least 1 hour before the first dose. Marked local swelling or erythema larger than 10 mm indicates an increased potential for severe systemic reaction (e.g., anaphylaxis).
- Monitor patient for signs of infection.
- ATG solutions must be filtered during administration; filters with pore sizes of 0.2 to 5 microns have been used.
- Drug should be infused over at least 4 hours.
- ATG concentrate is very heat-sensitive; refrigerate at 2° to 8° C. (do not freeze).
- Do not use solutions that are more than 12 hours old.

muromonab-CD3
Orthoclone OKT3

Pregnancy Risk Category: C

HOW SUPPLIED
Injection: 5 mg/5 ml in 5-ml ampules

Italicized adverse reactions are common or life-threatening.
*Liquid form contains alcohol.   **May contain tartrazine.

MECHANISM OF ACTION

Muromonab-CD3 is an IgG antibody that reacts in the T-lymphocyte membrane with a molecule (CD3) needed for antigen recognition. This drug depletes the blood of CD3-positive T cells, which leads to restoration of allograft function and reversal of rejection.

INDICATIONS & DOSAGE

Treatment of acute allograft rejection in renal transplant patients—
Adults: 5 mg I.V. bolus once daily for 10 to 14 days.
Children: 2.5 mg I.V. bolus once daily for 10 to 14 days.

ADVERSE REACTIONS

CV: *chest pain.*
GI: *nausea, vomiting,* diarrhea.
Other: *severe pulmonary edema, fever, chills, tremors, dyspnea, infection.*

INTERACTIONS

None reported.

NURSING CONSIDERATIONS

• Contraindicated in patients with fluid overload, as evidenced by chest X-ray or a weight gain greater than 3% within the week before treatment.
• Muromonab-CD3 is a monoclonal antibody preparation. Patients develop antibodies to this preparation that can lead to loss of effectiveness and more severe adverse reactions if a second course of therapy is attempted. Therefore, experts believe that this drug should be used for only a single course of treatment.
• Most adverse reactions develop within ½ hour to 6 hours after the first dose.
• Treatment should begin in a facility where the patient can be monitored closely and that is equipped and staffed for cardiopulmonary resuscitation.

• Assess patient for signs of fluid overload before treatment.
• Chest X-ray must be taken within 24 hours before starting drug treatment.
• Inform patient of expected adverse reactions. Reassure him that they will be less severe as treatment progresses.
• Administering an antipyretic before giving the drug may help lower incidence of expected pyrexia and chills. Corticosteroids may also be administered before first injection to help decrease incidence of adverse reactions. Methylprednisolone sodium succinate (1mg/kg) preinjection, followed by hydrocortisone sodium succinate (100 mg) 30 minutes postinjection, have been recommended to alleviate the severity of the first dose reaction.

74

Vaccines and toxoids

BCG vaccine
cholera vaccine
diphtheria and tetanus toxoids, adsorbed
diphtheria and tetanus toxoids and pertussis vaccine
Haemophilus b conjugate vaccines
hepatitis B vaccine, plasma derived
hepatitis B vaccine, recombinant
influenza virus vaccine, 1990-1991 trivalent types A & B (purified surface antigen)
influenza virus vaccine, 1990-1991 trivalent types A & B (sub virion or split virion)
influenza virus vaccine, 1990-1991 trivalent types A & B (whole virion)
measles, mumps, and rubella virus vaccine, live
measles (rubeola) and rubella virus vaccine, live attenuated
measles (rubeola) virus vaccine, live attenuated
meningitis vaccines
mumps virus vaccine, live
plague vaccine
pneumococcal vaccine, polyvalent
poliovirus vaccine, live, oral, trivalent
rabies vaccine, human diploid cell
rubella and mumps virus vaccine, live
rubella virus vaccine, live attenuated
tetanus toxoid, adsorbed
tetanus toxoid, fluid

typhoid vaccine
yellow fever vaccine

COMBINATION PRODUCTS
None.

BCG vaccine
Pregnancy Risk Category: C

HOW SUPPLIED
Intradermal vaccine: 3 to 26 million colony-forming units (CFU)/ml
Percutaneous vaccine: 1 to 8×10^8 CFU/vial

MECHANISM OF ACTION
Promotes active immunity to tuberculosis.

INDICATIONS & DOSAGE
Tuberculosis exposure, cancer immunotherapy—
Adults and children 3 months and over: 0.1 ml (intradermal vaccine) or 0.2 to 0.3 ml (percutaneous vaccine) applied to cleansed area of skin followed by application of multiple puncture disk.
Children under 3 months: 0.05 ml (intradermal vaccine).

ADVERSE REACTIONS
Local: lymphangitis, lymph node and skin abscess, ulceration at site of injection (2 to 3 weeks after injection), lupus reaction.
Other: urticaria of trunk and limbs, lymphadenitis, osteomyelitis, *anaphylaxis*.

Italicized adverse reactions are common or life-threatening.
*Liquid form contains alcohol.   **May contain tartrazine.

INTERACTIONS

Immunosuppressive therapy: may reduce response to BCG vaccine. Avoid if possible.

Isoniazid, rifampin, streptomycin : inhibited multiplication of BCG. Avoid using together.

Theophylline: BCG vaccine may impair theophylline elimination.

NURSING CONSIDERATIONS

• Contraindicated in hypogammaglobulinemia, positive tuberculin reaction (when meant for use as immunoprophylactic after exposure to tuberculosis), immunosuppression, fresh smallpox vaccination, burns, and in patients receiving corticosteroid therapy. Use cautiously in chronic skin disease. Inject in area of healthy skin only.

• Obtain history of allergies and reaction to immunization.

• Vaccine is of no value as immunoprophylactic in patients with positive tuberculin test.

• Keep epinephrine 1:1,000 available to treat anaphylaxis.

• Recommended injection site is over insertion of deltoid muscle.

• Do not shake vial following reconstitution.

• Expected lesion forms in 7 to 10 days.

• Allow an interval of at least 3 weeks between BCG and rubella vaccination.

• Don't administer to children with febrile illness.

• Live vaccine; destroy by autoclaving or formaldehyde solution before disposal.

• Patient should have tuberculin skin test 2 to 3 months after BCG vaccination to determine success of vaccine.

• Use of BCG has shown some value in treatment of various cancers, such as leukemia, some lung cancers, malignant melanoma, multiple myeloma, and some breast tumors. Currently, researchers are trying to find ways of augmenting the immune system's response to cancer. They hope to stimulate the body to destroy tumor cells.

---

cholera vaccine

Pregnancy Risk Category: C

HOW SUPPLIED

Injection: suspension of killed *Vibrio cholerae* (each milliliter contains 8 units of Inaba and Ogawa serotypes) in 1-ml, 1.5-ml, and 20-ml vials

MECHANISM OF ACTION

Promotes active immunity to cholera.

INDICATIONS & DOSAGE

Primary immunization—

Adults and children over 10 years: two doses of 0.5 ml I.M. or 1 ml S.C., 1 week to 1 month apart, before traveling in cholera area. Booster is 0.5 ml q 6 months as long as protection is needed.

Children 5 to 10 years: 0.3 ml I.M. or S.C.

Children 6 months to 4 years: 0.2 ml I.M. or S.C. Boosters of same dose should be given q 6 months as long as protection is needed.

ADVERSE REACTIONS

Systemic: malaise, fever, flushing, urticaria, tachycardia, hypotension, diarrhea, headache, *anaphylaxis*.
Local: erythema, swelling, pain, induration.

INTERACTIONS

Yellow fever vaccine: simultaneous administration may interfere with immune response to cholera vaccine and yellow fever vaccine. Administer 3 weeks apart.

NURSING CONSIDERATIONS

• Contraindicated in corticosteroid therapy or in immunosuppression. Defer in acute illness.

- Obtain history of allergies and reaction to immunization.
- Keep epinephrine 1:1,000 available.
- May be given intradermally, but I.M. and S.C. routes give higher levels of protection.
- Administer I.M. in deltoid muscle in adults and children over 3 years.

diphtheria and tetanus toxoids, adsorbed

Pregnancy Risk Category: C

HOW SUPPLIED
Available in pediatric (DT) and adult (Td) strengths
Injection (for pediatric use): diphtheria toxoid 6.6 Lf units and tetanus toxoid 5 Lf units per 0.5 ml; diphtheria toxoid 10 Lf units and tetanus toxoid 5 Lf units per 0.5 ml; diphtheria toxoid 12.5 Lf units and tetanus toxoid 5 Lf units per 0.5 ml; diphtheria toxoid 15 Lf units and tetanus toxoid 10 Lf units per 0.5 ml
Injection (for adult use): diphtheria toxoid 1.5 Lf units and tetanus toxoid 5 Lf units per 0.5 ml; diphtheria toxoid 2 Lf units and tetanus toxoid 5 Lf units per 0.5 ml; diphtheria toxoid 2 Lf units and tetanus toxoid 10 Lf units per 0.5 ml

MECHANISM OF ACTION
Promotes immunity to diphtheria and tetanus by inducing production of antitoxins.

INDICATIONS & DOSAGE
Primary immunization—
Adults and children over 7 years: use adult strength; 0.5 ml I.M. 4 to 6 weeks apart for two doses and a third dose 1 year later. Booster is 0.5 ml I.M. q 10 years.
Children 1 to 6 years: use pediatric strength; 0.5 ml I.M. at least 4 weeks apart for two doses. Give booster dosage 6 to 12 months after the second

injection. If the final immunizing dose is given after the 7th birthday, use the adult strength.
Infants 6 weeks to 1 year: use pediatric strength; 0.5 ml I.M. at least 4 weeks apart for three doses. Give booster dose 6 to 12 months after third injection.

ADVERSE REACTIONS
Systemic: chills, fever, malaise, *anaphylaxis*.
Local: stinging, edema, erythema, pain, induration.

INTERACTIONS
None significant.

NURSING CONSIDERATIONS
- Contraindicated in immunosuppression, radiation, or corticosteroid therapy. Defer in respiratory illness or polio outbreaks, or acute illness except in emergency. Use single antigen during polio risks. In children under 6 years, use only when diphtheria, tetanus, and pertussis combination is contraindicated because of pertussis component.
- Verify strength (pediatric or adult) of toxoid used.
- Obtain history of allergies and reaction to immunization.
- Keep epinephrine 1:1,000 available.
- Give in site not recently used for vaccines or toxoids.

diphtheria and tetanus toxoids and pertussis vaccine (DPT)
Tri-Immunol

HOW SUPPLIED
Injection: 12.5 Lf units inactivated diphtheria, 5 Lf units inactivated tetanus, and 4 protective units pertussis per 0.5 ml, in 7.5-ml vials

---

Italicized adverse reactions are common or life-threatening.
*Liquid form contains alcohol. **May contain tartrazine.

MECHANISM OF ACTION
Promotes active immunity to diphtheria, tetanus, and pertussis by inducing production of antitoxins and antibodies.

INDICATIONS & DOSAGE
Primary immunization—
Children 6 weeks to 6 years: 0.5 ml I.M. 2 months apart for three doses and a fourth dose 1 year later. Booster is 0.5 ml I.M. when starting school.

Not advised for adults or children over 6 years.

ADVERSE REACTIONS
Systemic: slight fever, chills, malaise, *seizures, encephalopathy, anaphylaxis,* anorexia, vomiting.
Local: *soreness, redness,* expected nodule remaining several weeks.
Other: *sudden infant death syndrome.*

INTERACTIONS
Immunosuppressive therapy: may reduce response to DPT vaccine. Avoid if possible.

NURSING CONSIDERATIONS
• Contraindicated in corticosteroid therapy, immunosuppression, and history of seizures. Defer in acute febrile illness.
• Children with preexisting neurologic disorders should not receive pertussis component. Also, children who react to any DPT injection by exhibiting neurologic signs shouldn't receive pertussis component in any succeeding injections. Diphtheria and tetanus toxoids (DT) should be given instead.
• DPT injection may be given at same time as trivalent oral polio vaccine.
• Obtain history of allergies and reaction to immunization.
• Keep epinephrine 1:1,000 available.
• Not to be used for active infection.
• Don't give subcutaneously.
• Shake before using. Refrigerate.

• Administer only by deep I.M. injection, preferably in thigh or deltoid muscle.

Haemophilus b conjugate vaccines (Hemophilus b conjugate vaccines)

Haemophilus b conjugate vaccine, diphtheria CRM$_{197}$ protein conjugate
HibTITER

Haemophilus b conjugate vaccine, diphtheria toxoid conjugate
ProHIBiT

Haemophilus b conjugate vaccine, meningococcal protein conjugate
PedvaxHIB

HOW SUPPLIED
conjugate vaccine, diphtheria CRM$_{197}$ protein conjugate
Injection: 10 mcg purified Haemophilus b saccharide and approximately 25 mcg CRM$_{197}$ protein per 0.5 ml
conjugate vaccine, diphtheria toxoid conjugate
Injection: 25 mcg of *Haemophilus influenzae* type B (Hib) capsular polysaccharide and 18 mcg of diphtheria toxoid protein per 0.5 ml
conjugate vaccine, meningococcal protein conjugate
Powder for injection: 15 mcg Haemophilus b PRP, 250 mcg *Neisseria meningitidis* OMPC per dose

MECHANISM OF ACTION
Promotes active immunity to Hib.

INDICATIONS & DOSAGE
Immunization against Hib infection—
Children 15 months to 5 years: 0.5 ml I.M.

ADVERSE REACTIONS
Systemic: fever, *anaphylaxis*.
Local: *erythema and pain at injection site*.

INTERACTIONS
Immunosuppressive agents: may suppress antibody response to Hib vaccine.

NURSING CONSIDERATIONS
• Contraindicated in immunosuppression. Defer immunization in acute illness.
• *Hib* is an important cause of meningitis in infants and preschool children.
• The conjugate vaccine is formed when Hib is chemically bound to other protein antigens. It produces a stronger immune response in most patients.
• Don't administer intradermally or I.V. Must administer I.M..
• Administer into the anterolateral aspect of the upper thigh in small children. Injections can be made into the deltoid of larger children if sufficient muscle mass is present.
• This vaccine will *not* protect children against any other microorganisms that cause meningitis. Will protect against Hib only.
• This vaccine and DPT can be given simultaneously, but should be administered at different sites.
• Don't administer to children with febrile illness.
• Not routinely given to adults or children over 5 years unless they are at high risk for infection (including patients with chronic conditions such as functional asplenia, splenectomy, Hodgkin's disease, or sickle cell anemia).
• Keep epinephrine 1:1,000 available in case of a severe allergic reaction.
• Children vaccinated with nonconjugated vaccine (no longer available in the United States) need not be routinely revaccinated if the primary immunization occurred at 24 months. However, if the first vaccination occurred at 18 to 23 months, the child should be revaccinated wtih conjugate vaccine, provided at least 2 months has elapsed.

---

hepatitis B vaccine, plasma derived
Heptavax-B

hepatitis B vaccine, recombinant
Engerix-B, Recombivax HB, Recombivax HB Dialysis Formulation

Pregnancy Risk Category: C

HOW SUPPLIED
plasma-derived form
Injection: 20 mcg hepatitis B surface antigen (Hb_xAg)/ml in 3-ml vials (Heptavax-B, adult formulation); 10 mcg Hb_xAg/0.5 ml in 0.5-ml vials (Heptavax-B, pediatric formulation)
recombinant form
Injection: 5 mcg HB_xAg/0.5 ml (Recombivax HB, pediatric injection); 10 mcg HB_xAg/0.5 ml (Engerix-B, pediatric injection); 10 mcg HB_xAg/ml (Recombivax HB); 20 mcg HB_xAg/ml (Engerix-B); 40 mcg HB_xAg/ml (Recombivax HB Dialysis Formulation)

MECHANISM OF ACTION
Promotes active immunity to hepatitis B.

INDICATIONS & DOSAGE
Immunization against infection from all known subtypes of hepatitis B; primary preexposure prophylaxis against hepatitis B; or postexposure prophylaxis (when given with hepatitis B immune globulin)—
Plasma-derived form (Heptavax-B)
Adults and children over 10 years: initially, give 20 mcg (1-ml adult formulation) I.M., followed by a second dose of 20 mcg I.M. 30 days later.

Italicized adverse reactions are common or life-threatening.
*Liquid form contains alcohol.   **May contain tartrazine.

Give a third dose of 20 mcg I.M. 6 months after the initial dose.
Neonates and children up to 10 years: initially, give 10 mcg (0.5-ml pediatric formulation) I.M., followed by a second dose of 10 mcg I.M. 30 days later. Give a third dose of 10 mcg I.M. 6 months after the initial dose.

Recombinant form (Engerix-B)
Adults and children over 10 years: initially, give 20 mcg (1-ml adult formulation) I.M., followed by a second dose of 20 mcg I.M. 30 days later. Give a third dose of 20 mcg I.M. 6 months after the initial dose.
Neonates and children up to 10 years: initially, give 10 mcg (0.5-ml pediatric formulation) I.M., followed by a second dose of 10 mcg I.M. 30 days later. Give a third dose of 10 mcg I.M. 6 months after the initial dose.
Adults undergoing dialysis or receiving immunosuppressant therapy: initially, give 40 mcg I.M. (divided into two 20-mcg doses and administered at different sites). Follow with a second dose of 40 mcg I.M. in 30 days, and a final dose of 40 mcg I.M. 6 months after the initial dose.

Note: Certain populations (neonates born to infected mothers, persons recently exposed to the virus, and travelers to high-risk areas) may receive the vaccine on an abbreviated schedule, with the initial dose followed by a second dose in 1 month, and the third dose after 2 months. For prolonged maintenance of protective antibody titers, a booster dose is recommended 12 months after the initial dose.

Recombinant form (Recombivax HB)
Adults: initially, give 10 mcg (1-ml adult formulation) I.M., followed by a second dose of 10 mcg I.M. 30 days later. Give a third dose of 10 mcg I.M. 6 months after the initial dose.

Children 11 to 19 years: initially, give 5 mcg (0.5-ml pediatric formulation) I.M., followed by a second dose of 5 mcg I.M. 30 days later. Give a third dose of 5 mcg I.M. 6 months after the initial dose.
Neonates (born to HB,Ag-negative mothers) and children to 11 years: initially, give 2.5 mcg (0.25-ml pediatric formulation) I.M., followed by a second dose of 2.5 mcg I.M. 30 days later. Give a third dose of 2.5 mcg I.M. 6 months after the initial dose.
Neonates born to HB,Ag-positive mothers: initially, give 5 mcg (0.5-ml pediatric formulation) I.M., followed by a second dose of 5 mcg I.M. 30 days later. Give a third dose of 5 mcg I.M. 6 months after the initial dose.
Adults undergoing dialysis or receiving immunosuppressant therapy: initially, give 40 mcg I.M. (use dialysis formulation, which contains 40 mcg/ml). Follow with a second dose of 40 mcg I.M. in 30 days, and give a final dose of 40 mcg I.M. 6 months after the initial dose.

ADVERSE REACTIONS
Systemic: slight fever, transient malaise, headache, dizziness, nausea, vomiting, flu-like symptoms, myalgia.
Local: discomfort at injection site, local inflammation.

INTERACTIONS
None reported.

NURSING CONSIDERATIONS
• Use cautiously in any serious, active infections; compromised cardiac or pulmonary status; and in those for whom a febrile or systemic reaction could pose a serious risk.
• Hepatitis B vaccine has *not* been associated with an increased incidence of AIDS (acquired immunodeficiency syndrome).
• The Centers for Disease Control re-

ports that response to hepatitis B vaccine is significantly better when administered in the arm rather than the buttock.

• May be administered S.C., but only to persons, such as hemophiliacs, who are at risk of hemorrhage.

• Although anaphylaxis has not been reported, epinephrine should always be available when administering this drug to counteract any possible reaction.

• The recommended dosage regimen provides immunity for at least 5 years.

• The following persons are at increased risk of infection and should be considered for the vaccine: certain health care personnel (especially those working with dialysis patients, in blood banks, and in emergency medicine); selected patients and patient contacts; certain endemic populations (Alaskan Eskimos, Indo-Chinese and Haitian refugees); certain military personnel; morticians and embalmers; sexually active homosexuals; prostitutes; prisoners; and users of illicit injectable drugs.

• Thoroughly agitate vial just before administration to restore suspension.

• Store both opened and unopened vials in the refrigerator. Don't freeze.

• Recombivax HB and Engerix-B are manufactured by recombinant DNA technology. Human plasma is *not* used.

influenza virus vaccine, 1990-1991 trivalent types A & B (purified surface antigen)
Flu-Imune

influenza virus vaccine, 1990-1991 trivalent types A & B (subvirion or split virion)
Fluogen Split, Fluzone Split, Influenza Virus Vaccine (Split)

influenza virus vaccine, 1990-1991 trivalent types A & B (whole virion)
Fluzone (Whole)

Pregnancy Risk Category: C

HOW SUPPLIED
Injection: 15 mcg A/Taiwan/1/86 (H1N1), 15 mcg A/Shanghai/11/87 (H3N2), and 15 mcg B/Yamagata/16/88 hemagglutinin antigens per 0.5 ml

MECHANISM OF ACTION
Promotes immunity to influenza by inducing production of antibodies.

INDICATIONS & DOSAGE
Influenza prophylaxis—
Adults and children over 12 years: 0.5 ml whole or split virus I.M. Only one dose is required.
Children 3 to 12 years: 0.5 ml split virus I.M. Repeat dose in 4 weeks unless child has been previously vaccinated.
Children 6 to 35 months: 0.25 ml split virus I.M. Repeat dose in 4 weeks unless child has been previously vaccinated.

ADVERSE REACTIONS
Systemic: fever, malaise, myalgia, *Guillain-Barré syndrome* (rare), *anaphylaxis*.
Local: erythema, induration, soreness at the injection site.
  Fever and malaise reactions occur

Italicized adverse reactions are common or life-threatening.
*Liquid form contains alcohol.   **May contain tartrazine.

most often in children and in others not exposed to influenza viruses. Severe reactions in adults are rare.

INTERACTIONS
Theophylline, warfarin: clearance may be impaired.

NURSING CONSIDERATIONS
• Contraindicated in egg allergy. Defer in acute respiratory or other active infection.
• Obtain history of allergies, especially to eggs, and reaction to immunization. Use cautiously in patients with a history of sulfite allergy.
• Ideally, vaccinations should be performed in November, since outbreaks of influenza generally don't occur until December. Try to avoid administering the vaccine too early in the season because antibody titers may begin to decline prior to the flu season.
• Patients should understand that annual vaccination using the current vaccine is necessary because immunity to influenza decreases in the year following the injection.
• Note that the combination of antigens used to create influenza vaccine changes annually even though some antigens may be the same as previous years. It is important that leftover supplies of 1989-1990 vaccine not be used to immunize patients for the 1990-1991 flu season.
• Children 12 years and under should receive their second dose in December, if possible.
• Vaccines could be given to both children and adults throughout the flu season, even as late as April.
• Give injections for adults and older children in deltoid muscle; in anterolateral aspect of thigh for infants and children under 3 years.
• Keep epinephrine 1:1,000 available.
• Strongly recommended for anyone over 6 months, and patients with chronic disease, metabolic disorders, or medical conditions that put them at risk of complications from influenza. Also strongly recommended for health care workers and household members that may come in contact with persons at high risk of medical complications of influenza.
• Influenza vaccine available as whole virus, split virus, and purified surface antigen preparations. Split virus and purified surface antigen vaccines cause somewhat fewer adverse reactions than whole virus in children.
• Fever, malaise, and myalgia may begin 6 to 12 hours after vaccination and persist 1 to 2 days.
• Allergic reactions, which occur immediately, are extremely rare.
• Paralysis associated with Guillain-Barré syndrome is rare, and has only been associated with the 1976 vaccine.
• Patient should be made aware of risk as compared with risk of influenza and its complications.
• Children should not be given pertussis vaccine within 3 days of influenza virus vaccine. However, they may receive Haemophilus b vaccine, oral polio vaccine, measles-mumps-rubella vaccine, or pneumococcal vaccine at the same time. Injections should be made at different sites.

measles, mumps, and rubella virus vaccine, live
M-M-RII

Pregnancy Risk Category: X

HOW SUPPLIED
Injection: single-dose vial containing not less than 1,000 TCID$_{50}$ (tissue culture infective doses) of attenuated measles virus derived from Enders' attenuated Edmonston strain (grown in chick embryo culture), 5,000 TCID$_{50}$ of the Jeryl Lynn (B level) mumps strain (grown in chick embryo culture), and the Wistar RA 27/3

strain of rubella virus (propagated in human diploid cell culture)

MECHANISM OF ACTION
Promotes immunity to measles, mumps, and rubella virus by inducing production of antibodies.

INDICATIONS & DOSAGE
Routine vaccination—
Children: administer 1 vial S.C. A two-dose schedule is recommended, with the first dose given at 15 months (12 months in high-risk areas) and the second dose given at the entry of school (kindergarten or first grade).
Measles outbreak control—
Children: if cases are occurring in children under 1 year, vaccinate children as young as 6 months. All students and their siblings should be revaccinated if they are without documentation of measles immunity.
Adults: school personnel born in or after 1957 should be revaccinated if they are without proof of measles immunity. If the outbreak is in a medical facility, all workers born in or after 1957 should be revaccinated if they are without proof of immunity. Revaccination should be considered for persons born before 1957 as well.

ADVERSE REACTIONS
Systemic: fever, rash, regional lymphadenopathy, urticaria, *anaphylaxis*.
Local: erythema.

INTERACTIONS
Immune serum globulin, whole blood, plasma: antibodies in serum may interfere with immune response. Don't use vaccine within 3 months of transfusion.

NURSING CONSIDERATIONS
• Contraindicated in immunosuppression; cancer; blood dyscrasias; corticosteroid or radiation therapy; gamma globulin disorders; fever; or active, untreated tuberculosis. Use cautiously in patients with hypersensitivity to neomycin, chickens, ducks, eggs, or feathers. Defer immunization in acute illness.
• Presence of maternal antibodies may prevent response in children under 12 months.
• Treat fever with antipyretics.
• Store in refrigerator; protect from light. Solution may be used if red, pink, or yellow, but must be clear.
• Use only diluent supplied. Discard 8 hours after reconstituting.
• Obtain history of allergies, especially to ducks, rabbits, antibiotics, and reaction to immunization.
• Inject in outer aspect of upper arm. Don't give I.V.
• Keep epinephrine 1:1,000 available.
• Because of a recent rise in the incidence of measles, the Immunization Practices Advisory Committee (ACIP) recommends that colleges and other post–high school educational institutions, as well as medical institutions employing health care providers, obtain documentation of the receipt of two doses of vaccine after age 1 (or other proof of immunity, such as infection, documented by a physician). Combined measles, mumps, and rubella (MMR) vaccine is preferred.
• The Centers for Disease Control (CDC) recommends that, during a measles outbreak in a health care facility, susceptible personnel exposed to the measles virus (whether or not they received measles vaccine or immunoglobulin) avoid patient contact for days 5 through 21 after such exposure. If they become ill, they should avoid patient contact for at least 7 days after developing rash.

Italicized adverse reactions are common or life-threatening.
*Liquid form contains alcohol.   **May contain tartrazine.

measles (rubeola) and rubella virus vaccine, live attenuated
M-R-Vax II

Pregnancy Risk Category: X

HOW SUPPLIED
Injection: single-dose vial containing not less than $1,000$ $TCID_{50}$ (tissue culture infective doses) per 0.5 ml of attenuated measles virus derived from Enders' attenuated Edmonston strain (grown in chick embryo culture); $1,000$ $TCID_{50}$ of the Wistar RA 27/3 strain of rubella virus

MECHANISM OF ACTION
Promotes immunity to measles and rubella virus by inducing production of antibodies.

INDICATIONS & DOSAGE
Immunization—
Children 15 months to puberty: 1 vial (1,000 units) S.C.

ADVERSE REACTIONS
Systemic: fever, rash, lymphadenopathy, *anaphylaxis.*

INTERACTIONS
Immune serum globulin, whole blood, plasma: antibodies in serum may interfere with immune response. Don't use vaccine within 3 months of transfusion.
Tuberculin skin test: may temporarily decrease response to test. Defer skin testing.

NURSING CONSIDERATIONS
• Contraindicated in immunosuppression; cancer; blood dyscrasias; corticosteroid or radiation therapy; gamma globulin disorders; fever; or active, untreated tuberculosis. Use cautiously in patients with hypersensitivity to neomycin, chickens, ducks, eggs, or feathers; when there is a history of febrile seizures; or in cerebral injury. Defer immunization in acute illness.
• Do not give within 1 month of other live virus vaccines, except oral poliovirus vaccine.
• Allow an interval of at least 3 weeks between BCG and rubella vaccines.
• Store in refrigerator and protect from light. Solution may be used if red, pink, or yellow, but must be clear (with no precipitation).
• Use only diluent supplied. Discard 8 hours after reconstituting.
• Inject in outer aspect of upper arm. Don't inject I.V.
• Keep epinephrine 1:1,000 available.

measles (rubeola) virus vaccine, live attenuated
Attenuvax

Pregnancy Risk Category: X

HOW SUPPLIED
Injection: single-dose vial containing not less than $1,000$ $TCID_{50}$ (tissue culture infective doses) of attenuated measles virus derived from Enders' attenuated Edmonston strain (grown in chick embryo culture)

MECHANISM OF ACTION
Promotes immunity to measles virus by inducing production of antibodies.

INDICATIONS & DOSAGE
Immunization—
Adults and children 15 months or over: 0.5 ml (1,000 units) S.C. A two-dose schedule is recommended, with the first dose given at 15 months (12 months in high-risk areas) and the second dose given at the entry of school (kindergarten or first grade).
Measles outbreak control—
Children: if cases are occurring in children under 1 year, vaccinate children as young as 6 months. All students and their siblings should be re-

vaccinated if they are without documentation of measles immunity.

Adults: school personnel born in or after 1957 should be revaccinated if they are without proof of measles immunity. If the outbreak is in a medical facility, all workers born in or after 1957 should be revaccinated if they are without proof of immunity. Revaccination should be considered for persons born before 1957 as well.

ADVERSE REACTIONS

Systemic: fever, rash, lymphadenopathy, *anaphylaxis,* febrile seizures in susceptible children, anorexia, leukopenia.

Local: erythema, swelling, tenderness.

INTERACTIONS

Immune serum globulin, whole blood, plasma: antibodies in serum may interfere with immune response. Don't use vaccine within 3 months of transfusion.

Tuberculin skin test: may temporarily decrease response to test. Defer skin testing.

NURSING CONSIDERATIONS

• Contraindicated in immunosuppression; cancer; blood dyscrasias; corticosteroid or radiation therapy; gamma globulin disorders; or active, untreated tuberculosis; fever. Use with caution in patients with hypersensitivity to neomycin, chickens, eggs, or feathers. Defer in acute illness or after administration of blood or plasma.

• Warn patient to avoid pregnancy for 3 months after vaccination.

• Do not give I.V.

• Obtain history of allergies, especially to eggs, and reaction to immunization.

• Keep epinephrine 1:1,000 available.

• Store in refrigerator and protect from light. Solution may be used if

red, pink, or yellow, but must be clear (with no precipitation).

• Use only diluent supplied. Discard 8 hours after reconstituting.

• May be given with oral poliovirus vaccine.

• Because of a recent rise in the incidence of measles, the Immunization Practices Advisory Committee (ACIP) recommends that colleges and other post–high school educational institutions, as well as medical institutions employing health care providers, obtain documentation of the receipt of two doses of vaccine after age 1 (or other proof of immunity, such as infection, documented by a physician). Combined measles, mumps, and rubella (MMR) vaccine is preferred.

• The Centers for Disease Control (CDC) recommends that, during a measles outbreak in a health care facility, susceptible personnel exposed to the measles virus (whether or not they received measles vaccine or immunoglobulin) avoid patient contact for days 5 through 21 after such exposure. If they become ill, they should avoid patient contact for at least 7 days after developing rash.

meningitis vaccines
Menomune-A/C, Menomune-A/C/Y/W-135

Pregnancy Risk Category: C

HOW SUPPLIED

Injection: a killed bacterial vaccine in 10-dose and 50-dose vials with vial of diluent

MECHANISM OF ACTION

Promotes active immunity to meningitis.

INDICATIONS & DOSAGE

Meningococcal meningitis prophylaxis—

Adults and children over 2 years: 0.5 ml S.C.

ADVERSE REACTIONS
Systemic: headache, malaise, chills, fever, cramps, *anaphylaxis.*
Local: pain, erythema, induration.

INTERACTIONS
None significant.

NURSING CONSIDERATIONS
• Contraindicated in immunosuppression. Defer in acute illness.
• Tell patient to avoid pregnancy for 3 months after vaccination.
• Obtain history of allergies and reaction to immunization.
• Do not give I.V.
• Keep epinephrine 1:1,000 available.

mumps virus vaccine, live
Mumpsvax

Pregnancy Risk Category: X

HOW SUPPLIED
Injection: single-dose vial containing not less than 5,000 TCID$_{50}$ (tissue culture infective doses) of attenuated mumps virus derived from Jeryl Lynn mumps strain (grown in chick embryo culture), and vial of diluent

MECHANISM OF ACTION
Promotes active immunity to mumps.

INDICATIONS & DOSAGE
Immunization—
Adults and children over 1 year: 1 vial (5,000 units) S.C.

ADVERSE REACTIONS
Systemic: *slight fever,* rash, malaise, mild allergic reactions, febrile seizures (rare).

INTERACTIONS
Immune serum globulin, whole blood, plasma: antibodies in serum may interfere with immune response. Don't use vaccine within 3 months of transfusion.

Tuberculin skin test: may temporarily decrease response to test. Defer skin testing.

NURSING CONSIDERATIONS
• Contraindicated in immunosuppression; cancer; blood dyscrasias; corticosteroid or radiation therapy; gamma globulin disorders; active, untreated tuberculosis; or pregnancy. Use cautiously in patients with hypersensitivity to neomycin, chickens, ducks, eggs, or feathers. Defer in acute or febrile illness and for 3 months following transfusions or treatment with immune serum globulin.
• Keep epinephrine 1:1,000 available.
• Mumpsvax should not be given less than 1 month before or after immunization with other live virus vaccines, with the exception of Attenuvax, Meruvax, and/or monovalent or trivalent live, oral poliovirus vaccine, which may be administered simultaneously.
• The vaccine will not protect if given after exposure to natural mumps.
• Not recommended for infants under 12 months because retained maternal mumps antibodies may interfere with the immune response.
• Stress importance of avoiding pregnancy for 3 months after immunization. If necessary, provide contraceptive information.
• Treat fever with antipyretics.
• Do not give I.V.
• Store in refrigerator and protect from light. Solution may be used if red, pink, or yellow (but must be clear).
• Use only diluent supplied. Discard 8 hours after reconstituting.
• Obtain history of allergies, especially to antibiotics, and reaction to immunization.

plague vaccine
Pregnancy Risk Category: C

HOW SUPPLIED
Injection: 2 billion killed plague bacilli (*Yersinia pestis*)/ml in 20-ml vials

MECHANISM OF ACTION
Promotes active immunity to plague.

INDICATIONS & DOSAGE
Primary immunization and booster—
Adults and children over 10 years: 1 ml I.M. followed by 0.2 ml in 4 weeks, then 0.2 ml 6 months after the first dose. Booster is 0.1 to 0.2 ml q 6 months while in plague area.
Children 5 to 10 years: ⅗ adult primary or booster dose.
Children 1 to 4 years: ⅖ adult primary or booster dose.
Children under 1 year: ⅕ adult primary or booster dose.

ADVERSE REACTIONS
Systemic: malaise, headache, slight fever, lymphadenopathy, *anaphylaxis.*
Local: swelling, *induration, erythema.*

INTERACTIONS
None significant.

NURSING CONSIDERATIONS
• Contraindicated in immunosuppression. Defer in respiratory infection.
• Deltoid area is the preferred injection site.
• Obtain history of allergies and reaction to immunization.
• Keep epinephrine 1:1,000 available.

pneumococcal vaccine, polyvalent
Pneumovax 23, Pnu-Imune 23
Pregnancy Risk Category: C

HOW SUPPLIED
Injection: 25 mcg each of 23 polysaccharide isolates/0.5 ml

MECHANISM OF ACTION
Promotes active immunity to infections caused by *Streptococcus pneumoniae.*

INDICATIONS & DOSAGE
Pneumococcal immunization—
Adults and children over 2 years: 0.5 ml I.M. or S.C.
   Not recommended for children under 2 years.

ADVERSE REACTIONS
Systemic: *slight fever, anaphylaxis.*
Local: soreness, severe, local reaction can occur when revaccination takes place within 3 years.

INTERACTIONS
None significant.

NURSING CONSIDERATIONS
• Check immunization history carefully to avoid revaccination within 3 years.
• Inject in deltoid or midlateral thigh. Don't inject I.V.
• Keep refrigerated. Reconstitution or dilution not necessary.
• Treat fever with mild antipyretics.
• Protects against 23 pneumococcal types, which account for 90% of pneumococcal disease.
• Also may be administered to children to prevent pneumococcal otitis media.
• Obtain history of allergies and reaction to immunization.
• Keep epinephrine 1:1,000 available.

Italicized adverse reactions are common or life-threatening.
*Liquid form contains alcohol.   **May contain tartrazine.

poliovirus vaccine, live, oral, trivalent
Orimune

Pregnancy Risk Category: C

HOW SUPPLIED
Oral vaccine: mixture of three viruses (types 1, 2, and 3), grown in monkey kidney tissue culture, in 0.5-ml single-dose Dispettes

MECHANISM OF ACTION
Promotes immunity to poliomyelitis by inducing humoral antibodies and antibodies in the lymphatic tissue.

INDICATIONS & DOSAGE
Poliovirus immunization—
Children and nonimmunized adults: two 0.5-ml doses should be administered 8 weeks apart. Give third 0.5-ml dose 6 to 12 months after second dose. A reinforcing dose of 0.5 ml should be given before entry to school.
Infants: administer 0.5-ml dose at age 2 months, 4 months, and 18 months. Optional dose may be given at 6 months.

ADVERSE REACTIONS
Systemic: *paralytic poliomyelitis.*

INTERACTIONS
Immune serum globulin, whole blood, plasma: antibodies in serum may interfere with immune response. Don't use vaccine within 3 months of transfusion.
Tuberculin skin test: skin test may be suppressed. Don't test for 6 weeks.

NURSING CONSIDERATIONS
• Contraindicated in immunosuppression, cancer, immunoglobulin abnormalities and in radiation, antimetabolite, alkylating agent, or corticosteroid therapy. Defer in acute illness, vomiting, or diarrhea.
• Should not be administered to newborns younger than 6 weeks.
• Use with caution in siblings of child with known immunodeficiency syndrome.
• This vaccine is not effective in modifying or preventing existing or incubating poliomyelitis.
• Check the parents' immunization history when they bring in child for vaccine; this is an excellent time for parents to receive booster immunizations.
• Keep frozen until used. Once thawed, if unopened, may store refrigerated up to 30 days. Opened vials may be refrigerated up to 7 days. Thaw before administration.
• Color change from pink to yellow has no effect on the efficacy of the vaccine. Yellow color results from vaccine being stored at low temperatures.
• Obtain history of allergies and reaction to immunization.
• Not for parenteral use.

rabies vaccine, human diploid cell (HDCV)
Imovax

Pregnancy Risk Category: C

HOW SUPPLIED
Intradermal injection: 0.25 IU rabies antigen/dose.
Intramuscular injection: 2.5 IU of rabies antigen/ml, in single-dose vial with diluent

MECHANISM OF ACTION
Promotes active immunity to rabies.

INDICATIONS & DOSAGE
Postexposure antirabies immunization—
Adults and children: five 1-ml doses of HDCV I.M. (for example, in the deltoid region). Give first dose as soon as possible after exposure; give

an additional dose on each of days 3, 7, 14, and 28 after first dose.
Preexposure prophylaxis immunization for persons in high-risk groups—
Adults and children: three 1-ml injections administered I.M. Give first dose on day 0 (the first day of therapy), second dose on day 7, and third dose on either day 21 or 28. Alternatively, give 0.1 ml intradermally on the same dosage schedule.

ADVERSE REACTIONS
Systemic: headache, nausea, abdominal pain, muscle aches, dizziness, fever, diarrhea, *anaphylaxis, serum sickness.*
Local: *pain, erythema, swelling or itching at injection site.*

INTERACTIONS
Corticosteroids, immunosuppressive agents, antimalarial drugs: decreased response to rabies vaccine. Avoid concomitant use.

NURSING CONSIDERATIONS
• Stop corticosteroids during immunizing period.
• When postexposure immunization is indicated, pregnancy is not a contraindication.
• Persons with a history of hypersensitivity should be given rabies vaccine with caution.
• Some patients who receive booster doses experience serum sickness–like allergic reactions. These reactions usually respond to antihistamines.
• Keep epinephrine 1:1,000 available.
• The Centers for Disease Control recommends a booster dose with Imovax for all persons who have been potentially exposed to rabies since October 15, 1984, and who have received postexposure prophylaxis with Wyvac unless acceptable titers were proven.
• The alternative regimen of 0.1-ml doses is only for *preexposure* prophylaxis. For postexposure prophylaxis, only the 1-ml doses should be used.

rubella and mumps virus vaccine, live
Biavax II
Pregnancy Risk Category: X

HOW SUPPLIED
Injection: single-dose vial containing not less than 1,000 TCID$_{50}$ (tissue culture infective doses) of the Wistar RA 27/3 rubella virus (propagated in human diploid cell culture) and not less than 5,000 TCID$_{50}$ of the Jeryl Lynn mumps strain (grown in chick embryo cell culture)

MECHANISM OF ACTION
Promotes immunity to rubella and mumps by inducing production of antibodies.

INDICATIONS & DOSAGE
Measles and mumps immunization—
Adults and children over 1 year: 1 vial (1,000 units) S.C.

ADVERSE REACTIONS
Systemic: fever, rash, thrombocytopenic purpura, urticaria, arthritis, arthralgia, polyneuritis, *anaphylaxis.*
Local: pain, erythema, induration, lymphadenopathy.

INTERACTIONS
Immune serum globulin, whole blood, plasma: antibodies in serum may interfere with immune response. Don't give vaccine within 3 months of transfusion.
Tuberculin skin test: may temporarily decrease response to test. Defer skin testing.

NURSING CONSIDERATIONS
• Contraindicated in immunosuppression; cancer; blood dyscrasias; corticosteroid or radiation therapy; gamma globulin disorders; active, untreated

---

Italicized adverse reactions are common or life-threatening.
*Liquid form contains alcohol.   **May contain tartrazine.

tuberculosis; fever; or pregnancy. Use with caution in patients with hypersensitivity to neomycin, chickens, ducks, eggs, or feathers. Defer in acute illness and after administration of immune serum globulin, blood, or plasma.

• Stress importance of avoiding pregnancy for 3 months after immunization. If necessary, provide contraceptive information.

• Store in refrigerator and protect from light. Solution may be used if red, pink, or yellow (but must be clear).

• Use only diluent supplied. Discard 8 hours after reconstituting.

• Obtain history of allergies, especially to ducks, rabbits, and antibiotics, and reaction to immunization.

• Inject into outer aspect of upper arm. Don't inject I.V.

• Keep epinephrine 1:1,000 available.

• Allow an interval of at least 3 weeks between BCG and rubella vaccines.

---

rubella virus vaccine, live attenuated (RA 27/3)
Meruvax II

Pregnancy Risk Category: X

HOW SUPPLIED
Injection: single-dose vial containing not less than 1,000 TCID$_{50}$ (tissue culture infective doses) of the Wistar RA 27/3 strain of rubella (virus propagated in human diploid cell culture)

MECHANISM OF ACTION
Promotes immunity to rubella by inducing production of antibodies.

INDICATIONS & DOSAGE
Measles immunization—
Adults and children over 1 year: 1 vial (1,000 units) S.C.

ADVERSE REACTIONS
Systemic: *joint pain,* fever, rash, thrombocytopenic purpura, urticaria, arthritis, arthralgia, polyneuritis, *anaphylaxis.*
Local: pain, erythema, induration, lymphadenopathy.

INTERACTIONS
Immune serum globulin, whole blood, plasma: antibodies in serum may interfere with immune response. Don't use vaccine within 3 months of transfusion.
Tuberculin skin test: may temporarily decrease response to test. Defer skin testing.

NURSING CONSIDERATIONS
• Contraindicated in immunosuppression; cancer; blood dyscrasias; corticosteroid or radiation therapy; gamma globulin disorders; active, untreated tuberculosis; or fever. Use cautiously in patients with hypersensitivity to neomycin, chickens, ducks, eggs, or feathers. Defer in acute illness and after administration of human immune serum globulin, blood, or plasma.

• Stress importance of avoiding pregnancy for 3 months after immunization. If necessary, provide contraceptive information.

• Store in refrigerator and protect from light. Solution may be used if red, pink, or yellow (but must be clear).

• Use only diluent supplied. Discard 8 hours after reconstituting.

• Obtain history of allergies, especially to ducks and rabbits, and reaction to immunization.

• Inject into outer aspect of upper arm. Don't inject I.V.

• Keep epinephrine 1:1,000 available.

• Allow an interval of at least 3 weeks between BCG and rubella vaccines.

---

tetanus toxoid, adsorbed

tetanus toxoid, fluid
Pregnancy Risk Category: C

HOW SUPPLIED
adsorbed
Injection: 5 to 10 Lf units of inactivated tetanus/0.5-ml dose, in 0.5-ml syringes and 5-ml vials
fluid
Injection: 4 to 5 Lf units of inactivated tetanus/0.5-ml dose, in 0.5-ml syringes and 7.5-ml vials

MECHANISM OF ACTION
Promotes immunity to tetanus by inducing production of antitoxin.

INDICATIONS & DOSAGE
Primary immunization—
Adults and children: 0.5 ml (adsorbed) I.M. 4 to 6 weeks apart for two doses, then third dose 1 year after the second; 0.5 ml (fluid) I.M. or S.C. 4 to 8 weeks apart for three doses, then fourth dose of 0.5 ml 6 to 12 months after third dose. Booster is 0.5 ml I.M. at 10-year intervals.

ADVERSE REACTIONS
Systemic: slight fever, chills, malaise, aches and pains, flushing, urticaria, pruritus, tachycardia, hypotension, *anaphylaxis.*
Local: erythema, induration, nodule.

INTERACTIONS
Chloramphenicol: may interfere with response to tetanus toxoid.

NURSING CONSIDERATIONS
• Contraindicated in immunosuppression and immunoglobulin abnormalities. Defer in acute illness and polio outbreaks, except in emergencies.
• For prevention, not treatment, of tetanus infections.
• Determine date of last tetanus immunization.
• Don't use hot or cold compresses; may increase severity of local reaction.
• Obtain history of allergies and reaction to immunization.
• Keep epinephrine 1:1,000 available.
• Adsorbed form produces longer duration of immunity. Fluid form provides quicker booster effect in patients actively immunized previously.
• Do not confuse this drug with tetanus immune globulin, human.

typhoid vaccine
Pregnancy Risk Category: C

HOW SUPPLIED
Injection: suspension of killed Ty-2 strain of *Salmonella typhi;* provides 8 units/ml in 5-ml, 10-ml, and 20-ml vials

MECHANISM OF ACTION
Provides active immunity to typhoid fever.

INDICATIONS & DOSAGE
Primary immunization—
Adults and children over 10 years: 0.5 ml S.C.; repeat in 4 weeks. Booster is the same dose as primary immunization q 3 years.
Children 6 months to 10 years: 0.25 ml S.C.; repeat in 4 weeks. Booster is the same dose as primary immunization q 3 years.

ADVERSE REACTIONS
Systemic: *fever,* malaise, headache, nausea, *anaphylaxis.*
Local: swelling, pain, inflammation.

INTERACTIONS
None significant.

NURSING CONSIDERATIONS
• Contraindicated in corticosteroid therapy. Defer in acute illness.
• Treat fever with antipyretics.

Italicized adverse reactions are common or life-threatening.
*Liquid form contains alcohol.   **May contain tartrazine.

- Do not give intradermally.
- Obtain history of allergies and reaction to immunization.
- Keep epinephrine 1:1,000 available.
- Store at 35.6° to 50° F. (2° to 10° C.).
- Shake thoroughly before withdrawing from vial.

yellow fever vaccine
YF-Vax

Pregnancy Risk Category: D

HOW SUPPLIED
Injection: live, attenuated 17D yellow fever virus in 1- and 5-dose vials, with diluent; supplied only to designated yellow fever vaccination centers authorized to issue yellow fever vaccination certificates

MECHANISM OF ACTION
Provides active immunity to yellow fever.

INDICATIONS & DOSAGE
Primary vaccination—
Adults and children over 6 months: 0.5 ml deep S.C. booster is 0.5 ml S.C. q 10 years.

ADVERSE REACTIONS
Systemic: fever, malaise, *anaphylaxis.*
Local: mild swelling, pain.

INTERACTIONS
Cholera vaccine: concurrent administration may interfere with immune response to both yellow fever vaccine and cholera vaccine. Administer 3 weeks apart.

NURSING CONSIDERATIONS
- Contraindicated in gamma globulin deficiency, immunosuppression, cancer, corticosteroid or radiation therapy, allergies to chickens or eggs, or in pregnancy. Also contraindicated in infants under 9 months except in high-risk areas.
- Reconstitute with sodium chloride injection that contains no preservatives (preservatives decrease potency).
- Must be kept frozen. Don't use unless shipping case contains some dry ice upon arrival. Avoid vigorous shaking; carefully swirl mixture until suspension is uniform. Use within 1 hour after reconstitution. Discard remainder.
- Obtain history of allergies, especially to eggs, and reaction to immunization.
- Don't give within 1 month of other live virus vaccines.
- Keep epinephrine 1:1,000 available.

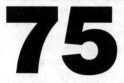

Antitoxins and antivenins

black widow spider antivenin
botulism antitoxin, bivalent
  equine
crotaline antivenin, polyvalent
diphtheria antitoxin, equine
***Micrurus fulvius* antivenin**
tetanus antitoxin (TAT), equine

COMBINATION PRODUCTS
None.

black widow spider antivenin

Antivenin *(Latrodectus mactans)*
Pregnancy Risk Category: C

HOW SUPPLIED
Injection: combination package—1 vial of antivenin (6,000 units/vial), one 2.5-ml vial of diluent (sterile water for injection), and one 1-ml vial of normal equine (horse) serum (1:10 dilution) for sensitivity testing

MECHANISM OF ACTION
Neutralizes and binds venom.

INDICATIONS & DOSAGE
Black widow spider bite—
Adults and children: 2.5 ml I.M. in deltoid. Second dose may be needed.

ADVERSE REACTIONS
Systemic: hypersensitivity, *anaphylaxis, neurotoxicity*.

INTERACTIONS
None significant.

NURSING CONSIDERATIONS
• Immobilize patient; splint the bitten limb to prevent spread of venom.
• Test for sensitivity before giving. Use 0.2 ml of a 1:10 dilution in normal saline solution.
• Epinephrine 1:1,000 should be available in case of adverse reaction.
• Venom is neurotoxic and may cause respiratory paralysis and seizures. Watch patient carefully for 2 to 3 days.
• Obtain accurate patient history of allergies, especially to horses, and reaction to immunization.
• Earliest possible use of antivenin recommended for best results.
• Antivenin may be given I.V. in severe cases (when patient is in shock), in 10 to 50 ml of saline solution over 15 minutes.

botulism antitoxin, bivalent equine

Pregnancy Risk Category: D

HOW SUPPLIED
Available through your state health department or the office of the state epidemiologist.

MECHANISM OF ACTION
Neutralizes and binds toxin.

INDICATIONS & DOSAGE
Botulism—
Adults and children: 1 vial I.V. stat and q 4 hours, p.r.n., until patient's condition improves. Dilute antitoxin 1:10 in dextrose 5% or 10% in water

---

Italicized adverse reactions are common or life-threatening.
*Liquid form contains alcohol.   **May contain tartrazine.

or normal saline solution before giving. Give first 10 ml of dilution over 5 minutes; after 15 minutes, rate may be increased.

ADVERSE REACTIONS
Systemic: hypersensitivity, *anaphylaxis,* serum sickness (urticaria, pruritus, fever, malaise, arthralgia) may occur in 5 to 13 days.

INTERACTIONS
None significant.

NURSING CONSIDERATIONS
• Test for sensitivity before giving.
• Epinephrine 1:1,000 should be available in case of adverse reaction. Bivalent antitoxin contains antibodies against types A and B *Clostridium botulinum.* Antitoxins against all other types available only from Centers for Disease Control in Atlanta: Monday to Friday, 8 a.m. to 4:30 p.m. (E.S.T.), (404) 329-3670; nights, weekends, and holidays (emergencies only), (404) 329-2888.
• Obtain accurate patient history of allergies, especially to horses, and reaction to immunization.
• Earliest possible use of antitoxin is recommended for best results.

---

crotaline antivenin, polyvalent
Pregnancy Risk Category: D

HOW SUPPLIED
Injection: combination package—one vial of lyophilized serum, one vial of diluent (10 ml bacteriostatic water for injection), and one 1-ml vial of normal horse serum (diluted 1:10) for sensitivity testing

MECHANISM OF ACTION
Neutralizes and binds venom.

INDICATIONS & DOSAGE
Crotalid (rattlesnake) bites—

Adults and children: initially, 10 to 50 ml or more I.M. or S.C., depending on severity of bite and patient response. If large amount of venom, 70 to 100 ml I.V. directly into superficial vein. Subsequent doses based on patient's response; may give 10 ml q ½ to 2 hours, p.r.n. If bite is in extremity, inject part of initial dose at various sites around limb above swelling; don't inject in finger or toe. The smaller the patient, the larger the initial dose.

ADVERSE REACTIONS
Systemic: hypersensitivity, *anaphylaxis, neurotoxicity, serum sickness.*

INTERACTIONS
Antihistamines: enhanced toxicity of crotaline venoms. Don't use together.

NURSING CONSIDERATIONS
• Test for sensitivity before giving. Give 0.02 to 0.03 ml of a 1:10 dilution in 0.9% normal saline solution intradermally. Read results after 5 to 10 minutes.
• Immobilize patient immediately. Splint the bitten extremity.
• Epinephrine 1:1,000 should be available in case of adverse reaction.
• Type and cross match blood as soon as possible since hemolysis from venom prevents accurate cross matching.
• Early use of antivenin is recommended for best results.
• Watch patient carefully for delayed allergic reaction or relapse.
• Children, who have less resistance and less body fluid to dilute venom, may need twice the adult dose.
• Obtain accurate patient history of allergies, especially to horses, and reaction to immunization.
• Discard unused reconstituted drug.

---

†Available in Canada only.   ‡Available in Australia only.   ◇ Available OTC.

diphtheria antitoxin, equine
Pregnancy Risk Category: D

HOW SUPPLIED
Injection: not less than 500 units/ml in 10,000-unit and 20,000-unit vials

MECHANISM OF ACTION
Neutralizes and binds toxin.

INDICATIONS & DOSAGE
Diphtheria prevention—
Adults and children: 1,000 to 5,000 units I.M.
Diphtheria treatment—
Adults and children: 20,000 to 80,000 units or more slow I.V. Additional doses may be given in 24 hours. I.M. route may be used in mild cases.

ADVERSE REACTIONS
Systemic: hypersensitivity, *anaphylaxis,* serum sickness (urticaria, pruritus, fever, malaise, arthralgia) may occur in 7 to 12 days.

INTERACTIONS
None significant.

NURSING CONSIDERATIONS
• Test for sensitivity before giving.
• Epinephrine 1:1,000 should be available in case of adverse reaction.
• Obtain accurate patient history of allergies, especially to horses, and reaction to immunization.
• Therapy should begin immediately, without delay for culture reports, if patient has symptoms of diphtheria (sore throat, fever, tonsillar membrane).
• For storage, refrigerate antitoxin at 35.6° to 50° F. (2° to 10° C.). Before administering, warm to 90° to 95° F. (32.2° to 35° C.), never higher.

Micrurus fulvius antivenin
Pregnancy Risk Category: D

HOW SUPPLIED
Injection: combination package with 10 ml diluent

MECHANISM OF ACTION
Neutralizes and binds venom.

INDICATIONS & DOSAGE
Eastern and Texas coral snake bite—
Adults and children: 3 to 5 vials slow I.V. through running I.V. of 0.9% normal saline solution. Give first 1 to 2 ml over 3 to 5 minutes, and watch for signs of allergic reaction. If no signs develop, continue injection. Up to 10 vials may be needed. Not effective for Sonoran or Arizona coral snake bites.

ADVERSE REACTIONS
Systemic: hypersensitivity, *anaphylaxis.*

INTERACTIONS
None significant.

NURSING CONSIDERATIONS
• Test for sensitivity before giving.
• Immobilize patient or splint bitten limb to prevent spread of venom.
• Early use of antivenin recommended for best results.
• Venom is neurotoxic and may cause respiratory paralysis. Watch patient carefully for 24 hours. Have epinephrine 1:1,000 available in case of adverse reaction.
• Obtain accurate patient history of allergies, especially to horses, and reaction to immunization.

Italicized adverse reactions are common or life-threatening.
*Liquid form contains alcohol.   **May contain tartrazine.

tetanus antitoxin (TAT), equine

Pregnancy Risk Category: D

HOW SUPPLIED
Injection: not less than 400 units/ml in 1,500-unit and 20,000-unit vials

MECHANISM OF ACTION
Neutralizes and binds toxin.

INDICATIONS & DOSAGE
Tetanus prophylaxis—
Patients over 30 kg: 3,000 to 5,000 units I.M. or S.C.
Patients under 30 kg: 1,500 to 3,000 units I.M. or S.C.
Tetanus treatment—
All patients: 10,000 to 20,000 units injected into wound. Give additional 40,000 to 100,000 units I.V. Start tetanus toxoid at same time but at different site and with a different syringe.

ADVERSE REACTIONS
Systemic: joint pain, hypersensitivity,
Local: pain, numbness, skin rash.
anaphylaxis, serum sickness.

INTERACTIONS
None significant.

NURSING CONSIDERATIONS
• Test for sensitivity before giving. Give 0.1 ml as a 1:1,000 dilution in normal saline solution intradermally.
• Use only when tetanus immune globulin (human) not available.
• Obtain accurate patient history of allergies, especially to horses, and reaction to immunization. If respiratory difficulty develops, give 0.4 ml of 1:1,000 solution epinephrine.
• Give preventive dose to those who have had two or fewer injections of tetanus toxoid and who have tetanus-prone injuries more than 24 hours old.

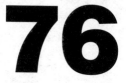

76

Immune serums

antirabies serum, equine
hepatitis B immune globulin, human
immune globulin intramuscular
immune globulin intravenous
rabies immune globulin, human
Rh$_o$(D) immune globulin, human
tetanus immune globulin, human
varicella-zoster immune globulin

COMBINATION PRODUCTS
None.

---

antirabies serum, equine
Pregnancy Risk Category: C

HOW SUPPLIED
Injection: 125 IU/ml

MECHANISM OF ACTION
Provides passive immunity to rabies.

INDICATIONS & DOSAGE
Rabies exposure—
Adults and children: 40 to 55 IU/kg at time of first dose of rabies vaccine. Use half of dose to infiltrate wound area. Give remainder I.M. Don't give rabies vaccine and antirabies serum in same syringe or at same site.

For wounds, including mucous membranes, the entire dose should be administered I.M.

ADVERSE REACTIONS
Systemic: within 6 to 12 days serum sickness occurs in 15% to 25% of patients. Symptoms are skin eruptions, arthralgia, pruritus, lymphadenopa-

thy, fever, headache, malaise, abdominal pain, *anaphylaxis*.
Local: pain at injection site.

INTERACTIONS
Corticosteroids and immunosuppressive agents: interferes with response. Avoid during postexposure immunization period.

NURSING CONSIDERATIONS
● In hypersensitivity to equine serum, use rabies immune globulin, human, instead. If unavailable, desensitize before giving. Consult doctor or pharmacist.
● Do sensitivity test on all patients before giving. Dilute serum 1:100 or 1:1,000 with normal saline solution for injection. Inject intradermally on inner forearm. Inject other arm with 0.1 ml of normal saline solution for injection intradermally as a control. Read within 20 minutes. Positive reaction: wheal 10 mm or more and erythematous flare 20 mm × 20 mm.
● Use only when rabies immune globulin, human, is not available.
● Obtain history of animal bite, allergies (especially to equine serum and to eggs), and reaction to immunizations.
● Epinephrine solution 1:1,000 should always be available when administering this drug.
● This immune serum provides immediate passive immunity (short-term).
● Do not confuse this drug with rabies vaccine, which is a suspension of attenuated or killed microorganisms

---

Italicized adverse reactions are common or life-threatening.
*Liquid form contains alcohol.   **May contain tartrazine.

used to confer long-term active immunity. These two drugs are often administered together prophylactically after exposure to known or suspected rabid animals.

• Ask patient when he received last tetanus immunization, since many doctors order a booster at this time.

hepatitis B immune globulin, human
H-BIG, Hep-B-Gammagee, HyperHep

Pregnancy Risk Category: C

HOW SUPPLIED
Injection: 1-ml, 4-ml, 5-ml vials

MECHANISM OF ACTION
Provides passive immunity to hepatitis B.

INDICATIONS & DOSAGE
Hepatitis B exposure—
Adults and children: 0.06 ml/kg I.M. within 7 days after exposure. Repeat 28 days after exposure.
Neonates born to women who test positive for hepatitis B surface antigen (HB$_s$Ag): 0.5 ml within 12 hours of birth. Repeat dose at ages 3 months and 6 months.

ADVERSE REACTIONS
Systemic: *anaphylaxis.*

INTERACTIONS
Other vaccines: Hepatitis B immune globulin may interfere with response to live virus vaccines. Defer administration for 3 months.

NURSING CONSIDERATIONS
• Anterolateral aspect of thigh or deltoid areas are the preferred injection sites in adults; anterolateral aspect of thigh is preferred for neonates and children under 3 years.
• Health-care personnel should receive immunization if exposed to hepatitis B (for example, needle-stick, direct contact).
• Obtain history of allergies and reaction to immunizations.

immune globulin intramuscular (IGIM, IG, gamma globulin)
Gamastan, Gammar

immune globulin intravenous (IGIV)
Gamimine N, Gammagard, Sandoglobulin, Venoglobulin-I

Pregnancy Risk Category: C

HOW SUPPLIED
intramuscular
Injection: 2-ml, 10-ml vials
intravenous
Injection: 5% in 10-ml, 50-ml, 100-ml vials (Gamimune N)
Powder for injection: 50 mg protein/ml in 0.5-g, 2.5-g, 5-g, 10-g vials (Gammagard); 1-g, 3-g, 6-g vials (Sandoglobulin); 2.5-g, 5-g vials (Venoglobulin-I)

MECHANISM OF ACTION
Provides passive immunity by increasing antibody titer.

INDICATIONS & DOSAGE
Agammaglobulinemia or hypogammaglobulinemia—
Adults: 30 to 50 ml I.M. monthly. Alternatively, administer 100 mg/kg I.V. (Gamimune N) once a month. Infuse at 0.01 to 0.02 ml/kg/min for 30 minutes. For Sandoglobulin, administer 200 mg/kg I.V. once a month. Infuse at 0.5 to 1 ml/min. After 15 to 30 minutes, increase infusion rate to 1.5 to 2.5 ml/min.
Children: 20 to 40 ml I.M. monthly.
Hepatitis A exposure—
Adults and children: 0.02 to 0.04 ml/kg I.M. as soon as possible after exposure. Up to 0.1 ml/kg may be

given after prolonged or intense exposure.

Post-transfusion hepatitis B—
Adults and children: 10 ml I.M. within 1 week after transfusion and 10 ml I.M. 1 month later.

Measles exposure—
Adults and children: 0.02 ml/kg I.M. within 6 days after exposure.

Modification of measles—
Adults and children: 0.04 ml/kg I.M. within 6 days after exposure.

Measles vaccine complications—
Adults and children: 0.02 to 0.04 ml/kg I.M.

Poliomyelitis exposure—
Adults and children: 0.3 to 0.4 ml/kg I.M. within 7 days after exposure.

Chicken pox exposure—
Adults and children: 0.2 to 1.3 ml/kg I.M. as soon as exposed.

Rubella exposure in first trimester of pregnancy—
Women: 0.2 to 0.4 ml/kg I.M. as soon as exposed.

Prophylaxis in primary immunodeficiencies—
Adults and children: 100 mg/kg by I.V. infusion monthly (Gamimune only). Infusion rate is 0.01 to 0.02 ml/kg/minute for 30 minutes. Rate can then be increased to 0.04 ml/minute for remainder of infusion.

Idiopathic thrombocytopenic purpura—
Adults: 0.4 g/kg Gamimune N or Sandoglobulin I.V. for 5 consecutive days; or 1,000 mg/kg Gammagard. Additional doses may be given based on response. Give up to three doses (every other day) if necessary. Or, give Venoglobulin-1,500 mg/kg/day for 2 to 7 days.

ADVERSE REACTIONS
Skin: urticaria.
Systemic: angioedema, headache, malaise, fever, nephrotic syndrome, *anaphylaxis.*
Local: pain, erythema, muscle stiffness.

INTERACTIONS
Live virus vaccines: don't administer within 3 months after administration of immune globulin.

NURSING CONSIDERATIONS
- Obtain history of allergies and reaction to immunizations.
- Have drugs available for anaphylactoid reaction.
- Inject into different sites, preferably anterolateral aspect of thigh or deltoid muscle for adults and anterolateral aspect of thigh for neonates and children under 3 years. Do not inject more than 3 ml per injection site.
- Do not give for hepatitis A exposure if 6 weeks or more have elapsed since exposure or after onset of clinical illness.

---

rabies immune globulin, human
Hyperab, Imogam
Pregnancy Risk Category: C

HOW SUPPLIED
Injection: 150 IU/ml in 2-ml, 10-ml vials

MECHANISM OF ACTION
Provides passive immunity to rabies.

INDICATIONS & DOSAGE
Rabies exposure—
Adults and children: 20 IU/kg I.M. at time of first dose of rabies vaccine. Use half of dose to infiltrate wound area. Give remainder I.M. Don't give rabies vaccine and rabies immune globulin in same syringe or at same site.

ADVERSE REACTIONS
Local: pain, redness, induration at injection site.
Other: slight fever, *anaphylaxis, angioedema.*

Italicized adverse reactions are common or life-threatening.
*Liquid form contains alcohol.   **May contain tartrazine.

INTERACTIONS
Corticosteroids and immunosuppressive agents: interferes with response. Avoid during postexposure immunization period.
Live virus vaccines (measles, mumps, rubella, or polio): response to these vaccines may not be reliable because of antibodies present in rabies immune globulin. Don't administer live vaccines within 3 months of rabies immune globulin.

NURSING CONSIDERATIONS
• Repeated doses contraindicated after rabies vaccine is started.
• Use only with rabies vaccine and immediate local treatment of wound. Give regardless of interval between exposure and initiation of therapy.
• Obtain history of animal bites, allergies, and reaction to immunizations.
• Don't administer more than 5 ml I.M. at one injection site; divide I.M. doses greater than 5 ml, and administer at different sites.
• This immune serum provides passive immunity.
• Do not confuse this drug with rabies vaccine, which is a suspension of attenuated or killed microorganisms used to confer active immunity. These two drugs are often given together prophylactically after exposure to known or suspected rabid animals.
• Ask the patient when he received his last tetanus immunization, since many doctors order a booster at this time.

$Rh_o(D)$ immune globulin, human
Gamulin Rh, HypRho-D, MICRhoGAM, Mini-Gamulin Rh, Rhesonativ, RhoGAM

Pregnancy Risk Category: C

HOW SUPPLIED
Injection: 300 mcg of $Rh_o(D)$ immune globulin/vial (standard dose); 50 mcg of $Rh_o(D)$ immune globulin/vial (microdose)

MECHANISM OF ACTION
Suppresses the active antibody response and formation of anti-$Rh_o(D)$ in $Rh_o(D)$-negative, D^u-negative individuals, exposed to Rh-positive blood.

INDICATIONS & DOSAGE
Rh exposure—
Women (postabortion, postmiscarriage, ectopic pregnancy, or postpartum): transfusion unit or blood bank determines fetal packed red blood cell (RBC) volume entering woman's blood, then gives one vial I.M. if fetal packed RBC volume is less than 15 ml. More than one vial I.M. may be required if there is large fetomaternal hemorrhage. Must be given within 72 hours after delivery or miscarriage.
Transfusion accidents—
Adults and children: consult blood bank or transfusion unit at once. Must be given within 72 hours.
Postabortion or postmiscarriage to prevent Rh antibody formation—
Women: consult transfusion unit or blood bank. One microdose vial will suppress immune reaction to 2.5 ml $Rh^o(D)$-positive RBCs. Ideally should be given within 3 hours, but may be given up to 72 hours after abortion or miscarriage.

ADVERSE REACTIONS
Local: discomfort at injection site.
Other: slight fever.

INTERACTIONS
Live virus vaccines: may interfere with response. Defer vaccination for 3 months after administration of $Rh_o(D)$ immune globulin.

NURSING CONSIDERATIONS
• Contraindicated in $Rh_o(D)$-positive

---

or D^u-positive patients and those previously immunized to $Rh_o(D)$ blood factor.

• Immediately after delivery, send a sample of infant's cord blood to laboratory for typing and cross matching. Confirm if mother is $Rh_o(D)$-negative and D^u-negative. Infant must be $Rh_o(D)$-positive or D^u-positive.

• Obtain history of allergies and reaction to immunization.

• MICRhoGAM is recommended for every woman undergoing abortion or miscarriage up to 12 weeks' gestation unless she is $Rh_o(D)$-positive or D^u-positive, has Rh antibodies, or the father and/or fetus is Rh-negative.

• Store at 36° to 46° F. (2° to 8° C.).

• This immune serum provides passive immunity to the woman exposed to Rh_o-positive fetal blood during pregnancy. Prevents formation of maternal antibodies (active immunity), which would endanger future Rh_o-positive pregnancies.

• Explain to the patient how drug protects future Rh_o-positive infants.

tetanus immune globulin, human
Homo-Tet, Hu-Tet, Hyper-Tet†
Pregnancy Risk Category: C

HOW SUPPLIED
Injection: 250 units per vial or syringe

MECHANISM OF ACTION
Provides passive immunity to tetanus.

INDICATIONS & DOSAGE
Tetanus exposure—
Adults and children: 250 to 500 units I.M.
Tetanus treatment—
Adults and children: single doses of 3,000 to 6,000 units I.M. have been used. Optimal dosage schedules have not been established. Don't give at same site as toxoid.

ADVERSE REACTIONS
Local: pain, stiffness, erythema.
Other: slight fever, allergy, *anaphylaxis.*

INTERACTIONS
None significant.

NURSING CONSIDERATIONS
• Use tetanus immune globulin only if wound is over 24 hours old or patient has had less than two previous tetanus toxoid injections.

• Obtain history of injury, tetanus immunizations, last tetanus toxoid injection, allergies, and reaction to immunizations.

• Thoroughly cleanse and remove all foreign matter from wound.

• Antibodies remain at effective levels for 3 weeks or longer, which is several times the duration of antitoxin-induced antibodies. Protects the patient for the incubation period of most tetanus cases.

• Human globulin is not a substitute for tetanus toxoid, which should be given at the same time to produce active immunization.

• Inject into the deltoid muscle for adults and children 3 years and older and into the anterolateral aspect of the thigh in neonates and children under 3 years.

• Do not confuse this drug with tetanus toxoid.

varicella-zoster immune globulin (VZIG)
Pregnancy Risk Category: C

HOW SUPPLIED
Injection: 10% to 18% solution of the globulin fraction of human plasma containing 125 units of varicella-zoster virus antibody (volume is about 1.25 ml)

Italicized adverse reactions are common or life-threatening.
*Liquid form contains alcohol.   **May contain tartrazine.

MECHANISM OF ACTION
Provides passive immunity to varicella-zoster virus.

INDICATIONS & DOSAGE
Passive immunization of susceptible immunodeficient patients after exposure to varicella (chicken pox or herpes zoster)—
Children to 10 kg: 125 units I.M.
Children 10.1 to 20 kg: 250 units I.M.
Children 20.1 to 30 kg: 375 units I.M.
Children 30.1 to 40 kg: 500 units I.M.
Adults and children over 40 kg: 625 units I.M.

ADVERSE REACTIONS
Systemic: gastrointestinal distress, malaise, headache, respiratory distress, *anaphylaxis.*
Local: discomfort at injection site, rash.

INTERACTIONS
Live virus vaccines: may interfere with response. Defer vaccination for 3 months after administration of VZIG.

NURSING CONSIDERATIONS
• Contraindicated in patients with a history of severe reaction to human immune serum globulin or severe thrombocytopenia.
• For maximum benefit, administer as soon as possible after presumed exposure.
• VZIG is not recommended for non-immunosuppressed patients.
• VZIG should not be administered indiscriminately because supplies are limited.
• Although usually restricted to children under 15 years, VZIG may be administered to adolescents and adults if necessary.
• Not commercially distributed. Available only from 20 regional distribution centers throughout the United States. These centers will distribute to Canada and overseas. Call the Centers for Disease Control for the distribution center in your area: Monday to Friday, 8 a.m. to 4:30 p.m. (E.S.T.), (404) 329-3670; weekends, nights, and holidays (emergencies only), (404) 329-2888.
• Should be administered only by deep I.M. injection. Never administer I.V.
• Store vial in refrigerator.

77

Biological response modifiers

epoetin alfa
interferon alfa-2a, recombinant
interferon alfa-2b, recombinant
interferon alfa-n3
interleukin-2, recombinant

COMBINATION PRODUCTS
None.

---

epoetin alfa (erythropoietin)
Epogen

HOW SUPPLIED
Injection: 2,000 units/ml, 4,000 units/ml, 6,000 units/ml

MECHANISM OF ACTION
A naturally occurring hormone, produced by recombinant DNA techniques. Epoetin alfa is one of the factors controlling the rate of red cell production. It acts on the erythroid tissues in the bone marrow stimulating the mitotic activity of erythroid progenitor cells and early precursor cells. It functions as a growth factor and as a differentiating factor.

INDICATIONS & DOSAGE
Anemia due to reduced production of endogenous erythropoietin, end-stage renal disease—
Adults: dosage is individualized. Starting dose is 50 to 100 units/kg I.V. three times weekly. (Nondialysis patients with chronic renal failure may receive the drug by S.C. injection or I.V.) Reduce dosage when target hematocrit is reached or if the hematocrit rises more than 4 points in any 2-

week period. Increase dosage if hematocrit does not increase by 5 to 6 points after 8 weeks of therapy. Maintenance dose is usually 25 units/kg three times weekly.

ADVERSE REACTIONS
Blood: iron deficiency, elevated platelet count.
CNS: headache, *seizures.*
CV: hypertension.
GI: nausea, vomiting, diarrhea.
Skin: rash.
Other: increased clotting of arteriovenous grafts.

INTERACTIONS
None reported.

NURSING CONSIDERATIONS
• Contraindicated in patients with uncontrolled hypertension. Reduce dosage in patients who exhibit a rapid rise in hematocrit (more than 4 points in any 2-week period) because of the risk of hypertension.
• Blood count should be monitored during therapy. Hematocrit may rise and cause excessive clotting.
• Monitor blood pressure before initiating therapy. Up to 80% of patients with chronic renal failure have hypertension. Blood pressure may rise, especially when the hematocrit is increasing in the early part of therapy. Diet restrictions or drug therapy may be required to control blood pressure.
• Patients should avoid hazardous activities, such as driving or operating heavy machinery, during the initiation of therapy. There may be a relation-

---

Italicized adverse reactions are common or life-threatening.
*Liquid form contains alcohol.   **May contain tartrazine.

ship between excessively rapid hematocrit rise and seizures.

• Patients treated with epoetin alfa may require additional heparin to prevent clotting during dialysis treatments.

• After injection (usually within 2 hours), some patients complain of pain or discomfort in their limbs (long bones) and pelvis. Coldness and sweating may also occur. These symptoms may persist up to 12 hours and then disappear.

• Patients with end-stage renal disease may experience an improved appetite and enhanced well-being as a result of increased hematocrit.

• Epoetin alfa has also been used to correct the hemostatic defect associated with uremia.

• Additional clinical trials are investigating epoetin alfa for treatment of the anemia of AIDS patients receiving zidovudine, of cancer patients undergoing chemotherapy, and of patients with rheumatoid arthritis. It is also being investigated for facilitating autologous transfusion by helping to produce more units of blood before surgery.

• Advise the patient that blood specimens will be drawn weekly for blood counts and, depending on their results, dosage adjustments may be necessary.

interferon alfa-2a, recombinant (rIFN-A)
Roferon-A

Pregnancy Risk Category: C

HOW SUPPLIED
3 million IU/vial; 18 million IU/multiple-dose vial for injection

MECHANISM OF ACTION
Interferon alfa-2a is a sterile protein product produced by recombinant DNA techniques. Its exact mechanism of action is unknown, but appears to involve direct antiproliferative action against tumor cells or viral cells to inhibit replication, and modulation of host immune response by enhancing the phagocytic activity of macrophages and by augmenting specific cytotoxicity of lymphocytes for target cells.

INDICATIONS & DOSAGE
Treatment of hairy-cell leukemia—
Adults: for induction, give 3 million units S.C. or I.M. daily for 16 to 24 weeks. For maintenance, 3 million units S.C. or I.M. three times a week.
Treatment of AIDS-related Kaposi's sarcoma—
Adults: for induction, give 36 million units S.C. or I.M. daily for 10 to 12 weeks. For maintenance, 36 million units S.C. or I.M. three times a week.

ADVERSE REACTIONS
Blood: leukemia, mild thrombocytopenia.
CNS: *dizziness,* confusion, paresthesias, numbness, lethargy, depression, nervousness, difficulty in thinking or concentrating, insomnia, sedation, apathy, anxiety, irritability, fatigue, vertigo, gait disturbances, poor coordination.
CV: hypotension, chest pain, dysrhythmias, palpitations, syncope, *CHF,* hypertension, edema.
EENT: visual disturbances, dryness or inflammation of the oropharynx, rhinorrhea, sinusitis, conjunctivitis, earache, eye irritation, rhinitis.
GI: *anorexia, nausea, diarrhea,* vomiting, abdominal fullness, abdominal pain, flatulence and constipation, hypermotility, gastric distress, dysgeusia.
GU: transient impotence.
Hepatic: hepatitis.
Respiratory: bronchospasm, coughing, dyspnea, tachypnea.
Skin: *rash,* dryness, *pruritus,* partial alopecia, urticaria, flushing.

Local: inflammation at injection site (rare).

Other: *flu-like syndrome (fever, fatigue, myalgias, headache, chills, arthralgia),* diaphoresis, hot flashes, excessive salivation, cyanosis.

INTERACTIONS

Aminophylline: may reduce the clearance of aminophylline.
CNS depressants: enhanced CNS effects.

NURSING CONSIDERATIONS

• Information based on current literature. Dosage, indications, and adverse reactions profile may change with additional clinical experience.
• Neurotoxicity and cardiotoxicity are more common in elderly patients, especially those with underlying CNS or cardiac impairment.
• Use with blood dyscrasia-causing medications, bone marrow suppressant therapy, or radiation therapy may increase bone marrow suppressant effects. Dosage reduction may be required.
• Use cautiously in severe hepatic or renal function impairment, seizure disorders, compromised CNS function, cardiac disease, and myelosuppression.
• S.C. administration route should be used in patients whose platelet count is below 50,000/mm³.
• Different brands of interferon may not be equivalent and may require different dosage.
• Almost all patients experience flu-like symptoms at the beginning of therapy. These effects tend to diminish with continued therapy. Premedication with acetaminophen minimizes flu-like symptoms.
• Patients should be well hydrated, especially during initial stages of treatment.
• Administer at bedtime to minimize daytime drowsiness.
• Severe adverse reactions may re-

quire reduction of dosage to one-half or discontinuation of therapy until reactions subside.
• Advise patient that laboratory tests will be performed before and periodically during therapy. Such tests will include a complete blood cell count with differential, platelet count, blood chemistry and electrolyte studies, liver function tests, and if the patient has a preexisting cardiac disorder or advanced stages of cancer, ECGs.
• Interferons may decrease hemoglobin, hemotocrit, leukocytes, platelets, and neutrophils; increase prothrombin and partial thromboplastin time; and increase serum levels of AST (SGOT), ALT (SGPT), LDH, alkaline phosphatase calcium, phosphorus, and fasting glucose. These effects are dose-related and reversible; recovery occurs within several days or weeks after withdrawal of interferon.
• Monitor for CNS adverse reactions, such as decreased mental status and dizziness. Periodic neuropsychiatric monitoring is recommended during therapy.
• Special precautions required for patients who develop thrombocytopenia: exercise extreme care in performing invasive procedures; inspect injection site and skin frequently for signs of bruising; limit frequency of I.M. injections; test urine, emesis fluid, stool, and secretions for occult blood.
• Instruct patient in proper oral hygiene during treatment, because the bone marrow suppressant effects of interferon may lead to microbial infection, delayed healing, and gingival bleeding. Interferon may also decrease salivary flow.
• Advise patient to check with doctor for further instructions after missing a dose.
• If patient is to self-administer drug, teach patient how to prepare and administer the injection and how to use disposable syringe. Give information on drug stability.

Italicized adverse reactions are common or life-threatening.
*Liquid form contains alcohol.   **May contain tartrazine.

- Store drug in refrigerator.
- Emphasize need to follow doctor's instructions about taking and recording temperature, and how and when to take acetaminophen.
- Concurrent use with a live virus vaccine may potentiate replication of vaccine virus, increase adverse reactions, and decrease patient's antibody response.
- Warn patient not to have any immunization without doctor's approval and to avoid contact with persons who have taken oral polio vaccine. Because interferon may decrease antibody response and potentiate replication of vaccine viruses, the patient is at special risk for infection during therapy.
- Tell patient drug may cause temporary loss of some hair. Normal hair growth should return when drug is withdrawn.

interferon alfa-2b recombinant (IFN-alpha 2)
Intron A

Pregnancy Risk Category: C

HOW SUPPLIED
3 million IU/vial with diluent for injection, 5 million IU/vial with diluent for injection, 10 million IU/vial with diluent for injection, 25 million IU/vial with diluent for injection, 50 million IU/vial with diluent for injection

MECHANISM OF ACTION
Interferon alfa-2b is a sterile protein product produced by recombinant DNA techniques. Its exact mechanism of action is unknown, but appears to involve direct antiproliferative action against tumor cells or viral cells to inhibit replication, and modulation of host immune response by enhancing the phagocytic activity of macrophages and by augmenting specific cytotoxicity of lymphocytes for target cells.

INDICATIONS & DOSAGE
Treatment of hairy-cell leukemia—
Adults: 2 million units/m² I.M. or S.C. three times a week.
Treatment of condylomata acuminata (genital or venereal warts)—
Adults: 1 million units/lesion intralesionally three times a week for 3 weeks.
Treatment of AIDS-related Kaposi's sarcoma—
Adults: 30 million units/m² S.C. or I.M. three times a week.

ADVERSE REACTIONS
Blood: leukemia, mild thrombocytopenia.
CNS: dizziness, confusion, paresthesias, lethargy, depression, difficulty in thinking or concentrating, insomnia, sedation, anxiety, *fatigue,* hypoesthesia, amnesia, agitation, weakness.
CV: hypotension, chest pain.
EENT: visual disturbances, hearing disorders, stye, pharyngitis, nasal congestion, sinusitis, rhinitis.
GI: *anorexia, nausea,* diarrhea, vomiting, abdominal pain, dyspepsia, constipation, loose stools, eructation, dry mouth, dysgeusia.
GU: transient impotence, gynecomastia.
Respiratory: dyspnea, coughing.
Skin: rash, dryness, pruritus, partial alopecia, urticaria, moniliasis, flushing, dermatitis.
Other: *flu-like symptoms (fever, fatigue, headache, chills, muscle aches), arthralgia,* asthenia, rigors, leg cramps, arthrosis, bone disorders, back pain, increased sweating, stomatitis, gingivitis, decreased libido, hypertonia, migraine, thirst.

INTERACTIONS
CNS depressants: CNS effects enhanced.

NURSING CONSIDERATIONS
- Information based upon current lit-

---

erature. Dosage, indications, and adverse reactions profile may change with additional clinical experience.

• Neurotoxicity and cardiotoxicity are more common in elderly patients, especially those with underlying CNS or cardiac impairment.

• Use cautiously in history of cardiovascular disease, pulmonary disease, diabetes mellitus, coagulation disorders, and severe myelosuppresion.

• Concurrent use with a live virus vaccine may potentiate replication of vaccine virus, increase adverse reactions, and decrease patient's antibody response.

• Use with blood dyscrasia-causing medications, bone marrow suppressant therapy, or radiation therapy may increase bone marrow supressant effects. Dosage reduction may be required.

• S.C. administration route should be used in patients whose platelet count is below 50,000/mm³.

• Different brands of interferon may not be equivalent and may require different dosage.

• Almost all patients experience flu-like symptoms at the beginning of therapy. These effects tend to diminish with continued therapy. Premedicate with acetaminophen to minimize flu-like symptoms.

• Patients should be well hydrated, especially during initial stages of treatment.

• Administer at bedtime to minimize daytime drowsiness.

• Severe adverse reactions may require reduction of dosage to one-half or discontinuation of therapy until reactions subside.

• Advise patient that laboratory tests will be performed before and periodically during therapy. Such tests will include a complete blood cell count with differential, platelet count, blood chemistry and electrolyte studies, liver function tests, and if the patient

has a preexisting cardiac disorder or advanced stages of cancer, ECGs.

• When administering interferon for condylomata acuminata, use only 10-million-IU vial since dilution of other strengths required for intralesional use results in a hypertonic solution. Do not reconstitute 10-million-IU vial with more than 1 ml diluent. Use tuberculin or similar syringe and 25G to 30G needle. Do not inject too deeply beneath lesion or too superficially. As many as five lesions can be treated at one time. To ease discomfort, administer in evening with acetaminophen.

• Maximum response usually occurs 4 to 8 weeks after initiation of therapy. If results are not satisfactory after 12 to 16 weeks, a second course may be instituted. Patients with six to ten condylomata may receive a second course of treatment; patients with more than ten condylomata may receive additional courses.

• Interferons may decrease hemoglobin, hemotocrit, leukocytes, platelets, and neutrophils; increase prothrombin and partial thromboplastin time; and increase serum levels of AST (SGOT), ALT (SGPT), LDH, alkaline phosphatase calcium, phosphorus, and fasting glucose. These effects are dose-related and reversible; recovery occurs within several days or weeks after withdrawal of interferon.

• Monitor for adverse CNS reactions, such as decreased mental status and dizziness. Periodic neuropsychiatric monitoring is recommended during therapy.

• Special precautions required for patients who develop thrombocytopenia: exercise extreme care in performing invasive procedures; inspect injection site and skin frequently for signs of bruising; limit frequency of I.M. injections; test urine, emesis fluid, stool, and secretions for occult blood.

• Instruct patient in proper oral hygiene during treatment, because the bone marrow suppressant effects of

---

Italicized adverse reactions are common or life-threatening.
*Liquid form contains alcohol.   **May contain tartrazine.

interferon may lead to microbial infection, delayed healing, and gingival bleeding. Interferon may also decrease salivary flow.
• Advise patient to check with doctor for further instructions after missing a dose.
• If patient is to self-administer drug, teach patient how to prepare the injection and how to use disposable syringe. Give information on drug stability.
• Store drug in refrigerator.
• Emphasize need to follow doctor's instructions about taking and recording temperature, and how and when to take acetaminophen.
• Warn patient not to have any immunization without doctor's approval, and to avoid contact with persons who have taken oral polio vaccine. Because interferon may decrease antibody response and potentiate replication of vaccine viruses, the patient is at risk for infection during therapy.
• Tell patient drug may cause temporary loss of some hair. Normal hair growth should return when drug is withdrawn.

---

interferon alfa-n3
Alferon N

Pregnancy Risk Category: C

HOW SUPPLIED
Injection: 5 million units/ml in 1-ml vials

MECHANISM OF ACTION
Interferon alfa-n3 is a naturally occurring antiviral agent derived from human leukocytes. It attaches to membrane receptors and causes cellular changes, including increased protein synthesis.

INDICATIONS & DOSAGE
Treatment of condylomata acuminata—
Adults: 0.05 ml/wart by intralesional

injection. Treatment usually continues twice weekly for 8 weeks. Dosage should not exceed 0.5 ml (2.5 million units)/session.

ADVERSE REACTIONS
CNS: dizziness, light-headedness.
GI: dyspepsia, heartburn, vomiting, nausea.
Other: *mild to moderate flu-like syndrome (myalgia, fever, headache), arthralgia, back pain, malaise.*

INTERACTIONS
None reported.

NURSING CONSIDERATIONS
• Contraindicated in patients hypersensitive to interferon alpha and in patients with a history of anaphylactic reactions to murine immunoglobulin, egg protein, or neomycin.
• Although anaphylaxis hasn't been reported, be prepared to treat acute hypersensitivity reactions. Teach patients how to recognize symptoms associated with hypersensitivity reactions (hives or urticaria, tightness of the chest, wheezing, shortness of breath). Tell patients they should report these symptoms immediately.
• Use cautiously in patients with debilitating illnesses (including uncontrolled CHF, unstable angina, severe pulmonary disease, coagulation disorders, seizure disorders, severe myelosuppression, or diabetes mellitus with ketoacidosis) because of the association of interferon administration and a "flu-like" syndrome.
• Flu-like symptoms may be relieved with acetaminophen.
• Explain to the patient that the warts will continue to disappear after the 8 weeks of therapy are complete and the drug has been discontinued.
• The drug should be injected into each lesion at the base of the wart using a 30G needle.
• Do not change brands of interferon once during the course of therapy be-

cause dosage changes may be necessary.

interleukin-2, recombinant

HOW SUPPLIED
Available only through investigational protocol.

MECHANISM OF ACTION
Interleukin-2 is a lymphokine that stimulates proliferation of T-lymphocytes and thus amplifies immune response to an antigen; it also acts on B-lymphocytes and induces production of interferon-gamma and the activation of natural killer cells.

INDICATIONS & DOSAGE
Adoptive immunotherapy of malignant neoplasms, such as renal cell carcinoma, melanoma, and non-Hodgkin's lymphoma—
Adults: administer with lymphokine-activated killer (LAK) cells. Dilute interleukin-2 in 50 ml of 0.9% sodium chloride solution containing 5% human serum albumin. Give 10,000, 30,000, or 100,000 units I.V. q 8 hours, and continue for several days, depending on tolerance.
To restore immune response in patients with AIDS—
Adults: up to 2.5 million units daily by continuous 24 hour I.V. infusion, for 5 days per week over 4 to 8 weeks.

ADVERSE REACTIONS
Blood: anemia, thrombocytopenia, eosinophilia.
CNS: headache, confusion, disorientation, drowsiness, restlessness, parathesias, coma, psychosis, hallucinations.
CV: hypotension, decreased vascular resistance and increased capillary permeability, myocardial infarction, arrhythmias, CHF, edema.
GI: nausea, vomiting, diarrhea, stomatitis.
GU: uremia, oliguria, decreased urine output, elevated serum creatinine.
Hepatic: elevated serum transaminase and bilirubin.
Skin: rashes, itching.
Other: fluid retention, weight gain, fever, fatigue, chills, dyspnea.

INTERACTIONS
None reported.

NURSING CONSIDERATIONS
• Information based upon current literature. Dosage, indications, and adverse reactions profile may change with additional clinical experience.
• Advise patient that adverse reactions usually subside after completion of therapy.
• If chills occur, I.V. meperidine may be administered. Nausea may be controlled with antiemetics such as prochlorperazine; headache may be treated with acetaminophen.
• Advise patients that laboratory tests will be performed before and periodically during therapy. Such tests will include complete blood count and liver function studies. Monitor results of these tests and notify the doctor of abnormalities.
• In various clinical trials, interleukin-2 has been given by I.V. bolus, by continuous I.V. infusion, by subcutaneous injection, and by intrahepatic or peritoneal infusion. It has also been administered I.V. piggyback three times daily, by 24 hour infusions twice a week, by weekly I.V. bolus injection, or by continuous I.V. infusion over 5 to 6 days.
• Special precautions required for patients who develop thrombocytopenia: exercise extreme care in performing invasive procedures; inspect injection site and skin frequently for signs of bruising; limit frequency of I.M. injections; test urine, emesis fluid, stool, and secretions for occult blood.

Italicized adverse reactions are common or life-threatening.
*Liquid form contains alcohol.   **May contain tartrazine.

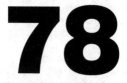

Ophthalmic anti-infectives

bacitracin
boric acid
chloramphenicol
erythromycin
gentamicin
gentamicin sulfate
idoxuridine
natamycin
polymyxin B sulfate
silver nitrate 1%
sulfacetamide sodium 10%
sulfacetamide sodium 15%
sulfacetamide sodium 30%
tetracycline
tetracycline hydrochloride
tobramycin
trifluridine
vidarabine

COMBINATION PRODUCTS

BLEPHAMIDE S.O.P. STERILE OPHTHALMIC OINTMENT: sulfacetamide sodium 10% and prednisolone acetate 0.2%.

CETAPRED OINTMENT: sulfacetamide sodium 10% and prednisolone acetate 0.25%.

CHLOROMYCETIN-HYDROCORTISONE OPHTHALMIC: chloramphenicol 0.25% and hydrocortisone acetate 0.5% (as the prepared solution).

CORTISPORIN OPHTHALMIC OINTMENT: polymyxin B sulfate 10,000 units, bacitracin zinc 400 units, neomycin sulfate 0.35%, and hydrocortisone 1%.

CORTISPORIN OPHTHALMIC SUSPENSION: polymyxin B sulfate 10,000 units, neomycin sulfate 0.35%, and hydrocortisone 1%.

ISOPTO CETAPRED: sulfacetamide sodium 10% and prednisolone acetate 0.25%.

MAXITROL OINTMENT/OPHTHALMIC SUSPENSION: dexamethasone 0.1%, neomycin sulfate 0.35%, and polymyxin B sulfate 10,000 units.

METIMYD OPHTHALMIC OINTMENT/ SUSPENSION: sulfacetamide sodium 10% and prednisolone acetate 0.5%.

MYCITRACIN OPHTHALMIC OINTMENT: polymyxin B sulfate 5,000 units, neomycin sulfate 3.5 mg, and bacitracin 500 units.

NEODECADRON OPHTHALMIC OINTMENT: dexamethasone phosphate 0.1% and neomycin sulfate 0.35%.

NEOSPORIN OPHTHALMIC: polymyxin B sulfate 10,000 units, neomycin sulfate 1.75 mg, and gramicidin 0.025 mg.

NEOSPORIN OPHTHALMIC OINTMENT: polymyxin B sulfate 10,000 units, neomycin sulfate 3.5 mg, and bacitracin zinc 400 units/g.

NEOTAL: polymyxin B sulfate 5,000 units, neomycin sulfate 5 mg, and bacitracin zinc 400 units.

OPHTHA P/S OPHTHALMIC SUSPENSION: prednisolone acetate 0.5%, sulfacetamide sodium 10%.

OPHTHOCORT: chloramphenicol 1.0%, polymyxin B sulfate 10,000 units, and hydrocortisone acetate 0.5%.

OPTIMYD: prednisolone phosphate 0.5% and sulfacetamide sodium 10%.

POLYSPORIN OPHTHALMIC OINTMENT: polymyxin B sulfate 10,000 units, and bacitracin zinc 500 units.

STATROL: neomycin sulfate 3.5 mg and polymyxin B sulfate 10,000 units.

SULFAPRED: sulfacetamide sodium 10%, prednisolone acetate 0.25%, and phenylephrine hydrochloride 0.125%.

VASOCIDIN OPHTHALMIC OINTMENT: sulfacetamide sodium 10%, prednisolone acetate 0.5%, and phenylephrine hydrochloride 0.125%.

VASOCIDIN OPHTHALMIC SOLUTION: sulfacetamide sodium 10%, prednisolone phosphate 0.25%.

VASOSULF: sulfacetamide sodium 15% and phenylephrine hydrochloride 0.125%.

---

bacitracin
Pregnancy Risk Category: C

HOW SUPPLIED
Ophthalmic ointment: 500 units/g

MECHANISM OF ACTION
Inhibits protein synthesis. Bactericidal or bacteriostatic, depending on concentration and infection.

INDICATIONS & DOSAGE
Ocular infections—
Adults and children: apply small amount of ointment into conjunctival sac several times daily or p.r.n. until favorable response is observed.

ADVERSE REACTIONS
Eye: slowed corneal wound healing, temporary visual haze.
Other: overgrowth of nonsusceptible organisms.

INTERACTIONS
Heavy metals (e.g., silver nitrate): inactivate bacitracin. Don't use together.

NURSING CONSIDERATIONS
• Use cautiously in patients with hereditary predisposition to antibiotic hypersensitivity.
• Warn patient to avoid sharing washcloths and towels with family members during infection.
• Always wash hands before and after applying ointment.
• Cleanse eye area of excessive exudate before application.
• Tell patient to watch for signs of sensitivity, such as itching lids, swelling, or constant burning. Patient who develops such signs should stop drug and notify doctor immediately.
• Teach patient how to apply. Advise him to wash his hands before and after administering and not to touch tip of tube or dropper to eye or surrounding tissue.
• Stress importance of compliance with recommended therapy.
• Warn patient that ointment may cause blurred vision.
• Solution not commercially available but may be prepared by pharmacy. May be stored up to 3 weeks in refrigerator.
• Store in tightly closed, light-resistant container.
• Tell patient not to share eye medications with family members. If a family member develops the same symptoms, instruct him to contact the doctor.

---

boric acid
Blinx◇, Collyrium◇, Neo-Flo◇
Pregnancy Risk Category: C

HOW SUPPLIED
Ophthalmic ointment: 5%◇, 10%◇
Ophthalmic solution: 30 ml◇, 120 ml◇, 180 ml◇

MECHANISM OF ACTION
Unknown. However, drug has fungistatic and bacteriostatic properties.

INDICATIONS & DOSAGE
For irrigation following tonometry, gonioscopy, foreign body removal, or use of fluorescein; used to soothe and cleanse the eye—

Italicized adverse reactions are common or life-threatening.
*Liquid form contains alcohol.   **May contain tartrazine.

Adults: apply 5% or 10% ointment, p.r.n.

ADVERSE REACTIONS
Note: Toxic if absorbed from abraded skin areas, granulating wounds, or ingestion.

INTERACTIONS
Idoxuridine, polyvinyl alcohol (Liquifilm): may form insoluble complex. Check with pharmacy on contents in other eye drugs and contact lens wetting solutions.

NURSING CONSIDERATIONS
• Contraindicated in eye lacerations.
• Don't apply to abraded cornea.
• Always wash hands before and after instilling solution or ointment.
• Not for use with soft contact lenses.
• Tell patient not to share eye solution with family members.
• Avoid contaminating solution container.

---

chloramphenicol
AK-Chlor, Chloromycetin Ophthalmic, Chloroptic, Chloroptic S.O.P., Chlorsig‡, Fenicol†, Isopto Fenicol†, Ophthoclor Ophthalmic, Pentamycetin†

Pregnancy Risk Category: C

HOW SUPPLIED
Ophthalmic ointment: 1%
Ophthalmic solution: 0.5%

MECHANISM OF ACTION
Inhibits protein synthesis.

INDICATIONS & DOSAGE
Surface bacterial infection involving conjunctiva or cornea—
Adults and children: instill 1 drop of solution in eye q 1 to 4 hours until condition improves, or instill q.i.d., depending on severity of infection. Apply small amount of ointment to lower conjunctival sac at bedtime as

supplement to drops. May use ointment alone by applying a small amount of ointment to lower conjunctival sac q 3 to 6 hours or more frequently, if necessary. Continue until condition improves.

ADVERSE REACTIONS
Note: systemic adverse reactions have not been reported with short-term topical use.
Blood: *bone marrow hypoplasia with prolonged use, aplastic anemia.*
Eye: optic atrophy in children, stinging or burning of eye after instillation, blurred vision (with ointment).
Other: overgrowth of nonsusceptible organisms; hypersensitivity, including itching and burning eye, dermatitis, angioedema.

INTERACTIONS
None significant.

NURSING CONSIDERATIONS
• Not for long-term use. Notify doctor if no improvement in 3 days.
• If patient has more than a superficial infection, systemic therapy should also be used.
• One of the safest topical ocular antibiotics, especially for endophthalmitis.
• Warn patient to avoid sharing washcloths and towels with family members during infection.
• Cleanse eye area of excessive exudate before application.
• Tell patient to watch for signs of sensitivity, such as itching lids, swelling, or constant burning. Patient who develops such signs should stop drug and notify doctor immediately.
• Teach patient how to instill. Advise him to wash hands before and after administering ointment or solution, and warn him not to touch tip of applicator to eye or surrounding tissue. Tell him to apply light finger-pressure on lacrimal sac for 1 minute after drops are instilled. Stress importance

---

of compliance with recommended therapy.
• If chloramphenicol drops are to be given q 1 hour, then tapered, follow order closely to ensure adequate anterior chamber levels.
• Store in tightly closed, light-resistant container.
• Tell patient not to share eye medications with family members. If a family member develops the same symptoms, instruct him to contact the doctor.

erythromycin
Ilotycin Ophthalmic

Pregnancy Risk Category: C

HOW SUPPLIED
Ophthalmic ointment: 5 mg/g

MECHANISM OF ACTION
Inhibits protein synthesis. Bacteriostatic, but may be bactericidal in high concentrations or against highly susceptible organisms.

INDICATIONS & DOSAGE
Acute and chronic conjunctivitis, trachoma, other eye infections—
Adults and children: apply 0.5% ointment 1 or more times daily, depending upon severity of infection.
Prophylaxis of ophthalmia neonatorum—
Neonates: a ribbon of ointment approximately 0.5 to 1 cm long placed in the lower conjunctival sacs shortly after birth.

ADVERSE REACTIONS
Eye: slowed corneal wound healing, blurred vision.
Other: overgrowth of nonsusceptible organisms with long-term use; hypersensitivity, including itching and burning eyes, urticaria, dermatitis, angioedema.

INTERACTIONS
None significant.

NURSING CONSIDERATIONS
• Has a limited antibacterial spectrum. Use only when sensitivity studies show it is effective against infecting organisms. Don't use in infections of unknown etiology.
• For prophylaxis of ophthalmia neonatorum, apply ointment no later than 1 hour after birth.
• Warn patient to avoid sharing washcloths and towels with family members during infection.
• Cleanse eye area of excessive exudate before application.
• Tell patient to watch for signs of sensitivity, such as itching lids, swelling, or constant burning. Patient who develops such signs should stop drug and notify doctor immediately.
• Teach patient how to apply. Advise him to wash hands before and after administering ointment and warn patient not to touch tip of applicator to eye or surrounding tissue. Tell him to apply light finger-pressure on lacrimal sac for one minute after administering. Stress importance of compliance with recommended therapy.
• Warn patient that ointment may cause blurred vision.
• Store at room temperature in tightly closed, light-resistant container.
• Tell patient not to share eye medications with family members. If a family member develops the same symptoms, instruct him to contact the doctor.

gentamicin
Gentacidin

gentamicin sulfate
Garamycin Ophthalmic, Genoptic

Pregnancy Risk Category: C

HOW SUPPLIED
gentamicin
Ophthalmic ointment: 3 mg/g
gentamicin sulfate
Ophthalmic ointment: 3 mg/g

Italicized adverse reactions are common or life-threatening.
*Liquid form contains alcohol.   **May contain tartrazine.

Ophthalmic solution: 3 mg/ml

MECHANISM OF ACTION
Inhibits protein synthesis.

INDICATIONS & DOSAGE
External ocular infections (conjunctivitis, keratoconjunctivitis, corneal ulcers, blepharitis, blepharoconjunctivitis, meibomianitis, and dacryocystitis) caused by susceptible organisms, especially Pseudomonas aeruginosa, Proteus, Klebsiella pneumoniae, Escherichia coli, *and other gram-negative organisms—*
Adults and children: instill 1 to 2 drops in eye q 4 hours. In severe infections, may use up to 2 drops q 1 hour. Apply ointment to lower conjunctival sac b.i.d. or t.i.d.

ADVERSE REACTIONS
Note: systemic absorption from excessive use may cause systemic toxicities.
Eye: burning, stinging or blurred vision (with ointment), transient irritation (from solution).
Other: hypersensitivity, overgrowth of nonsusceptible organisms with long-term use.

INTERACTIONS
None significant.

NURSING CONSIDERATIONS
• Contraindicated in aminoglycoside hypersensitivity. Use cautiously in impaired renal function.
• Solution is not for injection in conjunctiva or anterior chamber of the eye.
• Have culture taken before giving drug.
• If ophthalmic gentamicin is administered concomitantly with systemic gentamicin, be sure to carefully monitor serum gentamicin.
• Stress importance of following recommended therapy. *Pseudomonas* infections can cause complete vision

loss within 24 hours if infection is not controlled.
• Warn patient to avoid sharing washcloths and towels with family members during infection.
• Always wash hands before and after applying ointment or solution.
• Cleanse eye area of excessive exudate before application.
• Tell patient to watch for signs of sensitivity, such as itching lids, swelling, or constant burning. Patient who develops such signs should stop drug and notify doctor immediately.
• Teach patient how to instill. Advise him to wash hands before and after administering ointment or solution, and not to touch tip of tube or dropper to eye or surrounding tissue. Tell him to apply light finger-pressure on lacrimal sac for 1 minute after drops are instilled. Stress importance of compliance with recommended therapy.
• Store away from heat.
• Tell patient not to share eye medications with family members. If a family member develops the same symptoms, instruct him to contact the doctor.

idoxuridine (IDU)
Herplex, Stoxil
Pregnancy Risk Category: C

HOW SUPPLIED
Ophthalmic ointment: 0.5%
Ophthalmic solution: 0.1%

MECHANISM OF ACTION
Interferes with DNA synthesis.

INDICATIONS & DOSAGE
Herpes simplex keratitis—
Adults and children: instill 1 drop of solution into conjunctival sac q 1 hour during day and q 2 hours at night, or apply ointment to conjunctival sac q 4 hours or 5 times daily, with last dose at bedtime. A response should be seen in 7 days; if not, discontinue and be-

gin alternate therapy. Therapy should not be continued longer than 21 days.

ADVERSE REACTIONS
Eye: temporary visual haze; blurred vision (with ointment); irritation, pain, burning, or inflammation of eye; mild edema of eyelid or cornea; photophobia; small punctate defects in corneal epithelium, corneal ulceration; slowed corneal wound healing (with ointment).
Other: hypersensitivity.

INTERACTIONS
Boric acid: precipitate formation; increased risk of ocular toxicity.

NURSING CONSIDERATIONS
• Contraindicated in deep ulceration.
• Not for long-term use.
• Idoxuridine should not be mixed with other topical eye medications.
• Don't use old solution; causes ocular burning and has no antiviral activity.
• Warn patient to avoid sharing washcloths and towels with family members during infection.
• Tell patient to watch for signs of sensitivity, such as itching lids, swelling, or constant burning. Patient who develops such signs should stop drug and notify doctor immediately.
• Teach patient how to instill. Advise him to wash hands before and after administering and warn him not to touch dropper or tip to eye or surrounding tissue. Tell him to apply light finger-pressure on lacrimal sac for 1 minute after drops are instilled.
• Cleanse eye area of excessive exudate before application. Stress importance of compliance with recommended therapy.
• Refrigerate idoxuridine 0.1% solution. Store in tightly closed, light-resistant container.
• Tell patient not to share eye medications with family members. If a family member develops the same symptoms, instruct him to contact the doctor.
• If photophobia develops, patient should wear sunglasses. Avoid prolonged exposure to sunlight.

natamycin
Natacyn
Pregnancy Risk Category: C

HOW SUPPLIED
Ophthalmic suspension: 5%
Limited availability requires that orders be placed with manufacturer directly.

MECHANISM OF ACTION
Increases fungal cell-membrane permeability.

INDICATIONS & DOSAGE
Treatment of fungal keratitis—
Adults: initial dosage is 1 drop instilled in conjunctival sac q 1 to 2 hours. After 3 to 4 days, reduce dosage to 1 drop 6 to 8 times daily.
Treatment of blepharitis or fungal conjunctivitis—
Adults: instill 1 drop q 4 to 6 hours.

ADVERSE REACTIONS
Eye: ocular edema, hyperemia.

INTERACTIONS
None significant.

NURSING CONSIDERATIONS
• Only antifungal available as ophthalmic preparation.
• Treatment of choice for fungal keratitis. May also be used to treat fungal blepharitis and conjunctivitis.
• Therapy should be continued for 14 to 21 days, or until active disease subsides.
• Reduce dosage gradually at 4- to 7-day intervals to ensure that organism has been eliminated.
• If infection does not improve with 7

Italicized adverse reactions are common or life-threatening.
*Liquid form contains alcohol.   **May contain tartrazine.

to 10 days of therapy, clinical and laboratory reevaluation is recommended.
• Warn patient to avoid sharing washcloths and towels with family members during infection.
• Cleanse eye area of excessive exudate before application.
• Teach patient how to instill. Advise him to wash hands before and after administering ointment or solution, to apply light finger-pressure on lacrimal sac for 1 minute after drops are instilled, and not to touch tip of dropper to eye or surrounding tissue. Stress importance of compliance with recommended therapy.
• Tell patient not to share eye medications with family members. If a family member develops the same symptoms, instruct him to contact the doctor.
• Shake well before use. May be kept in refrigerator or at room temperature.

polymyxin B sulfate

Pregnancy Risk Category: B

HOW SUPPLIED
Ophthalmic sterile powder for solution: 500,000-unit vials to be reconstituted to 20 to 50 ml

MECHANISM OF ACTION
Inhibits protein synthesis.

INDICATIONS & DOSAGE
Used alone or in combination with other agents for treating corneal ulcers resulting from Pseudomonas *infection or other gram-negative organism infections—*
Adults and children: instill 1 to 3 drops of 0.1% to 0.25% (10,000 to 25,000 units/ml) q 1 hour. Increase interval according to patient response; or up to 10,000 units subconjunctivally daily by doctor. Do not exceed 2,000,000 units daily.

ADVERSE REACTIONS
Eye: eye irritation, conjunctivitis.
Other: overgrowth of nonsusceptible organisms, hypersensitivity (local burning, itching).

INTERACTIONS
None significant.

NURSING CONSIDERATIONS
• One of the most effective antibiotics against gram-negative organisms, especially *Pseudomonas.*
• Often used in combination with neomycin sulfate.
• In severe, life-threatening *Pseudomonas* infections, polymyxin B may be used as an ocular irrigant.
• Warn patient to avoid sharing washcloths and towels with family members during infection.
• Tell patient to watch for signs of sensitivity, such as itching lids, swelling, or constant burning. Patient who develops such signs should stop drug and notify doctor immediately.
• Cleanse eye area of excessive exudate before application.
• Teach patient how to instill. Advise him to wash hands before and after administering solution, and warn patient not to touch tip of dropper to eye or surrounding tissue. Apply light finger-pressure on lacrimal sac for 1 minute after drops are instilled. Stress importance of compliance with recommended therapy.
• Reconstitute carefully to ensure correct drug concentration in solution.
• Tell patient not to share eye medications with family members. If a family member develops the same symptoms, instruct him to contact the doctor.

silver nitrate 1%

Pregnancy Risk Category: C

HOW SUPPLIED
Ophthalmic solution: 1%

MECHANISM OF ACTION
Causes protein denaturation, which prevents gonorrheal ophthalmia neonatorum. Bacteriostatic, germicidal, and astringent.

INDICATIONS & DOSAGE
Prevention of gonorrheal ophthalmia neonatorum—
Neonates: cleanse lids thoroughly; instill 1 drop of 1% solution into each eye.

ADVERSE REACTIONS
Eye: periorbital edema, temporary staining of lids and surrounding tissue, conjunctivitis (with concentrations of 1% or greater).

INTERACTIONS
Bacitracin: inactivates silver nitrate. Don't use together.

NURSING CONSIDERATIONS
• Legally required for neonates in most states.
• Don't use repeatedly.
• If 2% solution is accidentally used in eye, prompt irrigation with normal saline solution is advised to prevent eye irritation.
• Solution may stain skin and utensils. Handle carefully.
• May delay instillation slightly to allow neonate to bond with mother.
• Always wash hands before instilling solution.
• Store wax ampules away from light and heat.
• Don't irrigate eyes after instillation.

sulfacetamide sodium 10%
Bleph-10 Liquifilm Ophthalmic, Cetamide Ophthalmic, Sodium Sulamyd 10% Ophthalmic, Sulf-10 Ophthalmic

sulfacetamide sodium 15%
Isopto Cetamide Ophthalmic, Sulfacel-15 Ophthalmic

sulfacetamide sodium 30%
Sodium Sulamyd 30% Ophthalmic

Pregnancy Risk Category: C

HOW SUPPLIED
Ophthalmic ointment: 10%
Ophthalmic solution: 10%, 15%, 30%

MECHANISM OF ACTION
Prevents uptake of para-aminobenzoic acid, a metabolite of bacterial folic-acid synthesis.

INDICATIONS & DOSAGE
Inclusion conjunctivitis, corneal ulcers, trachoma, chlamydial infection—
Adults and children: instill 1 to 2 drops of 10% solution into lower conjunctival sac q 2 to 3 hours during day, less often at night; or instill 1 to 2 drops of 15% solution into lower conjunctival sac q 1 to 2 hours initially, increasing interval as condition responds; or instill 1 drop of 30% solution into lower conjunctival sac q 2 hours. Instill ½" to 1" of 10% ointment into conjunctival sac q.i.d. and h.s. May use ointment at night along with drops during the day.

ADVERSE REACTIONS
Eye: slowed corneal wound healing (ointment), *pain on instilling eyedrop,* headache or brow pain, photophobia.
Other: hypersensitivity (including itching or burning), overgrowth of nonsusceptible organisms, *Stevens-*

Johnson syndrome, sensitivity to light.

INTERACTIONS
Local anesthetics (procaine, tetracaine), para-aminobenzoic acid derivatives: decreased sulfacetamide sodium action. Wait ½ to 1 hour after instilling anesthetic or para-aminobenzoic acid derivative before instilling sulfacetamide.
Silver preparations: precipitate formation. Avoid using together.

NURSING CONSIDERATIONS
• Contraindicated in sulfonamide hypersensitivity.
• Often used with systemic tetracycline in treating trachoma and inclusion conjunctivitis.
• Replaced by other antibiotics in treating major ocular infections; still used in minor ocular infections.
• Purulent exudate interferes with sulfacetamide action. Remove as much exudate as possible from lids before instilling sulfacetamide.
• Incompatible with silver preparations.
• Warn patient eyedrop burns slightly.
• Warn patient to avoid sharing washcloths and towels with family members during infection.
• Tell patient to watch for signs of sensitivity, such as itching lids, swelling, or constant burning. Patient who develops such signs should stop drug and notify doctor immediately.
• Teach patient how to instill. Advise him to wash hands before and after administering ointment or solution, not to touch tip of dropper to eye or surrounding tissues, and to apply light finger-pressure on lacrimal sac for 1 minute after drops are instilled. Stress importance of compliance with recommended therapy.
• Wait at least 5 minutes before administering other eyedrops.
• Warn patient not to touch tip of tube or dropper to eye or surrounding tissue.
• Warn patient that solution may stain clothing.
• Store in tightly closed, light-resistant container away from heat.
• Don't use discolored (dark brown) solution.
• Tell patient not to share eye medications with family members. If a family member develops the same symptoms, instruct him to contact the doctor.
• Tell patient he may minimize photophobia by wearing sunglasses. He should avoid prolonged exposure to sunlight.

tetracycline
Achryomycin Ophthalmic

tetracycline hydrochloride
Achromycin

Pregnancy Risk Category: D

HOW SUPPLIED
tetracycline
Ophthalmic suspension: 10 mg/ml
tetracycline hydrochloride
Ophthalmic ointment: 10mg/g

MECHANISM OF ACTION
Inhibits protein synthesis.

INDICATIONS & DOSAGE
Superficial ocular infections and inclusion conjunctivitis—
Adults and children: instill 1 to 2 drops in eye b.i.d., q.i.d., or more often, depending on severity of infection.
Trachoma—
Adults and children: instill 2 drops in each eye b.i.d., t.i.d., or q.i.d. Continue for 1 to 2 months or longer, or use 1% ointment t.i.d. or q.i.d. for 30 days.
Prophylaxis of ophthalmia neonatorum—
Neonates: 1 to 2 drops into each eye shortly after delivery.

ADVERSE REACTIONS
Eye: itching, blurred vision (with ointment).
Other: hypersensitivity (eye itching and dermatitis), overgrowth of non-susceptible organisms with long-term use.

INTERACTIONS
None significant.

NURSING CONSIDERATIONS
• Tell patient or family that trachoma therapy should continue for 1 to 2 months or longer. Trachoma may cause blindness if left untreated or if not treated properly.
• Tell patient that gnats and flies are vectors of *Chlamydia trachomatis.* Warn patient with trachoma not to let them settle around eye area. Also explain that infection is spread by direct contact, so handwashing is essential to prevent spread.
    Severe trachoma may require oral therapy as well.
• For prophylaxis of ophthalmia neonatorum, apply ointment no later than 1 hour after birth.
• Warn patient to avoid sharing washcloths and towels with family members during infection.
• Tell patient to watch for signs of sensitivity, such as itching lids, swelling, or constant burning. Patient who develops such signs should stop drug and notify doctor immediately.
• Cleanse eye area of excessive exudate before application.
• Teach patient how to instill. Advise him to wash hands before and after administering ointment or solution and not to touch tip of dropper to eye or surrounding tissue. Apply light finger-pressure on lacrimal sac for 1 minute after drops are instilled. Stress importance of compliance with recommended therapy.
• Store in tightly closed, light-resistant container.

• Remind patient to shake suspension well before use.
• Tell patient not to share eye medications with family members. If a family member develops the same symptoms, instruct him to contact the doctor.
• Ophthalmic ointment may be used with suspension to provide prolonged drug contact with affected area at night.

---

tobramycin
Tobrex
Pregnancy Risk Category: B

HOW SUPPLIED
Ophthalmic ointment: 0.3%
Ophthalmic solution: 0.3%

MECHANISM OF ACTION
Inhibits protein synthesis.

INDICATIONS & DOSAGE
Treatment of external ocular infections caused by susceptible gram-negative bacteria—
Adults and children: In mild to moderate infections, instill 1 or 2 drops into the affected eye q 4 hours or a thin strip of ointment q 8 to 12 hours. In severe infections, instill 2 drops into the infected eye hourly until condition improves; then reduce frequency. Or, apply thin strip of ointment q 3 to 4 hours until improvement then reduce frequency.

ADVERSE REACTIONS
Eye: burning or stinging upon instillation, lid itching, lid swelling, blurred vision (with ointment).
Other: hypersensitivity.

INTERACTIONS
Tetracycline-containing eye preparations: incompatible with tyloxapol, an ingredient in Tobrex. Don't use together.

NURSING CONSIDERATIONS

• Prolonged use may result in overgrowth of nonsusceptible organisms, including fungi.

• If topical ocular tobramycin is administered concomitantly with systemic tobramycin, be sure to carefully monitor serum levels.

• Clinical symptoms of tobramycin overdose include keratitis, erythema, increased lacrimation, edema, and lid itching. Stop drug and notify doctor if any of these occur.

• Warn patient to avoid sharing washcloths and towels with family members during infection.

• Tell patient to watch for signs of sensitivity, such as itching lids, swelling, or constant burning. Patient who develops such signs should discontinue drug and notify doctor immediately.

• Cleanse eye area of excessive exudate before application.

• Teach patient how to instill. Advise him to wash hands before and after administering ointment or solution and warn patient not to touch tip of dropper to eye or surrounding tissue. Apply light finger-pressure on lacrimal sac for 1 minute after drops are instilled. Stress importance of compliance with recommended therapy.

• Often used to combat gram-negative organisms that are resistant to gentamicin.

• When two different ophthalmic solutions are used, allow at least 5 minutes before instillation.

---

trifluridine
Viroptic Ophthalmic Solution 1%

Pregnancy Risk Category: C

HOW SUPPLIED
Ophthalmic solution: 1%

MECHANISM OF ACTION
Interferes with DNA synthesis.

INDICATIONS & DOSAGE
Primary keratoconjunctivitis and recurrent epithelial keratitis caused by herpes simplex virus, types I and II—
Adults: 1 drop of solution q 2 hours while patient is awake, to a maximum of 9 drops daily until re-epithelialization of the corneal ulcer occurs; then 1 drop q 4 hours (minimum 5 drops daily) for an additional 7 days.

ADVERSE REACTIONS
Eye: *stinging upon instillation,* edema of eyelids, increased intraocular pressure.
Other: hypersensitivity.

INTERACTIONS
None significant.

NURSING CONSIDERATIONS
• Should be prescribed only for those patients with clinical diagnosis of herpetic keratitis.

• Consider another form of therapy if improvement doesn't occur after 7 days' treatment or complete re-epithelialization after 14 days' treatment. Trifluridine shouldn't be used more than 21 days continuously due to potential ocular toxicity.

• Watch for signs of increased intraocular pressure.

• Reassure patient that mild local irritation of the conjunctiva and cornea that occurs when solution is instilled is usually temporary.

• More effective drug than vidarabine or idoxuridine with fewer adverse reactions.

• Warn patient to avoid sharing washcloths and towels with family members during infection.

• Cleanse eye area of excessive exudate before application.

• Teach patient how to instill. Advise him to wash hands before and after administering solution. Warn patient not to touch tip of dropper to eye or surrounding tissue. Apply light finger-pressure on lacrimal sac for 1 minute

after drops are instilled. Stress importance of complying with recommended therapy.
• Tell patient not to share eye medications with family members. If a family member develops the same disease symptoms, instruct him to contact the doctor.
• If steroids are administered concomitantly, continue trifluridine for several days after discontinuation of steroid therapy.
• Keep refrigerated. Do not use if outdated.

---

vidarabine
Vira-A Ophthalmic

Pregnancy Risk Category: C

HOW SUPPLIED
Ophthalmic ointment: 3% in 3.5-g tube (equivalent to 2.8% vidarabine)

MECHANISM OF ACTION
Interferes with DNA synthesis.

INDICATIONS & DOSAGE
Acute keratoconjunctivitis, superficial keratitis, and recurrent epithelial keratitis resulting from herpes simplex types I and II—
Adults and children: instill ½″ ointment into lower conjunctival sac 5 times daily at 3-hour intervals.

ADVERSE REACTIONS
Eye: temporary burning, itching, mild irritation of eye, lacrimation, foreign body sensation, conjunctival injection, superficial punctate keratitis, eye pain, photophobia.
Other: hypersensitivity.

INTERACTIONS
None significant.

NURSING CONSIDERATIONS
• Not for long-term use.
• Warn patient not to exceed recom-

mended frequency or duration of dosage.
• Not effective against RNA virus, adenoviral ocular infections, or bacterial, fungal, or chlamydial infections.
• Warn patient to avoid sharing washcloths and towels with family members during infection.
• Tell patient to watch for signs of sensitivity, such as itching lids, swelling, or constant burning. Patient who develops such signs should stop drug and notify doctor immediately.
• Cleanse eye area of excessive exudate before application.
• Teach patient how to instill. Advise him to wash hands before and after administering ointment and warn him not to touch tip of tube to eye or surrounding tissue. Apply light finger-pressure on lacrimal sac for 1 minute after drops are instilled. Stress importance of compliance with recommended therapy.
• Store in tightly closed, light-resistant container.
• Tell patient not to share eye medications with family members. If a family member develops the same symptoms, instruct him to contact the doctor.
• Explain to patient that the ointment may produce a temporary visual haze.
• If photophobia develops, patient should wear sunglasses. He should avoid prolonged exposure to sunlight.
• Treatment should not exceed 21 days, or 3 to 5 days after healing is complete.
• If steroids are administered concomitantly, continue vidarabine for several days after discontinuation of steroid therapy.

Italicized adverse reactions are common or life-threatening.
*Liquid form contains alcohol.   **May contain tartrazine.

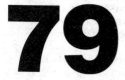

Ophthalmic anti-inflammatory agents

dexamethasone
dexamethasone sodium
  phosphate
fluorometholone
flurbiprofen sodium
medrysone
prednisolone acetate
  (suspension)
prednisolone sodium phosphate
  (solution)

COMBINATION PRODUCTS
Corticosteroids for ophthalmic use are commonly combined with antibiotics and sulfonamides. See Chapter 78, OPHTHALMIC ANTI-INFECTIVES.

dexamethasone
Maxidex Ophthalmic Suspension

dexamethasone sodium phosphate
Decadron Phosphate Ophthalmic, Maxidex Ophthalmic

Pregnancy Risk Category: C

HOW SUPPLIED
dexamethasone
Ophthalmic suspension: 0.01%
dexamethasone sodium phosphate
Ophthalmic ointment: 0.05%
Ophthalmic solution: 0.1%

MECHANISM OF ACTION
Decreases the infiltration of leukocytes at the site of inflammation.

INDICATIONS & DOSAGE
Uveitis; iridocyclitis; inflammatory conditions of eyelids, conjunctiva, cornea, anterior segment of globe; corneal injury from chemical or thermal burns, or penetration of foreign bodies; allergic conjunctivitis—
Adults and children: instill 1 to 2 drops of 0.01% suspension or 0.1% solution into conjunctival sac. In severe disease, drops may be used hourly, tapering to discontinuation as condition improves. In mild conditions, drops may be used up to four to six times daily or ointment applied q.i.d. As condition improves, taper dosage to b.i.d. then once daily. Treatment may extend from a few days to several weeks.

ADVERSE REACTIONS
Eye: increased intraocular pressure; thinning of cornea, interference with corneal wound healing, increased susceptibility to viral or fungal corneal infection, corneal ulceration; with excessive or long-term use, glaucoma exacerbations, cataracts, defects in visual acuity and visual field, optic nerve damage; mild blurred vision; burning, stinging, or redness of eyes; watery eyes.
Other: systemic effects and adrenal suppression with excessive or long-term use.

INTERACTIONS
None significant.

NURSING CONSIDERATIONS
• Contraindicated in acute superficial herpes simplex (dendritic keratitis), vaccinia, varicella, or other fungal or viral diseases of cornea and conjunc-

---

†Available in Canada only.   ‡Available in Australia only.   ◊ Available OTC.

tiva; ocular tuberculosis, or any acute, purulent, untreated infection of the eye. Use cautiously in corneal abrasions, since these may be infected (especially with herpes); in glaucoma (any form), because of possibility of increasing intraocular pressure (glaucoma medications may need to be increased to compensate).

• Viral and fungal infections of the cornea may be exacerbated by the application of steroids.

• Warn patient to call doctor immediately and to stop drug if visual acuity changes or visual field diminishes.

• Not for long-term use.

• May use eye pad with ointment.

• Teach patient how to instill. Advise him to wash hands before and after administering and warn him not to touch dropper tip to eye or surrounding tissue. Apply light finger-pressure on lacrimal sac for 1 minute following instillation.

• Watch for corneal ulceration; may require stopping drug.

• Dexamethasone has greater anti-inflammatory effect than dexamethasone sodium phosphate.

• Warn patient not to use leftover medication for a new eye inflammation; may cause serious problems.

• Tell patient not to share eye medications with family members. If a family member develops similar symptoms, instruct him to contact the doctor.

• Shake suspension well before use.

---

fluorometholone
FML Liquifilm Ophthalmic,
FML S.O.P.

Pregnancy Risk Category: C

HOW SUPPLIED
Ophthalmic ointment: 0.1%
Ophthalmic suspension: 0.1%, 0.25%

MECHANISM OF ACTION
Decreases the infiltration of leukocytes at the site of inflammation.

INDICATIONS & DOSAGE
Inflammatory and allergic conditions of cornea, conjunctiva, sclera, anterior uvea—
Adults and children: instill 1 to 2 drops in conjunctival sac b.i.d. to q.i.d. May use q hour during first 1 to 2 days if needed. Alternatively, apply thin strip of ointment to conjunctiva q 4 hours, decreasing to one to three times a day as inflammation subsides.

ADVERSE REACTIONS
Eye: increased intraocular pressure, thinning of cornea, interference with corneal wound healing, corneal ulceration, increased susceptibility to viral or fungal corneal infections; with excessive or long-term use, glaucoma exacerbations, cataracts, decreased visual acuity, diminished visual field, optic nerve damage.
Other: systemic effects and adrenal suppression in excessive or long-term use.

INTERACTIONS
None significant.

NURSING CONSIDERATIONS
• Contraindicated in vaccinia, varicella, acute superficial herpes simplex (dendritic keratitis), or other fungal or viral eye diseases; ocular tuberculosis; or any acute, purulent, untreated eye infection. Use cautiously in corneal abrasions since these may be contaminated (especially with herpes).

• Not for long-term use.

• Less likely to cause increased intraocular pressure with long-term use than other ophthalmic anti-inflammatory drugs (except medrysone).

• Store in tightly covered, light-resistant container.

• Warn patient to call doctor immedi-

Italicized adverse reactions are common or life-threatening.
*Liquid form contains alcohol.   **May contain tartrazine.

ately and to stop drug if visual acuity decreases or visual field diminishes.
• Shake well before using.
• Teach patient how to instill. Advise him to wash hands before and after administering ointment or solution, and warn him not to touch dropper or tip to eye or surrounding tissue. Apply light finger-pressure on lacrimal sac for 1 minute following instillation.
• Warn patient not to use leftover medication for a new eye inflammation; may cause serious problems.
• Tell patient not to share eye medications with family members. If a family member develops similar symptoms, instruct him to contact the doctor.

flurbiprofen sodium
Ocufen

Pregnancy Risk Category: C

HOW SUPPLIED
Ophthalmic solution: 0.03%

MECHANISM OF ACTION
Constricts the iris sphincter, thereby inhibiting miosis. The mechanism is independent of cholinergic action.

INDICATIONS & DOSAGE
Inhibition of intraoperative miosis—
Adults: instill 1 drop approximately every ½ hour, beginning 2 hours before surgery. Give a total of 4 drops.

ADVERSE REACTIONS
Eye: transient burning and stinging upon instillation, ocular irritation.

INTERACTIONS
Acetylcholine, carbachol: may be rendered ineffective.
Epinephrine or other antiglaucoma agents: reduced ability to lower intraocular pressure.

NURSING CONSIDERATIONS
• Contraindicated in epithelial herpes simplex keratitis.
• This is an NSAID. Use cautiously in patients who may be allergic to aspirin and other NSAIDs.
• Use cautiously in patients with bleeding tendencies and those who are receiving medications that may prolong clotting times.
• Wound healing may be delayed.

medrysone
HMS Liquifilm Ophthalmic

Pregnancy Risk Category: C

HOW SUPPLIED
Ophthalmic suspension: 1%

MECHANISM OF ACTION
Decreases the infiltration of leukocytes at the site of inflammation.

INDICATIONS & DOSAGE
Allergic conjunctivitis, vernal conjunctivitis, episcleritis, ophthalmic epinephrine sensitivity reaction—
Adults and children: instill 1 drop in conjunctival sac b.i.d. to q.i.d. May use q hour during first 1 to 2 days if needed.

ADVERSE REACTIONS
Eye: thinning of cornea, interference with corneal wound healing, increased susceptibility to viral or fungal corneal infection, corneal ulceration; with excessive or long-term use, glaucoma exacerbations, cataracts, visual acuity and visual field defects, optic nerve damage.
Other: systemic effects and adrenal suppression with excessive or long-term use.

INTERACTIONS
None significant.

NURSING CONSIDERATIC
• Contraindicated in vaccinia

cella, acute superficial herpes simplex (dendritic keratitis), viral diseases of conjunctiva and cornea, ocular tuberculosis, fungal or viral eye diseases, iritis, uveitis, or any acute, purulent, untreated eye infection. Use cautiously in corneal abrasions since these may be contaminated (especially with herpes).

• Shake well before using. Don't freeze.

• Teach patient how to instill. Advise him to wash hands before and after applying ointment or solution, and warn him not to touch dropper or tip to eye or surrounding tissue. Apply light finger-pressure on lacrimal sac for 1 minute following instillation.

• Warn patient not to use leftover medication for a new eye inflammation; may cause serious problems.

• Tell patient not to share eye medications with family members. If a family member develops similar symptoms, instruct him to contact the doctor.

prednisolone acetate (suspension)
Econopred Ophthalmic, Econopred Plus Ophthalmic, Pred-Forte, Pred Mild Ophthalmic

prednisolone sodium phosphate (solution)
AK-Pred, Hydeltrasol Ophthalmic, Inflamase Forte, Inflamase Ophthalmic, Ocu-Pred, Predsol Eye Drops‡

Pregnancy Risk Category: C

HOW SUPPLIED
prednisolone acetate
Ophthalmic suspension: 0.12%, 0.125%, 0.25%, 1%
prednisolone sodium phosphate
Ophthalmic solution: 0.125%, 0.5%, 1%

MECHANISM OF ACTION
Decreases the infiltration of leukocytes at the site of inflammation.

INDICATIONS & DOSAGE
Inflammation of palpebral and bulbar conjunctiva, cornea, and anterior segment of globe—
Adults and children: instill 1 to 2 drops in eye of 0.12% to 1% suspension (acetate) or 0.125% to 1% solution (phosphate). In severe conditions, may be used hourly, tapering to discontinuation as inflammation subsides. In mild conditions, may be used up to four to six times daily.

ADVERSE REACTIONS
Eye: increased intraocular pressure; thinning of cornea, interference with corneal wound healing, increased susceptibility to viral or fungal corneal infection, corneal ulceration; with excessive or long-term use, glaucoma exacerbations, cataracts, visual acuity and visual field defects, optic nerve damage.
Other: systemic effects and adrenal suppression with excessive or long-term use.

INTERACTIONS
None significant.

NURSING CONSIDERATIONS
• Contraindicated in acute, untreated, purulent, ocular infections; acute superficial herpes simplex (dendritic keratitis); vaccinia, varicella, or other viral or fungal eye diseases; or ocular tuberculosis. Use cautiously in corneal abrasions since these may be contaminated (especially with herpes).

• Tell patient on long-term therapy to have frequent tonometric examinations.

• Shake suspension before using, and store in tightly covered container.

• Teach patient how to instill. Advise patient to wash hands before and after applying, and warn him not to touch dropper or tip to eye or surrounding area. Apply light finger-pressure on lacrimal sac for 1 minute following instillation.

• Warn patient not to use leftover medication for a new eye inflammation; may cause serious problems.

• Tell patient not to share eye medications with family members. If a family member develops similar symptoms, instruct him to contact the doctor.

• Check dosage before administering to ensure using the correct strength.

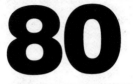

80

Miotics

acetylcholine chloride
carbachol (intraocular)
carbachol (topical)
demecarium bromide
echothiophate iodide
isoflurophate
physostigmine
pilocarpine hydrochloride
pilocarpine nitrate

COMBINATION PRODUCTS
E-PILO: epinephrine bitartrate 1%
and pilocarpine hydrochloride 1%,
2%, 3%, 4%, or 6%.
ISOPTO P-ES: pilocarpine hydrochloride 2% and physostigmine salicylate
0.25%.
P_1E_1, P_2E_1, P_3E_1, P_4E_1, P_6E_1: epinephrine bitartrate 1% and pilocarpine hydrochloride 1%, 2%, 3%, 4%, or 6%.

---

acetylcholine chloride
Miochol

Pregnancy Risk Category: C

HOW SUPPLIED
Ophthalmic solution: 1%

MECHANISM OF ACTION
A cholinergic drug that causes contraction of the sphincter muscles of
the iris, resulting in miosis. Also produces ciliary spasm, deepening of the
anterior chamber, and vasodilation of
conjunctival vessels of the outflow
tract.

INDICATIONS & DOSAGE
Anterior segment surgery—
Adults and children: doctor instills

0.5 to 2 ml of 1% solution gently in
anterior chamber of eye.

ADVERSE REACTIONS
Note: None reported with 1% concentration.
Eye: iris atrophy possible (with
higher concentrations).

INTERACTIONS
None significant.

NURSING CONSIDERATIONS
• Reconstitute immediately before
using.
• Shake vial gently until clear solution is obtained.
• Discard any unused solution.
• Complete miosis within seconds.
• Don't gas-sterilize vial. Ethylene
oxide may produce formic acid.

---

carbachol (intraocular)
Miostat

carbachol (topical)
Carbacel, Isopto Carbachol

Pregnancy Risk Category: C

HOW SUPPLIED
Intraocular solution: 0.01%
Topical ophthalmic solution: 0.75%,
1.5%, 2.25%, 3%

MECHANISM OF ACTION
A cholinergic drug that causes contraction of the sphincter muscles of
the iris, resulting in miosis. Also produces ciliary spasm, deepening of the
anterior chamber, and vasodilation of

Italicized adverse reactions are common or life-threatening.
*Liquid form contains alcohol.   **May contain tartrazine.

conjunctival vessels of the outflow tract.

INDICATIONS & DOSAGE
Ocular surgery (to produce pupillary miosis)—
Adults: doctor gently instills 0.5 ml (intraocular form) into the anterior chamber for production of satisfactory miosis. It may be instilled before or after securing sutures.
Open-angle glaucoma—
Adults: instill 1 drop (topical form) into eye daily, b.i.d., t.i.d., or q.i.d.

ADVERSE REACTIONS
CNS: headache.
Eye: accommodative spasm, blurred vision, conjunctival vasodilation, eye and brow pain.
GI: abdominal cramps, diarrhea.
Other: sweating, flushing, asthma.

INTERACTIONS
Pilocarpine: additive effect.

NURSING CONSIDERATIONS
• Contraindicated in acute iritis, corneal abrasion. Use cautiously in acute heart failure, bronchial asthma, peptic ulcer, hyperthyroidism, GI spasm, urinary tract obstruction, Parkinson's disease.
• Used in open-angle glaucoma, especially when patient is resistant or allergic to pilocarpine hydrochloride or nitrate.
• Teach patient how to instill. Advise him to wash hands before and after administering ointment or solution, and to apply light finger-pressure on lacrimal sac for 1 minute after drops are instilled. Warn him not to exceed recommended dosage.
• Tell glaucoma patient that long-term use may be necessary. Stress compliance. Tell him to remain under medical supervision for periodic tonometric readings.
• In case of toxicity, atropine should be given parenterally.

• Caution patient not to drive for 1 or 2 hours after administration until effect on vision is determined.
• Reassure patient that blurred vision usually diminishes with prolonged use.
• Patients with dark eyes (hazel or brown irides) may require stronger solutions or more frequent instillation to produce the desired reduction of intraocular pressure because the drug may be absorbed by the eye pigment.
• Tolerance to the drug effect may develop, which may be restored by switching to another miotic for a short period of time.

---

demecarium bromide
Humorsol

Pregnancy Risk Category: X

HOW SUPPLIED
Ophthalmic solution: 0.125%, 0.25% (with benzalkonium chloride 1:5,000)

MECHANISM OF ACTION
An anticholinesterase drug that inhibits the enzymatic destruction of acetylcholine by inactivating cholinesterase. This leaves acetylcholine free to act on the effector cells of the iridic sphincter and ciliary muscles, causing pupillary constriction and accommodation spasm.

INDICATIONS & DOSAGE
Angle-closure glaucoma after iridectomy, primary open-angle glucoma—
Adults: instill 1 drop of 0.125% or 0.25% solution once or twice/day.
Treatment of accommodative esotropia (uncomplicated)—
Adults: instill 1 drop of 0.125% or 0.25% solution q.d for 2 to 3 weeks then reduce to 1 drop q 2 days for 3 to 4 weeks. After reevaluation, 1 drop once or twice/week to once q 2 days as determined by patient's condition. Reevaluate q 4 to 12 weeks, adjusting dose as needed. Discontinue after 4

months if dose required is 1 drop q 2 days.

Diagnostic use—
Adults: 1 drop q.d. for 2 weeks then 1 drop q 2 days for 2 to 3 weeks.

ADVERSE REACTIONS
CNS: browache, unusual fatigue or weakness, headache.
CV: slow or irregular heartbeat.
Eye: eye pain, retinal detachment, iris cysts, conjunctival thickening, lens opacities, paradoxical increase in intraocular pressure, *lacrimation,* obstruction of nasolacrimal canals, burning, redness, stinging, irritation, twitching of eyelids, *blurred vision,* visual disturbances.
GI: nausea, vomiting, diarrhea, stomach cramps or pain.
GU: loss of bladder control.

INTERACTIONS
Anticholinergics, antimyasthenics, other cholinesterase inhibitors: potential for additive toxicity.
Carbamate or organophosphate-type insecticides: increased risk of systemic effects through respiratory tract or skin. Protective measures advised.
Cocaine: increased risk of cocaine toxicity; anticholinesterase effects may last weeks or months.
Edrophonium: worsening of patient's condition.
Local anesthetics, ophthalmic tetracaine: increased risk of systemic toxicity, prolonged ocular anesthetic effect.
Ophthalmic adrenocorticoids: increased intraocular pressure, decreased effectiveness of antiglaucoma agent.
Ophthalmic belladonna alkaloids, cyclopentolate: may antagonize miotic effects.
Succinylcholine: enhanced neuromuscular blockade, possible cardiovascular collapse, prolonged respiratory depression or apnea; effects may occur

for several weeks or months after demecarium is discontinued.

NURSING CONSIDERATIONS
• Contraindicated in patients with bronchial asthma, pronounced bradycardia and hypotension, Down's syndrome, epilepsy, spastic GI disturbances, angle-closure glaucoma before iridectomy, Parkinson's disease, uveitis, marked vagotonia, myocardial infarction, history of retinal detachment.
• Toxicity is cumulative; toxic systemic symptoms may not appear for weeks or months after start of therapy.
• Phenylephrine may be administered concurrently to reduce incidence of iris cyst formation.
• Tolerance may develop after prolonged use. Restore effectiveness by changing to another miotic for a short time then resuming demecarium.
• Concurrent use with epinephrine has additive effect, resulting in better control and lower dosage of both drugs.
• Regular medical supervision required to check ocular pressure.
• Patient should carry medical alert card or identification at all times during therapy.
• Instruct patient in correct administration techniques and dosages. Warn against using more than prescribed. Instruct patient to wash hands before and after application; avoid touching applicator tip to any surface; remove excess solution around eyes with clean tissue and without touching eye.
• If dose is missed, patient should not double dose. If schedule is every other day, apply as soon as possible if remembered same day; if remembered later, do not apply until next day then skip a day and resume regular schedule. If once a day, apply as soon as possible. If not remembered until next day, do not double dose; skip previous day's (missed) dose and resume

---

Italicized adverse reactions are common or life-threatening.
*Liquid form contains alcohol.   **May contain tartrazine.

schedule. If more than once daily, apply as soon as possible. If close to time for next dose, skip missed dose and resume regular schedule.

• Atropine sulfate I.V. or I.M. is antidote of choice for systemic cholinergic effects.

echothiophate iodide (ecotiophate iodide)
Phospholine Iodide

Pregnancy Risk Category: C

HOW SUPPLIED
Ophthalmic powder for solution: for reconstitution to make 0.03%, 0.06%, 0.125%, and 0.25% solutions

MECHANISM OF ACTION
An anticholinesterase drug that inhibits the enzymatic destruction of acetylcholine by inactivating cholinesterase. This leaves acetylcholine free to act on the effector cells of the iridic sphincter and ciliary muscles, causing pupillary constriction and accommodation spasm.

INDICATIONS & DOSAGE
Primary open-angle glaucoma, conditions obstructing aqueous outflow—
Adults and children: instill 1 drop of 0.03% to 0.125% solution into conjunctival sac daily. Maximum 1 drop b.i.d. Use lowest possible dosage to continuously control intraocular pressure.
Diagnosis of accommodative esotropia—
Adults: instill 1 drop of 0.125% solution daily at h.s. for 2 to 3 weeks.
Accommodative esotropia (treatment)—
Adults: instill 1 drop of 0.03% to 0.125% solution q.d. or q.o.d. at h.s.

ADVERSE REACTIONS
CNS: fatigue, muscle weakness, paresthesias, headache.
CV: bradycardia, hypotension.
Eye: ciliary or accommodative spasm, ciliary or conjunctival injection, nonreversible cataract formation (time- and dose-related), reversible iris cysts, pupillary block, blurred or dimmed vision, eye or brow pain, lid twitching, hyperemia, photophobia, lens opacities, lacrimation, retinal detachment.
GI: diarrhea, nausea, vomiting, abdominal pain, intestinal cramps, salivation.
GU: frequent urination.
Other: flushing, sweating, bronchial constriction.

INTERACTIONS
Anticholinergics, ophthalmic belladonna alkaloids (such as atropine), cyclopentolate: antagonized miotic effects.
Cocaine: increased risk of cocaine toxicity.
Local anesthetics, ophthalmic tetracaine: increased rate of systemic toxicity; prolonged ocular anesthesia.
Ophthalmic adrenocorticoids: increased intraocular pressure and decreased antiglaucoma effect.
Other cholinesterase inhibitors, edrophonium, organophosphorus insecticides (parathion, malathion): may have an additive effect that could cause systemic effects. Warn patient exposed to insecticides of this danger.
Succinylcholine: respiratory and cardiovascular collapse. Don't use together.
Systemic anticholinesterase for myasthenia gravis, pilocarpine: effects may be additive. Monitor patient for signs of toxicity.

NURSING CONSIDERATIONS
• Contraindicated in narrow-angle glaucoma, epilepsy, vasomotor instability, parkinsonism, iodide hypersensitivity, active uveal inflammation, bronchial asthma spastic GI conditions, urinary tract obstruction, peptic ulcer, severe bradycardia or hypoten-

sion, vascular hypertension, myocardial infarction, history of retinal detachment. Use cautiously in patients routinely exposed to organophosphorus insecticides. May cause nausea, vomiting, and diarrhea, progressing to muscle weakness and respiratory difficulty. Use cautiously in patients with myasthenia gravis receiving anticholinesterase therapy.

• Toxicity is cumulative. Toxic systemic symptoms don't appear for weeks or months after initiating therapy.
• Reconstitute powder carefully to avoid contamination. Use only diluent provided. Discard refrigerated, reconstituted solution after 6 months; discard solution at room temperature after 1 month.
• Warn patient that transient brow pain or dimmed or blurred vision is common at first but usually disappears within 5 to 10 days.
• Instill at bedtime since drug causes transient blurred vision.
• Tell patient to remain under constant medical supervision. Warn him not to exceed recommended dosage.
• Report salivation, diarrhea, profuse sweating, urinary incontinence, or muscle weakness.
• Stop drug at least 2 weeks preoperatively if succinylcholine is to be used in surgery.
• Atropine sulfate (S.C., I.M., or I.V.) is antidote of choice.
• A potent, long-acting, irreversible drug. Carry medical alert card or identification during therapy.
• Teach patient how to instill. Advise him to wash hands before and after administering ointment or solution, and to apply light finger-pressure on lacrimal sac for 1 minute following instillation. Warn him not to touch tip of dropper to eye or surrounding tissue.

isoflurophate
Floropryl
Pregnancy Risk Category: X

HOW SUPPLIED
Ophthalmic ointment: 0.025%

MECHANISM OF ACTION
Inhibits the enzymatic destruction of acetylcholine by inactivating cholinesterase, leaving the acetylcholine free to act on effector cells of iridic sphincter and ciliary muscles, causing pupillary constriction and accommodation spasm.

INDICATIONS & DOSAGE
Antiglaucoma agent—
Adults: apply thin strip of ointment to conjunctiva once q 3 days to t.i.d.
Treatment of accommodative esotropia (uncomplicated); diagnostic—
Adults: apply thin strip of ointment to conjunctiva h.s. for 2 weeks.
Treatment of accommodative esotropia—
Adults: apply thin strip of ointment to conjunctiva h.s. for 2 weeks then once a week to once q 2 days depending on patient's condition, for 2 months. If patient cannot be maintained on q 2 days dosage, discontinue drug.

ADVERSE REACTIONS
CNS: headache, browache, unusual fatigue or weakness.
CV: slow or irregular heartbeat.
Eye: eye pain, retinal detachment, iris cysts, conjunctival thickening, lens opacity, obstruction of nasolacrimal canals, paradoxical increase in intraocular pressure, *burning,* redness, stinging, irritation, twitching of eye lids, *blurred vision,* visual disturbances.
GI: nausea, vomiting, diarrhea, stomach cramps or pain.
GU: loss of bladder control.
Other: sweating, flushing.

Italicized adverse reactions are common or life-threatening.
*Liquid form contains alcohol.   **May contain tartrazine.

INTERACTIONS

Anticholinergics, antimyasthenics, other cholinesterase inhibitors: potential for additive toxicity.

Carbamate or organophosphate-type insecticides: increased risk of systemic effects through respiratory tract or skin. Protective measures advised.

Cocaine: increased risk of cocaine toxicity; anticholinesterase effects may last weeks or months.

Edrophonium: worsening of patient's condition.

Local anesthetics, ophthalmic tetracaine: increased risk of systemic toxicity, prolonged ocular anesthetic effect.

Ophthalmic adrenocorticoids: increased intraocular pressure, decreased effectiveness of antiglaucoma agent.

Ophthalmic belladonna alkaloids, cyclopentolate: may antagonize miotic effects.

Ophthalmic physostigmine: may shorten duration of action.

Succinylcholine: enhanced neuromuscular blockade, possible cardiovascular collapse, prolonged respiratory depression or apnea; effects may occur for several weeks or months after isoflurophate is discontinued.

NURSING CONSIDERATIONS

• Contraindicated in patients with bronchial asthma, pronounced bradycardia and hypotension, Down's syndrome, epilepsy, spastic GI disturbances, angle-closure glaucoma before iridectomy, Parkinson's disease, uveitis, marked vagotonia, myocardial infarction, history of retinal detachment.

• Toxicity is cumulative; toxic systemic symptoms may not appear for weeks or months after isoflurophate therapy is discontinued.

• Phenylephrine may be used concurrently to reduce incidence of iris cyst formation.

• Tolerance may develop after prolonged use. Restore effectiveness by changing to another miotic for a short time then resuming isoflurophate.

• Concurrent use with epinephrine has additive effect, resulting in better control and lower dosage of both drugs.

• Regular medical supervision required to check ocular pressure.

• Patient should carry medical alert card or identification at all times during therapy.

• Instruct patient in correct administration techniques and dosages. Warn against using more than prescribed. Instruct patient to wash hands before and after application; avoid touching applicator tip to any surface; avoid washing applicator tip or touching it to moist surface, which will cause medication to lose efficacy; and wipe tip with clean tissue.

• If dose is missed, patient should not double dose. If schedule is every other day, apply as soon as possible if remembered same day; if remembered later, do not apply until next day then skip a day and resume regular schedule. If once a day, apply as soon as possible. If not remembered until next day, skip missed dose and resume schedule. If more than once daily, apply as soon as possible. If close to time for next dose, skip missed dose and resume regular schedule.

• Atropine sulfate I.V. or I.M. is antidote of choice for systemic cholinergic effects.

physostigmine
Eserine, Isopto-Eserine
Pregnancy Risk Category: C

HOW SUPPLIED
Ophthalmic ointment: 0.25%
Ophthalmic solution: 0.25%, 0.5%

MECHANISM OF ACTION
Contraction of iris sphincter muscles results in miosis. Contraction of cili-

ary muscle increases outflow of aqueous humor and decreases intraocular pressure.

INDICATIONS & DOSAGE

Treatment of open-angle glaucoma—
Adults and children: 1 drop of 0.25% to 0.5% solution b.i.d. to t.i.d. or thin strip of ointment once daily to t.i.d.

ADVERSE REACTIONS

CNS: headache, weakness.
CV: slow or irregular heartbeats.
Eye: blurred vision, eye pain, burning, redness, stinging, eye irritation, twitching of eyelids, watering of eyes.
GI: nausea, vomiting, diarrhea.
GU: loss of bladder control.
Other: increased sweating, muscle weakness, shortness of breath.

INTERACTIONS

Echothiophate, isoflurophate: duration of action may be shortened.
Ophthalmic belladonna alkaloids: may antagonize miotic actions.

NURSING CONSIDERATIONS

• Contraindicated in patients with intolerance to physostigmine, active uveitis, corneal injury.
• Instruct patient in correct administration techniques and dosages. Warn patient against using more than prescribed. Instruct patient to wash hands immediately before and after application and avoid touching applicator tip to any surface.
• Tolerance may develop with prolonged use. Restore effectiveness by changing to another miotic for a short time then resuming physostigmine.
• Ointment form may be used at night to prolong contact with medication.

pilocarpine hydrochloride

Adsorbocarpine, Isopto Carpine, Miocarpine†, Ocusert Pilo, Pilocar, Pilocel, Pilomiotin, Pilopine HS, Pilopt‡

pilocarpine nitrate

P.V. Carpine Liquifilm

Pregnancy Risk Category: C

HOW SUPPLIED

hydrochloride
Ophthalmic solution: 0.25%, 0.5%, 1%, 2%, 3%, 4%, 5%, 6%, 8%, 10%
Ophthalmic gel: 4%
Releasing-system insert: 20 mcg/hr, 40 mcg/hr
nitrate
Ophthalmic solution: 1%, 2%, 4%

MECHANISM OF ACTION

A cholinergic drug that causes contraction of the sphincter muscles of the iris, resulting in miosis. Also produces ciliary spasm, deepening of the anterior chamber, and vasodilation of conjunctival vessels of the outflow tract.

INDICATIONS & DOSAGE

Primary open-angle glaucoma—
Adults and children: instill 1 to 2 drops in eye q.d. to q.i.d., as directed by doctor. Or, may apply 4% gel (Pilopine HS) once daily.
  Alternatively, apply one Ocusert Pilo system (20 or 40 mcg/hour) q 7 days.
Emergency treatment of acute narrow-angle glaucoma—
Adults and children: 1 drop of 2% solution q 5 minutes for three to six doses, followed by 1 drop q 1 to 3 hours until pressure is controlled.

ADVERSE REACTIONS

Eye: suborbital headache, *myopia,* ciliary spasm, *blurred vision,* conjunctival irritation, lacrimation, changes in visual field, *brow pain.*

Italicized adverse reactions are common or life-threatening.
*Liquid form contains alcohol.   **May contain tartrazine.

GI: nausea, vomiting, abdominal cramps, diarrhea, salivation.
Other: bronchiolar spasm, pulmonary edema, hypersensitivity.

INTERACTIONS
Carbachol, echothiophate: additive effect. Don't use together.
Ophthalmic belladona alkaloids (such as atropine, scopolamine), cyclopentolate: decreased antiglaucoma effects of pilocarpine; mydriatic effects of these agents blocked by pilocarpine.
Phenylephrine: decreased dilation by phenylephrine. Don't use together.

NURSING CONSIDERATIONS
• Contraindicated in acute iritis, acute inflammatory disease of anterior segment of eye, secondary glaucoma. Use cautiously in bronchial asthma and hypertension.
• Warn patient that vision will be temporarily blurred. Warn patient to avoid hazardous activities until this effect subsides.
• Transient brow pain and myopia are common at first; usually disappear in 10 to 14 days.
• Teach patient how to instill. Advise him to wash hands before and after administering gel or solution, and to apply light finger-pressure on lacrimal sac for 1 minute following instillation of drops. Warn him not to touch dropper to eye or surrounding tissue.
• Widely used drug to treat primary open-angle glaucoma.
• Used to counteract effects of mydriatics and cycloplegics after surgery or ophthalmoscopic examination.
• May be used alternately with atropine to break adhesions.
• In acute narrow-angle glaucoma before surgery, may be used alone or with mannitol, urea, glycerol, or acetazolamide.
• If the Ocusert Pilo system falls out of the eye during sleep, patient should wash hands, rinse the system in cool tap water, and reposition it in the eye. Tell patient not to use it if deformed.
• Instruct patient to apply gel at bedtime, as it will blur vision.

Mydriatics

atropine sulfate
cyclopentolate hydrochloride
epinephrine bitartrate
epinephrine hydrochloride
epinephryl borate
homatropine hydrobromide
phenylephrine hydrochloride
scopolamine hydrobromide
tropicamide

COMBINATION PRODUCTS

CYCLOMYDRIL OPHTHALMIC: cyclopentolate hydrochloride 0.2% and phenylephrine hydrochloride 1%.
MUROCOLL-2: scopolamine hydrobromide 0.3% and phenylephrine hydrochloride 10%.

---

atropine sulfate
Atropisol, Atropt‡, BufOpto
Atropine, Isopto Atropine

Pregnancy Risk Category: C

HOW SUPPLIED
Ophthalmic ointment: 0.5%, 1%
Ophthalmic solution: 1%, 2%, 3%

MECHANISM OF ACTION
Anticholinergic action leaves the pupil under unopposed adrenergic influence, causing it to dilate.

INDICATIONS & DOSAGE
Treatment of acute iritis; treatment of uveitis—
Adults and children: instill 1 drop of 1% solution or small amount of ointment q.d. to b.i.d.
Cycloplegic refraction—

Adults: instill 1 to 2 drops of 1% solution 1 hour before refracting.
Children: instill 1 to 2 drops of 0.5% to 1% solution in each eye b.i.d. for 1 to 3 days before eye examination and 1 hour before refraction, or instill small amount of ointment daily or b.i.d. 2 to 3 days before examination.

ADVERSE REACTIONS
Eye: ocular congestion in long-term use, conjunctivitis, contact dermatitis, edema, *blurred vision,* eye dryness, *photophobia.*
Systemic: flushing, dry skin and mouth, fever, tachycardia, abdominal distention in infants, ataxia, irritability, confusion, somnolence.

INTERACTIONS
None significant.

NURSING CONSIDERATIONS
• Contraindicated in angle-closure glaucoma (narrow-angle). Use cautiously in infants, children, and elderly or debilitated patients. Children with blond hair and blue eyes, patients with Down's syndrome, or patients with brain damage may be more susceptible to atropine or experience higher incidence of adverse reactions.
• Warn patient vision will be temporarily blurred. Dark glasses ease discomfort of photophobia.
• Not for internal use. Treat drops and ointment as poison. Signs of poisoning are disorientation and confusion. Physostigmine salicylate I.V. or I.M. may be used as an antidote.
• Watch for signs of glaucoma: in-

Italicized adverse reactions are common or life-threatening.
*Liquid form contains alcohol.   **May contain tartrazine.

creased intraocular pressure, ocular pain, headache, progressive blurring of vision.

• Most potent mydriatic and cycloplegic available; long duration.

• Systemic adverse reactions most commonly occur in children and elderly patients.

• Warn patient to avoid hazardous activities such as operating machinery or driving a car until the temporary visual impairment caused by this drug wears off.

• Teach patient how to instill. Advise him to wash hands before and after administering solution, and to apply light finger-pressure on lacrimal sac for 1 minute following instillation. Warn patient not to touch dropper or tip of tube to eye or surrounding tissue.

• Advise patient to use sugarless hard candy or gum if dry mouth is a problem.

cyclopentolate hydrochloride
AK-Pentolate, Cyclogyl

Pregnancy Risk Category: C

HOW SUPPLIED
Ophthalmic solution: 0.5%, 1%, 2%

MECHANISM OF ACTION
Anticholinergic action leaves the pupil under unopposed adrenergic influence, causing it to dilate.

INDICATIONS & DOSAGE
Diagnostic procedures requiring mydriasis and cycloplegia—
Adults: instill 1 drop of 1% solution in eye, followed by 1 more drop in 5 minutes. Use 2% solution in heavily pigmented irises.
Children: instill 1 drop of 0.5%, 1%, or 2% solution in each eye, followed in 5 minutes with 1 drop 0.5% or 1% solution, if necessary.

ADVERSE REACTIONS
Eye: burning sensation on instillation, blurred vision, eye dryness, *photophobia,* ocular congestion, contact dermatitis, conjunctivitis.
Systemic: flushing, tachycardia, urine retention, dry skin, fever, ataxia, irritability, confusion, somnolence, hallucinations, seizures, behavioral disturbances in children.

INTERACTIONS
Carbachol, pilocarpine: may counteract mydriatic effect.
Long-acting cholinergic antiglaucoma agents: Miotic actions may be inhibited.

NURSING CONSIDERATIONS
• Contraindicated in narrow-angle glaucoma. Use cautiously in elderly patients and in children with spastic paralysis.

• Potent drug with mydriatic and cycloplegic effect; superior to homatropine hydrobromide and has shorter duration of action. Physostigmine is antidote of choice.

• Instruct patient to wear dark glasses to ease discomfort of photophobia.

• Warn patient drug will burn when instilled.

• Warn patient to avoid hazardous activities such as operating machinery or driving until the temporary visual impairment caused by this drug subsides.

• Teach patient how to instill. Advise him to wash hands before and after administering, and to apply light finger-pressure on lacrimal sac for 1 minute following instillation. Warn patient not to touch tip of dropper to eye or surrounding tissue.

---

†Available in Canada only.   ‡Available in Australia only.   ◊Available OTC.

epinephrine bitartrate
Epitrate, Mytrate

epinephrine hydrochloride
Epifrin, Glaucon

epinephryl borate
Epinal, Eppy/N

Pregnancy Risk Category: C

HOW SUPPLIED
epinephrine bitartrate
Ophthalmic solution: 2%
epinephrine hydrochloride
Ophthalmic solution: 0.1%, 0.25%,
0.5%, 1%, 2%
epinephryl borate
Ophthalmic solution: 0.5%, 1%, 2%

MECHANISM OF ACTION
An adrenergic that dilates the pupil by
contracting the dilator muscle.

INDICATIONS & DOSAGE
Open-angle glaucoma—
Adults: instill 1 to 2 drops of 1% or
2% bitartrate solution in eye with frequency determined by tonometric
readings (once q 2 to 4 days up to
q.i.d.), or instill 1 drop of 0.5%, 1%,
or 2% hydrochloride solution (or
0.5% or 1% epinephryl borate solution) in eye b.i.d.
During surgery—
Adults: instill 1 or more drops of
0.1% solution up to three times.

ADVERSE REACTIONS
Eye: corneal or conjunctival pigmentation or corneal edema in long-term
use; follicular hypertrophy; chemosis;
conjunctivitis; iritis; hyperemic conjunctiva; maculopapular rash; *severe
stinging,* burning, and tearing upon
instillation; browache.
Systemic: palpitations, *tachycardia.*

INTERACTIONS
Cyclopropane or halogenated hydro-
carbons: arrhythmias, tachycardia.
Use together cautiously, if at all.
Digitalis glycosides: increased risk of
cardiac arrhythmias.
Local or systemic sympathomimetics:
additive toxic effects.
MAO inhibiters: exaggerated adrenergic effects. Adjust dose of epinephrine carefully.
Pilocarpine: additive effect in lowering intraocular pressure.
*Tricyclic antidepressants, antihista-
mines (diphenhydramine, dexchlorpheniramine):* potentiated cardiac effects of epinephrine.

NURSING CONSIDERATIONS
• Contraindicated in shallow anterior
chamber or narrow-angle glaucoma.
• Use cautiously in diabetes mellitus,
hypertension, Parkinson's disease, hyperthyroidism, aphakia (eye without
lens), cardiac disease, or cerebral arteriosclerosis; in elderly patients or
pregnant women.
• May stain soft contact lenses.
• Monitor blood pressure and other
systemic effects.
• Don't use darkened solution.
• Also used during surgery to control
local bleeding, or injected into the anterior chamber to produce rapid mydriasis during cataract removal.
• Teach patient how to instill. Advise
him to wash hands before and after
administering and to apply light finger-pressure on lacrimal sac for 1
minute following instillation. Warn
patient not to touch dropper to eye or
surrounding tissue.
• Epinephrine salts are not interchangeable. Don't substitute one salt
if another one is ordered.

homatropine hydrobromide
Homatrine, Homatropine, Isopto

Pregnancy Risk Category: C

HOW SUPPLIED
Ophthalmic solution: 2%, 5%

Italicized adverse reactions are common or life-threatening.
*Liquid form contains alcohol.   **May contain tartrazine.

MECHANISM OF ACTION
Anticholinergic action leaves the pupil under unopposed adrenergic influence, causing it to dilate.

INDICATIONS & DOSAGE
Cycloplegic refraction—
Adults and children: instill 1 to 2 drops of 2% or 5% solution in eye; repeat in 5 to 10 minutes if needed, for two or three doses.
Uveitis—
Adults and children: instill 1 to 2 drops of 2% or 5% solution in eye up to q 3 to 4 hours.

ADVERSE REACTIONS
Eye: irritation, *blurred vision, photophobia.*
Systemic: flushing, dry skin and mouth, fever, tachycardia, ataxia, irritability, confusion, somnolence.

INTERACTIONS
None significant.

NURSING CONSIDERATIONS
• Contraindicated in angle-closure glaucoma (narrow-angle). Use cautiously in infants and elderly or debilitated patients; children with blond hair and blue eyes; patients with cardiac disease; or patients with increased intraocular pressure.
• Patients who are hypersensitive to atropine will also be hypersensitive to homatropine.
• Warn patient that vision will be temporarily blurred after instillation. Tell patient to avoid hazardous activities such as operating machinery or driving a car until blurring subsides. Patient should wear dark glasses to ease discomfort of photophobia.
• May produce symptoms of atropine poisoning, such as severe dryness of mouth, tachycardia.
• Similar to atropine but weaker, with a shorter duration of action.
• Not for internal use.
• Teach patient how to instill. Advise

him to wash hands before and after administering and to apply light finger-pressure on lacrimal sac for 1 minute following instillation. Warn patient not to touch dropper tip to eye or surrounding tissue.
• Advise patient to use sugarless hard candy or gum if dry mouth is a problem.

phenylephrine hydrochloride
AK-Dilate, AK-Nefrin Ophthalmic◊, I-Phrine 2.5%, Isopto Frin◊, Mydfrin, Neo-Synephrine, Prefrin Liquifilm

Pregnancy Risk Category: C

HOW SUPPLIED
Ophthalmic solution: 0.12%◊, 2.5%, 10%

MECHANISM OF ACTION
An adrenergic that dilates the pupil by contracting the dilator muscle of the pupil.

INDICATIONS & DOSAGE
Mydriasis (without cycloplegia)—
Adults and children: instill 1 drop of 2.5% or 10% solution in eye before examination.
Mydriasis and vasoconstriction—
Adults and adolescents: instill 1 drop of 2.5% or 10% solution in eye; repeat in 1 hour if needed.
Children: instill 1 drop of 2.5% solution in eye; repeat in 1 hour if needed.
To relieve eye redness—
Adults: instill 1 to 2 drops of 0.12% solution in eye daily up to q.i.d.
Chronic mydriasis—
Adults and adolescents: instill 1 drop of 2.5% or 10% solution in eye b.i.d. or t.i.d.
Children: instill 1 drop of 2.5% solution in eye b.i.d. or t.i.d.
Posterior synechia (adhesion of iris)—
Adults and children: instill 1 drop of 10% solution in eye.

Do not use 10% concentration in infants; use cautiously in elderly patients.

ADVERSE REACTIONS
CNS: headache, browache.
CV: *hypertension* (with 10% solution), tachycardia, palpitations, premature ventricular contractions.
Eye: transient burning or stinging on instillation, blurred vision, reactive hyperemia, allergic conjunctivitis, iris floaters, narrow-angle glaucoma, rebound miosis, dermatitis.
Other: pallor, trembling, sweating.

INTERACTIONS
Guanethidine: increased mydriatic and pressor effects of phenylephrine. Use together cautiously.
Levodopa (systemic): reduced mydriatic effect of phenylephrine. Use together cautiously.
MAO inhibitors and beta blockers: may cause arrhythmias due to increased pressor effect. Use together cautiously.
Tricyclic antidepressants: potentiated cardiac effects of epinephrine. Use together cautiously.

NURSING CONSIDERATIONS
• Contraindicated in narrow-angle glaucoma, soft contact lens use. Avoid 10% solution and use cautiously in marked hypertension, cardiac disorders, and in children of low body weight.
• Should be avoided in patients with idiopathic orthostatic hypotension. May produce high blood pressure.
• Protect from light and heat.
• Warn patient not to exceed recommended dosage. Systemic effects can result. Monitor blood pressure and pulse rate.
• Potential for systemic adverse reactions less severe with 2.5% solution. Adverse reactions and toxicity much more likely with 10% solution.
• Teach patient how to instill. Advise

him to wash hands before and after administering and to apply light finger-pressure on lacrimal sac for 1 minute following instillation. Warn patient not to touch dropper tip to eye or surrounding tissue.
• May cause blurred vision. Warn patient to avoid driving a car or operating machinery until this effect subsides.
• May cause photophobia. Advise patient to wear dark sunglasses and to contact physician if condition persists longer than 12 hours after discontinuation of the drug.
• Do not use brown solutions or solutions that contain a precipitate.

---

scopolamine hydrobromide
Isopto Hyoscine
Pregnancy Risk Category: C

HOW SUPPLIED
Ophthalmic solution: 0.25%

MECHANISM OF ACTION
Anticholinergic action leaves the pupil under unopposed adrenergic influence, causing it to dilate.

INDICATIONS & DOSAGE
Cycloplegic refraction—
Adults: instill 1 to 2 drops of 0.25% solution in eye 1 hour before refraction.
Children: instill 1 drop of 0.25% solution or ointment b.i.d. for 2 days before refraction.
Iritis, uveitis—
Adults: instill 1 to 2 drops of 0.25% solution daily b.i.d. or t.i.d.
Children: instill 1 drop once daily to t.i.d.

ADVERSE REACTIONS
Eye: ocular congestion with prolonged use, conjunctivitis, *blurred vision,* eye dryness, increased intraocular pressure, *photophobia,* contact dermatitis.

Italicized adverse reactions are common or life-threatening.
*Liquid form contains alcohol.   **May contain tartrazine.

Systemic: flushing, fever, dry skin and mouth, tachycardia, hallucinations, ataxia, irritability, confusion, delirium, somnolence, acute psychotic reactions.

INTERACTIONS
None significant.

NURSING CONSIDERATIONS
• Contraindicated in angle-closure glaucoma (shallow anterior chamber or narrow-angle). Use cautiously in cardiac disease, increased intraocular pressure, and in elderly patients.
• Observe patient closely for systemic effects (disorientation, delirium).
• Warn patient that vision will be temporarily blurred; tell patient to avoid hazardous activities such as driving or operating machinery until this effect subsides.
• Instruct patient to wear dark glasses to ease discomfort of photophobia.
• May be used when patient is sensitive to atropine. Faster acting and has shorter duration of action and fewer adverse reactions.
• Teach patient how to instill. Advise him to wash hands before and after administering and to apply light finger-pressure on lacrimal sac for 1 minute following instillation. Warn him not to touch dropper tip to eye or surrounding tissue.

---

tropicamide
Mydriacyl, Tropicacyl

Pregnancy Risk Category: C

HOW SUPPLIED
Ophthalmic solution: 0.5%, 1%

MECHANISM OF ACTION
Anticholinergic action leaves the pupil under unopposed adrenergic influence, causing it to dilate.

INDICATIONS & DOSAGE
Cycloplegic refractions—

Adults: instill 1 drop of 1% solution; repeat in 5 minutes. Additional drop may be instilled in 20 to 30 minutes.
Children: instill 1 drop of 0.5% to 1% solution; may repeat in 5 minutes.
Fundus examinations—
Adults and children: instill 1 to 2 drops of 0.5% solution in each eye 15 to 20 minutes before examination.

ADVERSE REACTIONS
Eye: *transient stinging on instillation,* increased intraocular pressure (less than with other mydriatic agents because of shorter duration of action), *blurred vision, photophobia.*
Systemic: flushing, fever, dry skin, dry mouth and throat, ataxia, irritability, confusion, somnolence, hallucinations, behavioral disturbances in children.

INTERACTIONS
None significant.

NURSING CONSIDERATIONS
• Contraindicated in narrow-angle and shallow anterior chamber glaucoma. Use cautiously in elderly patients.
• Physostigmine is the antidote of choice.
• Shortest acting cycloplegic, but mydriatic effect greater than cycloplegic effect.
• Causes transient stinging; vision temporarily blurred. Warn patient to avoid driving and other hazardous activities that require good vision.
• Instruct patient to wear dark glasses if photophobia occurs (lasts about 2 hours).
• Teach patient how to instill. Advise him to wash hands before and after administering and to apply light finger-pressure on lacrimal sac for 1 minute following instillation. Warn him not to touch dropper to eye or surrounding tissue.

82

Ophthalmic vasoconstrictors

naphazoline hydrochloride
phenylephrine hydrochloride (See
Chapter 81, MYDRIATICS.)
tetrahydrozoline hydrochloride
zinc sulfate

COMBINATION PRODUCTS
ALBALON-A LIQUIFILM: naphazoline
hydrochloride 0.05% and antazoline
phosphate 0.5%.
BLEPHAMIDE LIQUIFILM SUSPENSION:
phenylephrine hydrochloride 0.12%,
sulfacetamide sodium 10%, and prednisolone acetate 0.2%. EDTA, 1.4%
polyvinyl alcohol, polysorbate 80, sodium thiosulfate, and benzalkonium
chloride.
PHENYLZIN◇: zinc sulfate 0.25% and
phenylephrine hydrochloride 0.12%.
PREFRIN-A: phenylephrine hydrochloride 0.12%, pyrilamine maleate
0.1%, and antipyrine 0.1%.
VASOCIDIN OPHTHALMIC OINTMENT:
phenylephrine hydrochloride
0.125%, sulfacetamide sodium 10%,
and prednisolone acetate 0.5%.
VASOCIDIN OPHTHALMIC SOLUTION:
phenylephrine hydrochloride
0.125%, sulfacetamide sodium 10%,
and prednisolone sodium phosphate
0.25%.
VASOCON-A OPHTHALMIC SOLUTION:
naphazoline hydrochloride 0.05% and
antazoline phosphate 0.5%.
ZINCFRIN◇: phenylephrine hydrochloride 0.12% and zinc sulfate 0.25%.

naphazoline hydrochloride
AK-Con, Albalon Liquifilm,
Allerest◇, Clear Eyes◇, Degest 2◇,
Estivin II, Naphcon◇, Naphcon
Forte, Optazine‡, Vasoclear◇,
Vasocon Regular

Pregnancy Risk Category: C

HOW SUPPLIED
Ophthalmic solution: 0.012%◇,
0.02%, 0.03%, 0.05%, 0.1%

MECHANISM OF ACTION
Produces vasoconstriction by local
adrenergic action on the blood vessels
of the conjunctiva.

INDICATIONS & DOSAGE
Ocular congestion, irritation, itch-
ing—
Adults: instill 1 to 2 drops of 0.1%
solution in eye q 3 to 4 hours or 1 drop
of 0.012% to 0.05% solution up to
q.i.d.

ADVERSE REACTIONS
Eye: transient stinging, pupillary dilation, irritation, photophobia.
Other: dizziness, headache, increased sweating, nausea, nervousness, weakness.

INTERACTIONS
Tricyclic antidepressants, MAO inhib-
itors: hypertensive crisis if naphazoline is systemically absorbed. Use together cautiously.

NURSING CONSIDERATIONS
• Contraindicated in narrow-angle

Italicized adverse reactions are common or life-threatening.
*Liquid form contains alcohol.   **May contain tartrazine.

glaucoma, hypersensitivity to any ingredients. Use cautiously in patients with hyperthyroidism, cardiac disease, hypertension, and diabetes mellitus, and in elderly patients.
• Not recommended for use in infants and children.
• Can produce marked sedation and coma if ingested by child.
• Advise patient that photophobia may follow pupil dilation if he is sensitive to drug. Tell patient to report this to the doctor if it occurs.
• Warn patient not to exceed recommended dosage. Rebound congestion and conjunctivitis may occur with frequent or prolonged use. Patient should not use nonprescription drops for more than 72 hours without the direction of a physician.
• Notify doctor if blurred vision, pain, or lid edema develops.
• Store in tightly closed container.
• Most widely used ocular decongestant.
• Teach patient how to instill. Advise him to wash hands before and after administering, and to apply light finger-pressure on lacrimal sac for 1 minute after instillation. Warn him not to touch tip of dropper to eye or surrounding tissues.

---

tetrahydrozoline hydrochloride
Murine Plus◊, Optigene◊, Soothe◊, Tetrasine◊, Visine◊

Pregnancy Risk Category: C

HOW SUPPLIED
Ophthalmic solution: 0.05%◊

MECHANISM OF ACTION
Produces vasoconstriction by local adrenergic action on the blood vessels of the conjunctiva.

INDICATIONS & DOSAGE
Ocular congestion, irritation, and allergic conditions—

Adults and children over 2 years: instill 1 to 2 drops of 0.05% solution in eye b.i.d. or t.i.d., or as directed by doctor.

ADVERSE REACTIONS
Eye: transient stinging, pupillary dilation, increased intraocular pressure, irritation, iris floaters in elderly.
Systemic: drowsiness, CNS depression, cardiac irregularities, headache, dizziness, tremors, insomnia.

INTERACTIONS
Tricyclics, guanethidine, MAO inhibitors: hypertensive crisis if tetrahydrozoline is systemically absorbed. Don't use together.

NURSING CONSIDERATIONS
• Contraindicated in patients receiving MAO inhibitors, and in those with hypersensitivity to any ingredients or narrow-angle glaucoma. Use cautiously in patients with hyperthyroidism, heart disease, hypertension, and diabetes mellitus and in the elderly.
• Do not exceed recommended dosage. Rebound congestion may occur with frequent or prolonged use.
• Warn patient to stop drug and notify doctor if relief is not obtained within 48 hours, or if redness or irritation persists or increases.
• Teach patient how to instill. Advise him to wash hands before and after administering, and to apply light finger-pressure on lacrimal sac for 1 minute after instillation. Warn patient not to touch dropper tip to eye or surrounding tissues.
• Caution patient not to share eye medications with others.

---

zinc sulfate
Bufopto Zinc Sulfate◇, Eye-Sed
Ophthalmic◇, Op-Thal-Zin◇

Pregnancy Risk Category: C

HOW SUPPLIED
Ophthalmic solution: 0.2%◇

MECHANISM OF ACTION
Produces astringent action on the conjunctiva.

INDICATIONS & DOSAGE
Ocular congestion, irritation—
Adults and children: instill 1 to 2 drops of 0.2% solution in eye b.i.d. or t.i.d.

ADVERSE REACTIONS
Eye: irritation.

INTERACTIONS
None significant.

NURSING CONSIDERATIONS
• Use cautiously in patients with a shallow anterior chamber or predisposition to narrow-angle glaucoma.
• A decongestant astringent.
• Store in tightly closed container.
• Teach patient how to instill. Advise him to wash hands before and after administering, and to apply light finger-pressure on lacrimal sac for 1 minute after instillation. Warn patient not to touch dropper tip to eye or surrounding tissues.

Italicized adverse reactions are common or life-threatening.
*Liquid form contains alcohol.   **May contain tartrazine.

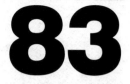

83

Topical ophthalmic anesthetics

proparacaine hydrochloride
tetracaine
tetracaine hydrochloride

COMBINATION PRODUCTS
None.

proparacaine hydrochloride
Alcaine, Ophthaine, Ophthetic

Pregnancy Risk Category: C

HOW SUPPLIED
Ophthalmic solution: 0.5%

MECHANISM OF ACTION
Produces anesthesia by preventing initiation and transmission of impulses at the nerve-cell membrane.

INDICATIONS & DOSAGE
Anesthesia for tonometry, gonioscopy; suture removal from cornea, removal of corneal foreign bodies—
Adults and children: instill 1 to 2 drops of 0.5% solution in eye just before procedure.
Anesthesia for cataract extraction, glaucoma surgery—
Adults and children: instill 1 drop of 0.5% solution in eye q 5 to 10 minutes for five to seven doses.

ADVERSE REACTIONS
Eye: occasional conjunctival redness, transient pain.
Other: hypersensitivity.

INTERACTIONS
None significant.

NURSING CONSIDERATIONS
• Use cautiously in patients with cardiac disease and hyperthyroidism.
• *Not* for long-term use; may delay wound healing.
• Warn patient not to rub or touch eye while cornea is anesthetized, since this may cause corneal abrasion and greater discomfort when anesthesia wears off.
• Warn patient with corneal abrasion that pain is relieved only temporarily.
• Systemic reactions unlikely when used in recommended doses.
• Equal in potency to tetracaine, but less irritating.
• Topical ophthalmic anesthetic of choice in diagnostic and minor surgical procedures.
• Don't use discolored solution.
• Store in tightly closed container.
• Ophthaine brand packaged in bottle that looks similar in size and shape to Hemoccult. When taking bottle from shelf, check label carefully.
• Opened containers should be refrigerated.

tetracaine
Pontocaine Eye

tetracaine hydrochloride
Pontocaine

Pregnancy Risk Category: C

HOW SUPPLIED
tetracaine
Ophthalmic ointment: 0.5%
tetracaine hydrochloride
Ophthalmic solution: 0.5%

MECHANISM OF ACTION

Produces anesthesia by preventing initiation and transmission of impulses at the nerve-cell membrane.

INDICATIONS & DOSAGE

Anesthesia for tonometry, gonioscopy; removal of corneal foreign bodies, suture removal from cornea; other diagnostic and minor surgical procedures—

Adults and children: instill 1 to 2 drops of 0.5% solution or a small strip of ointment in eye just before procedure.

ADVERSE REACTIONS

Eye: transient stinging in eye 30 seconds after initial instillation, epithelial damage in excessive or long-term use.

Other: sensitization in repeated use (allergic skin rash, urticaria).

INTERACTIONS

Cholinesterase inhibitors: prolonged ocular anesthesia and increased risk of toxicity.

Sulfonamides: interference with sulfonamide antibacterial activity. Wait ½ hour after anesthesia before instilling sulfonamide.

NURSING CONSIDERATIONS

- Systemic absorption unlikely in recommended doses.
- Avoid repeated use.
- Does not dilate the pupil, paralyze accommodation, or increase intraocular pressure.
- Don't use discolored solution. Keep container tightly closed.
- Warn patient not to touch or rub the eye while the cornea is anesthetized. This may cause corneal abrasion and greater discomfort when the anesthetic wears off.

Italicized adverse reactions are common or life-threatening.
*Liquid form contains alcohol.   **May contain tartrazine.

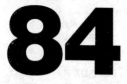

84

Miscellaneous ophthalmics

apraclonidine hydrochloride
artificial tears
betaxolol hydrochloride
botulinum toxin type A
cromolyn sodium
dipivefrin
eye irrigation solutions
fluorescein sodium
glycerin, anhydrous
isosorbide
levobunolol hydrochloride
sodium chloride, hypertonic
timolol maleate

COMBINATION PRODUCT
FLURESS: sodium fluorescein 0.25%
and benoxinate hydrochloride 0.4%.

---

apraclonidine hydrochloride
Iopidine

Pregnancy Risk Category: C

HOW SUPPLIED
Ophthalmic solution: 1%

MECHANISM OF ACTION
An alpha-adrenergic agonist that reduces intraocular pressure, possibly
by decreasing production of aqueous
humor.

INDICATIONS & DOSAGE
*Prevention or control of intraocular
pressure elevations after argon laser
trabeculoplasty or iridotomy—*
Adults: instill 1 drop in the eye 1 hour
before initiation of laser surgery on
the anterior segment, followed by 1

drop immediately after completion of
surgery.

ADVERSE REACTIONS
CNS: insomnia, irritability, dream
disturbances, headache.
CV: bradycardia, vasovagal attack,
palpitations, hypotension, orthostatic
hypotension.
EENT: upper eyelid elevation, conjunctival blanching, mydriasis, burning, discomfort, foreign body sensation, eye dryness and itching, blurred
vision, allergic response, conjunctival
microhemorrhage, taste disturbances,
dry mouth, nasal burning or dryness,
increased pharyngeal secretions.
GI: abdominal pain, discomfort,
diarrhea, vomiting.
Skin: pruritus not associated with
rash.
Other: sweaty palms, body heat sensation, decreased libido, extremity
pain or numbness.

INTERACTIONS
None reported.

NURSING CONSIDERATIONS
• Contraindicated in patients with hypersensitivity to apraclonidine or
clonidine.
• Patients who tend to develop exaggerated decreases in intraocular pressure after drug therapy should be
monitored closely.
• Onset of action is usually less than
1 hour, and drug effects usually peak
within 4 to 5 hours.
• Systemic effects of the drug (altered
heart rate and blood pressure) are un-

---

common after usual dose, but patients with severe systemic disease, including hypertension, should be monitored closely.
• Observe patient closely for vasovagal attack during laser surgery.

artificial tears
Adsorbotear◇, Hypotears◇, Isopto Alkaline◇, Isopto Plain◇, Isopto Tears◇, Lacril◇, Lacrisert, Liquifilm Forte◇, Liquifilm Tears◇, Lyteers◇, Methulose◇, Moisture Drops◇, Neo-Tears◇, Refresh◇, Tearisol◇, Tears Naturale◇, Tears Plus◇, Ultra Tears◇, Visculose◇

Pregnancy Risk Category: C

HOW SUPPLIED
Ophthalmic solution: 2-ml◇, 15-ml◇, 30-ml◇ bottles
Ocular insert: 5-mg (hydroxypropyl cellulose) insert

MECHANISM OF ACTION
Augments insufficient tear production.

INDICATIONS & DOSAGE
Insufficient tear production—
Adults and children: instill 1 to 2 drops of solution in eye t.i.d., q.i.d., or p.r.n.
Moderate to severe dry eye syndromes, including keratoconjunctivitis sicca—
Adults: insert 1 Lacrisert rod daily into inferior cul-de-sac. Some patients may require twice daily use.

ADVERSE REACTIONS
Eye: discomfort; burning, pain on instillation; blurred vision (especially with Lacrisert); crust formation on eyelids and eyelashes in products with high viscosity, such as Adsorbotear, Isopto Tears, and Tearisol.

INTERACTIONS
Borate external irrigation solutions: may form gummy deposits on the lid when used with artificial tear products containing polyvinyl alcohol (Liquifilm Forte, Liquifilm Tears). Keep patient's eyelids clean.

NURSING CONSIDERATIONS
• Contraindicated in patients with hypersensitivity to active product or preservatives. Do not use with contact lense in place unless product is designated for this use.
• Teach patient how to instill. Warn him not to touch dropper to eye or surrounding tissue. Advise him to wash hands before and after administration.
• To avoid contamination of solution, warn patient not to touch tip of container to eye, surrounding tissue, or other surface.
• Instruct patient that product should be used by one person only.
• Lacrisert rod should be inserted with special applicator that is included in the package. Familiarize patient with illustrated instructions that are also included.
• If no improvement or condition worsens, discontinue use and contact physician.

betaxolol hydrochloride
Betoptic

Pregnancy Risk Category: C

HOW SUPPLIED
Ophthalmic solution: 5 mg/ml (0.5%) in 5-ml, 10-ml dropper bottles

MECHANISM OF ACTION
Reduces formation and possibly increases outflow of aqueous humor. A cardioselective beta-blocker.

INDICATIONS & DOSAGE
Chronic open-angle glaucoma and ocular hypertension—
Adults: instill 1 drop of 0.5% solution in eyes b.i.d.

Italicized adverse reactions are common or life-threatening.
*Liquid form contains alcohol.   **May contain tartrazine.

ADVERSE REACTIONS
CNS: insomnia, confusion.
Eye: *stinging upon instillation,* occasional tearing, photophobia.

INTERACTIONS
Calcium channel blocking agents: AV conduction disturbances, ventricular failure, hypotension if significant systemic absorption occurs.
Cocaine: may inhibit betaxolol's effects.
Digitalis glycosides: excessive bradycardia; may require ECG monitoring if significant systemic absorption occurs.
Dipivefrin, ophthalmic epinephrine: may produce mydriasis.
Inhalational hydrocarbon anesthetics: prolonged severe hypotension if significant systemic absorption occurs.
Insulin, oral hypoglycemics: dosage adjustments or hypoglycemic medication may be necessary because of the risk of hypoglycemia or hyperglycemia if significant systemic absorption occurs.
Phenothiazines: additive hypotensive effects, increased risk of side effects if significant systemic absorption occurs.
Reserpine: excessive beta blockade.
Systemic beta blockers: additive effects.

NURSING CONSIDERATIONS
• Contraindicated in sinus bradycardia, greater than first-degree AV block, cardiogenic shock, or patients with overt heart failure.
• Use cautiously in patients with a history of heart failure; patients with restricted pulmonary function; patients with diabetes mellitus.
• Betaxolol differs from timolol and levobunolol in that it is a cardioselective beta-adrenergic blocker. Its pulmonary systemic effects are considerably milder than those of timolol and levobunolol.
• Betaxolol is intended for twice-daily dosage. Encourage your patient to comply with this regimen.
• In some patients, a few weeks' treatment may be required to stabilize pressure-lowering response. Determine intraocular pressure after 4 weeks of treatment.
• Teach patient how to instill. Advise him to wash hands before and after administering and to apply light finger-pressure on lacrimal sac for 1 minute following instillation. Warn patient not to touch dropper to eye or surrounding tissue.
• May cause photophobia. Advise patient to wear dark sunglasses on bright, sunny days.

---

botulinum toxin type A
Oculinum
Pregnancy Risk Category: C

HOW SUPPLIED
Powder for injection: 100 units/vial

MECHANISM OF ACTION
Produces a neuromuscular paralysis by binding to acetylcholine receptors on the motor end-plate; it may also inhibit the release of acetylcholine from presynaptic nerve endings.

INDICATIONS & DOSAGE
Treatment of strabismus—
Adults and children 12 years and over: injections should be made only by doctors familiar with the technique, which involves surgical exposure of the region as well as electromyographic guidance of the injection needle.
Dosage varies with the degree of deviation (lower doses are used for small deviations). For vertical muscles and for horizontal strabismus of <20 prism diopters, the usual dosage is 1.25 to 2.5 units in any one muscle. For horizontal strabismus of 20 to 50 prism diopters, dosage is 2.5 to 5 units injected into any one muscle.

For persistent VI nerve palsy of greater than 1 months' duration, dosage is 1.25 to 2.5 units injected into the medial rectus muscle.

Subsequent injections for recurrent or residual strabismus should not be made unless 7 to 14 days have elapsed after the initial dose, and substantial function has returned to the injected and adjacent muscles. Dosage may be increased up to twice the initial dose for patients experiencing incomplete paralysis; subsequent doses in patients with adequate response should not be increased. The maximum single dose for any one muscle is 25 units.

Treatment of blepharospasm—
Adults: initially, 1.25 to 2.5 units injected into the medial and lateral pretarsal orbicularis oculi of the upper lid and into the lateral pretarsal orbicularis oculi of the lower lid. Effects should be apparent within 3 days and peak in 1 to 2 weeks after treatment. At subsequent treatments, dosage may be doubled if inadequate paralysis is achieved; however, exceeding 5 units/site produces no apparent benefit. Each treatment lasts about 3 months and can be repeated indefinitely.

ADVERSE REACTIONS
EENT: double vision, blurred vision, spacial disorientation, *ptosis, vertical deviation (after treatment of strabismus), irritation (after treatment of blepharospasm), swelling of eyelid.*
Skin: diffuse skin rash, ecchymosis.

INTERACTIONS
None reported.

NURSING CONSIDERATIONS
• Contraindicated in patients hypersensitive to any ingredient in the formulation (which includes human albumin).
• Because the drug is a protein, epinephrine should be readily available in case of an anaphylactic reaction.

• The drug should be stored in the freezer at or below 23° F. (− 5° C.).
• Reconstitute the drug with normal saline solution (0.9% sodium chloride) without a preservative. The vacuum in the vial should be noticeable when reconstituting. Inject the diluent into the vial gently, because severe agitation can denature the protein.
• When treating strabismus, injection volume should be 0.05 to 0.15 ml/muscle; when treating blepharospasm, injection volumes are maintained at 0.05 to 0.1 ml/site. Dosage adjustments are made by altering the volume of diluent used to reconstitute the drug.
• Reconstituting with 1 ml of saline solution produces a concentration of 10 units/0.1 ml, adding 2 ml yields 5 units/0.1 ml. Adding more diluent (such as 4 ml to produce 2.5 units/0.1 ml or 8 ml to yield 1.25 units/0.1 ml) or using different injection volumes are common methods of adjusting dosage.
• Reconstituted drug should be clear, colorless, and free of particulate matter. It must be administered within 4 hours of removal from the freezer. Reconstituted drug should be kept in the refrigerator until use. Be sure to record the date and time of reconstitution.
• When treating strabismus, several drops of an ocular decongestant and a topical anesthetic should be applied before the procedure.
• Prepare the injection by drawing slightly more volume than needed into a sterile 1-ml syringe. Expel air bubbles in the barrel of the syringe, and attach an electromyographic injection needle (if treating strabismus), such as a 1.5-inch, 27G needle. Expel excess drug (into an appropriate waste container) while checking for leakage around the needle. Be sure to use a new needle and syringe for each injection.
• Muscle paralysis becomes evident 1

---

or 2 days after injection and increases in intensity over the first week. The paralysis lasts for 2 to 6 weeks and eventually resolves.

• The cumulative dosage of botulinum toxin type A should not exceed 200 units/month.

cromolyn sodium
Opticrom 4%

Pregnancy Risk Category: B

HOW SUPPLIED
Ophthalmic solution: 4%

MECHANISM OF ACTION
Inhibits degranulation of sensitized mast cells that follows exposure to specific antigens. Also inhibits release of histamine and slow-reacting substance of anaphylaxis (SRS-A).

INDICATIONS & DOSAGE
Treatment and prevention of allergic ocular disorders such as vernal keratoconjunctivitis and conjunctivitis, giant papillary conjunctivitis, vernal keratitis, and allergic keratoconjunctivitis—
Adults and children: 1 to 2 drops in each eye four to six times a day at regular intervals.

ADVERSE REACTIONS
Eye: transient stinging or burning upon instillation.

INTERACTIONS
None significant.

NURSING CONSIDERATIONS
• Because preparation contains benzalkonium chloride as a preservative, advise patient not to wear soft contact lenses during treatment period. Patient may resume wearing them a few hours after the drug's discontinued.
• Advise patient to instill medication at regular intervals.

• Tell patient that relief of symptoms may take several days to a week.
• Cromolyn is a safe treatment for some types of allergic conjunctivitis and keratitis and may be as effective as steroids.
• Teach patient how to instill. Advise him to wash hands before and after administering and to apply light finger-pressure on lacrimal sac for 1 minute following instillation. Warn patient not to touch dropper to eye or surrounding tissue.

dipivefrin
Propine

Pregnancy Risk Category: B

HOW SUPPLIED
Ophthalmic solution: 0.1%

MECHANISM OF ACTION
A prodrug of epinephrine (in the eye, dipivefrin is converted to epinephrine). The liberated epinephrine appears to decrease aqueous production and increase aqueous outflow.

INDICATIONS & DOSAGE
To reduce intraocular pressure in chronic open-angle glaucoma—
Adults: for initial glaucoma therapy, 1 drop in eye q 12 hours.

ADVERSE REACTIONS
CV: tachycardia, hypertension.
Eye: burning, stinging.

INTERACTIONS
Digitalis glycosides, inhalational hydrocarbon anesthetics, tricyclic antidepressants: increased risk of cardiac side effects if significant systemic absorption occurs.
Ophthalmic beta blockers: monitor for potential adverse effects.
Systemic sympathomimetics: possible additive effects if significant systemic absorption occurs.

NURSING CONSIDERATIONS
• Contraindicated in narrow-angle glaucoma.
• Use cautiously in patients with aphakia.
• Dipivefrin is a prodrug of epinephrine: It's converted to epinephrine when it enters the eye.
• May have fewer adverse reactions than conventional epinephrine therapy.
• Often used concomitantly with other antiglaucoma drugs.
• Teach patient how to instill. Advise him to wash hands before and after administration. Warn him not to touch dropper to eye or surrounding tissue.

eye irrigation solutions
Blinx◊, Collyrium◊, Dacriose◊, Eye-Stream◊, I-Lite Eye Drops◊, Lauro Eye Wash◊, Lavoptik Eye Wash◊, Murine Eye Drops◊, Neo-Flo◊, Sterile Normal Saline (0.9%)◊

HOW SUPPLIED
Ophthalmic solution: 15 ml◊, 30 ml◊, 120 ml◊, 180 ml◊

MECHANISM OF ACTION
Cleans the eye.

INDICATIONS & DOSAGE
Eye irrigation—
Adults and children: flush eye with 1 to 2 drops of solution t.i.d., q.i.d., or p.r.n.

ADVERSE REACTIONS
None reported.

INTERACTIONS
Products containing polyvinyl alcohol: may form gel and gummy deposits on the eye. Keep eyelids clean.

NURSING CONSIDERATIONS
• Contraindicated in patients with hypersensitivity to active ingredient or preservatives.

• To avoid contamination, don't touch tip of container to eye, surrounding tissue, or other surface.
• Check date of expiration to make sure solution is potent.
• Store in tightly closed, light-resistant container.
• Teach patient how to instill. Advise him to wash hands before and after administration.
• Should be used by one person only.
• When irrigating, have patient turn his head to side and irrigate from inner to outer canthus. Have tissues handy.

fluorescein sodium
Fluorescite, Fluor-I-Strip, Fluor-I-Strip A.T., Ful-Glo, Funduscein Injections

Pregnancy Risk Category: C

HOW SUPPLIED
Ophthalmic solution: 2%
Ophthalmic strips: 0.6 mg, 1 mg, 9 mg
Parenteral injection: 10%, 25%

MECHANISM OF ACTION
Produces an intense green fluorescence in alkaline solution (pH 5.0 or less) or a bright yellow if viewed under cobalt blue illumination.

INDICATIONS & DOSAGE
Diagnostic in corneal abrasions and foreign bodies; fitting hard contact lenses; lacrimal patency; fundus photography; applanation tonometry—
Topical solution:
Adults and children: instill 1 drop of 2% solution followed by irrigation, or moisten strip with sterile water. Touch conjunctiva or fornix with moistened tip. Flush eye with irrigating solution. Patient should blink several times after application.
Retinal angiography—
Intravenous:
Adults: 5 ml of 10% solution (500

Italicized adverse reactions are common or life-threatening.
*Liquid form contains alcohol.   **May contain tartrazine.

mg) or 3 ml of 25% solution (750 mg) injected rapidly into antecubital vein, by doctor or a specially trained nurse. **Children:** 0.077 ml of 10% solution (7.7 mg/kg body weight) or 0.044 ml of 25% solution (11 mg/kg body weight) injected rapidly into antecubital vein by doctor.

ADVERSE REACTIONS
Topical use:
Eye: stinging, burning, yellow streaks from tears.
Intravenous use:
CNS: headache persisting for 24 to 36 hours, dizziness, syncope, seizures.
CV: hypotension, shock, cardiac arrest.
GI: nausea, vomiting.
GU: bright yellow urine (persists for 24 to 36 hours).
Skin: yellow skin discoloration (fades in 6 to 12 hours).
Local: extravasation at injection site, thrombophlebitis.
Other: hypersensitivity, including urticaria and *anaphylaxis.*

INTERACTIONS
None significant.

NURSING CONSIDERATIONS
• Use with caution in patients with history of allergy or bronchial asthma.
• Never instill while patient is wearing soft contact lens. Drug will ruin it.
• Use topical anesthetic before instilling to partially relieve burning and irritation.
• Always use aseptic technique. Easily contaminated by *Pseudomonas.*
• Yellow skin discoloration may persist 6 to 12 hours.
• Warn patient that urine will be bright yellow after I.V. injection.
• Routine urinalysis will be abnormal within 1 hour after I.V. injection.
• A water-soluble dye.
• Don't freeze; store below 80° F. (26.7° C.).

• Defects appear green under normal light, or bright yellow under cobalt blue illumination. Foreign bodies are surrounded by a green ring. Similar lesions of the conjunctiva are delineated in orange-yellow.
• Always keep an emergency tray with an antihistamine, epinephrine, and oxygen available when giving parenterally.

---

glycerin, anhydrous
Ophthalgan
Pregnancy Risk Category: C

HOW SUPPLIED
Ophthalmic solution: 7.5-ml containers

MECHANISM OF ACTION
Removes excess fluid from the cornea.

INDICATIONS & DOSAGE
Corneal edema before ophthalmoscopy or gonioscopy in acute glaucoma and bullous keratitis—
Adults and children: instill 1 to 2 drops glycerin solution after instilling a local anesthetic.

ADVERSE REACTIONS
Eye: pain if instilled without topical anesthetic.

INTERACTIONS
None significant.

NURSING CONSIDERATIONS
• Use topical tetracaine or proparacaine before instilling to prevent discomfort.
• Don't touch tip of dropper to eye, surrounding tissues, or tear-film; glycerin will absorb moisture.
• Used to temporarily restore corneal transparency when cornea is too edematous to permit diagnosis.
• Store in tightly closed container.

---

isosorbide
Ismotic

Pregnancy Risk Category: C

HOW SUPPLIED
Oral solution: 45% (100 g/225 ml) in 220-ml containers

MECHANISM OF ACTION
Acts as an osmotic agent by promoting redistribution of water and thereby producing diuresis.

INDICATIONS & DOSAGE
Short-term reduction of intraocular pressure due to glaucoma—
Adults: initially, 1.5 g/kg P.O. Usual dosage range is 1 to 3 g/kg.

ADVERSE REACTIONS
CNS: vertigo, light-headedness, lethargy, headache, confusion.
GI: gastric discomfort, diarrhea, anorexia, nausea, vomiting.
Metabolic: hypernatremia, hyperosmolality, thirst.

INTERACTIONS
None significant.

NURSING CONSIDERATIONS
• Contraindicated in anuria due to severe renal disease, severe dehydration, in frank or impending acute pulmonary edema, and in hemorrhagic glaucoma.
• Monitor patient closely for 5 to 10 minutes after administration.
• Tell patient that this medication may make him feel thirsty.
• Repetitive doses should be used cautiously, especially in patients with diseases associated with salt retention, such as congestive heart failure. Carefully monitor patient's fluid and electrolyte balance.
• Pour over cracked ice, and tell patient to sip the medication. This improves palatability.
• Especially useful for rapid reduc-

tion in intraocular pressure. May be used to interrupt acute attack of glaucoma before laser surgery.

levobunolol hydrochloride
Betagan

Pregnancy Risk Category: C

HOW SUPPLIED
Ophthalmic solution: 0.5%

MECHANISM OF ACTION
Reduces formation and possibly increases outflow of aqueous humor. A nonselective beta-blocker.

INDICATIONS & DOSAGE
Chronic open-angle glaucoma and ocular hypertension—
Adults: instill 1 drop in eyes once daily or b.i.d..

ADVERSE REACTIONS
CNS: headache, dizziness, depression.
CV: slight reduction in resting heart rate.
Eye: *transient stinging and burning.* Long-term use may decrease corneal sensitivity.
GI: nausea.
Skin: urticaria.
Other: evidence of beta blockade and systemic absorption (*hypotension, bradycardia, syncope, exacerbation of asthma,* and *congestive heart failure*).

INTERACTIONS
Propranolol, metoprolol, and other oral beta-adrenergic blocking agents: increased ocular and systemic effect. Use together cautiously.
Reserpine and other catecholomine-depleting drugs: enhanced hypotensive and bradycardiac effects.

NURSING CONSIDERATIONS
• Contraindicated in bronchial asthma, a history of bronchial asthma or severe chronic obstructive pulmo-

---

Italicized adverse reactions are common or life-threatening.
*Liquid form contains alcohol.   **May contain tartrazine.

nary disease; sinus bradycardia; second-degree and third-degree AV block; cardiac failure; cardiogenic shock.
• Use cautiously in patients with chronic bronchitis and emphysema, diabetes mellitus, and hyperthyroidism.
• Levobunolol is faster acting than timolol. The onset of action occurs within 1 hour; maximum effect is between 2 and 6 hours.
• Teach patient how to instill. Advise him to wash hands before and after administering and to apply light finger-pressure on lacrimal sac for 1 minute after instillation. Warn patient not to touch dropper to eye or surrounding tissue.

sodium chloride, hypertonic
Adsorbonac Ophthalmic Solution, Muro-128 Ointment, Sodium Chloride Ointment 5%

Pregnancy Risk Category: C

HOW SUPPLIED
Ophthalmic ointment: 5%
Ophthalmic solution: 2%, 5%

MECHANISM OF ACTION
Removes excess fluid from the cornea.

INDICATIONS & DOSAGE
Corneal edema (postoperative) after cataract extraction or corneal transplantation; also in trauma or bullous keratopathy—
Adults and children: instill 1 to 2 drops q 3 to 4 hours, or apply ointment at bedtime.

ADVERSE REACTIONS
Eye: slight stinging.
Other: hypersensitivity.

INTERACTIONS
None significant.

NURSING CONSIDERATIONS
• Discontinue immediately if patient experiences severe headache, pain, rapid change in vision, acute redness of eyes, sudden appearance of floating spots, pain on exposure to light, or double vision.
• An osmotic agent used to reduce corneal edema when repeated instillation is indicated.
• May use a few drops of sterile irrigation solution inside bottle cap to prevent caking on dropper bottle tip.
• Store in tightly closed container.
• Ointment may cause blurred vision.
• Teach patient how to instill. Advise him to wash hands before and after administering and to apply light finger-pressure on lacrimal sac for 1 minute after drops are instilled. Warn patient not to touch dropper to eye or surrounding tissue.

timolol maleate
Timoptic Solution

Pregnancy Risk Category: C

HOW SUPPLIED
Ophthalmic solution: 0.25%, 0.5%

MECHANISM OF ACTION
Reduces aqueous formation and possibly increases aqueous outflow. A beta-blocker.

INDICATIONS & DOSAGE
Chronic open-angle glaucoma, secondary glaucoma, aphakic glaucoma, ocular hypertension—
Adults: initially, instill 1 drop of 0.25% solution in each eye b.i.d.; reduce to 1 drop daily for maintenance. If patient doesn't respond, instill 1 drop of 0.5% solution in each eye b.i.d. If intraocular pressure is controlled, dosage may be reduced to 1 drop in each eye daily.

ADVERSE REACTIONS
CNS: headache, depression, fatigue.

CV: slight reduction in resting heart rate.
Eye: minor irritation. Long-term use may decrease corneal sensitivity.
GI: anorexia.
Other: apnea in infants, *evidence of beta blockade and systemic absorption (hypotension, bradycardia, syncope, exacerbation of asthma, and congestive heart failure).*

INTERACTIONS
General anesthetics, fentanyl: excessive hypotension.
Propranolol, metoprolol tartrate, other oral beta-adrenergic blocking agents: increased ocular and systemic effect. Use together cautiously.

NURSING CONSIDERATIONS
• Use cautiously in bronchial asthma, sinus bradycardia, second- and third-degree heart block, cardiogenic shock, right ventricular failure resulting from pulmonary hypertension, congestive heart failure, severe cardiac disease, and in infants with congenital glaucoma. Systemic beta blocking effects can mask some signs of hypoglycemia in diabetic patients.
• In some patients, a few weeks may be required to stabilize pressure-lowering response. Determine intraocular pressure after 4 weeks of treatment.
• Warn patient not to touch dropper to eye or surrounding tissue.
• Can be used safely in patients with glaucoma who wear conventional (PMMA) hard contact lenses.
• Teach patient how to instill. Advise him to wash hands before and after administering and to apply light finger-pressure on lacrimal sac for 1 minute following instillation. Warn him not to touch dropper to eye or surrounding tissue.

Italicized adverse reactions are common or life-threatening.
*Liquid form contains alcohol.   **May contain tartrazine.

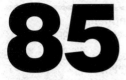

Otics

acetic acid
boric acid
carbamide peroxide
chloramphenicol
triethanolamine polypeptide
    oleate-condensate

COMBINATION PRODUCTS
COLY-MYCIN S OTIC: each ml contains neomycin SO_4 3.3 mg, colistin SO_4 3 mg, hydrocortisone acetate 10 mg, and thonzonium bromide 0.05%.
CORTISPORIN OTIC: each ml contains neomycin SO_4 5 mg, polymyxin B 10,000 units, and hydrocortisone 1%.

---

acetic acid
Domeboro Otic, VoSol Otic
Pregnancy Risk Category: C

HOW SUPPLIED
Otic solution: 2% in aluminum acetate, 2% in propylene glycol, 3%

MECHANISM OF ACTION
Inhibits or destroys bacteria present in the ear canal.

INDICATIONS & DOSAGE
External ear canal infection—
Adults and children: 4 to 6 drops into ear canal t.i.d. or q.i.d., or insert saturated wick for first 24 hours, then continue with instillations.
Prophylaxis of swimmer's ear—
Adults and children: 2 drops in each ear b.i.d.

ADVERSE REACTIONS
Ear: irritation or itching.

Skin: urticaria.
Other: overgrowth of nonsusceptible organisms.

INTERACTIONS
None significant.

NURSING CONSIDERATIONS
• Use cautiously in perforated eardrum.
• Has anti-infective, anti-inflammatory, and antipruritic effects.
• *Pseudomonas aeruginosa* particularly sensitive to drug.
• Reculture persistent drainage.
• Avoid touching ear with dropper.

---

boric acid
Aurocaine 2◇, Auro-Dri◇, Dri/Ear◇, Ear-Dry◇, Swim Ear◇
Pregnancy Risk Category: C

HOW SUPPLIED
Otic solution: 2.75% boric acid in isopropyl alcohol

MECHANISM OF ACTION
Inhibits or destroys bacteria present in the ear canal. Weak bacteriostatic action; also fungistatic agent.

INDICATIONS & DOSAGE
External ear canal infection—
Adults and children: 3 to 6 drops in ear canal and plug with cotton. Repeat t.i.d. or q.i.d.

ADVERSE REACTIONS
Ear: irritation or itching.
Skin: urticaria.

Other: overgrowth of nonsusceptible organisms.

INTERACTIONS
None significant.

NURSING CONSIDERATIONS
• Contraindicated in perforated eardrum or excoriated membranes in ear.
• Watch for signs of superinfection (continual pain, inflammation, fever).
• If cotton plug used, always moisten with medication.
• Avoid touching ear with dropper.

carbamide peroxide
Debrox◇

Pregnancy Risk Category: C

HOW SUPPLIED
Otic solution: 6.5% carbamide in glycerin or glycerin and propylene glycol

MECHANISM OF ACTION
Emulsifies and disperses accumulated cerumen. A ceruminolytic.

INDICATIONS & DOSAGE
Impacted cerumen—
Adults and children: 5 to 10 drops into ear canal b.i.d. for 3 to 4 days.

ADVERSE REACTIONS
None reported.

INTERACTIONS
None significant.

NURSING CONSIDERATIONS
• Contraindicated in perforated eardrum.
• Tell patient to call doctor if redness, pain, or swelling persists.
• Irrigation of ear may be necessary to aid in removal of cerumen.
• Avoid touching ear with dropper.

chloramphenicol
Chloromycetin Otic, Sopamycetin†

Pregnancy Risk Category: C

HOW SUPPLIED
Otic solution: 0.5%

MECHANISM OF ACTION
Inhibits or destroys bacteria present in the ear canal.

INDICATIONS & DOSAGE
External ear canal infection—
Adults and children: 2 to 3 drops into ear canal t.i.d. or q.i.d.

ADVERSE REACTIONS
Ear: itching or burning.
Local: pruritus, burning, urticaria, vesicular or maculopapular dermatitis.
Systemic: sore throat, angioedema.
Other: overgrowth of nonsusceptible organisms.

INTERACTIONS
None significant.

NURSING CONSIDERATIONS
• Avoid prolonged use.
• Obtain history of use and reaction to drug.
• Watch for signs of superinfection (continued pain, inflammation, fever).
• Reculture persistent drainage.
• Watch for signs of sore throat (early sign of toxicity).
• Avoid touching ear with dropper.

triethanolamine polypeptide oleate-condensate
Cerumenex

Pregnancy Risk Category: C

HOW SUPPLIED
Otic solution: 10% in 6-ml, 12-ml bottles with droppers

Italicized adverse reactions are common or life-threatening.
*Liquid form contains alcohol.   **May contain tartrazine.

MECHANISM OF ACTION
Emulsifies and disperses accumulated cerumen. A ceruminolytic.

INDICATIONS & DOSAGE
Impacted cerumen—
Adults and children: fill ear canal with solution and insert cotton plug. After 15 to 30 minutes, flush ear with warm water.

ADVERSE REACTIONS
Ear: erythema, pruritus.
Skin: severe eczema.

INTERACTIONS
None significant.

NURSING CONSIDERATIONS
• Contraindicated in perforated eardrum, otitis media, and allergies. Do patch test by placing 1 drop of drug on inner forearm; cover with small bandage. Read in 24 hours. If any reaction (redness, swelling) occurs, don't use drug.
• Tell patient not to use drops more often than prescribed. Flush ear gently with warm water, using soft rubber bulb ear syringe, within 30 minutes after instillation.
• Moisten cotton plug with medication before insertion.
• Keep container tightly closed and away from moisture.
• Avoid touching ear with dropper.

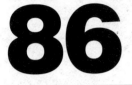

Nasal agents

beclomethasone dipropionate
dexamethasone sodium
   phosphate
ephedrine sulfate
epinephrine hydrochloride
flunisolide
naphazoline hydrochloride
oxymetazoline hydrochloride
phenylephrine hydrochloride
tetrahydrozoline hydrochloride
xylometazoline hydrochloride

COMBINATION PRODUCT
4-WAY NASAL SPRAY◇: phenylephrine hydrochloride 0.5%, naphazoline
hydrochloride 0.05%, and pyrilamine
maleate 0.2%.

---

beclomethasone dipropionate
Aldecin Aqueous Nasal Spray,
Beconase AQ Nasal Spray,
Beconase Nasal Inhaler,
Vancenase AQ Nasal Spray,
Vancenase Nasal Inhaler

Pregnancy Risk Category: C

HOW SUPPLIED
Nasal aerosol: 42 mcg/metered spray,
50 mcg/metered spray‡
Nasal spray: 0.042%, 50 mcg/me-
tered spray‡

MECHANISM OF ACTION
Decreases inflammation, mainly by
stabilizing leukocyte lysosomal membranes.

INDICATIONS & DOSAGE
Relief of symptoms of seasonal or pe-
rennial rhinitis; prevention of recur-
rence of nasal polyps after surgical re-
moval—
Adults and children over 12 years:
usual dosage is 1 spray (42 mcg) in
each nostril two to four times daily
(total dosage 168 to 336 mcg daily).
Most patients require 1 spray in each
nostril t.i.d. (252 mcg daily).
  Not recommended for children under 12 years.

ADVERSE REACTIONS
CNS: headache.
EENT: *mild transient nasal burning*
and stinging, nasal congestion, sneez-
ing, epistaxis, watery eyes.
GI: nausea and vomiting.
Other: development of nasopharyn-
geal fungal infections.

INTERACTIONS
None reported.

NURSING CONSIDERATIONS
• Use cautiously, if at all, in patients
with active or quiescent respiratory
tract tubercular infections or in untreated fungal, bacterial, or systemic
viral or ocular herpes simplex infections.
• Use cautiously in patients who have
recently had nasal septal ulcers or nasal surgery or trauma.
• Recommended dosages will not
suppress hypothalamic-pituitary-adrenal (HPA) function. Warn patient
not to exceed this dosage.
• Indicated when conventional treatment (antihistamines, decongestants)
fails.

Italicized adverse reactions are common or life-threatening.
*Liquid form contains alcohol.   **May contain tartrazine.

• Beclomethasone is not effective for active exacerbations. Nasal decongestants or oral antihistamines may be needed instead.

• Advise patients to use drug regularly, as prescribed; its effectiveness depends on regular use.

• Explain that the therapeutic effects of this corticosteroid, unlike those of decongestants, are not immediate. Most patients achieve benefit within a few days, but some may need 2 to 3 weeks for maximum benefit.

• If symptoms don't improve within 3 weeks or if nasal irritation persists, patient should stop drug and notify doctor.

• Observe for fungal infections.

• Teach patient good nasal and oral hygiene.

• Teach patient how to use. Shake container and invert. After clearing nasal passages, tilt head back, insert nozzle into nostril pointing away from septum. While holding other nostril closed, inspire and spray. Shake container again and repeat in other nostril.

---

dexamethasone sodium phosphate
Decadron Phosphate, Turbinaire

Pregnancy Risk Category: C

HOW SUPPLIED
Nasal aerosol: 84 mcg/metered spray, 170 doses/canister

MECHANISM OF ACTION
Decreases inflammation, mainly by stabilizing leukocyte lysosomal membranes.

INDICATIONS & DOSAGE
Allergic or inflammatory conditions, nasal polyps—
Adults: 2 sprays in each nostril b.i.d. or t.i.d. Maximum 12 sprays daily.
Children 6 to 12 years: 1 or 2 sprays in each nostril b.i.d. Maximum 8 sprays daily.

Each spray delivers 0.1 mg dexamethasone sodium phosphate equal to 0.084 mg dexamethasone.

ADVERSE REACTIONS
EENT: nasal irritation, dryness, rebound nasal congestion.
Other: hypersensitivity, systemic effects with prolonged use (pituitary-adrenal suppression, sodium retention, congestive heart failure, hypertension, hypokalemia, headaches, convulsions, peptic ulcer, ecchymoses, petechiae, masking of infection).

INTERACTIONS
None significant.

NURSING CONSIDERATIONS
• Contraindicated in cutaneous tuberculosis, fungal and herpetic lesions. Use cautiously in diabetes mellitus, peptic ulcer, or tuberculosis, as systemic absorption can activate disease.

• Mothers should not breast-feed, as systemic absorption can occur.

• Control underlying bacterial infection with anti-infectives.

• Irritation or sensitivity may require stopping drug.

• Don't break, incinerate, or store in extreme heat; contents under pressure.

• Gradually reduce dose as nasal condition improves.

• Fluid retention can occur as a result of systemic absorption.

• Teach patient how to use according to directions in package. Patient should shake container and invert. After cleaning nasal passages, tilt head back, insert nozzle into nostril, pointing away from septum. While holding other nostril closed, inspire and spray. Shake container again and repeat in other nostril.

• Only one person should use nasal spray.

• Hypertension and hypokalemia can occur with systemic absorption. Monitor blood pressure, serum potassium frequently.
• Should not be used for prolonged periods.
• Teach patient good nasal and oral hygiene.

ephedrine sulfate
Efedron Nasal Jelly◇, Va-tro-nol Nose Drops◇

Pregnancy Risk Category: C

HOW SUPPLIED
Nasal jelly: 0.5%◇
Nasal solution: 0.5%◇

MECHANISM OF ACTION
Produces local vasoconstriction of dilated arterioles to reduce blood flow and nasal congestion.

INDICATIONS & DOSAGE
Nasal congestion—
Adults and children: apply 3 to 4 drops of 0.5% solution or apply a small amount of jelly to nasal mucosa. Use no more frequently than q 4 hours.

ADVERSE REACTIONS
CNS: nervousness, excitation.
CV: *tachycardia.*
EENT: rebound nasal congestion with long-term or excessive use.
Local: mucosal irritation.

INTERACTIONS
MAO inhibitors: hypertensive crisis if ephedrine is absorbed. Don't use together.

NURSING CONSIDERATIONS
• Use cautiously in hyperthyroidism, coronary artery disease, hypertension, or diabetes mellitus, as systemic absorption can occur.
• Tell patient not to exceed recommended dose. Use only when needed.

• Teach patient how to apply. Only one person should use dropper bottle.

epinephrine hydrochloride
Adrenalin Chloride

Pregnancy Risk Category: C

HOW SUPPLIED
Nasal solution: 0.1%

MECHANISM OF ACTION
Produces local vasoconstriction of dilated arterioles to reduce blood flow and nasal congestion.

INDICATIONS & DOSAGE
Nasal congestion, local superficial bleeding—
Adults and children: apply 0.1% solution to oral or nasal mucosa.

ADVERSE REACTIONS
CNS: nervousness, excitation.
CV: *tachycardia.*
EENT: rebound nasal congestion, slight sting upon application.

INTERACTIONS
None significant.

NURSING CONSIDERATIONS
• Use cautiously in hyperthyroidism, coronary artery disease, hypertension, or diabetes mellitus, as systemic absorption can occur.
• Tell patient not to exceed recommended dose. Use only when needed.
• Teach patient how to apply. Only one person should use dropper bottle.

flunisolide
Nasalide, Rhinalar Nasal Mist‡

Pregnancy Risk Category: C

HOW SUPPLIED
Nasal inhalant: 25 mcg/metered spray, 200 doses/bottle
Nasal solution: 0.25 mg/ml in pump spray bottle

Italicized adverse reactions are common or life-threatening.
*Liquid form contains alcohol.   **May contain tartrazine.

MECHANISM OF ACTION
Decreases inflammation, mainly by stabilizing leukocyte lysosomal membranes.

INDICATIONS & DOSAGE
Relief of symptoms of seasonal or perennial rhinitis—
Adults: starting dose is 2 sprays (50 mcg) in each nostril b.i.d. Total daily dosage is 200 mcg. If necessary, dose may be increased to 2 sprays in each nostril t.i.d. Maximum total daily dosage is 8 sprays in each nostril (400 mcg daily).
Children 6 to 14 years: starting dose is 1 spray (25 mcg) in each nostril t.i.d. or 2 sprays (50 mcg) in each nostril b.i.d. Total daily dosage is 150 to 200 mcg. Maximum total daily dosage is 4 sprays in each nostril (200 mcg daily).

Not recommended for children under age 6.

ADVERSE REACTIONS
CNS: headache.
EENT: *mild, transient nasal burning and stinging,* nasal congestion, sneezing, epistaxis, watery eyes.
GI: nausea, vomiting.
Other: development of nasopharyngeal fungal infections.

INTERACTIONS
None reported.

NURSING CONSIDERATIONS
• Use cautiously, if at all, in patients with active or quiescent respiratory tract tubercular infections or in untreated fungal, bacterial, or systemic viral or ocular herpes simplex infections.
• Use cautiously in patients who have recently had nasal septal ulcers or nasal surgery or trauma.
• Recommended dosages will not suppress hypothalamic-pituitary-adrenal (HPA) function. Warn patient not to exceed this dosage.

• Indicated when conventional treatment (antihistamines, decongestants) fails.
• Flunisolide is not effective for acute exacerbations. Nasal decongestants or oral antihistamines may be needed instead.
• Advise patient to use drug regularly, as prescribed; its effectiveness depends on regular use.
• Explain that the therapeutic effects of this corticosteroid, unlike those of decongestants, are not immediate. Most patients achieve benefit within a few days, but some may need 2 to 3 weeks for maximum benefit.
• Patients with dryness and crusting of the nasal mucosa may prefer the liquid spray of flunisolide to the aerosolized powder of beclomethasone.
• If symptoms don't improve within 3 weeks or if nasal irritation persists, patient should stop drug and notify doctor.
• Teach patient how to apply. Clear nasal passages. After priming inhaler, tilt head slightly forward, insert spray tip into nostril pointing away from septum. While holding other nostril closed, inspire and spray. Repeat in other nostril.

---

naphazoline hydrochloride
Privine◇

Pregnancy Risk Category: C

HOW SUPPLIED
Nasal drops: 0.05% solution
Nasal sprays: 0.05% solution

MECHANISM OF ACTION
Produces local vasoconstriction of dilated arterioles to reduce blood flow and nasal congestion.

INDICATIONS & DOSAGE
Nasal congestion—
Adults: apply 2 drops or sprays of 0.05% solution to nasal mucosa q 3 to 4 hours.

Children 6 to 12 years: 1 to 2 drops or sprays of 0.05% solution. Repeat q 3 to 6 hours, p.r.n. Use no longer than 3 to 5 days.

ADVERSE REACTIONS
EENT: rebound nasal congestion with excessive or long-term use, sneezing, stinging, dryness of mucosa.
Other: systemic effects in children after excessive or long-term use; marked sedation.

INTERACTIONS
None significant.

NURSING CONSIDERATIONS
• Contraindicated in narrow-angle glaucoma. Use cautiously in hyperthyroidism, heart disease, hypertension, or diabetes mellitus, as systemic absorption can occur.
• Warn patient not to exceed recommended dosage.
• Tell patient to notify doctor if nasal congestion persists after 5 days.
• Teach patient how to apply. Hold spray container and head upright. Only one person should use dropper bottle or nasal spray.
• Do not shake container.

---

oxymetazoline hydrochloride
Afrin◇, Afrin Children's Strength Nose Drops◇, Allerest 12-Hour Nasal◇, Chlorphed-LA◇, Coricidin Nasal Mist◇, Dristan Long Lasting◇, Drixine Nasal‡, Duramist Plus◇, Duration◇, 4-Way Long-Acting Nasal, Genasal Spray◇, Neo-Synephrine 12 Hour◇, Nostrilla◇, NTZ Long Acting Nasal◇, Sinarest 12-Hour◇, Sinex Long-Acting◇, Twice-A-Day Nasal◇

Pregnancy Risk Category: C

HOW SUPPLIED
Nasal solution: 0.025%◇, 0.05%◇

MECHANISM OF ACTION
Produces local vasoconstriction of dilated arterioles to reduce blood flow and nasal congestion.

INDICATIONS & DOSAGE
Nasal congestion—
Adults and children over 6 years: apply 2 to 4 drops or sprays of 0.05% solution to nasal mucosa b.i.d.
Children 2 to 6 years: apply 2 to 3 drops 0.025% solution to nasal mucosa b.i.d. Use no longer than 3 to 5 days. Dosage for younger children has not been established.

ADVERSE REACTIONS
CNS: headache, drowsiness, dizziness, insomnia, possible sedation.
CV: palpitations, *hypotension with cardiovascular collapse,* hypertension.
EENT: rebound nasal congestion or irritation with excessive or long-term use, dryness of nose and throat, increased nasal discharge, stinging, sneezing.
Other: systemic effects in children with excessive or long-term use.

INTERACTIONS
None significant.

NURSING CONSIDERATIONS
• Use cautiously in hyperthyroidism, cardiac disease, hypertension, or diabetes mellitus, as systemic absorption can occur.
• Tell patient not to exceed recommended dose. Use only when needed.
• Warn patient that excessive use may cause bradycardia, hypotension, dizziness, and weakness.
• Teach patient how to apply. Have patient hold head upright and sniff spray briskly. Only one person should use dropper bottle or nasal spray.

Italicized adverse reactions are common or life-threatening.
*Liquid form contains alcohol.   **May contain tartrazine.

phenylephrine hydrochloride

Alconefrin 12◇, Alconefrin 25◇, Alconefrin 50◇, Doktors◇, Duration◇, Neo-Synephrine◇, Nostril◇, Rhinall◇, Rhinall-10◇, Sinex◇, St. Joseph Measured Dose Nasal Decongestant◇

Pregnancy Risk Category: C

HOW SUPPLIED
Nasal jelly: 0.5%
Nasal solution: 0.125%, 0.16%, 0.2%, 0.25%, 0.5%, 1%

MECHANISM OF ACTION
Produces local vasoconstriction of dilated arterioles to reduce blood flow and nasal congestion.

INDICATIONS & DOSAGE
Nasal congestion—
Adults: 1 to 2 drops or sprays of 0.125% to 1% solution; apply jelly or spray to nasal mucosa.
Children 6 to 12 years: apply 1 to 2 drops or sprays of 0.25% solution.
Children under 6 years: apply 2 to 3 drops or sprays of 0.125% solution.
   Drops, spray, or jelly can be given q 4 hours, p.r.n.

ADVERSE REACTIONS
CNS: headache, tremors, dizziness, nervousness.
CV: *palpitations, tachycardia,* premature ventricular contractions, hypertension, pallor.
EENT: transient burning, stinging; dryness of nasal mucosa; rebound nasal congestion may occur with continued use.
GI: nausea.

INTERACTIONS
None significant.

NURSING CONSIDERATIONS
• Contraindicated in narrow-angle glaucoma. Use cautiously in hyperthyroidism, hypertension, diabetes mellitus, or ischemic cardiac disease, as systemic absorption may occur.
• Tell patient not to exceed recommended dose. Use only when needed.
• Teach patient how to apply. Have patient hold head erect to minimize swallowing of medication. Only one person should use dropper bottle or nasal spray.

tetrahydrozoline hydrochloride

Tyzine Drops, Tyzine Pediatric Drops

Pregnancy Risk Category: C

HOW SUPPLIED
Nasal solution: 0.05%, 0.1%

MECHANISM OF ACTION
Produces local vasoconstriction of dilated arterioles to reduce blood flow and nasal congestion.

INDICATIONS & DOSAGE
Nasal congestion—
Adults and children over 6 years: apply 2 to 4 drops of 0.1% solution or spray to nasal mucosa q 4 to 6 hours, p.r.n.
Children 2 to 6 years: apply 2 to 3 drops of 0.05% solution to nasal mucosa q 4 to 6 hours, p.r.n.

ADVERSE REACTIONS
EENT: transient burning, stinging; sneezing, rebound nasal congestion in excessive or long-term use.

INTERACTIONS
None significant.

NURSING CONSIDERATIONS
• Contraindicated in narrow-angle glaucoma. Use cautiously in hyperthyroidism, hypertension, diabetes mellitus.
• Don't use 0.1% solution in children under 6 years.

---

†Available in Canada only.   ‡Available in Australia only.   ◇Available OTC.

• Tell patient not to exceed recommended dose. Use only as needed.
• Show patient how to apply. Only one person should use dropper or nasal spray.

• Teach patient how to apply. Have patient hold head upright and sniff spray briskly. Only one person should use dropper bottle or nasal spray.

xylometazoline hydrochloride
4-Way Long Acting, Neo-Synephrine II, Otrivin, Sine-Off Nasal Spray, Sinex-L.A.

Pregnancy Risk Category: C

HOW SUPPLIED
Nasal solution: 0.05%, 0.1%

MECHANISM OF ACTION
Produces local vasoconstriction of dilated arterioles to reduce blood flow and nasal congestion.

INDICATIONS & DOSAGE
Nasal congestion—
Adults and children over 12 years: apply 2 to 3 drops or 1 to 2 sprays of 0.1% solution to nasal mucosa q 8 to 10 hours.
Children under 12 years: apply 2 to 3 drops or 1 spray of 0.05% solution to nasal mucosa q 8 to 10 hours.

ADVERSE REACTIONS
EENT: rebound nasal congestion or irritation with excessive or long-term use; transient burning, stinging; dryness or ulceration of nasal mucosa; sneezing.

INTERACTIONS
None significant.

NURSING CONSIDERATIONS
• Contraindicated in narrow-angle glaucoma. Use cautiously in hyperthyroidism, cardiac disease, hypertension, diabetes mellitus, and advanced arteriosclerosis, as systemic absorption can occur.
• Tell patient not to exceed recommended dose.

Italicized adverse reactions are common or life-threatening.
*Liquid form contains alcohol.   **May contain tartrazine.

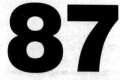

Local anti-infectives

acyclovir
amphotericin B
bacitracin
butoconazole nitrate
carbol-fuchsin solution
chloramphenicol
chlortetracycline hydrochloride
ciclopirox olamine
clindamycin phosphate
clotrimazole
econazole nitrate
erythromycin
gentamicin sulfate
gentian violet
haloprogin
iodochlorhydroxyquin
ketoconazole
mafenide acetate
metronidazole (topical)
miconazole nitrate
mupirocin
naftifine
neomycin sulfate
nitrofurazone
nystatin
oxiconazole nitrate
silver sulfadiazine
sulconazole nitrate
terconazole
tetracycline hydrochloride
tioconazole
tolnaftate
undecylenic acid and zinc
  undecylenate

COMBINATION PRODUCTS

BENZAMYCIN GEL: erythromycin 3% and benzoyl peroxide 5%.
CORDRAN-N CREAM, OINTMENT: flurandrenolide 0.05% and neomycin sulfate 0.5%.
LANABIOTIC◊: polymyxin B sulfate 5,000 units, neomycin sulfate 5 mg, bacitracin 500 units, and lidocaine 40 mg/g.
LOTRISONE CREAM: clotrimazole 1% and betamethasone dipropionate 0.05%.
MYCITRACIN OINTMENT◊: polymyxin B sulfate 5,000 units, bacitracin 500 units, and neomycin sulfate 3.5 mg/g.
MYCOLOG II CREAM, OINTMENT: triamcinolone acetonide 0.1%, and nystatin 100,000 units/g.
NEO-CORTEF OINTMENT: hydrocortisone acetate 1% and neomycin sulfate 0.5%.
NEODECADRON CREAM: dexamethasone phosphate 0.1% and neomycin sulfate 0.5%.
NEO-POLYCIN OINTMENT◊: polymyxin B sulfate 5,000 units, neomycin sulfate 5 mg, and zinc bacitracin 400 units/g.
NEOSPORIN CREAM†◊: polymyxin B sulfate 10,000 units, neomycin sulfate 5 mg.
NEOSPORIN OINTMENT◊: polymyxin B sulfate 5,000 units, bacitracin zinc 400 units, and neomycin sulfate 5 mg/g.
POLYSPORIN OINTMENT◊: polymyxin B sulfate 10,000 units and zinc bacitracin 500 units/g.
SULFACET-R LOTION: sulfacetamide sodium 10% and sulfur 5%.
VIOFORM-HYDROCORTISONE MILD CREAM, RACET CREAM: iodochlorhydroxyquin 3% and hydrocortisone 0.5%.

†Available in Canada only.   ‡Available in Australia only.   ◊Available OTC.

acyclovir
Zovirax

Pregnancy Risk Category: C

HOW SUPPLIED
Ointment: 5%

MECHANISM OF ACTION
Inhibits herpes virus DNA synthesis by interfering with the action of viral DNA polymerase.

INDICATIONS & DOSAGE
Initial herpes genitalis; limited, non–life-threatening mucocutaneous herpes simplex virus infections in immunocompromised patients—
Adults and children: apply sufficient quantity to adequately cover all lesions q 3 hours six times daily for 7 days.

ADVERSE REACTIONS
Skin: transient burning and stinging, rash, pruritus.

INTERACTIONS
None reported.

NURSING CONSIDERATIONS
• For cutaneous use only. Don't apply to the eye.
• Although the dose size for each application will vary depending upon the total lesion area, use approximately a ½″ ribbon of ointment on each 4-inch square of surface area.
• Ointment must thoroughly cover all lesions.
• Apply with a finger cot or rubber glove to prevent autoinoculation of other body sites and transmission of infection to other persons.
• Therapy should be initiated as early as possible following onset of signs and symptoms of herpes.
• Most studies show that acyclovir is not effective when used to treat *recurrent* genital herpes.

• Emphasize importance of compliance for successful therapy.
• Teach patient that he may transmit the virus even during treatment.

amphotericin B
Fungizone Cream, Lotion, Ointment

Pregnancy Risk Category: B

HOW SUPPLIED
Cream: 3%
Lotion: 3%
Ointment: 3%

MECHANISM OF ACTION
Alters the permeability of the cell membrane of fungi. Fungistatic.

INDICATIONS & DOSAGE
Cutaneous or mucocutaneous candidal infections—
Adults and children: apply liberally b.i.d., t.i.d., or q.i.d. for 1 to 3 weeks; up to several months for interdigital lesions and paronychias.

ADVERSE REACTIONS
Skin: possible drying, contact sensitivity, erythema, burning, pruritus.

INTERACTIONS
None significant.

NURSING CONSIDERATIONS
• Cream or lotion preferred for such areas as folds of groin, armpit, and neck creases.
• Cream discolors skin slightly when rubbed in; lotion or ointment doesn't. Lotion may stain nail lesions.
• Watch for and report signs of local irritation.
• Avoid occlusive dressings.
• Store at room temperature; avoid freezing.
• Well tolerated, even by infants, for long periods.
• Tell patient to continue using medication for full length of time pre-

---

Italicized adverse reactions are common or life-threatening.
*Liquid form contains alcohol.   **May contain tartrazine.

scribed, even if condition has improved.

bacitracin
Baciguent◇, Bacitin†
Pregnancy Risk Category: C

HOW SUPPLIED
Ointment: 500 units/g

MECHANISM OF ACTION
Inhibits bacterial cell-wall synthesis.

INDICATIONS & DOSAGE
Topical infections, impetigo, abrasions, cuts, and minor burns or wounds—
Adults and children: apply thin film b.i.d. or t.i.d. or more often, depending on severity of condition.

ADVERSE REACTIONS
Skin: stinging, rashes, and other allergic reactions; itching, burning, swelling of lips or face.
Other: *possible systemic adverse reactions when used over large areas for prolonged periods: potentially nephrotoxic and ototoxic; allergic reactions;* tightness in chest, hypotension.

INTERACTIONS
None significant.

NURSING CONSIDERATIONS
• Contraindicated for application in the external ear canal if the eardrum is perforated.
• Patients allergic to neomycin may also be allergic to bacitracin.
• Consider alternative treatment for burns that cover more than 20% of body surface, especially if patient suffers impaired renal function.
• If no improvement or if condition worsens, stop using and notify doctor.
• Prolonged use may result in overgrowth of nonsusceptible organisms.

butoconazole nitrate
Femstat
Pregnancy Risk Category: C

HOW SUPPLIED
Vaginal cream: 2% supplied with applicators

MECHANISM OF ACTION
Controls or destroys fungus by disrupting cell membrane permeability and reducing osmotic resistance.

INDICATIONS & DOSAGE
Local treatment of vulvovaginal mycotic infections caused by Candida *species—*
Adults (nonpregnant): one applicatorful intravaginally at bedtime for 3 days.
Adults (pregnant): one applicatorful intravaginally at bedtime for 6 days. Use only during second and third trimester.

ADVERSE REACTIONS
Skin: vulvar itching, soreness, and swelling; itching of the fingers.

INTERACTIONS
None significant.

NURSING CONSIDERATIONS
• Contraindicated during first trimester of pregnancy.
• Butoconazole may be used with oral contraceptive and antibiotic therapy.
• Diagnosis of *Candida* vulvaginal infection should be confirmed by smears or cultures.
• Symptom resolution comparable to 7-day miconazole cream therapy. Antifungal effect of butoconazole therapy is apparent after only 3 days of therapy.
• Teach patient how to apply. Tell patient not to use tampons during treatment.
• The patient's sexual partner should wear a condom during intercourse un-

til treatment is complete. He should consult his doctor if he experiences penile itching, redness, or discomfort.
• Advise patient to do the following to prevent reinfection: Keep cool and dry, wear loose-fitting cotton clothing, avoid feminine hygiene sprays, wash daily with unscented soap, dry thoroughly with clean towel, and maintain proper bowel hygiene by wiping from front to back.

carbol-fuchsin solution (Castellani's paint)
Castaderm

Pregnancy Risk Category: C

HOW SUPPLIED
Topical solution: 0.3% basic fuchsin, 4.5% phenol, 10% resorcinol, 5% acetone, and 10% alcohol.

MECHANISM OF ACTION
Disrupts protein synthesis. A fungicidal and bactericidal agent.

INDICATIONS & DOSAGE
Tinea, dermatophytosis, skin infections—
Adults and children: apply liberally once daily to b.i.d.

ADVERSE REACTIONS
Blood: possibility of bone marrow hypoplasia with use over long periods or at frequent intervals.
Skin: *contact dermatitis.*

INTERACTIONS
None significant.

NURSING CONSIDERATIONS
• Warn patient to expect a stinging sensation.
• An initial test application over a small area is recommended. If contact dermatitis or sensitivity occurs, discontinue use.
• Discontinue use after 1 week if no improvement shown; consult doctor.

Toxicities may develop in long-term use.
• Poisonous; warn against swallowing. Store in tight, light-resistant container.
• Instruct patient to continue using for full treatment period prescribed, even if condition has improved.
• Don't apply to eroded skin or over extensive areas.
• Will stain clothing.
• Clean skin with soap and water before application.

chloramphenicol
Chloromycetin

Pregnancy Risk Category: C

HOW SUPPLIED
Cream: 1%

MECHANISM OF ACTION
Disrupts protein synthesis.

INDICATIONS & DOSAGE
Superficial skin infections caused by susceptible bacteria—
Adults and children: after thorough cleansing, apply t.i.d. or q.i.d.

ADVERSE REACTIONS
Skin: possible contact sensitivity; itching, burning, urticaria, angioneurotic edema in patients hypersensitive to any of the components.
Other: *blood dyscrasias.*

INTERACTIONS
None significant.

NURSING CONSIDERATIONS
• If no improvement or if condition worsens, stop using and report to doctor.
• Prolonged use may result in overgrowth of nonsusceptible organisms.
• For all but very superficial infections, topical use of this drug should be supplemented by appropriate systemic medication.

Italicized adverse reactions are common or life-threatening.
*Liquid form contains alcohol.   **May contain tartrazine.

• Discontinue if signs of hypersensitivity develop.
• Tell patient to continue using for full treatment period prescribed, even if condition has improved.

---

chlortetracycline hydrochloride
Aureomycin 3%◊

Pregnancy Risk Category: D

HOW SUPPLIED
Ointment: 3% in 14.2-g, 30-g tubes◊

MECHANISM OF ACTION
Disrupts protein synthesis.

INDICATIONS & DOSAGE
Superficial infections of the skin caused by susceptible bacteria—
Adults and children: rub into affected area b.i.d. or t.i.d.

ADVERSE REACTIONS
Skin: *dermatitis*, drying.

INTERACTIONS
None significant.

NURSING CONSIDERATIONS
• Drug has lanolin base. Don't use in persons allergic to wool.
• Prolonged use may result in overgrowth of nonsusceptible organisms.
• If no improvement or if condition worsens, stop using and report to doctor.
• Treated skin fluoresces under ultraviolet light.

---

ciclopirox olamine
Loprox

Pregnancy Risk Category: B

HOW SUPPLIED
Cream: 1%

MECHANISM OF ACTION
Depletes essential intracellular substrates of fungi.

INDICATIONS & DOSAGE
Treatment of tinea pedis, tinea cruris, tinea corporis, and tinea versicolor; cutaneous candidiasis—
Adults and children over 10 years: massage gently into the affected and surrounding areas b.i.d., in the morning and evening.

ADVERSE REACTIONS
Local: pruritus, burning.

INTERACTIONS
None reported.

NURSING CONSIDERATIONS
• If sensitivity or chemical irritation occurs, discontinue treatment.
• Use the drug for the full treatment period even though symptoms may have improved. Notify doctor if there's no improvement after 4 weeks.
• Don't use occlusive dressings.
• Hypopigmentation from *tinea versicolor* will resolve gradually.

---

clindamycin phosphate
Cleocin T Gel, Lotion, Solution

Pregnancy Risk Category: B

HOW SUPPLIED
Gel: 1%
Lotion: 1%
Topical solution: 1%

MECHANISM OF ACTION
Suppresses growth of susceptible organisms in sebaceous glands.

INDICATIONS & DOSAGE
Treatment of acne vulgaris, grades II and III—
Adults and adolescents: apply to skin b.i.d., morning and evening; solutions have been used once daily to q.i.d.

ADVERSE REACTIONS
GI: GI disturbance, diarrhea, bloody diarrhea, abdominal pain, colitis (including pseudomembranous colitis).
Skin: *dryness,* rash, redness, itching, swelling, irritation.

INTERACTIONS
Abrasive or medicated soaps or cleansers; acne preparations or any containing a peeling agent (benzoyl peroxide, salicylic acid, sulfur, resorcinol, tretinoin); alcohol-containing products (after-shave, perfumed toiletries, shaving creams or lotions, cosmetics); soaps or cosmetics with strong drying effect; isotretinoin; medicated cosmetics or "cover-ups": may cause cumulative drying or irritation, resulting in excessive skin irritation.

NURSING CONSIDERATIONS
• May be used concurrently with tretinoin and/or benzoyl peroxide as well as systemic antibiotics. Caution patient to notify physician if skin becomes excessively dry.
• Noticeable improvement is usually seen within 6 weeks; however, 8 to 12 weeks may be required for maximum benefit.
• Instruct patient to wash area with warm water and soap, rinse and pat dry before application; and allow 30 minutes after washing or shaving to apply. Warn patient to avoid too frequent washing of area. Tell patient to cover entire affected area, but to avoid contact with eyes, nose, mouth, and other mucous membranes.
• Patient should not smoke while applying.
• Use only as prescribed.
• Tell patient to check with doctor or pharmacist before using antidiarrheal if diarrhea occurs.
• Use with caution in patients with GI disease, especially ulcerative colitis, regional enteritis, or antibiotic-related colitis.
• Explain correct use of applicator—

tip bottle: use dabbing motion rather than rolling action. If tip becomes dry, invert bottle and depress tip several times to moisten.

---

clotrimazole
Canesten†, Gyne-Lotrimin, Lotrimin (1% clotrimazole), Mycelex, Mycelex-G

Pregnancy Risk Category: B

HOW SUPPLIED
Lozenges: 1%
Cream: 1%
Topical lotion: 1%
Topical solution: 1%
Vaginal cream: 1%
Vaginal tablets: 100 mg, 500 mg

MECHANISM OF ACTION
Alters fungal cell wall permeability.

INDICATIONS & DOSAGE
Superficial fungal infections (tinea pedis, tinea cruris, tinea corporis, tinea versicolor, candidiasis)—
Adults and children: apply thinly and massage into affected and surrounding area, morning and evening, 1 to 8 weeks.
Candidal vulvovaginitis—
Adults: insert 1 applicatorful or 1 tablet intravaginally daily for 7 to 14 days at bedtime. Alternatively, insert two 100-mg tablets once daily for 3 consecutive days or one 500-mg tablet one time only at bedtime.
Oropharyngeal candidiasis—
Adults and children: dissolve lozenge in mouth five times daily for 14 consecutive days.

ADVERSE REACTIONS
GI: nausea and vomiting (with lozenges).
GU: (with vaginal use) *mild vaginal burning, irritation.*
Hepatic: elevated AST (SGOT) levels (from lozenges).
Skin: blistering, *erythema,* edema,

Italicized adverse reactions are common or life-threatening.
*Liquid form contains alcohol.   **May contain tartrazine.

pruritus, burning, stinging, peeling, urticaria, skin fissures, general irritation.

INTERACTIONS
None significant.

NURSING CONSIDERATIONS
• Not for ophthalmic use.
• Watch for and report irritation or sensitivity. Discontinue use.
• Improvement usually within a week; if no improvement in 4 weeks, diagnosis should be reviewed.
• Emphasize the need to continue treatment for full course even if symptoms have improved.
• Warn patients not to use occlusive wrappings or dressings.
• Shortened dosage schedule with tablets may be used when compliance is a problem.
• Hypopigmentation from *tinea versicolor* will resolve gradually.

econazole nitrate
Ecostatin, Spectazole
Pregnancy Risk Category: C

HOW SUPPLIED
Cream: 1%

MECHANISM OF ACTION
Alters fungal cell wall permeability.

INDICATIONS & DOSAGE
Treatment of tinea pedis, tinea cruris, and tinea corporis; cutaneous candidiasis—
Adults and children: apply sufficient quantity to cover affected areas b.i.d., in the morning and evening.
Tinea versicolor—
Adults and children: apply once daily.

ADVERSE REACTIONS
Local: burning, itching, stinging, erythema.

INTERACTIONS
Topical corticosteroids: may inhibit antifungal effect.

NURSING CONSIDERATIONS
• If condition persists or worsens or if irritation (burning, itching, stinging, redness) occurs, discontinue use and report this to doctor.
• Use medication for entire treatment period, even though symptoms may have improved. Notify doctor if there is no improvement; after 2 weeks (tinea cruris, corporis and versicolor) or 4 weeks (tinea pedis).
• Cleanse affected area before applying.
• Don't use occlusive dressings.
• Hypopigmentation from *tinea versicolor* will resolve gradually.

erythromycin
A/T/S, Erycette, EryDerm, EryGel, Staticin
Pregnancy Risk Category: B

HOW SUPPLIED
Ointment: 2%
Topical gel: 2%

MECHANISM OF ACTION
Disrupts protein synthesis.

INDICATIONS & DOSAGE
Superficial skin infections due to susceptible organisms, acne vulgaris—
Adults and children: clean affected area; apply t.i.d. or q.i.d.

ADVERSE REACTIONS
Skin: sensitivity reactions, erythema, burning, *dryness, pruritus*.

INTERACTIONS
None significant.

NURSING CONSIDERATIONS
• Prolonged use may result in overgrowth of nonsusceptible organisms.

• If no improvement or if condition worsens, stop using and notify doctor.
• Wash, rinse, and dry affected areas before application.
• Don't use near eyes, nose, mouth, or other mucous membranes.

gentamicin sulfate
Garamycin

Pregnancy Risk Category: C

HOW SUPPLIED
Cream: 0.1%
Ointment: 0.1%

MECHANISM OF ACTION
Disrupts protein synthesis.

INDICATIONS & DOSAGE
Primary and secondary bacterial infections, superficial burns, skin ulcers, infected insect bites and stings, infected lacerations and abrasions, wounds from minor surgery—
Adults and children over 1 year: rub in small amount gently t.i.d. or q.i.d., with or without gauze dressing.

ADVERSE REACTIONS
Skin: minor skin irritation; possible photosensitivity; allergic contact dermatitis.

INTERACTIONS
None significant.

NURSING CONSIDERATIONS
• If no improvement or if condition worsens, stop using and report to doctor.
• Should be used in selected patients. Widespread use may lead to resistant organisms.
• Avoid use on large skin lesions or over a wide area because of possible systemic toxic effects.
• Prolonged use may result in overgrowth of nonsusceptible organisms.
• May treat bacterial infections that

have not responded to other antibacterial agents.
• Store in cool place.
• Remove crusts before application of gentamicin in impetigo contagiosa.

gentian violet (methylrosaniline chloride, crystal violet)
Genapax

Pregnancy Risk Category: C

HOW SUPPLIED
Tampons: 5 mg
Topical solution: 1%◊, 2%◊

MECHANISM OF ACTION
Fungistatic and antibacterial activity.

INDICATIONS & DOSAGE
Superficial infections of skin; lesions, except ulcerative lesions of face, particularly Candida albicans—
Adults and children: apply with swab b.i.d. or t.i.d. Keep affected area clean, dry, and exposed to air to prevent spread of infection.
Vaginal fungal infections—
Adults: insert 1 tampon intravaginally for 3 to 4 hours once daily to b.i.d. for 12 days. An additional tampon may be used overnight for resistant infections.

ADVERSE REACTIONS
Skin: *permanent discoloration if applied to granulation tissue;* irritation or ulceration of mucous membranes.

INTERACTIONS
None significant.

NURSING CONSIDERATIONS
• Do not use on ulcerative lesions of the face.
• Apply carefully to avoid undue staining. Will stain skin and clothing.
• Do not use occlusive dressings.
• Tattooing of the skin may occur if applied to granulation tissue.

Italicized adverse reactions are common or life-threatening.
*Liquid form contains alcohol.   **May contain tartrazine.

haloprogin
Halotex

Pregnancy Risk Category: B

HOW SUPPLIED
Cream: 1%
Topical solution: 1%

MECHANISM OF ACTION
Fungistatic and fungicidal activity.

INDICATIONS & DOSAGE
Superficial fungal infections (tinea pedis, tinea cruris, tinea corporis, tinea manuum, and tinea versicolor)—
Adults and children: apply liberally b.i.d. for 2 to 3 weeks.

ADVERSE REACTIONS
Skin: burning sensation, irritation, vesicle formation, increased maceration, *pruritus or exacerbation of pre-existing lesions.*

INTERACTIONS
None significant.

NURSING CONSIDERATIONS
• Diagnosis should be reconsidered if no improvement in 4 weeks.
• Tell patient to continue using for full treatment period prescribed, even if condition has improved.
• Tell patient to notify doctor if increased irritation occurs.
• Don't allow drug to come in contact with the eyes.

iodochlorhydroxyquin (clioquinol)
Torofor◇, Vioform◇

Pregnancy Risk Category: C

HOW SUPPLIED
Cream: 3%
Ointment: 3%

MECHANISM OF ACTION
Fungistatic and fungicidal activity.

INDICATIONS & DOSAGE
Inflamed skin conditions, including eczema, athlete's foot, and other fungal infections; cutaneous or mucocutaneous mycotic infections caused by Candida *species (monilia)—*
Adults and children over 2 years: apply a thin layer b.i.d. or t.i.d., or as directed. Continue for 1 week after cessation of symptoms.

ADVERSE REACTIONS
Skin: *possible burning, itching, acneiform eruptions,* allergic contact dermatitis.

INTERACTIONS
Systemic corticosteroids: possible increased absorption. Use together cautiously.

NURSING CONSIDERATIONS
• Contraindicated in patients with hypersensitivity to iodine or iodine-containing preparations. Contraindicated in tuberculosis, vaccinia, and varicella.
• Don't use to treat diaper rash.
• Note all adverse reactions and precautions of each component in the combination antifungals.
• Presence in urine may cause false-positive result for phenylketonuria (PKU) or inaccurate thyroid function tests. Discontinue at least 1 month before thyroid function tests.
• Drug will stain fabric and hair.

ketoconazole
Nizoral

Pregnancy Risk Category: C

HOW SUPPLIED
Cream: 2%

MECHANISM OF ACTION
Inhibits yeast growth by altering the permeability of the cell membrane.

INDICATIONS & DOSAGE
Treatment of tinea corporis, tinea cruris, and tinea versicolor caused by susceptible organisms—
Adults: apply once daily to cover the affected and immediate surrounding area. Apply twice daily, if necessary, in the more resistant cases.

ADVERSE REACTIONS
Skin: severe irritation, pruritus, stinging.
Systemic: localized allergic reaction.

INTERACTIONS
None reported.

NURSING CONSIDERATIONS
• Discontinue if sensitivity or chemical irritation occurs.
• Most patients show improvement soon after treatment begins. However, treatment of tinea cruris or tinea corporis should continue for at least 2 weeks to reduce the possibility of recurrence.
• Check with doctor if condition worsens. The drug may have to be discontinued and diagnosis redetermined.

---

mafenide acetate
Sulfamylon

Pregnancy Risk Category: C

HOW SUPPLIED
Cream: 8.5%

MECHANISM OF ACTION
Interferes with bacterial cellular metabolism.

INDICATIONS & DOSAGE
Adjunctive treatment of second- and third-degree burns—
Adults and children: apply ⅟₁₆″

thickness of cream daily or b.i.d. to cleansed, debrided wounds. Reapply p.r.n. to keep burned area covered.

ADVERSE REACTIONS
Blood: eosinophilia.
Skin: pain, *burning sensation,* rash, itching, swelling, hives, blisters, erythema, facial edema.
Other: *metabolic acidosis.*

INTERACTIONS
None significant.

NURSING CONSIDERATIONS
• Use with caution in acute renal failure and in patients with known hypersensitivity to sulfonamides.
• Closely monitor acid-base balance, especially in the presence of pulmonary and renal dysfunction.
• If acidosis occurs, discontinue use for 24 to 48 hours.
• Can cause pain and burning at application site; if they occur, notify doctor. Severe and prolonged pain may indicate allergy. If other allergic reactions occur, treatment may have to be temporarily discontinued.
• Sometimes difficult to distinguish between adverse reactions and effects of severe burn.
• Cleanse area before applying. Mafenide washes off with water.
• Keep burn areas medicated at all times.
• Bathe patient daily, if possible.
• Using reverse isolation technique with sterile gloves and instruments to apply cream minimizes risk of further wound contamination.

---

metronidazole (topical)
MetroGel

Pregnancy Risk Category: B

HOW SUPPLIED
Topical gel: 0.75%

Italicized adverse reactions are common or life-threatening.
*Liquid form contains alcohol.   **May contain tartrazine.

MECHANISM OF ACTION

Exact mechanism of action is unknown. Probably exerts an antiinflammatory effect through its antibacterial and antiprotozoal actions.

INDICATIONS & DOSAGE

Topical treatment of acne rosacea—
Adults: apply a thin film b.i.d. to affected area during the morning and evening. Significant results should appear within 3 weeks and continue for the first 9 weeks of therapy.

ADVERSE REACTIONS

EENT: lacrimation (if drug applied in area around the eyes).

INTERACTIONS

Oral anticoagulants: may potentiate anticoagulant effect. Monitor patient for potential adverse reactions.

NURSING CONSIDERATIONS

• Contraindicated in patients with hypersensitivity to metronidazole or its other ingredients (such as parabens).
• Instruct patient to avoid use of the drug around the eyes.
• If local reactions occur, advise patient to apply less frequently or to discontinue and contact doctor.
• Use cautiously in patients with history or evidence of blood dyscrasias because chemically related compounds are associated with blood dyscrasias.
• Topical metronidazole therapy has not been associated with the adverse effects observed with parenteral or oral metronidazole therapy (including disulfiram-like reactions after alcohol ingestion). However, some of the drug can be absorbed following topical use. Limited clinical experience hasn't shown any of these adverse effects.
• Advise patient to cleanse area thoroughly before use. Patient may use cosmetics after applying the drug.

miconazole nitrate

Micatin◊, Monistat-Derm Cream and Lotion, Monistat 7 Vaginal Cream, Monistat 7 Vaginal Suppository, Monistat 3 Vaginal Suppository

Pregnancy Risk Category: C

HOW SUPPLIED

Cream: 2%◊
Lotion: 2%◊
Powder: 2%◊
Spray: 2%◊
Vaginal cream: 2%
Vaginal suppositories: 100 mg, 200 mg

MECHANISM OF ACTION

Controls or destroys fungus by disrupting fungal cell membrane permeability.

INDICATIONS & DOSAGE

Tinea pedis, tinea cruris, tinea corporis, tinea versicolor, cutaneous candidiasis (moniliasis), infections from common dermatophytes—
Adults and children: apply or spray sparingly b.i.d. for 2 to 4 weeks.
Vulvovaginal candidiasis—
Adults: insert 1 applicatorful or suppository (Monistat 7) intravaginally for 7 days at bedtime; repeat course if necessary. Alternatively, insert suppository (Monistat 3) intravaginally for 3 days at bedtime.

ADVERSE REACTIONS

Skin: isolated reports of irritation, burning, maceration.
Other: (with vaginal cream) vulvovaginal burning, itching, or irritation.

INTERACTIONS

None significant.

NURSING CONSIDERATIONS

• For perineal or intravaginal use only. Keep out of eyes.

• Discontinue if sensitivity or chemical irritation occurs.

• Tell patient to continue using for full treatment period prescribed, even if condition has improved.

• Do not use occlusive dressings.

• When using intravaginal forms, tell patient to cautiously insert high into the vagina with applicator provided.

• Concurrent use of intravaginal forms and certain latex products, such as vaginal contraceptive diaphragms are not recommended because of possible interaction.

mupirocin
Bactroban

Pregnancy Risk Category: C

HOW SUPPLIED
Ointment: 2%

MECHANISM OF ACTION
Inhibits bacterial protein and RNA synthesis.

INDICATIONS & DOSAGE
Treatment of common bacterial skin infections caused by susceptible bacteria—
Adults and children: apply to affected areas b.i.d. to t.i.d.

ADVERSE REACTIONS
Local: burning, itching, stinging, rash.

INTERACTIONS
None reported.

NURSING CONSIDERATIONS
• Mupirocin has proven especially useful in the treatment of impetigo in early clinical trials.

• Local reactions appear to be from the polyethylene glycol vehicle.

• If no improvement or condition worsens, notify doctor immediately.

• Prolonged use may cause overgrowth of nonsusceptible bacteria and fungi.

• Not intended for use on burns.

• Do not use in eye.

naftifine
Naftin

Pregnancy Risk Category: B

HOW SUPPLIED
Cream: 1%

MECHANISM OF ACTION
Inhibits sterol biosynthesis in susceptible fungi by blocking the actions of the enzyme squalene 2,3 epoxidase. A broad spectrum fungicidal agent.

INDICATIONS & DOSAGE
Treatment of tinea corporis and tinea cruris—
Adults: Apply to affected area b.i.d.

ADVERSE REACTIONS
Local: burning, dryness, itching, stinging, local irritation.

INTERACTIONS
None significant.

NURSING CONSIDERATIONS
• Not for ophthalmic use. Instruct patient to keep cream away from mucous membranes (eyes, nose, and mouth).

• Instruct patient to wash hands after application.

• Therapy should be reevaluated if there is not improvement after 4 weeks.

• Instruct patient to discontinue therapy and notify doctor if irritation or sensitivity develops.

• Cultures should be done to confirm diagnosis before therapy.

neomycin sulfate
Mycifradin†, Myciguent◇

Pregnancy Risk Category: C

HOW SUPPLIED
Cream: 0.5%◇
Ointment: 0.5%◇

MECHANISM OF ACTION
Disrupts protein synthesis.

INDICATIONS & DOSAGE
Topical bacterial infections, minor burns, wounds, skin grafts, following surgical procedure, primary pyodermas, pruritus, trophic ulcerations, otitis externa—
Adults and children: rub in small quantity gently b.i.d., t.i.d., or as directed.

ADVERSE REACTIONS
Skin: *rashes, contact dermatitis,* urticaria.
Other: *possible nephrotoxicity, ototoxicity, and neuromuscular blockade; possible systemic absorption when used on extensive areas of the body.*

INTERACTIONS
None significant.

NURSING CONSIDERATIONS
• If no improvement or if condition worsens, stop using and report to doctor.
• Don't use on more than 20% of the body surface and on patient with impaired renal function unless risk/benefit ratio has been assessed.
• Prolonged use may result in overgrowth of nonsusceptible organisms.
• In those combination products that contain corticosteroids, use of occlusive dressings increases corticosteroid absorption and the likelihood of systemic effects.
• Enhanced systemic absorption occurs on denuded or abraded areas.

• Watch for signs of hypersensitivity and contact dermatitis.
• Evaluate patient for signs of ototoxicity with prolonged or extended use.

nitrofurazone
Furacin

Pregnancy Risk Category: C

HOW SUPPLIED
Cream: 0.2%
Ointment: 0.2% (soluble dressing)
Topical solution: 0.2%

MECHANISM OF ACTION
Inhibits bacterial enzymes.

INDICATIONS & DOSAGE
Adjunctive treatment of second- and third-degree burns (especially when resistance to other antibiotics and sulfonamides occurs); prevention of skin allograft rejection—
Adults and children: apply directly to lesion daily or every few days, depending on severity of burn.

ADVERSE REACTIONS
GU: possible renal toxicity.
Skin: *erythema, pruritus,* burning, edema, severe reactions (vesiculation, denudation, ulceration), *allergic contact dermatitis.*

INTERACTIONS
None significant.

NURSING CONSIDERATIONS
• Use cautiously in patients with known or suspected renal impairment. Monitor serum creatinine regularly.
• If irritation, sensitization, or infection occurs, discontinue use.
• When using wet dressing, protect skin around wound with zinc oxide ointment.
• Cleanse wound as indicated by doctor before reapplying dressings.
• Solution should be stored in tight,

---

light-resistant containers (brown bottles). Avoid exposure of solution at all times to direct light, prolonged heat, and alkaline materials.
• Drug may discolor in light but is still usable because it retains its potency.
• Discard cloudy solutions if warming to 55° to 60° C. (131° to 140° F.) does not restore clarity.
• Use reverse isolation and/or sterile application technique to prevent further wound contamination.

nystatin
Mycostatin, Nadostine†, Nilstat
Pregnancy Risk Category: B

HOW SUPPLIED
Cream: 100,000 units/g
Ointment: 100,000 units/g
Powder: 100,000 units/g
Vaginal tablets: 100,000 units

MECHANISM OF ACTION
Alters the permeability of the cell membrane of fungi.

INDICATIONS & DOSAGE
Infant eczema, pruritus ani and vulvae, localized forms of candidiasis—
Adults and children: apply to affected area b.i.d. for 2 weeks.
Vulvovaginal candidiasis—
Adults: one vaginal tablet daily or b.i.d. for 14 days.

ADVERSE REACTIONS
Skin: occasional contact dermatitis from preservatives present in some formulations.

INTERACTIONS
None significant.

NURSING CONSIDERATIONS
• Generally well tolerated by all age-groups, including debilitated infants.
• Preparation does not stain skin or mucous membranes.

• Cream is recommended for intertriginous areas; powder, for very moist areas; ointment, for dry areas.
• Tell patient to continue using for full treatment period prescribed, even if condition has improved. Immunosuppressed patients may use the drug chronically.
• Do not use occlusive dressings.
• Store vaginal tablets in the refrigerator.

oxiconazole nitrate
Oxistat
Pregnancy Risk Category: B

HOW SUPPLIED
Cream: 1%

MECHANISM OF ACTION
Inhibits ergosterol synthesis in susceptible fungal organisms, thereby weakening cytoplasmic membrane integrity.

INDICATIONS & DOSAGE
Topical treatment of dermal infections caused by tinea rubrum and tinea mentagrophytes (tinea pedis, tinea cruris, and tinea corporis)—
Adults: apply to affected area once daily (in the evening) for 2 weeks (1 month for tinea pedis).

ADVERSE REACTIONS
Skin: itching, burning, irritation, maceration, erythema, fissuring.

INTERACTIONS
None reported.

NURSING CONSIDERATIONS
• Contraindicated in patients with hypersensitivity to oxiconazole nitrate.
• Be sure patient understands that drug is for external use only. Instruct him to avoid using it near the eyes.
• Animal studies have shown that oxiconazole is excreted in breast milk.

Italicized adverse reactions are common or life-threatening.
*Liquid form contains alcohol.   **May contain tartrazine.

Drug should be used with caution in breast-feeding women.

silver sulfadiazine
Flamazine†, Flint SSD, Silvadene, Thermazene

Pregnancy Risk Category: C

HOW SUPPLIED
Cream: 1%

MECHANISM OF ACTION
Acts upon cell membrane and cell wall.

INDICATIONS & DOSAGE
Prevention and treatment of wound infection especially for second- and third-degree burns—
Adults and children: apply 1/16″ thickness of cream to cleansed and debrided burn wound, then apply daily or b.i.d.

ADVERSE REACTIONS
Blood: *neutropenia (in 3% to 5%) of those receiving extensive applications.*
Skin: pain, burning, rashes, itching.

INTERACTIONS
Topical proteolytic enzymes: inactivity of enzymes when used together. Do not use together.

NURSING CONSIDERATIONS
• Contraindicated in premature and newborn infants during first month of life. (Drug may increase possibility of kernicterus.) Use with caution in hypersensitivity to sulfonamides.
• If hepatic or renal dysfunction occurs, consider discontinuing drug.
• Inspect patient's skin daily, and note any changes. Notify doctor if burning or excessive pain develops.
• Use only on affected areas. Keep medicated at all times.
• For patients with extensive burns, monitor serum sulfadiazine concentrations and renal function, and check urine for sulfa crystals.
• Bathe patient daily, if possible.
• Discard darkened cream.
• Reverse isolation and/or sterile application technique recommended to prevent wound contamination.

sulconazole nitrate
Exelderm

Pregnancy Risk Category: C

HOW SUPPLIED
Topical solution: 1%

MECHANISM OF ACTION
Unknown. An imidazole derivitive that inhibits the growth of both fungi and yeast.

INDICATIONS & DOSAGE
Treatment of tinea cruris and tinea corporis caused by Trichophyton mentagrophytes, Epidermophyton floccosum, *and* Microsporum canis; *treatment of tinea versicolor (caused by* Malassezia furfur)—
Adults: massage a small amount of solution into affected area daily to b.i.d.

ADVERSE REACTIONS
Local: itching, burning, stinging.

INTERACTIONS
None reported.

NURSING CONSIDERATIONS
• Contraindicated in patients hypersensitive to any component of the product. Efficacy against athlete's foot (tinea pedis) has not been proven.
• Treatment should continue for at least 3 weeks. If irritation develops during treatment, drug should be discontinued and patient should contact the doctor. If no improvement after 4 weeks, diagnosis should be reconsidered.
• Clinical improvement is usually ap-

parent within a week, with symptomatic relief in just a few days. Explain to the patient that he should complete the full course of therapy, even after symptoms subside, to prevent recurrence.

• Patient should avoid contact with the eyes and should wash hands thoroughly after applying.

terconazole
Terazol 3 Vaginal Suppositories, Terazol 7 Vaginal Cream

Pregnancy Risk Category: C

HOW SUPPLIED
Vaginal cream: 0.4%
Vaginal suppositories: 80 mg

MECHANISM OF ACTION
Exact mechanism unknown; may increase fungal cell membrane permeability (*Candida* species only).

INDICATIONS & DOSAGE
Local treatment of vulvovaginal candidiasis—
Adults: insert 1 applicatorful of cream into vagina h.s. for 7 days; or 1 suppository intravaginally h.s. for 3 days; may repeat course if necessary after reconfirmation by smear and/or culture

ADVERSE REACTIONS
CNS: headache.
Skin: vulvovaginal burning, irritation.
Other: fever, chills, body aches.

INTERACTIONS
None.

NURSING CONSIDERATIONS
• Contraindicated in patients with known sensitivity to terconazole or any inactive ingredients in formulations.
• Discontinue and do not retreat if

patient develops fever, chills, other flu-like symptoms, or sensitivity.
• Some photosensitivity reactions were observed after dermal use; none observed with vaginal use.
• Vaginal burning or itching is reportedly less frequent with terconazole than with miconazole or clotrimazole.
• Therapeutic effect of terconazole is unaffected by menstruation. However, tell patient not to use tampons during treatment.
• Tell patient to use for full treatment period prescribed. Explain how to prevent reinfection.

tetracycline hydrochloride
Topicycline

Pregnancy Risk Category: D

HOW SUPPLIED
Ointment: 3%
Topical solution: 2.2 mg/ml

MECHANISM OF ACTION
Disrupts protein synthesis.

INDICATIONS & DOSAGE
Acne vulgaris—
Adults and children over 12 years: apply generously to affected areas b.i.d. until skin is thoroughly covered.

ADVERSE REACTIONS
Skin: temporary stinging or burning on application; slight yellowing of treated skin, especially in patients with light complexions; severe dermatitis; treated skin areas fluoresce under black lights.

INTERACTIONS
None significant.

NURSING CONSIDERATIONS
• If no improvement or if condition worsens, stop using and notify doctor.
• Prolonged use may result in overgrowth of nonsusceptible organisms.

Italicized adverse reactions are common or life-threatening.
*Liquid form contains alcohol.   **May contain tartrazine.

- Patient may continue normal use of cosmetics.
- Store at room temperature, away from excessive heat.
- Medication to be used by one person only. Tell patient not to share with family members.
- Apply in morning and evening. Warn that drug should be used or discarded within 2 months.
- Explain that floating plug in bottle of Topicycline—an inert and harmless result of proper reconstitution of the preparation—shouldn't be removed.
- Serum levels with topical tetracycline hydrochloride are much lower than those for orally administered drug, so significant systemic effects are unlikely.
- To control flow rate of solution, increase or decrease pressure of the applicator against the skin.

ment, open the applicator just before using it.
- Review proper use of the drug with the patient. Instruct the patient to insert drug high into the vagina. Written instructions for the patient are available with the product.
- Watch for irritation or sensitivity. If it occurs, discontinue drug and report adverse reaction to the doctor.
- Emphasize to the patient the need to complete the full course of therapy, even after symptoms have improved. The patient should continue using the drug even during her menstrual period.
- Patient should use a sanitary napkin to avoid staining of clothing.
- Patient should avoid sexual intercourse during therapy or advise partner to use a condom to prevent reinfection.

tioconazole
Vagistat

Pregnancy Risk Category: C

HOW SUPPLIED
Vaginal ointment: 6.5%

MECHANISM OF ACTION
A fungicidal imidazole that alters cell wall permeability.

INDICATIONS & DOSAGE
Treatment of vulvovaginal candidiasis—
Women: insert 1 applicatorful (about 4.6 g) intravaginally h.s.

ADVERSE REACTIONS
GU: *burning, itching,* discharge, vulvar edema and swelling, irritation.

INTERACTIONS
None reported.

NURSING CONSIDERATIONS
- To avoid contamination of the oint-

tolnaftate
Aftate for Athlete's Foot◇, Aftate for Jock Itch◇, Footwork◇, Fungatin◇, Genaspor◇, NP-27◇, Tinactin◇, Zeasorb-AF◇

Pregnancy Risk Category: C

HOW SUPPLIED
Aerosol liquid: 1% (with 36% alcohol)◇
Aerosol powder: 1% (with 14% alcohol)◇
Cream: 1%◇
Gel: 1%◇
Powder: 1%◇
Pump spray liquid: 1% (with 36% alcohol)◇
Topical solution: 1%◇

MECHANISM OF ACTION
Fungistatic and fungicidal activity.

INDICATIONS & DOSAGE
Superficial fungal infections of the skin, infections due to common pathogenic fungi, tinea pedis, tinea cruris, tinea corporis, tinea versicolor—

Adults and children: ¼″ to ½″ ribbon of cream or 3 drops of lotion to cover about the size of one hand; same amount of cream or 3 drops of lotion to cover the toes and interdigital webs of one foot; or a sufficient amount of gel, powder, or spray to cover affected area. Apply and massage gently into skin b.i.d. for 2 weeks, up to 6 weeks.

ADVERSE REACTIONS
None significant.

INTERACTIONS
None significant.

NURSING CONSIDERATIONS
• Discontinue if condition worsens. Check with doctor.
• Odorless, greaseless. Won't stain or discolor skin, hair, nails, or clothing.
• Only a small quantity of cream or lotion is needed; area should not be wet with solution when application is completed.
• Commonly available product used to treat athlete's foot (tinea pedis). If no improvement after 10 days, consult doctor.
• Tell patient to continue using for full treatment period prescribed, even if condition has improved.
• Don't use as a side agent to treat hair or nail infections. Will not eradicate fungus from these structures.
• Powder or aerosol may continue to be used inside socks and shoes of persons susceptible to tinea infections.

---

undecylenic acid and zinc undecylenate
Cruex◊, Desenex◊, Desenex Aerosol◊, Quinsana Plus◊, Ting Spray◊

Pregnancy Risk Category: C

HOW SUPPLIED
Powder: 2% undecylenic acid and 20% zinc undecylenate◊

MECHANISM OF ACTION
Fungistatic and fungicidal activity.

INDICATIONS & DOSAGE
Athlete's foot and ringworm of the body exclusive of nails and hairy areas—
Adults and children: apply b.i.d. to thoroughly cleansed area.

ADVERSE REACTIONS
Skin: possible irritation in hypersensitive person.

INTERACTIONS
None significant.

NURSING CONSIDERATIONS
• Tell patient to continue using for full treatment period prescribed, even if condition has improved.
• Apply for at least 2 weeks to minimize risk of relapse.
• Liquids are preferable for hairy areas while powders are preferable in moist areas, for example, between skin folds.

Italicized adverse reactions are common or life-threatening.
*Liquid form contains alcohol.   **May contain tartrazine.

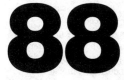

Scabicides and pediculicides

benzyl benzoate lotion
crotamiton
lindane
permethrin
pyrethrins

COMBINATION PRODUCTS
None.

---

benzyl benzoate lotion
Scabanca†

Pregnancy Risk Category: C

HOW SUPPLIED
Lotion: 14% (with benzocaine 2%)

MECHANISM OF ACTION
Unknown.

INDICATIONS & DOSAGE
Parasitic infestation (scabies, Phthirus pubis)—
Adults and children: first, scrub entire body with soap and water. Remove scales or crusts. Then apply the lotion undiluted over entire body, except the face and scalp, while still damp. Be sure to apply around nails. Let dry. Apply second coat on the most involved areas. Bathe after 24 hours.

ADVERSE REACTIONS
Skin: *irritation, itching; contact dermatitis with repeated applications.*

INTERACTIONS
None significant.

NURSING CONSIDERATIONS
• Contraindicated when skin is raw or inflamed. Notify doctor immediately if skin irritation or hypersensitivity develops; tell patient to discontinue drug and to wash it off skin.
• If live mites or new lesions occur, retreatment may be indicated in 7 to 10 days.
• Preferred over lindane for treatment of infants, young children, and pregnant or breast-feeding women.
• Do not apply to face, eyes, mucous membranes, or urethral meatus. If accidental contact with eyes does occur, flush with water and notify doctor.
• Instruct patient to change and sterilize (boil, launder, dry clean, or apply very hot iron) all clothing and bed linen after drug is washed off.
• Itching may continue for several weeks; this does not indicate that therapy is ineffective. Reassure patient that itching will cease.
• Topical corticosteroids may be needed if dermatitis develops from scratching.
• After application for lice infestation, use a fine comb dipped in white vinegar on hair to remove nits from hairy areas.
• Instruct patient to reapply if drug is washed off during treatment time.
• Don't apply to infant's or small children's hands because they will put hands in their mouths.
• Hospitalized patients should be placed in isolation with linen-handling precautions until treatment is completed.
• Store drug in light-resistant con-

---

tainer; avoid exposure to excessive heat.

crotamiton
Eurax

Pregnancy Risk Category: C

HOW SUPPLIED
Cream: 10%

MECHANISM OF ACTION
Unknown.

INDICATIONS & DOSAGE
Parasitic infestation (scabies)—
Adults and children: scrub entire body with soap and water. Then, apply a thin layer of cream over entire body, from chin down (with special attention to folds, creases, interdigital spaces, and genital area). Apply second coat in 24 hours. Wait additional 48 hours, then wash off.
Itching—
Adults and children: apply locally b.i.d. or t.i.d.

ADVERSE REACTIONS
Skin: *irritation.*

INTERACTIONS
None significant.

NURSING CONSIDERATIONS
• Contraindicated when skin is raw or inflamed. Notify doctor immediately if skin irritation or hypersensitivity develops; tell patient to discontinue drug and to wash it off skin.
• Do not apply to face, eyes, mucous membranes, or urethral meatus. If accidental contact with eyes does occur, flush with water and notify doctor.
• Instruct patient to change and sterilize (boil, launder, dry clean, or apply very hot iron) all clothing and bed linen after drug is washed off.
• Topical corticosteroids may be needed if dermatitis develops from scratching.

• Tendency to overuse scabicides. Estimate amount needed.
• Question other family members and sexual contacts about infestation.
• Instruct patient to reapply if drug is washed off during treatment time.
• Hospitalized patients should be placed in isolation with special linen-handling precautions until treatment is completed.

lindane
gBh†, Kwell, Kwellada†, Scabene

Pregnancy Risk Category: C

HOW SUPPLIED
Cream: 1%
Lotion: 1%
Shampoo: 1%

MECHANISM OF ACTION
Appears to inhibit neuronal membrane function in arthropods.

INDICATIONS & DOSAGE
Parasitic infestation (scabies, pediculosis)—
Adults and children: scrub entire body with soap and water.
*Cream or lotion—*apply thin layer over entire skin surface (with special attention to folds, creases, interdigital spaces, and genital area) for scabies, or to hairy areas for pediculosis. After 12 hours, wash off drug. If second application is needed, wait 1 week before repeating, but never more than twice in a week.
*Shampoo—*apply 30 ml undiluted to affected area and work into lather for 4 to 5 minutes. Rinse thoroughly and rub with dry towel.

ADVERSE REACTIONS
CNS: *dizziness, seizures.*
Skin: irritation with repeated use.

INTERACTIONS
None significant.

Italicized adverse reactions are common or life-threatening.
*Liquid form contains alcohol.   **May contain tartrazine.

NURSING CONSIDERATIONS
• Contraindicated when skin is raw or inflamed. Notify doctor immediately if skin irritation or hypersensitivity develops; tell patient to discontinue drug and to wash it off skin.
• Use cautiously in infants and young children as there's a greater risk for CNS toxicity in this group.
• Do not apply to open areas or acutely inflamed skin, or to face, eyes, mucous membranes, or urethral meatus. If accidental contact with eyes does occur, flush with water and notify doctor. Avoid inhaling vapors.
• Discourage repeated use, which can lead to skin irritation and systemic toxicity. Repeat use only if live lice or nits are found after 1 week.
• Warn patient that itching may continue for several weeks after effective treatment, especially in scabies.
• Topical corticosteroids or oral antihistamines may be needed for itching.
• Instruct patient to change and sterilize (boil, launder, dry clean, or apply very hot iron) all clothing and bed linen after drug is washed off.
• After application, use a fine comb dipped in white vinegar on hair to remove nits.
• Lindane shampoo can be used to clean combs or brushes; wash them thoroughly afterward. Warn patient not to use routinely.
• Instruct patient to reapply if drug is washed off during treatment time.
• Hospitalized patients should be placed in isolation with special linen-handling precautions until treatment is completed.
• Extremely toxic to CNS if accidentally swallowed.

---

permethrin
Nix

Pregnancy Risk Category: B

HOW SUPPLIED
Topical liquid: 1%

MECHANISM OF ACTION
Acts on the parasites' nerve cells to disrupt the sodium channel current, causing paralysis of the parasite.

INDICATIONS & DOSAGE
Treatment of infestation with Pediculus humanus capitis (head lice) and its nits—

Adults and children: use after hair has been washed with shampoo, rinsed with water, and towel-dried. Apply a sufficient amount (25 to 50 ml) of liquid to saturate the hair and scalp. Allow to remain on hair for 10 minutes before rinsing off with water.

ADVERSE REACTIONS
Skin: itching, burning, stinging, tingling, numbness or scalp discomfort, mild erythema, rash on the scalp.

INTERACTIONS
None reported.

NURSING CONSIDERATIONS
• Contraindicated in patients hypersensitive to pyrethrins or chrysanthemums.
• Don't use in infants because their skin is more permeable than that of children or adults.
• A single treatment is usually all that is necessary. Combing of nits is not required for effectiveness, but drug package supplies a fine-tooth comb for cosmetic use as desired.
• A second application may be necessary if lice are observed 7 days after the initial application.
• Head lice infestation is frequently accompanied by pruritus, erythema, and edema. Explain to the patient that treatment with permethrin may temporarily worsen these symptoms.
• Permethrin has been shown to be at least as effective as lindane (Kwell) in treating head lice.
• Not indicated to treat scabies.

---

†Available in Canada only.   ‡Available in Australia only.   ◇ Available OTC.

pyrethrins

A-200 Pyrinate◇, Barc◇, Pyrinyl◇,
RID◇, TISIT◇, Triple X◇

Pregnancy Risk Category: C

HOW SUPPLIED

Shampoo: pyrethrins 0.17% and piperonyl butoxide 2%; pyrethrins 0.3%
and piperonyl butoxide 3%
Topical gel: pyrethrins 0.18% and piperonyl butoxide 2.2%; pyrethrins
0.33% and piperonyl butoxide 3%;
pyrethrins 0.3% and piperonyl butoxide 4%
Topical solution: pyrethrins 0.18%
and piperonyl butoxide 2%; pyrethrins 0.2%, piperonyl butoxide 2%,
and deodorized kerosene 0.8%; pyrethrins 0.3% and piperonyl butoxide
3%

MECHANISM OF ACTION

Acts as contact poison that disrupts
the parasite's nervous system, causing
the parasite's paralysis and death.

INDICATIONS & DOSAGE

*Treatment of infestations of head,
body, and pubic (crab) lice and their
eggs—*
Adults and children: apply to hair,
scalp, or other infested area until en-
tirely wet. Allow to remain for 10
minutes, but no longer. Wash thoroughly with warm water and soap, or
shampoo. Remove dead lice and eggs
with fine-toothed comb. Treatment
may be repeated, if necessary, but
don't exceed two applications within
24 hours. May repeat in 7 to 10 days
to kill newly hatched lice.

ADVERSE REACTIONS

Skin: *irritation with repeated use.*

INTERACTIONS

None significant.

NURSING CONSIDERATIONS

• Contraindicated when skin is raw or
inflamed. Notify doctor immediately
if skin irritation develops; tell patient
to discontinue drug and to wash it off
skin. All preparations contain petroleum distillates. Also contraindicated
in patients allergic to ragweed. Use
cautiously in infants and small children.
• Do not apply to open areas or
acutely inflamed skin, or to face,
eyes, mucous membranes, or urethral
meatus. If accidental contact with
eyes does occur, flush with water and
notify doctor.
• Discourage repeated use, which can
lead to skin irritation and possible systemic toxicity.
• Topical corticosteroids or oral antihistamines may be needed if dermatitis develops from scratching.
• Instruct patient to change and sterilize (boil, launder, dry clean, or apply
very hot iron) all clothing and bed
linen after drug is washed off.
• Some authorities believe pyrethrins
and lindane (Kwell) are equally effective for lice infestation and that pyr-
ethins are less hazardous.
• Not effective against scabies.

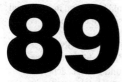

Topical corticosteroids

alclometasone dipropionate
amcinonide
betamethasone benzoate
betamethasone dipropionate
betamethasone valerate
clobetasol propionate
clocortolone pivalate
desonide
desoximetasone
dexamethasone
dexamethasone sodium
   phosphate
diflorasone diacetate
fluocinolone acetonide
fluocinonide
flurandrenolide
halcinonide
hydrocortisone
hydrocortisone acetate
hydrocortisone valerate
methylprednisolone acetate
mometasone furoate
triamcinolone acetonide

COMBINATION PRODUCTS
Corticosteroids for topical use are
commonly combined with antibiotics,
antifungals, and sulfonamides. (See
also Chapter 15, SULFONAMIDES, and
Chapter 70, ANTIBIOTIC ANTINEO-
PLASTIC AGENTS.)

alclometasone dipropionate
Alclovate, Logoderm‡

Pregnancy Risk Category: C

HOW SUPPLIED
Cream: 0.05%
Ointment: 0.05%

MECHANISM OF ACTION
Diffuses across cell membranes to
form complexes with specific cytoplasmic receptors.

INDICATIONS & DOSAGE
*Inflammation of corticosteroid-respon-
sive dermatoses—*
Adults: apply a thin film to affected
areas b.i.d. or t.i.d. Gently massage
until the medication disappears.

ADVERSE REACTIONS
Skin: burning, itching, irritation, dryness, folliculitis, striae, acneiform
eruptions, perioral dermatitis, hypopigmentation, hypertrichosis, allergic
contact dermatitis. With occlusive
dressings: *secondary infection, maceration, atrophy, striae, miliaria.*

INTERACTIONS
None significant.

NURSING CONSIDERATIONS
• Use cautiously in viral skin diseases, such as varicella, vaccinia, and
herpes simplex; in fungal infections;
and in bacterial skin infections.
• Avoid application near eyes or mucous membranes. Do not apply to
face, armpits, groin, or under breasts
unless specifically ordered.
• Systemic absorption especially
likely with occlusive dressings, prolonged treatment, or application to extensive body surface.
• Stop drug and notify doctor if patient develops signs of systemic absorption, skin irritation or ulceration,
hypersensitivity, or infection. (If anti-

fungals or antibiotics are being used concurrently, and infection does not respond immediately, corticosteroids should be discontinued until infection is controlled.)
• Before applying, wash skin gently. To prevent damage to skin, rub medication in gently, leaving a thin coat. When treating hairy sites, part hair and apply directly to lesion.
• Occlusive dressing (if ordered): Apply cream, then cover with a thin, pliable, nonflammable plastic film; seal to adjacent normal skin with hypoallergenic tape. Minimize adverse reactions by using occlusive dressing intermittently. Don't leave in place longer than 16 hours each day. Occlusive dressings should not be used in presence of infections or with weeping or exudative lesions.
• Notify doctor and remove occlusive dressing if fever develops.
• Change dressings as ordered by doctor. Inspect skin for infection, striae, and atrophy. Discontinue drug and notify doctor if these occur.
• Treatment should be continued for a few days after clearing of lesions to prevent recurrence.

---

amcinonide
Cyclocort

Pregnancy Risk Category: C

HOW SUPPLIED
Cream: 0.1%
Ointment: 0.1%

MECHANISM OF ACTION
Diffuses across cell membranes and complexes with specific cytoplasmic receptors.

INDICATIONS & DOSAGE
Inflammation of corticosteroid-responsive dermatoses—
Adults and children: apply a light film to affected areas b.i.d. or t.i.d.

Cream should be rubbed in gently and thoroughly until it disappears.

ADVERSE REACTIONS
Skin: burning, itching, irritation, dryness, folliculitis, striae, acneiform eruptions, perioral dermatitis, hypopigmentation, hypertrichosis, allergic contact dermatitis. With occlusive dressings: *secondary infection, maceration, atrophy, striae, miliaria.*

INTERACTIONS
None significant.

NURSING CONSIDERATIONS
• Use cautiously in viral diseases of skin, such as varicella, vaccinia, herpes simplex; fungal infections; bacterial skin infections.
• Avoid application near eyes or mucous membranes. Do not use on face, armpits, groin, in ear canal, or under breasts unless specifically ordered.
• Systemic absorption especially likely with occlusive dressings, prolonged treatment, or extensive body-surface treatment.
• When used in young children, avoid the use of plastic pants or tight-fitting diapers in treated areas.
• Stop drug and notify doctor if patient develops signs of systemic absorption, skin irritation or ulceration, hypersensitivity, or infection. (If antifungals or antibiotics are being used with corticosteroids and infection does not respond immediately, corticosteroids should be stopped until infection is controlled.)
• Before applying, gently wash skin. To prevent damage to skin, rub medication in gently, leaving a thin coat. When treating hairy sites, part hair and apply directly to lesion.
• Occlusive dressing (if ordered): apply cream, then cover with a thin, pliable, nonflammable plastic film; seal to adjacent normal skin with hypoallergenic tape. Minimize adverse reactions by using occlusive dressing in-

---

Italicized adverse reactions are common or life-threatening.
*Liquid form contains alcohol.   **May contain tartrazine.

termittently. Don't leave in place longer than 16 hours each day. Occlusive dressings should not be used in presence of infections or with weeping or exudative lesions.

• For patient with eczematous dermatitis who may develop irritation with adhesive material, hold dressing in place with gauze, elastic bandages, stockings, or stockinette.

• Notify doctor and remove occlusive dressing if fever develops.

• Change dressings as ordered by doctor. Inspect skin for infection, striae, and atrophy. Discontinue drug and notify doctor if these occur.

• Treatment should be continued for a few days after clearing of lesions to prevent recurrence.

---

betamethasone benzoate
Benisone, Uticort

betamethasone dipropionate
Alphatrex, Diprolene, Diprolene AF, Diprosone

betamethasone valerate
Betatrex, Beta-Val, Betnovate†‡, Valisone

Pregnancy Risk Category: C

HOW SUPPLIED
benzoate
Cream: 0.025%
Gel: 0.025%
Lotion: 0.025%
Ointment: 0.025%
dipropionate
Aerosol: 0.1%
Cream: 0.05%
Lotion: 0.05%
Ointment: 0.05%
valerate
Aerosol: 0.1%
Cream: 0.01%, 0.1%
Lotion: 0.1%
Ointment: 0.1%

MECHANISM OF ACTION
Diffuses across cell membranes and complexes with specific cytoplasmic receptors.

INDICATIONS & DOSAGE
Inflammation of corticosteroid-responsive dermatoses—
Adults and children: clean area; apply cream, lotion, spray, or gel sparingly daily to q.i.d.

ADVERSE REACTIONS
Skin: burning, itching, irritation, dryness, folliculitis, striae, acneiform eruptions, perioral dermatitis, hypopigmentation, hypertrichosis, allergic contact dermatitis. With occlusive dressings: *secondary infection, maceration, atrophy, striae, miliaria.*

INTERACTIONS
None significant.

NURSING CONSIDERATIONS
• Use cautiously in viral diseases of skin, such as varicella, vaccinia, herpes simplex; fungal infections; bacterial skin infections.

• Avoid application near eyes, mucous membranes, or in ear canal.

• Due to alcohol content of vehicle, gel preparations may cause mild, transient stinging, especially if used on or near excoriated skin.

• Systemic absorption especially likely with occlusive dressings, prolonged treatment, or extensive body-surface treatment.

• When used in young children, avoid the use of plastic pants or tight-fitting diapers in treated areas.

• Stop drug and notify doctor if patient develops signs of systemic absorption, skin irritation or ulceration, hypersensitivity, or infection. (If antifungals or antibiotics are being used with corticosteroids and infection does not respond immediately, corticosteroids should be stopped until infection is controlled.)

• Before applying, gently wash skin. To prevent damage to skin, rub medication in gently, leaving a thin coat. When treating hairy sites, part hair and apply directly to lesion.

• Occlusive dressing (if ordered): Apply cream, then cover with a thin, pliable, nonflammable plastic film; seal to adjacent normal skin with hypoallergenic tape. Minimize adverse reactions by using occlusive dressing intermittently. Don't leave in place longer than 16 hours each day. Occlusive dressings should not be used in presence of infections or with weeping or exudative lesions.

• For patient with eczematous dermatitis who may develop irritation with adhesive material, hold dressing in place with gauze, elastic bandages, stockings, or stockinette.

• Notify doctor and remove occlusive dressing if fever develops.

• Change dressings as ordered by doctor. Inspect skin for infection, striae, and atrophy. Discontinue drug and notify doctor if these occur.

• Treatment should be continued for a few days after clearing of lesions to prevent recurrence.

• Note that Diprolene and Diprolene AF may not be substituted generically because other products have different potencies.

clobetasol propionate
Dermovate†, Temovate

Pregnancy Risk Category: C

HOW SUPPLIED
Cream: 0.05%
Ointment: 0.05%

MECHANISM OF ACTION
Diffuses across cell membranes and forms complexes with specific cytoplasmic receptors.

INDICATIONS & DOSAGE
Inflammation of corticosteroid-responsive dermatoses—
Adults: apply a thin layer to affected skin areas b.i.d., once in the morning and once at night. Do not use more than 50 g of cream or ointment/week. Therapy should be limited to a maximum of 14 days.

ADVERSE REACTIONS
Skin: burning, itching, irritation, dryness, folliculitis, perioral dermatitis, allergic contact dermatitis, hypopigmentation, hypertrichosis, acneiform eruptions.

INTERACTIONS
None significant.

NURSING CONSIDERATIONS
• Use cautiously in viral skin diseases, such as varicella, vaccinia, herpes simplex; fungal infections; bacterial skin infections. Not recommended for children under 12 years.

• Clobetasol is a potent, fluoridated corticosteroid. Warn patient not to use for longer than 14 consecutive days.

• Avoid application near eyes, mucous membranes, or in ear canal.

• Occlusive dressings should not be used. Treated areas of skin should not be bandaged, covered, or wrapped.

• Stop drug and notify doctor if patient develops signs of systemic absorption, skin irritation or ulceration, hypersensitivity, or infection. (If antifungals or antibiotics are being used with corticosteroids and infection does not respond immediately, corticosteroids should be stopped until infection is controlled.)

• Before applying, gently wash skin. To prevent damage to skin, rub medication in gently, leaving a thin coat. When treating hairy sites, part hair and apply directly to lesions.

• Inspect skin for infection, striae,

Italicized adverse reactions are common or life-threatening.
*Liquid form contains alcohol.   **May contain tartrazine.

and atrophy. Discontinue drug and notify doctor if these occur.
• Do not refrigerate.

clocortolone pivalate
Cloderm

Pregnancy Risk Category: C

HOW SUPPLIED
Cream: 0.1%

MECHANISM OF ACTION
Diffuses across cell membranes and complexes with specific cytoplasmic receptors.

INDICATIONS & DOSAGE
Inflammation of corticosteroid-responsive dermatoses, such as atopic dermatitis, contact dermatitis, seborrheic dermatitis—
Adults and children: apply cream sparingly to affected areas once daily to q.i.d. and rub in gently.

ADVERSE REACTIONS
Skin: burning, itching, irritation, dryness, folliculitis, striae, acneiform eruptions, perioral dermatitis, hypertrichosis, hypopigmentation, allergic contact dermatitis. With occlusive dressings: *secondary infection, maceration, atrophy, striae, miliaria.*

INTERACTIONS
None significant.

NURSING CONSIDERATIONS
• Use cautiously in viral diseases of skin, such as varicella, vaccinia, herpes simplex; fungal infections; bacterial skin infections.
• Avoid application near eyes or mucous membranes.
• Systemic absorption especially likely with occlusive dressings, prolonged treatment, or extensive body-surface treatment.
• When used in young children, avoid the use of plastic pants or tight-fitting diapers in treated areas.
• Stop drug and notify doctor if patient develops signs of systemic absorption, skin irritation or ulceration, hypersensitivity, or infection. (If antifungals or antibiotics are being used with corticosteroids and infection does not respond immediately, corticosteroids should be stopped until infection is controlled.)
• Before applying, gently wash skin. To prevent damage to skin, rub medication in gently, leaving a thin coat. When treating hairy sites, part hair and apply directly to lesion.
• Occlusive dressing (if ordered): Apply cream, then cover with a thin, pliable, nonflammable plastic film; seal to adjacent normal skin with hypoallergenic tape. Minimize adverse reactions by using occlusive dressing intermittently. Don't leave in place longer than 16 hours each day. Occlusive dressings should not be used in presence of infections or with weeping or exudative lesions.
• For patient with eczematous dermatitis who may develop irritation with adhesive material, hold dressing in place with gauze, elastic bandages, or stockinette.
• Notify doctor and remove occlusive dressing if fever develops.
• Change dressings as ordered by doctor. Inspect skin for infection, striae, and atrophy. Discontinue drug and notify doctor if these occur.
• Treatment should be continued for a few days after clearing of lesions to prevent recurrence.

desonide
DesOwen, Tridesilon

Pregnancy Risk Category: C

HOW SUPPLIED
Cream: 0.05%
Ointment: 0.05%

MECHANISM OF ACTION
Diffuses across cell membranes and complexes with specific cytoplasmic receptors.

INDICATIONS & DOSAGE
Adjunctive therapy for inflammation in acute and chronic corticosteroid-responsive dermatoses—
Adults and children: clean area; apply cream or lotion sparingly b.i.d. to q.i.d.

ADVERSE REACTIONS
Skin: burning, itching, irritation, dryness, folliculitis, perioral dermatitis, allergic contact dermatitis, hypertrichosis, hypopigmentation, acneiform eruptions. With occlusive dressings: *maceration of skin, secondary infection, atrophy, striae, miliaria.*

INTERACTIONS
None significant.

NURSING CONSIDERATIONS
• Use cautiously in viral diseases of skin, such as varicella, vaccinia, herpes simplex; fungal infections; bacterial skin infections.
• Avoid application near eyes, mucous membranes, or in ear canal.
• Systemic absorption especially likely with occlusive dressings, prolonged treatment, or extensive body-surface treatment.
• When used in young children, avoid the use of plastic pants or tight-fitting diapers in treated areas.
• Stop drug and notify doctor if patient develops signs of systemic absorption, skin irritation or ulceration, hypersensitivity, or infection. (If antifungals or antibiotics are being used with corticosteroids and infection does not respond immediately, corticosteroids should be stopped until infection is controlled.)
• Before applying, gently wash skin. To prevent damage to skin, rub medication in gently, leaving a thin coat.

When treating hairy sites, part hair and apply directly to lesion.
• Occlusive dressing (if ordered): Apply cream or ointment, then cover with a thin, pliable, nonflammable plastic film; seal to adjacent normal skin with hypoallergenic tape. Minimize adverse reactions by using occlusive dressing intermittently. Don't leave in place longer than 16 hours each day. Occlusive dressings should not be used in presence of infection or with weeping or exudative lesions.
• For patient with eczematous dermatitis who may develop irritation with adhesive material, hold dressing in place with gauze, elastic bandages, stockings, or stockinette.
• Notify doctor and remove occlusive dressing if fever develops.
• Change dressing as ordered by doctor. Inspect skin for infection, striae, and atrophy. Discontinue drug and notify doctor if these occur.
• Treatment should be continued for a few days after clearing of lesions to prevent recurrence.

desoximetasone
Topicort
Pregnancy Risk Category: C

HOW SUPPLIED
Cream: 0.05%, 0.25%
Gel: 0.05%
Ointment: 0.25%

MECHANISM OF ACTION
Diffuses across cell membranes and complexes with specific cytoplasmic receptors.

INDICATIONS & DOSAGE
Inflammation of corticosteroid-responsive dermatoses—
Adults and children: clean area; apply cream, gel, or ointment sparingly once daily to b.i.d.

Italicized adverse reactions are common or life-threatening.
*Liquid form contains alcohol.   **May contain tartrazine.

ADVERSE REACTIONS
Skin: burning, itching, irritation, dryness, folliculitis, hypertrichosis, acneiform eruptions, perioral dermatitis, hypopigmentation, allergic contact dermatitis. With occlusive dressings: *maceration of skin, secondary infection, atrophy, striae, miliaria.*

INTERACTIONS
None significant.

NURSING CONSIDERATIONS
• Use cautiously in viral diseases of skin, such as varicella, vaccinia, herpes simplex; fungal infections; bacterial skin infections.
• Avoid application near eyes, mucous membranes, or in ear canal.
• Systemic absorption especially likely with occlusive dressings, prolonged treatment, or extensive body-surface treatment.
• When used in young children, avoid the use of plastic pants or tight-fitting diapers in treated areas.
• Stop drug and notify doctor if patient develops signs of systemic absorption, skin irritation or ulceration, hypersensitivity, or infection. (If antifungals or antibiotics are being used with corticosteroids and infection does not respond immediately, corticosteroids should be stopped until infection is controlled.)
• Before applying, gently wash skin. To prevent damage to skin, rub medication in gently, leaving a thin coat. When treating hairy sites, part hair and apply directly to lesions.
• Occlusive dressing (if ordered): Apply cream, then cover with a thin, pliable, nonflammable plastic film; seal to adjacent normal skin with hypoallergenic tape. To minimize adverse reactions, use occlusive dressing intermittently. Don't leave in place longer than 16 hours each day. Occlusive dressings should not be used in presence of infection or with weeping or exudative lesions.

• For patient with eczematous dermatitis who may develop irritation with adhesive material, hold dressing in place with gauze, elastic bandages, stockings, or stockinette.
• Notify doctor and remove occlusive dressing if fever develops.
• Change dressing as ordered by doctor. Inspect skin for infection, striae, and atrophy. Discontinue drug and notify doctor if these occur.
• Treatment should be continued for a few days after clearing of lesions to prevent recurrence.
• Gel contains alcohol and may cause burning or irritation in open lesions.
• Store in tightly sealed containers.

---

dexamethasone
Aeroseb-Dex, Decaderm, Decaspray

dexamethasone sodium phosphate
Decadron Phosphate

Pregnancy Risk Category: C

HOW SUPPLIED
dexamethasone
Aerosol: 0.01%, 0.04%
Gel: 0.1%
dexamethasone sodium phosphate
Cream: 0.1%

MECHANISM OF ACTION
Diffuses across cell membranes and complexes with specific cytoplasmic receptors.

INDICATIONS & DOSAGE
Inflammation of corticosteroid-responsive dermatoses—
Adults and children: clean area; apply cream, gel, or aerosol sparingly b.i.d. to q.i.d.

*Aerosol use on scalp—*shake can well and apply to dry scalp after shampooing. Hold can upright. Slide applicator tube under hair so that it touches scalp. Spray while moving tube to all affected areas, keeping tube under hair and in contact with scalp throughout spraying, which should take about 2 seconds. Inadequately covered areas may be spot sprayed. Slide applicator tube through hair to touch scalp, press and immediately release spray button. Don't massage medication into scalp or spray forehead or eyes.

ADVERSE REACTIONS
Skin: burning, itching, irritation, dryness, folliculitis, hypertrichosis, acneiform eruptions, perioral dermatitis, hypopigmentation, allergic contact dermatitis. With occlusive dressings: *maceration of skin, secondary infection, atrophy, striae, miliaria.*

INTERACTIONS
None significant.

NURSING CONSIDERATIONS
• Use cautiously in viral diseases of skin, such as varicella, vaccinia, herpes simplex; fungal infections; bacterial skin infections.
• Avoid application near eyes, mucous membranes, or in ear canal.
• Systemic absorption especially likely with occlusive dressings, prolonged treatment, or extensive body-surface treatment.
• When used in young children, avoid the use of plastic pants or tight-fitting diapers in treated areas.
• Stop drug and notify doctor if patient develops signs of systemic absorption, skin irritation or ulceration, hypersensitivity, or infection. (If antifungals or antibiotics are being used with corticosteroids and infection does not respond immediately, corticosteroids should be stopped until infection is controlled.)
• Before applying, gently wash skin. To prevent damage to skin, rub medication in gently, leaving a thin coat. When treating hairy sites, part hair and apply directly to lesions.

• For patient with eczematous dermatitis who may develop irritation with adhesive material, hold dressing in place with gauze, elastic bandages, stockings, or stockinette.
• Notify doctor and remove occlusive dressing if fever develops.
• Change dressing as ordered by doctor. Inspect skin for infection, striae, and atrophy. Discontinue drug and notify doctor if these occur.
• Occlusive dressings should not be used in presence of infection or with weeping or exudative lesions.
• Aerosol preparation contains alcohol and may produce irritation or burning in open lesions. When using about the face, cover patient's eyes and warn against inhalation of the spray. To avoid freezing tissues, do not spray longer than 3 seconds or closer than 6″ (15 cm).
• Treatment should be continued for a few days after clearing of lesions to prevent recurrence.

---

diflorasone diacetate
Florone, Flutone, Maxiflor, psorcon
Pregnancy Risk Category: C

HOW SUPPLIED
Cream: 0.05%
Ointment: 0.05%

MECHANISM OF ACTION
Diffuses across cell membranes and complexes with specific cytoplasmic receptors.

INDICATIONS & DOSAGE
Inflammation of corticosteroid-responsive dermatoses—
Adults and children: clean area; apply ointment daily to t.i.d.; apply cream b.i.d. to q.i.d. Apply sparingly in a thin film.

ADVERSE REACTIONS
Skin: burning, itching, irritation, dryness, folliculitis, perioral dermatitis,

---

Italicized adverse reactions are common or life-threatening.
*Liquid form contains alcohol.   **May contain tartrazine.

hypertrichosis, hypopigmentation, acneiform eruptions. With occlusive dressings: *maceration, secondary infection, atrophy, striae, miliaria.*

INTERACTIONS
None significant.

NURSING CONSIDERATIONS
• Use cautiously in viral diseases of skin, such as varicella, vaccinia; herpes simplex; fungal infections; bacterial skin infections.
• Use very cautiously in young children. A high-potency corticosteroid.
• Avoid application near eyes, mucous membranes, or in ear canal.
• Systemic absorption especially likely with occlusive dressings, prolonged treatment, or extensive body-surface treatment.
• When used in young children, avoid the use of plastic pants or tight-fitting diapers in treated areas.
• Stop drug and notify doctor if patient develops signs of systemic absorption, skin irritation or ulceration, hypersensitivity, or infection. (If antifungals or antibiotics are being used concomitantly, corticosteroids should be stopped until infection is controlled.)
• Before applying, gently wash skin. To prevent damage to skin, rub medication in gently, leaving a thin coat. When treating hairy sites, part hair and apply directly to lesion.
• Occlusive dressing (if ordered): Apply cream or ointment, then cover with a thin, pliable, nonflammable plastic film; seal to adjacent normal skin with hypoallergenic tape. Minimize adverse reactions by using occlusive dressing intermittently. Don't leave in place longer than 16 hours each day. Occlusive dressings should not be used in presence of infection or with weeping or exudative lesions.
• For patient with eczematous dermatitis who may develop irritation with adhesive material, hold dressing in place with gauze, elastic bandages, stockings, or stockinette.
• Notify doctor and remove occlusive dressing if fever develops.
• Change dressing as ordered by doctor. Inspect skin for infection, striae, and atrophy. Discontinue drug and notify doctor if these occur.
• Occlusive dressings should not be used with psorcon.
• Diflorasone is often effective with once-daily application.

---

fluocinolone acetonide
Fluocet, Fluonid, Flurosyn, Synalar, Synemol
Pregnancy Risk Category: C

HOW SUPPLIED
Cream: 0.01%, 0.025%, 0.2%
Ointment: 0.025%
Topical solution: 0.01%

MECHANISM OF ACTION
Diffuses across cell membranes and complexes with specific cytoplasmic receptors.

INDICATIONS & DOSAGE
Inflammation of corticosteroid-responsive dermatoses—
Adults and children over 2 years: clean area; apply cream, ointment, or solution sparingly b.i.d. to q.i.d. Treat multiple or extensive lesions sequentially, applying to only small areas at any one time.

ADVERSE REACTIONS
Skin: burning, itching, irritation, dryness, folliculitis, hypertrichosis, hypopigmentation, acneiform eruptions, perioral dermatitis, allergic contact dermatitis. With occlusive dressings: *maceration of skin, secondary infection, atrophy, striae, miliaria.*

INTERACTIONS
None significant.

NURSING CONSIDERATIONS
• Use cautiously in viral diseases of skin, such as varicella, vaccinia, herpes simplex; fungal infections; bacterial skin infections.
• Avoid application near eyes, mucous membranes, or in ear canal.
• Systemic absorption especially likely with occlusive dressings, prolonged treatment, or extensive body-surface treatment.
• When used in young children, avoid the use of plastic pants or tight-fitting diapers in treated areas.
• Stop drug and notify doctor if patient develops signs of systemic absorption, skin irritation or ulceration, hypersensitivity, or infection. (If antifungals or antibiotics are being used with corticosteroids and infection does not respond immediately, corticosteroids should be stopped until infection is controlled.)
• Before applying, gently wash skin. To prevent damage to skin, rub medication in gently, leaving a thin coat. When treating hairy sites, part hair and apply directly to lesion.
• Occlusive dressing (if ordered): Apply gently and sparingly to the lesion until cream disappears. Then reapply, leaving a thin coat. Cover with a thin, pliable, nonflammable plastic film; seal to adjacent normal skin with hypoallergenic tape. To minimize adverse reactions, use occlusive dressing intermittently. Don't leave in place longer than 16 hours each day. Occlusive dressings should not be used in presence of infection or with weeping or exudative lesions.
• For patient with eczematous dermatitis who may develop irritation with adhesive material, hold dressing in place with gauze, elastic bandages, stockings, or stockinette.
• Notify doctor and remove occlusive dressing if fever develops.
• Change dressing as ordered by doctor. Inspect skin for infection, striae,

and atrophy. Discontinue drug and notify doctor if these occur.
• Fluonid solution on dry lesions may increase dryness, scaling, or itching; on denuded or fissured areas, may produce burning or stinging. If burning or stinging persists and dermatitis has not improved, solution should be discontinued.

---

fluocinonide
Lidemol†, Lidex, Lidex-E, Topsyn
Pregnancy Risk Category: C

HOW SUPPLIED
Cream: 0.05%
Gel: 0.05%
Ointment: 0.05%
Topical solution: 0.05%

MECHANISM OF ACTION
Diffuses across cell membranes and complexes with specific cytoplasmic receptors.

INDICATIONS & DOSAGE
Inflammation of corticosteroid-responsive dermatoses—
Adults and children: clean area; apply cream, ointment, solution, or gel sparingly t.i.d. or q.i.d.

ADVERSE REACTIONS
Skin: burning, itching, irritation, dryness, folliculitis, hypertrichosis, hypopigmentation, acneiform eruptions, perioral dermatitis, allergic contact dermatitis. With occlusive dressings: *maceration of skin, secondary infection, atrophy, striae, miliaria.*

INTERACTIONS
None significant.

NURSING CONSIDERATIONS
• Use cautiously in viral diseases of skin, such as varicella, vaccinia, and herpes simplex; untreated purulent bacterial skin infections; fungal infections; bacterial skin infections.

Italicized adverse reactions are common or life-threatening.
*Liquid form contains alcohol.   **May contain tartrazine.

- Avoid application near eyes, mucous membranes, or in ear canal.
- Systemic absorption especially likely with occlusive dressings, prolonged treatment, or extensive body-surface treatment.
- When used in young children, avoid the use of plastic pants or tight-fitting diapers in treated areas.
- Stop drug and notify doctor if patient develops signs of systemic absorption, skin irritation or ulceration, hypersensitivity, or infection. (If antifungals or antibiotics are being used with corticosteroids and infection does not respond immediately, corticosteroids should be stopped until infection is controlled.)
- Before applying, gently wash skin. To prevent damage to skin, rub medication in gently, leaving a thin coat. When treating hairy sites, part hair and apply directly to lesion.
- Occlusive dressing (if ordered): Apply cream or ointment heavily, then cover with a thin, pliable, nonflammable plastic film; seal to adjacent normal skin with hypoallergenic tape. To minimize adverse reactions, use occlusive dressing intermittently. Don't leave in place longer than 16 hours each day. Occlusive dressings should not be used in presence of infection or with weeping or exudative lesions.
- For patient with eczematous dermatitis who may develop irritation with adhesive material, hold dressing in place with gauze, elastic bandages, stockings, or stockinette.
- Notify doctor and remove occlusive dressing if fever develops.
- Change dressing as ordered by doctor. Inspect skin for infection, striae, and atrophy. Discontinue drug and notify doctor if these occur.
- Treatment should be continued for a few days after clearing of lesions to prevent recurrence.

flurandrenolide
Cordran, Cordran SP, Cordran Tape, Drenison†, Drenison 1/4†, Drenison Tape†

Pregnancy Risk Category: C

HOW SUPPLIED
Cream: 0.025%, 0.05%
Lotion: 0.05%
Ointment: 0.025%, 0.05%
Tape: 4 mcg/cm²

MECHANISM OF ACTION
Diffuses across cell membranes and complexes with specific cytoplasmic receptors.

INDICATIONS & DOSAGE
Inflammation of corticosteroid-responsive dermatoses—
Adults and children: clean area; apply cream, lotion, or ointment sparingly b.i.d. or t.i.d. Apply tape q 12 to 24 hours. Before applying tape, cleanse skin carefully, removing scales, crust, and dried exudates. Allow skin to dry for 1 hour before applying new tape. Shave or clip hair to allow good contact with skin and comfortable removal. If tape ends loosen prematurely, trim off and replace with fresh tape. Lowest incidence of adverse reactions if tape is replaced q 12 hours, but may be left in place for 24 hours if well tolerated and adheres satisfactorily.
Drenison 1/4—for maintenance therapy of widespread or chronic lesions.

ADVERSE REACTIONS
Skin: burning, itching, irritation, dryness, folliculitis, hypertrichosis, hypopigmentation, acneiform eruptions, allergic contact dermatitis. With occlusive dressings: *maceration of skin, secondary infection, atrophy, striae, miliaria.* With tape: purpura, stripping of epidermis, furunculosis.

INTERACTIONS
None significant.

NURSING CONSIDERATIONS
• Use cautiously in viral diseases of skin, such as varicella, vaccinia, herpes simplex; fungal infections; bacterial skin infections.
• Tape not advised for exudative lesions or those in intertriginous areas.
• Tape should be cut with scissors. Don't tear.
• Avoid application near eyes, mucous membranes, or in ear canal.
• Systemic absorption especially likely with occlusive dressings, prolonged treatment, or extensive body-surface treatment.
• When used in young children, avoid the use of plastic pants or tight-fitting diapers in treated areas.
• Stop drug and notify doctor if patient develops signs of systemic absorption, skin irritation or ulceration, hypersensitivity, or infection. (If antifungals or antibiotics are being used with corticosteroids and infection does not respond immediately, corticosteroids should be stopped until infection is controlled.)
• Before applying, gently wash skin. To prevent damage to skin, rub medication in gently, leaving a thin coat. When treating hairy sites, part hair and apply directly to lesion.
• Occlusive dressing (if ordered): Apply cream heavily, then cover with a thin, pliable, nonflammable plastic film; seal to adjacent normal skin with hypoallergenic tape. To minimize adverse reactions, use occlusive dressing intermittently. Don't leave in place longer than 16 hours each day. Occlusive dressings should not be used in presence of infection or with weeping or exudative lesions.
• For patient with eczematous dermatitis who may develop irritation with adhesive material, hold dressing in place with gauze, elastic bandages, stockings, or stockinette.

• Notify doctor and remove occlusive dressing if fever develops.
• Inspect skin for infection, striae, and atrophy. Discontinue drug and notify doctor if these occur.
• Treatment should be continued for a few days after clearing of lesions to prevent recurrence.

---

halcinonide
Halciderm, Halog
Pregnancy Risk Category: C

HOW SUPPLIED
Cream: 0.025%, 0.1%
Ointment: 0.1%
Topical solution: 0.1%

MECHANISM OF ACTION
Diffuses across cell membranes and complexes with specific cytoplasmic receptors.

INDICATIONS & DOSAGE
Inflammation of acute and chronic corticosteroid-responsive dermatoses—
Adults and children: clean area; apply cream, ointment, or solution sparingly b.i.d. or t.i.d.

ADVERSE REACTIONS
Skin: burning, itching, irritation, dryness, folliculitis, hypertrichosis, hypopigmentation, acneiform eruptions, allergic contact dermatitis. With occlusive dressings: *maceration of skin, secondary infection, atrophy, striae, miliaria.*

INTERACTIONS
None significant.

NURSING CONSIDERATIONS
• Use cautiously in viral diseases of skin, such as varicella, vaccinia, herpes simplex; fungal infections; bacterial skin infections.
• Avoid application near eyes, mucous membranes, or in ear canal.

Italicized adverse reactions are common or life-threatening.
*Liquid form contains alcohol.   **May contain tartrazine.

- Systemic absorption especially likely with occlusive dressings, prolonged treatment, or extensive body-surface treatment.
- When used in young children, avoid the use of plastic pants or tight-fitting diapers in treated areas.
- Stop drug and notify doctor if patient develops signs of systemic absorption, skin irritation or ulceration, hypersensitivity, or infection. (If antifungals or antibiotics are being used with corticosteroids and infection does not respond immediately, corticosteroids should be stopped until infection is controlled.)
- Before applying, gently wash skin. To prevent damage to skin, rub medication in gently, leaving a thin coat. When treating hairy sites, part hair and apply directly to lesion.
- Occlusive dressing with cream: Gently rub small amount into lesion until it disappears. Reapply, leaving a thin coating on lesion, and cover with occlusive dressing. With ointment: Apply to lesion and cover with occlusive dressing. Cover with a thin, pliable, nonflammable plastic film; seal to adjacent normal skin with hypoallergenic tape. To minimize adverse reactions, use occlusive dressing intermittently. Don't leave in place longer than 16 hours each day.
- Good results have been obtained by applying occlusive dressings in the evening and removing them in the morning (that is, 12-hour occlusion). Medication should then be reapplied in the morning, without using the occlusive dressings during the day.
- For patient with eczematous dermatitis who may develop irritation with adhesive material, hold dressing in place with gauze, elastic bandages, stockings, or stockinette.
- Notify doctor and remove occlusive dressing if fever develops.
- Occlusive dressings should not be used in presence of infection or with weeping or exudative lesions.

- Change dressing as ordered by doctor. Inspect skin for infection, striae, and atrophy. Discontinue drug and notify doctor if these occur.
- Treatment should be continued for a few days after clearing of lesions to prevent recurrence.

---

hydrocortisone

Acticort, Aeroseb-HC, Carmol HC, Cetacort, Cort-Dome, Cortef◇, Cortinal, Cortizone 5◇, Cortril, Cremesone, Delacort, DermiCort◇, Dermolate◇, Durel-Cort, Ecosone, HC Cream, HI-Cor-2.5, Hycortole, Hydrocortex, Hytone, Ivocort, Maso-Cort, Microcort, Orabase HCA, Penecort, Proctocort, Rhus Tox HC, Rocort, Squibb-HC‡, Unicort

hydrocortisone acetate

Cortaid◇, Cortamed†, Cortef, Corticreme†, Cortifoam, Dermacort‡, Dermacort Ointment‡, Epifoam, Hydrocortisone Acetate, MyCort Lotion, Proctofoam-HC

hydrocortisone valerate

Westcort Cream

Pregnancy Risk Category: C

HOW SUPPLIED
hydrocortisone
Aerosol: 0.5%
Cream: 0.25%◇, 0.5%◇, 1%, 2.5%
Gel: 1%
Lotion: 0.125%, 0.25%, 0.5%◇, 1%, 2%, 2.5%
Ointment: 0.5%◇, 1%, 2.5%
Topical solution: 1%
hydrocortisone acetate
Cream: 0.5%◇
Lotion: 0.5%◇
Ointment: 0.5%◇, 1%
Rectal foam: 90 mg/application
hydrocortisone valerate
Cream: 0.2%
Ointment: 0.2%

---

†Available in Canada only.   ‡Available in Australia only.   ◇Available OTC.

MECHANISM OF ACTION
Diffuses across cell membranes and complexes with specific cytoplasmic receptors.

INDICATIONS & DOSAGE
Inflammation of corticosteroid-responsive dermatoses; adjunctive typical management of seborrheic dermatitis of scalp; may be safely used on face, groin, armpits, and under breasts—

Adults and children: clean area; apply cream, gel, lotion, ointment, topical solution, or aerosol sparingly daily to q.i.d.
Aerosol—shake can well. Direct spray onto affected area from a distance of 6″ (15 cm). Apply for only 3 seconds (to avoid freezing tissues). Apply to dry scalp after shampooing; no need to massage or rub medication into scalp after spraying. Apply daily until acute phase is controlled, then reduce dosage to 1 to 3 times a week as needed to maintain control.
Rectal form— shake can well. One applicatorful daily to b.i.d. for 2 to 3 weeks, then every other day as necessary.

ADVERSE REACTIONS
Skin: burning, itching, irritation, dryness, folliculitis, hypertrichosis, hypopigmentation, acneiform eruptions, allergic contact dermatitis. With occlusive dressings: *maceration of skin, secondary infection, atrophy, striae, miliaria.*

INTERACTIONS
None significant.

NURSING CONSIDERATIONS
• Use cautiously in viral diseases of skin, such as varicella, vaccinia, herpes simplex; fungal infections; bacterial skin infections.
• Avoid application near eyes, mucous membranes, or in ear canal.
• Systemic absorption especially likely with occlusive dressings, prolonged treatment, or extensive body-surface treatment.
• When used in young children, avoid the use of plastic pants or tight-fitting diapers in treated areas.
• Stop drug and notify doctor if patient develops signs of systemic absorption, skin irritation or ulceration, hypersensitivity, or infection. (If antifungals or antibiotics are being used with corticosteroids and infection does not respond immediately, corticosteroids should be stopped until infection is controlled.)
• Before applying, gently wash skin. To prevent damage to skin, rub medication in gently, leaving a thin coat. When treating hairy sites, part hair and apply directly to lesion.
• Occlusive dressing (if ordered): Apply cream heavily, then cover with a thin, pliable, nonflammable plastic film; seal to adjacent normal skin with hypoallergenic tape. To minimize adverse reactions, use occlusive dressing intermittently. Don't leave in place longer than 16 hours each day. Occlusive dressings should not be used in presence of infection or with weeping or exudative lesions.
• For patient with eczematous dermatitis who may develop irritation with adhesive material, it may be helpful to hold dressing in place with gauze, elastic bandages, stockings, or stockinette.
• Notify doctor and remove occlusive dressing if fever develops.
• Aerosol preparation contains alcohol and may produce irritation or burning in open lesions. When using about the face, cover patient's eyes and warn against inhalation of the spray. To avoid freezing tissues, do not spray longer than 3 seconds or closer than 6″ (15 cm).
• Change dressing as ordered by doctor. Inspect skin for infection, striae, and atrophy. Discontinue drug and notify doctor if these occur.

Italicized adverse reactions are common or life-threatening.
*Liquid form contains alcohol.   **May contain tartrazine.

• Treatment should be continued for a few days following clearing of lesions to prevent recurrence.

methylprednisolone acetate
Medrol

Pregnancy Risk Category: C

HOW SUPPLIED
Ointment: 0.25%, 1%

MECHANISM OF ACTION
Diffuses across cell membranes and complexes with specific cytoplasmic receptors.

INDICATIONS & DOSAGE
Inflammation of corticosteroid-responsive dermatoses—
Adults and children: clean area; apply ointment daily to q.i.d.

ADVERSE REACTIONS
Skin: burning, itching, irritation, dryness, folliculitis, hypertrichosis, hypopigmentation, acneiform eruptions, allergic contact dermatitis. With occlusive dressings: *maceration of skin, secondary infection, atrophy, striae, miliaria.*

INTERACTIONS
None significant.

NURSING CONSIDERATIONS
• Use cautiously in viral diseases of skin, such as varicella, vaccinia, herpes simplex; fungal infections; bacterial skin infections.
• Avoid application near eyes, mucous membranes, or in ear canal.
• Systemic absorption especially likely with occlusive dressings, prolonged treatment, or extensive body-surface treatment.
• When used in young children, avoid the use of plastic pants or tight-fitting diapers in treated areas.
• Stop drug and notify doctor if patient develops signs of systemic absorption, skin irritation or ulceration, hypersensitivity, or infection. (If antifungals or antibiotics are being used with corticosteroids and infection does not respond immediately, corticosteroids should be stopped until infection is controlled.)
• Before applying, gently wash skin. To prevent damage to skin, rub medication in gently, leaving a thin coat. When treating hairy sites, part hair and apply directly to lesion.
• Occlusive dressing (if ordered): Apply ointment heavily, then cover with a thin, pliable, nonflammable plastic film; seal to adjacent normal skin with hypoallergenic tape. To minimize adverse effects, use occlusive dressing intermittently. Don't leave in place longer than 16 hours each day. Occlusive dressings should not be used in presence of infection or with weeping or exudative lesions.
• For patient with eczematous dermatitis who may develop irritation with adhesive material, hold dressing in place with gauze, elastic bandages, stockings, or stockinette.
• Notify doctor and remove occlusive dressing if fever develops.
• Change dressing as ordered by doctor. Inspect skin for infection, striae, and atrophy. Discontinue drug and notify doctor if these occur.
• Treatment should be continued for a few days after clearing of lesions to prevent recurrence.

mometasone furoate
Elocon

Pregnancy Risk Category: C

HOW SUPPLIED
Cream: 0.1%
Ointment: 0.1%

MECHANISM OF ACTION
Diffuses across cell membranes and complexes with specific cytoplasmic receptors.

INDICATIONS & DOSAGE

Inflammatory and pruritic manifestations of corticosteroid-responsive dermatoses—
Adults: apply cream or ointment to affected areas once daily. Do not use occlusive dressings.

ADVERSE REACTIONS

Skin: burning, pruritus, atrophy, irritation, acneiform eruptions, hypopigmentation, allergic contact dermatitis.
Other: HPA axis suppression, Cushing's syndrome.

INTERACTIONS

None reported.

NURSING CONSIDERATIONS

• Use cautiously in viral diseases of skin, such as varicella, vaccinia, herpes simplex; fungal infections; bacterial skin infections.
• Use very cautiously in young children. A high-potency corticosteroid.
• Avoid application near eyes, mucous membranes, or in ear canal.
• Systemic absorption especially likely with occlusive dressings, prolonged treatment, or extensive body-surface treatment.
• Stop drug and notify doctor if patient develops signs of systemic absorption, skin irritation or ulceration, hypersensitivity, or infection. (If antifungals or antibiotics are being used concomitantly, corticosteroids should be stopped until infection is controlled.)
• Before applying, gently wash skin. To prevent damage to skin, rub medication in gently, leaving a thin coat. When treating hairy sites, part hair and apply directly to lesion.

triamcinolone acetonide

Aristocort, Kenalog, Kenalone‡

Pregnancy Risk Category: C

HOW SUPPLIED

Aerosol: 0.2 mg/2-second spray
Cream: 0.02%‡, 0.025%, 0.1%, 0.5%
Lotion: 0.025%, 0.1%
Ointment: 0.02%‡, 0.025%, 0.1%, 0.5%

MECHANISM OF ACTION

Diffuses across cell membranes and complexes with specific cytoplasmic receptors.

INDICATIONS & DOSAGE

Inflammation of corticosteroid-responsive dermatoses—
Adults and children: clean area; apply aerosol, cream, lotion, or ointment sparingly b.i.d. to q.i.d.
Aerosol—shake can well. Direct spray onto affected area from a distance of approximately 6″ (15 cm) and apply for only 3 seconds.

ADVERSE REACTIONS

Skin: burning, itching, irritation, dryness, folliculitis, hypertrichosis, hypopigmentation, acneiform eruptions, perioral dermatitis, allergic contact dermatitis. With occlusive dressings: *maceration of skin, secondary infection, atrophy, striae, miliaria.*

INTERACTIONS

None significant.

NURSING CONSIDERATIONS

• Use cautiously in viral diseases of skin, such as varicella, vaccinia, herpes simplex; fungal infections; bacterial skin infections.
• Avoid application near eyes, mucous membranes, or in ear canal.
• Systemic absorption especially likely with occlusive dressings, pro-

---

Italicized adverse reactions are common or life-threatening.
*Liquid form contains alcohol.   **May contain tartrazine.

longed treatment, or extensive body-surface treatment.

• When used in young children, avoid the use of plastic pants or tight-fitting diapers in treated areas.

• Stop drug and notify doctor if patient develops signs of systemic absorption, skin irritation or ulceration, hypersensitivity, or infection. (If antifungals or antibiotics are being used with corticosteroids and infection does not respond immediately, corticosteroids should be stopped until infection is controlled.)

• Before applying, gently wash skin. To prevent damage to skin, rub medication in gently, leaving a thin coat. When treating hairy sites, part hair and apply directly to lesion.

• Aerosol preparation contains alcohol and may produce irritation or burning in open lesions. When using about the face, cover patient's eyes and warn against inhalation of the spray. To avoid freezing tissues, do not spray longer than 3 seconds or closer than 6″ (15 cm).

• Occlusive dressing (if ordered): Apply cream or ointment heavily, then cover with a thin, pliable, nonflammable plastic film; seal to adjacent normal skin with hypoallergenic tape. To minimize adverse reactions, use occlusive dressing intermittently. Don't leave in place longer than 16 hours each day.

• Change dressing as ordered by doctor. Inspect skin for infection, striae, and atrophy.

• Treatment should be continued for a few days after clearing of lesions to prevent recurrence.

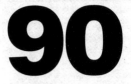
Local anesthetics

**bupivacaine hydrochloride
chloroprocaine hydrochloride
etidocaine hydrochloride
lidocaine hydrochloride
mepivacaine hydrochloride
procaine hydrochloride
tetracaine hydrochloride**

COMBINATION PRODUCTS
None, although epinephrine is added to some solutions to prolong effect.

---

bupivacaine hydrochloride
Marcain‡, Marcaine, Sensorcaine
Pregnancy Risk Category: C

HOW SUPPLIED
Injection: 0.25%, 0.5%, 0.75%; also available with epinephrine 1:200,000

MECHANISM OF ACTION
A local anesthetic of the amide type. Blocks depolarization by interfering with sodium-potassium exchange across the nerve cell membrane, preventing the nerve generation and conduction of the nerve impulse. When combined with epinephrine, action is prolonged.

INDICATIONS & DOSAGE
Dosages given are for drug without epinephrine.
Epidural:

Sol.	Vol. (ml)	Dose (mg)
0.25%	10 to 20	25 to 50
0.5%	10 to 20	50 to 100

Caudal:

Sol.	Vol. (ml)	Dose (mg)
0.25%	15 to 30	37.5 to 75
0.5%	15 to 30	75 to 150

Peripheral nerve block:

Sol.	Vol. (ml)	Dose (mg)
0.5%	5 to 80	25 to 400 (max.)

May repeat dose q 3 hours. Dosage and interval may be increased with epinephrine. Maximum 400 mg daily.

ADVERSE REACTIONS
Skin: dermatologic reactions.
Other: edema, status asthmaticus, *anaphylaxis,* anaphylactoid reactions.
The following systemic effects may result from high blood levels of the drug:
CNS: anxiety, nervousness, seizures followed by drowsiness, unconsciousness, tremors, twitches, shivering, *respiratory arrest.*
CV: myocardial depression, *arrhythmias, cardiac arrest.*
EENT: blurred vision, tinnitus.
GI: nausea, vomiting.

INTERACTIONS
Chloroprocaine: may lessen bupivacaine's action. Don't use together.
Enflurane, halothane, and related drugs: cardiac arrhythmias when used with bupivacaine *with* epinephrine. Use with extreme caution.
MAO inhibitors, cyclic antidepressants: severe, sustained hypertension when used with bupivacaine *with* epinephrine. Use with extreme caution.

NURSING CONSIDERATIONS
• Contraindicated in children under 12 years and for spinal, paracervical block, or topical anesthesia. Use cautiously in debilitated, elderly, or

---

Italicized adverse reactions are common or life-threatening.
*Liquid form contains alcohol.   **May contain tartrazine.

acutely ill patients; and in patients with severe hepatic disease or drug allergies.

• Although the 0.75% solution is still available, it is not to be used for obstetrical surgery. According to the FDA, lower concentrations are effective and much less hazardous.

• For epidural use, test doses are administered to verify needle or catheter placement. Initially, 2 to 3 ml is given to check for subarachnoid injection (which would cause extensive motor paralysis of the lower limbs and excessive sensory deficit). After about 5 minutes and in the absence of symptoms, a second, larger test dose of about 5 ml is given to check for intravascular injection (which would cause tinnitus, numbness around the lips, metallic taste, dysphoria, lethargy, or hypotension).

• Use solutions with epinephrine cautiously in cardiovascular disorders and in body areas with limited blood supply (ears, nose, fingers, toes).

• Keep resuscitative equipment and drugs available.

• Don't use solution with preservatives for caudal or epidural block.

• Onset in 4 to 17 minutes; duration is 3 to 6 hours.

• Discard partially used vials without preservatives.

• Check solution for particles.

chloroprocaine hydrochloride
Nesacaine, Nesacaine MPF

Pregnancy Risk Category: C

HOW SUPPLIED
Nesacaine
Injection (for infiltration and regional anesthesia): 1%, 2%
Nesacaine MPF
Injection (preservative-free, for caudal and epidural anesthesia): 2%, 3%

MECHANISM OF ACTION
A local anesthetic of the ester type. Blocks depolarization by interfering with sodium-potassium exchange across the nerve cell membrane, preventing generation and conduction of the nerve impulse.

INDICATIONS & DOSAGE
Infiltration and nerve block:
Adults: dosage limit is 11 mg/kg (14 mg/kg when used with epinephrine).

Sol.	Vol. (ml)	Dose (mg)
1%	3 to 20	30 to 200
2%	2 to 40	40 to 800

Caudal and epidural:

Sol.	Vol. (ml)	Dose (mg)
2% to 3%	15 to 25	300 to 750

May repeat with smaller doses q 40 to 50 minutes. Dose and interval may be increased with epinephrine. Maximum adult dosage is 800 mg, or 1 g when mixed with epinephrine.

ADVERSE REACTIONS
Skin: dermatologic reactions.
Other: edema, status asthmaticus, *anaphylaxis,* anaphylactoid reactions. The following systemic effects may result from high blood levels of the drug:
CNS: anxiety, nervousness, seizures followed by drowsiness, unconsciousness, tremors, twitches, shivering, *respiratory arrest.*
CV: myocardial depression, *arrhythmias, cardiac arrest.*
EENT: blurred vision, tinnitus.
GI: nausea, vomiting.

INTERACTIONS
None significant.

NURSING CONSIDERATIONS
• Contraindicated in hypersensitivity to procaine, tetracaine, or other para-aminobenzoic acid derivatives, and for spinal or topical anesthesia. Epidural and caudal blocks are contraindicated in CNS disease. Use cautiously in debilitated, elderly, or

---

acutely ill patients; in children; and in patients with drug allergies, paracervical block, or cardiovascular disease.
• For epidural use, test doses are administered to verify needle or catheter placement. Initially, 2 to 3 ml is given to check for subarachnoid injection (which would cause extensive motor paralysis of the lower limbs and excessive sensory deficit). After about 5 minutes and in the absence of symptoms, a second, larger test dose of about 5 ml is given to check for intravascular injection (which would cause tinnitus, numbness around the lips, metallic taste, dysphoria, lethargy, or hypotension).
• Repeat the test dose if patient is moved in a way that might displace the epidural catheter.
• At least 5 minutes should elapse after each test before proceeding further.
• Don't use solution with preservatives for caudal or epidural block.
• Don't use discolored solution.
• Keep resuscitative equipment and drugs available.
• Duration is 30 to 60 minutes.
• Discard partially used vials without preservatives.
• Check solution for particles.

etidocaine hydrochloride
Duranest

Pregnancy Risk Category: B

HOW SUPPLIED
Injection: 1%; also available with epinephrine 1:200,000 as a 1% or 1.5% solution

MECHANISM OF ACTION
A local anesthetic of the amide type. Blocks depolarization by interfering with sodium-potassium exchange across the nerve cell membrane, preventing generation and conduction of the nerve impulse. When combined with epinephrine, action is prolonged.

INDICATIONS & DOSAGE
Doses cited are for drug with epinephrine. Dose and interval are decreased without epinephrine.
Adults: Dose limit is 4 mg/kg or 300 mg per injection. When combined with epinephrine, dose limit is 5.5 mg/kg or 400 mg/injection.

Peripheral nerve block:

Sol.	Vol. (ml)	Dose (mg)
0.5%	5 to 40	25 to 200
1%	5 to 40	50 to 400

Central neural block:
Lower limbs, cesarean section, lumbar peridural

Sol.	Vol. (ml)	Dose (mg)
1%	10 to 30	100 to 300
1.5%	10 to 20	150 to 300

Vaginal:

Sol.	Vol. (ml)	Dose (mg)
1%	5 to 20	50 to 200

Caudal:

Sol.	Vol. (ml)	Dose (mg)
1%	10 to 30	100 to 300

ADVERSE REACTIONS
Skin: dermatologic reactions.
Other: edema, status asthmaticus, *anaphylaxis,* anaphylactoid reactions.
  The following systemic effects may result from high blood levels of the drug:
CNS: anxiety, apprehension, nervousness, seizures followed by drowsiness, unconsciousness, tremors, twitches, shivering, and *respiratory arrest.*
CV: myocardial depression, *arrhythmias, cardiac arrest.*
EENT: blurred vision, tinnitus.
GI: nausea, vomiting.

INTERACTIONS
Enflurane, halothane, and related drugs: cardiac arrhythmias when used with etidocaine *with* epinephrine. Use with extreme caution.
MAO inhibitors, cyclic antidepressants, phenothiazines: severe, sustained hypertension or hypotension when used with etidocaine solution

---

Italicized adverse reactions are common or life-threatening.
*Liquid form contains alcohol.   **May contain tartrazine.

with epinephrine. Use with extreme caution.

NURSING CONSIDERATIONS
• Contraindicated in inflammation or infection in puncture region, children under 14 years, septicemia, severe hypertension, spinal deformities, neurologic disorders, and spinal block. Use cautiously in debilitated, elderly, or acutely ill patients; severe shock; heart block; epidural block in obstetrics; general drug allergies; and hepatic and renal disease.
• For epidural use, test doses are administered to verify needle or catheter placement. Initially, 2 to 3 ml is given to check for subarachnoid injection (which would cause extensive motor paralysis of the lower limbs and excessive sensory deficit). After about 5 minutes and in the absence of symptoms, a second, larger test dose of about 5 ml is given to check for intravascular injection (which would cause tinnitus, numbness around the lips, metallic taste, dysphoria, lethargy, or hypotension).
• Use solutions with epinephrine cautiously in cardiovascular disease and in body areas with limited blood supply (ears, nose, fingers, toes).
• Don't use solution with preservatives for caudal or epidural block.
• Keep resuscitative equipment and drugs available.
• Onset in 2 to 8 minutes; duration is 3 to 6 hours.
• Check solution for particles.

---

lidocaine hydrochloride (lignocaine hydrochloride)
Caine-2, Dalcaine, Dilocaine, Duo-Trach Kit, Lidoject-2, Nervocaine 2%, Octocaine, Xylocaine

Pregnancy Risk Category: B

HOW SUPPLIED
Injection: 2%, 4%, 10%, 20%

Injection (with dextrose 7.5%): 1.5%, 5%
Injection (with epinephrine 1:50,000): 2% (for dental use)
Injection (with epinephrine 1:100,000): 1%, 2%
Injection (with epinephrine 1:200,000): 1%, 1.5%, 2%

MECHANISM OF ACTION
A local anesthetic of the amide type. Blocks depolarization by interfering with sodium-potassium exchange across the nerve cell membrane, preventing generation and conduction of the nerve impulse. When combined with epinephrine, action is prolonged.

INDICATIONS & DOSAGE
Doses cited are for drug without *epinephrine except where indicated.*
For anesthesia other than spinal—
maximum single adult dose is 4.5 mg/kg or 300 mg.
With epinephrine for anesthesia other than spinal—
maximum single adult dose is 7 mg/kg or 500 mg. Don't repeat dose more often than q 2 hours.
Caudal (obstetrics) *or epidural* (thoracic):

Sol.	Vol. (ml)	Dose (mg)
1%	20 to 30	200 to 300

Caudal (surgery):

Sol.	Vol. (ml)	Dose (mg)
1.5%	15 to 20	225 to 300

Epidural (lumbar anesthesia):

Sol.	Vol. (ml)	Dose (mg)
1.5%	15 to 20	225 to 300
2%	10 to 15	200 to 300

Maximum dose 200 to 300 mg/hour.
Spinal surgical anesthesia:

Sol.	Vol. (ml)	Dose (mg)
5% with 7.5% dextrose	1.5 to 2	75 to 100

Dosage and interval are increased with epinephrine.
For anesthesia other than spinal—
maximum single adult dose is 4.5 mg/kg or 300 mg.

With epinephrine for anesthesia other than spinal—
maximum single adult dose is 7 mg/kg or 500 mg. Don't repeat dose more often than q 2 hours.

ADVERSE REACTIONS
Skin: dermatologic reactions.
Other: edema, status asthmaticus, *anaphylaxis,* anaphylactoid reactions.
   The following systemic effects may result from high blood levels of the drug:
CNS: anxiety, nervousness, seizures followed by drowsiness, unconsciousness, tremors, twitches, shivering, *respiratory arrest.*
CV: myocardial depression, *arrhythmias, cardiac arrest.*
EENT: blurred vision, tinnitus.
GI: nausea, vomiting.

INTERACTIONS
Enflurane, halothane, and related drugs: cardiac arrhythmias when used with lidocaine *with* epinephrine. Use with extreme caution.
MAO inhibitors, cyclic antidepressants: severe, sustained hypertension when used with lidocaine *with* epinephrine. Use with extreme caution.

NURSING CONSIDERATIONS
• Contraindicated in inflammation or infection in puncture region, septicemia, severe hypertension, spinal deformities, and neurologic disorders. Use cautiously in debilitated, elderly, or acutely ill patients; severe shock; heart block; obstetrics; general drug allergies; and paracervical block.
• For epidural use, test doses are administered to verify needle or catheter placement. Initially, 2 to 3 ml is given to check for subarachnoid injection (which would cause extensive motor paralysis of the lower limbs and excessive sensory deficit). After 5 minutes and in the absence of symptoms, a second, larger test dose of about 5 ml is given to check for intra-

vascular injection (which would cause tinnitus, numbness around the lips, metallic taste, dysphoria, lethargy, or hypotension).
• Use solutions with epinephrine cautiously in cardiovascular disorders and in body areas with limited blood supply (ears, nose, fingers, toes).
• Keep resuscitative equipment and drugs available.
• Solutions containing preservatives should not be used for spinal, epidural, or caudal block.
• Discard partially used vials without preservatives.
• Check solution for particles.

mepivacaine hydrochloride
Carbocaine, Cavacaine, Isocaine
Pregnancy Risk Category: C

HOW SUPPLIED
Injection: 1%, 1.5%, 2%, 3% (dental injection); 2% injection also available with levonordefrin 1:200,000

MECHANISM OF ACTION
A local anesthetic of the amide type. Blocks depolarization by interfering with sodium-potassium exchange across the nerve cell membrane, preventing generation and conduction of the nerve impulse. When combined with levonordefrin, action is prolonged.

INDICATIONS & DOSAGE
Doses cited are for drug without levonordefrin.
Nerve block:

Sol.	Vol. (ml)	Dose (mg)
1%	5 to 20	50 to 200
2%	5 to 20	100 to 400

Transvaginal block or infiltration (maximum dose):

Sol.	Vol. (ml)	Dose (mg)
1%	40	400

Paracervical block (obstetrics):

Sol.	Vol. (ml)	Dose (mg)
1%	10	100

Italicized adverse reactions are common or life-threatening.
*Liquid form contains alcohol.   **May contain tartrazine.

Give on each side (200 mg total) per 90-minute period.

Caudal and epidural:

Sol.	Vol. (ml)	Dose (mg)
1%	15 to 30	150 to 300
1.5%	10 to 25	150 to 375
2%	10 to 20	200 to 400

Therapeutic block (pain management):

Sol.	Vol. (ml)	Dose (mg)
1%	1 to 5	10 to 50
2%	1 to 5	20 to 100

Adults: maximum single dose 7 mg/kg up to 550 mg. Don't repeat more often than q 90 minutes. Maximum dosage 1,000 mg daily.

Children: maximum dose 5 to 6 mg/kg. In children under 3 years or weighing less than 14 kg, use 0.5% or 1.5% solution only. Dose and interval may be increased with levonordefrin.

ADVERSE REACTIONS

Skin: dermatologic reactions.

Other: edema, status asthmaticus, *anaphylaxis,* anaphylactoid reactions.

The following systemic effects may result from high blood levels of the drug:

CNS: anxiety, nervousness, seizures followed by drowsiness, unconsciousness, tremors, twitches, shivering, *respiratory arrest.*

CV: myocardial depression, *arrhythmias, cardiac arrest.*

EENT: blurred vision, tinnitus.

GI: nausea, vomiting.

INTERACTIONS

Enflurane, halothane, and related drugs: cardiac arrhythmias when used with mepivacaine *with* levonordefrin. Use with extreme caution.

MAO inhibitors, cyclic antidepressants: severe, sustained hypertension when used with mepivacaine *with* levonordefrin. Use with extreme caution.

NURSING CONSIDERATIONS

• Contraindicated in sensitivity to methylparaben, in heart block, or for spinal anesthesia. Use cautiously in debilitated, elderly, or acutely ill patients, and for paracervical block.

• For epidural use, test doses are administered to verify needle or catheter placement. Initially, 2 to 3 ml is given to check for subarachnoid injection (which would cause extensive motor paralysis of the lower limbs and excessive sensory deficit). After about 5 minutes and in the absence of symptoms, a second, larger test dose of about 5 ml is given to check for intravascular injection (which would cause tinnitus, numbness around the lips, metallic taste, dysphoria, lethargy, or hypotension).

• Use solutions with levonordefrin cautiously in cardiovascular disease and in body areas with limited blood supply (ears, nose, fingers, toes).

• Monitor fetal heart rate when paracervical block is used in delivery.

• Keep resuscitative equipment and drugs available.

• Don't use solutions with preservatives for caudal or epidural block.

• Onset in 15 minutes; duration is 3 hours.

• Discard partially used vials without preservatives.

• Check solution for particles.

---

procaine hydrochloride
Novocain

Pregnancy Risk Category: C

HOW SUPPLIED
Injection: 1%, 2%, 10%

MECHANISM OF ACTION
A local anesthetic of the ester type. Blocks depolarization by interfering with sodium-potassium exchange across the nerve cell membrane, preventing generation and conduction of the nerve impulse.

INDICATIONS & DOSAGE

Spinal anesthesia—
Maximum dose is 11 mg/kg (14 mg/kg when mixed with epinephrine).

Before using, dilute 10% solution with 0.9% sodium chloride injection, sterile distilled water, or cerebrospinal fluid.

For hyperbaric technique, use dextrose solution.

Perineum: use 0.5 ml 10% solution and 0.5 ml diluent injected at fourth lumbar interspace.

Perineum and lower extremities: use 1 ml 10% solution and 1 ml diluent injected at third or fourth lumbar interspace.

Up to costal margin: use 2 ml 10% solution and 1 ml diluent injected at second, third, or fourth lumbar interspace.

Epidural block:

Sol.	Vol. (ml)	Dose (mg)
1.5%	25	375

Peripheral nerve block:

Sol.	Vol. (ml)	Dose (mg)
1%	50	500
2%	25	500

Infiltration: use 250 to 600 mg 0.25% to 0.5% solution. Maximum initial dose 1 g. Dose and interval may be increased with epinephrine. Maximum dosage 11 mg/kg to 14 mg/kg or epinephrine.

ADVERSE REACTIONS

Skin: dermatologic reactions.
Other: edema, status asthmaticus, *anaphylaxis,* anaphylactoid reactions.

The following systemic effects may result from high blood levels of the drug:

CNS: anxiety, nervousness, seizures followed by drowsiness, unconsciousness, tremors, twitches, shivering, *respiratory arrest.*
CV: myocardial depression, *arrhythmias, cardiac arrest.*
EENT: blurred vision, tinnitus.
GI: nausea, vomiting.

INTERACTIONS

Echothiophate iodide: reduced hydrolysis of procaine. Use together cautiously.

NURSING CONSIDERATIONS

• Contraindicated in traumatized urethra and in hypersensitivity to chloroprocaine, tetracaine, or other para-aminobenzoic acid derivatives. Use cautiously in hyperexcitable patients and in CNS diseases, infection at puncture site, shock, profound anemia, cachexia, sepsis, hypertension, hypotension, GI hemorrhage, bowel perforation or strangulation, peritonitis, cardiac decompensation, massive pleural effusions, and increased intraabdominal pressure.
• Contraindications in obstetric use are pelvic disproportion, placenta previa, abruptio placentae, floating fetal head, and intrauterine manipulation.
• Keep resuscitative equipment and drugs available.
• For epidural use, test doses are administered to verify needle or catheter placement. Initially, 2 to 3 ml is given to check for subarachnoid injection (which would cause extensive motor paralysis of the lower limbs and excessive sensory deficit). After about 5 minutes and in the absence of symptoms, a second, larger test dose of about 5 ml is given to check for intravascular injection (which would cause tinnitus, numbness around the lips, metallic taste, dysphoria, lethargy, or hypotension).
• Use solution without preservatives for epidural block.
• Onset in 2 to 5 minutes; duration 60 minutes.
• Discard partially used vials without preservatives.
• Check solution for particles.

Italicized adverse reactions are common or life-threatening.
*Liquid form contains alcohol. **May contain tartrazine.

tetracaine hydrochloride
Pontocaine

Pregnancy Risk Category: C

HOW SUPPLIED
Injection: 1%
Injection (with dextrose, 6%): 0.2%, 0.3%
Powder for reconstitution: 20 mg/ampule

MECHANISM OF ACTION
A local anesthetic of the ester type. Blocks depolarization by interfering with sodium-potassium exchange across the nerve cell membrane, preventing generation and conduction of the nerve impulse.

INDICATIONS & DOSAGE
Low spinal (saddle block) in vaginal delivery—
give 2 to 5 mg as hyperbaric solution (in 10% dextrose).
Perineum and lower extremities: give 5 to 10 mg.
Up to costal margin: give 15 to 20 mg.

ADVERSE REACTIONS
Skin: dermatologic reactions.
Other: edema, status asthmaticus, *anaphylaxis,* anaphylactoid reactions.
The following systemic effects may result from high blood levels of the drug:
CNS: anxiety, nervousness, seizures followed by drowsiness, unconsciousness, tremors, twitches, shivering, and *respiratory arrest*.
CV: myocardial depression, *arrhythmias, cardiac arrest*.
EENT: blurred vision, tinnitus.
GI: nausea, vomiting.

INTERACTIONS
None significant.

NURSING CONSIDERATIONS
• Contraindicated in infection at injection site, serious CNS diseases, and in hypersensitivity to procaine, chloroprocaine, tetracaine, or other para-aminobenzoic acid derivatives. Use cautiously in shock, profound anemia, cachexia, hypertension, hypotension, peritonitis, cardiac decompensation, massive pleural effusion, increased intracranial pressure, infection, and in highly nervous patients.
• Saddle block contraindicated in cephalopelvic disproportion, placenta previa, abruptio placentae, intrauterine manipulation, and floating fetal head.
• Don't use cloudy, discolored, or crystallized solutions.
• Keep resuscitative equipment and drugs available.
• 10 times as strong as procaine hydrochloride.
• Onset in 15 minutes; duration up to 3 hours.
• When cerebrospinal fluid is added to powdered drug or drug solution during spinal anesthesia, solution may be cloudy.
• Protect from light; store in refrigerator.

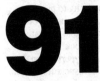

General anesthetics

droperidol
etomidate
fentanyl citrate with droperidol
ketamine hydrochloride
methohexital sodium
propofol
thiopental sodium

COMBINATION PRODUCTS
None.

droperidol
Droleptan‡, Inapsine
Pregnancy Risk Category: C

HOW SUPPLIED
Tablets: 10 mg‡
Oral solution: 1 mg/ml‡
Injection: 2.5 mg/ml, 5 mg/ml‡

MECHANISM OF ACTION
Acts at subcortical levels to produce sedation.

INDICATIONS & DOSAGE
Premedication—
Adults: 2.5 to 10 mg (1 to 4 ml) I.M. 30 to 60 minutes preoperatively.
Children 2 to 12 years: 1 to 1.5 mg (0.4 to 0.6 ml)/20 to 25 lb body weight I.M.
As an induction agent—
Adults: 2.5 mg (1 ml)/20 to 25 lb body weight I.V. with analgesic and/ or general anesthetic.
Children 2 to 12 years: 1 to 1.5 mg (0.4 to 0.6 ml)/20 to 25 lb I.V. Dosage should be titrated.
Elderly and debilitated patients: initial dose should be decreased.

Maintenance dosage in general anesthesia—
Adults: 1.25 to 2.5 mg (0.5 to 1 ml) I.V.
To suppress nystagmus, nausea, vomiting, and vertigo associated with an acute attack of Meniere's disease—
Adults: 5 mg I.M. as a single dose.
Management of severe agitation of psychotic disorders‡—
Adults: 10 to 25 mg P.O. daily in divided doses.

ADVERSE REACTIONS
Blood: *agranulocytosis.*
CNS: extrapyramidal reactions (dystonia, akathisia), upward rotation of eyes and oculogyric crises, extended neck, flexed arms, fine tremor of limbs, dizziness, chills or shivering, facial sweating, restlessness, decreased seizure threshold.
CV: *hypotension,* tachycardia.
Respiratory: *laryngospasm, bronchospasm.*

INTERACTIONS
None significant.

NURSING CONSIDERATIONS
• Use cautiously in elderly or debilitated patients and in patients with hypotension or other cardiovascular disease, impaired hepatic or renal function, and Parkinson's disease.
• Watch for extrapyramidal reactions. Call doctor at once if any occur.
• Droperidol has been used as an I.V. antiemetic in cancer chemotherapy.
• A butyrophenone compound, related to haloperiodol; has greater ten-

---

Italicized adverse reactions are common or life-threatening.
*Liquid form contains alcohol.   **May contain tartrazine.

dency to cause extrapyramidal reactions than other antipsychotics.
• Keep I.V. fluids and vasopressors available for treatment of hypotension.
• Monitor vital signs frequently; notify doctor of any changes immediately.
• Give I.V. injections slowly.
• Do not place patient in Trendelenburg's position (that is, shock position); severe hypotension and deeper anesthesia may result, causing respiratory arrest.

etomidate
Amidate, Hypnomidate
Pregnancy Risk Category: C

HOW SUPPLIED
Injection: 2 mg/ml

MECHANISM OF ACTION
Inhibits the firing rate of neurons within the ascending reticular-activating system.

INDICATIONS & DOSAGE
Induction of general anesthesia—
Adults and children over 10 years:
0.2 to 0.6 mg/kg I.V. over a period of 30 to 60 seconds.

ADVERSE REACTIONS
CNS: *myoclonic movements, averting movements, tonic movements, transient apnea, hyperventilation, hypoventilation.*
CV: hypertension, hypotension, tachycardia, bradycardia.
EENT: *eye movements,* laryngospasms.
GI: nausea or vomiting following induction of anesthesia.
Skin: inhibition of adrenal steroid production.
Local: *transient venous pain.*
Other: hiccups, snoring.

INTERACTIONS
None significant.

NURSING CONSIDERATIONS
• Should not be used during labor and delivery, including cesarean sections.
• Smaller increments of I.V. etomidate may be administered to adults during short operations to supplement subpotent anesthetic agents, such as nitrous oxide.
• Other commonly used preanesthesia drugs may be given before etomidate is used.
• Etomidate has a rapid onset of action (about 1 minute). Duration of effect is short (3 to 5 minutes).
• Transient muscle movements can be decreased by first administering 0.1 mg of fentanyl.
• Muscle movements seem more common in patients who feel transient venous pain after injection.
• Monitor vital signs before, during, and after anesthesia.
• Have resuscitative equipment and drugs ready. Maintain airway.
• Corticosteroid supplementation may be ordered to counteract reported inhibition of adrenal steroid production.
• Etomidate has a much lower incidence of cardiovascular and respiratory effects; therefore, it is advantageous for inducing anesthesia in high-risk surgical patients.

fentanyl citrate with droperidol
Innovar
Controlled Substance Schedule II
Pregnancy Risk Category: C

HOW SUPPLIED
Injection: 0.5 mg fentanyl and 2.5 mg droperidol per ml

MECHANISM OF ACTION
Acts as a CNS depressant to produce a

---

general calming effect, reduced motor activity, and analgesia.

INDICATIONS & DOSAGE

Dosages vary depending on application; use of other agents; and patient's age, body weight, and clinical status. *Anesthesia*—

Adults:

Premedication—0.5 to 2 ml I.M. 45 to 60 minutes before surgery.

Adjunct to general anesthesia—Induction: 1 ml/20 to 25 lb body weight by slow I.V. to produce neuroleptanalgesia.

   Maintenance: not indicated as sole agent for maintenance of surgical anesthesia. Used in combination with other agents. To prevent excessive accumulation of the relatively long-acting droperidol component, fentanyl alone should be used in increments of 0.025 to 0.05 mg (0.5 to 1 ml) for maintenance of analgesia. However, during prolonged surgery, additional 0.5- to 1-ml amounts of Innovar may be given with caution.

Diagnostic procedures—0.5 to 2 ml I.M. 45 to 60 minutes before procedure. In prolonged procedure, give 0.5 to 1 ml I.V. with caution and without a general anesthetic.

Adjunct in regional anesthesia—1 to 2 ml I.M. or slow I.V.

Children:

Premedication—0.25 ml/20 lb body weight I.M. 45 to 60 minutes before surgery.

Adjunct to general anesthesia—0.5 ml/20 lb body weight I.V. (total combined dose for induction and maintenance). Following induction with Innovar, fentanyl alone in a dose of ¼ to ⅓ of adult dosage should be used to avoid accumulation of droperidol. However, during prolonged surgery, additional amounts of Innovar may be administered with caution. Safety of use in children under 2 years has not been established.

ADVERSE REACTIONS

CNS: emergence delirium and hallucinations, postoperative drowsiness.

CV: vasodilation, *hypotension*, decreased pulmonary arterial pressure, bradycardia, tachycardia.

EENT: blurred vision, *laryngospasms*.

GI: *nausea, vomiting*.

Respiratory: *respiratory depression, apnea*, or *arrest*.

Other: drug dependence, muscle rigidity, chills, *shivering*, diaphoresis.

INTERACTIONS

CNS depressants (such as barbiturates, tranquilizers, narcotics, and general anesthetics): additive or potentiating effect. Dosage should be reduced.

MAO inhibitors: severe and unpredictable potentiation of Innovar. Do not use together or within 2 weeks of MAO inhibitor therapy.

NURSING CONSIDERATIONS

• Contraindicated in intolerance to either component. Use with caution in patients with head injuries and increased intracranial pressure, chronic obstructive pulmonary disease, hepatic and renal dysfunction, bradyarrhythmias, and in elderly or debilitated patients.

• Hypotension is a common adverse reaction. However, if blood pressure drops, also consider hypovolemia as a possible cause. Use appropriate parenteral fluids to help restore blood pressure.

• Vital signs should be monitored frequently.

• Be aware that respiratory depression, rigidity of respiratory muscles, and respiratory arrest can occur. Have narcotic antagonist and resuscitative equipment available.

• Maintain airway.

• Postoperative EEG pattern may return to normal slowly.

• If narcotic analgesics are required

Italicized adverse reactions are common or life-threatening.
*Liquid form contains alcohol.   **May contain tartrazine.

postoperatively, use initially in reduced doses, as low as ¼ to ⅓ those usually recommended.

• When Innovar is given for anesthesia induction, fentanyl (Sublimaze) should be used for maintenance analgesia during procedure.

• Premedication with Innovar has sometimes been associated with patient agitation and refusal of surgery. Administration of diazepam may relieve this.

ketamine hydrochloride
Ketalar

Pregnancy Risk Category: C

HOW SUPPLIED
Injection: 10 mg/ml, 50 mg/ml, 100 mg/ml

MECHANISM OF ACTION
Interrupts association pathways in the brain, causing dissociative anesthesia, a feeling of dissociation from the environment.

INDICATIONS & DOSAGE
Induce anesthesia for procedures, especially short-term diagnostic or surgical, not requiring skeletal muscle relaxation; before giving other general anesthetics or to supplement low-potency agents, such as nitrous oxide—

Adults and children: 1 to 4.5 mg/kg I.V., administered over 60 seconds; or 6.5 to 13 mg/kg I.M. To maintain anesthesia, repeat in increments of half to full initial dose.

ADVERSE REACTIONS
CNS: *tonic and clonic movements resembling seizures, respiratory depression, apnea when administered too rapidly.*
CV: *increased blood pressure and pulse rate,* hypotension, bradycardia.
EENT: diplopia, nystagmus, slight increase in intraocular pressure, *laryngospasms, salivation.*
GI: mild anorexia, nausea, vomiting.
Skin: transient erythema, measles-like rash.
Other: *dream-like states, hallucinations, confusion, excitement,* irrational behavior, psychic abnormalities.

INTERACTIONS
Thyroid hormones: may elevate blood pressure and cause tachycardia. Give cautiously.

NURSING CONSIDERATIONS
• Contraindicated in patients with history of CVA; patients who would be endangered by a significant rise in blood pressure; and in severe hypertension, severe cardiac decompensation, or surgery of the pharynx, larynx, or bronchial tree (unless used with muscle relaxants). Use with caution in chronic alcoholism, alcohol-intoxicated patients, and in patients with cerebrospinal fluid pressure elevated before anesthesia.

• Because of rapid induction, patient should be physically supported during administration.

• Do not inject barbiturates and ketamine from same syringe, as they are chemically incompatible.

• Monitor vital signs before, during, and after anesthesia.

• Check cardiac function in patients with hypertension or cardiac depression.

• Maintain airway.

• Resuscitative equipment should be available and ready for use.

• Start supportive respiration if respiratory depression occurs. Use mechanical support if possible rather than administering analeptics.

• Keep verbal, tactile, and visual stimulation at a minimum during recovery phase to reduce incidence of emergent reactions.

• Hallucinations and excitement can

occur on emergence from anesthesia; they can be abated by administering diazepam.

• A potent hallucinogen that can readily produce dissociative anesthesia (patient feels detached from environment). Dissociative effect and hallucinatory adverse reactions have made this a popular drug of abuse among young people.

---

methohexital sodium (methohexitone sodium)

Brevital Sodium, Brietal Sodium†‡
Controlled Substance Schedule IV

Pregnancy Risk Category: D

HOW SUPPLIED
Powder for injection: 500 mg, 2.5 g, 5 g

MECHANISM OF ACTION
Inhibits the firing rate of neurons within the ascending reticular-activating system.

INDICATIONS & DOSAGE
General anesthetic for short-term procedures (oral surgery, gynecologic and genitourinary examinations); reduction of fractures; before electroconvulsive therapy; for prolonged anesthesia when used with gaseous anesthetics—
Adults and children: 5 to 12 ml 1% solution (50 to 120 mg) I.V. at 1 ml/5 seconds. Dose required for induction may vary from 50 to 120 mg or more; average about 70 mg. Induction dose provides anesthesia for 5 to 7 minutes.
Maintenance—
Intermittent injection: 2 to 4 ml 1% solution (20 to 40 mg) q 4 to 7 minutes.
Continuous I.V. drip: administer 0.2% solution (1 drop/second).

ADVERSE REACTIONS
CNS: *muscular twitching,* headache, emergence delirium.
CV: *transient hypotension, tachycardia,* circulatory depression, *peripheral vascular collapse.*
GI: excessive salivation, *nausea, vomiting.*
Respiratory: *laryngospasm, bronchospasm, respiratory depression, apnea.*
Skin: tissue necrosis with extravasation.
Local: thrombophlebitis, pain at injection site, injury to nerves adjacent to injection site.
Other: hiccups, coughing, acute allergic reactions. Extended use may cause cumulative effect.

INTERACTIONS
None significant.

NURSING CONSIDERATIONS
• Contraindicated in severe hepatic dysfunction, hypersensitivity to barbiturates, or porphyria; in shock or impending shock; and in patients for whom general anesthetics would be hazardous. Use with caution in debilitated patients; in asthma, respiratory obstruction, severe hypertension or hypotension, myocardial disease, CHF, severe anemia, and extreme obesity.
• Maintain pulmonary ventilation.
• Avoid extravascular or intraarterial injections.
• Monitor vital signs before, during, and after anesthesia.
• Have resuscitative equipment and drugs ready.
• Reduce postoperative nausea by having patient fast before administration.
• Incompatible with silicone; avoid contact with rubber stoppers or parts of syringes that have been treated with silicone.
• Incompatible with lactated Ringer's solution.

Italicized adverse reactions are common or life-threatening.
*Liquid form contains alcohol.   **May contain tartrazine.

- Do not mix with acid solutions, such as atropine sulfate.
- Solvents recommended are 5% dextrose solution or normal saline solution instead of distilled water.
- Rate of flow must be individualized for each patient.
- Solutions may be stored and used as long as they remain clear and colorless. Solutions cannot be heated for sterilization.
- Has potential for abuse.

propofol
Diprivan

Pregnancy Risk Category: D

HOW SUPPLIED
Injection: 10 mg/ml in 20-ml ampules

MECHANISM OF ACTION
Propofol produces a dose-dependent CNS depression similar to benzodiazepines and barbiturates. However, it can be used to maintain anesthesia through careful titration of infusion rate.

INDICATIONS & DOSAGE
Induction of anesthesia—
Adults: doses must be individualized according to patient's condition and age. Most patients classified as American Society of Anesthesiologists (ASA) Physical Status category (PS) I or II under 55 years require 2 to 2.5 mg/kg I.V. The drug is usually administered in 40-mg boluses q 10 seconds until the desired response is obtained.

Elderly, debilitated, or hypovolemic patients, or patients in ASA PS III or IV should receive half of the usual induction dose (20 mg-boluses q 10 seconds).
Maintenance of anesthesia—
Adults: propofol may be given as a variable rate infusion, titrated to clinical effect. Most patients may be maintained with 0.1 to 0.2 mg/kg/minute (6 to 12 mg/kg/hr).

Elderly, debilitated, or hypovolemic patients, or patients in ASA PS III or IV should receive half of the usual maintenance dose (0.05 to 0.1 mg/kg/minute, or 3 to 6 mg/kg/hr).

ADVERSE REACTIONS
CNS: headache, dizziness, twitching, clonic/myoclonic movement.
CV: hypotension, bradycardia, hypertension.
GI: nausea, vomiting, abdominal cramping.
Respiratory: apnea, cough.
Skin: flushing.
Local: burning/stinging, pain, tingling or numbness, and coldness at injection site.
Other: fever, hiccups.

INTERACTIONS
Inhalational anesthetics (such as enflurane, isoflurane, and halothane) or supplemental anesthetics (such as nitrous oxide and opiates): may be expected to enhance the anesthetic and cardiovascular actions of propofol.
Opiate analgesics, sedatives: may cause a more pronounced decrease of systolic, diastolic, and mean arterial pressure and of cardiac output; may also decrease the induction dose requirements.

NURSING CONSIDERATIONS
- Contraindicated in patients hypersensitive to propofol or any components of the emulsion, including soybean oil, egg lecithin, and glycerol. Because the drug is administered as an emulsion, administer with caution to patients with a history of disorders of lipid metabolism, such as pancreatitis or primary hyperlipoproteinemia, and in patients with diabetic hyperlipidemia. Use cautiously in patients who are elderly or debilitated and in patients with circulatory disorders. Although the hemodynamic effects of the drug can vary, its major effect in patients maintaining sponta-

neous ventilation is arterial hypotension (arterial pressure can decrease as much as 30%) with little or no change in heart rate and cardiac output. Cardiac output may be markedly depressed in patients undergoing assisted or controlled positive-pressure ventilation.

• Propofol is not recommended for use in obstetric anesthesia because the safety to the fetus has not been established. It is not recommended for use in patients with increased intracranial pressure or impaired cerebral circulation because the drug's effect in reducing systemic arterial pressure may substantially reduce cerebral perfusion pressure.

• Propofol should be administered under direct medical supervision by persons familiar with airway management and the administration of I.V. anesthetics.

• Patients should be closely monitored for signs of significant hypotension or bradycardia. Treatment of such effects may include increased rate of fluid administration, pressor agents, elevation of lower extremities, or atropine. Apnea, which may occur during induction, may persist for longer than 60 seconds and require ventilatory support.

• Pharmacokinetics of propofol are not altered by chronic hepatic cirrhosis, chronic renal failure, or gender.

• Propofol has no vagolytic activity. Premedication with anticholinergics such as glycopyrrolate or atropine may help manage potential increases in vagal tone caused by other drugs or surgical manipulations.

• Propofol should not be mixed with other drugs or blood products. If it is to be diluted before infusion, use only 5% dextrose in water, and do not dilute to a concentration less than 2 mg/ml. After dilution, it appears to be more stable in glass containers as compared to plastic.

• When administered into a running

I.V. catheter, propofol emulsion is compatible with 5% dextrose in water, lactated Ringer's injection, lactated Ringer's and 5% dextrose injection, 5% dextrose and 0.45% sodium chloride injection, and 5% dextrose and 0.2% sodium chloride injection.

• Propofol emulsion should be stored above 40° F. (4° C.) and below 72° F. (22° C.). Refrigeration is not recommended.

• Propofol is excreted in breast milk and is not recommended for use by breast-feeding mothers.

thiopental sodium (thiopentone sodium)
Intraval Sodium‡, Pentothal Sodium
Controlled Substance Schedule III
Pregnancy Risk Category: C

HOW SUPPLIED
Injection: 250-mg, 400-mg, 500-mg syringes; 500-mg/1-g vial with diluent; 1-g (2.5%), 2.5-g (2.5%), 5-g (2.5%), 2.5-g (2%), and 5-g (2%) kits
Rectal suspension: 2-g disposable syringe (400 mg/g of suspension)

MECHANISM OF ACTION
Inhibits the firing rate of neurons within the ascending reticular-activating system.

INDICATIONS & DOSAGE
Induce anesthesia before administering other anesthetics—
Adults: 210 to 280 mg (3 to 4 ml/kg) usually required for average adult (70 kg).
General anesthetic for short-term procedures—
Adults: 2 to 3 ml 2.5% solution (50 to 75 mg) administered I.V. only at intervals of 20 to 40 seconds, depending on reaction. Dose may be repeated with caution, if necessary.
Seizures following anesthesia—

Italicized adverse reactions are common or life-threatening.
*Liquid form contains alcohol.   **May contain tartrazine.

Adults: 75 to 125 mg (3 to 5 ml of 2.5% solution) immediately.
Psychiatric disorders (narcoanalysis, narcosynthesis)—
Adults: 100 mg/minute (4 ml/minute 2.5% solution) until confusion occurs and before sleep.
Basal anesthesia by rectal administration—
Adults and children: administer up to 1 g/22.5 kg (50 lb) body weight, or 0.5 ml 10% solution/kg body weight. Maximum 1 to 1.5 g (children weighing 34 kg or more) and 3 to 4 g (adults weighing 91 kg or more).
  Note: Thiopental is rarely administered rectally for basal sedation or anesthesia because of variable absorption from the rectum.

ADVERSE REACTIONS
CNS: *prolonged somnolence,* retrograde amnesia.
CV: *myocardial depression, arrhythmias.*
Skin: tissue necrosis with extravasation.
Respiratory: *respiratory depression (momentary apnea following each injection is typical), bronchospasm, laryngospasm.*
Local: pain at injection site.
Other: sneezing, coughing, *shivering.*

INTERACTIONS
None significant.

NURSING CONSIDERATIONS
• Contraindicated in absence of suitable veins for I.V. administration, hypersensitivity to barbiturates, status asthmaticus, porphyria, respiratory depression or obstruction, decompensated cardiac disease, severe anemia, hepatic cirrhosis, shock, renal dysfunction, myxedema.
• Give test dose (1 to 3 ml 2.5% solution) to assess reaction to drug.
• When used as general anesthetic, give atropine sulfate as premedication to diminish laryngeal reflexes and to prevent laryngeal spasm.
• Have resuscitative equipment and oxygen available. Maintain airway.
• Avoid extravasation.
• Monitor vital signs before, during, and after anesthesia.
• Solutions of atropine sulfate, d-tubocurarine, or succinylcholine may be given concurrently.
• Do not heat solutions for sterilization. Solutions should be used within 24 hours.
• Has potential for abuse.

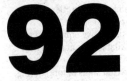

Vitamins and minerals

COMBINATION PRODUCTS
B complex vitamins◇
B complex vitamins with iron◇
B complex with vitamin C◇
B vitamin combinations◇
Calcium and vitamin products◇
Fluoride with vitamins◇
Geriatric supplements with multivitamins and minerals◇
Miscellaneous vitamins and minerals◇
Multivitamins◇
Multivitamins and minerals with hormones◇
Multivitamins with B₁₂◇
Vitamin A and D combinations◇

vitamin A (retinol)
Acon, Aquasol A

Pregnancy Risk Category: A (X if > RDA)

HOW SUPPLIED
Tablets: 10,000 IU
Capsules: 10,000 IU◇, 25,000 IU, 50,000 IU
Drops: 30 ml with dropper (5,000 IU/0.1 ml)
Injection: 2-ml vials (5,000 IU/ml with 0.5% chlorobutanol, polysorbate 80, butylated hydroxyanisol, and butylated hydroxytoluene)

MECHANISM OF ACTION
Coenzyme necessary for retinal function, bone growth, and differentiation of epithelial tissues.

INDICATIONS & DOSAGE
Recommended daily allowance (RDA)—
Neonates and infants to 6 months: 2,100 IU
Infants 6 months to 1 year: 2,000 IU
Children over 1 year to 3 years: 2,000 IU
Children 4 to 6 years: 2,500 IU
Children 7 to 10 years: 3,500 IU

Italicized adverse reactions are common or life-threatening.
*Liquid form contains alcohol.   **May contain tartrazine.

Males over 11 years: 5,000 IU
Females over 11 years: 4,000 IU
Pregnant women: 5,000 IU
Lactating women: 6,000 IU
Severe vitamin A deficiency with xerophthalmia—
Adults and children over 8 years: 500,000 IU P.O. daily for 3 days, then 50,000 IU P.O. daily for 14 days, then maintenance with 10,000 to 20,000 IU P.O. daily for 2 months, followed by adequate dietary nutrition and RDA vitamin A supplements.
Severe vitamin A deficiency—
Adults and children over 8 years: 100,000 IU P.O. or I.M. daily for 3 days, then 50,000 IU P.O. or I.M. daily for 14 days, then maintenance with 10,000 to 20,000 IU P.O. daily for 2 months, followed by adequate dietary nutrition and RDA vitamin A supplements.
Children 1 to 8 years: 17,500 to 35,000 IU I.M. daily for 10 days.
Infants under 1 year: 7,500 to 15,000 IU I.M. daily for 10 days.
Maintenance only—
Children 4 to 8 years: 15,000 IU I.M. daily for 2 months, then adequate dietary nutrition and RDA vitamin A supplements.
Children under 4 years: 10,000 IU I.M. daily for 2 months, then adequate dietary nutrition and RDA vitamin A supplements.

ADVERSE REACTIONS
Adverse effects are usually seen only with toxicity (hypervitaminosis A).
Blood: hypoplastic anemia, leukopenia.
CNS: irritability, headache, increased intracranial pressure, fatigue, lethargy, malaise.
EENT: miosis, papilledema, exophthalmos.
GI: anorexia, epigastric pain, diarrhea.
GU: hypomenorrhea.
Hepatic: jaundice, hepatomegaly.
Skin: alopecia; drying, cracking, scaling of skin; pruritus; lip fissures; massive desquamation; increased pigmentation; night sweating.
Other: skeletal—slow growth, decalcification of bone, fractures, hyperostosis, painful periostitis, premature closure of epiphyses, migratory arthralgia, cortical thickening over the radius and tibia, bulging fontanelles; splenomegaly.

INTERACTIONS
Mineral oil, cholestyramine resin: reduced GI absorption of fat-soluble vitamins. If needed, give mineral oil at bedtime.

NURSING CONSIDERATIONS
• Oral administration contraindicated in malabsorption syndrome; if malabsorption is from inadequate bile secretion, oral route may be used with concurrent administration of bile salts (dehydrocholic acid). Also contraindicated in hypervitaminosis A. I.V. administration contraindicated except for special water-miscible forms intended for infusion with large parenteral volumes. I.V. push of vitamin A of any type is also contraindicated (anaphylaxis or anaphylactoid reactions and death have resulted).
• Evaluate patient's vitamin A intake from fortified foods, dietary supplements, self-administered drugs, and prescription drug sources.
• In pregnant women, avoid doses exceeding RDA.
• To avoid toxicity, discourage patient self-administration of megavitamin doses without specific indications. Also stress that the patient should not share prescribed vitamins with family members or others. If family member feels vitamin therapy may be of value, have him contact his doctor.
• Watch for adverse reactions if dosage is high.
• Acute toxicity has resulted from single doses of 25,000 IU/kg of body weight; 350,000 IU in infants and

over 2,000,000 IU in adults have also proved acutely toxic.

• Chronic toxicity in infants (3 to 6 months) has resulted from doses of 18,500 IU daily for 1 to 3 months. In adults, chronic toxicity has resulted from doses of 50,000 IU daily for over 8 months; 500,000 IU daily for 2 months, and 1,000,000 IU daily for 3 days.

• Monitor patient closely during vitamin A therapy for skin disorders since high dosages may induce chronic toxicity.

• Liquid preparations available if nasogastric administration is necessary. May be mixed with cereal or fruit juice.

• Record eating and bowel habits. Report abnormalities to doctor.

• Adequate vitamin A absorption requires suitable protein intake, bile (give supplemental salts if necessary), concurrent RDA doses of vitamin E, and zinc (multivitamins usually supply zinc, but supplements may be necessary in long-term total parenteral nutrition).

• Absorption is fastest and most complete with water-miscible preparations, intermediate with emulsions, and slowest with oil suspensions.

• In severe hepatic dysfunction, diabetes, and hypothyroidism, use vitamin A rather than carotenes for vitamin therapy because the vitamin itself is more easily absorbed and the diseases adversely affect conversion of carotenes into vitamin A. If carotenes are prescribed, dosage should be doubled.

• Because of the potential for additive toxicity, vitamin supplements containing vitamin A should be used cautiously in patients taking isotretinoin (Accutane).

• Protect from light and heat.

cyanocobalamin (vitamin B$_{12}$)

Anacobin†, Bedoce, Bedoz†, Betalin 12, Bioglan B$_{12}$ Plus‡, Crystamine, Cyanabin†, Cyanocobalamin, Cyano-Gel, Dodex, Kaybovite, Poyamin, Redisol, Rubesol-1000, Rubion†, Rubramin, Sigamine

hydroxocobalamin (vitamin B$_{12a}$)

Alpha-Ruvite, Codroxomin, Droxomin, Rubesol-L.A.

Pregnancy Risk Category: A (C if > RDA)

HOW SUPPLIED
Tablets: 25 mcg◊, 50 mcg◊, 100 mcg◊, 250 mcg◊, 500 mcg, 1,000 mcg
Injection: 30-ml vials (30 mcg/ml, 100 mcg/ml, 120 mcg/ml with benzyl alcohol, 1,000 mcg/ml, 1,000 mcg/ml with benzyl alcohol), 10-ml vials (100 mcg/ml, 100 mcg/ml with benzyl alcohol, 1,000 mcg/ml, 1,000 mcg/ml with benzyl alcohol, 1,000 mcg/ml with methyl and propyl parabens), 5-ml vials (1,000 mcg/ml with benzyl alcohol), 1-ml vials (1,000 mcg/ml with benzyl alcohol), 1-ml unimatic (1,000 mcg/ml with benzyl alcohol)

MECHANISM OF ACTION
Coenzyme for various metabolic functions. Necessary for cell replication and hematopoiesis.

INDICATIONS & DOSAGE
Recommended daily allowance (RDA) for cyanocobalamin—
Neonates and infants to 6 months: 0.5 mcg
Infants 6 months to 1 year: 1.5 mcg
Children over 1 year to 3 years: 2 mcg
Children 4 to 6 years: 2.5 mcg

Italicized adverse reactions are common or life-threatening.
*Liquid form contains alcohol.   **May contain tartrazine.

Adults and children 7 years and over: 3 mcg

Pregnant and lactating women: 4 mcg

Vitamin B_{12} deficiency caused by inadequate diet, subtotal gastrectomy, or any other condition, disorder, or disease except malabsorption related to pernicious anemia or other GI disease—

Adults: 25 mcg P.O. daily as dietary supplement, or 30 to 100 mcg S.C. or I.M. daily for 5 to 10 days, depending on severity of deficiency. Maintenance dosage is 100 to 200 mcg I.M. once monthly. For subsequent prophylaxis, advise adequate nutrition and daily RDA vitamin B_{12} supplements.

Children: 30 to 100 mcg S.C. or I.M. daily for 5 to 10 days, depending on severity of deficiency. Maintenance dosage is at least 60 mcg/month I.M. or S.C. For subsequent prophylaxis, advise adequate nutrition and daily RDA vitamin B_{12} supplements.

Pernicious anemia or vitamin B_{12} malabsorption—

Adults: initially, 100 to 1,000 mcg I.M. daily for 2 weeks, then 100 to 1,000 mcg I.M. once monthly for life. If neurologic complications are present, follow initial therapy with 100 to 1,000 mcg I.M. once q 2 weeks before starting monthly regimen.

Children: 1,000 to 5,000 mcg I.M. or S.C. given over 2 or more weeks in 100-mcg increments; then 60 mcg I.M. or S.C. monthly for life.

Methylmalonic aciduria—

Neonates: 1,000 mcg I.M. daily for 11 days with a protein-restricted diet.

Schilling test flushing dose—

Adults and children: 1,000 mcg I.M. in a single dose.

ADVERSE REACTIONS

CV: peripheral vascular thrombosis.
GI: transient diarrhea.
Skin: itching, transitory exanthema, urticaria.

Local: pain, burning at S.C. or I.M. injection sites.
Other: *anaphylaxis,* anaphylactoid reactions with parenteral administration.

INTERACTIONS

Neomycin, colchicine, para-aminosalicylic acid and salts, chloramphenicol: malabsorption of vitamin B_{12}. Don't use together.

NURSING CONSIDERATIONS

• Parenteral administration contraindicated in hypersensitivity to vitamin B_{12} or cobalt. Alternate use of large oral doses of vitamin B_{12} is controversial and should not be considered routine; combined with intrinsic factor increases risk of hypersensitive reactions and should be avoided. Therapeutic dosage contraindicated before proper diagnosis; vitamin B_{12} therapy may mask folate deficiency.

• Use cautiously in anemic patients with coexisting cardiac, pulmonary, or hypertensive disease; in early Leber's disease; in severe vitamin B_{12}–dependent deficiencies, especially those receiving cardiotonic glycosides (monitor closely the first 2 to 3 days for hypokalemia, fluid overload, pulmonary edema, CHF, and hypertension); and in gouty conditions (monitor serum uric acid for hyperuricemia).

• I.V. administration may cause anaphylactoid reactions. Use cautiously and only if other routes are ruled out.

• Don't mix parenteral liquids in same syringe with other medications.

• Protect from light and heat.

• Infection, tumors, or renal, hepatic, and other debilitating diseases may reduce therapeutic response.

• Deficiencies are more common in strict vegetarians and their breast-fed infants.

• Stress need for patients with pernicious anemia to return for monthly injections. Although total body stores

---

may last 3 to 6 years, anemia will recur if not treated monthly.

• May cause false-positive intrinsic factor antibody test.

• Hydroxocobalamin is approved for I.M. use only. Only advantage of hydroxocobalamin over vitamin B_{12} is its longer duration.

• 50% to 98% of injected dose may appear in urine within 48 hours. Major portion of drug is excreted within first 8 hours after injection.

• Closely monitor serum potassium for first 48 hours. Give potassium if necessary.

• Physically incompatible with dextrose solutions, alkaline or strongly acidic solutions, oxidizing and reducing agents, and many other drugs.

---

folic acid (vitamin B_9)
Folvite, Novofolacid†

Pregnancy Risk Category: A (C if > RDA)

HOW SUPPLIED
Tablets: 0.1 mg, 0.4 mg, 0.8 mg, 1 mg
Injection: 10-ml vials (5 mg/ml with 1.5% benzyl alcohol or 10 mg/ml with 1.5% benzyl alcohol and 0.2% EDTA)

MECHANISM OF ACTION
Necessary for normal erythropoiesis and nucleoprotein synthesis.

INDICATIONS & DOSAGE
Recommended daily allowance (RDA)—
Neonates and infants to 6 months: 30 mcg
Infants 6 months to 1 year: 45 mcg
Children over 1 year to 3 years: 100 mcg
Children 4 to 6 years: 200 mcg
Children 7 to 11 years: 300 mcg
Adults and children over 11 years: 400 mcg
Pregnant women: 800 mcg

Lactating women: 500 mcg
Megaloblastic or macrocytic anemia secondary to folic acid or other nutritional deficiency, hepatic disease, alcoholism, intestinal obstruction, excessive hemolysis—
Pregnant and lactating women: 0.8 mg P.O., S.C., or I.M. daily.
Adults and children over 4 years: 1 mg P.O., S.C., or I.M. daily for 4 to 5 days. After anemia secondary to folic acid deficiency is corrected, proper diet and RDA supplements are necessary to prevent recurrence.
Children under 4 years: up to 0.3 mg P.O., S.C., or I.M. daily.
Prevention of megaloblastic anemia of pregnancy and fetal damage—
Women: 1 mg P.O., S.C., or I.M. daily throughout pregnancy.
Nutritional supplement—
Adults: 0.1 mg P.O., S.C., or I.M. daily.
Children: 0.05 mg P.O. daily.
Treatment of tropical sprue—
Adults: 3 to 15 mg P.O. daily.
Test of megaloblastic anemia patients to detect folic acid deficiency without masking pernicious anemia—
Adults and children: 0.1 to 0.2 mg P.O. or I.M. for 10 days while maintaining a diet low in folate and vitamin B_{12}.
(Reticulosis, reversion to normoblastic hematopoiesis, and return to normal hemoglobin indicate folic acid deficiency.)

ADVERSE REACTIONS
Skin: allergic reactions (rash, pruritus, erythema).
Other: *allergic bronchospasms,* general malaise.

INTERACTIONS
Chloramphenicol: antagonism of folic acid. Monitor for decreased folic acid effect. Use together cautiously.

NURSING CONSIDERATIONS
• Contraindicated in normocytic, re-

Italicized adverse reactions are common or life-threatening.
*Liquid form contains alcohol.   **May contain tartrazine.

refractory, or aplastic anemias; as sole agent in treating pernicious anemia (because it may mask neurologic effects); in treating methotrexate, pyrimethamine, or trimethoprim overdose; and in undiagnosed anemia (because it may mask pernicious anemia).

• Patients with small-bowel resections and intestinal malabsorption may require parenteral administration routes.

• Don't mix with other medications in same syringe for I.M. injections.

• Protect from light and heat.

• May use concurrent folic acid and vitamin B_{12} therapy if supported by diagnosis.

• Proper nutrition is necessary to prevent recurrence of anemia.

• Peak folate activity occurs in the blood in 30 to 60 minutes.

• Patients with pernicious anemia should avoid multivitamins containing folic acid.

• Hematologic response to folic acid in patients receiving chloramphenicol concurrently with folic acid should be carefully monitored.

---

leucovorin calcium (citrovorum factor or folinic acid)
Wellcovorin

Pregnancy Risk Category: C

HOW SUPPLIED
Tablets: 5 mg, 25 mg
Injection: 1-ml ampule (3 mg/ml with 0.9% benzyl alcohol or 5 mg/ml, with methyl and propyl parabens); 50-mg vial (10 mg/ml after reconstitution, contains no preservatives); 5-ml ampule (5 mg/ml, with methyl and propyl parabens)

MECHANISM OF ACTION
A reduced form of folic acid that is readily converted to other folic acid derivatives.

INDICATIONS & DOSAGE
Overdose of folic acid antagonist—
Adults and children: P.O., I.M., or I.V. dose equivalent to the weight of the antagonist given.
Leucovorin rescue after high methotrexate dose in treatment of malignancy—
Adults and children: dose at doctor's discretion within 6 to 36 hours of last dose of methotrexate.
Toxic effects of methotrexate used to treat severe psoriasis—
Adults and children: 4 to 8 mg I.M. 2 hours after methotrexate dose.
Hematologic toxicity caused by pyrimethamine therapy—
Adults and children: 5 mg P.O. or I.M. daily.
Hematologic toxicity caused by trimethoprim therapy—
Adults and children: 400 mcg to 5 mg P.O. or I.M. daily.
Megaloblastic anemia caused by congenital enzyme deficiency—
Adults and children: 3 to 6 mg I.M. daily, then 1 mg P.O. daily for life.
Folate-deficient megaloblastic anemia—
Adults and children: up to 1 mg of leucovorin I.M daily. Duration of treatment depends on hematologic response.

ADVERSE REACTIONS
Skin: allergic reactions (rash, pruritus, erythema).
Other: *allergic bronchospasms.*

INTERACTIONS
None significant.

NURSING CONSIDERATIONS
• Contraindicated in treating undiagnosed anemia, since it may mask pernicious anemia. Use cautiously in pernicious anemia; a hemolytic remission may occur while neurologic manifestations remain progressive.
• Do not confuse leucovorin (folinic acid) with folic acid.

---

†Available in Canada only.   ‡Available in Australia only.   ◊ Available OTC.

- Follow leucovorin rescue schedule and protocol closely to maximize therapeutic response. Generally, leucovorin should not be administered simultaneously with systemic methotrexate.
- Treat overdosage of folic acid antagonists; administer within 1 hour if possible; usually ineffective after 4-hour delay.
- Protect from light and heat, especially reconstituted parenteral preparations.
- Since allergic reactions have been reported with folic acid, the possibility of allergic reactions to leucovorin should be considered.

---

niacin (vitamin B₃, nicotinic acid)

Niac, Nico-400, Nicobid◇, Nicolar**, Ni-Span◇

niacinamide (nicotinamide)◇

Pregnancy Risk Category: A (C if > RDA)

HOW SUPPLIED
niacin
Tablets: 20 mg◇, 25 mg◇, 50 mg◇, 100 mg◇, 500 mg
Tablets (timed-release): 150 mg
Capsules (timed-release): 125 mg◇, 250 mg◇, 300 mg◇, 400 mg◇, 500 mg
Elixir: 50 mg/5 ml◇
Injection: 30-ml vials, 100 mg/ml
niacinamide
Tablets: 50 mg◇, 100 mg◇, 500 mg◇
Tablets (timed-release): 1,000 mg◇
Injection: 100 mg/ml

MECHANISM OF ACTION
Necessary for lipid metabolism, tissue respiration, and glycogenolysis. Also (niacin only) decreases synthesis of low-density lipoproteins and inhibits lipolysis in adipose tissue.

INDICATIONS & DOSAGE
Recomended daily allowance (RDA)—
Neonates and infants to 6 months: 6 mg
Infants 6 months to 1 year: 8 mg
Children over 1 year to 3 years: 8 mg
Children 4 to 6 years: 11 mg
Children 7 to 10 years: 16 mg
Males 11 to 18 years: 18 mg
Males 19 to 22 years: 19 mg
Males 23 to 50 years: 18 mg
Males over 50 years: 16 mg
Females 11 to 14 years: 15 mg
Females 15 to 22 years: 14 mg
Females 23 years and over: 13 mg
Pregnant women: 15 mg
Lactating women: 18 mg
Pellagra—
Adults: 10 to 20 mg P.O., S.C., I.M., or I.V. infusion daily, depending on severity of niacin deficiency. Maximum daily dosage recommended is 500 mg; should be divided into 10 doses, 50 mg each.
Children: up to 300 mg P.O. or 100 mg I.V. infusion daily, depending on severity of niacin deficiency.

After symptoms subside, advise adequate nutrition and RDA supplements to prevent recurrence.
Peripheral vascular disease and circulatory disorders—
Adults: 250 to 800 mg P.O. daily in divided doses.
Adjunctive treatment of hyperlipidemias, especially with hypercholesterolemia—
Adults: 1.5 to 3 g P.O. daily in three divided doses with or after meals, increased at intervals to 6 g daily.

ADVERSE REACTIONS
Most adverse reactions are dose-dependent.
CNS: dizziness, transient headache.
CV: *excessive peripheral vasodilation (especially niacin).*
GI: *nausea, vomiting, diarrhea,* possible activation of peptic ulcer, epigastric or substernal pain.

Italicized adverse reactions are common or life-threatening.
*Liquid form contains alcohol.   **May contain tartrazine.

Hepatic: hepatic dysfunction.
Metabolic: hyperglycemia, hyperuricemia.
Skin: *flushing,* pruritus, dryness.

INTERACTIONS

Antihypertensive drugs (sympathetic blocking type): may have an additive vasodilating effect and cause postural hypotension. Use together cautiously. Warn patient about postural hypotension.

NURSING CONSIDERATIONS

• Contraindicated in hepatic dysfunction, active peptic ulcer disease, severe hypotension, or arterial hemorrhage. Use with caution in gallbladder disease, diabetes mellitus, and gout.
• Monitor hepatic function and blood glucose early in therapy.
• Give with meals to minimize GI side effects.
• Aspirin may reduce the flushing response to niacin.
• Timed-release niacin or niacinamide may avoid excessive flushing effects with large doses.
• Give slow I.V. (no faster than 2 mg/minute). Explain harmlessness of flushing syndrome to ease patient's mind.
• Stress that medication used to treat hyperlipoproteinemia or to dilate peripheral vessels is not "just a vitamin." Explain importance of adhering to therapeutic regimen.

pyridoxine hydrochloride (vitamin B₆)

Beesix, Hexa-Betalin, Hexacrest, Nestrex◊

Pregnancy Risk Category: A (C if > RDA)

HOW SUPPLIED

Tablets◊: 10 mg, 25 mg, 50 mg, 100 mg, 200 mg, 250 mg, 500 mg
Tablets (time-release): 500 mg
Injection: 100 mg/ml.

MECHANISM OF ACTION

Acts as coenzyme for various metabolic functions. Required for amino acid metabolism.

INDICATIONS & DOSAGE

Recommended daily allowance (RDA)—
Neonates and infants to 6 months: 0.3 mg
Infants 6 months to 1 year: 0.6 mg
Children over 1 year to 3 years: 0.9 mg
Children 4 to 6 years: 1.3 mg
Children 7 to 10 years: 1.6 mg
Males 11 to 14 years: 1.8 mg
Males 15 to 18 years: 2 mg
Males 19 years and over: 2.2 mg
Females 11 to 14 years: 1.8 mg
Females 15 years and over: 2 mg
Pregnant women: 2.6 mg
Lactating women: 2.5 mg
Dietary vitamin B₆ deficiency—
Adults: 10 to 20 mg P.O., I.M., or I.V. daily for 3 weeks, then 2 to 5 mg daily as a supplement to a proper diet.
Children: 100 mg P.O., I.M., or I.V. to correct deficiency, then an adequate diet with supplementary RDA doses to prevent recurrence.
Seizures related to vitamin B₆ deficiency or dependency—
Adults and children: 100 mg I.M. or I.V. in single dose.
Vitamin B₆–responsive anemias or dependency syndrome (inborn errors of metabolism)—
Adults: up to 600 mg P.O., I.M., or I.V. daily until symptoms subside, then 50 mg daily for life.
Children: 100 mg I.M. or I.V., then 2 to 10 mg I.M. or 10 to 100 mg P.O. daily.
Prevention of vitamin B₆ deficiency during isoniazid therapy—
Adults: 25 to 50 mg P.O. daily.
Children: at least 0.5 to 1.5 mg P.O. daily.
Infants: at least 0.1 to 0.5 mg P.O. daily.
If neurologic symptoms develop in pe-

diatric patients, increase dosage as
necessary.
*Treatment of vitamin B₆ deficiency
secondary to isoniazid—*
Adults: 100 mg P.O. daily for 3
weeks, then 50 mg daily.

ADVERSE REACTIONS
CNS: drowsiness, paresthesias.

INTERACTIONS
None significant.

NURSING CONSIDERATIONS
• Contraindicated in hypersensitivity
to parenteral pyridoxine and in doses
larger than 5 mg for patients also receiving levodopa. Caution patient to
check dosage, especially in multivitamins.
• Protect from light. Do not use injection solution if it contains a precipitate. Slight darkening is acceptable.
• Excessive protein intake increases
daily pyridoxine requirements.
• If sodium bicarbonate is required to
control acidosis in isoniazid toxicity,
do not mix in same syringe with pyridoxine.
• If prescribed for maintenance therapy to prevent deficiency recurrence,
stress importance of compliance and
of good nutrition. Explain that pyridoxine in combination therapy with
isoniazid has a specific therapeutic
purpose and is not "just a vitamin."
Explain importance of adhering to
therapeutic regimen.
• Patients receiving levodopa alone
(not with carbidopa) shouldn't take
pyridoxine.
• Used to treat seizures and coma as a
result of acute isoniazid overdosage.
Dosage equal to amount of isoniazid
ingested.

riboflavin (vitamin B₂)◊
*Pregnancy Risk Category: A (C if >
RDA)*

HOW SUPPLIED
Tablets: 5 mg◊, 10 mg◊, 25 mg◊
Tablets (sugar-free): 50 mg◊, 100
mg◊

MECHANISM OF ACTION
Converted to two other coenzymes
that are necessary for normal tissue
respiration.

INDICATIONS & DOSAGE
*Recommended Daily Allowance
(RDA):*
Neonates and infants to 6 months:
0.4 mg
Infants 6 months to 1 year: 0.6 mg
Children over 1 year to 3 years: 0.8
mg
Children 4 to 6 years: 1 mg
Children 7 to 10 years: 1.4 mg
Males 11 to 14 years: 1.6 mg
Males 15 to 22 years: 1.7 mg
Males 23 to 50 years: 1.6 mg
Males 51 years and over: 1.4 mg
Females 11 to 22 years: 1.3 mg
Females 23 years and over: 1.2 mg
Pregnant women: +0.3 mg
Lactating women: +0.5 mg
*Riboflavin deficiency or adjunct to
thiamine treatment for polyneuritis or
cheilosis secondary to pellagra—*
Adults and children over 12 years: 5
to 50 mg P.O. daily, depending on se-
verity.
Children under 12 years: 2 to 10 mg
P.O. daily, depending on severity.
  For maintenance, increase nutri-
tional intake and supplement with vi-
tamin B complex.

ADVERSE REACTIONS
GU: high doses turn urine bright yellow.

INTERACTIONS
None significant.

NURSING CONSIDERATIONS
• Protect from light.
• Stress proper nutritional habits to prevent recurrence of deficiency.
• Riboflavin deficiency usually accompanies other vitamin B complex deficiencies and may require multivitamin therapy.
• Since food increases absorption of riboflavin, encourage patient to take with meals.
• May be given I.M. or I.V. as a component of multiple vitamins.

---

thiamine hydrochloride (vitamin B₁)
Apatate Drops, Betalin S◇, Betamin‡, Beta-Sol‡, Biamine, Thia

Pregnancy Risk Category: A (C if > RDA)

HOW SUPPLIED
Tablets◇: 5 mg, 10 mg, 25 mg, 50 mg, 100 mg, 250 mg, 500 mg
Elixir: 2.25 mg/5 ml (with alcohol 10%)◇
Injection: 100 mg/ml

MECHANISM OF ACTION
Combines with adenosine triphosphate to form a coenzyme necessary for carbohydrate metabolism.

INDICATIONS & DOSAGE
Recommended Daily Allowance (RDA)—
Neonates and infants to 6 months: 0.3 mg
Infants 6 months to 1 year: 0.5 mg
Children over 1 year to 3 years: 0.7 mg
Children 4 to 6 years: 0.9 mg
Children 7 to 10 years: 1.2 mg
Males 11 to 18 years: 1.4 mg
Males 19 to 22 years: 1.5 mg
Males 23 years and over: 1.4 mg
Females 11 to 22 years: 1.1 mg
Females 23 years and over: 1 mg
Pregnant women: +0.4 mg
Lactating women: +0.5 mg

Beriberi—
Adults: 10 to 500 mg, depending on severity, I.M. t.i.d. for 2 weeks, followed by dietary correction and multivitamin supplement containing 5 to 10 mg thiamine daily for 1 month.
Children: 10 to 50 mg, depending on severity, I.M. daily for several weeks with adequate dietary intake.
Anemia secondary to thiamine deficiency; polyneuritis secondary to alcoholism, pregnancy, or pellagra—
Adults: 100 mg P.O. daily.
Children: 10 to 50 mg P.O. daily in divided doses.
Wernicke's encephalopathy—
Adults: up to 500 mg to 1 g I.V. for crisis therapy, followed by 100 mg b.i.d. for maintenance.
"Wet beriberi," with myocardial failure—
Adults and children: 100 to 500 mg I.V. for emergency treatment.

ADVERSE REACTIONS
CNS: restlessness.
CV: *hypotension after rapid I.V. injection,* angioneurotic edema, cyanosis.
EENT: tightness of throat (allergic reaction).
GI: nausea, hemorrhage, diarrhea.
Skin: feeling of warmth, pruritus, urticaria, sweating.
Other: *anaphylactoid reactions,* weakness, pulmonary edema.

INTERACTIONS
None significant.

NURSING CONSIDERATIONS
• Contraindicated in hypersensitivity to thiamine products. I.V. push is contraindicated, except when treating life-threatening myocardial failure in "wet beriberi." Use with caution in I.V. administration of large doses; give patient skin test if he has a history of hypersensitivity before therapy. Have epinephrine on hand to

---

†Available in Canada only.   ‡Available in Australia only.   ◇Available OTC.

treat anaphylaxis should it occur after a large parenteral dose.

• Thiamine malabsorption is most likely in alcoholism, cirrhosis, or GI disease.

• Use parenteral administration only when P.O. route is not feasible.

• Clinically significant deficiency can occur in approximately 3 weeks of totally thiamine-free diet. Thiamine deficiency usually requires concurrent treatment for multiple deficiencies.

• Doses larger than 30 mg t.i.d. may not be fully utilized. After tissue saturation with thiamine, it is excreted in urine as pyrimidine.

• If beriberi occurs in a breast-fed infant, both mother and child should be treated with thiamine.

• Unstable in alkaline solutions; should not be used with materials that yield alkaline solutions.

vitamin C (ascorbic acid)
Ascorbicap◊, Cebid Timecelles◊, Cetane, Cevalin◊, Cevi-Bid, Ce-Vi-Sol*, Cevita◊, C-Span◊, Dull-C◊, Flavettes‡, Redoxon†, Solucap C, Vita C Crystals◊

Pregnancy Risk Category: A (C if > RDA)

HOW SUPPLIED
Tablets◊: 25 mg, 50 mg, 100 mg, 250 mg, 500 mg, 1,000 mg, 1,500 mg
Tablets (chewable): 100 mg◊, 250 mg◊, 500 mg◊
Tablets (effervescent): 1,000 mg sugar-free◊
Tablets (timed-release): 500 mg◊, 750 mg◊, 1,000 mg◊, 1,500 mg
Capsules (timed-release): 500 mg◊
Crystals: 100 g (4 g/tsp)◊, 1,000 g (4 g/tsp, sugar-free)◊
Oral liquid: 50 ml (35 mg/0.6 ml)◊
Oral solution: 50 ml (100 mg/ml)◊
Powder: 100 g (4 g/tsp)◊, 500 g (4 g/tsp)◊, 1,000 g (4 g/tsp, sugar-free)◊
Syrup: 20 mg/ml in 120 ml and 480

ml◊; 500 mg/5ml in 5 ml◊, 10 ml◊, 120 ml◊, 473 ml◊
Injection: 100 mg/ml in 2-ml, 10-ml ampules; 250 mg/ml in 10-ml ampules and 10-ml, 30-ml, 50-ml vials; 500 mg/ml in 2-ml, 5-ml ampules and 50-ml vials; 500 mg/ml (with mono-thioglycerol) in 1-ml ampules

MECHANISM OF ACTION
Necessary for collagen formation and tissue repair; involved in oxidation-reduction reactions throughout the body.

INDICATIONS & DOSAGE
Recommended Daily Allowance (RDA)—
Neonates and infants 6 months to 1 year: 35 mg
Children over 1 year to 10 years: 45 mg
Males 11 to 14 years: 50 mg
Males 15 years and over: 60 mg
Females 11 to 14 years: 50 mg
Females 15 years and over: 60 mg
Pregnant women: + 20 mg
Lactating women: + 40 mg
Frank and subclinical scurvy—
Adults: 100 mg to 2 g, depending on severity, P.O., S.C., I.M., or I.V. daily, then at least 50 mg daily for maintenance.
Children: 100 to 300 mg, depending on severity, P.O., S.C., I.M., or I.V. daily, then at least 35 mg daily for maintenance.
Infants: 50 to 100 mg P.O., I.M., I.V., or S.C. daily.
Extensive burns, delayed fracture or wound healing, postoperative wound healing, severe febrile or chronic disease states—
Adults: 200 to 500 mg S.C., I.M., or I.V. daily.
Children: 100 to 200 mg P.O., S.C., I.M., or I.V. daily.
Prevention of vitamin C deficiency in those with poor nutritional habits or increased requirements—

Italicized adverse reactions are common or life-threatening.
*Liquid form contains alcohol.   **May contain tartrazine.

Adults: at least 45 mg P.O., S.C., I.M., or I.V. daily.
Pregnant and lactating women: at least 60 mg P.O., S.C., I.M., or I.V. daily.
Children: at least 40 mg P.O., S.C., I.M., or I.V. daily.
Infants: at least 35 mg P.O., S.C., I.M., or I.V. daily.
Potentiation of methenamine in urine acidification—
Adults: 4 to 12 g P.O. daily in divided doses.

ADVERSE REACTIONS
CNS: faintness or dizziness with fast I.V. administration.
GI: diarrhea, epigastric burning.
GU: acid urine, oxaluria, renal calculi, renal failure.
Skin: discomfort at injection site.

INTERACTIONS
None significant.

NURSING CONSIDERATIONS
• Use cautiously in G6PD deficiency.
• Administer I.V. infusion cautiously in patients with renal insufficiency.
• Avoid rapid I.V. administration.
• When administering for urine acidification, check urine pH to ensure efficacy.
• Protect solution from light.

vitamin D

cholecalciferol (vitamin D₃)
Delta-D◊, Vitamin D₃◊

ergocalciferol (vitamin D₂)
Calciferol, Drisdol, Radiostol†, Radiostol Forte†, Vitamin D

Pregnancy Risk Category: A (D if > RDA)

HOW SUPPLIED
Tablets: 1.25 mg (50,000 IU)
Capsules: 0.625 mg (25,000 IU), 1.25 mg (50,000 IU)

Oral liquid: 8,000 IU/ml in 60-ml dropper bottle
Injection: 12.5 mg (500,000 IU)/ml

MECHANISM OF ACTION
Promotes absorption and utilization of calcium and phosphate. Helps to regulate calcium concentration.

INDICATIONS & DOSAGE
Recommended Daily Allowance (RDA)—
Neonates, infants, and children to 10 years: 400 IU
Males 11 to 22 years: 400 IU
Males 23 years and over: 200 IU
Females 11 to 22 years: 400 IU
Females 19 to 22 years: 300 IU
Females 23 years and over: 200 IU
Pregnant and lactating women: + 200 IU
Rickets and other vitamin D deficiency diseases; renal osteodystrophy—
Adults: initially, 12,000 IU P.O. or I.M. daily, increased as indicated by response up to 500,000 IU daily in most cases and up to 800,000 IU daily for vitamin D–resistant rickets.
Children: 1,500 to 5,000 IU P.O. or I.M. daily for 2 to 4 weeks, repeated after 2 weeks, if necessary. Alternatively, a single dose of 600,000 IU may be given.
   Monitor serum calcium daily to guide dosage. After correction of deficiency, maintenance includes adequate dietary nutrition and RDA supplements.
Hypoparathyroidism—
Adults and children: 50,000 to 200,000 IU P.O. or I.M. daily, with 4-g calcium supplement.

ADVERSE REACTIONS
Side effects listed are usually seen in vitamin D toxicity only.
CNS: headache, dizziness, ataxia, weakness, somnolence, decreased libido, overt psychosis, seizures.
CV: calcifications of soft tissues, including the heart.

---

†Available in Canada only.   ‡Available in Australia only.   ◊Available OTC.

EENT: dry mouth, metallic taste, rhinorrhea, conjunctivitis (calcific), photophobia, tinnitus.
GI: anorexia, nausea, constipation, diarrhea.
GU: polyuria, albuminuria, hypercalciuria, nocturia, impaired renal function, renal calculi.
Metabolic: hypercalcemia, hyperphosphatemia.
Skin: pruritus.
Other: bone and muscle pain, bone demineralization, weight loss.

INTERACTIONS
Mineral oil, cholestyramine resin: inhibited GI absorption of oral vitamin D. Space doses. Use together cautiously.

NURSING CONSIDERATIONS
• Contraindicated in hypercalcemia, hypervitaminosis A, or renal osteodystrophy with hyperphosphatemia.
• If I.V. route is necessary, use only water-miscible solutions intended for dilution in large-volume parenterals. Use cautiously in cardiac patients, especially those receiving digitalis glycosides.
• Monitor eating and bowel habits; dry mouth, nausea, vomiting, metallic taste, and constipation may be early signs and symptoms of toxicity.
• Patients with hyperphosphatemia require dietary phosphate restrictions and binding agents to avoid metastatic calcifications and renal calculi.
• When high therapeutic dosages are used, serum and urine calcium, potassium, and urea should be monitored frequently.
• Malabsorption from inadequate bile or hepatic dysfunction may require addition of exogenous bile salts to oral vitamin D.
• I.M. injection of vitamin D dispersed in oil is preferable in patients who are unable to absorb the oral form.
• This vitamin is fat-soluble. Warn patient of the dangers of increasing dosage without consulting the doctor.
• Dosages of 60,000 IU/day can cause hypercalcemia.
• Patients taking vitamin D should restrict their intake of magnesium-containing antacids.

vitamin E
Aquasol E*◊, Eprolin◊, Pertropin◊, Solucap E◊, Tocopher◊

Pregnancy Risk Category: A (C if > RDA)

HOW SUPPLIED
Tablets◊: 100 IU, 200 IU, 400 IU, 500 IU, 600 IU, 1,000 IU
Tablets (chewable): 100 IU◊, 200 IU◊, 400 IU◊
Capsules◊: 50 IU, 100 IU, 200 IU, 400 IU, 600 IU, 1,000 IU
Oral solution: 50 IU/ml◊

MECHANISM OF ACTION
Acts as a cofactor and an antioxidant.

INDICATIONS & DOSAGE
Recommended Daily Allowance (RDA)—
Neonates and infants to 6 months: 4 IU
Infants 6 months to 1 year: 6 IU
Children over 1 year to 3 years: 7 IU
Children 4 to 6 years: 9 IU
Children 7 to 10 years: 10 IU
Males 11 to 14 years: 12 IU
Males 15 years and over: 15 IU
Females 11 and over: 12 IU
Pregnant women: + 3 IU
Lactating women: + 4 IU
Vitamin E deficiency in premature infants and in patients with impaired fat absorption—
Adults: 60 to 75 IU, depending on severity, P.O. or I.M. daily.
Children: 1 mg equivalent/0.6 g of dietary unsaturated fat P.O. or I.M. daily.

Italicized adverse reactions are common or life-threatening.
*Liquid form contains alcohol.   **May contain tartrazine.

ADVERSE REACTIONS
None reported.

INTERACTIONS
Mineral oil, cholestyramine resin: inhibited GI absorption of oral vitamin E. Space doses. Use together cautiously.

NURSING CONSIDERATIONS
• Water-miscible forms more completely absorbed in GI tract than other forms.
• Adequate bile is essential for absorption.
• Requirements increase with rise in dietary polyunsaturated acids.
• May protect other vitamins against oxidation.
• Megadoses can cause thrombophlebitis.
• This vitamin is fat-soluble. Discourage patient from self-medication with megadoses.

menadione/menadiol sodium diphosphate (vitamin K₃)
Synkavite†, Synkayvite

Pregnancy Risk Category: C (X near term)

HOW SUPPLIED
Tablets: 5 mg
Injection: 5 mg/ml, 10 mg/ml, 37.5 mg/ml

MECHANISM OF ACTION
Promotes hepatic formation of active prothrombin.

INDICATIONS & DOSAGE
Hypoprothrombinemia secondary to vitamin K malabsorption or drug therapy, or when oral administration is desired and bile secretion is inadequate—
Adults: 5 to 15 mg P.O. or parenterally, titrated to patient's requirements.

ADVERSE REACTIONS
CNS: headache, kernicterus.
GI: nausea, vomiting.
Skin: allergic rash, pruritus, urticaria.
Local: pain, hematoma at injection site.

INTERACTIONS
Mineral oil, cholestyramine resin: inhibited GI absorption of oral vitamin K. Space doses. Use together cautiously.

NURSING CONSIDERATIONS
• Contraindicated in treatment of hereditary hypoprothrombinemia (because vitamin K₃ can paradoxically worsen it); in hepatocellular disease, unless it is caused by biliary obstruction; in treatment of heparin-induced bleeding; and during last weeks of pregnancy to avoid toxic reactions in neonates. Use cautiously in G6PD deficiency to avoid hemolysis. In severe bleeding, do not delay other measures, such as giving fresh frozen plasma or whole blood. Use large dosages cautiously in severe hepatic disease.
• Failure to respond to vitamin K₃ may indicate coagulation defects.
• Excessive use of vitamin K₃ may temporarily defeat oral anticoagulant therapy. Higher doses of oral anticoagulant or interim use of heparin may be required.
• Protect parenteral products from light.
• When I.V. route must be used, rate shouldn't exceed 1 mg/minute.
• Effects of I.V. injections are more rapid but shorter lived than S.C. or I.M. injections.
• Monitor prothrombin time to determine dosage effectiveness.
• Observe for signs of adverse reactions and report them to doctor.
• Use caution in handling bulk menadione powder. It is irritating to the skin and the respiratory tract.

• This vitamin is fat-soluble.

---

phytonadione (vitamin K₁)

AquaMEPHYTON, Konakion, Mephyton

Pregnancy Risk Category: C

HOW SUPPLIED

Tablets: 5 mg
Injection (aqueous colloidal solution): 2 mg/ml, 10 mg/ml
Injection (aqueous dispersion): 2 mg/ml, 10 mg/ml

MECHANISM OF ACTION

Promotes hepatic formation of active prothrombin.

INDICATIONS & DOSAGE

Hypoprothrombinemia secondary to vitamin K malabsorption, drug therapy, or excess vitamin A—
Adults: 2.5 to 25 mg, depending on severity, P.O. or parenterally, repeated and increased up to 50 mg, if necessary.
Children: 5 to 10 mg P.O. or parenterally.
Infants: 2 mg P.O. or parenterally. I.V. injection rate for children and infants should not exceed 3 mg/m²/minute or a total of 5 mg.
Hypoprothrombinemia secondary to effect of oral anticoagulants—
Adults: 2.5 to 10 mg P.O., S.C., or I.M., based on prothrombin time, repeated, if necessary, within 12 to 48 hours after oral dose or within 6 to 8 hours after parenteral dose. In emergency, give 10 to 50 mg slow I.V., rate not to exceed 1 mg/minute, repeated q 4 hours, p.r.n.
Prevention of hemorrhagic disease in neonates—
Neonates: 0.5 to 1 mg S.C. or I.M. immediately after birth, repeated within 6 to 8 hours, if needed, especially if mother received oral anticoagulants or long-term anticonvulsant therapy during pregnancy.
Differentiation between hepatocellular disease or biliary obstruction as source of hypoprothrombinemia—
Adults and children: 10 mg I.M. or S.C.
Prevention of hypoprothrombinemia related to vitamin K deficiency in long-term parenteral nutrition—
Adults: 5 to 10 mg S.C. or I.M. weekly.
Children: 2 to 5 mg S.C. or I.M. weekly.
Prevention of hypoprothrombinemia in infants receiving less than 0.1 mg/liter vitamin K in breast milk or milk substitutes—
Infants: 1 mg S.C. or I.M. monthly.

ADVERSE REACTIONS

CNS: dizziness, seizure-like movements.
CV: transient hypotension after I.V. administration, rapid and weak pulse, cardiac irregularities.
GI: nausea, vomiting.
Skin: sweating, flushing, erythema.
Local: pain, swelling, and hematoma at injection site.
Other: bronchospasms, dyspnea, cramp-like pain, *anaphylaxis and anaphylactoid reactions (usually after rapid I.V. administration).*

INTERACTIONS

Mineral oil, cholestyramine resin: inhibited GI absorption of oral vitamin K. Space doses. Use together cautiously.

NURSING CONSIDERATIONS

• Contraindicated in hereditary hypoprothrombinemia; bleeding secondary to heparin therapy or overdose; hepatocellular disease, unless caused by biliary obstruction (vitamin K can paradoxically worsen the hypoprothrombinemia). Oral administration is contraindicated if bile secretion is inadequate, unless supplemented with

---

Italicized adverse reactions are common or life-threatening.
*Liquid form contains alcohol.   **May contain tartrazine.

bile salts. Use cautiously, if at all, during last weeks of pregnancy to avoid toxic reactions in neonates and in G6PD deficiency to avoid hemolysis. Use large dosages cautiously in severe hepatic disease.

• Failure to respond to vitamin K may indicate coagulation defects.

• In severe bleeding, don't delay other measures, such as fresh frozen plasma or whole blood.

• Protect parenteral products from light. Wrap infusion container with aluminum foil.

• Effects of I.V. injections more rapid but shorter lived than S.C. or I.M. injections.

• Monitor prothrombin time to determine dosage effectiveness.

• Observe for signs of adverse reactions and report them to the doctor.

• Phytonadione therapy for hemorrhagic disease in infants causes fewer adverse reactions than do other vitamin K analogs.

• Check brand name labels for administration route restrictions.

• Administer I.V. by slow infusion (over 2 to 3 hours). Mix in normal saline solution, dextrose 5% in water, or dextrose 5% in normal saline solution. Observe patient closely for signs of flushing, weakness, tachycardia, and hypotension; may progress to shock.

• This vitamin is fat-soluble.

• Weekly addition of 5 to 10 mg to TPN solutions may be ordered.

sodium fluoride
Fluor-A-Day†, Fluoritab, Flura, Flura-Drops, Karidium, Luride, Pediaflor, Phos-Flur

sodium fluoride, topical
ACT◇, Checkmate, Fluorigard◇, Fluorinse, Flura-Drops, Gel II, Gel-Kam, Gel-Tin, Home Treatment Fluoride Gelution, Karigel, Karigel-N, Listermint with Fluoride◇, Minute-Gel, Point-Two, PreviDent, Stop, Thera-Flur, Thera-Flur N

Pregnancy Risk Category: C

HOW SUPPLIED
sodium fluoride
Tablets: 0.5 mg, 1 mg (sugar-free)
Tablets (chewable): 0.25 mg (sugar-free)
Drops: 0.125 mg/drop (30 ml), 0.125 mg/drop (60 ml, sugar-free), 0.25 mg/drop (19 ml), 0.25 mg/drop (24 ml, sugar-free), 0.5 mg/ml (50 ml)
Rinse: 0.01%◇ (180 ml, 260 ml, 540 ml, 720 ml); 0.02%◇ (180 ml, 300 ml, 360 ml, 480 ml)
sodium fluoride, topical
Gel: 0.5% (24 g, 30 g, 60 g, 120 g, 125 g, 130 g), 0.5% (250 g, sugar-free), 1.23% (480 g)
Gel drops: 0.5% (24 ml, 60 ml)
Rinse: 0.02%◇ (250 ml, 480 ml, 500 ml), 0.09% (250 ml, 480 ml), 0.09% (480 ml, sugar-free)

MECHANISM OF ACTION
May catalyze bone remineralization.

INDICATIONS & DOSAGE
Aid in the prevention of dental caries—
Children over 3 years: 1 mg P.O. daily.
Children under 3 years: 0.5 mg P.O. daily.
Topical: use once daily after thoroughly brushing teeth and rinsing mouth. Rinse around and between teeth for 1 minute, then spit out.

Adults and children over 12 years:
10 ml of 0.01% to 0.02% solution.
Children 6 to 12 years: 5 ml of 0.2%
solution.
Topical: use once daily after thoroughly brushing teeth and rinsing
mouth. Rinse around and between
teeth for 1 minute, then spit out.

ADVERSE REACTIONS
CNS: headaches, weakness.
GI: gastric distress.
Skin: hypersensitivity reactions, such
as atopic dermatitis, eczema, and ur-
ticaria.

INTERACTIONS
None significant.

NURSING CONSIDERATIONS
• Contraindicated when fluoride intake from drinking water exceeds 0.7
parts/million.
• Chronic toxicity (fluorosis) may result from prolonged use of higher-
than-recommended doses.
• Advise patient to notify dentist if
tooth mottling occurs.
• Tablets may be dissolved in mouth,
chewed, or swallowed whole.
• Drops may be administered orally
undiluted or mixed with fluids or
food.
• Topical forms (rinses and gels)
should not be swallowed. Most effective when used immediately after
brushing teeth.
• Tell patient to dilute drops or rinses
in plastic containers rather than glass.
• The presence of fluoride in prenatal
vitamins has been shown to produce
healthier teeth in infants.
• Used investigationally in treating
osteoporosis.

trace elements

**chromium (chromic
chloride)**
Chrometrace

**copper (cupric chloride,
cupric sulfate)**
Coppertrace

iodine (sodium iodide)
Iodopen

**manganese (mangenese
chloride, manganese
sulfate)**
Mangatrace

selenium (selenious acid)
Selenitrace

**zinc (zinc chloride, zinc
sulfate)**
Zinctrace

Pregnancy Risk Category: C

HOW SUPPLIED
chromium
Injection: 4 mcg/ml
copper
Injection: 0.4 mg/ml
iodine
Injection: 100 mcg/ml
manganese
Injection: 0.1 mg/ml, 0.5 mg/ml
selenium
Injection: 40 mcg/ml, 50 mcg/ml
zinc
Injection: 1 mg/ml, 5 mg/ml

MECHANISM OF ACTION
Participate in synthesis and stabiliza-
tion of proteins and nucleic acids in
subcellular and membrane transport
systems.

INDICATIONS & DOSAGE
*Prevention of individual trace element
deficiencies in patients receiving long-
term total parenteral nutrition—*

Italicized adverse reactions are common or life-threatening.
*Liquid form contains alcohol.   **May contain tartrazine.

Chromium—
Adults: 10 to 15 mcg I.V. daily.
Children: 0.14 to 0.20 mcg/kg I.V.
daily.
Copper—
Adults: 0.5 to 1.5 mg I.V. daily.
Children: 0.05 to 0.2 mg/kg I.V.
daily.
Iodine—
Adults: 1 mcg/kg I.V. daily.
Manganese—
Adults: 1 to 3 mg I.V. daily.
Selenium—
Adults: 40 to 120 mcg I.V. daily.
Children: 3 mcg/kg I.V. daily.
Zinc—
Adults: 2 to 4 mg I.V. daily.
Children: 0.05 mg/kg I.V. daily.

ADVERSE REACTIONS
None reported.

INTERACTIONS
None significant at recommended
dosages.

NURSING CONSIDERATIONS
• Check serum levels of trace elements in patients who have received
total parenteral nutrition for 2 months
or longer. Give supplement if ordered.
Call doctor's attention to low serum
levels of these elements.
• Normal serum levels are 0.07 to
0.15 mg/ml copper; 0.05 to 0.15 mg/
100 ml zinc; 4 to 20 mcg/100 ml manganese; selenium 0.1 to 0.19 mcg/ml.
• Solutions of trace elements are
compounded by pharmacy for addition to total parenteral nutrition solutions according to various formulas.
One common trace element solution is
Shil's solution, which contains copper
1 mg/ml, iodide 0.06 mg/ml, manganese 0.4 mg/ml, and zinc 2 mg/ml.

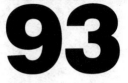
Calorics

amino acid injection
amino acid solution
corn oil
dextrose
essential crystalline amino acid
    solution
fat emulsions
fructose
invert sugar
medium-chain triglycerides

COMBINATION PRODUCTS
Various products contain dextrose, fructose, or invert sugar in combination with electrolytes.

---

amino acid injection
FreAmine HBC, HepatAmine

Pregnancy Risk Category: C

HOW SUPPLIED
Injection: sulfur-containing amino acid—10-ml additive syringe (50 mg/ml)
Injection (with electrolytes): 1,000 ml (3%, 3.5%); 500 ml (3.5%, 5.5%, 7%, 8%, 8.5%)
Injection (without electrolytes): 1,000 ml (3.5%, 5%, 8.5%, 10%, 11.4%); 500 ml (5%, 5.5%, 7%, 8.5%, 10%, 11.4%); 250 ml (5%, 10%, 11.4%)

MECHANISM OF ACTION
Provides a substrate for protein synthesis or enhances conservation of existing body protein.

INDICATIONS & DOSAGE
Treatment of hepatic encephalopathy in patients with cirrhosis or hepatitis; nutritional support—
Adults: 80 to 120 g of amino acids (12 to 18 g of nitrogen)/day. Typically, 500 ml is mixed with 500 ml dextrose 50% in water and administered over a 24-hour period. Add electrolytes, vitamins, and trace elements p.r.n.

ADVERSE REACTIONS
CNS: mental confusion, unconsciousness, headache, dizziness.
CV: hypervolemia, CHF (in susceptible patients), *pulmonary edema,* exacerbation of hypertension (in predisposed patients).
GI: nausea, vomiting.
GU: glycosuria, osmotic diuresis.
Hepatic: fatty liver.
Metabolic: *rebound hypoglycemia* (when long-term infusions are abruptly stopped), *hyperglycemia,* metabolic acidosis, alkalosis, hypophosphatemia, *hyperosmolar nonketotic syndrome,* hyperammonemia, *electrolyte imbalances,* dehydration (if hyperosmolar solutions are used).
Skin: chills, flushing, feeling of warmth.
Local: tissue sloughing at infusion site due to extravasation, *catheter sepsis, thrombophlebitis,* thrombosis.
Other: allergic reactions.

INTERACTIONS
None significant.

NURSING CONSIDERATIONS
• Contraindicated in anuria and in those with inborn errors of amino

---

Italicized adverse reactions are common or life-threatening.
*Liquid form contains alcohol.   **May contain tartrazine.

acid metabolism, especially involving branched-chain amino acid metabolism, such as maple syrup urine disease and isovaleric acidemia.

• Monitor serum electrolytes, and glucose, BUN, and renal and hepatic function.

• Administer cautiously to diabetic patients. To prevent hyperglycemia, insulin may be required. Administer cautiously in cardiac insufficiency. May cause circulatory overload. Patients with fluid restriction may only tolerate 1 to 2 liters.

• Monitor for extraordinary electrolyte losses that may occur during nasogastric suction, vomiting, or drainage from GI fistula.

• Control infusion rate carefully with infusion pump.

• If infusion rate falls behind, do not attempt to catch up. Notify doctor.

• Peripheral infusions should be limited to 2.5% amino acids and dextrose 10%. Check infusion site frequently for erythema, inflammation, irritation, tissue sloughing, necrosis, and phlebitis. Change peripheral I.V. sites routinely to prevent irritation and infection. If a subclavian catheter is used, the solution is administered into the midsuperior vena cava.

• Check fractional urine every 6 hours for glycosuria initially, then every 12 to 24 hours in stable patients. Abrupt onset of glycosuria may be an early sign of impending sepsis.

• Assess body temperature every 4 hours; elevation may indicate sepsis or infection.

• If patient has chills, fever, or other signs of sepsis, replace I.V. tubing and bottle, and send them to the laboratory to be cultured.

amino acid solution (crystalline amino acid solution)

Aminosyn II, FreAmine III, Novamine, Travasol

Pregnancy Risk Category: C

HOW SUPPLIED

Injection: sulfur-containing amino acid—10-ml additive syringe (50 mg/ml)

Injection (with electrolytes): 1,000 ml (3%, 3.5%); 500 ml (3.5%, 5.5%, 7%, 8%, 8.5%)

Injection (without electrolytes): 1,000 ml (3.5%, 5%, 8.5%, 10%, 11.4%); 500 ml (5%, 5.5%, 7%, 8.5%, 10%, 11.4%); 250 ml (5%, 10%, 11.4%)

MECHANISM OF ACTION

Used for protein synthesis of the viscera and skeletal muscles in the protein-depleted patient.

INDICATIONS & DOSAGE

Total, supportive, or supplemental and protein-sparing parenteral nutrition when gastrointestinal system must rest during healing, or when patient can't, shouldn't, or won't eat at all or eat enough to maintain normal nutrition and metabolism—

Adults: 1 to 1.5 g/kg I.V. daily.

Children: 2 to 3 g/kg I.V. daily. Individualize dosage to metabolic and clinical response as determined by nitrogen balance and body weight corrected for fluid balance. Add electrolytes, vitamins, and nonprotein caloric solutions as needed.

ADVERSE REACTIONS

CNS: mental confusion, unconsciousness, headache, dizziness.

CV: hypervolemia, CHF (in susceptible patients), *pulmonary edema,* exacerbation of hypertension (in predisposed patients).

GI: nausea, vomiting.

GU: glycosuria, osmotic diuresis.

Hepatic: fatty liver.
Metabolic: *rebound hypoglycemia* (when long-term infusions are abruptly stopped), *hyperglycemia,* metabolic acidosis, alkalosis, hypophosphatemia, *hyperosmolar nonketotic syndrome,* hyperammonemia, *electrolyte imbalances,* dehydration (if hyperosmolar solutions are used).
Skin: chills, flushing, feeling of warmth.
Local: tissue sloughing at infusion site due to extravasation, *catheter sepsis, thrombophlebitis, thrombosis.*
Other: allergic reactions.

INTERACTIONS
None significant.

NURSING CONSIDERATIONS
• Contraindicated in severe uncorrected electrolyte or acid-base imbalances, hyperammonemia, and decreased circulating blood volume. Use cautiously in renal insufficiency or failure, cardiac disease, and hepatic impairment. Long-term use for infants and children must be closely monitored.
• Monitor serum electrolytes, magnesium, and glucose; BUN; and renal and hepatic function. Check serum calcium frequently to avoid bone demineralization in children.
• If long-term therapy is needed, doctor may order trace element and vitamin supplements.
• Don't mix medications, except electrolytes, vitamins, and trace elements, with total parenteral nutrition solution without first consulting pharmacist.
• Control infusion rate carefully with infusion pump.
• If infusion rate falls behind, do not attempt to catch up. Notify doctor.
• Peripheral infusions should be limited to 2.5% amino acids and dextrose 10%. Check infusion site frequently for erythema, inflammation, irritation, tissue sloughing, necrosis, and phlebitis. Change I.V. sites routinely

to prevent irritation and infection. I.V. catheter is usually introduced into subclavian vein.
• Watch closely for signs of fluid overload. Notify doctor promptly.
• Some crystalline amino acid solutions contain large amounts of acetates and lactates; use cautiously in alkalosis or hepatic insufficiency.
• Most adverse reactions result from mixing amino acids with hypertonic dextrose solutions.
• Initially, check every 12 to 24 hours in stable patients, check fractional urines every 6 hours for glycosuria (if present, the doctor may order insulin coverage).
• Assess body temperature every 4 hours; elevation may indicate sepsis or infection.
• If patient has chills, fever, or other signs of sepsis, replace I.V. tubing and bottle, and send them to the laboratory to be cultured.

corn oil
Lipomul

Pregnancy Risk Category: C

HOW SUPPLIED
Liquid: 473-ml container with 10 g corn oil/15 ml (sugar-free)

MECHANISM OF ACTION
Source of calories.

INDICATIONS & DOSAGE
To increase caloric intake—
Adults: 45 ml P.O. b.i.d. to q.i.d. after or between meals, alone or with proteins, milk, or other energy sources.
Children: 30 ml P.O. daily to q.i.d. after or between meals, alone or with proteins, milk, or other energy sources.

ADVERSE REACTIONS
GI: nausea, vomiting, diarrhea.

Italicized adverse reactions are common or life-threatening.
*Liquid form contains alcohol.   **May contain tartrazine.

INTERACTIONS
Griseofulvin: increased GI absorption of griseofulvin. A beneficial interaction.

NURSING CONSIDERATIONS
• Contraindicated in gallbladder calculi or complete GI obstructions. Use cautiously in steatorrhea, partial GI obstruction, and enterostomies.
• To minimize nausea, diarrhea, and vomiting, give more frequent, smaller doses with meals or mixed with milk.
• The dosage varies greatly with individual requirements; 30 ml of the emulsion provides 180 calories.

dextrose (D-glucose)

Pregnancy Risk Category: C

HOW SUPPLIED
Injection: 1,000 ml (2.5%, 5%, 10%, 20%, 30%, 40%, 50%, 60%, 70%); 650 ml (38.5%); 500 ml (5%, 10%, 20%, 30%, 40%, 50%, 60%, 70%); 400 ml (5%); 250 ml (5%, 10%); 100 ml (5%); 70-ml pin-top vial (70% for additive use only); 50 ml (5% and 50% available in vial, ampule, and Bristoject); 10 ml (25%); 5-ml ampule (10%); 3-ml ampule (10%)

MECHANISM OF ACTION
Minimizes glyconeogenesis and promotes anabolism in patients who can't receive sufficient oral caloric intake.

INDICATIONS & DOSAGE
Fluid replacement and caloric supplementation in patient who can't maintain adequate oral intake or who is restricted from doing so—
Adults and children: dosage depends on fluid and caloric requirements. Use peripheral I.V. infusion of 2.5%, 5%, or 10% solution, central I.V. infusion of 20% solution for minimal fluid needs. Use 50% solution to treat insulin-induced hypoglycemia. Solutions from 40% to 70% are used diluted in admixtures, normally with amino acid solutions, for total parenteral nutrition given through a central vein.

ADVERSE REACTIONS
CNS: mental confusion, unconsciousness in hyperosmolar nonketotic syndrome.
CV: (with fluid overload) pulmonary edema, exacerbated hypertension, and CHF in susceptible patients. *Prolonged or concentrated infusions may cause phlebitis, venous sclerosis, especially with peripheral route of administration.*
GU: glycosuria, osmotic diuresis.
Metabolic: (with rapid infusion of concentrated solution or prolonged infusion) hyperglycemia, hypervolemia, hyperosmolarity. Rapid termination of long-term infusions may cause hypoglycemia from rebound hyperinsulinemia.
Skin: sloughing and tissue necrosis, if extravasation occurs with concentrated solutions.

INTERACTIONS
None significant.

NURSING CONSIDERATIONS
• Contraindicated in hyperglycemia, diabetic coma, intracranial or intraspinal hemorrhage, or delirium tremens. Use cautiously in cardiac or pulmonary disease, hypertension, renal insufficiency, urinary obstruction, and hypovolemia.
• Control infusion rate carefully. Maximal rate for dextrose infusion is 0.5 g/kg hourly. Use infusion pump when infusing dextrose with amino acids for total parenteral nutrition.
• Never infuse concentrated solutions rapidly; may cause hyperglycemia and fluid shift.
• Monitor serum glucose carefully. Prolonged therapy with dextrose 5% in water solution can cause depletion of pancreatic insulin production and secretion.

• Never stop hypertonic solutions abruptly. If necessary, have dextrose 10% in water solution available to treat hypoglycemia if rebound hyperinsulinemia occurs.

• Take care to prevent extravasation. Check injection site frequently to prevent irritation, tissue sloughing, necrosis, and phlebitis.

• Watch closely for signs of fluid overload, especially if fluid intake is restricted.

• Monitor intake/output and weight carefully, especially when renal function is impaired.

• Check vital signs frequently. Report adverse effects promptly.

• Don't give dextrose solutions without saline solution in blood transfusions; may cause clumping of red blood cells. Use central veins to infuse dextrose solutions with concentrations greater than 10%.

---

essential crystalline amino acid solution
Aminess 5.2%, Aminosyn-RF 5.2%, NephrAmine 5.4%, RenAmin

Pregnancy Risk Category: C

HOW SUPPLIED
Injection: 5.2%, 5.4%, 6.5% amino acids

MECHANISM OF ACTION
Enhances conservation of existing body protein.

INDICATIONS & DOSAGE
Management of potentially reversible renal decompensation—
Adults: 0.3 to 0.5 g/kg I.V., up to 26 g total daily (250 ml with 500 ml dextrose 70% injection), and infuse through central I.V. line at initial rate of 20 to 30 ml/hour, increased in steps of 10 ml/hour q 24 hours, to a maximum of 60 to 100 ml/hour. Individualize dosage and infusion rate to patient's tolerance for glucose, fluid,

and nitrogen. Add electrolytes and vitamins p.r.n.
Children: up to 1 g/kg daily, individualized to patient's tolerance for glucose, fluid, and nitrogen. Add electrolytes, trace elements, and vitamins p.r.n.

ADVERSE REACTIONS
CNS: mental confusion, dizziness, unconsciousness, headache.
CV: hypervolemia, CHF (in susceptible patients), *pulmonary edema,* exacerbation of hypertension (in predisposed patients).
GI: nausea, vomiting.
GU: glycosuria, osmotic diuresis.
Metabolic: *rebound hypoglycemia* (when long-term infusions are abruptly stopped), *hyperglycemia,* metabolic acidosis, alkalosis, hypophosphatemia, *hyperosmolar nonketotic syndrome,* hyperammonemia, *electrolyte imbalances,* dehydration (if hyperosmolar solutions are used).
Skin: chills, flushing, feeling of warmth.
Local: tissue sloughing at infusion site due to extravasation, *catheter sepsis, thrombophlebitis.*
Other: allergic reactions.

INTERACTIONS
None significant.

NURSING CONSIDERATIONS
• Contraindicated in severe uncorrected electrolyte or acid-base imbalances, hyperammonemia, and decreased circulating blood volume.
• Monitor serum electrolytes, magnesium, and glucose; BUN; and renal and hepatic function. Check serum calcium frequently to avoid bone demineralization in children.
• In long-term therapy, doctor may order trace element and vitamin supplements. Avoid overuse of fat-soluble vitamins.
• Refrigerate solution until half an hour before it will be infused.

Italicized adverse reactions are common or life-threatening.
*Liquid form contains alcohol.   **May contain tartrazine.

- Don't mix medications, except electrolytes, vitamins, and trace elements with total parenteral nutrition solution without first consulting pharmacist.
- Control infusion rate carefully with infusion pump.
- If infusion rate falls behind, do not attempt to catch up. Notify doctor.
- Peripheral infusions should be limited to 2.5% amino acids and dextrose 10%. Check infusion site frequently for erythema, inflammation, irritation, tissue sloughing, necrosis, and phlebitis. Change I.V. sites routinely to prevent irritation. I.V. catheter is usually placed in subclavian vein.
- Watch closely for signs of fluid overload. Notify doctor promptly.
- Essential amino acid solution is used identically to other crystalline amino acid solutions, except that it contains only the essential amino acids. By controlling amino acid content, patients with impaired renal function have decreases in BUN and minimized deterioration of serum potassium, magnesium, and phosphorus balances. May lead to earlier return of renal function in patients with potentially reversible acute renal failure and may decrease morbidity associated with acute renal failure.
- Most adverse reactions result from mixing essential crystalline amino acid solution with hypertonic dextrose solutions.
- Check blood glucose every 6 hours. Doctor may need to order insulin.
- Assess body temperature every 4 hours; elevation may indicate sepsis or infection.
- If patient has chills, fever, or other signs of sepsis, replace I.V. tubing and bottle, and send them to the laboratory to be cultured.

fat emulsions
Intralipid 10%, Intralipid 20%, Liposyn 10%, Liposyn 20%, Liposyn II 10%, Liposyn II 20%, Soyacal 10%, Soyacal 20%, Travamulsion 10%, Travamulsion 20%

Pregnancy Risk Category: B for Soyacal 10%; C for all others

HOW SUPPLIED
Injection: 50 ml (10%, 20%), 100 ml (10%, 20%), 200 ml (10%, 20%), 250 ml (10%, 20%), 500 ml (10%, 20%); 50 ml (20%)

MECHANISM OF ACTION
Provides neutral triglycerides, predominantly unsaturated fatty acids.

INDICATIONS & DOSAGE
Intralipid:
Source of calories adjunctive to total parenteral nutrition—
Adults: 1 ml/minute I.V. for 15 to 30 minutes (10% emulsion); 0.5 ml/minute I.V. for 15 to 30 minutes (20% emulsion). If no adverse reactions, increase rate to deliver 500 ml over 4 to 8 hours. Total daily dosage should not exceed 2.5 g/kg.
Children: 0.1 ml/minute for 10 to 15 minutes (10% emulsion), 0.05 ml/minute I.V. for 10 to 15 minutes (20% emulsion). If no adverse reactions, increase rate to deliver 1 g/kg over 4 hours. Daily dosage should not exceed 4 g/kg. Equals 60% of daily caloric intake. Protein-carbohydrate total parenteral nutrition should supply remaining 40%.
Fatty acid deficiency—
Adults and children: 8% to 10% of total caloric intake I.V.
Liposyn:
Prevention of fatty acid deficiency—
Adults: 500 ml (10% emulsion) I.V. twice weekly. Infuse initially at a rate of 1 ml/minute for 30 minutes. Rate

may be increased but should not exceed 500 ml over 4 to 6 hours.

Children: 5 to 10 ml/kg (10% emulsion) I.V. daily. Infuse initially at a rate of 0.1 ml/minute for 30 minutes. Rate may be increased but should not exceed 100 ml/hour.

ADVERSE REACTIONS

Early reactions of fat overload:
Blood: hyperlipemia, hypercoagulability, thrombocytopenia in neonates (rare).
CNS: headache, sleepiness, dizziness.
EENT: pressure over eyes.
GI: nausea, vomiting.
Skin: flushing, diaphoresis.
Local: irritation at infusion site.
Other: fever, dyspnea, chest and back pains, cyanosis, allergic reactions, deposition of I.V. fat.
Delayed reactions:
Blood: thrombocytopenia, leukopenia, leukocytosis.
CNS: focal seizures.
CV: *shock.*
Hepatic: transient increased liver function test, hepatomegaly.
Other: fever, splenomegaly, fat accumulation in lungs.

INTERACTIONS
None significant.

NURSING CONSIDERATIONS
• Contraindicated in hyperlipemia, lipid nephrosis, or acute pancreatitis accompanied by hyperlipemia. Use cautiously in severe hepatic disease, pulmonary disease, anemia, blood coagulation disorders, and in patients at risk for fat embolism.
• Lipids support bacterial growth. Change all I.V. tubing at each infusion. Check injection site daily. Report signs of inflammation or infection promptly.
• Use cautiously in premature infants, as they are susceptible to I.V. fat overload. Carefully monitor tri-

glycerides and free fatty acids in these infants.
• May be mixed with amino acid solution, dextrose, electrolytes, and vitamins in the same I.V. container. Check with pharmacist for acceptable proportions and compatibility information.
• Do not use an in-line filter when administering this drug because the fat particles are larger than the 0.22-micron cellulose filter.
• Do not use fat emulsion if it separates or becomes oily.
• Refrigeration is not necessary.
• Avoid rapid infusion. Use an infusion pump to regulate rate.
• Watch closely for adverse reactions, especially during first half hour of infusion.
• Monitor serum lipids closely when patient is receiving fat emulsion therapy. Lipemia must clear between dosing.
• Check platelet count frequently in neonates receiving fat emulsions I.V.
• Monitor hepatic function carefully in long-term use.
• Intralipid, Travamulsion, and Liposyn differ mainly by their fatty acid components.

fructose (levulose)
Pregnancy Risk Category: C

HOW SUPPLIED
Injection: 1,000 ml (10% or 100 g/liter)

MECHANISM OF ACTION
Minimizes glyconeogenesis and promotes anabolism in patients who can't receive sufficient oral caloric intake.

INDICATIONS & DOSAGE
Source of carbohydrate calories primarily when fluid replacement is also indicated and as a dextrose substitute for patients with diabetes—
Adults and children: dosage depends

Italicized adverse reactions are common or life-threatening.
*Liquid form contains alcohol.   **May contain tartrazine.

on caloric needs. I.V. infusion rate should not exceed 1 g/kg hourly. Single liter 10% solution yields 375 calories.

ADVERSE REACTIONS
CV: increased pulse rate, precipitation or exacerbation of CHF in susceptible patients, *pulmonary edema*.
Hepatic: hepatomegaly.
Metabolic: metabolic acidosis, hypervolemia.
Local: extravasation at infusion site may cause sloughing of skin, thrombophlebitis.
Other: increased respiratory rate.

INTERACTIONS
None significant.

NURSING CONSIDERATIONS
• Contraindicated in hereditary fructose intolerance, in gout, or in patients receiving therapy for hypoglycemia. Use cautiously in cardiac disease, hypertension, pulmonary disease, hypervolemia, renal insufficiency, and urinary tract obstructions.
• Control infusion rate carefully. Make sure rate does not exceed 1 g/kg hourly for infants.
• Change infusion sites regularly to avoid irritation with prolonged therapy. Take care to avoid extravasation.
• Don't use unless the solution is clear and the seal is intact.
• Watch closely for signs of fluid overload, pulmonary edema, or CHF.

invert sugar
Travert

Pregnancy Risk Category: C

HOW SUPPLIED
Injection: 500 ml, 1,000 ml (10% or 100 g/liter)

MECHANISM OF ACTION
Minimizes glyconeogenesis and promotes anabolism in patients who can't

receive sufficient oral caloric intake. Composed of equal amounts of dextrose and fructose.

INDICATIONS & DOSAGE
Nonelectrolyte fluid replacement and caloric supplementation solution—
Adults and children: dosage depends on patient's age, weight, and clinical need. I.V. infusion rate should not exceed 1 g/kg hourly. A single liter of 5% invert sugar yields 375 calories.

ADVERSE REACTIONS
CNS: mental confusion.
CV: increased pulse rate, precipitation or exacerbation of CHF in susceptible patients, *pulmonary edema,* hypertension.
GU: glycosuria, osmotic diuresis.
Metabolic: metabolic acidosis, hypervolemia, hyperglycemia, hypoglycemia.
Local: extravasation at infusion site may cause sloughing of skin, thrombophlebitis.
Other: increased respiratory rate.

INTERACTIONS
None significant.

NURSING CONSIDERATIONS
• Contraindicated in hereditary fructose intolerance, hyperglycemia, diabetic coma, intracranial or intraspinal hemorrhage, or delirium tremens. Use cautiously in cardiac disease, hypertension, pulmonary disease, hypervolemia, renal insufficiency, and urinary tract obstructions.
• Control infusion rate carefully. Make sure rate does not exceed 1 g/kg hourly for infants.
• Change infusion sites regularly to avoid irritation with prolonged therapy. Take care to avoid extravasation.
• Watch closely for signs of fluid overload, pulmonary edema, or CHF. Monitor blood pressure frequently.
• Monitor serum glucose closely. Prolonged therapy can cause depletion

of pancreatic insulin production and secretion.
• Monitor intake/output and weight closely, especially if renal function is impaired.
• Check vital signs frequently. Tell doctor promptly if adverse reactions occur.

---

medium-chain triglycerides
M.C.T.◊

Pregnancy Risk Category: C

HOW SUPPLIED
Oil: 960 ml (115 calories/15 ml)◊

MECHANISM OF ACTION
Source of rapidly hydrolyzable lipid.

INDICATIONS & DOSAGE
Inadequate digestion or absorption of food fats—
Adults: 15 ml P.O. t.i.d. or q.i.d. Maximum of 100 ml/day.

ADVERSE REACTIONS
CNS: reversible coma in susceptible patients.
GI: *nausea, vomiting, diarrhea, abdominal distention, cramps.*

INTERACTIONS
None significant.

NURSING CONSIDERATIONS
• Contraindicated in advanced hepatic disease or abetalipoproteinemia. Use cautiously in patients with portacaval shunts.
• To minimize GI adverse reactions, give smaller doses more frequently with meals or mixed with salad dressing or chilled fruit juice.
• More easily absorbed than long-chain fats; not dependent on bile salts for emulsification.
• Rapid metabolism provides quick energy.
• May be useful in lowering choles-

terol levels. Also used in patients with short-bowel syndrome.
• Provides 7.7 calories/ml. No essential fatty acids are provided.

Italicized adverse reactions are common or life-threatening.
*Liquid form contains alcohol.   **May contain tartrazine.

94

Uricosurics

probenecid
sulfinpyrazone

COMBINATION PRODUCTS
COLBENEMID: probenecid 500 mg and colchicine 0.5 mg.
PROBEN-C: probenecid 500 mg and colchicine 0.5 mg.

---

probenecid
Benemid, Benn, Benuryl†, Probalan, Robenecid

Pregnancy Risk Category: B

HOW SUPPLIED
Tablets: 500 mg

MECHANISM OF ACTION
Blocks renal tubular reabsorption of uric acid, increasing excretion. Also inhibits active renal tubular secretion of many weak organic acids (for example, penicillins and cephalosporins).

INDICATIONS & DOSAGE
Adjunct to penicillin or cephalosporin therapy—
Adults and children over 50 kg: 500 mg P.O. q.i.d.
Children 2 to 14 years or under 50 kg: initially, 25 mg/kg P.O., then 40 mg/kg divided q.i.d.
Single-dose treatment of gonorrhea—
Adults: 3.5 g ampicillin P.O. with 1 g probenecid P.O. given together; or 1 g probenecid P.O. 30 minutes before dose of 4.8 million units of aqueous penicillin G procaine I.M., injected at two different sites.

Treatment of hyperuricemia of gout, gouty arthritis—
Adults: 250 mg P.O. b.i.d. for first week, then 500 mg b.i.d., to maximum of 2 g daily. Maintenance dosage is 500 mg daily for 6 months.

ADVERSE REACTIONS
Blood: *hemolytic anemia.*
CNS: *headache,* dizziness.
CV: hypotension.
GI: anorexia, nausea, vomiting, *gastric distress.*
GU: urinary frequency.
Skin: dermatitis, pruritus.
Other: flushing, sore gums, fever.

INTERACTIONS
Indomethacin: decreased indomethacin excretion. Lower indomethacin dosages may be required.
Salicylates: inhibited uricosuric effect of probenecid, causing urate retention. Do not use together.

NURSING CONSIDERATIONS
• Contraindicated in blood dyscrasias; acute gout attack; penicillin therapy in presence of known renal impairment; gouty nephropathy; urinary tract stones or obstruction; and azotemia or hyperuricemia secondary to cancer chemotherapy, radiation, or myeloproliferative neoplastic diseases. Use cautiously in peptic ulcer and renal impairment.
• Usually preferred over sulfinpyrazone because probenecid produces fewer and less severe GI and hematologic adverse reactions.
• Contains no analgesic or anti-in-

---

flammatory agent, and is of no value during acute gout attacks. Don't initiate therapy until acute attack subsides.

• Suitable for long-term use; no cumulative effects or tolerance.

• Not effective with chronic renal insufficiency (glomerular filtration rate less than 30 ml/minute).

• Periodic BUN and renal function tests recommended in long-term therapy.

• May increase frequency, severity, and length of acute gout attacks during first 6 to 12 months of therapy. Prophylactic colchicine or another anti-inflammatory agent is given during first 3 to 6 months.

• Tell patient with gout to avoid alcohol; it increases urate level.

• Patient with gout should avoid all medications that contain aspirin. These may precipitate gout. Acetaminophen may be used for pain.

• Force fluids to maintain minimum daily output of 2 to 3 liters. Alkalinize urine with sodium bicarbonate or potassium citrate as ordered by doctor. These measures will prevent hematuria, renal colic, urate stone development, and costovertebral pain.

• Give with milk, food, or antacids to minimize GI distress. Continued disturbances might indicate need to lower dosage.

• Patients with gout should restrict foods high in purine: anchovies, liver, sardines, kidneys, sweetbreads, peas, and lentils.

• Instruct patient and his family that drug must be taken regularly as ordered or gout attacks may result. Tell him to visit doctor regularly so uric acid can be monitored and dosage can be adjusted if necessary. Lifelong therapy may be required in patients with hyperuricemia.

• May produce false-positive glucose tests with Benedict's solution or Clinitest, but not with glucose oxidase

method (Clinistix, Diastix, Tes-Tape).

• Decreases urinary excretion of 17-ketosteroids, Bromsulphalein (BSP), aminohippuric acid, and iodine-related organic acids, interfering with laboratory procedures.

sulfinpyrazone
Anturan†, Anturane

Pregnancy Risk Category: C

HOW SUPPLIED
Tablets: 100 mg
Capsules: 200 mg

MECHANISM OF ACTION
Blocks renal tubular reabsorption of uric acid, increasing excretion. Also inhibits platelet aggregation.

INDICATIONS & DOSAGE
Inhibition of platelet aggregation, increase of platelet survival time in treatment of thromboembolic disorders, angina, myocardial infarction, transient cerebral ischemic attacks, peripheral arterial atherosclerosis—
Adults: 200 mg P.O. q.i.d.
Maintenance therapy for common gout: reduction, prevention of joint changes and tophi formation—
Adults: 100 to 200 mg P.O. b.i.d. first week, then 200 to 400 mg P.O. b.i.d. Maximum dosage is 800 mg daily.

ADVERSE REACTIONS
Blood: *agranulocytosis,* blood dyscrasias (rare).
CNS: dizziness, vertigo, tinnitus.
GI: *nausea, dyspepsia,* epigastric pain, blood loss, reactivation of peptic ulcers.
Skin: rash.

INTERACTIONS
Oral antidiabetic agents, anticoagulants: increased effects. Monitor closely.

Italicized adverse reactions are common or life-threatening.
*Liquid form contains alcohol.   **May contain tartrazine.

Probenecid: inhibited renal excretion of sulfinpyrazone. Use together cautiously.

Salicylates: inhibited uricosuric effect of sulfinpyrazone. Do not use together.

NURSING CONSIDERATIONS
• Contraindicated in hypersensitivity to pyrazole derivatives (including oxyphenbutazone and phenylbutazone); active peptic ulcer; gouty nephropathy; urolithiasis or urinary obstruction; bone marrow suppression; azotemia, hyperuricemia secondary to cancer chemotherapy, radiation, or myeloproliferative neoplastic diseases; blood dyscrasias; and during or within 2 weeks after gout attack. Use cautiously in diminished hepatic or renal function.
• Use in treating thromboembolic conditions is investigational and is most often directed at prevention of recurrent myocardial infarction.
• Recommended for patients unresponsive to probenecid. Suitable for long-term use; neither cumulative effects nor tolerance develops.
• Contains no analgesic or anti-inflammatory agent and is of no value during acute gout attacks.
• Periodic BUN, CBC, and renal function studies advised during long-term use.
• May increase frequency, severity, and length of acute gout attacks during first 6 to 12 months of therapy. Prophylactic colchicine or another anti-inflammatory agent is given during first 3 to 6 months.
• Therapy, especially at start, may lead to renal colic and formation of uric acid stones. Until acid levels are normal (about 6 mg/100 ml), monitor intake/output closely.
• Force fluids to maintain minimum daily output of 2 to 3 liters. Alkalinize urine with sodium bicarbonate or other agent ordered by doctor.

• Give with milk, food, or antacids to minimize GI disturbances.
• Patients with gout should restrict foods high in purine: anchovies, liver, sardines, kidneys, sweetbreads, peas, and lentils.
• Instruct patient and his family that drug must be taken regularly as ordered or gout attacks may result. Tell him to visit doctor regularly so blood levels can be monitored and dosage adjusted if necessary.
• Lifelong therapy may be required in patients with hyperuricemia.
• Decreases urinary excretion of aminohippuric acid, interfering with laboratory test results.
• Alkalinizing agents are used therapeutically to increase sulfinpyrazone activity, preventing urolithiasis.
• Warn patients with gout not to take any aspirin-containing medications since these may precipitate gout. Acetaminophen may be used for pain.

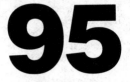

Enzymes

chymopapain
fibrinolysin and
   desoxyribonuclease
hyaluronidase

COMBINATION PRODUCTS
CHYMORAL-100: 100,000 units enzymatic activity; trypsin and chymotrypsin in ratio of 6:1.
GRANULEX AEROSOL: trypsin 0.1 mg, balsam Peru 72.5 mg, and castor oil 650 mg/0.82 ml.
ORENZYME BITABS ENTERIC-COATED TABLETS: 100,000 units trypsin and 8,000 units chymotrypsin.

chymopapain
Chymodiactin, Discase

Pregnancy Risk Category: C

HOW SUPPLIED
Powder for injection: 4,000 units/vial, 10,000 units/vial; each unit of chymopapain is also referred to as 1 pico-Katal (pKat)

MECHANISM OF ACTION
Hydrolyzes noncollagenous proteins in the chondromucoprotein of the nucleus pulposus.

INDICATIONS & DOSAGE
Treatment of herniated lumbar intervertebral disk—
Adults: 2,000 to 4,000 pKat units/disk injected intradiskally. Maximum dosage in a single patient with multiple disk herniation is 10,000 units.

ADVERSE REACTIONS
Systemic: *anaphylaxis, paraplegia, cerebral hemorrhage, acute transverse myelitis,* nausea, headache, dizziness, leg weakness, paresthesias, numbness of legs and toes.
Local: *back pain, stiffness, back spasm.*

INTERACTIONS
None significant.

NURSING CONSIDERATIONS
• Contraindicated in patients with history of allergy to papaya or meat tenderizer; patients who have previously received an injection of chymopapain; severe spondylolisthesis in addition to spinal stenosis; severe progressing paralysis; or evidence of spinal cord tumor or a cauda equina lesion. Most clinicians advocate pretreatment with antihistamine (both H_1 and H_2 blockers).
• Should be used only by doctors qualified by training and experience to perform laminectomy, diskectomy or other spinal procedures, and who have received specialized training in chemonucleolysis. Drug shouldn't be injected in any region other than the lumbar spine. Chymopapain is extremely toxic if injected into the subarachnoid space.
• A new test (ChymoFAST) can detect allergic sensitivity to chymopapain.
• Monitor very closely for anaphylactoid reaction (0.5% of patients). Can be immediate or delayed up to 1 hour after injection and can last for min-

---

Italicized adverse reactions are common or life-threatening.
*Liquid form contains alcohol.   **May contain tartrazine.

utes to several hours or longer. Watch for hypotension and bronchospasm. These may lead to laryngeal edema, arrhythmias, cardiac arrest, coma, and death. Other signs of allergic response include erythema, pilomotor erection, rash, pruritic urticaria, conjunctivitis, vasomotor rhinitis, angioedema, or various GI disturbances.

• Keep an I.V. line open to permit rapid management of anaphylaxis. Keep epinephrine and steroids readily available.

• Instruct patient to anticipate the possibility of delayed allergic reactions, such as rash, urticaria, or itching, which may occur as late as 15 days after injection. Patient should report these to doctor immediately.

• Patients may experience back pain or involuntary muscle spasm in the lower back for several days after injection. Reassure patient that this is common and will not be chronic.

• Use within 60 minutes after reconstitution. Discard unused drug.

---

fibrinolysin and desoxyribonuclease
Elase

Pregnancy Risk Category: C

HOW SUPPLIED
Dry powder: 25 units fibrinolysin and 15,000 units deoxyribonuclease in 30-ml vial
Ointment: 30 units fibrinolysin and 20,000 units deoxyribonuclease in 30-g tube

MECHANISM OF ACTION
Desoxyribonuclease attacks DNA and fibrinolysin attacks fibrin of blood clots and fibrinous exudates. Enzymatic action produces clean surfaces and promotes healing.

INDICATIONS & DOSAGE
Debridement of inflammatory and infected lesions (surgical wounds, ulcer-
ative lesions, second- and third-degree burns, circumcision, episiotomy, cervicitis, vaginitis, abscesses, fistulas, and sinus tracts)—
Intravaginally:
Adults and children: 5 ml ointment may be inserted using applicator supplied, once daily for vaginitis or cervicitis.
Topical use:
Adults and children: apply ointment at intervals as long as enzyme action is desired.
Irrigating agent for infected wounds, empyema cavities, abscesses, otorhinolaryngologic wounds, subcutaneous hematomas—
Adults and children: dilution for irrigation depends on extent and severity of wound.

ADVERSE REACTIONS
Local: hyperemia with high doses, allergic reactions.

INTERACTIONS
None significant.

NURSING CONSIDERATIONS
• Contraindicated for parenteral use.
• Dense, dry eschar must be removed surgically before enzymatic debridement. Enzyme must be in constant contact with substrate. Accumulated necrotic debris must be removed periodically and the enzyme replenished at least once daily.
• Cleanse wound with water, normal salines, or peroxide and dry gently; cover with thin layer of Elase. Cover with nonadhering dressing.
• Change dressing at least once and preferably two to three times daily. Flush away necrotic debris and reapply ointment. Frequency of application may be more important than the amount of drug used.
• Solution as wet to dry dressing: mix 1 vial of Elase powder with 10 to 50 ml saline solution; saturate strips of fine gauze with solution. Pack ulcer-

---

†Available in Canada only.   ‡Available in Australia only.   ◊Available OTC.

ated area with Elase gauze. Allow gauze to dry in contact with ulcerated lesion for about 6 to 8 hours. Remove dried gauze and repeat 3 to 4 times daily.

• Solution as irrigating agent: Drain cavity and replace Elase every 6 to 10 hours to reduce amount of by-product accumulation and to minimize loss of enzyme activity. Although parenteral use is contraindicated, Elase is used as an irrigating agent in certain specific conditions.

• Prepare solution just before use. Discard after 24 hours.

hyaluronidase
Wydase

Pregnancy Risk Category: C

HOW SUPPLIED
Injection: 150 units/vial, 1,500 units/vial; 150 units/ml in 1-ml, 10-ml vials

MECHANISM OF ACTION
Hydrolyzes hyaluronic acid, thereby promoting diffusion of fluids in the tissues.

INDICATIONS & DOSAGE
Adjunct to increase absorption and dispersion of other injected drugs—
Adults and children: 150 units to injection medium containing other medication.
Hypodermoclysis—
Adults and children over 3 years: 150 units injected S.C. before clysis or injected into clysis tubing near needle for each 1,000 ml clysis solution.
Excretory urography when contrast medium is given S.C.—
Adults and children: with patient in a prone position, give 75 units S.C. over each scapula, followed by injection of contrast medium at same sites.

ADVERSE REACTIONS
Skin: rash, urticaria.
Local: irritation.

INTERACTIONS
Local anesthetics: increased potential for toxic local reaction. Use together cautiously.

NURSING CONSIDERATIONS
• Use with caution in patients with blood-clotting abnormalities, severe hepatic or renal disease.

• Do not inject into acutely inflamed or cancerous areas.

• In hypodermoclysis, adjust dosage, rate of injection, and type of solution according to patient's response.

• Administration precautions: Perform a skin test for sensitivity. Avoid injecting into diseased areas (may spread infection). Observe injection site for local reactions.

• Avoid getting solution in eyes. If solution does get in eyes, flush with water at once.

• Protect from heat. Do not use cloudy or discolored solution.

• For children, 15 units are added to each 100 ml of solution. The drip rate should not exceed 2 ml/minute.

• Hyaluronidase is incompatible with epinephrine and heparin. Don't add to any solutions containing these drugs.

Italicized adverse reactions are common or life-threatening.
*Liquid form contains alcohol.   **May contain tartrazine.

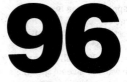

Oxytocics

carboprost tromethamine
dinoprostone
ergonovine maleate
methylergonovine maleate
oxytocin, synthetic injection
oxytocin, synthetic nasal
  solution

COMBINATION PRODUCTS
None.

---

carboprost tromethamine
Hemabate, Prostin/15 M

HOW SUPPLIED
Injection: 250 mcg/ml

MECHANISM OF ACTION
Produces strong, prompt contractions of uterine smooth muscle, possibly mediated by calcium and cyclic 3′,5′-adenosine monophosphate. A prostaglandin.

INDICATIONS & DOSAGE
Abort pregnancy between 13th and 20th weeks of gestation—
Adults: initially, 250 mcg is administered deep I.M. Subsequent doses of 250 mcg should be administered at intervals of 1½ to 3½ hours, depending on uterine response. Increments in dosage may be increased to 500 mcg if contractility is inadequate after several 250-mcg doses. Total dosage should not exceed 12 mg.
Postpartum hemorrhage caused by uterine atony that has not responded to conventional management—
Adults: 250 mcg by deep I.M. injec-

tion. May administer repeat doses at 15- to 90-minute intervals. Maximum total dosage is 2 mg.

ADVERSE REACTIONS
GI: *vomiting, diarrhea,* nausea.
Other: *fever,* chills.

INTERACTIONS
None significant.

NURSING CONSIDERATIONS
• Contraindicated in pelvic inflammatory disease or active cardiac, pulmonary, renal, or hepatic disease. Use cautiously in history of asthma; hypertension; cardiovascular, renal, or hepatic disease; anemia; jaundice; diabetes; epilepsy; and previous uterine surgery.
• I.M. injection of this drug is technically less difficult and poses fewer potential risks than other prostaglandin abortifacients.
• Unlike other prostaglandin abortifacients, carboprost tromethamine is administered by I.M. injection. Injectable form avoids risk of expelling vaginal suppositories, which may occur in the presence of profuse vaginal bleeding.
• Should be used only in a hospital setting by trained personnel.

---

dinoprostone
Prostin E₂

HOW SUPPLIED
Vaginal suppositories: 20 mg

MECHANISM OF ACTION
Produces strong, prompt contractions of uterine smooth muscle, possibly mediated by calcium and cyclic $3',5'$-adenosine monophosphate. A prostaglandin.

INDICATIONS & DOSAGE
Abort second trimester pregnancy, evacuate uterus in cases of missed abortion, intrauterine fetal deaths up to 28 weeks of gestation, or benign hydatidiform mole—
Adults: insert 20-mg suppository high into posterior vaginal fornix. Repeat q 3 to 5 hours until abortion is complete.

ADVERSE REACTIONS
CNS: headache, *dizziness.*
CV: hypotension (in large doses).
GI: *nausea, vomiting, diarrhea.*
GU: vaginal pain, vaginitis.
Other: *fever, shivering, chills, joint inflammation, nocturnal leg cramps, bronchospasm.*

INTERACTIONS
Alcohol (I.V. infusions of 500 ml of 10% over 1 hour): inhibited uterine activity.

NURSING CONSIDERATIONS
• Contraindicated in pelvic inflammatory disease or history of pelvic surgery, incisions, uterine fibroids, or cervical stenosis. Use cautiously in asthma, epilepsy, anemia, diabetes, hypertension or hypotension, jaundice, and cardiovascular, renal, or hepatic disease.
• Administer only when critical care facilities are readily available.
• Patient may be pretreated with an antiemetic and an antidiarrheal agent.
• Just before use, warm dinoprostone suppositories in their wrapping to room temperature.
• After administration, patient should remain supine for 10 minutes.

• Store suppositories in freezer at temperature of $-20°$ C. ($-4°$ F.).
• Dinoprostone-induced fever is self-limiting and transient and occurs in approximately 50% of all patients. Treat with water or alcohol sponging and increased fluid intake rather than with aspirin.
• Check vaginal discharge daily.
• Abortion should be complete within 30 hours.
• Dinoprostone is being investigated as an agent that promotes cervical inducibility (cervical "ripening") before induction of labor with oxytocin.

ergonovine maleate (ergometrine maleate)
Ergotrate Maleate

HOW SUPPLIED
Tablets: 0.2 mg
Injection: 0.2 mg/ml

MECHANISM OF ACTION
Increases motor activity of the uterus by direct stimulation. Prolonged uterine contraction helps control hemorrhage.

INDICATIONS & DOSAGE
Prevent or treat postpartum and post-abortion hemorrhage from uterine atony or subinvolution—
Adults: 0.2 mg I.M. q 2 to 4 hours, maximum of 5 doses; or 0.2 mg I.V. (only for severe uterine bleeding or other life-threatening emergency) over 1 minute while blood pressure and uterine contractions are monitored. I.V. dose may be diluted to 5 ml with normal saline injection. After initial I.M. or I.V. dose, may give 0.2 to 0.4 mg P.O. q 6 to 12 hours for 2 to 7 days. Decrease dosage if severe uterine cramping occurs.

ADVERSE REACTIONS
CNS: dizziness, headache.
CV: hypertension, chest pain.

Italicized adverse reactions are common or life-threatening.
*Liquid form contains alcohol.   **May contain tartrazine.

EENT: tinnitus.
GI: nausea, vomiting.
GU: uterine cramping.
Other: sweating, dyspnea, hypersensitivity.

INTERACTIONS
Regional anesthetics, dopamine, I.V. oxytocin: excessive vasoconstriction. Use together cautiously.

NURSING CONSIDERATIONS
• Contraindicated for induction or augmentation of labor, before delivery of placenta, in threatened spontaneous abortion, and in patients with allergy or sensitivity to ergot preparations. Use cautiously in hypertension, cardiac disease, venoatrial shunts, mitral valve stenosis, obliterative vascular disease, sepsis, and hepatic or renal impairment.
• Monitor blood pressure, pulse rate, and uterine response. Report sudden changes in vital signs, frequent periods of uterine relaxation, and/or character and amount of vaginal bleeding.
• If hypertension occurs, it may respond to chlorpromazine or hydralazine.
• Hypocalcemia may decrease patient response. If patient is not also taking digitalis, cautious administration of calcium gluconate I.V. may produce desired oxytocic action.
• Contractions begin 5 to 15 minutes after P.O. administration; immediately after I.V. injection. May continue 3 hours or more after P.O. or I.M. administration; 45 minutes after I.V. injection.
• Keep patient warm.
• Store in tightly closed, light-resistant container. Discard if discolored.
• Store I.V. solutions below 8° C. (46.4° F.). Daily stock may be kept at cool room temperature for 60 days.
• Have drug ready for immediate use if it is to be given postpartum.
• I.V. ergonovine is used to diagnose

coronary artery spasm (Prinzmetal's angina).

---

methylergonovine maleate
Methergine

HOW SUPPLIED
Tablets: 0.2 mg
Injection: 0.2 mg/ml

MECHANISM OF ACTION
Increases motor activity of the uterus by direct stimulation.

INDICATIONS & DOSAGE
Prevent and treat postpartum hemorrhage caused by uterine atony or subinvolution—
Adults: 0.2 mg I.M. q 2 to 5 hours for maximum of 5 doses; or I.V. (excessive uterine bleeding or other emergencies) over 1 minute while blood pressure and uterine contractions are monitored. I.V. dose may be diluted to 5 ml with normal saline solution. Following initial I.M. or I.V. dose, may give 0.2 to 0.4 mg P.O. q 6 to 12 hours for 2 to 7 days. Decrease dosage if severe cramping occurs.

ADVERSE REACTIONS
CNS: dizziness, headache.
CV: hypertension, transient chest pain, dyspnea, palpitation.
EENT: tinnitus.
GI: *nausea, vomiting.*
Other: sweating, hypersensitivity.

INTERACTIONS
Regional anesthetics, dopamine, I.V. oxytocin: excessive vasoconstriction.

NURSING CONSIDERATIONS
• Contraindicated for induction of labor; before delivery of placenta; in patients with hypertension, toxemia, or sensitivity to ergot preparations; and in threatened spontaneous abortion. Use cautiously in sepsis, obliter-

---

ative vascular disease, and hepatic, renal, or cardiac disease.

• Drug should not be routinely administered I.V. If it must be given by this route, administer slowly over 1 minute with careful blood pressure monitoring.

• Monitor and record blood pressure, pulse rate, and uterine response; report any sudden change in vital signs or frequent periods of uterine relaxation, and character and amount of vaginal bleeding.

• Contractions begin 5 to 15 minutes after P.O. administration; 2 to 5 minutes after I.M. injection; immediately following I.V. injection. May continue 3 hours or more after P.O. or I.M. administration; 45 minutes after I.V.

• Store in tightly closed, light-resistant containers. Discard if discolored.

• Store I.V. solutions below 8° C. (46.4° F.). Daily stock may be kept at room temperature for 60 to 90 days.

oxytocin, synthetic injection
Oxytocin, Pitocin, Syntocinon

HOW SUPPLIED
Injection: 10 units/ml

MECHANISM OF ACTION
Causes potent and selective stimulation of uterine and mammary gland smooth muscle.

INDICATIONS & DOSAGE
Induction or stimulation of labor—
Adults: initially, 1 ml (10 units) ampule in 1,000 ml of dextrose 5% injection or normal saline solution I.V. infused at 1 to 2 milliunits/minute. Increase rate at 15- to 30-minute intervals until normal contraction pattern is established. Maximum is 1 to 2 ml (20 milliunits)/minute. Decrease rate when labor is firmly established.
Reduction of postpartum bleeding after expulsion of placenta—

Adults: 10 to 40 units added to 1,000 ml of dextrose 5% in water or normal saline solution infused at rate necessary to control bleeding, usually 10 to 20 milliunits/minute. Also, 1 ml (10 units) can be given I.M. after delivery of the placenta.
Incomplete or inevitable abortion—
Adults: I.V. infusion with 10 units of oxytocin in 500 ml of normal saline solution or dextrose 5% in normal saline solution. Infuse at rate of 10 to 20 milliunits/minute.

ADVERSE REACTIONS
Maternal—
Blood: afibrinogenemia; may be related to increased postpartum bleeding.
CNS: subarachnoid hemorrhage resulting from hypertension; *seizures or coma resulting from water intoxication.*
CV: hypotension; increased heart rate, systemic venous return, and cardiac output; arrhythmias.
GI: nausea, vomiting.
Other: hypersensitivity, tetanic contractions, abruptio placentae, *impaired uterine blood flow, increased uterine motility.*
Fetal—
Blood: hyperbilirubinemia.
CV: bradycardia, tachycardia, premature ventricular contractions.
Other: *anoxia, asphyxia.*

INTERACTIONS
Cyclopropane anesthetics: less pronounced bradycardia; hypotension.
Thiopental anesthetics: delayed induction reported.
Vasoconstrictors: severe hypertension if oxytocin is given within 3 to 4 hours of vasoconstrictor in patient receiving caudal block anesthetic.

NURSING CONSIDERATIONS
• Contraindicated in cases of cephalopelvic disproportion or where delivery requires conversion, as in trans-

---

Italicized adverse reactions are common or life-threatening.
*Liquid form contains alcohol.   **May contain tartrazine.

verse lie; fetal distress, when delivery isn't imminent; severe toxemia; and other obstetric emergencies. Use cautiously in history of cervical or uterine surgery, grand multiparity, uterine sepsis, traumatic delivery, or overdistended uterus, and in primiparas over 35 years. Use with extreme caution during first and second stages of labor because cervical laceration, uterine rupture, and maternal and fetal death have been reported.

• Don't give by I.V. bolus injection. Must administer by infusion; give by piggyback infusion so the drug may be discontinued without interrupting the I.V. line. Use an infusion pump.

• Used to induce or reinforce labor only when pelvis is known to be adequate, when vaginal delivery is indicated, when fetal maturity is assured, and when fetal position is favorable. Should be used only in hospital where critical care facilities and doctor are immediately available.

• Oxytocin should never be given simultaneously by more than one route.

• Do the following every 15 minutes: monitor and record uterine contractions, heart rate, blood pressure, intrauterine pressure, fetal heart rate, and character of blood loss.

• May produce an antidiuretic effect; fluid overload can lead to seizures and coma. Monitor fluid intake/output.

• If contractions occur less than 2 minutes apart and if contractions above 50 mm Hg are recorded, or if contractions last 90 seconds or longer, stop infusion, turn patient on her side, and notify doctor.

• Not recommended for routine I.M. use. However, 10 units may be given I.M. after delivery of placenta to control postpartum uterine bleeding.

• Should have magnesium sulfate (20% solution) available for relaxation of the myometrium.

oxytocin, synthetic nasal solution
Syntocinon

HOW SUPPLIED
Nasal solution: 40 units/ml

MECHANISM OF ACTION
Stimulates impaired milk ejection.

INDICATIONS & DOSAGE
To promote initial milk ejection; may relieve postpartum breast engorgement—
Adults: 1 spray into one or both nostrils 2 or 3 minutes before breastfeeding or pumping breasts.

ADVERSE REACTIONS
None reported.

INTERACTIONS
None significant.

NURSING CONSIDERATIONS
• Instruct patient to clear nasal passages first. With patient's head in vertical position, hold squeeze bottle upright and eject solution into nostril.

97

Spasmolytics

flavoxate hydrochloride
oxybutynin chloride

COMBINATION PRODUCTS
None.

flavoxate hydrochloride
Urispas

Pregnancy Risk Category: C

HOW SUPPLIED
Tablets: 100 mg

MECHANISM OF ACTION
Has a direct spasmolytic effect on smooth muscles of the urinary tract. It also provides some local anesthesia and analgesia.

INDICATIONS & DOSAGE
Symptomatic relief of dysuria, frequency, urgency, nocturia, incontinence, and suprapubic pain associated with urologic disorders—
Adults and children over 12 years:
100 to 200 mg P.O. t.i.d. to q.i.d.

ADVERSE REACTIONS
CNS: *mental confusion* (especially in elderly), nervousness, dizziness, headache, drowsiness, difficulty with concentration.
CV: tachycardia, palpitations.
EENT: *dry mouth and throat, blurred vision,* disturbed eye accommodation.
GI: abdominal pain, constipation (with high doses), nausea, vomiting.
Skin: urticaria, dermatoses.
Other: fever.

INTERACTIONS
None significant.

NURSING CONSIDERATIONS
• Contraindicated in pyloric or duodenal obstruction, obstructive intestinal lesions or ileus, achalasia, GI hemorrhage, or obstructive uropathies of lower urinary tract. Use cautiously in patients suspected of having glaucoma.
• Check history for other drug use before giving drugs with anticholinergic adverse reactions.
• Warn about possible drowsiness, mental confusion, and blurred vision.
• Tell the patient to report adverse reactions or lack of response to drug.

oxybutynin chloride
Ditropan

Pregnancy Risk Category: C

HOW SUPPLIED
Tablets: 5 mg
Syrup: 5 mg/5 ml

MECHANISM OF ACTION
Has both a direct spasmolytic effect and an atropine-like effect on urinary tract smooth muscles. It increases urinary bladder capacity and provides some local anesthesia and mild analgesia.

INDICATIONS & DOSAGE
Antispasmodic for neurogenic bladder—
Adults: 5 mg P.O. b.i.d. to t.i.d., to maximum of 5 mg q.i.d.

Italicized adverse reactions are common or life-threatening.
*Liquid form contains alcohol.   **May contain tartrazine.

Children over 5 years: 5 mg P.O.
b.i.d., to maximum of 5 mg t.i.d.

ADVERSE REACTIONS
CNS: *drowsiness,* dizziness, insomnia, *dry mouth,* flushing.
CV: *palpitations, tachycardia.*
EENT: *transient blurred vision,* mydriasis, cycloplegia.
GI: nausea, vomiting, *constipation,* bloated feeling.
GU: impotence, *urinary hesitance or urine retention.*
Skin: urticaria, severe allergic reactions in patients sensitive to anticholinergics.
Other: decreased sweating, fever, suppression of lactation.

INTERACTIONS
None significant.

NURSING CONSIDERATIONS
• Contraindicated in myasthenia gravis, GI obstruction, glaucoma, adynamic ileus, megacolon, severe or ulcerative colitis, obstructive uropathy, or in elderly or debilitated patients with intestinal atony. Use cautiously in elderly patients and in autonomic neuropathy, reflux esophagitis, and hepatic or renal disease.
• May aggravate symptoms of hyperthyroidism, coronary artery disease, CHF, cardiac arrhythmias, tachycardia, hypertension, or prostatic hypertrophy.
• Therapy should be stopped periodically to determine whether patient can get along without it. Minimizes tendency toward tolerance.
• Rapid onset of action, peaks at 3 to 4 hours, and lasts 6 to 10 hours.
• Neurogenic bladder should be confirmed by cystometry before oxybutynin is given. Evaluate patient response to therapy periodically by cystometry.
• Rule out partial intestinal obstruction in patients with diarrhea, especially those with colostomy or ileostomy, before giving oxybutynin.
• If urinary tract infection is present, patient should receive antibiotics concomitantly.
• Warn patient that drug may impair alertness or vision.
• Since oxybutynin suppresses sweating, its use during very hot weather may precipitate fever or heatstroke.
• Store in tightly closed containers at 59° to 86° F. (15° to 30° C.).

98

Gold salts

**auranofin
aurothioglucose
gold sodium thiomalate**

COMBINATION PRODUCTS
None.

---

auranofin
Ridaura

Pregnancy Risk Category: C

HOW SUPPLIED
Capsules: 3 mg

MECHANISM OF ACTION
Unknown. Anti-inflammatory effects in rheumatoid arthritis are probably caused by inhibition of sulfhydryl systems, which alters cellular metabolism. Auranofin may also alter enzyme function and immune response and suppress phagocytic activity.

INDICATIONS & DOSAGE
Rheumatoid arthritis—
Adults: 6 mg P.O. daily, administered either as 3 mg b.i.d. or 6 mg once daily. After 6 months, may be increased to 9 mg daily.

ADVERSE REACTIONS
Blood: *thrombocytopenia* (with or without purpura), *aplastic anemia, agranulocytosis,* leukopenia, eosinophilia.
GI: *diarrhea, abdominal pain, nausea, vomiting, stomatitis, enterocolitis,* anorexia, metallic taste, dyspepsia, flatulence.
GU: *proteinuria,* hematuria.

Hepatic: jaundice, elevated liver enzymes.
Respiratory: interstitial pneumonitis.
Skin: *rash, pruritus, dermatitis, exfoliative dermatitis.*

INTERACTIONS
None significant.

NURSING CONSIDERATIONS
• Contraindicated in patients with history of necrotizing enterocolitis, pulmonary fibrosis, exfoliative dermatitis, bone marrow aplasia, or severe hematologic disorders. Use cautiously with other drugs that cause blood dyscrasias. Use cautiously in patients who have preexisting renal disease, liver disease, inflammatory bowel disease, and skin rash.
• Remind patients to see their doctors on schedule for monthly platelet counts. Auranofin should be stopped if platelet count falls below 100,000/mm³.
• Reassure patient that beneficial drug effect may be delayed as long as 3 months. However, if response is inadequate after 3 months and after maximum dose is reached, doctor will probably discontinue auranofin.
• Encourage patient to take the drug as prescribed and not to alter the dosage schedule.
• Diarrhea is the most common adverse reaction. Tell patient to continue taking this drug if he experiences mild diarrhea; however, if he notes blood in his stool he should contact the doctor immediately.
• Tell patient to continue taking con-

Italicized adverse reactions are common or life-threatening.
*Liquid form contains alcohol.   **May contain tartrazine.

comitant drug therapy, such as NSAIDs, if prescribed.

• Dermatitis is a common adverse reaction. Advise patient to report any rashes or other skin problems immediately. Pruritus often precedes dermatitis and should be considered a warning of impending skin reactions. Any pruritic skin eruption while a patient is receiving auranofin should be considered a reaction to this drug until proven otherwise. Therapy is stopped until reaction subsides.

• Stomatitis is another common adverse reaction. Tell patient that stomatitis is often preceded by a metallic taste. Advise him to report this symptom to his doctor immediately. Careful oral hygiene is recommended during therapy.

• Auranofin, like injectable gold preparations, should be prescribed only for selected rheumatoid arthritis patients. Warn your patient *not* to give the drug to others.

• Patient should receive a copy of the patient information supplied by the manufacturer.

aurothioglucose
Gold-50‡, Solganal

gold sodium thiomalate
Myochrysine

Pregnancy Risk Category: C

HOW SUPPLIED
aurothioglucose
Injection (suspension): 50 mg/ml in sesame oil with aluminum monostearate 2% and propylparaben 0.1% in a 10 ml container
gold sodium thiomalate
Injection: 10 mg/ml, 50 mg/ml with benzyl alcohol

MECHANISM OF ACTION
Unknown. Anti-inflammatory effects in rheumatoid arthritis are probably caused by inhibition of sulfhydryl systems, which alters cellular metabolism. Gold salts may also alter enzyme function and immune response and suppress phagocytic activity.

INDICATIONS & DOSAGE
Rheumatoid arthritis—
Adults: initially, 10 mg (aurothioglucose) I.M., followed by 25 mg for second and third doses at weekly intervals. Then, 50 mg weekly until 1 g has been given. If improvement occurs without toxicity, continue 25 to 50 mg at 3- to 4-week intervals indefinitely as maintenance therapy.
Children 6 to 12 years: ¼ usual adult dosage. Alternatively, 1 mg/kg I.M. once weekly for 20 weeks.
Rheumatoid arthritis—
Adults: initially, 10 mg (gold sodium thiomalate) I.M., followed by 25 mg in 1 week. Then, 50 mg weekly until 14 to 20 doses have been given. If improvement occurs without toxicity, continue 50 mg q 2 weeks for 4 doses; then, 50 mg q 3 weeks for 4 doses; then, 50 mg q month indefinitely as maintenance therapy. If relapse occurs during maintenance therapy, resume injections at weekly intervals.
Children: 1 mg/kg I.M. weekly for 20 weeks. If response is good, may be given q 3 to 4 weeks indefinitely.

ADVERSE REACTIONS
Adverse reactions to gold are considered severe and potentially life-threatening. Report any side effects to the doctor at once.
Blood: *thrombocytopenia* (with or without purpura), *aplastic anemia, agranulocytosis,* leukopenia, eosinophilia.
CNS: *dizziness,* syncope, sweating.
CV: bradycardia, hypotension.
EENT: corneal gold deposition, corneal ulcers.
GI: *metallic taste, stomatitis,* difficulty swallowing, nausea, vomiting.
GU: *albuminuria, proteinuria, ne-*

phrotic syndrome, nephritis, acute tubular necrosis.
Hepatic: hepatitis, jaundice.
Skin: *rash and dermatitis in 20% of patients. (If drug is not stopped, may lead to fatal exfoliative dermatitis.)*
Other: *anaphylaxis,* angioneurotic edema.

INTERACTIONS
None significant.

NURSING CONSIDERATIONS
• Contraindicated in severe uncontrollable diabetes, renal disease, hepatic dysfunction, marked hypertension, heart failure, systemic lupus erythematosus, Sjögren's syndrome, skin rash, and drug allergies or hypersensitivities. Use cautiously with other drugs that cause blood dyscrasias.
• Indicated only in active rheumatoid arthritis that has not responded adequately to salicylates, rest, and physical therapy.
• Should be administered only under constant supervision of a doctor who is thoroughly familiar with the drug's toxicities and benefits.
• Most adverse reactions are readily reversible if drug is stopped immediately.
• Administer all gold salts I.M., preferably intragluteally. Color of drug is pale yellow; don't use if it darkens.
• Observe patient for 30 minutes after administration because of possible anaphylactoid reaction.
• Inform patient that benefits of therapy may not appear for 3 to 4 months or longer.
• Increased joint pain may occur for 1 to 2 days after injection. This usually subsides after a few injections.
• Gold therapy may alter liver function studies.
• Aurothioglucose is a suspension. Immerse vial in warm water and shake vigorously before injecting.
• When giving gold sodium thioma-

late, advise patient to lie down and to remain recumbent for 10 to 20 minutes after injection to minimize adverse reactions of hypotension.
• CBC, including platelet count, should be performed before every second injection for the duration of therapy.
• Dermatitis is the most common adverse reaction of gold salts. Advise patient to report any skin rashes or problems immediately. Pruritus often precedes dermatitis and should be considered a warning of impending skin reactions. Any pruritic skin eruption while a patient is receiving gold therapy should be considered a reaction until proven otherwise. Therapy is stopped until reaction subsides.
• Exposure to sunlight or artificial ultraviolet light should be minimized.
• Stomatitis is the second most common adverse reaction of gold therapy. Advise patient that stomatitis is often preceded by a metallic taste. This warning should be reported to the doctor immediately.
• Careful oral hygiene is recommended during therapy.
• Advise patient of the importance of close medical follow-ups and the need for frequent blood and urine tests during therapy.
• Urine should be analyzed for protein and sediment changes before each injection.
• Platelet counts should be performed if patient develops purpura or ecchymoses.
• If adverse reactions are mild, some rheumatologists may order resumption of gold therapy after 2 to 3 weeks' rest.
• Dimercaprol should be kept on hand to treat acute toxicity.

Italicized adverse reactions are common or life-threatening.
*Liquid form contains alcohol.   **May contain tartrazine.

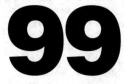

99

Diagnostic skin tests

coccidioidin
histoplasmin
mumps skin test antigen
tuberculin purified protein
   derivative
tuberculosis multiple-puncture
   tests

COMBINATION PRODUCTS
None.

---

coccidioidin
Spherulin

Pregnancy Risk Category: C

HOW SUPPLIED
Injection: 1:100 dilution (1 ml), 1:10 dilution (0.5 ml)

MECHANISM OF ACTION
Causes a cell-mediated immune response.

INDICATIONS & DOSAGE
Suspected coccidioidomycosis; to assess cell-mediated immunity—
Adults and children: 0.1 ml of 1:100 dilution intradermally into the flexor surface of the forearm. Use tuberculin syringe with 26G or 27G ⅝″ to ½″ needle. In persons nonreactive to this form, repeat test using 1:10 dilution.

ADVERSE REACTIONS
Local: hypersensitivity (vesiculation, ulceration, necrosis).
Other: *anaphylaxis,* Arthus reaction.

INTERACTIONS
None significant.

NURSING CONSIDERATIONS
• Test is read at 24 and 48 hours. Induration of 5 mm or more indicates a positive reaction (cell-mediated immune response). Erythema is not considered indicative of a delayed hypersensitivity reaction or positive response.
• Obtain history of allergies and reactions to skin tests. Patients allergic to thimerosal should not receive this skin test.
• Tell the patient not to wash off the circle marked on the the skin for serial skin tests, since this aids in the reading of the test results.
• Obtain history of any recent residence or travel to endemic areas— southern California, Arizona, New Mexico, and western Texas.
• Keep epinephrine 1:1,000 available.
• If a patient is suspected of having coccidioidomycosis because of clinical manifestations or X-ray findings and the 1:100 dilution is negative, the 1:10 dilution may be used.
• Reactivity to this test may be depressed or suppressed for as long as 4 to 6 weeks in individuals who have received concurrent or recent immunization with certain virus vaccines (for example, measles or influenza), in those who are receiving corticosteroid or immunosuppressive agents, in malnourished patients, and in those who have had viral infections (rubeola, influenza, mumps, and probably others).

---

histoplasmin
Histolyn-CYL

Pregnancy Risk Category: C

HOW SUPPLIED
Histolyn-CYL
Injection: vials containing 10 doses of 0.1 ml

MECHANISM OF ACTION
Causes a cell-mediated immune response.

INDICATIONS & DOSAGE
Suspected histoplasmosis; to assess cell-mediated immunity—
Adults and children: 0.1 ml intradermally into the flexor surface of the forearm. Use tuberculin syringe with 26G or 27G ⅝″ to ½″ needle.

ADVERSE REACTIONS
Local: urticaria, ulceration or necrosis in highly sensitive patients.
Other: *anaphylaxis.*

INTERACTIONS
None significant.

NURSING CONSIDERATIONS
• Read test within 24 to 48 hours. Induration of 5 mm or more is positive response. In some instances, maximum reactions may not be present until the fourth day.
• A positive reaction may indicate a past infection or a mild subacute or chronic infection with histoplasmosis or such immunologically related organisms as coccidioidomycosis or blastomycosis.
• Obtain history of allergies and reactions to skin tests.
• Histoplasmin should not be administered to known positive reactors because of severity of reaction.
• Cold packs or topical corticosteroids may relieve pain and itching if severe local reaction occurs.
• Serologic titers are often boosted by previous skin test. Draw serologic sample between 48 to 96 hours after skin test administration.
• Tuberculin skin test is advisable concurrently with histoplasmin test.
• Obtain history of any residence or recent travel to endemic areas—central (Ohio Valley) and eastern United States and Africa.
• Reactivity to this test may be depressed or suppressed for as long as 4 to 6 weeks in individuals who have received concurrent or recent immunization with certain virus vaccines (for example, measles or influenza), in those who are receiving corticosteroid or immunosuppressive agents, in malnourished patients, and in those who have had viral infections (rubeola, influenza, mumps, and probably others).

mumps skin test antigen
MSTA

HOW SUPPLIED
Injection (suspension): 20 complement-fixing units/ml

MECHANISM OF ACTION
Causes a cell-mediated immune response.

INDICATIONS & DOSAGE
To assess cell-mediated immunity—
Adults and children: 0.1 ml intradermally into the flexor surface of the forearm. Use tuberculin syringe with 26G or 27G ⅝″ to ½″ needle.

ADVERSE REACTIONS
Local: hypersensitivity (vesiculation, ulceration).
Other: *anaphylaxis,* Arthus reaction.

INTERACTIONS
None significant.

NURSING CONSIDERATIONS
• Test is read at 48- and 72-hour in-

Italicized adverse reactions are common or life-threatening.
*Liquid form contains alcohol.   **May contain tartrazine.

tervals. A positive reaction (cell-mediated immune response) is 5 mm or more of induration. Erythema is not considered indicative of a delayed hypersensitivity reaction.
• Obtain history of allergies and reactions to skin tests. In patients hypersensitive to eggs, feathers, and chicken, a severe reaction may follow administration.
• Don't administer to patients allergic to thimerosal.
• Keep epinephrine 1:1,000 available.
• Store vials in refrigerator.
• Mumps skin test antigen is *not* used to assess exposure to mumps. This antigen is used in assessing T cell function for immunocompetence.
• Reactivity to this test may be depressed or suppressed for as long as 4 to 6 weeks in individuals who have received concurrent or recent immunization with certain virus vaccines (for example, measles or influenza), in those who are receiving corticosteroid or immunosuppressive agents, in malnourished patients, and in those who have had viral infections (rubeola, influenza, mumps, and probably others).

tuberculin purified protein derivative (PPD)
Aplisol, PPD-stabilized Solution (Mantoux test), Tubersol

Pregnancy Risk Category: C

HOW SUPPLIED
Injection (intradermal): 1 tuberculin unit (TU)/0.1 ml, 5 TU/0.1 ml, 250 TU/0.1 ml

MECHANISM OF ACTION
Causes a cell-mediated immune response.

INDICATIONS & DOSAGE
Diagnosis of tuberculosis, evaluation of immunocompetence in patients with cancer, malnutrition—
Adults and children: initially, 1 TU (0.1 ml of appropriate solution) intradermally into flexor surface of the forearm. Use tuberculin syringe with 26G or 27G ⅝″ to ½″ needle. Retest with 5 TU and, if negative, 250 TU. If still no response, the individual is nonreactive.

ADVERSE REACTIONS
Local: pain, pruritus, vesiculation, ulceration, necrosis.
Other: *anaphylaxis,* Arthus reaction.

INTERACTIONS
None significant.

NURSING CONSIDERATIONS
• Contraindicated in known tuberculin-positive reactors; severe reactions may occur.
• Read test within 48 to 72 hours. An induration of 10 mm or greater indicates a significant reaction (formerly called positive reaction). Significance of a reaction is determined not only by the size of the reaction but by circumstances. For example, a reaction of 5 mm or more may be considered significant in a close relative of a person with known tuberculosis. A reaction of 2 mm or more may also be considered significant in infants and children. The amount of induration at the site—not erythema—determines the significance of the reaction.
• Report all known cases of tuberculosis to the appropriate public health agency.
• Obtain history of allergies and reactions to skin tests.
• Reactivity to this test may be depressed or suppressed for as long as 4 to 6 weeks in individuals who have received concurrent or recent immunization with certain virus vaccines (for example, measles or influenza), in those who are receiving corticosteroid or immunosuppressive agents, in

malnourished patients, and in those who have had viral infections (rubeola, influenza, mumps, and probably others).

• Keep epinephrine 1:1,000 available.

• S.C. injection invalidates test results. Bleb (6 to 10 mm in diameter) must form on skin upon intradermal injection.

• Cold packs or topical corticosteroids may relieve pain and itching of severe local reaction.

• Strongly positive tests can result in scarring at test site.

• Never give initial test with second test strength (250 tuberculin units). Use only when a patient has negative response to a 5–tuberculin unit PPD but has the clinical signs and symptoms of tuberculosis.

tuberculosis multiple-puncture tests

Aplitest (dried purified protein derivative [PPD]),
Mono-Vacc Test (liquid Old Tuberculin [OT]), Sclavo Test (dried PPD), Tine Test (dried OT, dried PPD)

Pregnancy Risk Category: C

HOW SUPPLIED
Test: 25 devices/pack, 5 tuberculin units/device

MECHANISM OF ACTION
Causes a cell-mediated immune response.

INDICATIONS & DOSAGE
Screening for tuberculosis—
Adults and children: cleanse skin thoroughly with alcohol; make skin taut on flexor surface of forearm and press points firmly into selected site. Hold device at injection site for about 3 seconds. This will ensure stabilizing the dried tuberculin B in tissue lymph.

ADVERSE REACTIONS
Local: hypersensitivity (vesiculation, ulceration, necrosis).
Other: *anaphylaxis.*

INTERACTIONS
Virus vaccine: tuberculosis skin-test reaction may be suppressed if test is given within 4 to 6 weeks after immunization with live or attenuated virus vaccines.

NURSING CONSIDERATIONS
• Contraindicated in known tuberculin-positive reactors.

• False-positive reaction can occur in sensitive patients.

• Reactivity to this test may be depressed or suppressed for as long as 4 to 6 weeks in individuals who have received concurrent or recent immunization with certain virus vaccines (for example, measles or influenza), in those who are receiving corticosteroid or immunosuppressive agents, in malnourished patients, and in those who have had viral infections (rubeola, influenza, mumps, and probably others), or miliary tuberculosis.

• Minimal bleeding can occur at the puncture site. This occurs infrequently and does not interfere with interpretation of the test results.

• Read test within 48 to 72 hours. Questionable or positive reactions to any multiple-puncture test must be verified by the Mantoux test. The amount of induration—not erythema—at the site determines significance of the reaction.

• Induration of 1 to 2 mm is significant.

• If vesiculation is present, the test may be interpreted as positive.

• Obtain history of allergies, especially to acacia (contained in the Tine Test as a stabilizer), and reactions to skin tests.

• Keep epinephrine 1:1,000 available.

• Report all known cases of tubercu-

Italicized adverse reactions are common or life-threatening.
*Liquid form contains alcohol.   **May contain tartrazine.

losis to appropriate public health agency.

• Cold packs or topical corticosteroids may relieve pain and itching if severe local reaction occurs after test.

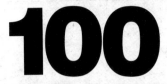

100

Miscellaneous antagonists and antidotes

Electrolyte depleting agents
sodium cellulose phosphate
sodium polystyrene sulfonate

Emetics
apomorphine hydrochloride
ipecac syrup

Heavy metal antagonists
deferoxamine mesylate
dimercaprol
D-penicillamine
edetate calcium disodium
edetate disodium
trientine hydrochloride

Opioid antagonists
naloxone hydrochloride
naltrexone hydrochloride

Respiratory stimulants
ammonia, aromatic spirits
doxapram hydrochloride

Miscellaneous
activated charcoal
aminocaproic acid
digoxin immune FAB (ovine)
pralidoxime chloride
protamine sulfate

(See also Chapter 36, CHOLINERGIC
BLOCKERS [PARASYMPATHOLYTICS].)
(See also Chapter 38, ADRENERGIC
BLOCKERS [SYMPATHOLYTICS].)

COMBINATION PRODUCTS
None.

---

activated charcoal
Actidose-Aqua◇, Charcoaide◇,
Charcocaps◇, Liqui-Char◇,
Superchar◇

Pregnancy Risk Category: C

HOW SUPPLIED
Tablets: 200 mg‡◇, 300 mg‡◇, 325
mg◇, 650 mg◇
Capsules: 260 mg◇
Powder: 30 g◇, 50 g◇
Oral suspension: 0.625 g/5 ml◇, 0.83
g/5 ml◇, 1 g/5 ml◇, 1.25 g/5 ml◇

MECHANISM OF ACTION
Adheres to many drugs and chemicals, inhibiting their absorption from
the GI tract. An adsorbent.

INDICATIONS & DOSAGE
Flatulence or dyspepsia—
Adults: 600 mg to 5 g P.O. t.i.d. or
q.i.d.
Poisoning—
Adults: initially, 1g/kg (30 to 100 g)
P.O. or 5 to 10 times the amount of
poison ingested as a suspension in 180
to 240 ml of water.
Children: 5 to 10 times estimated
weight of drug or chemical ingested.
Minimum dose is 30 g P.O. in 250 ml
water to make a slurry. Give orally,
preferably within 30 minutes of poisoning. Larger dose is necessary if
food is in the stomach. For treating
poisoning or overdosage with acetaminophen, amphetamines, aspirin,
antimony, atropine, arsenic, barbiturates, camphor, cocaine, cardiac glycosides, glutethimide, ipecac, mala-

---

Italicized adverse reactions are common or life-threatening.
*Liquid form contains alcohol.   **May contain tartrazine.

thion, morphine, poisonous mushrooms, opium, oxalic acid, parathion, phenol, phenothiazines, potassium permanganate, propoxyphene, quinine, strychnine, sulfonamides, or tricyclic antidepressants.

ADVERSE REACTIONS
GI: black stools, nausea.

INTERACTIONS
Acetylcysteine/ipecac: rendered ineffective. Don't administer together or lavage stomach until all charcoal is removed.

NURSING CONSIDERATIONS
• Don't use in semiconscious or unconscious persons.
• Because activated charcoal absorbs and inactivates syrup of ipecac, give after emesis is complete.
• Don't give in ice cream, milk, or sherbert. Reduces absorptive capacity.
• Powder form is most effective. Mix with tap water to form consistency of thick syrup. May add small amount of fruit juice or flavoring to make more palatable.
• May need to repeat dose if patient vomits shortly after administration.
• Space doses at least 1 hour apart from other drugs if activated charcoal is being used for any indication other than poisoning.
• Warn patient that feces will be black.

---

aminocaproic acid
Amicar

Pregnancy Risk Category: C

HOW SUPPLIED
Tablets: 500 mg
Syrup: 250 mg/ml
Injection: 5 g/20 ml for dilution, 24 g/96 ml for infusion

MECHANISM OF ACTION
Inhibits plasminogen activator substances. To a lesser degree, it blocks antiplasmin activity by inhibiting fibrinolysis.

INDICATIONS & DOSAGE
Excessive bleeding resulting from hyperfibrinolysis—
Adults: initially, 5 g P.O. or slow I.V. infusion, followed by 1 to 1.25 g hourly until bleeding is controlled. Maximum dosage is 30 g daily.

ADVERSE REACTIONS
Blood: generalized thrombosis.
CNS: dizziness, malaise, headache.
CV: hypotension, bradycardia, arrhythmias (with rapid I.V. infusion).
EENT: tinnitus, nasal stuffiness, conjunctival suffusion.
GI: nausea, cramps, diarrhea.
Skin: rash.
Other: malaise.

INTERACTIONS
Oral contraceptives, estrogens: increased probability of hypercoagulability. Use together cautiously.

NURSING CONSIDERATIONS
• Contraindicated in active intravascular clotting. Use cautiously in thrombophlebitis and cardiac, hepatic, or renal disease.
• Monitor coagulation studies, heart rhythm, and blood pressure. Notify doctor of any change immediately.
• Also used as antidote for streptokinase or urokinase toxicity; not beneficial in treating thrombocytopenia.
• Dilute solution with sterile water for injection, normal saline injection, dextrose 5% in water, or Ringer's injection.
• Drug is sometimes helpful as an adjunct in treating hemophilia.

---

ammonia, aromatic spirits◊

Pregnancy Risk Category: C

HOW SUPPLIED
Solution: 30 ml◊, 60 ml◊, 120 ml◊;
pints◊; gallons◊
Inhalant: 0.33 ml◊, 0.4 ml◊

MECHANISM OF ACTION
Irritates the sensory receptors in the
nasal membranes, producing reflex
stimulation of the respiratory centers.

INDICATIONS & DOSAGE
Fainting—
Adults and children: inhale as
needed.

ADVERSE REACTIONS
None reported.

INTERACTIONS
None significant.

NURSING CONSIDERATIONS
• Avoid inhaling vapors when administering drug.

apomorphine hydrochloride
Controlled Substance Schedule II
Pregnancy Risk Category: C

HOW SUPPLIED
Soluble tablets for injection: 6 mg

MECHANISM OF ACTION
Acts directly on the chemoreceptor
trigger zone in the medulla oblongata
to induce vomiting.

INDICATIONS & DOSAGE
To induce vomiting in poisoning—
Adults: 5 to 6 mg S.C. preceded by
200 to 300 ml water or, preferably,
evaporated milk. Don't repeat.
Children: 0.07 to 0.1 mg/kg S.C.
preceded by up to 2 glasses of water
or, preferably, evaporated milk.

ADVERSE REACTIONS
CNS: *depression, euphoria,* restlessness, tremor.
CV: *acute circulatory failure in elderly or debilitated patients,* tachycardia.
Other: *depressed respiratory center in
large or repeated doses.*

INTERACTIONS
*Antiemetics (such as antihistamines,
phenothiazines):* decreased emetic response, possibly with increased CNS
depression.

NURSING CONSIDERATIONS
• Contraindicated in patients with hypersensitivity to narcotics; impending
shock; corrosive poisoning; narcosis
resulting from opiates, barbiturates,
alcohol, or other CNS depressants;
and in patients too inebriated to stand
unaided. Use cautiously in children
and in patients who are debilitated,
have cardiac decompensation, or are
predisposed to nausea and vomiting.
• Don't give after ingestion of petroleum distillates (for example, kerosene, gasoline) or volatile oils; retching and vomiting may cause aspiration
and lead to bronchospasm, pulmonary
edema, or aspiration pneumonitis.
Vegetable oil will delay absorption of
these substances.
• Emetic action is increased if dosage
is followed immediately by water or
evaporated milk. Evaporated milk is
preferred because studies show that
water may increase absorption of
toxic substances.
• Don't give after ingestion of caustic
substances, such as lye; additional injury to the esophagus and mediastinum can occur.
• Keep narcotic antagonists, such as
naloxone, available to help stop vomiting and to alleviate drowsiness.
• If delay in giving emetic is expected, give activated charcoal P.O.
immediately. When absorbable poison
is ingested, give activated charcoal

Italicized adverse reactions are common or life-threatening.
*Liquid form contains alcohol.   **May contain tartrazine.

P.O. immediately after apomorphine hydrochloride.
• Vomiting occurs in 5 to 10 minutes in adults. If vomiting doesn't occur within 15 minutes, gastric lavage should begin. Apomorphine is emetic of choice when rapid removal of poisons is necessary, and when identification of enteric-coated tablets or other ingested toxic material in vomitus is important. Stomach contents are usually expelled completely; vomitus may also contain material from upper portion of intestinal tract.
• Don't administer if solution for injection is discolored green or precipitate is present.

deferoxamine mesylate
Desferal

Pregnancy Risk Category: C

HOW SUPPLIED
Powder for injection: 500 mg

MECHANISM OF ACTION
Chelates iron by binding ferric ions.

INDICATIONS & DOSAGE
Adjunctive treatment of acute iron intoxication—
Adults and children: 1 g I.M. or I.V. followed by 500 mg I.M. or I.V. for two doses, q 4 hours; then 500 mg I.M. or I.V. q 4 to 12 hours. Infusion rate shouldn't exceed 15 mg/kg hourly. Don't exceed 6 g in 24 hours.
Chronic iron overload resulting from multiple transfusions—
Adults and children: 500 mg to 1 g I.M. daily and 2 g slow I.V. infusion in separate solution along with each unit of blood transfused. Maximum dosage is 6 g daily. I.V. infusion rate shouldn't exceed 15 mg/kg hourly.
S.C.: 1 to 2 g via a subcutaneous infusion pump over 8 to 24 hours.

ADVERSE REACTIONS
Local: pain and induration at injection site.
Other: *after rapid I.V. administration: erythema, urticaria, hypotension, shock.*
With long-term use: sensitivity reaction (cutaneous wheal formation, pruritus, rash, *anaphylaxis), leg cramps, fever, tachycardia, dysuria, diarrhea, abdominal discomfort, blurred vision, cataracts.*

INTERACTIONS
None significant.

NURSING CONSIDERATIONS
• Contraindicated in severe renal disease or anuria. Use cautiously in impaired renal function.
• Monitor intake/output carefully.
• I.M. route preferred.
• Use I.V. only when patient has cardiovascular collapse or shock. For I.V. use, dissolve as for I.M. use; dilute in normal saline solution, dextrose 5% in water, or lactated Ringer's solution.
• If giving I.V., change to I.M. as soon as possible.
• For reconstitution, add 2 ml of sterile water for injection to each ampule. Make sure drug is completely dissolved. Reconstituted solution is good for 1 week at room temperature. Protect from light.
• Warn patient that urine may be red.
• Have epinephrine 1:1,000 readily available in case of allergic reaction.
• Recommend regular eye exams during long-term therapy.

digoxin immune FAB (ovine)
Digibind

Pregnancy Risk Category: C

HOW SUPPLIED
Injection: 40-mg vial

MECHANISM OF ACTION
Binds molecules of digoxin and digitoxin, making them unavailable for binding at site of action on cells in the body.

INDICATIONS & DOSAGE
Treatment of potentially life-threatening digoxin or digitoxin intoxication—
Adults and children: administered I.V. over 30 minutes or as a bolus if cardiac arrest is imminent. The dosage varies according to the amount of digoxin or digitoxin to be neutralized. Each vial binds about 0.6 mg digoxin or digitoxin. Average dosage is 10 vials (400 mg). However, if the toxicity resulted from acute digoxin ingestion, and neither a serum digoxin level nor an estimated ingestion amount is known, 20 vials (800 mg) should be administered. See package insert for complete, specific dosage instructions.

ADVERSE REACTIONS
CV: CHF, rapid ventricular rate (both caused by reversal of the cardiac glycoside's therapeutic effects).
Metabolic: hypokalemia.
Other: *hypersensitivity.*

INTERACTIONS
None reported.

NURSING CONSIDERATIONS
• Since digoxin immune FAB is derived from digoxin-specific antibody fragments obtained from immunized sheep, use cautiously in persons known to be allergic to ovine proteins. In these high-risk patients, skin testing is recommended. A limited supply of this drug is available at major medical centers or from the manufacturer (call Burroughs Wellcome at 1-800-334-4828 or, in North Carolina, 1-800-672-7223).
• This antidote should be used only for life-threatening overdose in patients in shock or cardiac arrest; with ventricular arrhythmias, such as ventricular tachycardia or fibrillation; with progressive bradycardia, such as severe sinus bradycardia; or with second- or third-degree AV block not responsive to atropine.
• Monitor potassium closely.
• In most patients, signs of digitalis toxicity disappear within a few hours.
• Best to infuse this drug through a 0.22-mcm membrane filter. However, give by bolus injection if cardiac arrest is considered imminent.
• Refrigerate powder for reconstitution. Reconstituted product should be used immediately, but it may be stored for up to 4 hours in the refrigerator.
• Digoxin immune FAB will interfere with digitalis immunoassay measurements, so standard serum digoxin levels will be misleading until the drug is cleared from the body (about 2 days).
• Total serum digoxin levels may rise after administration of this drug, but this reflects FAB-bound (inactive) digoxin.

---

dimercaprol
BAL in Oil

Pregnancy Risk Category: D

HOW SUPPLIED
Injection: 100 mg/ml

MECHANISM OF ACTION
Forms complexes with heavy metals.

INDICATIONS & DOSAGE
Severe arsenic or gold poisoning—
Adults and children: 3 mg/kg deep I.M. q 4 hours for 2 days, then q.i.d. on third day, then b.i.d. for 10 days.
Mild arsenic or gold poisoning—
Adults and children: 2.5 mg/kg deep I.M. q.i.d. for 2 days, then b.i.d. on third day, then once daily for 10 days.
Mercury poisoning—
Adults and children: 5 mg/kg deep

Italicized adverse reactions are common or life-threatening.
*Liquid form contains alcohol.   **May contain tartrazine.

I.M. initially, then 2.5 mg/kg daily or b.i.d. for 10 days.

Acute lead encephalopathy or lead level more than 100 mcg/ml—
Adults and children: 4 mg/kg deep I.M. injection, then q 4 hours with edetate calcium disodium (12.5 mg/kg I.M.). Use separate sites. Maximum dosage is 5 mg/kg per dose.

ADVERSE REACTIONS
CNS: pain or tightness in throat, chest, or hands; headache; paresthesias; muscle pain or weakness.
CV: *transient increase in blood pressure, returns to normal in 2 hours; tachycardia.*
EENT: blepharospasm, conjunctivitis, lacrimation, rhinorrhea, excessive salivation.
GI: *halitosis; nausea; vomiting; burning sensation in lips, mouth, and throat; abdominal pain.*
GU: *dysuria;* renal damage if alkaline urine not maintained.
Metabolic: decreased iodine uptake.
Local: sterile abscess, pain at injection site.
Other: *fever (especially in children),* sweating, pain in teeth.

INTERACTIONS
[131]I uptake thyroid tests: decreased; don't schedule patient for this test during course of dimercaprol therapy.
Iron: forms toxic metal complex; concurrent therapy contraindicated. Wait 24 hours after last dimercaprol dose.

NURSING CONSIDERATIONS
• Contraindicated in hepatic dysfunction (except postarsenical jaundice), or in acute renal insufficiency. Use cautiously in hypertension.
• Should not be used in pregnancy except to treat life-threatening poisoning.
• Don't use for iron, cadmium, or selenium toxicity. Complex formed is highly toxic, even fatal.
• Ephedrine or antihistamine may

prevent or relieve mild adverse reactions.
• Ineffective in arsine gas poisoning.
• Solution with slight sediment usable.
• Keep urine alkaline to prevent renal damage. Oral sodium bicarbonate may be ordered.
• Don't give I.V.; give by deep I.M. route only. The injection site can be massaged after drug is given.
• Drug has an unpleasant, garlic-like odor.
• Be careful when preparing and administering drug not to let drug come in contact with skin, as it may cause a skin reaction.

---

doxapram hydrochloride
Dopram
Pregnancy Risk Category: C

HOW SUPPLIED
Injection: 20 mg/ml (benzyl alcohol 0.9%)

MECHANISM OF ACTION
Acts either directly on the central respiratory centers in the medulla or indirectly on the chemoreceptors.

INDICATIONS & DOSAGE
Postanesthesia respiratory stimulation, drug-induced CNS depression, and chronic pulmonary disease associated with acute hypercapnia—
Adults: 0.5 to 1 mg/kg of body weight (up to 2 mg/kg in CNS depression), I.V. injection or infusion. Maximum dosage is 4 mg/kg, up to 3 g/day. Infusion rate is 1 to 3 mg/minute (initial: 5 mg/minute for postanesthesia).
Chronic obstructive pulmonary disease—
Adults: infusion, 1 to 2 mg/minute. Maximum is 3 mg/minute for a maximum duration of 2 hours.

ADVERSE REACTIONS
CNS: *seizures, headache,* dizziness, apprehension, disorientation, pupillary dilation, bilateral Babinski's signs, flushing, sweating, paresthesias.
CV: *chest pain and tightness, variations in heart rate, hypertension,* lowered T waves.
GI: nausea, vomiting, diarrhea.
GU: urine retention, or stimulation of the bladder with incontinence.
Other: sneezing, coughing, laryngospasm, bronchospasm, hiccups, rebound hypoventilation, pruritus.

INTERACTIONS
MAO inhibitors, sympathomimetics: potentiate adverse cardiovascular effects. Use together cautiously.

NURSING CONSIDERATIONS
• Contraindicated in seizure disorders; head injury; cardiovascular disorders; frank uncompensated heart failure; severe hypertension; CVA; respiratory failure or incompetence secondary to neuromuscular disorders, muscle paresis, flail chest, obstructed airway, pulmonary embolism, pneumothorax, restrictive respiratory disease, acute bronchial asthma, extreme dyspnea; or hypoxia not associated with hypercapnia. Use with caution in bronchial asthma, severe tachycardia or cardiac arrhythmias, cerebral edema or increased cerebrospinal fluid pressure, hyperthyroidism, pheochromocytoma, and metabolic disorders.
• Doxapram's use as an analeptic is strongly discouraged by most doctors.
• Establish adequate airway before administering drug. Prevent patient from aspirating vomitus by placing him on his side.
• Monitor blood pressure, heart rate, deep tendon reflexes, and arterial blood gases before giving drug and every 30 minutes afterward.
• Be alert for signs of overdosage: hypertension, tachycardia, arrhythmias, skeletal muscle hyperactivity, dyspnea. Discontinue if patient shows signs of increased arterial carbon dioxide or oxygen tension, or if mechanical ventilation is started. May give I.V. injection of anticonvulsant.
• Use only in surgical or emergency room situations.
• Do not combine with alkaline solutions such as thiopental sodium; doxapram is acidic.
• Extravasation may lead to thrombophlebitis and local skin irritation.
• Rapid infusion may cause hemolysis.

D-penicillamine
Cuprimine, Depen, D-Penamine‡
Pregnancy Risk Category: D

HOW SUPPLIED
Tablets: 125 mg‡, 250 mg
Capsules: 125 mg, 250 mg

MECHANISM OF ACTION
Mechanism of action in rheumatoid arthritis is unknown but is probably from inhibition of collagen formation. Also chelates heavy metals.

INDICATIONS & DOSAGE
Wilson's disease—
Adults: 250 mg P.O. q.i.d. 30 to 60 minutes before meals. Adjust dosage to achieve urinary copper excretion of 0.5 to 1 mg daily.
Children: 20 mg/kg P.O. daily divided q.i.d. before meals. Adjust dosage to achieve urinary copper excretion of 0.5 to 1 mg daily.
Cystinuria—
Adults: 250 mg to 1 g P.O. q.i.d. before meals. Adjust dosage to achieve urinary cystine excretion of less than 100 mg daily when renal calculi present, or 100 to 200 mg daily when no calculi present. Maximum dosage is 5 g daily.
Children: 30 mg/kg P.O. daily di-

---

vided q.i.d. before meals. Adjust dosage to achieve urinary cystine excretion of less than 100 mg daily when renal calculi present, or 100 to 200 mg daily when no calculi present.
Rheumatoid arthritis—
Adults: 125 to 250 mg P.O. daily initially, with increases of 250 mg q 2 to 3 months if necessary. Maximum dosage is 1.5 g daily.

ADVERSE REACTIONS
Blood: *leukopenia, eosinophilia, thrombocytopenia, monocytosis, granulocytopenia,* elevated sedimentation rate, lupus-like syndrome.
EENT: tinnitus.
GU: *nephrotic syndrome, glomerulonephritis, proteinuria.*
Hepatic: hepatotoxicity.
Metabolic: *decreased pyridoxine (may cause optic neuritis),* decreased zinc and mercury.
Skin: friability, especially at pressure spots; wrinkling; erythema; urticaria; ecchymoses.
Other: reversible taste impairment, especially of salts and sweets; hair loss. *About ⅓ of patients develop allergic reactions (rash, pruritus, fever), arthralgia, lymphadenopathy, or pneumonitis.* With long-term use, myasthenia gravis syndrome.

INTERACTIONS
Antacids, oral iron: decreased effectiveness of D-penicillamine. If used together, give at least 2 hours apart.

NURSING CONSIDERATIONS
• Contraindicated in pregnant women with cystinuria. Use cautiously in penicillin allergy; cross-sensitivity may occur. However, most penicillin-allergic patients can receive penicillamine.
• Rash and fever are important signs of toxicity and should be reported immediately.
• Patient should receive supplemental pyridoxine daily.

• Handle patient carefully to avoid skin damage if patient has a skin reaction.
• Antihistamines may be tried to manage skin reactions.
• Dose should be given on empty stomach to facilitate absorption, preferably 1 hour before or 3 hours after meals.
• Patient should drink large amounts of fluid, especially at night.
• Tell patient that therapeutic effect may be delayed up to 3 months in treatment of rheumatoid arthritis.
• Monitor CBC and renal and hepatic function regularly throughout therapy (every 2 weeks for the first 6 months, then monthly).
• Monitor urinalysis regularly for protein loss.
• Withhold drug and notify doctor if WBC count falls below 3,500/mm³ and/or platelet count falls below 100,000/mm³ (these are indications to stop drug). A progressive decline in platelet or WBC count in three successive blood tests may necessitate temporary cessation of therapy, even if these counts are within normal limits.
• Advise patient to report fever, sore throat, chills, bruising, and increased bleeding time; may be early signs of granulocytopenia.
• Provide appropriate health teaching for patients with Wilson's disease and cystinuria.
• Taste impairment usually resolves in 6 weeks without changes in dosage.

edetate calcium disodium
Calcium Disodium Versenate,
Calcium EDTA

Pregnancy Risk Category: C

HOW SUPPLIED
Injection: 200 mg/ml

MECHANISM OF ACTION
Forms stable, soluble complexes with metals, particularly lead.

INDICATIONS & DOSAGE
Lead poisoning (blood levels greater than 50 mcg/dl)—
Adults and children: 1 g/m² in dextrose 5% in water or normal saline solution I.V. over 1 to 2 hours daily for 3 to 5 days.
Acute lead encephalopathy or lead levels above 100 mcg/dl—
Adults and children: 1.5 g/m² I.V. daily for 3 to 5 days, usually in conjunction with dimercaprol. A second course may be administered at least 4 days later, but preferably 2 to 3 weeks should elapse between courses.

ADVERSE REACTIONS
CNS: headache, paresthesias, numbness.
CV: cardiac arrhythmias, hypotension.
GI: anorexia, nausea, vomiting.
GU: *proteinuria, hematuria; nephrotoxicity with renal tubular necrosis leading to fatal nephrosis.*
Other: arthralgia, myalgia, hypercalcemia.
   4 to 8 hours after infusion: sudden fever and chills, fatigue, excessive thirst, sneezing, nasal congestion.

INTERACTIONS
None significant.

NURSING CONSIDERATIONS
● Contraindicated in severe renal disease or anuria.
● I.V. use contraindicated in lead encephalopathy; may increase intracranial pressure. Use I.M. route instead.
● Force fluids to facilitate lead excretion in all patients except those with lead encephalopathy.
● Monitor intake/output, urinalysis, BUN, and ECGs daily.
● To avoid toxicity, use with dimercaprol.

● Procaine hydrochloride may be added to I.M. solutions to minimize pain. Watch for local reactions.
● Avoid rapid I.V. infusions. I.M. route preferred, especially for children.
● Do not confuse this drug with edetate disodium, which is used for treating hypercalcemia.

edetate disodium
Disodium EDTA, Disotate, Endrate
Pregnancy Risk Category: C

HOW SUPPLIED
Injection: 150 mg/ml

MECHANISM OF ACTION
Chelates with metals, such as calcium, to form a stable, soluble complex.

INDICATIONS & DOSAGE
Hypercalcemic crisis—
Adults: 50 mg/kg by slow I.V. infusion added to 500 ml of dextrose 5% in water or normal saline solution. Maximum dosage is 3 g/day.
Children: 40 to 70 mg/kg by slow I.V. infusion, diluted to a maximum concentration of 30 mg/ml in dextrose 5% in water or normal saline solution. Maximum dosage is 70 mg/kg/day.

ADVERSE REACTIONS
CNS: circumoral paresthesias, numbness, headache, malaise, fatigue, muscle pain or weakness.
CV: hypertension, thrombophlebitis, orthostatic hypotension.
GI: nausea, vomiting, diarrhea, anorexia, abdominal cramps.
GU: in excessive doses—nephrotoxicity with urgency, nocturia, dysuria, polyuria, proteinuria, renal insufficiency and failure, tubular necrosis.
Metabolic: *severe hypocalcemia,* decreased magnesium.
Local: pain at site of infusion, erythema, dermatitis.

Italicized adverse reactions are common or life-threatening.
*Liquid form contains alcohol.   **May contain tartrazine.

INTERACTIONS
None significant.

NURSING CONSIDERATIONS
• Contraindicated in anuria, known or suspected hypocalcemia, significant renal disease, active or healed tubercular lesions, history of seizures or intracranial lesions, and generalized arteriosclerosis associated with aging. Use cautiously in limited cardiac reserve, CHF, hypokalemia, and diabetes.
• Drug must be diluted before use. Avoid rapid I.V. infusion; profound hypocalcemia may occur, leading to tetany, seizures, cardiac arrhythmias, and respiratory arrest.
• Monitor ECG, and test renal function frequently.
• Obtain serum calcium after each dose.
• Keep I.V. calcium available.
• Monitor blood pressure closely.
• Keep patient in bed for 15 minutes after infusion to avoid orthostatic hypotension.
• Don't use to treat lead toxicity; use edetate calcium disodium instead.
• Record I.V. site used, and try to avoid repeated use of the same site, as this increases likelihood of thrombophlebitis.
• Generalized systemic reactions may occur 4 to 8 hours after drug administration; these include fever, chills, back pain, emesis, muscle cramps, and urinary urgency. Report such reactions to doctor. Treatment is usually supportive. Symptoms generally subside within 12 hours.
• Edetate disodium not currently drug of choice for treatment of hypercalcemia; other treatments are safer and more effective.
• EDTA chelation therapy has been inappropriately recommended for treatment of atherosclerosis and related disorders. There's no scientific evidence that the drug is either safe or effective for these indications.

ipecac syrup*
Pregnancy Risk Category:C

HOW SUPPLIED
Syrup: 70 mg powdered ipecac/ml ◊

MECHANISM OF ACTION
Induces vomiting by acting locally on the gastric mucosa and centrally on the chemoreceptor trigger zone.

INDICATIONS & DOSAGE
To induce vomiting in poisoning—
Adults and children over 12 years: 30 ml P.O., followed by 200 to 300 ml of water.
Children 1 year or older: 15 ml P.O., followed by about 200 ml of water or milk.
Children under 1 year: 5 to 10 ml P.O., followed by 100 to 200 ml of water or milk. May repeat dose once after 20 minutes, if necessary.

ADVERSE REACTIONS
CNS: depression.
CV: *cardiac arrhythmias, bradycardia, hypotension, atrial fibrillation, or fatal myocarditis after ingestion of excessive dose.*
GI: diarrhea.

INTERACTIONS
Activated charcoal: neutralized emetic effect. Don't give together but may give activated charcoal after vomiting has occurred.

NURSING CONSIDERATIONS
• Contraindicated in semicomatose or unconscious patients, or those with severe inebriation, seizures, shock, or loss of gag reflex.
• Don't give after ingestion of petroleum distillates (for example, kerosene, gasoline) or volatile oils; retching and vomiting may cause aspiration and lead to bronchospasm, pulmonary edema, or aspiration pneumonitis.

---

†Available in Canada only.   ‡Available in Australia only.   ◊ Available OTC.

Vegetable oil will delay absorption of these substances.

• Don't give after ingestion of caustic substances, such as lye; additional injury to the esophagus and mediastinum can occur.

• Clearly indicate ipecac *syrup*, not single word "ipecac," to avoid confusion with fluidextract. Fluidextract is 14 times more concentrated and, if inadvertently used instead of syrup, may cause death. This is unlikely in the United States, because the fluidextract is no longer commerically available.

• Induces vomiting within 30 minutes in more than 90% of patients; average time usually less than 20 minutes.

• Stomach is usually emptied completely; vomitus may contain some intestinal material as well.

• In antiemetic toxicity, ipecac syrup is usually effective if less than 1 hour has passed since ingestion of antiemetic.

• Recommend that 1 oz (30 ml) of syrup be readily available in the home when child becomes 1 year old for immediate use in case of emergency.

• No systemic toxicity with doses of 30 ml or less.

• If two doses do not induce vomiting, gastric lavage is necessary.

• Now commonly abused by bulimics who practice "binge-purge."

---

naloxone hydrochloride
Narcan

Pregnancy Risk Category: B

HOW SUPPLIED
Injection: 0.4 mg/ml, 1 mg/ml

MECHANISM OF ACTION
Displaces previously administered narcotic analgesics from their receptors (competitive antagonism). Has no pharmacologic activity of its own.

INDICATIONS & DOSAGE
Known or suspected narcotic-induced respiratory depression, including that caused by pentazocine and propoxyphene—
Adults: 0.4 to 2 mg I.V., S.C., or I.M. May repeat q 2 to 3 minutes, p.r.n. If no response is observed after 10 mg has been administered, the diagnosis of narcotic-induced toxicity should be questioned.
Postoperative narcotic depression—
Adults: 0.1 to 0.2 mg I.V. q 2 to 3 minutes, p.r.n. Adult concentration is 0.4 mg/ml.
Children: 0.01 mg/kg dose I.M., I.V., or S.C. May repeat q 2 to 3 minutes.
  Note: If initial dose of 0.01 mg/kg does not result in clinical improvement, up to 10 times this dose (0.1 mg/kg) may be needed to be effective.
Neonates (asphyxia neonatorum): 0.01 mg/kg I.V. into umbilical vein. May repeat q 2 to 3 minutes for 3 doses.

ADVERSE REACTIONS
With higher-than-recommended doses:
CV: tachycardia, hypertension.
GI: nausea, vomiting.
Other: tremors, withdrawal symptoms (in narcotic-dependent patients).

INTERACTIONS
None significant.

NURSING CONSIDERATIONS
• Use cautiously in cardiac irritability and narcotic addiction.

• Safest drug to use when cause of respiratory depression is uncertain.

• Monitor respiratory depth and rate. Be prepared to provide oxygen, ventilation, and other resuscitative measures.

• Respiratory rate increases within 1 to 2 minutes. Effect lasts 1 to 4 hours, but dosage may have to be repeated q 20 minutes.

• Duration of narcotic may exceed

Italicized adverse reactions are common or life-threatening.
*Liquid form contains alcohol.   **May contain tartrazine.

that of the naloxone. Patient may relapse into respiratory depression.
• May be administered by continuous I.V. infusion, which is often necessary to control the adverse effects of epidurally administered morphine.
• Can see "overshoot" effect—respiratory rate exceeds the rate before respiratory depression.
• Although generally believed to be ineffective in respiratory depression caused by nonnarcotics, recent reports indicate that it may reverse coma induced by alcohol intoxication.
• Does *not* reverse respiratory depression secondary to diazepam.
• May dilute adult concentration (0.4 mg) by mixing 0.5 ml with 9.5 ml sterile water or saline solution for injection to make neonatal concentration (0.02 mg/ml).
• Now available in 1-ml prefilled disposable syringes, 1-ml ampules, and 10-ml vials.
• Naloxone has been used investigationally to treat the senile dementia of Alzheimer's disease.
• Also has been shown to improve circulation in refractory shock.
• Used by some researchers to relieve certain kinds of chronic constipation.

naltrexone hydrochloride
Trexan

Pregnancy Risk Category: C

HOW SUPPLIED
Tablets: 50 mg

MECHANISM OF ACTION
Reversibly blocks the subjective effects of intravenously administered opioids by occupying opiate receptors in the brain.

INDICATIONS & DOSAGE
As an adjunct for maintenance of an opioid-free state in detoxified individuals—
Adults: initially, 25 mg P.O. If no

withdrawal signs occur within 1 hour, give an additional 25 mg. Once patient has been started on 50 mg q 24 hours, flexible maintenance schedule may be used. From 50 to 150 mg may be given daily, depending on the schedule prescribed.

ADVERSE REACTIONS
CNS: *insomnia, anxiety, nervousness, headache,* depression.
GI: *nausea, vomiting,* anorexia, *abdominal pain.*
Hepatic: *hepatotoxicity.*
Other: *muscle and joint pain.*

INTERACTIONS
None significant.

NURSING CONSIDERATIONS
• Contraindicated in patients receiving opioid analgesics, opioid-dependent patients, patients in acute opioid withdrawal, and in those with positive urine screen for opioids or acute hepatitis or liver failure.
• Treatment shouldn't begin until patient receives Narcan challenge, a provocative test of opioid dependency. If signs of opioid withdrawal persist after Narcan challenge, don't administer naltrexone.
• Use cautiously in mild liver disease or history of recent liver disease.
• Patients must be completely free of opioids before taking naltrexone, or they may experience severe withdrawal symptoms. Those who have been addicted to short-acting opioids (such as heroin and meperidine) must wait at least 7 days after the last opioid dose before starting naltrexone. Those who have been addicted to longer-acting opioids (such as methadone) should wait at least 10 days.
• In an emergency that requires opioid analgesia, a patient receiving naltrexone can be given an opioid analgesic. However, the dose must be higher than usual to surmount naltrexone's effect. Monitor for respiratory

depression from the opioid, which may be longer and deeper.

• Naltrexone should be used only as part of a comprehensive rehabilitation program.

• A suggested flexible maintenance dosage regimen: 100 mg on Monday and Wednesday; 150 mg on Friday. This schedule would be preferred for those expected to be poor compliers.

• Advise the patient to carry a medical identification card. Warn him to tell medical personnel that he is taking naltrexone, if he needs medical treatment.

• Give patient the names of nonopioid drugs that he can continue to take for pain, diarrhea, or cough.

---

pralidoxime chloride (pyridine-2-aldoxime methochloride; 2-PAM)
Protopam Chloride

Pregnancy Risk Category: C

HOW SUPPLIED
Tablets: 500 mg
Injection: 1-g/20-ml vial without diluent or syringe; 1-g/20-ml vial with diluent, syringe, needle, alcohol swab (emergency kit); 600-mg/2-ml autoinjector, parenteral

MECHANISM OF ACTION
Reactives cholinesterase that has been inactivated by organophosphorus pesticides and related compounds. It permits degradation of accumulated acetylcholine and facilitates normal functioning of neuromuscular junctions.

INDICATIONS & DOSAGE
Antidote for organophosphate poisoning—
Adults: I.V. infusion of 1 to 2 g in 100 ml of saline solution over 15 to 30 minutes. If pulmonary edema is present, give drug by slow I.V. push over 5 minutes. Repeat in 1 hour if muscle weakness persists. Additional

doses may be given cautiously. I.M. or S.C. injection can be used if I.V. is not feasible; or 1 to 3 g P.O. q 5 hours.
Children: 20 to 40 mg/kg I.V.
To treat cholinergic crisis in myasthenia gravis—
Adults: 1 to 2 g I.V., followed by increments of 250 mg I.V. q 5 minutes.

ADVERSE REACTIONS
CNS: dizziness, headache, drowsiness, excitement, and manic behavior following recovery of consciousness.
CV: tachycardia.
EENT: blurred vision, diplopia, impaired accommodation, laryngospasm.
GI: nausea.
Other: muscular weakness, muscle rigidity, hyperventilation.

INTERACTIONS
None significant.

NURSING CONSIDERATIONS
• Contraindicated in poisoning with Sevin, a carbamate insecticide, since it increases drug's toxicity. Use with extreme caution in renal insufficiency or myasthenia gravis (overdosage may precipitate myasthenic crisis); also in asthma or peptic ulcer.

• Use in hospitalized patients only; have respiratory and other supportive measures available. Obtain accurate medical history and chronology of poisoning if possible. Give as soon as possible after poisoning.

• I.V. preparation should be given slowly, as diluted solution.

• Initial measures should include removal of secretions, maintenance of patent airway, and artificial ventilation if needed. After dermal exposure to organophosphate, patient's clothing should be removed and his skin and hair should be washed with sodium bicarbonate, soap, water, and alcohol as soon as possible. A second washing may be necessary. When washing the

---

Italicized adverse reactions are common or life-threatening.
*Liquid form contains alcohol.   **May contain tartrazine.

patient, wear protective gloves and clothes to avoid exposure.

• Drug relieves paralysis of respiratory muscles but is less effective in relieving depression of respiratory center.

• Atropine along with pralidoxime should be given I.V., 2 to 4 mg, if cyanosis is not present. If cyanosis is present, atropine should be given I.M. Give atropine every 5 to 6 minutes until signs and symptoms of atropine toxicity appear (flushing, tachycardia, dry mouth, blurred vision, excitement, delirium, and hallucinations); maintain atropinization for at least 48 hours.

• Dilute with sterile water without preservatives.

• Not effective against poisoning due to phosphorus, inorganic phosphates, or organophosphates with no anticholinesterase activity.

• Difficult to distinguish between toxic effects produced by atropine or by organophosphate compounds and those resulting from pralidoxime. Observe patient for 48 to 72 hours if poison was ingested. Delayed absorption may occur from lower bowel.

• Caution patients treated for organophosphate poisoning to avoid contact with insecticides for several weeks.

• Patients with myasthenia gravis treated for overdose of cholinergic drugs should be observed closely for signs of rapid weakening. These patients can pass quickly from a cholinergic crisis to a myasthenic crisis, and require more cholinergic drugs to treat the myasthenia. Keep edrophonium (Tensilon) available in such situations for establishing differential diagnosis.

• Although not approved, subconjunctival injection of pralidoxime has been used to reverse adverse ocular reactions resulting from splashing into the eye or systemic overdose of organophosphates.

• Treatment is most effective if initiated within 24 hours after exposure.

• Draw blood for cholinesterase levels before giving pralidoxime.

---

protamine sulfate
Pregnancy Risk Category: C

HOW SUPPLIED
Injection: 10 mg/ml

MECHANISM OF ACTION
Forms a physiologically inert complex with heparin sodium.

INDICATIONS & DOSAGE
Heparin overdose—
Adults: dosage based on venous blood coagulation studies, usually 1 mg for each 90 to 115 units of heparin. Give diluted to 1% (10 mg/ml) slow I.V. injection over 1 to 3 minutes. Maximum dose is 50 mg/10 minutes.

ADVERSE REACTIONS
CV: fall in blood pressure, bradycardia.
Other: transitory flushing, feeling of warmth, dyspnea.

INTERACTIONS
None significant.

NURSING CONSIDERATIONS
• Use cautiously after cardiac surgery.
• Should be given slowly to reduce adverse reactions. Have equipment available to treat shock.
• Monitor patient continually. Check vital signs frequently.
• Watch for spontaneous bleeding (heparin "rebound"), especially in patients undergoing dialysis and those who have had cardiac surgery.
• Protamine sulfate may act as anticoagulant in very high doses.
• 1 mg of protamine neutralizes 90 to 115 units of heparin depending on the salt (hepardin calcium or heparin so-

---

dium) and the source of heparin (beef or pork).
• Heparin antagonist.

sodium cellulose phosphate
Calcibind

Pregnancy Risk Category: C

HOW SUPPLIED
Powder: 2.5-g packets or 300-g bulk. Inorganic phosphate content approximately 34%; sodium content approximately 11%.

MECHANISM OF ACTION
Binds calcium in the GI tract and decreases the amount absorbed.

INDICATIONS & DOSAGE
Treatment of absorptive hypercalciuria type I with recurrent calcium oxalate or calcium phosphate renal stones—
Adults: 15 g/day P.O. (5 g with each meal) in patients with urine calcium greater than 300 mg/day. When urine calcium declines to less than 150 mg/day, reduce dosage to 10 g/day (5 g with dinner, 2.5 g with two remaining meals).

ADVERSE REACTIONS
CNS: drowsiness, mood or mental changes, *seizures,* trembling.
GI: anorexia, nausea, vomiting, discomfort, diarrhea, dyspepsia.
GU: hyperoxaluria, hypomagnesuria.
Other: acute arthralgias.

INTERACTIONS
Magnesium-containing products: may bind drug. Separate doses by at least 1 hour.

NURSING CONSIDERATIONS
• Contraindicated in primary or secondary hyperparathyroidism, including renal hypercalciuria; hypomagnesemic states; bone disease; hypocalcemic states; normal or low intestinal

absorption; renal excretion of calcium; or enteric hyperoxaluria.
• Use cautiously in CHF or ascites.
• Recommended only for the type of absorptive hypercalciuria in which both intestinal calcium absorption and urine calcium remain abnormally high even with a calcium-restricted diet. When administered inappropriately, it can cause hypocalciuria. This could stimulate parathyroid function and lead to parathyroid bone disease.
• Patient should maintain a calcium-restricted diet and avoid all dairy products.
• Patient taking sodium cellulose phosphate may develop hyperoxaluria and hypomagnesuria, which predispose him to stone formation. Therefore, advise patient to restrict dietary intake of oxalate (found in spinach, rhubarb, chocolate, and tea).
• Avoid vitamin C because it can increase urine oxalate.
• Encourage fluid intake. Urine output should be at least 2 liters/day.
• Patient can mix the powder with 8 oz of fruit juice, water, or a soft drink and take it with meals. Patient should rinse glass and drink all of the fluid to get the full dose.
• Encourage a low-sodium diet. Tell patient to avoid salty foods and to avoid adding salt at the table.
• Because of the difficulty involved in managing sodium cellulose phosphate therapy, many doctors prefer to treat hypercalciuria with a low-calcium diet, high fluid intake, and thiazides, when necessary.

sodium polystyrene sulfonate
Kayexalate, Resonium A, SPS

Pregnancy Risk Category: C

HOW SUPPLIED
Oral powder: 1.25 g/5 ml suspension
Rectal: 1.25 g/5 ml suspension

Italicized adverse reactions are common or life-threatening.
*Liquid form contains alcohol.   **May contain tartrazine.

MECHANISM OF ACTION

The potassium-removing resin exchanges sodium ions for potassium ions in the intestine: 1 g of sodium polystyrene sulfonate is exchanged for 0.5 to 1 mEq of potassium. The resin is then eliminated. Much of the exchange capacity is used for cations other than potassium (calcium and magnesium) and possibly for fats and proteins.

INDICATIONS & DOSAGE

Hyperkalemia—
Adults: 15 g P.O. daily to q.i.d. in water or sorbitol (3 to 4 ml/g of resin).

For rectal administration, 30 to 50 g/100 ml of sorbitol q 6 hours as warm emulsion deep into sigmoid colon (20 cm). In persistent vomiting or paralytic ileus, high retention enema of sodium polystyrene sulfonate (30 g) suspended in 200 ml of 10% methylcellulose, 10% dextrose, or 25% sorbitol solution.

Children: 1 g of resin P.O. for each mEq of potassium to be removed.

Oral administration preferred since drug should remain in intestine for at least 6 hours; otherwise, consider nasogastric administration.

For nasogastric administration, mix dose with appropriate medium— aqueous suspension or diet appropriate for renal failure; instill in plastic tube.

ADVERSE REACTIONS

GI: *constipation,* fecal impaction (in elderly patients), anorexia, gastric irritation, nausea, vomiting, *diarrhea (with sorbitol emulsions).*
Other: *hypokalemia,* hypocalcemia, hypomagnesemia, sodium retention.

INTERACTIONS

Antacids and laxatives (nonabsorbable cation-donating type, including magnesium hydroxide): systemic alkalosis, reduced potassium exchange capability. Don't use together.

NURSING CONSIDERATIONS

• Use with caution in elderly patients and those on digitalis therapy, with severe congestive heart failure, severe hypertension, and marked edema.
• Treatment may result in potassium deficiency. Monitor serum potassium at least once daily. Usually stopped when potassium is reduced to 4 or 5 mEq/liter. Watch for other signs of hypokalemia: irritability, confusion, cardiac arrhythmias, ECG changes, severe muscle weakness and sometimes paralysis, and digitalis toxicity in digitalized patients.
• Monitor for symptoms of other electrolyte deficiencies (magnesium, calcium) since drug is nonselective. Monitor serum calcium in patients receiving sodium polystyrene therapy for more than 3 days. Supplementary calcium may be needed.
• Drug contains about 100 mg sodium/g. Watch for sodium overload. About ⅓ of resin's sodium is retained.
• Premixed forms are available (SPS and others).
• Do not heat resin. This will impair effectiveness of drug. Mix resin only with water or sorbitol for P.O. administration. Above all, *never* mix with orange juice (high potassium content) to disguise taste.
• Chill oral suspension for greater palatability.
• If sorbitol is given, it may be mixed with resin suspension.
• Consider solid form. Resin cookie and candy recipes are available; perhaps pharmacist or dietitian can supply.
• Watch for constipation in oral or nasogastric administration. Use sorbitol (10 to 20 ml of 70% syrup every 2 hours as needed) to produce one or two watery stools daily.
• If preparing manually, mix polystyrene resin only with water and sorbitol

for rectal use. Do not use other vehicles (that is, mineral oil) for rectal administration to prevent impactions. Ion exchange requires aqueous medium. Sorbitol content prevents impaction.
• Prevent fecal impaction in elderly by administering resin rectally. Give cleansing enema before rectal administration. Explain necessity of retaining enema to patient. Retention for 6 to 10 hours is ideal, but 30 to 60 minutes is acceptable.
• Prepare rectal dose at room temperature. Stir emulsion gently during administration.
• Use #28 French rubber tube for rectal dose; insert 20 cm into sigmoid colon. Tape tube in place. Alternatively, consider a Foley catheter with a 30-ml balloon inflated distal to anal sphincter to aid in retention. This is especially helpful for patients with poor sphincter control (for example, after cerebrovascular accident). Use gravity flow. Drain returns constantly through Y-tube connection. When giving rectally, place patient in knee-chest position or with hips on pillow for a while if back-leakage occurs.
• After rectal administration, flush tubing with 50 to 100 ml of nonsodium fluid to ensure delivery of all medication.
• Flush rectum to remove the resin.
• If hyperkalemia is severe, more drastic modalities should be added; for example, dextrose 50% with regular insulin I.V. push. Do not depend solely on polystyrene resin to lower serum potassium in severe hyperkalemia.

---

trientine hydrochloride
Cuprid

Pregnancy Risk Category: C

HOW SUPPLIED
Capsules: 250 mg

MECHANISM OF ACTION
Chelates copper and increases its urinary excretion.

INDICATIONS & DOSAGE
Treatment of Wilson's disease in patients who cannot tolerate penicillamine—
Adults: 750 to 2,000 mg P.O. daily in two, three, or four divided doses.
Children: 500 to 1,500 mg P.O. daily in two, three, or four divided doses.

The optimal long-term maintenance dosage should be determined q 6 to 12 months, according to serum copper analysis.

ADVERSE REACTIONS
Blood: iron deficiency anemia.
Other: hypersensitivity (rash), fever.

INTERACTIONS
Mineral supplements (including iron): may block trientine absorption. Administer at least 2 hours apart.

NURSING CONSIDERATIONS
• Patients (especially women) should be closely monitored for evidence of iron deficiency anemia throughout therapy.
• Observe patient for signs of hypersensitivity, such as skin rash.
• Tell patient to take trientine on an empty stomach at least 1 hour before meals or 2 hours after meals, and at least 1 hour apart from any other drug, food, or milk.
• Capsules should be swallowed whole with water and should not be opened or chewed.
• Exposure to capsule contents may cause contact dermatitis. If capsule is accidentally opened and contents spilled on the skin, tell patient to wash the site thoroughly.
• Trientine should be prescribed for only patients who cannot tolerate penicillamine, the standard treatment for Wilson's disease.
• Urge your patient to faithfully fol-

Italicized adverse reactions are common or life-threatening.
*Liquid form contains alcohol.   **May contain tartrazine.

low his trientine regimen and low-copper diet as prescribed.
• Patient should take his temperature every night and report any fevers or skin eruptions, especially during the first month of therapy.

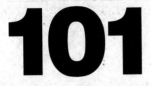

Uncategorized drugs

acetohydroxamic acid
allopurinol
alpha-1 proteinase inhibitor
  (human)
alprostadil
benzoyl peroxide cleansers
benzoyl peroxide creams
benzoyl peroxide gels
benzoyl peroxide lotions
bromocriptine mesylate
capsaicin
carbidopa-levodopa
clomiphene citrate
colchicine
cromolyn sodium
diazoxide, oral
disulfiram
etretinate
fluorouracil
isotretinoin
levocarnitine
levodopa
mesalamine
mesna
methoxsalen
minoxidil (topical)
nicotine polacrilex
octreotide acetate
pentoxifylline
pergolide mesylate
ritodrine hydrochloride
selegiline hydrochloride
sodium benzoate and sodium
  phenylacetate
tiopronin
tretinoin

COMBINATION PRODUCTS
COLBENEMID: probenecid 500 mg
and colchicine 0.5 mg.
PROBENECID WITH COLCHICINE: probenecid 500 mg and colchicine 0.5
mg.

---

acetohydroxamic acid
Lithostat

Pregnancy Risk Category: X

HOW SUPPLIED
Tablets (scored): 250 mg

MECHANISM OF ACTION
Prevents formation of renal stones by
inhibiting bacterial urease activity.

INDICATIONS & DOSAGE
*Treatment of infection-related kidney
stones—*
Adults: 250 mg P.O. t.i.d. or q.i.d.
Administer at 6- to 8-hour intervals at
a time when the stomach is empty.
Maximum daily dosage is 1.5 g.
Children: 10 mg/kg/day P.O. in two
or three divided doses.

ADVERSE REACTIONS
Blood: *hemolytic anemia.*
CNS: *mild headache, depression,
anxiety, nervousness.*
CV: *phlebitis, palpitations.*
GI: *nausea, vomiting, diarrhea, con-
stipation, anorexia.*
Skin: *nonpruritic, macular rash on
arms and face.*
Other: alopecia, deep vein thrombo-
sis, malaise.

INTERACTIONS
Methenamine: may produce synergis-
tic effects.
Oral iron supplements: reduce ab-

Italicized adverse reactions are common or life-threatening.
*Liquid form contains alcohol.   **May contain tartrazine.

sorption of acetohydroxamic acid. Check with doctor; he may request that iron be administered I.M.

NURSING CONSIDERATIONS

• Contraindicated in patients whose physical state and disease are amenable to surgery and appropriate antibiotics; in patients whose urine is infected by nonurease-producing organisms in pregnancy; and in poor renal function.

• Use cautiously in patients predisposed to deep vein thrombosis.

• Coombs'-negative hemolytic anemia has occurred in patients receiving acetohydroxamic acid.

• Monitor CBC, including a reticulocyte count, after 2 weeks of therapy. Thereafter, monitor at 3-month intervals for the duration of treatment. If laboratory findings indicate hemolytic anemia, discontinue drug.

• Skin rash more common during prolonged use and with concomitant use of alcoholic beverages. The rash appears 30 to 45 minutes after ingestion of alcoholic beverages; disappears spontaneously in 30 to 60 minutes. Although skin rash doesn't usually require treatment, advise patient to avoid alcohol.

• Reduced dosage may be necessary in renal impairment.

---

allopurinol

Alloremed‡, Capurate‡, Lopurin, Zyloprim

Pregnancy Risk Category: C

HOW SUPPLIED
Tablets (scored): 100 mg, 300 mg
Capsules: 100 mg‡, 300 mg‡

MECHANISM OF ACTION
Reduces uric acid production by inhibiting the biochemical reactions preceding its formation.

INDICATIONS & DOSAGE
Gout, primary or secondary to hyperuricemia; secondary to diseases such as acute or chronic leukemia, polycythemia vera, multiple myeloma, and psoriasis—
Dosage varies with severity of disease; can be given as single dose or divided, but doses larger than 300 mg should be divided.
Adults: mild gout, 200 to 300 mg P.O. daily; severe gout with large tophi, 400 to 600 mg P.O. daily. Same dosage for maintenance in secondary hyperuricemia.
Hyperuricemia secondary to malignancies—
Children 6 to 10 years: 300 mg P.O. daily or divided t.i.d.
Children under 6 years: 50 mg P.O. t.i.d.
Impaired renal function—
Adults: 200 mg P.O. daily if creatinine clearance is 10 to 20 ml/minute; 100 mg P.O. daily if creatinine is less than 10 ml/minute; 100 mg P.O. more than 24 hours apart if clearance is less than 3 ml/minute.
To prevent acute gouty attacks—
Adults: 100 mg P.O. daily; increase at weekly intervals by 100 mg without exceeding maximum dose (800 mg), until serum uric acid falls to 6 mg/100 ml or less.
To prevent uric acid nephropathy during cancer chemotherapy—
Adults: 600 to 800 mg P.O. daily for 2 to 3 days, with high fluid intake.
Recurrent calcium oxalate calculi—
Adults: 200 to 300 mg P.O. daily in single dose or divided doses.

ADVERSE REACTIONS
Blood: *agranulocytosis,* anemia, *aplastic anemia.*
CNS: drowsiness, headache.
EENT: cataracts, retinopathy.
GI: nausea, vomiting, diarrhea, abdominal pain.
Hepatic: altered liver function studies, hepatitis.

Skin: *rash, usually maculopapular; exfoliative,* urticarial, and purpuric lesions; erythema multiforme; severe furunculosis of nose; ichthyosis, *toxic epidermal necrolysis.*

INTERACTIONS

Alcohol, bumetanide, diazoxide, ethacrynic acid, furosemide, triamterene, mecamylamine, pyrazinamide: increased serum uric acid concentration; adjust dosage of allupurinol.

Ampicillin, bacampicillin, hetacillin: increased possibility of skin rash.

Anticoagulants: potentiation of anticoagulant effect. Dosage adjustments may be necessary.

Antineoplastic agents: increased potential for bone marrow suppression. Monitor patient carefully.

Chlorpropamide: possible increased hypoglycemic effect.

Uricosuric agents: additive effect; may be used to therapeutic advantage.

Urinary acidifying agents (ammonium chloride, ascorbic acid, potassium or sodium phosphate): may increase the possibility of kidney stone formation.

Xanthines: increased serum theophylline. Adjust dosage of theophyllines.

NURSING CONSIDERATIONS

• Contraindicated in hypersensitivity and in idiopathic hemochromatosis. Use cautiously in cataracts and hepatic or renal disease.

• Obtain accurate patient history.

• Discontinue at first sign of rash, which may precede severe hypersensitivity reaction or any other adverse reaction. Tell patient to report all adverse reactions immediately. Skin rash is more common in patients taking diuretics and in those with renal disorders.

• Monitor intake/output; daily urine output of at least 2 liters and maintenance of neutral or slightly alkaline urine are desirable. Patient should be encouraged to drink plenty of fluids

while taking this drug unless otherwise contraindicated.

• If renal insufficiency exists at any time during treatment, allopurinol dosage should be reduced.

• Periodically check CBC and hepatic and renal function, especially at start of therapy.

• If patient is taking allopurinol for treatment of recurrent calcium oxalate stones, advise him to also reduce his dietary intake of animal protein, sodium, refined sugars, oxalate-rich foods, and calcium.

• Acute gouty attacks may occur in first 6 weeks of therapy; concurrent use of colchicine may be prescribed prophylactically.

• Minimize GI adverse reactions by administering with meals or immediately after.

• Evaluate effectiveness, using serum uric acid level.

• Allopurinol may predispose patient to ampicillin-induced rash.

• Allopurinol may cause rash even weeks after discontinuation.

• Since drug may cause drowsiness, advise patient to refrain from driving car or performing tasks requiring mental alertness until CNS effects of the drug are known.

alpha-1 proteinase inhibitor (human)
Prolastin

Pregnancy Risk Category: C

HOW SUPPLIED
Injection: 500 mg, 1,000 mg

MECHANISM OF ACTION
Replaces alpha₁-proteinase in patients with alpha₁-antitrypsin deficiency.

INDICATIONS & DOSAGE
Chronic replacement therapy in patients with congenital alpha₁-antitrypsin deficiency and demonstrable panacinar emphysema—

Italicized adverse reactions are common or life-threatening.
*Liquid form contains alcohol.   **May contain tartrazine.

Adults: 60 mg/kg I.V. once weekly. May be given at the rate of 0.08 ml/kg/minute or greater.

ADVERSE REACTIONS
Blood: possible viral transmission.

INTERACTIONS
None reported.

NURSING CONSIDERATIONS
• Explain to the patient that the product has been treated to minimize the risk of transmission of hepatitis and AIDS.
• Many commercial assays for alpha$_1$-proteinase inhibitor measure immunoreactivity of the protein and not inhibitor activity. Monitoring serum level may not accurately reflect clinical response.

alprostadil
Prostin VR Pediatric

HOW SUPPLIED
Injection: 500 mcg/ml

MECHANISM OF ACTION
A prostaglandin derivative which relaxes the smooth muscle of the ductus arteriosus.

INDICATIONS & DOSAGE
Palliative therapy for temporary maintenance of patency of ductus arteriosus until surgery can be performed—
Infants: 0.05 to 0.1 mcg/kg/minute by I.V., intraarterial, or intraaortic infusion. When therapeutic response is achieved, reduce infusion rate to give lowest dosage that will maintain response. Maximum dosage is 0.4 mcg/kg/minute. Alternatively, administer through umbilical artery catheter placed at ductal opening.

ADVERSE REACTIONS
Blood: disseminated intravascular coagulation.

CNS: *seizures.*
CV: *flushing,* bradycardia, hypotension, tachycardia.
GI: diarrhea.
Other: *apnea, fever, sepsis.*

INTERACTIONS
None reported.

NURSING CONSIDERATIONS
• Contraindicated in neonatal respiratory distress syndrome.
• Because drug inhibits platelet aggregation, use cautiously in neonates with bleeding tendencies.
• Monitor arterial pressure by umbilical artery catheter, auscultation, or Doppler transducer. Slow rate of infusion if arterial pressure falls significantly.
• In infants with restricted pulmonary blood flow, measure drug's effectiveness by monitoring blood oxygenation. In infants with restricted systemic blood flow, measure drug's effectiveness by monitoring systemic blood pressure and blood pH.
• Drug must be diluted before being administered. Fresh solution must be prepared daily. Discard any solution more than 24 hours old.
• Apnea and bradycardia may reflect drug overdose. If the signs occur, stop infusion immediately.
• CV and CNS adverse reactions are more frequent in infants weighing less than 2 kg and in those receiving infusions for longer than 48 hours.
• Keep respiratory support available.
• Use a constant rate infusion pump to administer.
• If flushing occurs from peripheral vasodilation, reposition catheter.
• Reduce infusion rate if fever or significant hypotension occurs.
• Do not use diluents that contain benzyl alcohol. Fatal toxic syndrome may occur.

benzoyl peroxide cleansers
Benzac W Wash 5, Benzac W Wash 10, Desquam-X 5 Wash, Desquam-X 10 Wash, Fostex 10% BPO Cleansing◇, Fostex 10% BPO Wash◇, Oxy-10 Wash◇, PanOxyl 5◇, PanOxyl 10◇, Propa P.H. Liquid Acne Soap◇

benzoyl peroxide creams
Acne-Aid◇, Clearasil Maximum Strength◇, Cuticura Acne◇, Dry and Clear Double Strength, Fostex 10% BPO Tinted◇, Oxy 10 Cover◇, phisoAc BP◇

benzoyl peroxide gels
5 Benzagel, 10 Benzagel, Benzac 5, Benzac W 5, Benzac W 10, Benzac W 2 1/2, Ben-Aqua 5, Ben-Aqua 10, Buf-Oxal 10◇, Clear By Design◇, Del Aqua 5◇, Del Aqua 10◇, Desquam-E, Desquam-X 5, Desquam-X 10, Desquam-X 2.5, Fostex 5% BPO◇, Fostex 10% BPO◇, PanOxyl 5, PanOxyl 10, PanOxyl AQ 5, PanOxyl AQ 10, PanOxyl AQ 2 1/2, Persa-Gel, Persa-Gel W 5%, Persa-Gel W 10%, Xerac BP5◇, Xerac BP10◇, Zeroxin-5, Zeroxin-10,

benzoyl peroxide lotions
Acne-10◇, Ben-Aqua 5◇, Benoxyl 5◇, Benoxyl 10◇, Clearasil 10◇, Dry and Clear◇, Loroxide ◇, Oxy 5◇, Oxy 10◇, Vanoxide◇

Pregnancy Risk Category: C

HOW SUPPLIED
Cream: 5%◇, 10%◇
Gel: 2.5%◇, 5%◇, 10%◇
Liquid cleanser: 5%, 10%◇
Lotion: 5%◇, 5.5%◇, 10%◇
Soap (bar): 5%◇, 10%◇

MECHANISM OF ACTION
Antimicrobial and comedolytic.

INDICATIONS & DOSAGE
Acne—
Adults and children: apply once daily to q.i.d., depending on tolerance and effect.

ADVERSE REACTIONS
Skin: stinging on application, warmth, painful irritation, pruritus, vesicles, allergic contact dermatitis.

INTERACTIONS
Abrasives, medical soaps and cleansers, acne preparations and preparations containing peeling agents, topical alcohol preparations (including cosmetics, after-shave, cologne): cumulative irritation of skin or excessive drying of skin. Use together cautiously.

NURSING CONSIDERATIONS
• Contraindicated in sensitivity to any of the drug's ingredients.
• Initiate therapy with 2.5% or 5% preparation; change to 10% strength after 3 to 4 weeks or as tolerance develops.
• Patients with fair skin or patients living in very dry climates should begin with one application daily.
• Patient should wash face thoroughly 20 to 30 minutes before applying.
• Don't use near the eyes, on mucous membranes, or on denuded or highly inflamed skin.
• Dryness, redness, and peeling should occur 3 to 4 days after starting treatment. If these common reactions cause considerable discomfort, discontinue temporarily.
• If painful irritation or vesicles develop, discontinue use.
• May bleach hair or clothing.

Italicized adverse reactions are common or life-threatening.
*Liquid form contains alcohol.   **May contain tartrazine.

bromocriptine mesylate
Parlodel

Pregnancy Risk Category: C

HOW SUPPLIED
Tablets: 2.5 mg
Capsules: 5 mg

MECHANISM OF ACTION
Inhibits secretion of prolactin. It acts as a dopamine-receptor agonist by activating postsynaptic dopamine receptors.

INDICATIONS & DOSAGE
To treat amenorrhea and galactorrhea associated with hyperprolactinemia; treatment of female infertility—
Women: 1.25 to 2.5 mg P.O. daily. Increase dosage by 2.5 mg daily at 3- to 7-day intervals until desired effect is achieved. Safety and efficacy of doses greater than 100 mg daily have not been established.
Prevention of postpartum lactation—
Women: 2.5 mg P.O. b.i.d. with meals for 14 days. Treatment may be extended for up to 21 days, if necessary.
Treatment of Parkinson's disease—
Adults: 1.25 mg P.O. b.i.d. with meals. Dosage may be increased q 14 to 28 days, up to 100 mg daily.
Treatment of acromegaly—
Adults: 1.25 to 2.5 mg P.O. for 3 days. An additional 1.25 to 2.5 mg may be added q 3 to 7 days until patient receives therapeutic benefit.

ADVERSE REACTIONS
CNS: confusion, hallucinations, uncontrolled body movements, *dizziness, headache,* fatigue, mania, delusions, nervousness, insomnia, depression.
CV: *hypotension,* syncope.
EENT: nasal congestion, tinnitus, blurred vision.
GI: *nausea,* vomiting, *abdominal cramps,* constipation, diarrhea.
GU: urine retention, urinary frequency.
Other: *pulmonary infiltration and pleural effusion,* coolness and pallor of fingers and toes.

INTERACTIONS
Antihypertensive drugs: increased hypotensive effects. Adjust dosage of antihypertensive agent.
Haloperidol, loxapine, phenothiazines, methyldopa, metoclopramide, MAO inhibitors, reserpine: may interfere with bromocriptine's effects.
Levodopa: additive effects. Adjust dosage of levodopa.
Oral contraceptives, estrogens, progestins: interfere with effects of bromocriptine. Concurrent use not recommended.

NURSING CONSIDERATIONS
• Contraindicated in hypersensitivity to ergot derivatives.
• Use cautiously in preexisting psychiatric disorders.
• Patient should be examined carefully for pituitary tumor (Forbes-Albright syndrome). Use of bromocriptine will not affect tumor size although it may alleviate amenorrhea or galactorrhea.
• May lead to early postpartum conception. Test for pregnancy every 4 weeks or whenever period is missed after menses are reinitiated.
• Advise patient to use contraceptive methods other than oral contraceptives during treatment.
• Patients with impaired renal function may require dosage adjustments.
• Incidence of adverse reactions is high, particularly at beginning of therapy. Orthostatic hypotension is common. Adverse reactions can be minimized by gradually titrating doses to effective levels. Advise patients to avoid dizziness and fainting by rising slowly to an upright position and avoiding sudden position changes.
• Monitor blood pressure closely in

women who receive bromocriptine for suppression of postpartum lactation. In such patients, transient hypotension is common; however, hypertension, seizures, and stroke have also been reported.

• Incidence of adverse reactions is high (68%); however, most are mild to moderate, and only 6% of patients discontinue drug for this reason. Nausea is the most common adverse reaction.

• Recurrence rates when used to treat amenorrhea or galactorrhea associated with hyperprolactinemia are high (70% to 80%).

• Advise the patient that it may take 6 to 8 weeks or longer for menses to be reinstated and galactorrhea to be suppressed.

• Patient may experience mild to moderate rebound breast secretion, congestion, or engorgement when therapy is discontinued.

• Should be given with meals.

• When used to treat Parkinson's disease, bromocriptine is usually given in addition to either levodopa alone or levodopa-carbidopa combination (Sinemet).

• Adverse reactions are more frequent when drug is used for Parkinson's disease.

capsaicin
Axsain◊, Zostrix◊

Pregnancy Risk Category: C

HOW SUPPLIED
Cream: 0.025%◊ (Zostrix◊), 0.075%◊ (Axsain◊)

MECHANISM OF ACTION
Exact mechanism unknown, but the drug may deplete substance P (the principle neurotransmitter for pain) in peripheral type C sensory fibers.

INDICATIONS & DOSAGE
Temporary relief of pain after herpes zoster infections—

Adults and children 2 years and over: 0.025% cream applied to affected areas not more than q.i.d.
Relief of neuralgias, such as postsurgical pain and painful diabetic neuropathy—
Adults and children over 2 years: 0.075% cream applied to affected areas not more than q.i.d.

ADVERSE REACTIONS
Local: redness, *stinging or burning upon application.*

INTERACTIONS
None reported.

NURSING CONSIDERATIONS
• Avoid getting drug in the eyes or on broken skin.

• Note that the drug may cause transient burning or stinging with application. This is usually evident at initial therapy and will persist in patients who use the drug less than t.i.d.

• Do not bandage area tightly after applying drug.

• Tell patient who is self-medicating with capsaicin that he should contact the doctor if symptoms persist beyond 2 to 4 weeks or if they resolve and shortly reappear.

• Tell patient to wash hands frequently after applying drug.

carbidopa-levodopa
Sinemet

Pregnancy Risk Category: C

HOW SUPPLIED
Tablets: carbidopa 10 mg with levodopa 100 mg (Sinemet 10-100), carbidopa 25 mg with levodopa 100 mg (Sinemet 25-100), carbidopa 25 mg with levodopa 250 mg (Sinemet 25-250)

MECHANISM OF ACTION
Levodopa is decarboxylated to dopamine, countering the depletion of

---

Italicized adverse reactions are common or life-threatening.
*Liquid form contains alcohol. **May contain tartrazine.

striatal dopamine in extrapyramidal centers. Carbidopa inhibits the peripheral decarboxylation of levodopa without affecting levodopa's metabolism within the CNS. Therefore, more levodopa is available to be decarboxylated to dopamine in the brain.

INDICATIONS & DOSAGE
Treatment of idiopathic Parkinson's disease, postencephalitic parkinsonism, and symptomatic parkinsonism resulting from carbon monoxide or manganese intoxication—
Adults: 3 to 6 tablets of 25 mg carbidopa/250 mg levodopa daily given in divided doses. Do not exceed 8 tablets of 25 mg carbidopa/250 mg levodopa daily. Optimum daily dosage must be determined by careful titration for each patient.

ADVERSE REACTIONS
Blood: hemolytic anemia.
CNS: *choreiform, dystonic, dyskinetic movements; involuntary grimacing, head movements, myoclonic body jerks, ataxia,* tremors, muscle twitching; bradykinetic episodes; psychiatric disturbances, memory loss, nervousness, anxiety, disturbing dreams, euphoria, malaise, fatigue; severe depression, suicidal tendencies, dementia, delirium, hallucinations (may necessitate reduction or withdrawal of drug).
CV: *orthostatic hypotension,* cardiac irregularities, flushing, hypertension, phlebitis.
EENT: blepharospasm, blurred vision, diplopia, mydriasis or miosis, widening of palpebral fissures, activation of latent Horner's syndrome, oculogyric crises, nasal discharge.
GI: *nausea, vomiting, anorexia,* weight loss may occur at start of therapy; constipation; flatulence; diarrhea; *epigastric pain;* hiccups; sialorrhea; *dry mouth;* bitter taste.
GU: urinary frequency, urine retention, urinary incontinence, darkened urine, excessive and inappropriate sexual behavior, priapism.
Hepatic: hepatotoxicity.
Other: dark perspiration, hyperventilation.

INTERACTIONS
Antihypertensives: additive hypotensive effects.
Papaverine, phenothiazines and other antipsychotics, phenytoin: may antagonize antiparkinsonian actions. Use together cautiously.
Sympathomimetics: increased risk of cardiac arrhythmias.

NURSING CONSIDERATIONS
• Contraindicated in narrow-angle glaucoma, melanoma, or undiagnosed skin lesions. Use cautiously in cardiovascular, renal, hepatic, pulmonary disorders, in history of peptic ulcer, psychiatric illness, myocardial infarction with residual arrhythmias, bronchial asthma, emphysema, and endocrine disease.
• Carefully monitor patients also receiving antihypertensive medication, hypoglycemic agents. Discontinue MAO inhibitors at least 2 weeks before therapy is begun.
• Dosage is adjusted according to patient's response and tolerance to drug. Therapeutic and adverse reactions occur more rapidly with levodopa-carbidopa than with levodopa alone. Observe and monitor vital signs, especially while dosage is being adjusted; report significant changes.
• Instruct patient to report adverse reactions and therapeutic effects.
• Warn patient of possible dizziness and orthostatic hypotension, especially at start of therapy. Patient should change position slowly and dangle legs before getting out of bed. Elastic stockings may control this adverse reaction in some patients.
• Muscle twitching and blepharospasm (twitching of eyelids) may be

---

an early sign of drug overdosage; report immediately.

• Patients on long-term therapy should be tested regularly for diabetes and acromegaly; blood tests, liver and kidney function studies should be repeated periodically.

• If patient is being treated with levodopa, discontinue at least 8 hours before starting levodopa-carbidopa.

• This combination drug usually reduces the amount of levodopa needed by 75%, thereby reducing the incidence of adverse reactions.

• Pyridoxine (vitamin B_6) does not reverse the beneficial effects of Sinemet. Multivitamins can be taken without fear of losing control of symptoms.

• If therapy is interrupted temporarily, the usual daily dosage may be given as soon as patient resumes oral medication.

• The different ratios of carbidopa: levodopa facilitate dosage adjustments. At least 70 mg of the carbidopa component should be given daily to effectively block peripheral dopa decarboxylase.

• Carbidopa (Lodosyn) as a single agent is available from Merck Sharp & Dohme on doctor's request.

• Warn the patient and his family not to increase dosage without doctor's order.

---

clomiphene citrate
Clomid

Pregnancy Risk Category: X

HOW SUPPLIED
Tablets: 50 mg

MECHANISM OF ACTION
Appears to stimulate release of pituitary gonadotropins, follicle-stimulating hormone, and luteinizing hormone. This results in maturation of the ovarian follicle, ovulation, and development of the corpus luteum.

INDICATIONS & DOSAGE
To induce ovulation—
Women: 50 to 100 mg P.O. daily for 5 days, starting any time; or 50 to 100 mg P.O. daily starting on day 5 of menstrual cycle (first day of menstrual flow is day 1). Repeat until conception occurs or until three courses of therapy are completed.

ADVERSE REACTIONS
CNS: headache, restlessness, insomnia, dizziness, light-headedness, depression, fatigue, tension.
CV: hypertension.
EENT: blurred vision, diplopia, scotoma, photophobia (signs of impending visual toxicity).
GI: nausea, vomiting, bloating, distention, increased appetite, weight gain.
GU: urinary frequency and polyuria; ovarian enlargement and cyst formation, which regress spontaneously when drug is stopped.
Metabolic: hyperglycemia.
Skin: urticaria, rash, dermatitis.
Other: *hot flashes,* reversible alopecia, *breast discomfort*.

INTERACTIONS
None significant.

NURSING CONSIDERATIONS
• Contraindicated in undiagnosed abnormal genital bleeding, ovarian cyst, or hepatic disease or dysfunction, or in patients with a history of thrombophlebitis or thromboembolism. Use cautiously in hypertension, mental depression, migraines, seizures, diabetes mellitus, and gonadotropin sensitivity. Report the development or worsening of these conditions to doctor. May require stopping drug.

• Patient with visual disturbances should report symptoms to doctor immediately.

• Tell patient possibility of multiple births exists with this drug. Risk increases with higher doses.

Italicized adverse reactions are common or life-threatening.
*Liquid form contains alcohol.   **May contain tartrazine.

- Teach patient to take basal body temperature and chart on graph to ascertain whether ovulation has occurred.
- Advise patient to stop drug and contact doctor immediately if abdominal symptoms or pain occurs because these indicate ovarian enlargement or ovarian cyst.
- Reassure patient that response (ovulation) generally occurs after the first course of therapy. If pregnancy does not occur, course of therapy may be repeated twice.
- Since drug may cause dizziness or visual disturbances, caution patient not to perform hazardous tasks until CNS effects of the drug are known.
- Advise patient to stop drug and contact doctor immediately if she suspects she is pregnant (drug may have teratogenic effect).

colchicine
Colchicine MR‡, Colgout‡, Colsalide, Novocolchicine†

Pregnancy Risk Category: D

HOW SUPPLIED
Tablets: 0.5 mg (1/120 grain), 0.6 mg (1/100 grain) as sugar-coated granules
Injection: 1 mg (1/60 g)/2 ml

MECHANISM OF ACTION
As antigout agent, apparently decreases leukocyte motility, phagocytosis, and lactic acid production, thus decreasing urate crystal deposits and reducing inflammation. As antiosteolytic agent, apparently inhibits mitosis of osteoprogenitor cells and decreases the activity of osteoclasts.

INDICATIONS & DOSAGE
To prevent acute attacks of gout as prophylactic or maintenance therapy—
Adults: 0.5 or 0.6 mg P.O. daily; or 1 to 1.8 mg P.O. daily for more severe cases.
To prevent attacks of gout in patients undergoing surgery—
Adults: 0.5 to 0.6 mg P.O. t.i.d. 3 days before and 3 days after surgery.
To treat acute gout, acute gouty arthritis—
Adults: initially, 1 to 1.2 mg P.O., then 0.5 or 0.6 mg q hour, or 1 to 1.2 mg q 2 hours until pain is relieved or until nausea, vomiting, or diarrhea ensues. Or 2 mg I.V. followed by 0.5 mg q 6 hours if necessary. Total I.V. dosage over 24 hours (one course of treatment) not to exceed 4 mg.
Note: Give I.V. by slow I.V. push over 2 to 5 minutes. Avoid extravasation. Don't dilute colchicine injection with dextrose 5% injection or any other fluid that might change pH of colchicine solution. If lower concentration of colchicine injection is needed, dilute with normal saline solution or sterile water for injection and administer over 2 to 5 minutes by direct injection. Preferably, inject into the tubing of a free-flowing I.V. solution. However, if diluted solution becomes turbid, don't inject.
Familial Mediterranean fever suppression—
Adults: acute attack—P.O. 0.6 mg hourly for four doses, then q 2 hours for four doses on the first day. Then, give 1.2 mg P.O. q 12 hours for 2 days. Maintenance dosage is 0.5 to 0.6 mg P.O. b.i.d. to t.i.d.
Antiosteolytic treatment—
Adults: 0.6 mg t.i.d. Instruct patient in the proper methods of oral hygiene, including the use of a toothbrush, dental floss, and toothpicks.

ADVERSE REACTIONS
Blood: *aplastic anemia and agranulocytosis with prolonged use;* nonthrombocytopenic purpura.
CNS: peripheral neuritis.
GI: *nausea, vomiting, abdominal pain, diarrhea.*

Skin: urticaria, dermatitis.
Local: severe local irritation if extravasation occurs.
Other: alopecia.

INTERACTIONS
Alcohol: may impair efficacy of colchicine prophylaxis.
Loop diuretics: may decrease efficacy of colchicine prophylaxis.
Phenylbutazone: may increase risk of leukopenia or thrombocytopenia.
Vitamin B_{12}: impaired absorption of vitamin B_{12}.

NURSING CONSIDERATIONS
• Use cautiously in hepatic dysfunction, cardiac disease, blood dyscrasias, renal disease, GI disorders, and in elderly or debilitated patients.
• Reduce dosage if weakness, anorexia, nausea, vomiting, or diarrhea appears. First sign of acute overdosage may be GI symptoms, followed by vascular damage, muscle weakness, and ascending paralysis. Delirium and seizures may occur without the patient losing consciousness.
• Discontinue drug as soon as gout pain is relieved or at the first sign of GI symptoms.
• Colchicine has no effect on non-gouty arthritis.
• A course of I.V. colchicine should not be repeated for several weeks to avoid cumulative toxicity.
• Do not administer I.M. or S.C.; severe local irritation occurs. Administer I.V. over 2 to 5 minutes.
• As maintenance therapy, give with meals to reduce GI effects. May be used with uricosuric agents.
• Baseline laboratory studies, including CBC, should precede therapy and be repeated periodically.
• Monitor fluid intake/output. Keep output at 2,000 ml daily.
• Store in tightly closed, light-resistant container.
• Change needle before making direct I.V. injection.

cromolyn sodium (sodium cromoglycate)
Gastrocrom, Intal**, Intal Inhaler, Intal Spincaps†, Nalcrom, Nasalcrom, Opticrom, Rynacrom†

Pregnancy Risk Category: B

HOW SUPPLIED
Capsules (for oral solution): 100 mg
Aerosol: 800 mcg/metered spray
Capsules (for inhalation): 20 mg
Nasal solution: 5.2 mg/metered spray (40 mg/ml)
Solution: 20 mg/2 ml for nebulization
Ophthalmic solution: 4% (with benzalkonium chloride 0.01%, EDTA 0.01%, and phenylethyl alcohol 0.4%)

MECHANISM OF ACTION
Inhibits the degranulation of sensitized mast cells that occurs after a patient's exposure to specific antigens. It also inhibits release of histamine and slow-reacting substance of anaphylaxis (SRS-A).

INDICATIONS & DOSAGE
Adjunct in treatment of severe perennial bronchial asthma—
Adults and children over 5 years: contents of 20-mg capsule inhaled q.i.d. at regular intervals. Or administer 2 metered sprays using inhaler q.i.d. at regular intervals. Also available as an aqueous solution administered through a nebulizer.
Prevention and treatment of allergic rhinitis—
Adults and children over 5 years: 1 spray in each nostril t.i.d or q.i.d. May give up to 6 times daily.
Prevention of exercise-induced bronchospasm—
Adults and children over 5 years: contents of 20-mg capsule or 2 metered sprays inhaled no more than 1 hour before anticipated exercise.
Allergic ocular disorders—
Adults and children 4 years and

Italicized adverse reactions are common or life-threatening.
*Liquid form contains alcohol.   **May contain tartrazine.

older: 1 to 2 drops in each eye 4 to 6 times daily at regular intervals.
Systemic mastocytosis—
Adults: 100 to 200 mg P.O. q.i.d.
Food allergy—
Adults: 200 mg P.O. q.i.d. 15 to 20 minutes before meals. Dosage may be doubled in 2 to 3 weeks if results are not satisfactory.
Children 2 to 13 years: 100 mg P.O. q.i.d. 15 to 20 minutes before meals. Dosage may be doubled in 2 to 3 weeks if results are not satisfactory. Do not exceed 40 mg/kg daily.
Children under 2 years: up to 20 mg/kg P.O. daily.
Inflammatory bowel disease—
Adults: 200 mg P.O. q.i.d. 15 to 20 minutes before meals.
Children 2 to 14 years: 100 mg P.O. q.i.d. 15 to 20 minutes before meals.

ADVERSE REACTIONS
CNS: dizziness, headache.
EENT: *irritation of the throat and trachea, cough, bronchospasm following inhalation of dry powder; esophagitis;* nasal congestion; pharyngeal irritation; wheezing.
GI: nausea.
GU: dysuria, urinary frequency.
Skin: rash, urticaria.
Other: joint swelling and pain, lacrimation, swollen parotid gland, angioedema, *eosinophilic pneumonia.*

INTERACTIONS
None significant.

NURSING CONSIDERATIONS
• Contraindicated in acute asthma attacks and status asthmaticus because the drug is useful only in preventing attacks.
• Use cautiously in coronary artery disease or history of cardiac arrhythmias.
• Should be discontinued if patient develops eosinophilic pneumonia.
• Capsule for inhalation not to be swallowed; insert capsule into inhaler provided; follow manufacturer's directions.
• Watch for recurrence of asthmatic symptoms when dosage is decreased, especially when corticosteroids are also used.
• Use only when acute episode has been controlled; airway is cleared; and patient is able to inhale.
• Patient considered for cromolyn therapy should have pulmonary function tests to show significant bronchodilator-reversible component to his airway obstruction.
• Teach correct use of Spinhaler: insert capsule in device properly, exhale completely before placing mouthpiece between lips, then inhale deeply and rapidly with a steady, even breath; remove inhaler from mouth, hold breath a few seconds, and then exhale. Repeat until all powder has been inhaled.
• Store capsules for inhalation at room temperature in a tightly closed container; protect from moisture and temperatures higher than 40° C. (104° F.).
• Instruct patient to avoid excessive handling of capsule for inhalation.
• Esophagitis may be relieved by antacids or a glass of milk.
• Don't confuse capsules for oral solution with capsules for inhalation.
• Powder in capsules for oral dose must be dissolved in hot water. May be further diluted with cold water before ingestion. Do not mix with fruit juice, milk, or food.
• Use of oral forms is still investigational.

---

diazoxide, oral
Proglycem
Pregnancy Risk Category: C

HOW SUPPLIED
Capsules: 50 mg
Oral suspension: 50 mg/ml in 30-ml bottle

MECHANISM OF ACTION
Inhibits the release of insulin from the pancreas and decreases peripheral utilization of glucose.

INDICATIONS & DOSAGE
Management of hypoglycemia from a variety of conditions resulting in hyperinsulinism—
Adults and children: 3 to 8 mg/kg P.O. daily, in three equally divided doses q 8 hours.
Infants and newborns: 8 to 15 mg/kg P.O. daily, in two or three equally divided doses q 8 to 12 hours.

ADVERSE REACTIONS
Blood: *leukopenia, thrombocytopenia.*
CV: *cardiac arrhythmias.*
EENT: diplopia.
GI: nausea, vomiting, anorexia, taste alteration.
Metabolic: sodium and fluid retention, ketoacidosis and hyperosmolar nonketotic syndrome, hyperuricemia.
Other: *severe hypertrichosis (hair growth) in 25% of adults and higher percentage of children.*

INTERACTIONS
Alpha-adrenergic blocking agents: antagonize inhibition of insulin release by diazoxide.
Anticoagulants: increased anticoagulant effect. Adjust dosage of anticoagulant.
Antigout agents: increased serum uric acid. Adjust dosage of antigout agent.
Antihypertensive agents, peripheral vasodilators: additive hypotensive effects.
Beta-adrenergic blocking agents: increased hypotensive effect.
Hydantoin anticonvulsants: decreased anticonvulsant effects and decreased hyperglycemic effect of diazoxide. Don't use together.
Thiazide diuretics: may potentiate hyperglycemic, hyperuricemic, and hy-

potensive effects. Monitor appropriate laboratory values.

NURSING CONSIDERATIONS
• Contraindicated in thiazide hypersensitivity and functional hypoglycemia.
• Oral diazoxide does not significantly lower blood pressure in dosages used to treat hypoglycemia.
• Most important use is in management of hypoglycemia from hyperinsulinism in infants and children.
• Monitor urine regularly for glucose and ketones; report any abnormalities to doctor.
• If not effective after 2 or 3 weeks, drug should be stopped.
• Reassure patient that hair growth on arms and forehead is a common adverse reaction that subsides when drug treatment is completed.
• Explain importance of following dietary restrictions for successful therapy.
• Advise patient to report any adverse reactions, including excessive thirst, fruity breath odor, or urinary frequency.

disulfiram
Antabuse, Cronetal, Ro-Sulfiram-500

Pregnancy Risk Category: X

HOW SUPPLIED
Tablet: 250 mg, 500 mg

MECHANISM OF ACTION
Blocks oxidation of alcohol at the acetaldehyde stage. Excess acetaldehyde produces a highly unpleasant reaction in the presence of even small amounts of alcohol.

INDICATIONS & DOSAGE
Adjunct in management of chronic alcoholism—
Adults: maximum of 500 mg P.O. q morning for 1 to 2 weeks. Can be

---

Italicized adverse reactions are common or life-threatening.
*Liquid form contains alcohol.   **May contain tartrazine.

taken in evening if drowsiness occurs.
Maintenance: 125 to 500 mg P.O.
daily (average dose 250 mg) until permanent self-control is established.
Treatment may continue for months or years.

ADVERSE REACTIONS
CNS: drowsiness, headache, fatigue, delirium, depression, neuritis.
EENT: optic neuritis.
GI: metallic or garlic-like aftertaste.
GU: impotence.
Skin: acneiform or allergic dermatitis.
Other: disulfiram reaction, which may include flushing, throbbing headache, dyspnea, nausea, copious vomiting, sweating, thirst, chest pain, palpitations, hyperventilation, hypotension, syncope, anxiety, weakness, blurred vision, confusion. *In severe reactions, respiratory depression, cardiovascular collapse, arrhythmias, myocardial infarction, acute CHF, seizures, unconsciousness, and even death can occur.*

INTERACTIONS
Alfentanil: prolonged duration of effect.
Anticoagulants: increased anticoagulant effect. Adjust dosage of anticoagulant.
Ascorbic acid: may interfere with disulfiram-alcohol interaction.
Bacampicillin: use with caution, because its metabolism produces low concentrations of alcohol and acetaldehyde.
CNS depressants: increased CNS depression.
Isoniazid (INH): ataxia or marked change in behavior. Don't use together.
Metronidazole: psychotic reaction. Do not use together.
Midazolam: increased plasma levels of midazolam.
Paraldehyde: toxic levels of the acetaldehyde. Don't use together.

Tricyclic antidepressants, especially amitriptylene: transient delirium.

NURSING CONSIDERATIONS
• Contraindicated in alcohol intoxication, psychoses, myocardial disease, coronary occlusion, or in patients receiving metronidazole, paraldehyde, alcohol, or alcohol-containing preparations; and in pregnancy. Use cautiously in diabetes mellitus, hypothyroidism, epilepsy, cerebral damage, nephritis, hepatic cirrhosis or insufficiency, abnormal EEG, and multiple drug dependence.
• Used only under close medical and nursing supervision. Patient should clearly understand consequences of disulfiram therapy and give permission. Drug should be used only in patients who are cooperative, well motivated, and are receiving supportive psychiatric therapy.
• Complete physical examination and laboratory studies, including CBC, SMA-12, and transaminase, should precede therapy and be repeated regularly.
• Warn patient to avoid all sources of alcohol (for example, sauces and cough syrups). Even external application of liniments, shaving lotion, and back-rub preparations may precipitate disulfiram reaction. Tell him that alcohol reaction may occur as long as 2 weeks after single dosage of disulfiram; the longer the patient remains on drug, the more sensitive he will become to alcohol.
• Patient should wear a bracelet or carry a card supplied by drug manufacturer identifying him as disulfiram user.
Note: Mild reactions may occur in sensitive patients with blood alcohol level of 5 to 10 mg/100 ml; symptoms are fully developed at 50 mg/100 ml; unconsciousness usually occurs at 125 to 150 mg/100 ml level. Reaction may last half an hour to several hours, or as long as alcohol remains in blood.

---

†Available in Canada only.   ‡Available in Australia only.   ◊Available OTC.

• Caution patient's family that disulfiram should never be given to the patient without his knowledge; severe reaction or death could result if such a patient then ingested alcohol.
• Reassure patient that disulfiram-induced adverse reactions, such as drowsiness, fatigue, impotence, headache, peripheral neuritis, and metallic or garlic taste, subside after about 2 weeks of therapy.

---

etretinate
Tegison

Pregnancy Risk Category: X

HOW SUPPLIED
Capsules: 10 mg, 25 mg

MECHANISM OF ACTION
Unknown.

INDICATIONS & DOSAGE
Treatment of severe recalcitrant psoriasis, including the erythrodermic and generalized pustular types in patients unresponsive to standard therapy (topical tar plus UVB light, psoralens plus UVA light, systemic corticosteroids, and methotrexate)—
Adults: initially, 0.75 to 1 mg/kg P.O. daily in divided doses. Don't exceed maximum initial dose of 1.5 mg/kg daily. After initial response, begin maintenance dosage of 0.5 to 0.75 mg/kg daily (usually after 8 to 16 weeks).

ADVERSE REACTIONS
Blood: *blood dyscrasias,* anemia, altered prothrombin time.
CNS: *benign intracranial hypertension (pseudotumor cerebri), fatigue, headache,* dizziness, lethargy.
CV: thrombosis, edema.
EENT: *eye pain, sore tongue, chapped lips.*
GI: *appetite change, nausea, dry mouth.*

Hepatic: *hepatitis, elevated liver enzymes.*
GU: *white blood cells in urine,* proteinuria, hematuria.
Metabolic: *hypokalemia or hyperkalemia, hyperlipidemia.*
Skin: *skin peeling, itching.*
Other: *bone pain,* dyspnea, photosensitivity.

INTERACTIONS
Alcohol: increased risk of hypertriglyceridemia.
Hepatotoxic medications (including methotrexate): increased risk of hepatotoxicity.
Milk, high-fat diet: increases etretinate's absorption.
Tetracyclines: increased risk of pseudotumor cerebri.
Vitamin A: additive toxic effects. Avoid concomitant use.

NURSING CONSIDERATIONS
• Contraindicated in patients who are pregnant, who intend to become pregnant, or who may not use reliable contraception during and after treatment because drug causes severe birth defects.
• Significant residual blood levels of etretinate have been reported as long as 2.9 years after discontinuation of treatment. Consequently, the period of time after treatment during which pregnancy must be avoided to prevent teratogenicity is unknown.
• Women of childbearing age must not receive etretinate unless pregnancy is excluded by a pregnancy test within 2 weeks before initiating therapy. Therapy may begin on the 2nd or 3rd day of the next normal menstrual period.
• Patient should use effective contraception for 1 month before therapy begins, during treatment, and for an indefinite time after treatment is discontinued.
• Sugarless gum or hard candy or ice may help relieve dry mouth. Check

---

Italicized adverse reactions are common or life-threatening.
*Liquid form contains alcohol.   **May contain tartrazine.

with dentist if this continues beyond 2 weeks.

• Monitor liver function tests at 1- to 2-week intervals for the first 1 to 2 months of therapy, and thereafter at intervals of 1 to 3 months. Suspected hepatotoxicity requires discontinuation of etretinate.

• Monitor blood lipids every 1 to 2 weeks during treatment.

• Tell patient to promptly report headache, nausea and vomiting, and visual disturbances (possible early signs of pseudotumor cerebri). These reactions require immediate check for papilledema. If present, discontinue drug immediately.

• Advise patient not to take vitamin A supplements to avoid possible additive adverse reactions.

• Reassure patient that transient exacerbation of psoriasis is common during the beginning of therapy.

• Advise patient to expect dry skin and possible difficulty tolerating contact lenses during treatment.

• Advise patient to take this drug with milk or fatty food to enhance absorption. Otherwise, patient should follow a low-fat diet.

• Patient should take a missed dose as soon as possible, with milk or fatty food. If it's nearly time for the next dose, he should skip the missed dose and resume schedule. Never double dose.

• May cause photosensitivity. Patient should avoid excess bright sun and use a sunscreen.

• If a decrease in night vision occurs, patient should contact doctor.

• Diabetic patients should monitor blood glucose closely. Adjustments of hypoglycemic medications may be necessary.

fluorouracil
Efudex, Fluoroplex
Pregnancy Risk Category: D

HOW SUPPLIED
Cream: 1%, 5%
Solution: 1%, 2%, 5%

MECHANISM OF ACTION
Interferes with DNA synthesis by inhibiting thymidylate synthetase.

INDICATIONS & DOSAGE
Multiple actinic or solar keratoses; superficial basal cell carcinoma—
Adults and children: apply cream or solution b.i.d.

ADVERSE REACTIONS
Skin: erythema, pain, burning, scaling, pruritus, hyperpigmentation, contact dermatitis, soreness, suppuration, swelling.

INTERACTIONS
None significant.

NURSING CONSIDERATIONS
• Wash hands immediately after handling medication.
• Patient should avoid prolonged exposure to sunlight or ultraviolet light.
• Apply with caution near eyes, nose, and mouth.
• Warn patient that treated area may be unsightly during therapy and for several weeks after therapy. Complete healing may take 1 or 2 months.
• Ingestion and systemic absorption may cause leukopenia, thrombocytopenia, stomatitis, diarrhea, or GI ulceration, bleeding, and hemorrhage.
• Application to large ulcerated areas may cause systemic toxicity.
• Use 1% concentration on the face. Reserve higher concentrations for thicker-skinned areas or resistant lesions.
• For superficial basal cell carcinoma confirmed by biopsy, use 5% strength.

• Lesions resistant to fluorouracil should be biopsied.
• Avoid occlusive dressings as they increase the risk of inflammatory reactions in adjacent normal skin.

---

isotretinoin
Accutane, Roaccutane‡

Pregnancy Risk Category: X

HOW SUPPLIED
Capsules: 10 mg, 20 mg, 40 mg

MECHANISM OF ACTION
Normalizes keratinization, reversibly decreases the size of sebaceous glands, and alters the composition of sebum to a less viscous form that's less likely to cause follicular plugging.

INDICATIONS & DOSAGE
Severe cystic acne unresponsive to conventional therapy—
Adults and adolescents: 0.5 to 2 mg/ kg P.O. daily given in two divided doses and continued for 15 to 20 weeks.

ADVERSE REACTIONS
Blood: anemia, elevated platelet count.
CNS: headache, fatigue, *pseudotumor cerebri* (benign intracranial hypertension).
EENT: conjunctivitis, corneal deposits, dry eyes.
Endocrine: hyperglycemia.
GI: nonspecific GI symptoms, gum bleeding and inflammation.
Hepatic: elevated AST (SGOT), ALT (SPGT), and alkaline phosphatase.
Skin: *cheilosis, rash, dry skin,* peeling of palms and toes, skin infection, photosensitivity.
Other: *hypertriglyceridemia, musculoskeletal pain (skeletal hyperostosis),* thinning of hair.

INTERACTIONS
Abrasives, medicated soaps and cleansers, acne preparations containing peeling agents, topical alcohol preparations (including cosmetics, after-shave, cologne): cumulative irritation of skin or excessive drying of skin. Use together cautiously.
Alcohol: increased risk of hypertriglyceridemia
Tetracyclines: increased risk of pseudotumor cerebri.
Vitamin A and vitamin supplements containing vitamin A: increase in isotretinoin's toxic effects. Don't use together without doctor's permission.

NURSING CONSIDERATIONS
• Isotretinoin is contraindicated in women of childbearing age unless the patient has had a negative serum pregnancy test within 2 weeks before beginning therapy; will begin drug therapy on the 2nd or 3rd day of the next menstrual period; and will comply with stringent contraception measures for 1 month before therapy, during therapy, and for at least 1 month after therapy. *Severe fetal abnormalities may occur if used during pregnancy.*
• Contraindicated in patients hypersensitive to parabens, which are used as preservatives.
• If used with other photosensitivity agents may have additive effect. Avoid prolonged exposure to the sun; use sunscreen.
• Tell patient to immediately report any visual disturbances and bone or skeletal pain.
• Patients who experience headache, nausea and vomiting, or visual disturbances should be screened for papilledema. Signs and symptoms of pseudotumor cerebri require immediate discontinuation of therapy and prompt neurologic intervention.
• Perform serum lipid studies and liver function tests before therapy begins and then at regular intervals until response to drug is established, usually about 4 weeks.
• Monitor blood glucose regularly.

Italicized adverse reactions are common or life-threatening.
*Liquid form contains alcohol.   **May contain tartrazine.

• Monitor creatine phosphokinase levels in patients who undergo vigorous physical activity.

• Warn patient that contact lenses may feel uncomfortable during isotretinoin therapy.

• If a second course of therapy is needed, it shouldn't be started until at least 8 weeks after the completion of the first course because improvement may continue after withdrawal of the drug.

• Most adverse reactions appear to be dose-related, occurring at dosages greater than 1 mg/kg daily. They are generally reversible when therapy is discontinued or dosage is reduced.

• Advise patient to take drug with or shortly after meals to ensure adequate absorption.

---

levocarnitine (L-carnitine)
Carnitor, Vitacarn

Pregnancy Risk Category: B

HOW SUPPLIED
Tablets: 330 mg
Capsules: 250 mg
Oral liquid: 100 mg/ml

MECHANISM OF ACTION
Facilitates the transport of fatty acids into cellular mitochondria. The fatty acids are then used to produce energy.

INDICATIONS & DOSAGE
Primary systemic carnitine deficiency—
Adults: 990 mg (three tablets) P.O. b.i.d. or t.i.d. Alternatively, may give enteral liquid 10 to 30 ml (1 to 3 g) daily.
Children: 50 to 100 mg/kg/day P.O. in divided doses of either the tablet or enteral liquid form.

All dosages depend upon the clinical response. Higher dosages may be given. However, for children, the maximum dosage is 3 g/day.

ADVERSE REACTIONS
GI: *nausea, vomiting, cramps, diarrhea.*
Other: body odor.

INTERACTIONS
D,L-carnitine (sold as vitamin B_T in vitamin stores): inhibits levocarnitine and can cause deficiency.
Valproic acid: increased requirement for carnitine.

NURSING CONSIDERATIONS
• Monitor patient's tolerance during the first week of therapy and after increasing dosage.

• Monitor blood chemistries and plasma carnitine concentrations periodically, as well as vital signs and patient's overall clinical condition.

• May give enteral liquid alone or dissolved in drinks or liquid food.

• Space doses evenly every 3 to 4 hours if possible. Best to give with or after meals.

• Tell patient to consume enteral liquid slowly to minimize GI distress. If GI intolerance persists, dosage may have to be reduced.

• Warn patient to avoid so-called "vitamin B_T" in health food stores. This will interact with the drug and render it ineffective.

• Caution patient not to share drug with others. Some people have used it to improve athletic performance.

• The entire or partial contents of the containers of liquid should be used immediately after opening. Discard any unused contents of opened containers.

• Do not refrigerate solution.

---

levodopa
Dopar, Larodopa, Levopa, Parda, Rio-Dopa

Pregnancy Risk Category: C

HOW SUPPLIED
Tablets: 100 mg, 250 mg, 500 mg

Capsules: 100 mg, 250 mg, 500 mg

MECHANISM OF ACTION
Levodopa is decarboxylated to dopamine, countering the depletion of striatal dopamine in extrapyramidal centers, which is thought to produce parkinsonism.

INDICATIONS & DOSAGE
Treatment of idiopathic parkinsonism, postencephalitic parkinsonism, and symptomatic parkinsonism after carbon monoxide or manganese intoxication; or in association with cerebral arteriosclerosis—
Adults and children over 12 years: initially, 0.5 to 1 g P.O. daily, given b.i.d., t.i.d., or q.i.d. with food; increase by no more than 0.75 g daily q 3 to 7 days, until usual maximum of 8 g is reached. Carefully adjust dosage to individual requirements, tolerance, and response. Higher dosage requires close supervision.

ADVERSE REACTIONS
Blood: hemolytic anemia, leukopenia.
CNS: *aggressive behavior, choreiform, dystonic, and dyskinetic movements, involuntary grimacing, head movements, myoclonic body jerks, ataxia, tremors, muscle twitching, bradykinetic episode, psychiatric disturbances, memory loss, mood changes, nervousness, anxiety, disturbing dreams, euphoria, malaise, fatigue, severe depression, suicidal tendencies, dementia, delirium, hallucinations (may necessitate reduction or withdrawal of drug).*
CV: *orthostatic hypotension,* cardiac irregularities, flushing, hypertension, phlebitis.
EENT: blepharospasm, blurred vision, diplopia, mydriasis or miosis, widening of palpebral fissures, activation of latent Horner's syndrome, oculogyric crises, nasal discharge.
GI: *nausea, vomiting, anorexia,* weight loss may occur at start of therapy, constipation, flatulence, diarrhea, epigastric pain, hiccups, sialorrhea, dry mouth, bitter taste.
GU: urinary frequency, retention, incontinence; darkened urine; excessive and inappropriate sexual behavior; priapism.
Hepatic: hepatotoxicity.
Other: dark perspiration, hyperventilation.

INTERACTIONS
Antacids: increased absorption of levodopa.
Antihypertensives: additive hypertensive effect.
High-protein foods: decreased absorption of levodopa.
Metoclopramide: accelerated gastric emptying of levodopa.
Papaverine, phenothiazines and other antipsychotics, phenytoin: watch for decreased levodopa effect.
Pyridoxine: reduced efficacy of levodopa. Examine vitamin preparations and nutritional supplements for content of vitamin B_6 (pyridoxine).
Sympathomimetics: increased risk of cardiac arrhythmias.

NURSING CONSIDERATIONS
• Contraindicated in narrow-angle glaucoma, melanoma, or undiagnosed skin lesions. Use cautiously in cardiovascular, renal, hepatic, and pulmonary disorders, peptic ulcer, psychiatric illness, myocardial infarction with residual arrhythmias, bronchial asthma, emphysema, and endocrine disease.
• Carefully monitor patients also receiving antihypertensive medication and hypoglycemic agents. Stop MAO inhibitors at least 2 weeks before therapy is begun.
• Adjust dosage according to patient's response and tolerance. Observe and monitor vital signs, especially while adjusting dose. Report significant changes.

Italicized adverse reactions are common or life-threatening.
*Liquid form contains alcohol.   **May contain tartrazine.

- Instruct patient to report adverse reactions and therapeutic effects.
- Warn patient of possible dizziness and orthostatic hypotension, especially at start of therapy. Patient should change position slowly and dangle legs before getting out of bed. Elastic stockings may control this adverse reaction in some patients.
- Muscle twitching and blepharospasm (twitching of eyelids) may be early signs of drug overdosage; report immediately.
- Patients on long-term use should be tested regularly for diabetes and acromegaly; repeat blood tests and liver and kidney function studies periodically.
- Advise patient and family that multivitamin preparations, fortified cereals, and certain OTC medications may contain pyridoxine (vitamin B_6), which can reverse the effects of levodopa.
- If therapy is interrupted for a long time, drug should be adjusted gradually to previous level.
- Therapeutic response usually occurs following each dose and disappears within 5 hours but varies considerably.
- Patient who must undergo surgery should continue levodopa as long as oral intake is permitted, generally 6 to 24 hours before surgery. Drug should be resumed as soon as patient is able to take oral medication.
- Protect from heat, light, and moisture. If preparation darkens, it has lost potency and should be discarded.
- Coombs' test occasionally becomes positive during extended use. Expect uric acid elevations with colorimetric method but not with uricase method.
- Alkaline phosphatase, AST (SGOT), ALT (SGPT), lactate dehydrogenase, bilirubin, BUN, and protein-bound iodine show transient elevations in patients receiving levodopa; WBC, hemoglobin, and hematocrit show occasional reduction.

- A doctor-supervised period of drug discontinuance (called a drug holiday) may reestablish the effectiveness of a lower dosage regimen.
- Combination of levodopa-carbidopa usually reduces amount of levodopa needed by 75%, thereby reducing incidence of adverse reactions.
- Pills may be crushed and mixed with applesauce or baby food fruits for patients who have difficulty swallowing pills.
- Warn patient and family not to increase dosage without the doctor's orders (they may be tempted to do this as disease symptoms of parkinsonism progress). Daily dosage should not exceed 8 g.

mesalamine
Rowasa

Pregnancy Risk Category: B

HOW SUPPLIED
Rectal suspension: 4 g/60 ml.

MECHANISM OF ACTION
Exact mechanism unknown; mesalamine is one of the active metabolites of sulfasalazine. Probably acts topically by inhibiting prostaglandin production in the colon.

INDICATIONS & DOSAGE
Treatment of active mild to moderate distal ulcerative colitis, proctitis, or proctosigmoiditis—
Adults: 1 rectal unit as a retention enema once daily (preferably h.s.). Drug should be retained overnight (for about 8 hours). Usual course of therapy is 3 to 6 weeks.

ADVERSE REACTIONS
CNS: headache, dizziness, fatigue, malaise.
GI: abdominal pain, cramps, discomfort, flatulence, diarrhea, rectal pain, bloating, nausea, *pancolitis*.

---

†Available in Canada only.   ‡Available in Australia only.   ◊ Available OTC.

Skin: hives, itching, rash, urticaria, hair loss.
Other: wheezing, *anaphylaxis* (rare), fever.

INTERACTIONS
None significant.

NURSING CONSIDERATIONS
• Contraindicated in patients sensitive to the drug or its components.
• Mesalamine may rarely cause allergic reactions in patients sensitive to sulfites, becasue it contains potassium metabisulfite.
• Instruct patient to carefully follow instructions supplied with medication.
• Patients intolerant of sulfasalazine may also be hypersensitive to mesalamine. Instruct these patients to discontinue drug if they have a fever or rash.
• Use cautiously in renal impairment. Problems have not been documented, but the nephrotoxic potential from absorbed mesalamine exists. Patients on long-term mesalamine therapy should have periodic renal function studies.

---

mesna
Mesnex

Pregnancy Risk Category: B

HOW SUPPLIED
Injection: 100 mg/ml

MECHANISM OF ACTION
Prevents ifosfamide-induced hemorrhagic cystitis by reacting with urotoxic ifosfamide metabolites.

INDICATIONS & DOSAGE
Prophylaxis of hemorrhagic cystitis in patients receiving ifosfamide—
Adults: dosage varies with amount of ifosfamide administered. Usual dosage is 240 mg/m² administered as an I.V. bolus with administration of ifosfamide. Repeat dosage at 4 hours and 8 hours after administration of ifosfamide.

ADVERSE REACTIONS
Note: Because it is used concomitantly with ifosfamide and other chemotherapeutic agents, it is difficult to determine adverse reactions attributable solely to mesna.
EENT: dysgeusia.
GI: soft stools, nausea, vomiting, diarrhea.

INTERACTIONS
None reported.

NURSING CONSIDERATIONS
• Contraindicated in patients with hypersensitivity to mesna or thiol-containing compounds. Not effective in preventing hematuria from other causes (such as thrombocytopenia). Although formulated to prevent hemorrhagic cystitis from ifosfamide, it will not protect against other toxicities associated with ifosfamide therapy.
• Monitor urine samples in patients receiving mesna for hematuria daily.
• Up to 6% of patients may not respond to the drug's protective effects.
• May interfere with diagnostic tests for urine ketones.
• Prepare I.V. solutions by diluting commercially available ampules with dextrose 5% in water solution, dextrose 5% and normal saline injection, normal saline injection, or lactated Ringer's solution.
• Diluted solutions are stable for 24 hours at room temperature, but they should be refrigerated after preparation and used within 6 hours. After the ampule is opened, any unused drug should be discarded because it decomposes quickly into an inactive compound.
• Mesna I.V. is incompatible with cisplatin.

Italicized adverse reactions are common or life-threatening.
*Liquid form contains alcohol.   **May contain tartrazine.

methoxsalen
Oxsoralen, Oxsoralen-Ultra
Pregnancy Risk Category: C

HOW SUPPLIED
Capsules: 10 mg
Lotion: 1%

MECHANISM OF ACTION
May enhance melanogenesis, either directly or secondarily, to an inflammatory process.

INDICATIONS & DOSAGE
To induce repigmentation in vitiligo; psoriasis—
Adults and children over 12 years: 0.6 mg/kg P.O. 1.5 to 2 hours before measured periods of high-intensity long-wave ultraviolet exposure, 2 to 3 times weekly at least 48 hours apart.
Topical solution:
Apply to small, well-defined vitiliginous lesions and allow to dry (1 to 2 minutes) and reapply: 2 to 2.5 hours before measured periods of long-wave ultraviolet exposure. After exposure, wash lesions with soap and water. Protect area with opaque sunscreen. Although manufacturer recommends treatment weekly, some clinicians may treat q 3 to 5 days.

ADVERSE REACTIONS
CNS: nervousness, insomnia, depression, vertigo, headache.
GI: *discomfort, nausea, diarrhea.*
Skin: edema, erythema, painful blistering, burning, peeling, pruritus.

INTERACTIONS
Photosensitizing agents: do not use together. May increase toxicity.

NURSING CONSIDERATIONS
• Contraindicated in hepatic insufficiency, porphyria, acute lupus erythematosus, or hydromorphic and polymorphic light eruptions. Use with caution in patients with familial history of sunlight allergy, GI diseases, and chronic infection.
• Regulate therapy carefully. Overdosage or overexposure to light can cause serious burning or blistering. Patients should avoid excessive sunlight during therapy.
• Drug should be taken with meals or milk. Patient should avoid the following foods: limes, figs, parsley, parsnips, mustard, carrots, and celery.
• During light exposure treatments, protect eyes and lips.
• Monthly liver function tests should be done on patients with vitiligo (especially at beginning of therapy).

minoxidil (topical)
Rogaine
Pregnancy Risk Category: C

HOW SUPPLIED
Topical solution: 2%

MECHANISM OF ACTION
Stimulation of hair growth may be related to dilation of arterial microcapillaries around hair follicles.

INDICATIONS & DOSAGE
Treatment of male pattern baldness (alopecia androgenetica) of the vertex and scalp—
Adults: apply 1 ml of 2% solution to affected area twice daily. Total daily dosage should not exceed 2 ml.

ADVERSE REACTIONS
CNS: headache, dizziness, faintness, light-headedness.
CV: edema, chest pain, increased or decreased blood pressure, palpitations, increased or decreased pulse rate.
EENT: sinusitis.
GU: urinary tract infections, renal calculi, urethritis.
Metabolic: edema, weight gain.
Respiratory: bronchitis, upper respiratory infection.

Skin: irritant dermatitis, allergic contact dermatitis, eczema, hypertrichosis, local erythema, pruritus, dry skin or scalp, flaking, alopecia, exacerbation of hair loss.
Other: back pain, tendonitis.

INTERACTIONS
Topical corticosteroids, petrolatum, topical retinoids, or other drugs that may enhance skin absorption: increased risk of systemic effects of minoxidil. Do not apply minoxidil with other drugs.

NURSING CONSIDERATIONS
• Contraindicated in patients with hypersensitivity to any component of the topical solution. Adverse effects are uncommon.
• Tell patient to avoid inhalation of any spray or mist from the drug. Avoid spraying around the eyes, because the solution contains alcohol and may be irritating.
• Patient needs to have a normal, healthy scalp before beginning therapy, because absorption of the drug through irritated skin may cause adverse systemic effects.
• Treatment with topical minoxidil is most likely to be successful in patients with balding area smaller than 4″ (10 cm) within the last 10 years.
• Patients with a history of heart disease should be aware that this drug may exacerbate their illness.
• Teach patient to monitor pulse rate and body weight.
• Patients need medical follow-ups 1 month after initiation of therapy and every 6 months thereafter.
• Teach patient how to correctly apply topical minoxidil. Hair and scalp should be thoroughly dry before application, and the drug should not be applied to any other areas of the body. Patient should not use the drug on irritated or sunburned scalp, or with any other medication on the scalp.

Tell patient to thoroughly wash his hands after application.
• Advise patient that therapy will be prolonged and will continue for at least 4 months before clinical effects appear. About 40% of patients will see moderate to dense hair growth.
• Discontinuing the drug may result in the loss of new hair growth. New hair growth is usually fine and may be colorless, but will resemble existing hair after continued treatment.

---

nicotine polacrilex (nicotine resin complex)
Nicorette
Pregnancy Risk Category: X

HOW SUPPLIED
Chewing gum: 2 mg/square

MECHANISM OF ACTION
Stimulates receptors in the CNS and causes the release of catecholamines from the adrenal medulla.

INDICATIONS & DOSAGE
Temporary aid to the cigarette smoker seeking to give up smoking while participating in a behavior modification program under medical supervision—
Adults: chew one piece of gum slowly and intermittently for 30 minutes whenever the urge to smoke occurs. Most patients require approximately 10 pieces of gum daily during the first month. Don't exceed 30 pieces of gum daily.

ADVERSE REACTIONS
CNS: dizziness, light-headedness.
CV: atrial fibrillation.
EENT: throat soreness, jaw muscle ache (from chewing).
GI: nausea, vomiting, indigestion.
Other: hiccups.

INTERACTIONS
None significant.

NURSING CONSIDERATIONS

• Contraindicated in nonsmokers, during the immediate postmyocardial infarction period; in life-threatening arrhythmias, severe or worsening angina pectoris, and active temporomandibular joint disease; or in pregnancy.

• Use cautiously in with hyperthyroidism, pheochromocytoma, or insulin-dependent diabetes.

• Nicotine resin complex is the only smoking cessation aid that has been proven safe and effective.

• Smokers most likely to benefit from nicotine gum are those with a high "physical" nicotine dependence. Such smokers show the following characteristics: smoke more than 15 cigarettes daily; prefer brands of cigarettes with high nicotine levels; usually inhale the smoke; smoke the first cigarette within 30 minutes of arising; find the first morning cigarette the hardest to give up; smoke most frequently during the morning; find it difficult to refrain from smoking in places where it's forbidden; or smoke even when they are so ill that they are confined to bed during the day.

• Instruct patient to chew gum slowly and intermittently (chew several times, then place between cheek and gums) for about 30 minutes to promote slow and even buccal absorption of nicotine. Fast chewing tends to produce more adverse reactions.

• Successful abstainers will begin gradually withdrawing gum usage after 3 months. Use of the gum for longer than 6 months is not recommended. For gradual withdrawal, cut gum in halves or quarters and mix with other sugar-free gum.

• Emphasize the importance of withdrawing the gum gradually.

• The gum is sugar-free and usually doesn't stick to dentures.

• Patient who stops smoking may require dosage adjustments of propoxyphene, propranolol, beta-blocking agents, and xanthine bronchodilators because decreased metabolism of these agents may increase their therapeutic effects.

• A patient instruction sheet is included in the package dispensed to the patient.

---

octreotide acetate
Sandostatin

Pregnancy Risk Category: B

HOW SUPPLIED
Injection: 0.05 mg, 0.1 mg, 0.5 mg

MECHANISM OF ACTION
Mimics the action of naturally occurring somatostatin.

INDICATIONS & DOSAGE
Symptomatic treatment of flushing and diarrhea associated with carcinoid tumors—
Adults: initially, 0.1 to 0.6 mg daily S.C. in two to four divided doses for the first 2 weeks of therapy (usual daily dosage is 0.3 mg). Subsequent dosage is based upon individual response.
Symptomatic treatment of watery diarrhea associated with vasoactive intestinal peptide secreting tumors (VIPomas)—
Adults: initially, 0.2 to 0.3 mg daily S.C. in two to four divided doses for the first 2 weeks of therapy. Subsequent dosage is based upon individual response, but usually will not exceed 0.45 mg daily.

ADVERSE REACTIONS
CNS: dizziness, light-headedness, fatigue.
GI: *nausea, diarrhea, abdominal pain or discomfort,* loose stools, vomiting, fat malabsorption.
Metabolic: hyperglycemia, hypoglycemia, hypothyroidism.
Skin: flushing, edema, wheal, erythema or pain at injection site.

INTERACTIONS

Cyclosporine: may decrease plasma levels of cyclosporine.

NURSING CONSIDERATIONS

• Contraindicated in patients with hypersensitivity to the drug or any of its components.

• Octreotide therapy may be associated with the development of cholelithiasis by either altering gallbladder motility or fat absorption. Monitor patient regularly for gallbladder disease, and tell patient to report any signs of abdominal discomfort.

• Half-life may be altered in patients in end-stage renal failure who are receiving dialysis.

• Baseline and periodic tests of thyroid function are advised because of the drug's metabolic effects.

• Laboratory tests that are frequently monitored during therapy include urine 5-hydroxyindole acetic acid (5-HIAA), plasma serotonin, and plasma substance P (for carcinoid tumors); plasma vasoactive intestinal peptide for VIPomas.

• Mild, transient hypoglycemia or hyperglycemia may occur during octreotide therapy. Monitor closely for symptoms of glucose imbalance during therapy.

• Insulin-dependent diabetic patients and patients receiving oral hypoglycemics (sulfonylureas) or oral diazoxide may require dosage adjustments during therapy.

• Octreotide therapy may alter fluid and electrolyte balance and may require adjustment of other drugs used to control symptoms of the disease (such as beta blockers).

pentoxifylline
Trental

Pregnancy Risk Category: C

HOW SUPPLIED

Tablets (extended-release): 400 mg

MECHANISM OF ACTION

Improves capillary blood flow by increasing erythrocyte flexibility and lowering blood viscosity.

INDICATIONS & DOSAGE

Treatment of intermittent claudication caused by chronic occlusive vascular disease—
Adults: 400 mg P.O. t.i.d. with meals.

ADVERSE REACTIONS

CNS: headache, dizziness.
GI: dyspepsia, nausea, vomiting.

INTERACTIONS

Anticoagulants: increased anticoagulant effect.
Antihypertensives: increased hypotensive effect. Dosage adjustments may be necessary.

NURSING CONSIDERATIONS

• Contraindicated in patients who are intolerant to methylxanthines such as caffeine, theophylline, and theobromine.

• Pentoxifylline should be taken for a minimum of 8 weeks to achieve clinical effects. Tell patient not to discontinue the drug during this period unless directed by doctor.

• Advise patient to take with meals to minimize GI upset.

• Patient should report any GI or CNS adverse reactions. Doctor may reduce dosage.

• Pentoxifylline therapy is useful in patients who are not good surgical candidates.

• Patient should avoid smoking because nicotine causes vasoconstriction that can worsen the condition.

• Patient should swallow medication whole, without breaking, crushing, or chewing.

• Elderly patients may be more sensitive to this drug's effects.

Italicized adverse reactions are common or life-threatening.
*Liquid form contains alcohol.   **May contain tartrazine.

pergolide mesylate
Permax

Pregnancy Risk Category: B

HOW SUPPLIED
Tablets: 0.05 mg, 0.25 mg, 1 mg

MECHANISM OF ACTION
Directly stimulates dopamine receptors in the nigrostriatal system.

INDICATIONS & DOSAGE
Adjunctive treatment to carbidopa-levodopa in the management of the symptoms associated with Parkinson's disease—
Adults: initially, 0.05 mg P.O. daily for the first 2 days. Gradually increase dosage by 0.1 to 0.15 mg every third day over the next 12 days of therapy. Subsequent dosage can be increased by 0.25 mg every third day until optimum response is seen. The drug is usually administered in divided doses t.i.d. Gradual reductions in carbidopa-levodopa dosage may be made during dosage titration.

ADVERSE REACTIONS
CNS: headache, asthenia, *dyskinesia, dizziness, hallucinations,* dystonia, confusion, *somnolescence,* insomnia, anxiety, depression, tremor, abnormal dreams, personality disorder, psychosis, abnormal gait, akathisia, extrapyramidal syndrome, incoordination, paresthesias, akinesia, hypertonia, neuralgia, speech disorder.
CV: *orthostatic hypotension,* vasodilation, palpitations, hypotension, syncope, hypertension, arrhythmias, myocardial infarction.
EENT: *rhinitis,* epistaxis, abnormal vision, diplopia, eye disorder.
GI: abdominal pain, *nausea, constipation,* diarrhea, dyspepsia, anorexia, vomiting, dry mouth, taste alteration.
GU: urinary frequency, urinary tract infection, hematuria.
Skin: rash, sweating.

Other: accident or injury; chest, neck, and back pain; flu-like syndrome; chills; infection; facial, peripheral, or generalized edema; weight gain; arthralgia; bursitis; myalgia; twitching.
Note: The above adverse reactions, although not always attributable to the drug, occurred in 1% of the study population.

INTERACTIONS
Phenothiazines, butyrophenones, thioxanthines, metoclopramide, and other drugs that are dopamine antagonists: may antagonize the effects of pergolide.

NURSING CONSIDERATIONS
• Contraindicated in patients allergic to the drug or to ergot alkaloids. Symptomatic orthostatic or sustained hypotension may occur in some patients, especially at the start of therapy.
• Hallucinations may occur in some patients. Tolerance to this adverse reaction was not seen in early clinical trials.
• In premarketing trials, over 140 of approximately 2,300 patients died while taking pergolide. However, the drug did not appear to be responsible for these deaths because these patients were elderly, ill, and at high risk for death.
• In early clinical trials, 27% of the patients who attempted pergolide therapy did not finish the trial because of adverse reactions (primarily hallucinations and confusion). Inform patients of the potential adverse reactions. Warn them to avoid activities that could expose them to injury as a result of orthostatic hypotension and syncope.

---

†Available in Canada only.   ‡Available in Australia only.   ◊ Available OTC.

ritodrine hydrochloride
Yutopar

Pregnancy Risk Category: B

HOW SUPPLIED
Tablets: 10 mg
Injection: 10-mg/ml, 15-mg/ml ampules

MECHANISM OF ACTION
A beta-receptor agonist that stimulates the $beta_2$-adrenergic receptors in uterine smooth muscle, inhibiting contractility.

INDICATIONS & DOSAGE
Management of preterm labor—
I.V. therapy: dilute 150 mg (3 ampuls) in 500 ml of fluid, yielding a final concentration of 0.3 mg/ml. Usual initial dose is 0.1 mg/minute, to be gradually increased according to the results by 0.05 mg/minute q 10 minutes until desired result obtained. Effective dosage usually ranges from 0.15 and 0.35 mg/minute.

Note: I.V. infusion should be continued for 12 to 24 hours after contractions have stopped. Oral maintenance: 1 tablet (10 mg) may be given approximately 30 minutes before termination of I.V. therapy. Usual dosage for first 24 hours of oral maintenance is 10 mg q 2 hours. Thereafter, usual dosage is 10 to 20 mg q 4 to 6 hours. Total daily dosage should not exceed 120 mg.

ADVERSE REACTIONS
I.V.:
CNS: nervousness, anxiety, headache.
CV: *dose-related alterations in blood pressure, palpitations, pulmonary edema, tachycardia,* ECG changes.
GI: nausea, vomiting.
Metabolic: *hyperglycemia,* hypokalemia.
Other: erythema.
Oral:

CNS: tremors, nervousness.
CV: palpitations.
GI: nausea, vomiting.
Skin: rash.

INTERACTIONS
Beta blockers: may inhibit ritodrine's action. Avoid concurrent administration.
Corticosteroids: may produce pulmonary edema in mother. When these drugs are used concomitantly, monitor closely.
Inhalational anesthetics: potentiated adverse cardiac effects, arrhythmias, hypotension.
Sympathomimetics: additive effects. Use together cautiously.

NURSING CONSIDERATIONS
• Contraindicated before 20th week of pregnancy and in the following conditions: antepartum hemorrhage, eclampsia, intrauterine fetal death, chorioamnionitis, maternal cardiac disease, pulmonary hypertension, maternal hyperthyroidism, or uncontrolled maternal diabetes mellitus.
• Because cardiovascular responses are common and more pronounced during I.V. administration, cardiovascular effects—including maternal pulse rate and blood pressure, and fetal heart rate—should be closely monitored. A maternal tachycardia of over 140 or persistent respiratory rate of over 20/minute may be a sign of impending pulmonary edema.
• Monitor blood glucose concentrations during ritodrine infusions, especially in diabetic mothers.
• Discontinue drug if pulmonary edema develops.
• Monitor amount of fluids administered I.V., to prevent circulatory overload.
• Ritodrine decreases intensity and frequency of uterine contractions.
• Don't use ritodrine I.V. if solution is discolored or contains a precipitate.

Italicized adverse reactions are common or life-threatening.
*Liquid form contains alcohol.   **May contain tartrazine.

selegiline hydrochloride (L-deprenyl hydrochloride)
Eldepryl

Pregnancy Risk Category: C

HOW SUPPLIED
Tablets: 5 mg

MECHANISM OF ACTION
Probably acts by selectively inhibiting MAO type B (found mostly in the brain). At higher-than-recommended doses, it is a nonselective inhibitor of MAO, including MAO type A (found in the GI tract). It also may directly increase dopaminergic activity by decreasing the reuptake of dopamine into nerve cells. It has pharmacologically active metabolites (amphetamine and methamphetamine) that may contribute to this effect.

INDICATIONS & DOSAGE
Adjunctive treatment to carbidopa-levodopa in the management of the symptoms associated with Parkinson's disease—
Adults: 10 mg P.O. daily, taken as 5 mg at breakfast and 5 mg at lunch. After 2 or 3 days of therapy, begin gradual decrease of carbidopa-levodopa dosage.

ADVERSE REACTIONS
CNS: *dizziness,* increased tremor, chorea, loss of balance, restlessness, blepharospasm, increased bradykinesia, facial grimace, stiff neck, dyskinesia, involuntary movements, increased apraxia, behavioral changes, tiredness, headache.
CV: orthostatic hypotension, hypertension, hypotension, arrhythmias, palpitations, new or increased anginal pain, tachycardia, peripheral edema, syncope.
GI: *nausea,* vomiting, constipation, weight loss, anorexia or poor appetite, dysphagia, diarrhea, heartburn, dry mouth, taste alteration.
GU: slow urination, transient nocturia, prostatic hypertrophy, urinary hesitancy, urinary frequency, urine retention, sexual dysfunction.
Skin: rash, hair loss, sweating.
Other: malaise.

INTERACTIONS
Adrenergic agents: possible increased pressor response, particularly in patients that have taken an overdose of selegiline.

NURSING CONSIDERATIONS
• Contraindicated in patients hypersensitive to the drug.
• Warn patients to move about cautiously at the start of therapy because they may experience dizziness and risk falling.
• Some patients experience increased adverse reactions associated with levodopa (including muscle twitches) and require reduction of carbidopa-levodopa dosage. Such patients commonly reduce carbidopa-levodopa dosage by 10% to 30%.
• Because the drug is an MAO inhibitor, patients should be told about the possibility of an interaction with tyramine-containing foods. They should immediately report any signs or symptoms of hypertension, including severe headache. However, at recommended dosage, there is no evidence that this interaction occurs because, at 10 mg daily, the drug inhibits only MAO type B. No dietary restrictions appear necessary if the patient does not exceed the recommended dose.
• Advise patient not to take more than 10 mg daily, because there is no evidence that a greater amount improves efficacy and it may increase adverse reactions.

---

sodium benzoate and sodium phenylacetate
Ucephan

Pregnancy risk category: C

HOW SUPPLIED
Oral solution: 10 g sodium benzoate and 10 g sodium phenylacetate per 100 ml

MECHANISM OF ACTION
Activates metabolic pathways that are ineffective in patients with urea cycle enzymopathies, resulting in decreased ammonia formation.

INDICATIONS & DOSAGE
Prevention or treatment of hyperammonemia in patients with urea cycle enzymopathy—
Children: 2.5 ml/kg P.O. daily in three to six equally divided doses. Total daily dosage should not exceed 100 ml.

ADVERSE REACTIONS
GI: nausea and vomiting.

INTERACTIONS
Penicillin, probenecid: may impair renal excretion of conjugated metabolites.

NURSING CONSIDERATIONS
• Contraindicated in patients with hypersensitivity to sodium benzoate or sodium phenylacetate. Use cautiously in neonates with hyperbilirubinemia.
• Benzoic acid may compete with bilirubin for binding sites on serum albumin.
• Not intended as sole therapy for patients with urea cycle enzymopathies. Most effective when combined with dietary modification (low-protein diet) and amino acid supplementation.
• Dilute each dose in 4 to 8 oz of infant formula or milk and administer with meals. Inspect the mixture for compatibility if other liquids are used. The drug may precipitate in some solutions (especially acidic solutions like fruit juice), depending upon concentration and pH.
• Carefully measure the required dosage because the stock solution is very concentrated (10 g of sodium benzoate and 10 g of sodium phenylacetate per 100 ml).
• Avoid getting the solution on skin or clothing. The lingering odor of the drug may be offensive.
• Benzoic acid is structurally similar to salicylates.
• Watch for adverse reactions associated with salicylates, including mild respiratory alkalosis and exacerbation of peptic ulcers.

tiopronin
Thiola

Pregnancy Risk Category: C

HOW SUPPLIED
Tablets: 100 mg

MECHANISM OF ACTION
Forms a water-soluble chemical complex with cysteine in the urine, increasing cysteine solubility and preventing the formation of urinary cysteine stones.

INDICATIONS & DOSAGE
Prevention of urinary cysteine stone formation in patients with severe homozygous cysteinuria (urinary cysteine excretion exceeding 500 mg/day) unresponsive to other therapies—
Adults: 800 mg P.O. daily, divided t.i.d.
Children: 15 mg/kg P.O. daily, divided t.i.d.

ADVERSE REACTIONS
EENT: hypogeusia.
Skin: rash, pruritus, wrinkling and friability.
Other: drug fever, lupus erythematous-like reaction.

Italicized adverse reactions are common or life-threatening.
*Liquid form contains alcohol.   **May contain tartrazine.

INTERACTIONS
None reported.

NURSING CONSIDERATIONS
• Contraindicated in patients with a history of agranulocytosis, aplastic anemia, or thrombocytopenia with tiopronin therapy.
• Dosage is usually adjusted to keep urine cysteine levels below 250 mg/liter.
• Conservative measures to treat cysteinuria should be attempted before tiopronin is administered. Patients should drink at least 3 liters of fluid daily, including at least two 8-oz glasses of water at each meal and at bedtime. Patient's urine output should be at least 3 liters daily, and urine pH should be 6.5 to 7. Excessive alkalization of urine may precipitate calcium stones. Urine pH should not exceed 7.
• Whenever possible, tiopronin should be administered at least 1 hour before or 2 hours after meals.
• Routine monitoring tests are recommended at 3- to 6-month intervals during treatment, including CBC, platelet counts, hemoglobin, serum albumin, liver functions tests, 24-hour urine protein, and routine urinalysis.
• Urine cysteine should be frequently monitored during the first 6 months of treatment (to identify optimal dosage level) and then at least every 6 months.
• An abdominal X-ray is advised annually to assess for the presence of stones.
• Tell patient to report any signs or symptoms of hematologic abnormalities, including fever, sore throat, bleeding or bruising, and chills. Blood dyscrasias have been reported in patients receiving other drugs for cysteinuria.
• Rare complications seen with other drugs used to treat cysteinuria include Goodpasture's syndrome (evidenced by abnormal urine findings, pulmonary infiltrates, and hemoptysis), myasthenia (evidenced by severe muscle weakness), and pemphigus-like reactions (bullous skin eruptions).
• Drug fever may develop, especially during the first month of therapy. Discontinue drug until fever subsides, then therapy will probably be reinstituted at lower dosages.
• Skin rashes have been noted with tiopronin therapy. A generalized rash with mild pruritus that develops in the first few months of therapy may be controlled with antihistamines, and disappears after discontinuing the drug. A less common rash that appears after at least 6 months of therapy appears on the trunk and is accompanied by intense pruritus. This form of rash disappears slowly after discontinuing the drug.
• Some clinicians prefer to use penicillamine for cysteinuria therapy, but patients may not tolerate it well. Studies indicate about two-thirds of patients who cannot tolerate penicillamine will tolerate tiopronin.

---

tretinoin (vitamin A acid, retinoic acid)
Retin-A, StieVAA†

Pregnancy Risk Category: B

HOW SUPPLIED
Cream: 0.025%, 0.05%, 0.1%
Gel: 0.025%, 0.01%
Solution: 0.05%

MECHANISM OF ACTION
Inhibits comedones by increasing epidermal cell mitosis and turnover.

INDICATIONS & DOSAGE
Acne vulgaris (especially grades I, II, and III), treatment of fine wrinkles from photodamaged skin—
Adults and children: cleanse affected area and lightly apply solution once daily h.s.

ADVERSE REACTIONS
Skin: *feeling of warmth, slight stinging, local erythema, peeling,* chapping, swelling, blistering, crusting, temporary hyper- or hypopigmentation.

INTERACTIONS
None significant.

NURSING CONSIDERATIONS
• Contraindicated in hypersensitivity to any tretinoin component. Use with caution in eczema.
• If severe local irritation develops, discontinue temporarily and readjust dosage when application is resumed.
• Some redness and scaling are normal reactions.
• Beneficial effects should be seen within 6 weeks of treatment.
• Relapses generally occur within 3 to 6 weeks after treatment.
• Patient should wash face with a mild soap no more than two or three times a day. Warn against using strong or medicated cosmetics, soaps, or other skin cleansers. Patient should also avoid topical products containing alcohol, astringents, spices, and lime since these may interfere with drug.
• Exposure to sunlight or ultraviolet rays should be minimal during treatment. If patient is sunburned, delay therapy until sunburn subsides.
• Patient who can't avoid exposure to sunlight should use a SPF 15 sunscreen and protective clothing.
• Avoid contact with eyes, mouth, and mucous membranes.
• Patient may experience increased sensitivity to wind or cold temperatures.
• No medicated cosmetics may be used.
• Cleanse area thoroughly before application.

Italicized adverse reactions are common or life-threatening.
*Liquid form contains alcohol.   **May contain tartrazine.

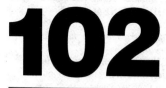

Investigational drugs

amsacrine
azacytidine
dipalmitoylphosphatidylcholine
domperidone
enoxacin
hexamethylmelamine
isradipine
ketotifen fumarate
loratidine
metformin
nedocromil sodium
semustine
teniposide
tolrestat
trimebutine maleate
vindesine sulfate

COMBINATION PRODUCTS
None.

amsacrine (m-AMSA)
Amsidyl†

HOW SUPPLIED
Available only through investigational protocols
Injection: 50 mg/ml

MECHANISM OF ACTION
Intercalates DNA and inhibits DNA synthesis, producing a cytotoxic effect.

INDICATIONS & DOSAGE
Ovarian carcinoma, lymphomas—
Adults: 30 to 50 mg/m²/day I.V. for 3 days, or 90 to 180 mg/m² as a single dose.
Acute myelogenous leukemia—
Adults: 75 to 120 mg/m²/day for 5 days given by I.V. or intraarterial infusion.

ADVERSE REACTIONS
Blood: *leukopenia (usually dose-limiting adverse reaction),* mild thrombocytopenia.
CNS: *seizures at dosages as low as 40 mg/m²/day.*
CV: *ventricular arrhythmias* (rare) *and cardiac arrests,* possibly caused by the diluent.
GI: infrequent and mild nausea and vomiting, stomatitis at higher doses.
Other: *local irritation and mild phlebitis,* abnormal liver function tests.

INTERACTIONS
Heparin: don't mix. May form a precipitate.

NURSING CONSIDERATIONS
• Use cautiously in impaired hepatic function.
• To prepare solution for administration, two sterile liquids are combined. Add 1.5 ml from the amsacrine ampule (50 mg/ml) to the vial containing 13.5 ml of lactic acid. The combined solution will contain 5 mg/ml of amsacrine and is stable for at least 48 hours at room temperature.
• Use glass syringes for combining the amsacrine and lactic acid. The diluent in the amsacrine may dissolve plastic syringes.
• The solution may be further diluted for infusion with dextrose 5% in water (D₅W) to minimize vein irritation. Administer doses of less than 100 mg in at least 100 ml of D₅W, doses from

100 to 199 mg in 250 ml D₅W, and doses 200 mg or greater in a minimum of 500 ml D₅W. Solutions for infusion are stable at least 48 hours at room temperature.
• Solutions should be infused slowly over several hours to minimize vein irritation.
• Do not add amsacrine to normal saline or other chloride-containing solution. Precipitation may occur.
• Do not administer amsacrine through membrane-type in-line filters. The diluent may dissolve the filter.
• Inform the patient that the drug may turn the urine orange.
• Monitor CBC and liver function tests.
• Monitor patient closely for CNS and cardiac toxicity during administration.
• Avoid direct contact of amsacrine with skin to prevent possible sensitization.
• Preparation of parenteral form is associated with carcinogenic, mutagenic, and teratogenic risks for personnel. Follow institutional policy to reduce risks.

azacytidine (5-azacytidine)

HOW SUPPLIED
Available only through investigational protocols
Injection: 100-mg vials

MECHANISM OF ACTION
An antimetabolite that disrupts the translation of nucleic acid sequences into protein.

INDICATIONS & DOSAGE
Acute lymphocytic and acute myelogenous leukemia—
Adults and children: 200 to 300 mg/m² I.V. daily for 5 to 10 days. Repeated at 2- to 3-week intervals.

ADVERSE REACTIONS
Blood: *leukopenia (usually dose-limiting adverse reaction), thrombocytopenia.*
CNS: infrequent neurologic toxicities, including generalized muscle pain and weakness.
CV: *hypotension from rapid infusion.*
GI: *severe nausea and vomiting, diarrhea.*
Other: rare hepatotoxicity and drug fever.

INTERACTIONS
None significant.

NURSING CONSIDERATIONS
• Information based upon current literature. Dosage, indications, and adverse effect profile may change with additional clinical experience.
• Contraindicated in liver disease.
• For stability reasons, azacytidine should be infused only in lactated Ringer's solution.
• After the drug is diluted for infusion, it is stable for 8 hours.
• The drug should be given by slow I.V. infusion to prevent severe hypotension.
• Blood pressure should be monitored before infusion and at 30-minute intervals during infusion. If systolic blood pressure falls below 90 mm Hg, stop infusion and notify doctor.
• Nausea and vomiting may be reduced with continuous infusions. Tolerance to nausea and vomiting develops during extended course of treatment.
• Instruct patient to report any signs of neurotoxicity; for example, muscle pain and weakness.
• If necessary, the drug may be given S.C. The drug should be mixed in a smaller quantity of diluent (3 to 5 ml for a 100-mg vial) for S.C. administration.
• Monitor temperature, CBC, and liver function tests.

Italicized adverse reactions are common or life-threatening.
*Liquid form contains alcohol.   **May contain tartrazine.

dipalmitoylphosphatidyl-choline (lung surfactant, synthetic)
Exosurf

Pregnancy Risk Category: C

HOW SUPPLIED
Sterile powder for endotracheal administration: 10-ml vials

MECHANISM OF ACTION
Lowers the surface tension of lung alveoli, permitting improved gas exchange.

INDICATIONS & DOSAGE
Prevention of respiratory distress syndrome (RDS) in premature infants at high risk—
Neonates: 5 ml/kg by endotracheal instillation.

ADVERSE REACTIONS
Respiratory: transient apnea.

INTERACTIONS
None reported.

NURSING CONSIDERATIONS
• Drug is available under treatment IND status for the prophylaxis of RDS in high-risk neonates weighing 1.5 to 2.5 lb. Infants who have RDS may receive the drug b.i.d.
• Drug should be administered only by persons familiar with airway management.
• Currently, this drug is being investigated for use in adults with adult respiratory distress syndrome (ARDS).

domperidone
Motilium†‡

HOW SUPPLIED
Tablets: 10 mg

MECHANISM OF ACTION
Blocks peripheral dopamine receptors, including those in the medullary chemoreceptor trigger zone (located outside the blood brain barrier). In the GI tract, it enhances motility in the stomach and small intestine.

INDICATIONS & DOSAGE
Symptomatic treatment of upper GI motility disorders associated with gastritis and diabetic gastroparesis; prevention of nausea and vomiting caused by antiparkinsonian medications—
Adults: 10 mg P.O. t.i.d. to q.i.d. 30 minutes before meals and h.s. Maximum dose is 20 mg P.O. q.i.d.

ADVERSE REACTIONS
CNS: headache.
GI: dry mouth.
Metabolic: galactorrhea, gynecomastia, menstrual irregularities, hot flashes.
Skin: rash.

INTERACTIONS
Antacids, H_2 antagonists: may impair absorption of domperidone.
Anticholinergic agents: decreased domperidone effectiveness.

NURSING CONSIDERATIONS
• Information based upon current literature. Dosage, indications, and adverse reactions profile may change with additional clinical experience.
• Contraindicated in patients with hypersensitivity to the drug, mechanical obstruction of the GI tract, or gastrointestinal hemorrhage.
• Parenteral domperidone has also been tested as an antiemetic for patients receivin chemotherapy. Dosage up to 1 mg/kg appears to be effective and well tolerated.
• Because domperidone enhances gastric emptying and small intestine motility, it may alter the absorption of other drugs orally administered and may require dosage adjustments.

---

enoxacin
Comprecin

HOW SUPPLIED
Tablets: 200 mg, 300 mg, 400 mg

MECHANISM OF ACTION
Inhibits bacterial DNA gyrase, preventing bacterial replication.

INDICATIONS & DOSAGE
Mild to moderate urinary tract infections—
Adults: 200 mg P.O. b.i.d. for 5 days.
Complicated to severe urinary tract infections—
Adults: 400 mg P.O. b.i.d. for 14 days.
Skin and skin structure infections—
Adults: 400 mg P.O. b.i.d. for 7 to 14 days.
Uncomplicated genital tract infections (urethral or endocervical gonorrhea caused by Neisseria gonorrhoeae*)—*
Adults: 400 mg P.O. for one dose.

ADVERSE REACTIONS
CNS: headache, insomnia, tremors, restlessness.
GI: nausea, vomiting, diarrhea.

INTERACTIONS
Antacids containing aluminum or magnesium: decreased enoxacin absorption. Separate administration times as far as possible.
NSAIDs: possible increased risk of seizures.
Theophylline, caffeine: decreased metabolism and clearance of these drugs.

NURSING CONSIDERATIONS
• Contraindicated during pregnancy and in children because similar compounds have been shown to cause arthropathy in immature animals.
• Crystalluria has been reported with other compounds of this class. Dehydration, alkaline urine, and high doses may be contributing factors.
• Photosensitivity and skin rashes have been reported with other quinolones. Advise patient to avoid unnecessary exposure to sunlight and to use a sunscreen.
• Use cautiously with known or suspected CNS conditions that may predispose the patient to seizures, including epilepsy and severe cerebral arteriosclerosis.
• Encourage the patient to drink caffeine-free beverages while taking enoxacin because the drug impairs the metabolism of caffeine, which may lead to such adverse reactions as tachycardia, nausea, and agitation.
• Obtain specimens for culture and sensitivity before starting therapy. First dose may be given before laboratory results are completed.

hexamethylmelamine (HMM, HXM)

HOW SUPPLIED
Available only through investigational protocols
Capsules: 50 mg, 100 mg

MECHANISM OF ACTION
Unknown.

INDICATIONS & DOSAGE
Ovarian carcinomas, lung cancer—
Adults: 4 to 8 mg/kg/day continuously, or 240 to 320 mg/m² daily for 21 days repeated q 6 weeks.

ADVERSE REACTIONS
Blood: *mild leukopenia,* thrombocytopenia.
CNS: *paresthesias, numbness,* sleep disturbances, confusion, hallucinations, seizures, and parkinsonian syndrome with ataxia.
GI: *severe GI toxicity including nausea and vomiting, anorexia,* and occasional abdominal cramps and diarrhea.

INTERACTIONS
None significant.

NURSING CONSIDERATIONS
• Information based upon current literature. Dosage, indications, and adverse reactions profile may change with additional clinical experience.
• GI toxicity may be decreased by giving the daily dosage in four divided doses. Antiemetics may be useful.
• Neurotoxicity is most common in patients receiving continuous daily therapy for longer than 3 months.
• Concomitant administration of pyridoxine 100 mg t.i.d. may decrease neurotoxicity.
• Instruct patient to report any signs of central nervous system or peripheral neuropathy.
• Monitor CBC.

isradipine
DynaCirc

HOW SUPPLIED
Capsules: 2.5 mg

MECHANISM OF ACTION
Decreases calcium ion movement across cardiac and smooth muscle cells. Israpidine appears to be selective for vascular smooth muscle.

INDICATIONS & DOSAGE
Mild to moderate hypertension—
Adults: 2.5 mg P.O. b.i.d. Early studies indicate that doses of 2.5 to 10 mg b.i.d. are effective, but most patients respond to 7.5 mg b.i.d. or less.

ADVERSE REACTIONS
CNS: headache, dizziness, fatigue.
CV: peripheral edema, flushing, tachycardia.
GI: abdominal discomfort, constipation.

INTERACTIONS
None reported.

NURSING CONSIDERATIONS
• Information is based upon current literature and may change with further clinical experience.
• Israpidine is similar to nifedipine in many respects, but it may produce less reflex tachycardia because of drug's direct effect on the SA node.
• Food may delay the rate, but not the extent, of absorption.
• Drug is secreted in breast milk.

ketotifen fumarate
Zaditen*

HOW SUPPLIED
Tablets: 1 mg
Capsules: 1 mg
Elixir: 1 mg/5 ml*

MECHANISM OF ACTION
Like cromolyn, ketotifen stabilizes mast cells. However, it has a number of other pharmacologic effects that may contribute to its action, including antihistamine, phosphodiesterase-inhibiting, and calcium channel blocking effects. It may also have some activity on beta$_2$-adrenergic receptors.

INDICATIONS & DOSAGE
Asthma prophylaxis; treatment of allergic rhinitis and conjunctivitis—
Adults: 1 mg P.O. b.i.d. with food. May be increased to 2 mg b.i.d.

ADVERSE REACTIONS
CNS: sedation, tiredness, dizziness, headache.
GI: dry mouth, nausea.
Other: increased appetite and weight gain, exacerbation of asthma, *bronchospasm, status asthmaticus.*

INTERACTIONS
Alcohol: may potentiate adverse reactions.

---

†Available in Canada only.   ‡Available in Australia only.   ◊ Available OTC.

Oral antidiabetic agents: reversible fall in platelet count has been reported. Avoid concomitant use.

NURSING CONSIDERATIONS
• Information is based upon current literature and may change with further clinical experience. Ketotifen is currently available in Europe.
• Long-term therapy is necessary for asthma prophylaxis. Studies lasting less than 4 weeks have not shown consistent benefits, but patients taking the drug for 3 months or more consider the drug effective.
• Ketotifen may produce drowsiness. Warn patients not to perform hazardous activities requiring alertness (such as operating heavy machinery or driving) until the adverse CNS effects of the drug are known.

loratidine
Claritin

HOW SUPPLIED
Capsules: 10 mg, 20 mg, 40 mg

MECHANISM OF ACTION
A selective histamine$_1$-receptor antagonist that has minimal CNS activity. A nonsedating antihistamine.

INDICATIONS & DOSAGE
Symptomatic treatment of seasonal and allergic rhinitis and of chronic urticaria—
Adults: 10 mg P.O. once daily. Preliminary trials have studied dosages as high as 40 mg daily.

ADVERSE REACTIONS
Early clinical trials indicate that the drug is well tolerated. Further study is necessary to obtain a complete adverse reactions profile.

INTERACTIONS
None reported.

NURSING CONSIDERATIONS
• Information is based upon current literature and may change with further clinical experience.
• Loratidine appears to be well tolerated in early trials with no sedation or performance impairment with dosage up to 20 mg/day and only minimal performance impairment with 40 mg/day. It may have a more rapid onset of action than other nonsedating antihistamines.
• Once a day dosing may be an advantage.
• Some studies indicate that loratidine with pseudoephedrine is an effective combination.

metformin
Glucophage†

HOW SUPPLIED
Tablets: 500 mg

MECHANISM OF ACTION
A substituted biguanide that produces its antidiabetic effects only in the presence of insulin. It facilitates insulin's action on peripheral receptor sites and may increase the number of insulin receptors. It has no effect on pancreatic beta cells.

INDICATIONS & DOSAGE
To control diabetes in stable, mild, nonketosis-prone type II diabetics—
Adults: Initially, 500 mg P.O. t.i.d., preferably with food. Adjust dosage upward as necessary, not to exceed 2.5 g daily.

ADVERSE REACTIONS
EENT: metallic taste.
GI: epigastric discomfort, nausea, vomiting, diarrhea, anorexia.
Other: *lactic acidosis.*

INTERACTIONS
Anticoagulants: metformin may increase the elimination of oral antico-

---

Italicized adverse reactions are common or life-threatening.
*Liquid form contains alcohol. **May contain tartrazine.

agulants. Monitor prothrombin times carefully during changes in metformin dosage.

Diuretics, corticosteroids, oral contraceptives, nicotinic acid: may produce hyperglycemia and reduce effectiveness of metformin therapy.

NURSING CONSIDERATIONS

• Information is based upon current literature and may change with further clinical experience.

• Contraindicated in patients allergic to the drug. It is also contraindicated in insulin-dependent diabetes; a history of ketoacidosis; liver disease; during periods of acute stress (surgery, severe infections, or trauma); lactic acidosis or a history of lactic acidosis; renal dysfunction; pregnancy; and in patients undergoing examinations that may involve pyelography or angiography, which may precipitate a temporary functional oliguria.

• Lactic acidosis is a potentially fatal complication of biguanide therapy. Phenformin (DBI), a similar compound, was withdrawn from the U.S. market in the mid 1970's after it was associated with this adverse effect. If vomiting occurs, drug should be discontinued immediately and patient assessed for the presence of lactic acidosis.

• Metformin should be discontinued 2 days before elective surgery or angiographic exams. Renal function should be assessed before the drug is restarted.

• Some patients may only need transient metformin therapy during periods of transient loss of blood glucose control.

• Metformin will not prevent the development of complications from diabetes mellitus.

• Patients should be advised of the importance of good dietary management to control their diabetes. Met-

formin therapy should not be used in place of good diet.

• Advise the patient to take metformin with food to minimize gastric irritation.

• Advise patients to avoid excessive alcohol consumption while taking metformin to prevent excessive elevation of blood lactate.

• Impaired absorption of vitamin B_{12} and folic acid have been reported in some patients on long-term therapy. Serum levels of these co-factors should be measured every 1 or 2 years.

• The drug should be temporarily discontinued once or twice a year to assess the patient's need for continued therapy.

nedocromil sodium
Tilade

HOW SUPPLIED
Inhaler: 2 mg/metered dose

MECHANISM OF ACTION
Inhibits activation and mediator release from inflammatory cells, such as mast cells. It may also act in the lung to attenuate local axon reflexes that are responsible for bronchoconstriction and edema.

INDICATIONS & DOSAGE
Prevention of symptomatic airway obstruction in patients with asthma—
Adults and children over age 12: 4 mg by inhalation (using metered-dose inhaler) two to four times a day.

ADVERSE REACTIONS
CNS: headache, dizziness.
EENT: unpleasant taste.
GI: nausea, vomiting.

INTERACTIONS
None reported.

NURSING CONSIDERATIONS

• Information is based upon current literature and may change with further clinical experience.

• Like cromolyn, nedocromil is contraindicated during an acute asthmatic attack. Beneficial effects are derived from regular daily use of the drug to prevent symptoms from appearing.

• Early studies indicate that nedocromil has both antiallergic and anti-inflammatory properties. Some patients have been able to reduce (but not eliminate) the use of both bronchodilators and inhaled corticosteroids without increasing asthma symptoms.

semustine
(methyl CCNU)

HOW SUPPLIED
Available only through investigational protocols.

MECHANISM OF ACTION
A nitrosourea compound that probably acts as an alkylating agent. The drug cross-links DNA and also inhibits several key enzymatic processes.

INDICATIONS & DOSAGE
Advanced GI tumors, brain tumors, Hodgkin's and non-Hodgkin's lymphomas—
Adults: 150 to 200 mg/m² P.O. q 6 to 8 weeks.

ADVERSE REACTIONS
Blood: *delayed thrombocytopenia (about 4 weeks) and leukopenia (about 6 weeks). Myelosuppression may be cumulative.*
GI: *acute nausea and vomiting 2 to 6 hours after administration, anorexia.*
GU: renal toxicity.
Hepatic: elevated liver enzymes.
Other: pulmonary fibrosis with prolonged use.

INTERACTIONS
None significant.

NURSING CONSIDERATIONS
• Use cautiously when other nephrotoxic drugs are also being administered.

• Monitor renal and liver function tests.

• Capsules are usually stored in the refrigerator but are stable for 1 year at room temperature. Avoid storage in high temperatures and excessive moisture.

• The drug should be taken on an empty stomach to ensure complete absorption.

• Monitor CBC for delayed myelosuppression, up to 4 weeks for the onset of thrombocytopenia and 6 weeks for leukopenia.

teniposide (VM-26)
Vumon‡

HOW SUPPLIED
Available only through investigational protocols.
Injection: 50 mg/5 ml ampules

MECHANISM OF ACTION
A semi-synthetic derivative of podophyllotoxin that arrests cell mitosis.

INDICATIONS & DOSAGE
Hodgkin's and non-Hodgkin's lymphomas, acute lymphocytic leukemia, bladder carcinoma—
Adults: 50 to 100 mg/m² I.V. once or twice weekly for 4 to 6 weeks, or 40 to 50 mg/m² daily I.V. for 5 days repeated every 3 to 4 weeks.

ADVERSE REACTIONS
Blood: *myelosuppression (dose-limiting), leukopenia,* some thrombocytopenia.
CV: hypotension from rapid infusion.
GI: nausea and vomiting.
Local: *phlebitis,* extravasation.

Italicized adverse reactions are common or life-threatening.
*Liquid form contains alcohol.   **May contain tartrazine.

Other: alopecia (rare), *anaphylaxis* (rare).

INTERACTIONS
None significant.

NURSING CONSIDERATIONS
• May be diluted for infusion in either dextrose 5% in water or normal saline solution, but cloudy solutions should be discarded.
• Infuse over 45 to 90 minutes to prevent hypotension.
• Don't administer through a membrane-type in-line filter because the diluent may dissolve the filter.
• Solutions containing 0.5 to 2 mg/ml are stable for 4 hours. Solutions containing 0.1 to 0.2 mg/ml are stable for 6 hours.
• Monitor blood pressure before infusion and at 30-minute intervals during infusion. If systolic blood pressure falls below 90 mm Hg, stop infusion and notify doctor.
• Have diphenhydramine, hydrocortisone, epinephrine, and airway available in case of anaphylaxis.
• Monitor CBC. Observe patient for signs of bone marrow suppression.
• Avoid extravasation.
• Drug may be given by local bladder instillation as a treatment for bladder cancer.
• Preparation of parenteral form is associated with carcinogenic, mutagenic, and teratogenic risks for personnel. Follow institutional policy to reduce risks.

tolrestat
Alderase

HOW SUPPLIED
Available only through investigational protocols.

MECHANISM OF ACTION
Blocks the enzyme aldose reductase, and prevents the intracellular formation of sorbitol from glucose and galactitol from galactose. This metabolic pathway is active in patients with diabetes and may be responsible for late diabetic complications.

INDICATIONS & DOSAGE
Prevention of late complications of diabetes, including diabetic retinopathy and neuropathy—
Adults: dosage not clearly established. Early studies have used 50 to 200 mg P.O. once or twice daily.

ADVERSE REACTIONS
CNS: dizziness.
Skin: rash.
Other: elevations of liver enzymes.

INTERACTIONS
Salicylates, tolbutamide: increased plasma levels of active tolrestat by displacing the drug from protein-binding sites.

NURSING CONSIDERATIONS
• Information is based upon current literature and may change with further clinical experience.
• Aldose reductase inhibitors have no effect on blood glucose, and patients must continue antidiabetic agents as instructed. The purpose of therapy is to prevent late complications of diabetes that may be secondary to chronic elevation of blood sugar.
• The benefits of tolrestat therapy have been difficult to establish because of the slow onset of complications of diabetes. The drug appears to be well tolerated in clinical trials.

trimebutine maleate
Modulon†

HOW SUPPLIED
Tablets: 100 mg
Injection: 50 mg/5 ml

---

†Available in Canada only.   ‡Available in Australia only.   ◊ Available OTC.

MECHANISM OF ACTION
Acts on intestinal opiate and serotonin receptors to regulate normal intestinal motility.

INDICATIONS & DOSAGE
Symptomatic relief of irritable bowel syndrome—
Adults: 100 to 200 mg P.O. t.i.d. before meals.
Treatment of postoperative paralytic ileus—
Adults: 50 to 100 mg I.M. t.i.d. May also be given by slow I.V. push, or infused I.V. over 1 hour.

ADVERSE REACTIONS
CNS: dizziness, syncope, drowsiness, tiredness, headache.
CV: hypotension.
GI: constipation, diarrhea, nausea, vomiting, abdominal pain.

INTERACTIONS
Antihypertensives: possibly excessive hypotension, especially after rapid I.V. injection of trimebutine maleate. Use together cautiously.
Tubocurarine: Animal studies have shown that trimebutine maleate may prolong neuromuscular blockade.

NURSING CONSIDERATIONS
• Information is based upon current literature and may change with further clinical experience.
• I.V. infusions may be mixed with normal saline solution or 5% dextrose in water.
• Rapid I.V. injection may cause hypotension. Inject drug over 1 minute.

vindesine sulfate
Eldisine†

HOW SUPPLIED
Available only through investigational protocols
Injection: 5-mg, 10-mg ampules

MECHANISM OF ACTION
Arrests mitosis in metaphase, blocking cell division.

INDICATIONS & DOSAGE
Acute lymphoblastic leukemia, breast cancer, malignant melanoma, lymphosarcoma, non–small cell lung carcinoma—
Adults: 3 to 4 mg/m² I.V. q 7 to 14 days, or continuous I.V. infusion of 1.2 to 1.5 mg/m² daily for 5 days q 3 weeks.

ADVERSE REACTIONS
Blood: *leukopenia, thrombocytopenia.*
CNS: *paresthesias, decreased deep tendon reflex, muscle weakness.*
GI: *constipation, abdominal cramping,* nausea, vomiting.
Local: *phlebitis,* necrosis on extravasation.
Other: *acute bronchospasm, reversible alopecia,* jaw pain, fever with continuous infusions.

INTERACTIONS
None significant.

NURSING CONSIDERATIONS
• Do not give as a continuous infusion unless patient has a central I.V. line.
• After administering, monitor for life-threatening acute bronchospasm reaction. If this occurs, notify doctor immediately. Reaction most likely to occur in patient who is also receiving mitomycin.
• To prevent paralytic ileus, encourage patient to drink fluids, increase ambulation, and use stool softeners.
• Instruct patient to report any symptoms of neurotoxicity: numbness and tingling of extremities, jaw pain, constipation (may be an early symptom).
• Assess for depression of Achilles tendon reflex, footdrop or wristdrop, and slapping gait (late signs of neurotoxicity).

Italicized adverse reactions are common or life-threatening.
*Liquid form contains alcohol.   **May contain tartrazine.

- Neuropathy may be assessed by recording patient signatures before each course of therapy and observing for deterioration of handwriting.
- Monitor CBC.
- Avoid extravasation. Drug is a painful vesicant. Give 10-ml normal saline solution flush before drug to test vein patency, and 10-ml normal saline solution flush to remove any remaining drug from tubing after drug is given.
- When reconstituted with the 10-ml diluent provided or normal saline solution, the drug is stable for 30 days under refrigeration.
- Do not mix vindesine with other drugs; compatibility with other drugs has not yet been determined.

Appendices
and Index

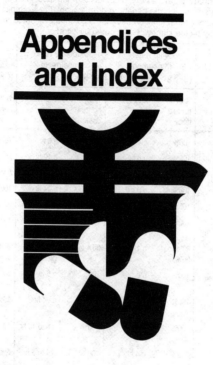

Recommended drug dosage in renal failure

This table lists recommended dosage adjustments in mild, moderate, and severe renal failure. These adjustments are necessary because impaired renal function may modify a drug's bioavailability, distribution, pharmacologic action, or elimination, thereby predisposing the patient to drug toxicity. For example, digoxin toxicity can follow impaired renal function because digoxin is eliminated from the body almost exclusively by the kidneys (via glomerular filtration).

Drug	Mild renal impairment (GFR* >50 ml/min)		Moderate renal impairment (GFR 10 to 50 ml/min)		Severe renal impairment (GFR <10 ml/min)	
	% of normal dose	Interval	% of normal dose	Interval	% of normal dose	Interval
acetaminophen	100%	q 4 hr	100%	q 6 hr	100%	q 8 hr
acetazolamide	100%	q 6 hr	100%	q 12 hr	Avoid	Avoid
acetohexamide	100%	q 12 hr	Avoid	Avoid	Avoid	Avoid
acyclovir	100%	q 8 hr	100%	q 24 hr	100%	q 48 hr
allopurinol	100%	q 8 hr	75%	q 8 hr	50%	q 8 hr
amantadine	100%	q 12 to 24 hr	100%	q 48 to 72 hr	100%	q 7 days
amikacin	60% to 90%	q 12 hr	30% to 70%	q 12 to 24 hr	20% to 30%	q 24 to 48 hr
amoxicillin	100%	q 6 hr	100%	q 6 to 12 hr	100%	q 12 to 16 hr
amphotericin B	100%	q 24 hr	100%	q 24 hr	100%	q 24 to 36 hr
ampicillin	100%	q 6 hr	100%	q 6 to 12 hr	100%	q 12 to 16 hr
aspirin	100%	q 4 hr	100%	q 4 to 6 hr	Avoid	Avoid
atenolol	100%	q 24 hr	100%	q 48 hr	100%	q 96 hr
azathioprine	100%	q 24 hr	100%	q 24 hr	100%	q 36 hr
azlocillin	100%	q 4 to 6 hr	100%	q 6 to 8 hr	100%	q 8 hr
bleomycin	100%	Varies	100%	Varies	50%	Varies
bretylium	100%	Continuous infusion	25% to 50%	Continuous infusion	Avoid	Avoid
captopril	100%	t.i.d.	100%	t.i.d.	50%	t.i.d.
carbamazepine	100%	q 6 to 8 hr	100%	q 6 to 8 hr	75%	q 6 to 8 hr
carbenicillin	100%	q 8 to 12 hr	100%	q 12 to 24 hr	100%	q 24 to 48 hr
cefaclor	100%	q 8 hr	50% to 100%	q 8 hr	50%	q 8 hr

*glomerular filtration rate

Recommended drug dosage in renal failure (continued)

Drug	Mild renal impairment (GFR* >50 ml/min)		Moderate renal impairment (GFR 10 to 50 ml/min)		Severe renal impairment (GFR <10 ml/min)	
	% of normal dose	Interval	% of normal dose	Interval	% of normal dose	Interval
cefadroxil	100%	q 12 hr	100%	q 12 to 24 hr	100%	q 24 to 48 hr
cefamandole	100%	q 6 hr	100%	q 6 to 8 hr	100%	q 12 hr
cefazolin	100%	q 8 hr	100%	q 12 hr	100%	q 24 to 48 hr
cefotaxime	100%	q 6 to 8 hr	100%	q 8 to 12 hr	100%	q 24 hr
cefoxitin	100%	q 8 hr	100%	q 8 to 12 hr	100%	q 24 to 48 hr
cephalexin	100%	q 6 hr	100%	q 6 to 8 hr	100%	q 8 to 12 hr
cephalothin	100%	q 6 hr	100%	q 6 to 8 hr	100%	q 12 hr
cephapirin	100%	q 6 hr	100%	q 6 to 8 hr	100%	q 12 hr
cephradine	100%	q 6 hr	50%	q 6 hr	25%	q 6 hr
chloral hydrate	100%	At bedtime	Avoid	Avoid	Avoid	Avoid
chlorpropamide	100%	q 24 hr	Avoid	Avoid	Avoid	Avoid
chlorthalidone	100%	q 24 hr	100%	q 24 hr	100%	q 48 hr
cimetidine	100%	q 6 hr	100%	q 8 hr	100%	q 12 hr
ciprofloxacin	100%	q 12 hr	100%	q 12 to 24 hr	100%	q 24 hr
cisplatin	100%	Varies	75%	Varies	50%	Varies
clofibrate	100%	q 6 to 12 hr	100%	q 12 to 18 hr	100%	q 24 to 48 hr
clonidine	100%	b.i.d.	100%	b.i.d.	50% to 75%	b.i.d.
colchicine	100%	Varies	100%	Varies	50%	Varies
cyclacillin	100%	q 6 hr	100%	q 6 to 12 hr	100%	q 12 to 24 hr
cyclophosphamide	100%	q 12 hr	100%	q 12 hr	100%	q 18 to 24 hr
diflunisal	100%	q 12 hr	100%	q 12 hr	50%	q 12 hr
digitoxin	100%	q 24 hr	100%	q 24 hr	50% to 75%	q 24 hr
digoxin	100%	q 24 hr	100%	q 36 hr	100%	q 48 hr
diphenhydramine	100%	q 6 hr	100%	q 6 to 9 hr	100%	q 9 to 12 hr

*glomerular filtration rate

(continued)

Recommended drug dosage in renal failure (continued)

Drug	Mild renal impairment (GFR* >50 ml/min)		Moderate renal impairment (GFR 10 to 50 ml/min)		Severe renal impairment (GFR <10 ml/min)	
	% of normal dose	Interval	% of normal dose	Interval	% of normal dose	Interval
disopyramide	100%	q 6 hr	100%	q 12 to 24 hr	100%	q 24 to 40 hr
doxycycline	100%	q 12 hr	100%	q 12 to 18 hr	100%	q 18 to 24 hr
ethacrynic acid	100%	q 6 hr	100%	q 6 hr	Avoid	Avoid
ethambutol	100%	q 24 hr	100%	q 24 to 36 hr	100%	q 48 hr
ethosuximide	100%	q 12 hr	100%	q 12 hr	75%	q 12 hr
flucytosine	100%	q 6 hr	100%	q 12 to 24 hr	100%	q 24 to 48 hr
gemfibrozil	100%	b.i.d.	50%	b.i.d.	25%	b.i.d.
gentamicin	60% to 90%	q 8 to 12 hr	30% to 70%	q 12 hr	20% to 30%	q 24 hr
guanethidine	100%	q 24 hr	100%	q 24 hr	100%	q 24 to 36 hr
hydralazine	100%	q 8 hr	100%	q 8 hr	100%	q 8 to 16 hr (fast acetylators) q 12 to 24 hr (slow acetylators)
hydroxyurea	100%	Varies	75%	Varies	50%	Varies
isoniazid	100%	q 24 hr	100%	q 24 hr	66% to 75%	q 24 hr
kanamycin	60% to 90%	q 8 to 12 hr	30% to 70%	q 12 hr	20% to 30%	q 24 to 48 hr
lincomycin	100%	q 6 hr	100%	q 12 hr	100%	q 24 hr
lithium carbonate	100%	t.i.d. to q.i.d.	50% to 75%	t.i.d. to q.i.d.	25% to 50%	t.i.d. to q.i.d.
lorazepam	100%	t.i.d. to q.i.d.	100%	t.i.d. to q.i.d.	50%	t.i.d. to q.i.d.
meprobamate	100%	q 6 hr	100%	q 9 to 12 hr	100%	q 12 to 18 hr
methadone	100%	q 6 to 8 hr	100%	q 6 to 8 hr	50% to 75%	q 6 to 8 hr
methenamine mandelate	100%	q.i.d.	Avoid	Avoid	Avoid	Avoid

*glomerular filtration rate

Recommended drug dosage in renal failure (continued)

Drug	Mild renal impairment (GFR* >50 ml/min)		Moderate renal impairment (GFR 10 to 50 ml/min)		Severe renal impairment (GFR <10 ml/min)	
	% of normal dose	Interval	% of normal dose	Interval	% of normal dose	Interval
methicillin	100%	q 4 hr	100%	q 4 to 8 hr	100%	q 8 to 12 hr
methotrexate	100%	Varies	50%	Varies	Avoid	Avoid
methyldopa	100%	q 6 hr	100%	q 8 to 12 hr	100%	q 12 to 24 hr
metoclopramide	100%	Varies	75%	Varies	50%	Varies
metronidazole	100%	q 8 hr	100%	q 8 to 12 hr	100%	q 12 to 24 hr
mezlocillin	100%	q 4 to 6 hr	100%	q 6 to 8 hr	100%	q 8 hr
mithramycin	100%	Varies	75%	Varies	50%	Varies
mitomycin C	100%	Varies	100%	Varies	75%	Varies
moxalactam	100%	q 8 hr	100%	q 12 hr	100%	q 12 to 24 hr
nadolol	100%	q 24 hr	50%	q 24 hr	25%	q 24 hr
nalidixic acid	100%	q.i.d.	Avoid	Avoid	Avoid	Avoid
neostigmine	100%	q 6 hr	100%	q 6 hr	100%	q 12 to 18 hr
netilmicin	60% to 90%	q 8 to 12 hr	30% to 70%	q 12 hr	20% to 30%	q 24 hr
nicotinic acid	100%	t.i.d.	50%	t.i.d.	25%	t.i.d.
nitrofurantoin	100%	q.i.d.	Avoid	Avoid	Avoid	Avoid
oxazepam	100%	q.i.d.	100%	q.i.d.	75%	q.i.d.
penicillin G	100%	q 6 to 8 hr	100%	q 8 to 12 hr	Avoid over 10 million units/day	q 12 to 16 hr
pentamidine isethionate (parenteral)	100%	q 24 hr	100%	q 24 to 36 hr	100%	q 48 hr
phenobarbital	100%	t.i.d.	100%	t.i.d.	100%	q 12 to 16 hr
phenylbutazone	100%	t.i.d. to q.i.d.	100%	t.i.d. to q.i.d.	Avoid	Avoid
piperacillin	100%	q 4 to 6 hr	100%	q 6 to 8 hr	100%	q 8 hr
plicamycin	100%	Varies	75%	Varies	50%	Varies

*glomerular filtration rate

(continued)

Recommended drug dosage in renal failure *(continued)*

Drug	Mild renal impairment (GFR* >50 ml/min)		Moderate renal impairment (GFR 10 to 50 ml/min)		Severe renal impairment (GFR <10 ml/min)	
	% of normal dose	Interval	% of normal dose	Interval	% of normal dose	Interval
probenecid	100%	q.i.d.	Avoid	Avoid	Avoid	Avoid
procainamide	100%	q 4 hr	100%	q 6 to 12 hr	100%	q 8 to 24 hr
propoxyphene	100%	q 4 hr	100%	q 4 hr	25%	q 4 hr
reserpine	100%	q 24 hr	100%	q 24 hr	Avoid	Avoid
spironolactone	100%	q 6 to 12 hr	100%	q 12 to 24 hr	Avoid	Avoid
streptomycin	100%	q 24 hr	100%	q 24 to 72 hr	100%	q 72 to 96 hr
streptozocin	100%	Varies	75%	Varies	50%	Varies
sulfamethoxazole	100%	q 12 hr	100%	q 18 hr	100%	q 24 hr
sulfisoxazole	100%	q 6 hr	100%	q 8 to 12 hr	100%	q 12 to 24 hr
sulindac	100%	b.i.d.	100%	b.i.d.	50%	b.i.d.
terbutaline	100%	t.i.d.	50%	t.i.d.	Avoid	Avoid
thiazides	100%	Daily to b.i.d.	100%	Daily to b.i.d.	Avoid	Avoid
ticarcillin	100%	q 8 to 12 hr	100%	q 12 to 24 hr	100%	q 24 to 48 hr
tobramycin	60% to 90%	q 8 to 12 hr	30% to 70%	q 12 hr	20% to 30%	q 24 hr
triamterene	100%	q 12 hr	100%	q 12 hr	Avoid	Avoid
trimethoprim	100%	q 12 hr	100%	q 18 hr	100%	q 24 hr
vancomycin	100%	q 1 to 3 days	100%	q 3 to 10 days	100%	q 10 days
vidarabine	100%	Continuous infusion	100%	Continuous infusion	75%	Continuous infusion

*glomerular filtration rate

Orphan drugs and biologicals

As defined by the Orphan Drug Act, an orphan drug is one that is useful for the diagnosis, treatment, or prevention of a rare disease or disorder. This act defines a rare disease as one that affects fewer than 200,000 persons in the United States, or one for which the expected sales will not recover the cost of developing and making the drug available. The following list includes the drugs and biologicals that have received orphan drug designation.

GENERIC NAME	TRADE NAME	DESIGNATED USE
Drugs		
aconiazide		Treatment of tuberculosis.
allopurinol	Zyloprim	Ex vivo preservation of cadaveric kidneys for transplantation.
allopurinol riboside		Treatment of cutaneous and visceral leishmaniasis and Chagas' disease.
4-aminopyridine (4-AP)		Relief of symptoms of multiple sclerosis.
4-amino salicylic acid		Treatment of mild to moderate ulcerative colitis in patients intolerant to sulfasalazine.
anagrelide		Treatment of polycythemia vera, essential thrombocytopenia, or thrombocytosis in chronic myelogenous leukemia.
ancrod	Arvin	Antithrombotic treatment in patients with heparin-induced thrombocytopenia or thrombosis who require continuous and immediate anticoagulation.
antiepilepsirine		Treatment of drug-resistant generalized tonic-clonic epilepsy in children and adults.
antipyrine		Antipyrine test as an index of hepatic drug-metabolizing capacity.
AS-101		Treatment of AIDS.
5-AZA-2'-deoxycytidine (DAC)		Treatment of acute leukemia.
3' azido-2,3'dideoxyuridine		Treatment of AIDS.
bacitracin zinc	Altracin	Treatment of antibiotic-associated pseudomembranous enterocolitis caused by toxins A and B and elaborated by *Clostridium difficile*.
baclofen (intrathecal)	Liorasal	Treatment of intractable spasticity of cord injury or multiple sclerosis.

(continued)

Orphan drugs and biologicals (continued)

GENERIC NAME	TRADE NAME	DESIGNATED USE
Drugs (continued)		
bethanidine sulfate		Prevention of recurrence of ventricular fibrillation.
bromhexine		Treatment of mild to moderate keratoconjunctivitis sicca in patients with Sjögren's syndrome.
BW B759U		Treatment of severe human cytomegalovirus (HCMV) infections in immunosuppressed patients (bone marrow transplant recipients and AIDS patients).
BW 12C		Treatment of sickle cell disease crisis.
caffeine		Treatment of apnea of prematurity.
calcium acetate	Phos-Lo	Treatment of hyperphosphatemia in end-stage renal disease (ESRD).
carbovir		Treatment of AIDS; treatment of symptomatic human immunodeficiency virus (HIV) infection.
carmustine polymer implant	Biodel containing BCNU	Treatment of recurrent malignant melanoma by local implant.
cetiedal citrate		Treatment of sickle cell disease crisis.
chlorhexidine gluconate mouth rinse	Peridex	Amelioration of oral mucositis associated with cytoreductive therapy used in conditioning patients for bone marrow transplantation therapy.
citric acid, glucono-delta-lactone and magnesium carbonate	Renacidin	Treatment of renal and bladder calculi of the apatite and struvite variety.
clonidine hydrochloride (epidural route)		Treatment of pain in cancer patients tolerant to or unresponsive to intraspinal opiates.
colchicine		Arresting progression of neurologic disability caused by chronic progressive multiple sclerosis.
cromolyn sodium	Cromoral, Gastrocrom	Treatment of mastocytosis.
cyclosporine ophthalmic	Optimmune	Treatment of severe keratoconjunctivitis sicca.
cyproterone acetate	Cyproteron, Androcur	Treatment of severe hirsutism.
cysteamine (2-aminoethanethiol)		Treatment of nephropathic cystinosis.

Orphan drugs and biologicals *(continued)*

GENERIC NAME	TRADE NAME	DESIGNATED USE
Drugs *(continued)*		
dantrolene sodium	Dantrium	Treatment of the neuroleptic malignant syndrome.
defibrotide		Treatment of thrombotic thrombocytopenic purpura.
deslorin	Somogard	Treatment of central precocious puberty.
dextran sulfate sodium (UA001)		Treatment of AIDS.
diaziquone		Treatment of primary brain cancers (grade III and IV astrocytomas).
2′-3′-dideoxyadenosine		Treatment of AIDS.
2′-3′-dideoxycytidine		Treatment of AIDS.
2′-3′dideoxyinosine		Treatment of AIDS.
diethyldithiocarbamate sodium	Imuthiol	Treatment of AIDS.
dihematoporphyrin ethers	Photofrin II	Photodynamic therapy of in situ transitional cell carcinoma of the bladder; photodynamic therapy of patients with primary or recurrent obstructing (either partially or completely) esophageal carcinoma.
24,25 dihydroxycholecalciferol		Treatment of uremic osteodystrophy.
2,3-dimercaptonsuccinic acid (DMSA)		Treatment of lead poisoning in children.
dimethyl sulfoxide (DMSO)	Sclerosol	Treatment of cutaneous manifestations of scleroderma.
dipalmitoyl-phosphatidylcholine (DPPC)/ phosphatidylglycerol (PG)	ALEC (Artificial Lung Expanding Compound)	Prevention and treatment of neonatal respiratory distress syndrome (RDS).
disodium silibinin dihemisuccinate	Legalon	Treatment of hepatic intoxication by *Amanita phalloides* (mushroom poisoning).
D,L-sotalol hydrochloride		Prevention and treatment of life-threatening ventricular tachyarrhythmias.
eflornithine hydrochloride (DFMO)	Ornidyl	Treatment of *Trypanosoma brucei gambiense* sleeping sickness, and of *Pneumocystis carinii* pneumonia (PCP) in AIDS patients.

(continued)

Orphan drugs and biologicals *(continued)*

GENERIC NAME	TRADE NAME	DESIGNATED USE
Drugs *(continued)*		
enisoprost		Reduction of organ transplant rejection and nephrotoxicity of cyclosporine in organ transplant recipients.
epoprostenol	Cyclo-Prostin	Replacement of heparin in patients who require hemodialysis and who are at increased risk of hemorrhage.
epoprostenol/ prostacyclin/PGI$_2$/PGX	Flolan	Replacement of heparin in patients who require hemodialysis and are at increased risk of hemorrhage; treatment of primary pulmonary hypertension (PPH).
ethinyl estradiol		Treatment of Turner's syndrome.
ethiofos	Ethyl	Chemoprotective agent for cisplatin and cyclophosphamide in treatment of ovarian cancer or for cisplatin in treatment of metastatic melanoma.
etidronate disodium	Didronel	Treatment of hypercalcemia of a cancer inadequately managed by dietary modification and/or oral hydration.
felbamate		Treatment of Lennox-Gastaut syndrome
fludarabine monophosphate		Treatment of chronic lymphocytic leukemia (CLL).
flumecinol	Zixoryn	Treatment of neonatal hyperbilirubinemia unresponsive to phototherapy.
flunarizine	Sibelium	Treatment of alternating hemiplegia.
fluorouracil		Treatment of esophageal carcinoma (in combination with interferon alfa-2a, recombinant).
gallium nitrate		Treatment of hypercalcemia of metastatic cancer.
ganciclovir (DHPG)		Treatment of serious life- or sight-threatening cytomegalovirus (CMV) infections in immunocompromised patients.
guanethidine monosulfate	Ismelin I.V.	Treatment of moderate to severe reflex sympathetic dystrophy and causalgia.
hexamethylmelamine	Hexastat	Treatment of advanced ovarian adenocarcinoma.

Orphan drugs and biologicals (continued)

GENERIC NAME	TRADE NAME	DESIGNATED USE

Drugs (continued)

histrelin		Treatment of central precocious puberty.
HPA-23		Treatment of AIDS.
4-hydroperoxy-cyclophosphamide	4-HC	Treatment of autologous bone marrow ex vivo (with subsequent reinfusion) in patients with acute nonlymphocytic leukemia (ANLL).
hydroxycobalamin/sodium thiosulfate		Treatment of severe acute cyanide poisoning.
idarubicin HCl		Treatment of acute myelogenous leukemia (AML), also referred to as acute nonlymphocytic leukemia (ANLL).
iloprost		Treatment of Raynaud's phenomenon secondary to systemic sclerosis.
inosine pranobex	Isoprinosine	Treatment of subacute sclerosing panencephalitis.
iodine 131I meta-iodobenzylguanidine		Diagnostic adjunct in patients with pheochromocytoma.
iodine 131I 6B-iodomethyl 19-norcholesterol		Adrenal cortical imaging.
L-alpha-acetyl-methadol (LAAM)		Treatment of heroin addicts suitable for maintenance on opiate agonists.
L-cycloserine		Treatment of Gaucher's disease.
L-leucine, L-isoleucine, L-valine		Treatment of amyotrophic lateral sclerosis (ALS).
leucovorin	Leucovorin Calcium, Wellcovorin	Treatment of a metastatic adenocarcinoma of the colon and rectum (with 5-fluorouracil). Rescue after high dose methotrexate therapy in treatment of osteosarcoma (Leucovorin Calcium only).
leuprolide acetate	Lupron injection	Treatment of central precocious puberty.
levocabastine hydrochloride		Treatment of vernal keratoconjunctivitis (VKC).
levocarnitine	Carnitor	Primary and secondary carnitine deficiency of genetic origin.
L-5 hydroxytryp-tophan (L-5HTP)		Treatment of postanoxic intention myoclonus.
l-threonine	Threostat	Treatment of amyotrophic lateral sclerosis (ALS).

(continued)

Orphan drugs and biologicals *(continued)*

GENERIC NAME	TRADE NAME	DESIGNATED USE
Drugs *(continued)*		
lysine acetylsalicylate	Aspegic	Treatment of pain and fever caused by sickle cell crisis.
mazindol	Sanorox	Treatment of Duchenne muscular dystrophy (DMD).
4-methylpyrazole (4-MP)		Treatment of methanol, ethylene glycol, 2-methoxy-ethanol and 2-butoxyethanol poisoning.
metronidazole (topical)	Flagyl	Topical treatment of Grade III and IV anaerobically infected decubitus ulcers.
midodrine hydrochloride	Midamine	Treatment of idiopathic orthostatic hypotension.
multi-vitamin infusion, neonatal formula		Maintenance of total parenteral nutrition (TPN) in low-birthweight neonates ($<$1,500 g).
nafarelin acetate		Treatment of central precocious puberty.
NG-29		Assessment of pituitary capacity to release growth hormone in children of short stature possibly due to growth hormone deficiency.
oxymorphone hydrochloride	Numorphan H.P.	Relief of severe, intractable pain in narcotic-tolerant patients.
pentostatin		Treatment of hairy cell leukemia.
phosphocysteamine		Treatment of cystinosis.
physostigmine salicylate	Antilirium	Treatment of Friedreich's and other inherited ataxias.
piracetam	Nootropil	Treatment of myoclonus.
piritrexim isethionate		Treatment of infections caused by *Pneumocystis carinii*, *Toxoplasma gondii*, and *Mycobacterium avium-intracellulare*.
poloxamer 188	Rheoth	Treatment of sickle cell crisis.
potassium citrate	Urocit-K	Prevention of calcium renal stones in patients with hypocitraturia and patients with uric acid nephrolithiasis.
potassium citrate/citric acid	Polycitra-K, Urocit-K	Dissolution and control of calcium, uric acid, and cystine calculi in the urinary tract.
prednimustine	Sterecyt	Treatment of malignant non-Hodgkin's lymphomas.

Orphan drugs and biologicals (continued)

GENERIC NAME	TRADE NAME	DESIGNATED USE
Drugs (continued)		
propamidine isethionate	Brolene Eye Drops	Treatment of acanthamoeba keratitis.
protirelin (TRH)	Thymone	Treatment of amyotrophic lateral sclerosis (ALS).
pulmonary surfactant replacement		Prevention and treatment of respiratory distress syndrome (RDS).
quinacrine hydrochloride		Prevention of recurrence of pneumothorax in patients at high risk.
rifabutin		Treatment of disseminated *Mycobacterium avium* complex (MAC) disease; prevention of MAC disease in patients with CD4 counts <200/mm^3.
rifampin	Rifadin I.V.	Antituberculosis treatment when use of the oral form of the drug is not feasible.
rifampin/isoniazid/pyrazinamide	Rifater V	Short-course treatment of tuberculosis.
sermorelin acetate [GRF (1-29) NH2]		Treatment of idiopathic and organic growth hormone deficiency in children with growth failure.
sodium monomercaptoundecahydro-*closo*-dodecaborate	Borolife	Treatment of glioblastoma multiforme as an alternative to conventional photon therapy.
sodium oxybate (sodium gamma hydroxybutyrate)		Treatment of narcolepsy and the auxiliary symptoms of cataplexy, sleep paralysis, hypnagogic hallucinations, and automatic behavior.
sodium pentosan polysulphate	Elmiron	Treatment of interstitial cystitis.
sodium tetradecyl sulfate	Sotradecol	Treatment of bleeding esophageal varices.
spiramycin	Rovamycine	Symptomatic relief and parasitic cure of chronic cryptosporidiosis in patients with immunodeficiency.
surface active extract of saline lavage of bovine lungs	Infasurf	Prevention and treatment of respiratory failure due to pulmonary surfactant deficiency in preterm infants.
surfactant (human) (amniotic fluid derived)	Human Surf	Prevention and treatment of neonatal respiratory distress syndrome (RDS).
surfactant TA (modified bovine lung surfactant extract)	Survanta	Prevention and treatment of neonatal respiratory distress syndrome (RDS).

(continued)

Orphan drugs and biologicals (continued)

GENERIC NAME	TRADE NAME	DESIGNATED USE
Drugs (continued)		
T4 endonuclease-V, liposome encapsulated (T4N5)		Prevention of skin tumors associated with xeroderma pigmentosum.
teriparatide	Parathar	Diagnostic agent in patients with clinical and laboratory evidence of hypocalcemia due to either hypoparathyroidism or pseudohypoparathyroidism.
terlipressin	Glypressin	Treatment of bleeding esophageal varices.
thalidomide		Prevention and treatment of graft-versus-host disease (GVHD) in patients receiving bone marrow transplantation (BMT); treatment and maintenance of reactional lepromatous leprosy.
thymoxamine		Reversal of phenylephrine-induced mydriasis in patients with narrow anterior angles, who are at risk of developing an acute attack of angle-closure glaucoma after mydriasis.
tocophersolan oral solution [(Vitamin E/d-alpha tocopheryl polylene glycol-1000 succinate (TPGS)]		Treatment of Vitamin E deficiency resulting from malabsorption due to prolonged cholestatic hepatobiliary disease.
tranexamic acid	Cyklokapron	Treatment of hereditary angioneurotic edema; treatment of patients undergoing prostatectomy who risk hemorrhage as a result of increased fibrinolysis or fibinogenolysis; treatment of surgical patients with congenital coagulopathies.
tretinoin		Treatment of squamous metaplasia of the ocular surface epithelia (conjunctive and/or cornea) with mucous deficiency and keratinization.
trientine hydrochloride	Cuprid	Treatment of patients with Wilson's disease who cannot tolerate or respond to penicillamine.
trimetrexate glucuonate		Treatment of metastatic colorectal adenocarcinoma, carcinoma of the head and neck; pancreatic adenocarcinoma; *Pneumocystis carinii* pneumonia (PCP) in AIDS patients; and non-small-cell lung cancer.

Orphan drugs and biologicals (continued)

GENERIC NAME	TRADE NAME	DESIGNATED USE
Drugs (continued)		
troleandomycin		Treatment of severe steroid-dependent asthma.
urofollitropin	Metrodin	Induction of ovulation in patients with polycystic ovarian disease who have an elevated LH/FSH ratio and who have failed to respond to adequate clomiphene citrate therapy.
viloxazine hydrochloride	Catatrol	Treatment of narcolepsy and cataplexy.
zinc acetate		Treatment of Wilson's disease.
Biologicals		
alpha-1 antitrypsin (recombinant DNA origin)		Treatment of alpha-1 antitrypsin deficiency in the ZZ phenotype population.
anti-J5mAb		Treatment of patients with gram-negative bacteremia that has progressed to endotoxin shock.
antimelanoma antibody XMMME-001-RTA		Treatment of Stage III melanoma not amenable to surgical resection.
anti-TAP-72 immunotoxin	XOMAZYME-791	Treatment of metastatic colorectal cancer adenocarcinoma.
antithrombin III (AT-III)		Replacement therapy in hereditary deficiency of AT-III for prevention and treatment of thrombosis and pulmonary emboli.
antithrombin III concentrate I.V.	Kybermin	Prophylaxis and treatment of thromboembolic episodes in patients with hereditary AT-III deficiency.
antithrombin III (human)	Antithrombin	Treatment of hereditary AT-III deficiency; prevention or arrest of thrombotic episodes in patients with hereditary AT-III deficiency; prevention of thrombosis in patients with AT-III deficiency after trauma or before surgery or parturition.
benzylpenicillin, benzylpenicilloic acid, and benzylpenilloic acid	Pre-Pen, MDM	Assessment of risk in administering penicillin when it is the drug of choice in adults with a history of hypersensitivity to it.
botulinum toxin	Ortholinum	Treatment of spasmodic torticollis.
CD4, human recombinant soluble	Receptin	Treatment of AIDS.

(continued)

Orphan drugs and biologicals *(continued)*

GENERIC NAME	TRADE NAME	DESIGNATED USE
Biologicals *(continued)*		
CD4, human truncated-369 AA polypeptide (recombinant CHO cells)	Soluble T4	Treatment of AIDS.
CD4, recombinant soluble		Treatment of AIDS resulting from infection with human immunodeficiency virus (HIV).
CD5-T lymphocyte immunotoxin	Xomazyme-H65	Ex vivo treatment to eliminate mature T cells from potential bone marrow grafts; in vivo treatment of bone marrow recipients to prevent graft rejection and graft-versus-host disease (GVHD); treatment of GVHD and/or rejection in patients who have received bone marrow transplants.
ceramide trihexosidase/alpha-galactosidase		Treatment of Fabry's disease.
clostridium botulinum Type A	Dysport	Treatment of essential blepharospasm.
copolymer 1 (COP1)		Treatment of multiple sclerosis.
corticotropin releasing hormone (ovine)	oCRH	Diagnostic agent for differentiating pituitary from ectopic adrenocorticotropic hormone (ACTH) in patients with ACTH-dependent Cushing's syndrome.
cytomegalovirus immune globulin (human)		Prevention or attenuation of primary cytomegalovirus disease in immunosuppressed recipients of organ transplants.
epidermal growth factor (human)		Acceleration of corneal epithelial regeneration and healing of stromal incisions from corneal transplant surgery; accleration of corneal epithelial regeneration and the healing of stromal tissue in nonhealing corneal defects; promotion of cutaneous wound healing in extreme burn treatment protocols.
erythropoietin (recombinant human)	Eprex	Treatment of anemia associated with end-stage renal disease (ESRD); treatment of anemia associated with prematurity in preterm infants; treatment of human immunodeficiency virus (HIV)–associated anemia.

Orphan drugs and biologicals (continued)

GENERIC NAME	TRADE NAME	DESIGNATED USE
Biologicals (continued)		
factor VIIa		Treatment of patients with hemophilia A & B with and without antibodies against factor VII/IX; treatment of patients with von Willebrand's disease.
factor XIII	Fibrogammin	Treatment of congenital factor XIII deficiency.
fibronectin (human plasma-derived)		Treatment of nonhealing corneal ulcers or epithelial defects that have been unresponsive to conventional therapy when the underlying cause has been eliminated.
gangliosides as sodium salts	Cronassial	Treatment of retinitis pigmentosa.
glucocerebrosidase/ beta-glucosidase (placenta-derived)		Replacement therapy in patients with Gaucher's disease type 1.
granulocyte-macrophage colony stimulating factor		Treatment of neutropenia associated with bone marrow transplant.
heme arginate	Normosang	Treatment of symptomatic stage of acute porphyria.
hemin	Panhematin	Amelioration of recurrent attacks of acute intermittent porphyria temporally related to the menstrual cycle in susceptible women and similar symptoms in other patients with acute intermittent porphyria, porphyria variegata, and hereditary coproporphyria.
human growth hormone (recombinant)		Treatment of children of short stature associated with chronic renal failure.
human growth hormone releasing factor		Long-term treatment of children with growth failure due to a lack of adequate endogenous growth hormone secretion.
human immunodeficiency virus (HIV-1) immune globulin I.V.		Treatment of AIDS.
human IgM monoclonal antibody (C-58) to cytomegalovirus (CMV)	Centovir	Treatment of cytomegalovirus (CMV) infections in bone marrow transplant patients; prophylaxis of CMV infections in bone marrow tranplant patients.

(continued)

Orphan drugs and biologicals (continued)

GENERIC NAME	TRADE NAME	DESIGNATED USE
Biologicals (continued)		
human T-lymphocytic virus type III gp160 antigens, recombinant vaccine	VaxSyn HIV-1	Treatment of AIDS.
indium ¹¹¹In antimelanoma antibody XMMME-0001-DTPA		Diagnostic imaging of systemic and nodal melanoma metastasis.
indium ¹¹¹In murine monoclonal antibody B72.3	OncoScint OV103	Detection of ovarian cancer.
indium ¹¹¹In murine monoclonal antibody Fab to myosin	Myoscint	Detection of necrosis as an indicator of rejection of cardiac transplants.
interferon alfa-n1	Wellferon	Treatment of AIDS-related Kaposi's sarcoma; treatment of human papillomavirus (HPV) in patients with severe resistant or recurrent respiratory (laryngeal) papillomatosis.
interferon alfa-2a (recombinant)	Roferon-A	Treatment of AIDS-related Kaposi's sarcoma, metastatic renal cell carcinoma, chronic myelogenous leukemia (CML); treatment of esophageal carcinoma (in combination with interferon alfa-2a).
interferon alfa-2b (recombinant)	Intron-A	Treatment of chronic myelogenous leukemia (CML), metastatic renal cell carcinoma, AIDS-related Kaposi's sarcoma, ovarian carcinoma, invasive carcinoma of cervix, primary malignant brain tumors, carcinoma in situ of urinary bladder, human papillomavirus (laryngeal), acute hepatitis B.
interferon beta (recombinant, human)	Betase	Treatment of AIDS; treatment of multiple sclerosis (MS).
interferon gamma-1b		Treatment of chronic granulomatous disease (CGD).
interleukin-2 (recombinant)	Proleukin	Treatment of metastatic renal cell carcinoma and primary immunodeficiency disease associated with T-cell defects.
iodine ¹²³I murine monoclonal antibody to human alpha-fetoprotein (AFP)		Detection of hepatocellular carcinoma hepatoblastoma; detection of AFP–producing germ cell tumors.

Orphan drugs and biologicals (continued)

GENERIC NAME	TRADE NAME	DESIGNATED USE
Biologicals (continued)		
iodine ^{123}I murine monoclonal antibody to human chorionic gonadotropin (hCG)		Detection of hCG-producing tumors, such as germ cell and trophoblastic cell tumors.
iodine ^{131}I Lym-1 monoclonal antibody		Treatment of B-cell lymphoma.
iodine ^{131}I murine monoclonal antibody to human alpha-fetoprotein (AFP)		Treatment of hepatocellular carcinoma and hepatoblastoma; treatment of AFP-producing germ cell tumors.
iodine ^{131}I murine monoclonal antibody to human chorionic gonadotropin (hCG)		Treatment of hCG-producing tumors such as germ cell and trophoblastic cell tumors.
iodine ^{131}I murine monoclonal antibody IgG_{2a} to B cell	ImmuRAIT, LL-2-I-131	Treatment of B-cell leukemia and B-cell lymphoma.
luteinizing hormone-releasing hormone (GnRH)		Induction of ovulation in women with hypothalamic amenorrhea due to a deficiency or absence in the quantity or pulse pattern of endogenous gonadotropin-releasing hormone (GnRH) secretion.
melanoma vaccine	Melaccine	Treatment of Stage III to Stage IV melanoma.
monoclonal antibodies (murine or human) recognizing B-cell lymphoma idiotypes		Treatment of B-cell lymphoma.
monoclonal antibody 17-1A	Panorex	Treatment of pancreatic cancer.
monoclonal antiendotoxin antibody XMMEN-OE5		Treatment of gram-negative sepsis that has progressed to shock.
monoclonal factor IX		Replacement treatment and prophylaxis of hemorrhagic complications of hemophilia B.
PEG-adenosine deaminase (PEG-ADA)	Imudon	Enzyme replacement therapy for ADA deficiency in patients with severe combined immunodeficiency (SCID).
PEG-L asparaginase		Treatment of acute lymphocytic leukemia.
pentastarch	Pentaspan	Adjunct in leukapheresis, to improve the harvesting and increase the yield of leukocytes by centrifugal means.

(continued)

Orphan drugs and biologicals (continued)

GENERIC NAME	TRADE NAME	DESIGNATED USE
Biologicals (continued)		
polyribonucleotide	Ampligen	Treatment of AIDS.
ricin (blocked) conjugated murine monoclonal antibody (anti-B4) to B cell (CD19)		Treatment of B-cell leukemia and B-cell lymphoma.
somatostatin	Reducin	Adjunct to the nonoperative management of secreting cutaneous fistulas of the stomach, duodenum, small intestine (jejunum and ileum), and pancreas.
somatrem	Protropin	Long-term treatment of children with growth failure resulting from inadequate secretion of endogenous growth hormone; treatment of short stature associated with Turner's syndrome.
somatropin	Saizen, Humatrope, Protropin II	Treatment of idiopathic or organic growth hormone deficiency in children with growth failure; enhancement of nitrogen retention in hospitalized patients with severe burns (Saizen only).
somatropin (recombinant, methionyl-free)	Norditropin	Treatment of growth failure in children with inadequate secretion of growth hormone; adjunct in the induction of ovulation in women with infertility resulting from hypogonadotropic hypogonadism as well as bilateral tubal occlusion or unexplained infertility, who are undergoing in vivo fertilization procedures or in vitro fertilization with embryo transfer, respectively, and who fail to ovulate in response to gonadotropin therapy alone; treatment of short stature associated with Turner's syndrome.
Serratia marcescens extract (polyribosomes)	ImuVert	Treatment of primary brain cancers.
ST1-RTA immunotoxin (SR 44163)		Prevention of acute graft-versus-host disease (GVHD) in allogenic bone marrow transplantation and treatment of patients with chronic lymphocytic leukemia (CLL).

Orphan drugs and biologicals (continued)

GENERIC NAME	TRADE NAME	DESIGNATED USE
Biologicals (continued)		
superoxide diamutase (recombinant human)		Protection of donor organ tissue from damage or injury mediated by oxygen-derived free radicals that are generated during the necessary periods of ischemia (hypoxia, anoxia) and reperfusion.
technetium 99m (Tc 99m) anti-melanoma murine monoclonal antibody kit		Imaging detection of metastases of malignant melanoma.
technetium Tc 99m murine monoclonal antibody to human alpha-fetoprotein	ImmuRAID, AFP-Tc 99m	Detection of hepatocellular carcinoma and hepatoblastoma; detection of AFP-producing germ cell tumors.
technetium Tc 99m murine monoclonal antibody to human chorionic gonadotropin (hCG)	ImmuRAID, hCG-Tc 99m	Detection of hCG-producing tumors such as germ cell tumors and trophoblastic cell tumors.
trisaccharides A and B		Treatment of neonatal hemolytic disease arising from placental transfer of antibodies against blood group substances A and B; treatment of ABO-incompatible solid organ transplantation; treatment of transfusion reactions arising from ABO-incompatible transfusion of blood products.

Topical agents

DRUG	INDICATIONS & DOSAGE

Antibacterials and antifungals

alcohol, ethyl and isopropyl

To disinfect skin, instruments, and ampules: disinfect as needed. Isopropyl alcohol is superior to ethyl alcohol as an anti-infective (70%).
Antipyresis: apply 25% solution.
Anhidrosis: apply 50% solution p.r.n.

hydrogen peroxide

Cleansing wounds: use 1.5% to 3% solution, p.r.n.
Mouthwash for necrotizing ulcerative gingivitis: gargle with 3% solution, p.r.n.
Cleansing douche: use 2% solution q.i.d., p.r.n.

salicyclic acid
(Calicyclic, Compound W, Derma-Soft Creme, Freezone, Gordofilm, Hydrisalic, Keralyt, Occlusal, Off-Ezy, Salacid, Salonil, Wart-Off)

Superficial fungal infections, acne, psoriasis, seborrheic dermatitis, other scaling dermatoses, hyperkeratosis, calluses, warts: apply to affected area and place under occlusion at night.

Antiseptics and germicidals

benzalkonium chloride
(Benza, Germicin, Spensomide, Zephiran)

Preoperative disinfection of unbroken skin: apply 1:750 tincture or spray.
Disinfection of mucous membranes and denuded skin: apply 1:10,000 to 1:5,000 aqueous solution.
Irrigation of vagina: instill 1:5,000 to 1:2,000 aqueous solution.
Irrigation of deep infected wounds: instill 1:20,000 to 1:3,000 aqueous solution.
Preservation of metallic instruments, ampules, thermometers, and rubber articles: wipe with or soak objects in 1:5,000 to 1:750 solution.
Disinfection of operating room equipment: wipe with 1:5,000 solution.

chlorhexidine gluconate
(Hibiclens, Hibistat, Peridex)

Surgical hand scrub, hand wash, hand rinse, skin wound cleanser: use p.r.n.
Gingivitis: use 0.12% strength (Peridex oral rinse), p.r.n.

hexachlorophene
(pHisoHex, pHisoScrub, Septisol, Septsoft)

Surgical scrub, bacteriostatic skin cleanser: use p.r.n. in 0.25% to 3% concentrations.

ACTION	SPECIAL CONSIDERATIONS
Antibacterial effect through reduction of surface tension of bacterial cell walls, inhibiting bacterial growth. Also antipyretic and astringent effects.	• Avoid contact with eyes and mucous membranes. • Contraindicated in patients taking disulfiram if used over large surface area. • Do not apply to open wounds.
Antibacterial effect through oxidation.	• Do not instill into closed body cavities or abscesses because gas generated cannot escape. • Store in tightly capped, dark container in cool, dry place. • Do not confuse with peroxide (6% to 20%) used for bleaching hair.
Causes desquamation of cornified epithelium by increasing hydration.	• Avoid use on eyes and mucous membranes. • Do not use in aspirin-sensitive patients. • Apply emollient to surrounding skin for protection. • Do not use on birth marks, moles, or areas with hair follicle involvement. • Wash off thoroughly, after overnight use.
Cationic surface action producing bacteriostatic or bacteriocidal effect depending on the concentration used.	• Do not use with occlusive dressings or packs. • Use only in proper diluted strength for each use. • Inactivated by anionic compounds such as soap. • Rinse area thoroughly after each application. • Skin inflammation and irritation may require lower concentration or discontinuation.
Persistent antimicrobial effect against gram-negative and gram-positive bacteria.	• Avoid contact with eyes, ears, and mucous membranes. Rinse well if drug enters eyes or ears. • May cause deafness if drug enters middle ear.
Bacteriostatic effect against staphylococci and other gram-positive bacteria, probably due to inhibition of bacterial membrane-bound enzymes.	• Do not use on broken skin, skin lesions, burns, wounds, or under occlusive dressings to prevent increased absorption and neurotoxicity. • Do not use around eyes or mucous membranes. • Use for at least 3 days preoperatively for optimum effect. • Rinse thoroughly after use. • Do not use in infants; use cautiously in children. • May be toxic if ingested.

(continued)

Topical agents *(continued)*

DRUG	INDICATIONS & DOSAGE

Antiseptics and germicidals *(continued)*

iodine
(Sepp)

Preoperative disinfection of skin (small wounds and abraded areas): apply p.r.n.

povidone-iodine
(Acu-dyne, Betadine, Biodine, Efodine, Frepp, Iodex, Iso-dine, Operand, Pharmadine, Polydine, Proviodine*, Sepp)

Preoperative skin preparation and scrub; germicide for surface wounds; postoperative application to incisions; prophylactic application to urinary meatus of catheterized patients; miscellaneous disinfection: apply p.r.n., or use as scrub p.r.n.

Astringents

calamine

Astringent and protectant; itching, poison ivy and poison oak, nonpoisonous insect bites, mild sunburn, minor skin irritations: apply p.r.n. three or four times a day.

hamamelis water, witch hazel
(Mediconet, Tucks)

Anal discomfort, itching, burning, minor external hemorrhoidal or outer vaginal discomfort, diaper rash: apply t.i.d. or q.i.d.

Emollients

petrolatum
(Vaseline)

Dry rough skin; temporary relief of discomfort due to sunburn, windburn, or any drying of epithelial tissue: topical protection and emollience: use alone or with other drugs, apply p.r.n.

Keratolytics

podophyllum resin
(Pod-Ben 25, Podoben, Pudofin)

Venereal warts: apply podophyllum resin preparation to the lesion, cover with waxed paper, and bandage. Leave covered for 4 to 6 hours, then wash lesion to remove medication. Repeat at weekly intervals, if indicated.
Multiple superficial epitheliomatosis and keratosis: apply daily with applicator and allow to dry. Remove necrotic tissue before each application.

Protectants

collodion, flexible collodion

Protectant; vehicle for other medicinal agents; sealant for small wounds: apply to dry skin, p.r.n., or use flexible collodion when a flexible noncontracting film is desired.

---

*Available in Canada only

ACTION	SPECIAL CONSIDERATIONS
Germicidal effect against bacteria, fungi, and viruses, probably due to disruption of micro-organism proteins.	• Cleanse area before applying. • Do not cover after application to avoid irritation. • Iodine stains skin and clothing. • Do not use near eyes or on mucous membranes. • Toxic if ingested; sodium thiosulfate is antidote.
Germicidal effect against bacteria, fungi, and viruses; has same action as iodine without its irritating effects.	• Contraindicated in known sensitivity to iodine. • Do not use around eyes; do not use full strength solution on mucous membranes. • May stain skin and mucous membranes.
Antipruritic and astringent activity through drying effect.	• Avoid use on eyes and mucous membranes. • Do not apply to raw, oozing areas. • Cleanse and dry area before each application.
Soothing, cooling effect of superficial irritation through astringent action.	• Avoid use around eyes. • Cleanse area before use.
Protective and emollient effect through formation of moisture barrier, increasing the natural retention of moisture.	• Avoid use in eyes. • May stain clothing. • May cause body surfaces to become slippery. • Apply sparingly; is not absorbed, so coating is all that is necessary.
Caustic and erosive action due to disruption of cell division of the epithelium.	• Avoid eye contact. • May be toxic if applied to large surface area or applied too frequently. • Should not be used in pregnant women. • Wash hands thoroughly after applying. • Protect surrounding area with petrolatum. • Wash off thoroughly with soap and water after prescribed time period. • May cause abnormal pigmentation.
Protects wounds from the environment by forming an occlusive seal and excluding air.	• Do not use on deep or puncture wounds; may promote growth of anaerobic bacteria. • Avoid use on eyes and mucous membranes. • May be painful on application or cause dry skin. • Use alcohol or acetone as solvent for removal.

(continued)

Topical agents *(continued)*

DRUG	INDICATIONS & DOSAGE

Protectants *(continued)*

compound benzoin tincture

Demulcent and protectant (cutaneous ulcers, bedsores, cracked nipples, fissures of lips and anus): apply locally once daily or b.i.d.

zinc gelatin
(Dome-Paste, Unna's Boot, Unna's Powder)

Protectant (lesions or injuries of lower legs or arms): Wrap the wet bandage in place and retain for about 1 week. Dome-Paste, in 3″ to 4″ (8 to 10 cm) bandages, can be applied directly to arm or leg.

Wet dressings/soaks

aluminum acetate, aluminum sulfate
(Bluboro Powder, Burow's solution, Domeboro powder, Pedi-Boro Soak Paks)

Mild skin irritation from exposure to soaps, detergents, chemicals, diaper rash, acne, scaly skin, eczema: apply p.r.n.
Skin inflammation, contact dermatoses: mix powder or tablet with 1 pint of lukewarm water. Apply to loose dressing q 15 to 30 minutes for 48 hours.

sulfurated lime solution
(Vlemasque, Vlem-Dome, Vleminckx's solution)

Acne vulgaris, seborrhea: dilute 1 packet in 1 pint hot water. Apply as hot dressing for 15 to 20 minutes daily; or as a mask to dry areas, and rinse with warm water after 15 to 20 minutes once daily.
Generalized furunculosis: add 30 to 60 ml to bath water.

Miscellaneous agents

hydroquinone
(Eldoquin, Esoterica, Porcelana, Solaquin Forte)

Treatment of hyperpigmentation in conditions such as freckling, inactive chloasma, lentigo, photosensitization: apply uniformly to desired area b.i.d., until desired depigmentation occurs, then as needed to maintain depigmentation.

methyl salicylate
(Ben-Gay, Icy Hot Balm/Cream, Deep Heating Rub)

Counterirritant (minor pains of osteoarthritis, rheumatism, sprains, muscle and tendon soreness and tightness, lumbago, sciatica): apply with gentle massage several times daily for adults.

para-aminobenzoic acid (PABA)
(Pabanol)

Topical protectant; sunburn protection, sun-sensitive skin, slow tanning: apply evenly to dry skin indoors before exposure to sun. Reapply after swimming.

selenium sulfide
(Exsel, Selsun, Selsun Blue)

Treatment of tinea versicolor: massage into affected area; rinse after 10 minutes. Apply daily for 7 days.
Dandruff, seborrheic scalp dermatitis: massage 1 to 2 teaspoonfuls into wet scalp. After 2 to 3 minutes, rinse thoroughly, and repeat application. Apply twice weekly for at least 2 weeks.

*Available in Canada only

ACTION	SPECIAL CONSIDERATIONS
Protects skin from external environment by coating action.	• Avoid contact with eyes and mucous membranes. • Cleanse and dry area before application. • Useful in protection of skin from adhesive.
Protects skin by forming occlusive barrier.	• Avoid contact with eyes and mucous membranes. • Watch for signs of infection. • Warn patient not to shower or bathe with gel on. • Remove by soaking in warm water. Remove all of previous application before reapplication. • Apply with nap of hair to avoid folliculitis. • Do not use with constrictive bandage.
Reduces friction and provides soothing relief through astringent action.	• Avoid use around eyes and mucous membranes. • Do not apply under occlusive dressings. • Discontinue if irritation occurs.
Sublimed sulfur products are germicidal through oxidation of the sulfur ion.	• Contraindicated in sulfur-sensitive patients. • Avoid use around eyes or with other acne preparations. • May discolor jewelry and other metals.
Depigmenting action.	• Avoid use near eyes and on broken skin. • Sunscreen and protective clothing should be used during and after use to prevent repigmentation. • Should not be used in children or pregnant women. • May be toxic if ingested.
Acts as counterirritant, replacing pain perception with another sensation that blocks pain temporarily.	• Avoid use in patients allergic to salicylates, around eyes, on mucous membranes, or on broken skin, or in children. • May be toxic if ingested. • Do not use with heating pad or hot water.
Provides sun screening action by absorbing ultraviolet rays.	• Avoid use in eyes and on mucous membranes. • May discolor clothing. • Not recommended for infants.
Antiseborrheic effect through cytostatic action on epithelial cells, which inhibits corneocyte production.	• Avoid use in eyes and on mucous membranes or inflamed areas. • May damage jewelry. • Should not be used in pregnant women. • May discolor hair or cause increased hair loss.

Index

t refers to a table.

t refers to a table.

t refers to a table.

t refers to a table.

t refers to a table.

t refers to a table.

t refers to a table.

t refers to a table.

t refers to a table.

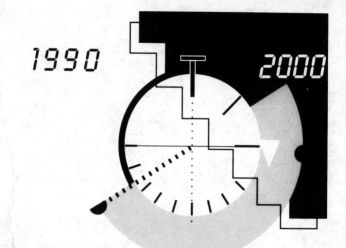

TABLE OF EQUIVALENTS

Frequently used equivalents in the metric system

Metric Weight
1 kilogram = 1,000 grams (g or gm)
1 gram = 1,000 milligrams (mg)
1 milligram = 1,000 micrograms (μg or mcg)

Metric Volume
1 liter (l or L) = 1,000 milliliters (ml)*
1 milliliter = 1,000 microliters (μl)

Frequently used equivalents in the apothecary system

Apothecary Weight
20 grains (gr)	=	1 scruple (℈)
3 scruples	=	1 dram (ʒ)
8 drams	=	1 ounce (℥)
12 ounces	=	1 pound (lb)

Apothecary Volume
60 minims (†)	=	1 fluidram (fʒ)
8 fluidrams	=	1 fluidounce (f℥)
16 fluidounces	=	1 pint (pt)
2 pints	=	1 quart (qt)
4 quarts	=	1 gallon (gal)

Approximate metric and apothecary weight equivalents

Metric		Apothecary	Metric		Apothecary
1 gram (g) (1000 mg)	=	15 grains	0.05 g (50 mg)	=	¾ grain
0.6 g (600 mg)	=	10 grains	0.03 g (30 mg)	=	½ grain
0.5 g (500 mg)	=	7½ grains	0.015 g (15 mg)	=	¼ grain
0.3 g (300 mg)	=	5 grains	0.001 g (1 mg)	=	1/60 grain
0.2 g (200 mg)	=	3 grains	0.6 mg	=	1/100 grain
0.1 g (100 mg)	=	1½ grains	0.5 mg	=	1/120 grain
0.06 g (60 mg)	=	1 grain	0.4 mg	=	1/150 grain

Approximate household, apothecary, and metric volume equivalents

Household		Apothecary		Metric
1 teaspoon (tsp)	=	1 fluidram (fʒ)	=	4 or 5 ml‡
1 tablespoon (T or tbs)	=	½ fluidounce (f℥)	=	15 ml
2 tablespoons	=	1 fluidounce	=	30 ml
1 measuring cupful	=	8 fluidounces	=	240 ml
1 pint (pt)	=	16 fluidounces	=	473 ml
1 quart (qt)	=	32 fluidounces	=	946 ml
1 gallon (gal)	=	128 fluidounces	=	3,785 ml

Conversions

Temperature Centigrade Fahrenheit   Fahrenheit Centigrade
(°C. x 9/5) + 32 = °F.   (°F. − 32) x 5/9 = °C.

Weight 1 oz = 30 g   1 lb = 453.6 g   2.2 lb = 1 kg

*1 ml = 1 cubic centimeter (cc); however, ml is the preferred measurement term today.

†A minim is *almost equal* to a drop. When a drug is prescribed in minims, it is best to measure it in minims. The minim is measured with a minim glass; a drop, with a medicine dropper.

‡Although the fluidram is approximately 4 ml, in prescriptions it is considered equivalent to the teaspoon (which is 5 ml).